CONTENTS

PHYSICAL
EXAMINATION
AND HEALTH
ASSESSMENT

PHYSICAL EXAMINATION AND HEALTH ASSESSMENT

THIRD EDITION

CAROLYN JARVIS, MSN, RN,C, FNP

Family Nurse Practitioner
Chestnut Health Systems
Bloomington, Illinois
and
Adjunct Assistant Professor of Nursing
School of Nursing
Illinois Wesleyan University
Bloomington, Illinois

Original Illustrations by

PAT THOMAS, CMI, FAMI

Oak Park, Illinois

• • •

Assessment Photographs by

KEVIN STRANDBERG

Associate Professor of Art
Illinois Wesleyan University
Bloomington, Illinois

W.B. SAUNDERS COMPANY

A Harcourt Health Sciences Company

Philadelphia   London   New York   St. Louis   Toronto   Sydney

W.B. SAUNDERS COMPANY
A Harcourt Health Sciences Company

The Curtis Center
Independence Square West
Philadelphia, Pennsylvania 19106

Library of Congress Cataloging-in-Publication Data

Jarvis, Carolyn.
Physical examination and health assessment / Carolyn Jarvis; original illustrations by Pat Thomas; assessment photographs by Kevin Strandberg.—3rd ed.

p. cm.

Includes bibliographical references and index.

ISBN 0–7216–8424–6

1. Physical diagnosis.   2. Nursing assessment.   I. Title.
[DNLM: 1. Physical Examination—methods Nurses' Instruction.
2. Nursing Assessment.   WB 205 J38p 2000]

RC76.J37   2000   616.07′54—dc21

DNLM/DLC   99–17267

NOTICE

Nursing is an ever-changing field. Standard safety precautions must be followed, but as new research and clinical experience broaden our knowledge, changes in treatment and drug therapy become necessary or appropriate. Readers are advised to check the product information currently provided by the manufacturer of each drug to be administered to verify the recommended dose, the method and duration of administration, and the contraindications. It is the responsibility of the treating physician, relying on experience and knowledge of the patient, to determine the dosages and the best treatment for the patient. Neither the publisher nor the editor assumes any responsibility for any injury and/or damage to persons or property.

THE PUBLISHER

To

Paul *and* ***Sarah*** *and* ***Julia***

About the Author

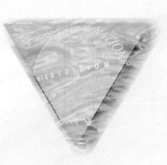

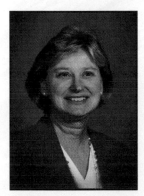

Carolyn Jarvis received her B.S.N. cum laude from the University of Iowa in 1968 and her M.S.N. from Loyola University (Chicago) in 1974. She has taught physical assessment and critical care nursing at Rush University (Chicago), University of Missouri (Columbia), and University of Illinois (Urbana), and she has taught physical assessment, pharmacology, and pathophysiology at Illinois Wesleyan University (Bloomington).

Ms. Jarvis is a recipient of the University of Missouri's Superior Teaching Award and has taught physical assessment to hundreds of baccalaureate students and nursing professionals, has held 150 continuing education seminars, and is the author of numerous articles and textbook contributions.

Ms. Jarvis has maintained a clinical practice in advanced practice roles—first as a cardiovascular clinical specialist in various critical care settings and, for the last 20 years, as a certified family nurse practitioner in primary care. She is currently a nurse practitioner at Chestnut Health Systems, Bloomington, Illinois.

Ms. Jarvis is currently a doctoral student at the University of Illinois in Chicago, with a research interest in the physiologic effect of alcohol on the cardiovascular system.

Contributors

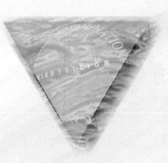

Margaret M. Andrews, PhD, RN, CTN
The contributor for Chapter 3, Transcultural Considerations in Assessment, is Chairperson and Professor in the Department of Nursing at Nazareth College of Rochester, New York and is certified by the Transcultural Nursing Society. In addition to her teaching experience, she is the author of many articles and books on transcultural nursing, has practiced nursing worldwide, and is a respected authority in that field.

Joyce K. Keithley, DNSc, RN, FAAN
The contributor for Chapter 7, Nutritional Assessment, is Practitioner-Teacher and Professor, Rush-Presbyterian-St. Luke's Medical Center and Rush University College of Nursing in Chicago. Because she has worked in both clinical and instructional settings, she is an experienced and well-known practitioner, teacher, researcher, and author in the area of clinical nutrition.

Constance Sinclair, MSN, CNM, CEN
The contributor for Chapter 25, The Pregnant Female, is a certified nurse midwife at Kaiser Permanente Medical Center in Santa Rosa, California, and a clinical preceptor for graduate nurse-midwifery students. She is the author of *Handbook of Obstetrical Emergencies* and numerous articles on emergency nursing and obstetrical nursing. She is currently writing a handbook for nurse-midwives.

Preface

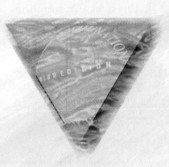

It is important to me that students develop, practice, and then learn to trust their health history and physical examination skills. In this book, I give you the tools to do that. Learn to listen to the patient—most often he or she will tell you what is wrong (and right) and what you can do to meet the health care needs. Then learn to inspect, examine, and listen to the person's body. The data are all there and are accessible to you by using just a few extra tools. "High-tech machinery" is a smart and sophisticated adjunct, but it cannot replace your own bedside assessment of your patient.

Whether you are a beginning examiner or an advanced-practice student, this book holds the content you need to develop and refine your clinical skills. The third edition of *Physical Examination and Health Assessment* continues to be a comprehensive textbook of health history–taking methods, physical examination skills, health promotion techniques, and clinical assessment tools. This text presents a firm foundation in these subjects and continues to be an excellent clinical reference.

I am grateful for the enthusiastic response of instructors and students to the earlier editions of *Physical Examination and Health Assessment*. I am also grateful for your encouragement and for your suggestions, which are incorporated wherever possible. In preparing this third edition, I have worked hard to build on the strengths of *Physical Examination and Health Assessment* while updating information and adding timely features.

NEW TO THE THIRD EDITION

All chapters are revised and updated, with expanded coverage in anatomy and physiology, as well as new nutrition screening tools, newborn assessments for gesta-tional age, tympanic membrane–thermometer measurements, classification of hypertension with risk stratification and treatment, pulse oximetry, and 12-minute distance walk to measure functional status.

A new chapter, **The Pregnant Female,** describes the physiologic adaptation of a woman's body to pregnancy, the history and physical examination throughout pregnancy, and the important abnormal findings to consider. Students in advanced practice who are primary care providers for pregnant women will appreciate this chapter, as will undergraduate students making their unique contribution to the health care team.

Abnormal Findings Tables, located at the end of the chapters, are fully revised with over 100 new full color photographs of abnormalities. New table content includes *Pneumocystis carinii* pneumonia, sites of referred abdominal pain, inflammatory arthritis/osteoarthritis/osteoporosis, and more. The goal for this section is to form a selected illustrated atlas of frequently encountered conditions.

Transcultural Considerations are revised and updated in each chapter, including new content on age of onset of puberty and incidence of coronary heart disease and prostate cancer. Together with a revised Chapter 3 on **Transcultural Considerations in Assessment,** this content reflects the importance of diversity and cultural awareness.

Full-color art of over 68 new illustrations shows shapes of skin lesions, head and neck overlays, lactation disorders, thorax configurations, tactile fremitus abnormalities, and joint abnormalities. All the art in Chapter 25, **The Pregnant Female,** is new.

Examination illustrations contain over 60 new full-color photographs located in Chapter 11: Head and Neck, Including Regional Lymphatics; Chapter 13: Ear; Chapter 15: Breast and Regional Lymphatics; Chapter 22: Male Genitalia; Chapter 24: Female Genitalia; Chapter 25: The Pregnant Female, and others.

Chapter bibliographies are thoroughly updated to include the best of clinical practice readings as well as basic science research and nursing research, with an emphasis on scholarship from the last five years.

Physical examination skills continue to be refined as the clinician notes what works in his or her own setting and then validates it through research.

Assessment video critical thinking questions are included in each body system chapter. These questions provide a connection to the *Saunders Physical Examination and Health Assessment Video Series,* which is developed from this textbook.

DUAL FOCUS AS TEXT AND REFERENCE

As mentioned, *Physical Examination and Health Assessment, 3rd edition,* is a text for beginning students of physical examination as well as a text and reference for advanced practitioners. The chapter progression and format permit this scope without sacrificing one use for the other.

Chapters 1 through 7 focus on health assessment of the whole person, including developmental tasks and health promotion for all age groups, cultural assessment, nutritional assessment, interviewing and complete health history gathering, and mental status assessment.

In Chapters 8 through 25, the focus turns to physical data–gathering techniques. The physical examination and related health history are presented in a body systems approach, the most efficient method of performing the examination and, thus, the most logical method for student learning and retrieval of data. Each chapter has four major sections: Structure and Function, Subjective Data (History), Objective Data (Examination and Findings), and Abnormal Findings. The beginning student can review anatomy and physiology in the Structure and Function sections and learn the skills, expected findings, and common variations for generally healthy people and selected abnormal findings in the Objective Data sections.

Students may continue to use this text in subsequent courses throughout their education and into advanced practice. As each course demands more advanced skills and techniques, students can review the detailed presentation and the Additional Techniques in the Objective Data sections as well as variations for different age levels. Students can also study the extensive pathology illustrations and detailed text in the Abnormal Findings sections.

This text is valuable to both advanced practice students and experienced clinicians because of its comprehensive approach. *Physical Examination and Health Assessment* can help clinicians to learn the skills for advanced practice, to refresh the memory, to review a specific examination technique when confronted with an unfamiliar clinical situation, and to compare and label a diagnostic finding.

Continuing education students who are learning or refining assessment techniques can appreciate the clear and orderly presentation, excellent full-color artwork, and use of space.

CONCEPTUAL APPROACH

Physical Examination and Health Assessment, 3rd edition, is written with the belief that practitioners must have a current and thorough knowledge base and highly developed examination skills to function effectively in a demanding, multidisciplinary inpatient setting, as well as in an independent, sometimes isolated, outpatient setting.

This book reflects commitment to

- **Holism,** in the focus on the individual as a whole, both in wellness needs and illness needs
- **Health promotion,** in the health history questions that elicit **self-care behaviors,** the **age-specific charts for periodic health examinations** (Chapter 2), and the **self-examination** teaching presented for skin, breast, and testicles, and for nutrition
- **Contracting with the person as active participant in health care,** by encouraging discussion of what the person currently is doing to promote health, and by engaging the person to participate in self-care
- **Transcultural considerations** that take into account this global society in which culturally diverse people seek health care
- **Individuals across the life cycle,** supported by the belief that a person's state of health must be considered in light of developmental stage. Chapter 2 presents a baseline of developmental tasks and topics expected for each age group, and subsequent chapters integrate relevant developmental content. Developmental anatomy, modifications of examination technique, and expected findings are given for infants and children, adolescents, pregnant females, and aging adults.

FEATURES FROM EARLIER EDITIONS

Physical Examination and Health Assessment, 3rd edition, is built on the previous edition strengths designed to engage students and enhance learning:

1. **Method of examination** (Objective Data section) is clear, orderly, and easy to follow. Hundreds of original examination illustrations are placed directly with the text to demonstrate the physical examination in a step-by-step format.
2. **Two-column format** begins in the Subjective Data section, where the running column highlights the ra-

tionales for asking history questions. In the Objective Data section, the running column highlights selected abnormal findings to show a clear relationship between normal and abnormal findings.

3. **Abnormal Findings tables** organize and expand on material in the examination section. The atlas format of these extensive collections of pathology and original illustrations helps students recognize, sort, and describe abnormal findings. When applicable, the text under a table entry is presented in Subjective Data—Objective Data format.

4. **Developmental approach** in each chapter presents prototypical content on the adult, then age-specific content for the infant, child, adolescent, pregnant female, and aging adult so that students can learn common variations for all age groups.

5. **Transcultural considerations** are extensive throughout and present the expected variations for culturally diverse people. In addition to Chapter 3, the organizational chapter on cultural content, this includes cultural customs to consider when planning the interview, cultural variations to consider when reviewing examination findings, and a Cultural Assessment Guide presented in Chapter 5.

6. **Stunning full-color art** shows detailed human anatomy, physiology, examination techniques, and abnormal findings.

7. **Health history (Subjective Data)** appears in two places: The Complete Health History in Chapter 5, and pertinent history questions that are repeated and expanded in each regional examination chapter, including history questions that highlight health promotion and self care. This presentation helps students understand the relationship between subjective and objective data. Considering the history and examination data together, as you do in the clinical setting, means that each chapter can stand on its own if a person has a specific problem related to that body system.

   Chapter 4, The Interview, has the most complete discussion available on the process of communication, interviewing skills, techniques and traps, and transcultural considerations (for example, how nonverbal behavior varies crossculturally and the use of an interpreter).

8. **Chapter outlines** on the first page of each chapter show the contents at a glance.

9. **Summary checklists** toward the end of each chapter provide a quick review of examination steps to help develop a mental checklist.

10. **Sample recordings** of normal findings show the written language you should use so that charting is complete, yet succinct.

11. **Clinical case studies** of frequently encountered situations show the application of assessment techniques to patients of different ages in differing clinical situations. These case histories, in SOAP format ending in diagnosis, are presented in language actually used in recording.

12. **Nursing Diagnosis boxes** in NANDA format show how nursing diagnoses are derived from assessment data by demonstrating the relationship between medical and nursing diagnoses. A list of nursing diagnoses commonly used with function or dysfunction of each body system is presented.

13. **Integration of the complete health assessment** for the adult, infant, and child is presented as an illustrated essay in Chapter 26. This approach integrates all the steps into a choreographed whole. Included is a complete write-up of a health history and physical examination.

14. **Critical Thinking in Health Assessment** (Chapter 27) describes the use of diagnostic reasoning in order to make clinical judgments.

15. **User-friendly design** makes the book easy to use. Frequent subheadings and instructional headings assist in easy retrieval of material.

16. **Spanish language translation chart** highlights important phrases for communication during the physical examination and appears on the inside back cover.

SUPPLEMENTS

- A dynamic new *Instructor's Manual and Test Questions* contains annotated learning objectives; key terms; teaching strategies for classroom, skills laboratory, and clinical setting; critical thinking exercises; as well as a testbank of over 850 multiple-choice questions. The critical thinking exercises are 8 to 10 case studies per chapter in which students study and discuss the developmental, age, socioeconomic and transcultural considerations that are addressed during the gathering of subjective and objective data and the implications for the provision of health care. A new section features reproducible worksheets with critical thinking questions related to the new video series that accompanies this text (see subsequent information).

- **EXAMaster,** an updated computerized testbank of the test questions, is found in the *Instructor's Manual.*

- The *Pocket Companion for Physical Examination and Health Assessment, 3rd edition,* continues to be a handy clinical reference that provides pertinent material and 100 illustrations from the textbook. It now also appears in full color.

- The *Student Laboratory Manual, 3rd edition,* with physical examination forms, is a workbook that includes for each chapter a student study guide, glossary of key terms, clinical objectives, regional write-up forms, and review test questions. All are on perforated pages so that students can use the regional write-up forms in the skills laboratory or in the clinical setting and turn them in to the instructor.

- *Saunders Physical Examination and Health Assessment Video Series* is a 17-tape package developed in conjunction with this text. There are 12 body-system videos and 5 head-to-toe videos, the latter containing complete examinations of the neonate, child, adult, older adult, and pregnant female.
- **LectureView,** a new CD-ROM presentation program with 300 illustrations and 200 text-based electronic slides, facilitates in-class instruction of this text.

Throughout all stages of manuscript preparation and book production, every effort has been made to develop a book that is readable, informative, instructive, and vital. Your comments and suggestions have been important to this task, and continue to be welcome for this third edition.

CAROLYN JARVIS
c/o Nursing Books
W.B. Saunders Company
The Curtis Center
Independence Square West
Philadelphia, PA 19106–3399

Acknowledgments

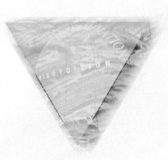

It is my pleasure to recognize the many wonderful friends and colleagues who helped make the revision of this textbook possible. For their help and support I send my gratitude:

To my colleagues, who were a willing resource of information and constructive comments. I am particularly grateful to Joyce Keithley, RN, DNSc, who contributed the chapter on nutritional assessment and who was always willing and responsive to my queries about content and photographs. Margaret Andrews, PhD, RN, contributed the chapter on transcultural considerations in assessment, sharing a wealth of pertinent content on diversity, and a global perspective. Connie Sinclair, MSN, CNM, CEN, brought her years of experience to the new chapter on The Pregnant Female. Through outlines and revisions, Connie was a delight to work with. Her contributions always reflected her commitment to the best of care for the pregnant female. Laura Berk, PhD, took time from her busy schedule of teaching and textbook writing to provide a valuable review of the lifespan development chapter, Chapter 2. Her sound suggestions were an important resource.

To my colleagues who provided advice on specific topics in this edition: David Chow, MD; Eileen Fowles, RN, PhD; Stephen Irwin, MD; Donna Hartweg, RN, PhD; Paul Jarvis, PhD; Sharie Metcalfe, RN, PhD; Mary Evelyn Moore, PhD; Marilyn Prasun, RN, MSN; Lawrence Raines, MD; and Margo Tennis, RN, EdD.

To my artistic colleagues, who made this book the vibrant visual display it is. Pat Thomas, medical illustrator, is a gifted artist with an eye for detail and clarity. Kevin Strandberg is a clever and careful photographer, who has endless patience for capturing the images of children and adults in just the right moment of the examination. Our team has worked together for three editions, providing an artistic unity and clarity to this latest textbook.

To my research assistants, whose tireless help enabled me to survive and proceed through manuscript preparation and revision. Julia Jarvis and Julie Hoerr worked hard to research in the libraries for thousands of articles and references. Marsha Van Etten read and reread endless copies of galley and page proofs, making astute suggestions and correcting errors.

To the faculty and students who took the time to write letters of encouragement and suggestions—your comments are gratefully received and are very helpful. To the reviewers who spent considerable time in reading the chapter manuscript and filling out response questionnaires—your suggestions and ideas are very important for this third edition.

Thank you to the remarkable professional team at W.B. Saunders Company—these are amazing people who love books and who love shepherding projects into print. I am grateful to Robin Carter, Senior Editor, Nursing Books, for the best of advice and for carefully guiding this edition in all stages. Thank you to Thomas Eoyang, Vice President and Editor-in-Chief, Nursing Books, for his wise counsel and witty insights. Fran Murphy, Assistant to the Developmental Editor, is the gem who tirelessly wound her way through a library of resources to find the hundred-plus pathology photographs needed for this 3rd edition. I am grateful to Mary D. McCoy, Copy Editor, for her careful scrutiny of manuscript and her excellent editing. Thanks to the Production Manager, Denise LeMelledo, who carefully directed the smooth flow of all stages of production. Lisa Lambert, Illustration Specialist, did an excellent job of preparing, sizing, proofing, and double checking the color on hundreds and hundreds of illustrations. I am grateful for her careful attention to detail. Leslie Roesler is the genius who set up all the chapter dummies. Her understanding of the goals of the project and her artistic layout make the final pages so conducive to reading and learning. I am grateful to Paul Fry, Designer, for his beautiful interior design and attractive cover. Finally, all my gratitude extends to Robin Levin Richman, Senior Developmental Editor. Throughout three editions now, she continues to be the glue that holds us all together. Her endless encouragement, loyalty to the project, and skill in solving all problems are amazing.

Most importantly, I am once again grateful to my wonderful family for their help and love and steadfast support—their constant belief in me and encouragement kept me going.

CAROLYN JARVIS

Contents

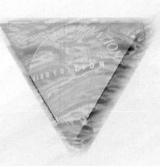

UNIT 1

Assessment of the Whole Person

Assessment for Health and Illness

Ellen K. is a 23-year-old white unemployed female who entered a substance abuse treatment program because of numerous drug-related driving offenses. After her admission, the examiner collected a health history and performed a complete physical examination. The actual preliminary list of significant findings looked like this:

- High school academic record strong (A−/B+) in first 3 years, grades fell senior year but did graduate
- Alcohol abuse, started age 16, heavy daily usage × 3 years PTA (prior to admission), last drink 4 days PTA
- Cigarette use, two PPD (packs per day) × 2 years, prior use one PPD × 4 years
- Elevated B/P (blood pressure; 142/100 at end of exam today)
- Diminished breath sounds, with moderate expiratory wheeze and scattered rhonchi at both bases
- Grade ii/vi systolic heart murmur, loudest at left lower sternal border
- Resolving hematoma, 2 to 3 cm, R (right) infraorbital ridge
- Missing R lower 1st molar, gums receding on lower incisors, multiple dark spots on all teeth
- Well-healed scar, 28 cm long × 2 cm wide, R lower leg, with R leg 3 cm shorter than L (left), sequela auto accident age 12
- Altered nutrition—omits breakfast, daily intake has no fruits, no vegetables, meals at fast food restaurants most days
- Oral contraceptives for birth control × 3 years, last pelvic exam 1 year PTA
- Unemployed × 6 months, previous work as cashier, bartender
- History of physically abusive relationship with boyfriend, today has orbital hematoma as a result of being hit; states, "It's OK, I probably deserved it"
- History of sexual abuse by father when Ellen was aged 12 to 16
- Relationships—estranged from parents, no close women friends, only significant relationship is with boyfriend of 2 years whom Ellen describes as physically abusive and alcoholic

The examiner analyzed and interpreted all the data, sorting out which data to refer and which to treat, and identified the diagnoses. Although the diagnostic process is discussed later (see Chapter 27), it is interesting now to note how many significant findings are derived from data the examiner collected. Not just physical data but cognitive, psychosocial, and behavioral data are significant for an analysis of Ellen's health state. Also, the findings are interesting when considered from a life cycle perspective, i.e., a young adult who normally should be concerned with the developmental tasks of emancipation from parents, building an independent lifestyle, establishing a vocation, and choosing a mate (see Chapter 2, p. 28). Many factors are important for a complete health assessment.

EXPANDING THE CONCEPT OF HEALTH

Assessment is the collection of data about an individual's health state. A clear idea of health is important because this determines which assessment data should be collected. In general, the list of data that must be collected has lengthened as our concept of health has broadened.

The **biomedical model** of Western tradition views health as the absence of disease. Health and disease are opposites, extremes on a linear continuum. Disease is caused by specific agents or pathogens. Thus, the biomedical focus is the diagnosis and treatment of those pathogens and the curing of disease. Assessment factors are a list of biophysical symptoms and signs. The person is certified as healthy when these symptoms and signs have been eliminated. When disease does exist, medical diagnosis is worded to identify and explain the cause of disease.

The accurate diagnosis and treatment of illness is an important part of health care. But the medical model has limiting boundaries. The public's concept of health has expanded since the 1950s. Now we view health in a wider context. We have an increasing interest in lifestyle, personal habits, exercise and nutrition, and the social and natural environment.

Halpert Dunn's view of health is **wellness** (Dunn, 1961). Wellness is a dynamic process, a move toward optimal functioning. Different levels of wellness exist; optimal health is high-level wellness. Wellness is a direction of progress. Health care providers serve to maximize the person's potential, to assist the person to grow toward high-level wellness.

Consideration of the whole person is the essence of **holistic health** (Dunn, 1961; Travis and Ryan, 1986). Holistic health views the mind, body, and spirit as interdependent and functioning as a whole within the environment. Health depends on all these factors working together. The basis of disease is multifaceted, originating both from within the person and from the external environment. Thus, the treatment of disease requires the services of numerous providers.

A natural progression to **health promotion and disease prevention** now rounds out our concept of health. Guidelines to prevention place emphasis on the link between health and personal behavior. The *Report of the U.S. Preventive Services Task Force* (1996) asserts that the majority of deaths among Americans under age 65 are preventable. Prevention can be achieved through counseling from primary care providers designed to change people's unhealthy behaviors related to smoking, alcohol and other drug use, lack of exercise, poor nutrition, injuries, and sexually transmitted diseases. This is a wider, more dynamic concept of health. Health promotion is a set of positive acts the consumer can take. In this model, the focus of the health professional is on teaching and helping the consumer choose a healthier lifestyle.

EXPANDING ASSESSMENT FACTORS

Nursing includes many aspects of the holistic model—the interaction of the mind and body, the oneness and unity of the individual. Both the individual human and the external environment are open systems, which are dynamic and continually changing and adapting to each other. Each person is responsible for his or her own personal health state, and should be considered an active participant in health care. Health promotion and disease prevention form the core of nursing practice.

In a holistic model, assessment factors must be expanded to include such things as culture and values, family and social roles, self-care behaviors, job-related stress, developmental tasks, and failures and frustrations of life. All are significant to health.

The nursing model of health care delivery fits nicely with the expanded view of health because nurses have long considered the whole person rather than just separate biologic systems. The consideration of the complete person in the nursing model is illustrated in the list of assessment factors nurses use to judge health:

- Growth and development
- Biophysical status
- Emotional status
- Cultural, religious, and socioeconomic background
- Performance of activities of daily living
- Patterns of coping
- Interaction patterns
- Client/patient perception of and satisfaction with his or her health status
- Client/patient health goals
- Environment (physical, social, emotional, ecological)
- Available and accessible human and material resources (American Nurses' Association, 1991)

Assessment is the collection of these data that relate to the individual's health state. These data can be grouped into **subjective** data, what the person *says* about himself or herself during history-taking; **objective** data, what the health professional *observes* by inspecting, percussing, palpating, and auscultating during the physical examination; and the person's record and laboratory studies. These elements form the **data base.**

From the data base, the health professional makes a judgment or diagnosis about the individual's health state. Thus, the *purpose* of assessment is to make a judgment or diagnosis.

Nurses from many institutions must be able to communicate with each other. They must speak a common language so that the health care consumer is assured of consistently efficient care. This list of assessment data provides a consistent data base that is adaptable to any nursing model and allows for nursing diagnoses. The use of nursing diagnoses and the companion classification systems for interventions and outcomes give nurses a common language with which to communicate nursing findings.

Nursing diagnoses are clinical judgments about a person's response to an actual or potential health state, which are amenable to primarily independent nursing interventions (North American Nursing Diagnosis Association [NANDA], 1990; Taptich, Iyer, and Bernocchi-Losey, 1994). The most recent approved NANDA list is given in Table 1–1. Note that the list includes three types of nursing diagnosis: 1) *actual diagnoses,* existing problems that are amenable to independent nursing interventions, 2) *risk diagnoses,* potential problems that an individual does not currently have but is particularly vulnerable to developing, and 3) *wellness diagnoses* that focus on strengths and reflect an individual's transition to a higher level of wellness. Throughout this book, appropriate diagnoses from this list are presented and developed as they pertain to related content in each chapter. In the final chapter, Chapter 27, Critical Thinking in Health Assessment, the steps in the diagnostic reasoning process are developed. Here, the list of findings for Ellen K. are analyzed and rewritten as diagnoses. For the best understanding, skim Chapter 27 next so that you begin to understand the framework of diagnostic reasoning. Then return to study diagnostic reasoning toward the end of your course, after you have had time to learn the physical examination and health assessment parameters.

FOCUS OF ASSESSMENT SKILLS AND DIAGNOSIS IN MEDICINE AND NURSING

Health care professionals need a common foundation of knowledge and many shared skills in order to collaborate. Most of the history-taking and physical examination skills taught in this book are shared by nurses and physicians in providing health care. The history-taking skills described in the mental health assessment are shared not only by physicians and nurses but by psychologists and psychiatric social workers. The physical examination skill of auscultating lung sounds may be shared by physicians, nurses, and respiratory therapists. Although health care professionals share knowledge and many skills, what differs is the *purpose* for which the knowledge and skills are used.

The medical diagnosis is used to evaluate the etiology (cause) of disease. The nursing diagnosis is used to evaluate the response of the whole person to actual or poten-

Table 1–1 • NANDA-Approved Nursing Diagnoses, 1999–2000

Activity Intolerance
Activity Intolerance, Risk for
Adaptive Capacity: Intracranial, Decreased
Adjustment, Impaired
Airway Clearance, Ineffective
Anxiety
†Anxiety, Death
Aspiration, Risk for
*Autonomic Dysreflexia, Risk for
†Bed Mobility, Impaired
Body Image Disturbance
Body Temperature, Risk for Altered
Breastfeeding, Effective
Breastfeeding, Ineffective
Breastfeeding, Interrupted
Breathing Pattern, Ineffective
Caregiver Role Strain
Caregiver Role Strain, Risk for
Communication, Impaired Verbal
Community Coping, Ineffective
Community Coping, Potential for Enhanced
Confusion, Acute
Confusion, Chronic
Constipation
Constipation, Perceived
†Constipation, Risk for
Decisional Conflict (specify)
Decreased Cardiac Output
Defensive Coping
Denial, Ineffective
†Dentition, Altered
Development, Risk for Altered
Diarrhea
Disuse Syndrome, Risk for
Diversional Activity Deficit
Dysfunctional Ventilatory Weaning Response
   (DVWR)
Energy Field Disturbance
Environmental Interpretation Syndrome, Im-
   paired
†Failure to Thrive, Adult
Family Coping: Compromised, Ineffective
Family Coping: Disabling, Ineffective
Family Coping: Potential for Growth
Family Processes: Altered
Family Processes: Alcoholism, Altered
Fatigue
Fear
Fluid Volume Deficit
Fluid Volume Deficit, Risk for
Fluid Volume Excess
†Fluid Volume Imbalance, Risk for
Gas Exchange, Impaired
Grieving, Anticipatory
Grieving, Dysfunctional

†Growth, Risk for Altered
Growth and Development, Altered
Health Maintenance, Altered
Health Seeking Behaviors (specify)
Home Maintenance Management, Impaired
Hopelessness
Hyperthermia
Hypothermia
Incontinence: Bowel
Incontinence: Functional
*Incontinence: Reflex Urinary
Incontinence: Stress
Incontinence: Total
Incontinence: Risk for Urinary Urge
Incontinence: Urge
Individual Coping, Ineffective
Infant Behavior, Disorganized
Infant Behavior, Potential for Enhanced
   Organized
Infant Behavior, Risk for Disorganized
Infant Feeding Pattern, Ineffective
Infection, Risk for
Injury, Risk for
Knowledge Deficit (specify)
†Latex Allergy
†Latex Allergy, Risk for
Loneliness, Risk for
Management of Therapeutic Regimen:
   Community, Ineffective
Management of Therapeutic Regimen:
   Families, Ineffective
Management of Therapeutic Regimen:
   Individual, Effective
Management of Therapeutic Regimen:
   Individual, Ineffective
Memory, Impaired
†Nausea
Noncompliance
Nutrition: Less than Body Requirements,
   Altered
Nutrition: More than Body Requirements,
   Altered
Nutrition: Potential for more than Body
   Requirements, Altered
Oral Mucous Membrane, Altered
Pain
Pain, Chronic
Parental Role Conflict
Parent/Infant/Child Attachment, Risk for
   Altered
Parenting, Altered
Parenting, Risk for Altered
Perioperative Positioning Injury, Risk for
Peripheral Neurovascular Dysfunction, Risk
   for

Personal Identity Disturbance
Physical Mobility, Impaired
Poisoning, Risk for
*Post-Trauma Syndrome
†Post-Trauma Syndrome, Risk for
Powerlessness
Protection, Altered
Rape-Trauma Syndrome
Rape-Trauma Syndrome: Compound Reaction
Rape-Trauma Syndrome: Silent Reaction
Relocation Stress Syndrome
Role Performance, Altered
Self-Care Deficit
   Bathing/Hygiene
   Feeding
   Dressing/Grooming
   Toileting
Self-Esteem, Chronic Low
Self-Esteem, Situational Low
Self-Esteem Disturbance
Self-Mutilation, Risk for
Sensory/Perceptual Alterations (specify:
   visual, auditory, kinesthetic, gustatory,
   tactile, olfactory)
Sexual Dysfunction
Sexuality Patterns, Altered
Skin Integrity, Impaired
Skin Integrity, Risk for Impaired
†Sleep Deprivation
Sleep Pattern Disturbance
Social Interaction, Impaired
Social Isolation
†Sorrow, Chronic
Spiritual Distress
†Spiritual Distress, Risk for
Spiritual Well-Being, Potential for Enhanced
Suffocation, Risk for
†Surgical Recovery, Delayed
Sustain Spontaneous Ventilation, Inability to
Swallowing, Impaired
Thermoregulation, Ineffective
Thought Processes, Altered
Tissue Integrity, Impaired
Tissue Perfusion, Altered (specify type: renal,
   cerebral, cardiopulmonary, gastrointes-
   tinal, peripheral)
Trauma, Risk for
Unilateral Neglect
Urinary Elimination, Altered
Urinary Retention
Violence, Risk for: Self-Directed or Directed
   at Others
†Walking, Impaired
†Wheelchair Mobility, Impaired
†Wheelchair Transfer Ability, Impaired

*Revised diagnoses with modified definitions, 1999–2000.
†New diagnoses, 1999–2000.
   From North American Nursing Diagnosis Association: NANDA Nursing Diagnoses: Definitions and Classifications 1999–2000. Philadelphia, NANDA, 1999. Used with permission.

tial health problems. For example, both the admitting nurse and later the physician auscultate Ellen's lung sounds and determine that they are diminished and that wheezing is present. This is both a medical and a nursing clinical problem. The physician listens to diagnose the cause of the abnormal sounds (in this case, asthma) and to order specific drug treatment. The nurse listens to detect abnormal sounds early, to monitor Ellen's response to treatment, and to initiate supportive measures and teaching, e.g., the nurse may teach Ellen which behavioral measures may help her to quit smoking and may recommend that Ellen initiate a walking program.

The medical and nursing diagnoses are independent but are interrelated; they should not be seen as isolated from each other (Field, 1987). It makes sense that the medical diagnosis of asthma be reflected in the nursing diagnoses, as interpreted by the nurse's knowledge of the person's response to asthma. In this book, common nursing diagnoses are presented along with medical diagnoses to illustrate common abnormalities. Please observe how these two types of diagnoses are interrelated.

Of further interest are *collaborative problems,* clinical problems that are amenable to interdependent management by medicine and nursing. Collaborative problems are "certain physiological complications that nurses monitor to detect their onset or changes in status; nurses manage collaborative problems using physician-prescribed and nursing-prescribed interventions to minimize the complications of events" (Carpenito, 1997). A list of collaborative problems is presented in Table 1–2.

COLLECTING FOUR TYPES OF DATA

Although the list of data is standard, the *amount* of the data varies depending on the patient's needs, the health care setting, and the nurse's role in that setting. Every examiner needs to collect four different kinds of data base depending on the clinical situation: complete, episodic or problem-centered, follow-up, and emergency.

1. Complete (Total Health) Data Base

This includes a complete health history and a full physical examination. It describes the current and past health state and forms a baseline against which all future changes can be measured. It yields the first diagnoses.

In primary care, the complete data base is collected in a primary care setting, such as a pediatric or family practice clinic, independent or group private practice, college health service, women's health care agency, visiting nurse agency, or community health agency. When you work in these settings, you are the first health professional to see the patient and have primary responsibility for monitoring the person's health care. For the well person, this data base must describe the person's health state, perception of health, strengths or assets such as health maintenance behaviors, individual coping patterns, support systems, current developmental tasks, and any risk factors or lifestyle changes. For the ill person, the data base also includes a description of the person's health problems, perception of illness, and response to the problems.

For well and ill people, the complete data base must screen for pathology as well as determine the ways people respond to that pathology or to any health problem. You must screen for pathology because you are the first, and often the only, health professional to see the patient. You will screen for pathology in order to refer the patient to another professional, to help the patient make decisions, and to perform appropriate treatments. But this data base also notes the human responses to health problems. This factor is important because it provides additional information about the person that leads to nursing diagnoses.

In acute hospital care, the complete data base also is gathered following admission to the hospital. In the hospital, data related specifically to pathology already may have been collected by the admitting physician. It makes little sense for you to ask the same questions; you can use the data the physician has collected. You will collect additional information on the patient's perception of illness, functional ability or patterns of living, activities of daily living, health maintenance behaviors, response to health problems, coping patterns, interaction patterns, and health goals. This approach completes the data base from which the nursing diagnoses can be made.

2. Episodic or Problem-Centered Data Base

This is for a limited or short-term problem. Here, you collect a "mini" data base, smaller in scope and more focused than the complete data base. It concerns mainly one problem, one cue complex, or one body system. It is used in all settings—hospital, primary care, or long-term care. For example, 2 days following surgery, a hospitalized person suddenly has a congested cough, shortness of breath, and fatigue. The history and examination focus primarily on the respiratory and cardiovascular systems. Or, in an outpatient clinic, a person presents with a rash. The history and examination follow the direction of this presenting concern, such as whether the rash had an acute or chronic onset, was associated with a fever, and was localized or generalized, and must include a clear description of the rash.

3. Follow-Up Data Base

The status of any identified problems should be evaluated at regular and appropriate intervals. What change has

Table 1-2 • Collaborative Problems

1. Potential Complication: Gastrointestinal/Hepatic/Biliary
   PC: Paralytic Ileus/Small Bowel Obstruction
   PC: Hepatorenal Syndrome
   PC: Hyperbilirubinemia
   PC: Evisceration
   PC: Hepatosplenomegaly
   PC: Curling's Ulcer
   PC: Ascites
   PC: Gastrointestinal Bleeding
   PC: Hepatic Insufficiency/Failure
2. Potential Complication: Metabolic/Immune/Hematopoietic
   PC: Hypoglycemia, Hyperglycemia
   PC: Opportunistic Infections
   PC: Negative Nitrogen Balance
   PC: Electrolyte Imbalances
   PC: Thyroid Dysfunction
   PC: Hypothermia (Severe)
   PC: Hyperthermia (Severe)
   PC: Sepsis
   PC: Acidosis
   PC: Alkalosis
   PC: Anemia
   PC: Thrombocytopenia
   PC: Hypothyroidism/Hyperthyroidism
   PC: Allergic Reaction
   PC: Sickling Crisis
   PC: Adrenal Insufficiency
3. Potential Complication: Neurologic/Sensory
   PC: Increased Intracranial Pressure
   PC: Stroke
   PC: Seizures
   PC: Spinal Cord Compression
   PC: Autonomic Dysreflexia
   PC: Retinal detachment
   PC: Hydrocephalus
   PC: Microcephalus
   PC: Meningitis
   PC: Cranial Nerve Impairment
   PC: Paresis/Paresthesia/Paralysis
   PC: Neuroleptic Malignant Syndrome
   PC: Increased Intraocular Pressure
   PC: Corneal Ulceration
   PC: Neuropathies
   PC: Alcohol Withdrawal
4. Potential Complication: Cardiac/Vascular
   PC: Dysrhythmias
   PC: Congestive Heart Failure
   PC: Cardiogenic Shock
   PC: Thromboemboli/Deep Vein Thrombosis
   PC: Hypovolemic Shock
   PC: Peripheral Vascular Insufficiency
   PC: Hypertension
   PC: Congenital Heart Disease
   PC: Decreased Cardiac Output
   PC: Cardiac Tamponade

    PC: Air Embolism
    PC: Disseminated Intravascular Coagulation
    PC: Endocarditis
    PC: Septic Shock
    PC: Embolism
    PC: Spinal Shock
    PC: Ischemic Ulcers
    PC: Angina
    PC: Compartmental Syndrome
5. Potential Complication: Respiratory
   PC: Atelectasis/Pneumonia
   PC: Tracheobronchial Constriction
   PC: Oxygen Toxicity
   PC: Pulmonary Embolism
   PC: Pleural Effusion
   PC: Tracheal Necrosis
   PC: Pneumothorax
   PC: Laryngeal Edema
   PC: Hypoxemia
6. Potential Complication: Renal/Urinary
   PC: Acute Urinary Retention
   PC: Renal Insufficiency
   PC: Bladder Perforation
   PC: Renal Calculi
7. Potential Complication: Reproductive
   PC: Reproductive Tract Infections
   PC: Fetal Distress
   PC: Postpartum Hemorrhage
   PC: Pregnancy-Associated Hypertension
   PC: Prenatal Bleeding
   PC: Preterm Labor
   PC: Hypermenorrhea
   PC: Polymenorrhea
   PC: Intrapartum Hemorrhage
   PC: Sexually Transmitted Disease
   PC: Dystocia
8. Potential Complication: Musculoskeletal
   PC: Pathologic Fractures
   PC: Osteoporosis
   PC: Joint Dislocation
   PC: Osteomyelitis
9. Potential Complication: Medication Therapy Adverse Effects
   PC: Adrenocorticosteroid Therapy Adverse Effects
   PC: Antianxiety Therapy Adverse Effects
   PC: Antiarrhythmic Therapy Adverse Effects
   PC: Anticoagulant Therapy Adverse Effects
   PC: Anticonvulsant Therapy Adverse Effects
   PC: Antidepressant Therapy Adverse Effects
   PC: Antihypertensive Therapy Adverse Effects
   PC: β-Adrenergic Blocker Therapy Adverse Effects
   PC: Calcium Channel Blocker Therapy Adverse Effects
   PC: Angiotensin-Converting Enzyme Therapy Adverse Effects
   PC: Antineoplastic Therapy Adverse Effects
   PC: Antipsychotic Therapy Adverse Effects

From Carpenito LJ: Nursing Diagnosis—Application to Clinical Practice, 7th ed. Philadelphia, J.B. Lippincott, 1997. Used with permission.

occurred? Is the problem getting better or worse? What coping strategies are used? This type of data base is used in all settings to follow up short-term or chronic health problems.

4. Emergency Data Base

This calls for a rapid collection of the data, often compiled concurrently with lifesaving measures. Diagnosis must be swift and sure. For example, in a hospital emergency department, a person is brought in with suspected substance overdose. One of the first history questions is "What did you take?" The person is questioned simultaneously while his or her airway, breathing, circulation, and disability are being assessed. Clearly, the emergency data base requires more rapid collection of data than the episodic data base.

FREQUENCY OF ASSESSMENT

The interval of assessment varies with the person's illness and wellness needs. Most ill people seek care because of pain or some abnormal signs and symptoms they have noticed. This prompts an assessment—gathering a complete, an episodic, or an emergency data base.

But for the well person, opinions are changing about assessment intervals. The term *annual checkup* is vague. What does it constitute? In practice, its extent varies considerably among physicians, nurses, and agencies. Is the annual checkup necessary? Is it cost effective? Does it sometimes give an implicit promise of health and thus provide false security? Many health professionals are aware of the classic situation of a person suffering a heart attack 2 weeks after a routine checkup and normal findings on electrocardiogram. The timing of some formerly accepted procedures is now being questioned, e.g., the annual Papanicolaou test for cervical cancer in women. The same annual routine physical examination cannot be recommended for all persons because health priorities vary among individuals in different age groups and risk categories and because some preventive services are effective only in certain populations (Report, 1996).

The Age-Specific Charts for the Periodic Health Examination are one example of a positive approach to health assessment (Report, 1996). These charts define a lifetime schedule of health care, organized into packages for four specific age groups (see Tables in Chapter 2). Each chart lists a frequency schedule for periodic health visits and preventive services for that age group. These services include screening factors to gather during the history, and age-specific items for physical examination and laboratory procedures, counseling topics, and immunizations. The charts focus on *major risk factors specific for each age group* based on lifestyle, health needs, and problems. These charts move away from an annual physical ritual and toward rational and varying periodicity. The charts incorporate health promotion and disease prevention at *every* health visit, not just at one annual physical examination. Health education and counseling are highlighted as the means to deliver health promotion.

For example, the routine periodic examination for Ellen K.'s age group (11 to 24 years old) would be recommended to include the following services for preventive health care:

1. **Screening history** for dietary intake, physical activity, tobacco/alcohol/drug use, and sexual practices
2. **Physical examination** for height and weight, blood pressure, and Papanicolaou test for sexually active females
3. **Counseling** for injury prevention (lap/shoulder belts, bicycle/motorcycle/ATV [all terrain vehicle] helmets, smoke detector, safe storage/removal of firearms), substance use (avoid tobacco, avoid underage drinking and illicit drug use, avoid alcohol/drug use while driving, swimming, boating), sexual behavior (STD [sexually transmitted disease] prevention, abstinence, avoidance of high-risk behavior, use of condoms/female barrier with spermicide, unintended pregnancy, contraception), diet and exercise (limit fat and cholesterol, maintain caloric balance, emphasize grains, fruits, vegetables, adequate calcium intake for females, regular physical activity), dental health (regular visits to provider, floss, brush with fluoride toothpaste)
4. **Immunizations** for tetanus-diphtheria (11 to 16 years); hepatitis B, MMR (measles-mumps-rubella), and varicella (11 to 12 years); and rubella (females over 12 years)
5. **Chemoprophylaxis** to include multivitamin with folic acid (females capable of/planning pregnancy)

Additionally, the **leading causes of death** in Ellen K.'s age group are listed as motor vehicle/other injuries, homicide, suicide, malignant neoplasms, and heart disease.

Obviously, Ellen's individual health problems demand immediate intervention and preclude a strict adherence to this preventive list. Indeed, many of Ellen's findings are seen as "red flags" based on predictable risk factors from this list.

ASSESSMENT THROUGHOUT THE LIFE CYCLE

It makes good sense to consider health assessment from a life cycle approach. First, the health professional must be familiar with the usual and expected developmental tasks for each age group (see Chapter 2). This alerts one to which physical, psychosocial, cognitive, and behavioral tasks are currently important for each person. For example, an adult in Ellen K.'s age group should have developmental tasks that include growing independent from the parents' home and care, establishing a career, forming an intimate bond with another, making friends, and establishing a social group (see complete lists on p. 28).

Next, once assessment skills are learned, they are more meaningful when considered from a developmental perspective. One's knowledge of communication skills and health history content is enhanced as one considers how they apply to individuals throughout the life cycle. The physical examination also is more relevant when one considers age-specific data about anatomy, method of examination, normal findings, and abnormal findings. For example, an average normal blood pressure for a woman Ellen K.'s age is 116/70 mm Hg (see Fig. 9–18 on p. 204).

For each age group, a holistic approach to health assessment arises from an orientation toward wellness and health maintenance. One learns to capitalize on the person's strengths. What is the person already doing that promotes health? What other areas are ripe for health teaching so that the person can further build his or her potential for health?

TRANSCULTURAL CONSIDERATIONS

In a holistic model of health care, assessment factors must include culture. An introduction to transcultural concepts follows in Chapter 3. These concepts are developed throughout the text as they relate to specific chapters.

Metaphors such as *melting pot, mosaic,* and *salad bowl* have been used to describe the cultural diversity that characterizes the United States. According to the U.S. Census Bureau, close to 50 percent of the population of the United States soon will consist of people from racial, ethnic, and cultural groups sometimes referred to as minorities (Table 1–3; Fig. 1–1). Because the term *minority* is perceived to connote inferiority, members of some groups object to its use and prefer terms such as *ethnicity* or *cultural diversity.*

If current demographic trends continue, the following cultural diversity is expected in the United States in the 21st century: Hispanics, 24.5%; blacks, 13.6%; and Asians, 8.2% (U.S. Bureau of the Census, 1990). The Hispanic and Asian populations will double between now and 2025. At the same time, the Native American popula-

tion is projected to remain close to 0.8% or perhaps decrease slightly because of intermarriage (U.S. Bureau of the Census, 1990).

As the 21st century begins, the steady flow of immigrants and refugees in the United States will increase. Because the United States is sometimes perceived as the mecca of advanced health care and technology, foreign nationals who return home after treatment have been inflating the census reports at many U.S. hospitals, with the more popular types of U.S. interventions being cardiovascular, neurological, and cancer treatments. For example, 35 percent of kidney transplant recipients at some U.S. hospitals have come from other countries. At the same time, U.S. health care providers go abroad to work in a wide variety of health care settings in the international market place. Furthermore, international interchanges are increasing among nurses and physicians, making attention to the cultural aspects of health and illness an even greater priority.

During your professional career, you may be expected to assess short-term foreign visitors, international university faculty, students from abroad studying in U.S. high schools and universities, family members of foreign diplomats, immigrants, refugees, members of more than 106 different ethnic groups, and Native Americans from 510 federally recognized tribes. A serious conceptual problem exists in that nurses and physicians are expected to know, understand, and meet the health needs of people from culturally diverse backgrounds without any formal preparation for doing so.

The inclusion of cultural considerations in health assessment is of paramount importance to gather data that are accurate and meaningful and to intervene with culturally sensitive and appropriate care. Members of some cultural groups are demanding culturally relevant health care that incorporates their specific beliefs and practices. An increasing expectation exists among members of certain cultural groups that health care providers will respect

Table 1–3 • Percent Distribution of the U.S. Population by Race and Ethnic Group: 1990 to 2050					
	Hispanic Origin*	White (Non-Hispanic)	Black (Non-Hispanic)	American Indian†	Asian‡
1990	9.0	75.6	11.8	0.7	2.8
1995	10.2	73.6	12.0	0.7	3.3
2000	11.4	71.6	12.2	0.7	3.9
2005	12.6	69.9	12.4	0.8	4.4
2010	13.8	68.0	12.6	0.8	4.8
2020	16.3	64.3	12.9	0.8	5.7
2030	18.9	60.5	13.1	0.8	6.6
2040	21.7	56.7	13.3	0.9	7.5
2050	24.5	52.6	13.6	0.9	8.2

*Persons of Hispanic origin may be of any race. The information was collected in the 50 states and the District of Columbia and, therefore, does not include residents of Puerto Rico.
†American Indian represents American Indian, Inuit, and Aleut.
‡Asian represents Asian and Pacific Islander.
Data from the U.S. Bureau of the Census: General Population Characteristics. Washington, DC, U.S. Government Printing Office, 1990.

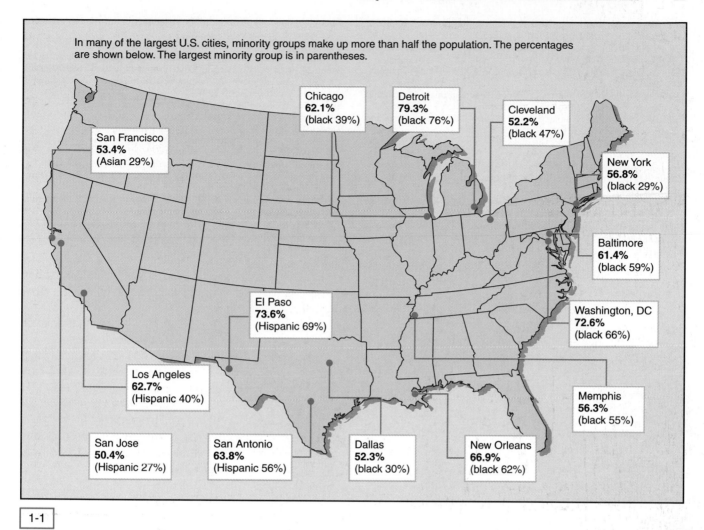

In many of the largest U.S. cities, minority groups make up more than half the population. The percentages are shown below. The largest minority group is in parentheses.

Chicago
62.1%
(black 39%)

Detroit
79.3%
(black 76%)

Cleveland
52.2%
(black 47%)

San Francisco
53.4%
(Asian 29%)

New York
56.8%
(black 29%)

Baltimore
61.4%
(black 59%)

El Paso
73.6%
(Hispanic 69%)

Washington, DC
72.6%
(black 66%)

Los Angeles
62.7%
(Hispanic 40%)

Memphis
56.3%
(black 55%)

San Jose
50.4%
(Hispanic 27%)

San Antonio
63.8%
(Hispanic 56%)

Dallas
52.3%
(black 30%)

New Orleans
66.9%
(black 62%)

1-1

their "cultural health rights," an expectation that frequently conflicts with the unicultural, Western, biomedical world view taught in American educational programs preparing nurses and other health care providers.

Given the multicultural composition of the United States and the projected increase in the number of individuals from diverse cultural backgrounds anticipated in the future, a concern for the cultural beliefs and practices of people is becoming increasingly important. Nursing is inherently a transcultural phenomenon in that the context and process of helping people involves at least two persons generally having different cultural orientations or intracultural lifestyles.

HIGH-LEVEL ASSESSMENT SKILLS

This attention to life cycle, holism, and culture does not detract from the importance of assessment skills themselves. Assessment skills must be practiced and refined to a high level. In many community settings, the

nurse is the first and often the only health professional to see an individual. In the hospital, the nurse is the only health professional continually present at the bedside.

Current efforts of cost containment result in a hospital population composed of people who have increased acuity, a shorter stay, and an earlier discharge than in the past. This situation requires faster, more efficient assessments from the nurse. Procedures that used to require a standard hospital stay of several days (e.g., surgery for inguinal hernia, insertion of a central intravenous line for total parenteral alimentation) now are done on an outpatient basis. As a result, nurses often go to people's homes for follow-up assessment and diagnosis. These situations require first-rate assessment skills, grounded in a holistic approach, with knowledge of age-specific problems.

Bibliography

American Nurses' Association: Standards of Clinical Nursing Practice. Washington, DC, American Nurses' Association, 1991.
Carpenito LJ: Nursing Diagnosis: Application to Clinical Practice, 7th ed. Philadelphia, Lippincott-Raven, 1997.

Cox RP: Family health care delivery for the 21st century. J Obstet Gynecol Neonatal Nurs 26(1):109–118, Jan–Feb 1997.

Crigger N: Defying denial: Clues to detecting alcohol abuse. Am J Nurs 98(8):20–21, Aug 1998.

Dunn H: High Level Wellness. Arlington VA, R.W. Beatty Company, 1961.

Dykeman M, Ervin NE: Nurses' attitudes towards primary health care: Development of an instrument. J Adv Nurs 18:1567–1572, 1993.

Field PA: The impact of nursing theory on the clinical decision making process. J Advanced Nurs 12:563–571, 1987.

Jensen L, Allen M: Wellness: The dialectic of illness. Image 25(3):220–224, 1993.

Joel LA: From NANDA to ICNP. Am J Nurs 98(7):7, July 1998.

Landis BJ: Employing prevention in practice. Am J Nurs 97(8):40–47, Aug 1997.

Leininger M: Transcultural Nursing: Concepts, Theories, and Practice, 2nd ed. New York, McGraw-Hill, 1995.

North American Nursing Diagnosis Association: News. Nurs Diagnosis 1(3):124, 1990.

Pender N: Health Promotion in Nursing Practice, 3rd ed. Norwalk, CT, Appleton & Lange, 1996.

Report of the U.S. Preventive Services Task Force: Guide to Clinical Preventive Services, 2nd ed. Baltimore, Williams & Wilkins, 1996.

Shoultz J, Hatcher PA: Looking beyond primary care to primary health care: An approach to community-based action. Nurs Outlook 45(1):23–26, Jan–Feb 1997.

Stolte KM: Wellness nursing diagnosis: Accentuating the positive. Am J Nurs 97(7):16B–16N, July 1997.

Taptich BJ, Iyer PW, Bernocchi-Losey D: Nursing Diagnosis and Care Planning, 2nd ed. Philadelphia, W.B. Saunders, 1994.

Travis JW, Ryan RS: Wellness Workbook, 2nd ed. Berkeley, CA, Ten Speed, 1986.

U.S. Bureau of the Census: General Population Characteristics. Washington DC, U.S. Government Printing Office, 1990.

Weber JR: Where are we going? Nursing diagnosis in education. Nurs Diagnosis 6(4):167–170, Oct–Dec 1995.

Woolf SH, Jonas S, Lawrence RS: Health Promotion and Disease Prevention in Clinical Practice. Baltimore, Williams & Wilkins, 1996.

CHAPTER TWO

Developmental Tasks and Health Promotion Across the Life Cycle

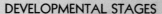

Application and
Critical Thinking

Much of this book details the method of collecting subjective and objective data about a person to construct a data base. The **data base** is used to assess the health state, to applaud health strengths and assets, and to uncover, diagnose, and treat health problems. To fit this data base into a meaningful frame, one must consider the developmental stage of that individual at that particular time. Appraising the life tasks that currently absorb the individual lets one appreciate the holistic frame of reference.

Consider a 66-year-old man who seeks health care for recurrent early morning insomnia: He falls asleep easily at night but awakens around 3:00 AM and spends hours unable to fall back asleep, sitting in his armchair. Among the data revealed in the interview is that 7 months ago this man was forced to retire because of his age from a powerful position as sales director for an appliance firm. The diagnosis and treatment of this presenting symptom are affected by the knowledge that the suicide rate among forced retirees is markedly greater than that for others in the same age group. Ask yourself—what interventions would you use had this same symptom been presented by a 38-year-old man who is considering whether to stay with his company or to set up his own business?

Growth is continuous and change is perpetual throughout the life cycle. A person progresses through a series of **stages,** not only in biologic growth but also in maturation of the physiologic systems, in cognitive development, and in personality development. Developmental stages are "qualitative changes in thinking, feeling, and behaving that characterize particular time periods of development" (Berk, 1998). During each of the stages, certain issues are dominant and consume more of the individual's attention and energy. The stages are not precisely distinct; transitions occur and overlap exists between stages.

A full consideration of developmental stages is beyond the scope of this text. You must refer to texts on child, adolescent, and lifespan development for a complete overview of the field. However, as you study health assessment, it helps to consider a few of the major frameworks of developmental theory to construct a holistic view of health assessment.

DEVELOPMENTAL STAGES

This section combines data from biologic growth and development and from the developmental theories to give a general portrayal of the individual in each stage of the life cycle. Each portrayal considers the physical, psychosocial, cognitive, and behavioral development of the person. Although they are not intended to be limiting, these portrayals offer a general framework. The stages are

1. Infancy (birth to 1 year)
2. Early childhood—Toddler (1 to 3 years)
3. Early childhood—Preschooler (3 to 5 or 6 years)
4. School child (6 to 10 or 12 years)
5. Preadolescent (10 to 12 or 13 years)
6. Adolescent (12 or 13 to 19 years)
7. Early adult (20 to 40 years)
8. Middle adult (40 to 64 years)
9. Late adult (65+ years)

Infancy (Birth to 1 Year)

The 1st year is the most dramatic and rapid period of growth and development. The baby changes from a totally dependent being into a person who interacts with the environment, and forms close relationships with other people (Fig. 2–1).

Physical Development

Growth. Weight, height, and head circumference reflect physical growth and are sensitive indicators of the infant's general health.

The average normal term infant weighs 3.4 kg (7½ lb), with 95 percent of full-term infants ranging from 2.5 to 4.6 kg (5½ to 10 lb). During the first few days, the baby loses a little weight but regains the birth weight by 10 days. Growth spurts double the birth weight by 4 to 6 months and triple the birth weight by 1 year. Length increases 50 percent by 1 year.

Head circumference reflects brain size; head growth shows brain growth. At birth, the average head circumference is 35 cm (13½ inches), with about 95 percent of infants within the range of 32.6 to 37.2 cm. Brain growth occurs rapidly during the first 2 years. Nutrition is essential, with the proper type and amount of fat calories and essential fatty acids required for brain development (see Chapter 7).

Physiologic Development. The development of each organ system through the life cycle is described in the corresponding physical examination chapter. But the central nervous system is worth mentioning here because during infancy it makes the most dramatic gains. Tremendous brain growth occurs during this period. Also, the

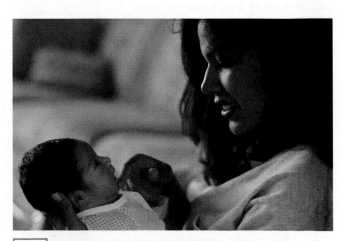

2–1

baby has numerous primitive reflexes that are present at birth or soon after and persist for specific time periods. These are under subcortical control; as the cerebral cortex grows and matures, it inhibits their expression. In a normal infant, these reflexes should disappear at specific times during the first year (see Chapter 21, Neurologic System). Certain protective reflexes (cough, gag, sneeze, eye-blink) are always present. Visual acuity is very poor at birth (about 20/800) and for the first few months, owing to immature and widely spaced foveas (i.e., the area on the retina of keenest vision). But acuity develops rapidly and is close to adult levels by the end of the first year (Barnard and Edgar, 1996).

Psychosocial Development

Stages of Ego Development. Erik Erikson (1902 to 1994) focused on cultural and societal influences as determinants of behavior. Erikson was concerned with the growth of the **ego,** the conscious, organized, rational part of the personality. He described eight stages of ego development that encompass the life span (Erikson, 1963).

Each stage is characterized by a distinct conflict, or **crisis,** relating to the person's physiologic maturation and to what society expects of a person at that age. Each crisis is a bipolar issue, a point at which personality development may go one way or another through the choices made by the individual. The bipolar aspect means that the crisis can have a positive or a negative outcome. The crisis must be resolved for the person to continue on to the next stage.

Erikson's Theory of Trust Versus Mistrust. Erikson's first stage has a broad psychosocial dimension. Erikson viewed the mother as the primary caregiver. The crucial element in this stage, then, is the *quality* of the mother-child relationship. The infant is completely helpless and depends on the mother for food, warmth, comfort, and companionship. When the mother is responsive and consistent in her nurturing, the infant learns **trust.** The security from this trust extends to trust in others and in the self. The infant learns that the world is a safe and reliable place and that he or she is welcome in it. If the mother is unresponsive, unnurturing, haphazard, or abusing, the infant learns **mistrust.** Since the infant never feels secure, he or she experiences anxiety and alienation. Without a trusting foundation, this individual will flounder in attempts to resolve future crises.

Absolute trust actually is not the healthy goal of this conflict. When resolution of this crisis is successful, the infant holds *relatively* more trust than mistrust. Total trust would impede survival in later years because not everyone or everything in the world *should* be trusted.

Cognitive Development

Jean Piaget (1896 to 1980) described stages of cognitive development in the growing child. Cognition is de-

fined as how the individual perceives and processes information about the world; it is the ability to know. Piaget believed that a child's thinking develops progressively from simple reflex behavior into complex logical and abstract thought. This development is biologically inherent in each maturing child and occurs independently of any special training.

The child's cognitive development proceeds through four definite and sequential stages. Each stage demonstrates a *qualitative* change, representing a new way of thinking and behaving. Although the ages of reaching the stages are approximate, the sequence of stages never varies. All children move through the same stages in the same order; no stage is skipped. Each stage is the foundation for the next, and the next stage builds on the stage before it. At each stage, the child's *scheme* (how the child views the world) becomes more intricate and complex.

According to Piaget, the first stage of **sensorimotor skills** (birth to 2 years) lasts longer than the 1st year of infancy. It is a time of intelligent activity, although full language skill has not yet developed. Infants perceive information through the five senses and learn to modify their behavior in response to these environmental stimuli. At birth, the only response is an array of reflexes (crying, rooting, sucking, grasping) that occur automatically. Gradually, the infant learns the important concept of **object permanence,** that objects and people continue to exist even when they are no longer in sight. This starts around 7 months when the infant searches for an object that is partly hidden but does not search for one completely out of sight. By 9 to 10 months, the infant looks behind a screen for an object, but only if it was seen to be hidden there. By 18 to 24 months, the concept is fully developed and the child conducts a true search in many places for objects hidden from sight. As this concept develops, the infant also learns that he or she is *separate* from objects in the environment.

Last, by age 2 the infant has acquired **mental representation** (or thought) and can think of an external event without actually experiencing it.

Behavioral Development

Gross Motor Skills. These skills include posture, head balance, sitting, crawling, and walking. Their development is predictable because it follows the direction of myelinization (laying down of myelin) in the nervous system; cephalocaudal (head-to-foot direction) and proximodistal (central-to-peripheral direction, or midline before extremities).*

Some head balance already is present at birth for protection; when prone, the baby can turn the head to the

---

*Tables summarizing growth and development milestones for infancy and for other age groups can be found in *Student Laboratory Manual for Physical Examination and Health Assessment,* 3rd ed.

side to avoid suffocation. Otherwise there is marked head lag, as when pulled to a sitting position from a lying position. By 3 months of age, the baby can raise the head *and* chest from a prone position with the arms extended for support. By 4 months of age, the head and chest are raised 90 degrees, and only slight head lag is demonstrated when the child is pulled to a sitting position. Sitting alone without support occurs at 6 to 7 months of age.

After 7 months, the baby ventures from the sitting position to explore the environment. Crawling usually begins around 7 months. At 8 months, the baby pulls to a stand and stands while holding onto an object for support. Between 9 and 11 months, the baby starts to "cruise" the room, walking upright while holding onto the furniture. Usually, the child can stand independently around 11 months, and by 12 months the child walks alone.

Fine Motor Skills. The development of fine motor skills involves using the hands and fingers for **prehension,** or the act of grasping. The infant is born with a grasp reflex; it fades at 2 months of age and is absent at 3 months of age. At 3 months the infant expresses interest in an object more with the eyes than with the hands. At 4 months, the infant inspects his or her hands, looks from object to hands and back, and may try to grasp an object with the hands but overshoots the mark. The voluntary two-handed grasp is present at 4 to 5 months.

Further distal refinement follows at 8 to 10 months with a crude pincer grasp using the index, fourth, and fifth fingers. By 10 months, the index finger is an apposition with the thumb for a neat pincer grasp, and the baby is absorbed in picking up raisins and finger foods. By 11 months the baby puts objects into a container and removes them. And at 13 months the baby builds a tower of two blocks.

Language Skills. Crying is the infant's first means of communication. Cries are undifferentiated at first, but by 1 month of age the infant alters the pitch and intensity of the cry to communicate different needs, such as hunger, discomfort, or loneliness. Vocal sounds build rapidly; the baby laughs out loud at 3 months, coos when he or she awakens or when someone talks to him or her at 2 to 4 months, and babbles at 6 months. At 9 to 10 months, the baby can imitate the sounds of others, although he or she may not necessarily understand them. At 12 months, a baby usually can say the first recognizable word with meaning.

Personal-Social Skills. Throughout the 1st year, the infant learns more and more social ties that bind her or him to other people. Early on, the baby shows a visual preference for the human face, and even in the first 30 to 60 minutes following birth watches the mother intently (see Fig. 2–1). The social smile erupts at 6 to 8 weeks, to the family's delight and continual reinforcement. At 4 months, the baby laughs and enjoys other people, and at 6 months extends arms to the parent to be picked up.

Imitation, or the copying of another person's behavior, is present in a limited way in newborns. Even the young baby will copy adult facial expressions such as opening the mouth, protruding the tongue, pursing the lips. As the neurologic system develops, at 7 months, the baby imitates others' actions, at 9 months their sounds, and at 10 months waves bye-bye and enjoys interactive games like pat-a-cake and peek-a-boo. At 11 months, the baby can help with feeding and dressing and follows simple directions. Emotions develop during the 1st year, and by 12 months, the baby will give a hug or kiss and show jealousy, fear, or anger.

Infant's Periodic Health Examination

Table 2–1 lists the services that you as health care provider should address during the infant's well-baby checkups. Note the aspects of screening at birth, the immunization schedule, and the parent counseling items regarding diet and injury prevention. Screening measures include those for high-risk groups, such as hearing impairment, and screening for lead poisoning. Note also that these tables are not intended to be a complete list of all the steps that *should* be included in the examination checkup. Instead, the table lists preventive services that were studied and shown to be clinically effective (U.S. Preventive Services Task Force, 1996).

Lead Poisoning. Lead poisoning prevalence had declined by 78 percent in the United States during the last decade. However, it is still a risk in central city communities and others that have exposure to lead sources, such as dilapidated, pre-1950 housing with peeling lead-based paint, lead water pipes, and lead in dust and soil from heavy traffic and factories (U.S. Task Force, 1996). Children are at risk because their bodies absorb four to five times greater amounts of the lead than adults do. Adverse effects of lead poisoning include below-average weight, developmental delays, learning disabilities, hearing deficits, hyperactivity and irritability, and physical symptoms of abdominal pain and constipation.

Sudden Infant Death Syndrome (SIDS). One important parent counseling measure is the "Back to Sleep" campaign that promotes sleeping on their backs for healthy infants as a way of decreasing the risk of SIDS (Gilbert-Barness and Barness, 1996; American Academy of Pediatrics, 1994). About 6000 infant deaths each year in the United States are attributed to SIDS, with the peak incidence occurring between 2 and 4 months. Although research has not identified the exact causes of SIDS, studies in Australia, New Zealand, and Great Britain reported striking reductions in SIDS deaths of over 50 percent after media campaigns that urged avoidance of prone (abdomen) sleeping. The mechanism of sudden

Table 2–1 • Periodic Health Examination: Birth to 10 Years

Interventions Considered and Recommended for the Periodic Health Examination	Leading Causes of Death
	Conditions originating in perinatal period
	Congenital anomalies
	Sudden infant death syndrome (SIDS)
	Unintentional injuries (nonmotor vehicle)
	Motor vehicle injuries

Interventions for the General Population

Screening	Limit fat and cholesterol; maintain caloric balance; emphasize grains, fruits, vegetables (age ≥2 yr)
Height and weight	Regular physical activity*
Blood pressure	Substance use
Vision screen (age 3–4 yr)	Effects of passive smoking*
Hemoglobinopathy screen (birth)[1]	Antitobacco message*
Phenylalanine level (birth)[2]	Dental Health
T_4 and/or TSH (birth)[3]	Regular visits to dental care provider*
Counseling	Floss, brush with fluoride toothpaste daily*
Injury Prevention	Advice about baby bottle tooth decay*
Child safety car seats (age <5 yr)	**Immunizations**
Lap-shoulder belts (age ≥5 yr)	Diphtheria-tetanus-pertussis (DTP)[4]
Bicycle helmet; avoid bicycling near traffic	Oral poliovirus (OPV)[5]
Smoke detector, flame retardant sleepwear	Measles-mumps-rubella (MMR)[6]
Hot water heater temperature <120–130°F	*H. influenzae* type b (Hib) conjugate[7]
Window/stair guards, pool fence	Hepatitis B[8]
Safe storage of drugs, toxic substances, firearms, and matches	Varicella[9]
Syrup of ipecac, poison control phone number	**Chemoprophylaxis**
CPR training for parents/caretakers	Ocular prophylaxis (birth)
Diet and Exercise	
Breastfeeding, iron-enriched formula and foods (infants and toddlers)	

Interventions for High-Risk Populations

Population	Potential Interventions (see detailed high-risk definitions)
Preterm or low birth weight	Hemoglobin/hematocrit (HR1)
Infants of mothers at risk for HIV	HIV testing (HR2)
Low income; immigrants	Hemoglobin/hematocrit (HR1); PPD (HR3)
TB contacts	PPD (HR3)
Native American/Alaska Native	Hemoglobin/hematocrit (HR1); PPD (HR3); hepatitis A vaccine (HR4); pneumococcal vaccine (HR5)
Travelers to developing countries	Hepatitis A vaccine (HR4)
Residents of long-term care facilities	PPD (HR3); hepatitis A vaccine (HR4); influenza vaccine (HR6)
Certain chronic medical conditions	PPD (HR3); pneumococcal vaccine (HR5); influenza vaccine (HR6)
Increased individual or community lead exposure	Blood lead level (HR7)
Inadequate water fluoridation	Daily fluoride supplement (HR8)
Family h/o skin cancer; nevi; fair skin, eyes, hair	Avoid excess/midday sun, use protective clothing* (HR9)

HR1 = Infants age 6–12 mo who are: living in poverty, black, Native American or Alaska Native, immigrants from developing countries, preterm or low birth weight infants, or infants whose principal dietary intake is unfortified cow's milk.

HR2 = Infants born to high-risk mothers whose HIV status is unknown. Women at high risk include: past or present injection drug use; persons who exchange sex for money or drugs, and their sex partners; injection drug-using, bisexual, or HIV-positive sex partners currently or in past; persons seeking treatment for STDs; blood transfusion during 1978–1985.

HR3 = Persons infected with HIV, close contacts of persons with known or suspected TB, persons with medical risk factors associated with TB, immigrants from countries with high TB prevalence, medically underserved low-income populations (including homeless), residents of long-term care facilities. See appropriate text for indications for BCG vaccine.

HR4 = Persons ≥2 yr living in or traveling to areas where the disease is endemic and where periodic outbreaks occur (e.g., countries with high or intermediate endemicity; certain Alaska Native, Pacific Island, Native American, and religious communities). Consider for institutionalized children aged ≥2 yr. Clinicians should also consider local epidemiology.

HR5 = Immunocompetent persons ≥2 yr with certain medical conditions, including chronic cardiac or pulmonary disease, diabetes mellitus, and anatomic asplenia. Immunocompetent persons ≥2 yr living in high-risk environments or social settings (e.g., certain Native American and Alaska Native populations).

HR6 = Annual vaccination of children ≥6 mo who are residents of chronic care facilities or who have chronic cardiopulmonary disorders, metabolic diseases (including diabetes mellitus), hemoglobinopathies, immunosuppression, or renal dysfunction. See appropriate text for indications for amantadine/rimantadine prophylaxis.

Continued

Table 2–1 • Periodic Health Examination: Birth to 10 Years *Continued*

Interventions for High-Risk Populations

HR7 = Children about age 12 mo who: 1) live in communities in which the prevalence of lead levels requiring individual intervention, including residential lead hazard control or chelation, is high or undefined; 2) live in or frequently visit a home built before 1950 with dilapidated paint or with recent or ongoing renovation or remodeling; 3) have close contact with a person who has an elevated lead level; 4) live near lead industry or heavy traffic; 5) live with someone whose job or hobby involves lead exposure; 6) use lead-based pottery; or 7) take traditional ethnic remedies that contain lead.

HR8 = Children living in areas with inadequate water fluoridation (<0.6 ppm).

HR9 = Persons with a family history of skin cancer, a large number of moles, atypical moles, poor tanning ability, or light skin, hair, and eye color.

---

[1]Whether screening should be universal or targeted to high-risk groups will depend on the proportion of high-risk individuals in the screening area, and other considerations. [2]If done during first 24 hr of life, repeat by age 2 wk. [3]Optimally between day 2 and 6, but in all cases before newborn nursery discharge. [4]2, 4, 6, and 12–18 mo, once between ages 4–6 yr (DTaP may be used at 15 mo and older). [5]2, 4, 6–18 mo, once between ages 4–6 yr. [6]12–15 mo and 4–6 yr. [7]2, 4, 6, and 12–15 mo, no dose needed at 6 mo if PRP-OMP vaccine is used for first 2 doses. [8]Birth, 1 mo, 6 mo; or, 0–2 mo, 1–2 mo later, and 6–18 mo. If not done in infancy: current visit, and 1 and 6 mo later. [9]12–18 mo; or older child without hx of chickenpox or previous immunization. Include information on risk in adulthood, duration of immunity, and potential need for booster doses.
*The ability of clinician counseling to influence this behavior is unproven.
CPR = cardiopulmonary resuscitation; HIV = human immunodeficiency virus; TB = tuberculosis; PPD = purified protein derivative; STDs = sexually transmitted diseases; BCG = bacille Calmette-Guérin.
From U.S. Preventive Services Task Force: Guide to Clinical Preventive Services, 2nd ed. Baltimore, MD, Williams & Wilkins, 1996.

death in a prone position may be an increased resistance to airflow, obstruction from displacement of the mandible, compression of the nose in soft bedding, or compromised blood supply to the brain stem (Gilbert-Barness and Barness, 1996). Although the new recommendations will not prevent all SIDS deaths, placing the baby on the back to sleep will decrease the risk of SIDS. Additional parent counseling strategies to help reduce SIDS risk include avoiding smoking around the infant, avoiding drugs and alcohol while pregnant, using a firm, flat mattress, avoiding overheating, avoiding crib bumpers, stuffed animals, waterbeds, and pillows, and continuing to breast feed the baby as long as possible.

Early Childhood, Toddler (1 to 3 Years)

With successful completion of 1st-year tasks, the child enters the 2nd year secure in a basic sense of trust. That security plus maturing muscles and developing language enable the child to launch into the process of exploring the environment (Fig. 2–2). The toddler explores everything, inhaling the world with the zeal of all first-time adventurers. Developmental tasks of this next stage include (Wong, 1999)

1. Differentiating self from others, particularly the mother
2. Tolerating separation from mother or parent
3. Withstanding delayed gratification
4. Controlling bodily functions
5. Acquiring socially acceptable behavior
6. Acquiring verbal communication
7. Interacting with others in a less egocentric manner

The child does not master all tasks during the toddler years, but a good foundation at this stage will facilitate successful completion of other tasks later.

Physical Development

Growth. The rate of growth decelerates during the 2nd year, with the child gaining an average of 2.5 kg (5½ lb) in body weight and 12 cm (4¾ in) in length.

Appearance. Toddler lordosis describes the normal upright posture of the toddler, with the potbelly, sway back, and short, slightly bowed legs. The increase in head circumference slows, and the head circumference equals the chest circumference between 1 and 2 years. After the 2nd year, the chest circumference exceeds individual head and abdominal measurements, and the extremities grow faster than the trunk.

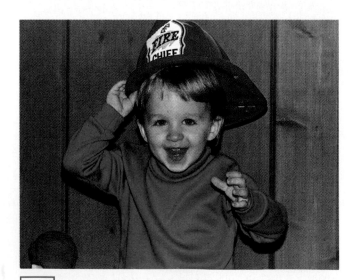

2–2

Physiologic Systems. Maturation of the physiologic systems is detailed in the corresponding physical examination chapters. Some neurologic advances are cited now because they permit developmental changes during the toddler years. For example, most brain growth occurs during the first 2 years, and changes in certain cortical areas permit language and motor development. In the spinal cord, myelination is almost complete by age 2, matching the gross motor achievements in locomotion. Visual acuity is close to 20/40 at 2 years and close to 20/30 by age 3 (Barnard and Edgar, 1996). The maturing convergence-accommodation mechanism matches the toddler's fascination with minute objects.

Psychosocial Development

Autonomy is the goal of all daily activities. The pursuit of independence occupies the toddler. For example, muscle maturation allows walking, exploring, and some self-care in feeding and dressing; refined visual acuity enhances close scrutiny and attention span; and language advances so the child can make known independent demands, such as "me do," "mommy way," or "me out." Between 12 and 18 months, the toddler ventures away from the parent to explore the immediate environment, still using her or him as a home base to come back to for support. Practice builds confidence, which encourages more exploration. Between 18 months and 3 years, it occurs to the child that he or she really has become quite separate from the parent. This creates some anxiety, which is manifested in the negativism, or the "terrible twos" behavior, normally seen at this age.

Autonomy Versus Shame and Doubt (1 to 3 Years). The quest for autonomy characterizes Erikson's second stage. The toddler wants to be autonomous and to govern his or her own body and experiences. The child wants to apply newly attained skills to explore the world. However, the child has not yet attained any sense of discrimination or judgment. The parent lives in the balance of letting the child explore but also firmly protecting the child from experiences that are dangerous or frustrating for the child's current ability level.

Erikson believed that toilet training symbolizes this stage. The toddler's muscle maturation has progressed to the "holding on" and "letting go" of things; this naturally extends to the sphincter muscles.

Cognitive Development

During the 2nd year, the toddler is still considered to be in Piaget's **sensorimotor period.** The readiness for independence is demonstrated between 12 and 18 months as the child now tries out new activities and new experiments to reach a goal. To reach a desired toy in her toybox, a girl at this age may try the various routes of taking out each object one by one, overturning the box and dumping the contents out, or climbing into the box herself. Learning comes by trial and error.

Between 18 and 24 months, the child develops **mental representation** for external events. This is a major achievement because the toddler can *think* through plans to reach a goal rather than merely perform them and observe the results by trial and error.

The concept of **object permanence** now is fully developed. The toddler comprehends both visible and invisible *displacements.* That means the child can search for an object in several places, even though it was not seen as it was hidden.

Around age 2, Piaget's **preoperational** stage begins. This use of symbols to represent objects and experiences is discussed in the next section on preschoolers.

Behavioral Development

Gross Motor Skills. Locomotion advances as the toddler usually walks alone at 12 months, runs stiffly at 18 months, and runs well without falling at 2 years. At 2 years, the child also can walk up and down stairs. The child jumps with both feet by 2 years.

Fine Motor Skills. Fine motor development shows increasing manual dexterity. At 15 months, the child can drop a pellet into a narrow-neck container and can hurl and retrieve objects. Fourteen-month-old hands hold a pencil and make scribbles, whereas by 2 years, the child can reproduce a vertical line from a demonstration.

Language Skills. Language progresses from a vocabulary of about two words at 1 year to a spurt to about 200 words by 2 years. Then the 2-year-old combines words into simple two-word phrases—"all gone," "me up," "baby crying." This is called **telegraphic speech,** which is usually a combination of a noun and a verb and includes only words that have concrete meaning. Interest in language is high during the 2nd year, and a 2-year-old seems to understand all that is said to him or her. A 3-year-old uses more complex sentences with more parts of speech.

Personal-Social Skills. Toddlers are usually compliant and cooperative with parents who are warm and sensitive and have reasonable expectations (Berk, 1998). However, parents often are surprised at the swift transformation of their loving affectionate child into a determined toddler who resists requests. Toddlers want their parents' approval but also want to assert themselves and do as many things for themselves as they can. As they test their powers, they sometimes clash with parents' restrictions, and a battle of wills results. "No" seems to be their favorite word.

This **negativism** is a normal part of the quest for autonomy. Although they protest vigorously, toddlers seem to fare better with firm, consistent limits. The thought of a limitless world and of personal untested powers is disabling to the child. Knowing where they stand, even if they disagree, is reassuring to toddlers.

Ritualism emerges along with the negativity. A 2-year-old wants things done in the same way; any change in schedule or habit is upsetting. A consistent routine assures the child that the world is predictable and orderly. Ritualism is heightened at age 2½, especially at bedtime, when the child insists on the same order of night-time tasks or the same order of colored blankets on the bed.

Although attachment to the parent is still strong, the toddler begins to play alone. Children 1 and 2 years of age venture away to explore but still need the reassurance of the parent's being there. Play with peers can be comical to the observer. Toddlers engage in **parallel** play, i.e., playing the same thing side by side without interaction and without trying to influence each other's behavior. The two children seemingly ignore each other yet unobtrusively check the other out to note what is happening. Imitation in play is apparent, both of peer activities and especially of parent activities such as sweeping, lawn mowing, or cooking. As the toddler is increasingly able to form mental images, play reveals increased imagination.

Toddler Periodic Health Examination

Study Table 2–1 for the immunization schedule, examination, screening measures, and parent counseling measures to address with parents of young children. Note the screening measures for high-risk categories of lead poisoning, tuberculosis exposure, and anemia.

Early Childhood, Preschool (3 to 5 or 6 Years)

Successful mastery of the toddler tasks plus a highly energized state make the preschooler ready for this time of developing initiative and purpose. Although parental relationships are still the most important, the preschooler begins to turn to other children and adults to broaden learning and play. Tasks during this period include

1. Realizing separateness as an individual
2. Identifying sex role and its functions
3. Developing a conscience
4. Developing a sense of initiative
5. Interacting with others in socially acceptable ways
6. Growing use of language for social interaction
7. Developing readiness for school

Physical Development

The rate of growth continues at a slower pace, and the average child gains about 2 kg (4½ lb) in weight and 7 cm (2¾ in) in height per year. The appearance changes as the "baby face" matures, the potbelly slims, and the legs elongate more than the trunk does. The preschooler looks taller, slimmer, and more graceful.

Most physiologic systems are now mature, but the musculoskeletal system is still developing. Muscles are growing, and cartilage is changing to bone at a faster rate than before. Nutrition is crucial for bone growth. A serious nutrient loss at this age alters the shape, thickness, and growth of bones.

Psychosocial Development

Although still primarily egocentric, the preschooler now broadens the scope to include some awareness of other people's interests, needs, and values. As this happens, the **conscience** or **superego** develops. The child learns right from wrong and their corresponding rewards and punishments.

Identifying the Gender Role. As children become aware of their separateness, they also learn that they belong to a further differentiated category—male or female. They are learning **gender,** or how males and females *do* differ. As early as age 2, children label themselves as "girl" or "boy" and assign their family members and pets to these basic gender categories. Then children begin to develop gender roles by a process called **gender typing,** or how society says males and females *should* differ. Children learn the behaviors and attitudes that their culture says are right for a man or a woman. The parents have a strong influence in gender typing, as is seen, for example, as a preschool girl imitates words and actions she has observed in her mother. But her social circle is enlarging, and the girl also picks up important messages from peers, teachers, books, and television about how girls and boys should differ. These messages can forge strong gender-stereotyping, and the preschooler often develops rigid rules about what boys and girls should wear and about what roles they can "be" when they play make-believe (Berk, 1998).

Learning at this stage has a broader scope, though, than just learning the appropriate gender role. As the girl mentioned earlier identifies with her mother, she assimilates and internalizes the mother's ideals and values. She learns the standards of society presented to her by the words and deeds of the mother. This is the development of the conscience, which now will direct the girl's behavior. Interaction with peers helps to develop the conscience too, as in play where children construct notions of justice and fair play.

Initiative Versus Guilt (4 to 5 Years). For this stage of ego development, Erikson believed that the child's chief task is to develop a sense of initiative. With increasing locomotor and mental power, the child now has an energy surplus, resulting in determination and enterprise. The child plans and attacks a new task with gusto and wants to stay with it. Any failures are easily forgotten in the quest to test the world. When the parent encourages, reassures, and cheers the child on (while protecting him or her from harm), the child learns self-assertion, spontaneity, self-sufficiency, direction, and purpose. But if the parent ridicules, punishes, or prevents the child from following through on tasks that could be done, the child feels guilty. The guilt exists not only when the child acts inappropriately but also when he or she is thinking of goals that the child would like to accomplish.

By nurturing successes and promoting a healthy self-image, the parents help the preschooler develop *self-esteem.* Self-esteem is the judgment the child makes about his or her own worth as well as any feelings about the judgment (Berk, 1998). Self-esteem is most important because it becomes the way we value our own competence. Our self-esteem affects our emotional experiences, future behavior, and long-term psychological adjustment (Berk, 1998).

Cognitive Development

Piaget's **preoperational stage** covers age 2 to 7 years, a longer span than the preschool years. It is characterized by **symbolic function,** because the child now uses symbols to represent people, objects, and events. This process is liberating. Now the child can conjure up thoughts of the father, for example, without actually seeing him or hearing his voice. The symbolic function is revealed in child's play, as in **delayed imitation.** That means a child can witness an event, form a mental representation of it, and imitate it later in the absence of the model. For example, a little boy watches his father dress and leave for work, then later in the day the boy wraps a tie around his neck, packs his "briefcase," and heads for the door.

Although representational thought is a great milestone, the preschooler's thinking continues to be limited. Thinking is concrete and literal. The preschooler focuses on only one aspect of a situation at a time and ignores others, a characteristic known as **centration.** For example, given a pile of blocks, a preschooler will sort by color (red, blue, yellow), or by shape (square, triangle, circle), but not by both. According to Piaget, a child in the preoperational stage is **egocentric.** This child cannot see another's point of view and feels no need to elaborate his or her own point of view, because the child assumes everyone else sees things as he or she does (Piaget, 1968). More recent research suggests that 4-year-olds can have an awareness of another's view (Berk, 1998).

Behavioral Development

Motor Skills. The physical bumbling of the toddler fades, and the preschool child demonstrates admirable gross motor and fine motor control. A 4-year-old child can hop on one foot. A 5-year-old child can skip on alternate feet and jump rope and may begin to swim and skate. Girls often achieve fine motor milestones ahead of boys of the same age. A 3-year-old child can draw a circle; a 4-year-old child can cut on a line with scissors, draw a person, and make crude letters. A 5-year-old can string beads, control a crayon well, and copy a square and letters and numbers, and has demonstrated preference for the right or left hand.

Language Skills. Between 3 and 4 years of age, the child uses three- to four-word **telegraphic** sentences containing only essential words. By 5 to 6 years, the sentences are six to eight words long, and grammar is well developed.

Piaget labeled the earlier speech pattern as egocentric (Piaget, 1975). Children at this age talk incessantly. They are wrapped up in their own thoughts and talk to themselves merely for the pleasure of hearing their own voices say the words. Piaget believed speech here is in the form of a *monologue* to the self, or a *collective monologue* between two children, in which they talk at each other but are still absorbed in themselves, and no communication has occurred.

However, more recent research challenges Piaget's views and demonstrates that this **private speech** is a problem-solving tool that is beneficial to all children as they try new tasks or work through unfamiliar situations (Berk, 1994). Children chatter to themselves between the ages of 4 and 6; this chatter becomes inaudible muttering during early elementary school; and then it mostly drops away. Researchers noted that when a child undertakes a new task, an adult usually explains the steps needed to perform the task, often in detail, as directions or strategies. When the child next works through the task alone, he or she uses private speech as a way of repeating the adult's expert advice as his or her own independent guidelines. This evolves into muttering because one often uses verbal shorthand with one's own self; that is, the child omits saying the words that refer to familiar steps and verbalizes only the words that refer to the still-confusing steps. Finally, as the child has mastered the skill, the air is silent because the mind has internalized the private speech into thinking inner speech. Private speech reemerges throughout life as we confront new tasks or unfamiliar or stressful situations (Berk, 1994).

Personal-Social Skills. The preschooler is self-assertive, but the negativism of the toddler years has diminished. This child wants to please others. By taking on the values of the family and developing a conscience, the child monitors his or her own behavior to maximize acceptance. The preschooler is proud of his or her self-sufficiency and accomplishes everyday self-care (dressing, feeding, toileting) almost completely. The world enlarges because the child's anxiety toward strangers and fear of separation decreases; the at-home preschooler is able to tolerate brief separations from the parents to enjoy visiting peers or preschool. Some preschoolers have already been in day care from an early age, and parental separations are less of an issue.

With their growing social regard, preschoolers enjoy **cooperative play** with each other. This means that they play the same game and interact while doing it. The child's imagination runs rampant, and this factor shows in the play. Preschoolers love to dress up and imitate the sex role behaviors of their parents as well as admired adult models, such as nurses, doctors, media heroes, fire-fighters, or police officers. Often this make-believe or fantasy play is a coping strategy: a sheltered workshop in which the preschooler can work out conflicts and fears or master life experiences.

It is easy for fantasy and reality to blur. Children experience the greatest number of new fears between 2 and 6 years of age. Visions of ghosts and monsters, fear of the dark, fear of being lost—all arise from the child's increased imagination as well as from some frightening experiences that the child really has had. Also, beginning around age 2½ or 3 years, children often invent imaginary playmates. The imaginary friend often serves as an alter ego and tries out behaviors that the child yearns to try or takes the blame when the child misbehaves. Although it is important for a time, the imaginary friend is easily given up when the child enters school.

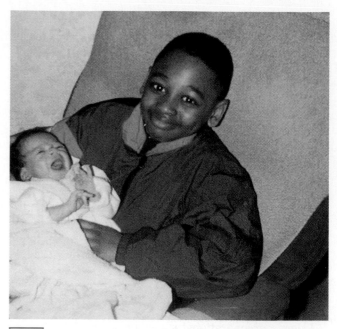

2–3

Middle Childhood, School-Age Child (6 to 10 or 12 Years)

The best preparation for this age is a firm foundation in trust, autonomy, and initiative (Fig. 2–3). Secure in these attributes, the child is able to move into a larger world and tackle these tasks:

1. Mastering skills that will be needed later as an adult
2. Winning approval from other adults and peers
3. Building self-esteem and a positive self-concept
4. Taking a place in a peer group
5. Adopting moral standards

Physical Development

Physical growth is slow but steady during the school years. The average child gains about 3 kg (6½ lb) and grows about 5.5 cm (2 in) per year. The growth rates in boys and girls are basically the same, with boys only slightly heavier and taller than girls. Black children are slightly larger and Asian children slightly smaller than white children of the same age. The preadolescent growth spurt occurs earlier in girls, at about age 10 years, as compared with age 12 for boys.

The physical appearance of the school-age child is relatively slimmer than that of the younger child because of the older child's proportionately longer legs, diminishing body fat, and a lower center of gravity. Although the cranium achieved most of its growth in the early years, now the bones of the face and jaw grow faster. During these years, primary teeth are lost, which the child hails as a big event and developmental milestone. The eruption

of large permanent teeth into a mouth and face that looks too small for them gives this child the ungainly, so-called ugly duckling appearance.

Body carriage is more agile and graceful. Bones continue to ossify during these years, and bone replaces cartilage. Muscles are stronger and more developed, though not yet fully mature. Neuromuscular control is more coordinated. All these refinements ready the school child for repetitive pursuit of activities requiring fine motor skills, such as writing, drawing, needlework, small model building, and playing instruments, and large muscle activities, such as running, throwing, jumping, biking, and swimming.

Psychosocial Development

Erikson highlights the directing of energy into learning skills when he characterizes middle childhood as a period focused on **industry versus inferiority.** In this stage, age 6 to 11 years, the child focuses much of the time at school. Now, the approval and esteem of people outside the immediate family become important. The child wins this recognition by working and producing. Play and fantasy give way to mastering the skills that the child will need later to compete in the adult world. This child values independence in tackling a new task and takes pleasure in carrying it through to completion. The young worker is eager, diligent, and absorbed. Also, the value of social relationships emerges as the child sees the benefits of working in an organized group. Children learn to divide labor and to cooperate to achieve a common goal.

Real achievement at this stage builds a feeling of confidence, competence, and industry. The child is rewarded by his or her own inner sense of satisfaction in achieving a skill and more importantly at this age by external rewards such as approval from teachers, parents, and peers in the form of grades, allowance, or special gifts. Problems arise when the child feels inferior. If the child believes that he or she cannot measure up to society's expectations, the child loses confidence and does not take pleasure in the work. A gnawing feeling of inferiority and incompetence grows and will continue to haunt this child.

The reality is that no one can master everything. There is bound to be something at which each child will feel inferior. Caring parents and teachers will try to balance these weaker skills with areas in which the child can excel. The problem is that, in some cultures, success in certain areas has a higher social value, particularly among peers. For example, in Western cultures, team sports are admired more than playing chess, or success in reading may be rewarded more than in drawing. The challenge to adults is to provide the successful experiences and positive reinforcement so that each child can achieve.

At this age, peer approval is beginning to be significant. During middle childhood, it is important to belong to a peer group. The peer group is a key socializing agent. Group solidarity is enhanced by secret codes or strict rules. The child conforms to group rules because acceptance is paramount. The child begins to prefer peer group activities to activities with the parents.

Cognitive Development

Piaget labels the stage of middle childhood, age 7 to 11 years, as the period in which the child focuses on **concrete operations.** At this age, the child can use symbols (mental representations) of objects and events in more logical ways. This means a child can experience mentally what she or he would have had to do physically before. For example, to describe the classic hopscotch maneuvers to you, a girl now can articulate them ("first you hop on one foot . . .") rather than merely performing them.

Armed with the ability to use thinking to experience things or events, the school child can

- Use numbers. While counting with numbers begins in preschool years, the school-age child has the combinational skill to add and subtract, multiply and divide.
- Read. By using printed symbols (words) for objects and events, the child can process a significant amount of information. Also, reading fosters independence in learning.
- Serialize. While this begins in preschool years, the school-age child can order objects by an increasing or decreasing scale, such as according to number size (smallest to largest) or weight (lightest to heaviest).
- Classify. This is the ability to sort objects by something they have in common. While young children can

do this, the school-age child is able to organize a hierarchy of classes and subclasses. It shows in the school-age child's penchant for collections: rocks, shells, novelty cards, cars, and dolls. A child spends many hours sorting the collections, and the logic of the classification system gets more complex as the child grows.

- Understand conservation principles. Understanding conservation of matter is the ability to tell the difference between how things seem and how they really are. It is the ability to see that mass or quantity stays constant even though shape or position is transformed. For example, the child who can conserve sees that two equal amounts of water remain the same even if one is poured into a different-shaped beaker (see Fig. 2–4).

At this age, thinking is more stable and logical. The school-age child can *decenter* and consider all sides of a situation to form a conclusion. The school-age child is able to reason, but this reasoning capacity still is limited because he or she cannot yet deal with abstract ideas.

Preadolescence (10 to 12 or 13 Years)

This period covers fifth to eighth grades, ending with puberty. Although this stage is still part of childhood, children in this group have common skills and interests that set them apart. It becomes more difficult now to

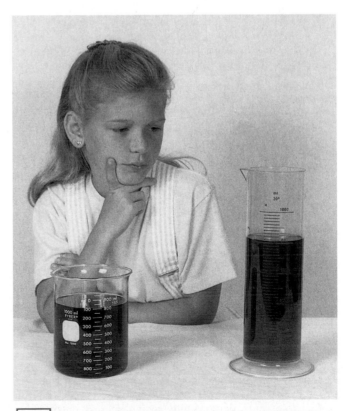

2–4

typify characteristics of a single year. Because of rapid growth, the age levels start to blend and overlap. A child may be at one level physically and intellectually but at another level socially. Children of the same age show diverse development levels.

Physical Development

Physical growth is markedly different at this stage; boys show slow and steady growth, whereas girls have rapid growth. On the average, the growth spurt begins in girls at age 10 years and reaches its greatest velocity at 12, whereas in boys the growth spurt begins at 12 and attains its maximum velocity at 14 years.

Even among girls, growth is varied. In a group of 11-year-old girls, each girl looks different from the others. Some look like children, and some are starting to look like adolescents. At 10 years, some girls have begun their growth spurt and have begun to grow pubic hair and to have breast development. At age 12 years, girls demonstrate the most rapid growth in height and weight. The breasts enlarge, the areolae darken, growth of axillary hair begins, and menarche occurs.

Physical size among 11-year-old boys is fairly uniform. At 12 years, boys show a wider range of growth. Most demonstrate the onset of secondary sex characteristics with initial genital growth, appearance of pubic hair, and the occurrence of erections and nocturnal emissions.

Boys and girls both exhibit a great amount of physical restlessness. Their activity is well directed into individual and team sports. Their percolating energy makes it hard for them to sit still, and it shows by tapping the foot or drumming the finger.

Psychosocial Development

Parent-child ties exhibit some strain as the child gradually starts to drift away from the family. The parents continue to set standards and values, but the child begins to challenge authority and to reject their standards. Parents decrease in stature in the child's eyes as the child learns that parents are not perfect and do not know everything. Yet the child loves the parents. He or she needs and wants some restrictions. Making up one's own rules is too frightening.

At 9 to 10 years, the child demonstrates a new ability to love by establishing a relationship with a best friend. This is important because the best friend is the first one outside the family that the child loves as being as important as himself or herself. By sharing interests, goals, and secret ideas with the best friend, the child learns a lot about himself or herself. This is comforting because the child realizes that he or she is not so different from other children after all. This yields a valuable lesson in self-acceptance.

Preadolescents demonstrate social interest outside the family. There is strong identity with the peer group by a small *clique* or a larger, more loosely organized *crowd* formation. Girls and boys stay within their own sex group. The clique has an exclusive membership, and one is privileged to belong. The code of the clique is important, with rules for dressing, speaking, and behaving in common. The child merges his or her identity with that of the peer group. The child is substituting conformity with the family to that with the peers because he or she needs the security of a temporary identity before formulating a clear sense of self (Berk, 1998).

Despite the fact that peer groupings are composed of the same sex, some preadolescents show an emerging interest in mixed groups, an interest that will flourish in adolescence.

Adolescence (12 or 13 to 19 Years)

This is a transition stage between childhood and adulthood (Fig. 2–5). Beginning at puberty and extending through the teenage years, the most important task of adolescence is the **search for identity,** "who I really am." With successful mastery of skills from the previous stage, childhood ends. Now, the adolescent must process the information from earlier stages and assume a personal identity that is more than just the sum of childhood experiences. The search for identity is the motive behind all the other tasks of the period:

1. Searching for one's identity
2. Appreciating one's achievements
3. Growing independent from parents
4. Forming close relationships with peers
5. Developing analytic thinking
6. Evolving one's own value system

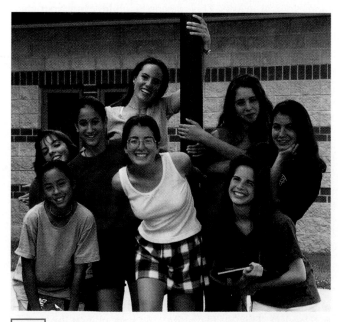

2–5

7. Developing a sexual identity
8. Beginning to choose a career

Physical Development

Adolescence begins with puberty. Puberty is a time of dramatic physiologic change. It includes the growth spurt—rapid growth in height, weight, and muscular development; development of primary and secondary sex characteristics; and maturation of the reproductive organs.

A changing body affects a person's self-concept. With bodies that are changing so rapidly, it is difficult for boys and girls to adjust. Their self-awareness peaks; they continually compare how their body looks with that of their peers and to some ideal standard of attractiveness. They are keenly attuned to the appearance of secondary sex characteristics but are embarrassed if these appear too early or too late. It is best when their own development parallels that of close friends and peers. Being an early maturer or, especially, a late maturer adds to normal self-doubts that they experience.

Physical health is generally good. Childhood illnesses are behind them, and the risks of adult illnesses are not yet present. What does place their health at risk are episodes of poor or immature judgment resulting in accidents, drug or alcohol abuse, sexually transmitted disease (STD), and unwanted pregnancy. Psychological dysfunction may occur, such as anorexia nervosa or depression. Suicide acts and attempts affect an increasing number of adolescents. Suicide is a leading cause of death in this age group. Its incidence would probably be higher if more accidental deaths were investigated.

Adolescent's Periodic Health Examination

Study Table 2–2 for screening procedures and counseling measures. The physical examination now should include self-care on skin self-examination, breast self-examination or testicular self-examination, and frequency of pelvic examinations (see Chapters 10, 15, 22, 24 for details). It is particularly important to include counseling on substance use, unwanted pregnancy prevention, and STD risk reduction.

Psychosocial Development

Theoretical views of adolescence vary. Psychologist G. Stanley Hall (1916) saw adolescence as a transitional stage fraught with turbulence and vacillating emotions. He called it in German *Sturm und Drang,* or storm and stress. In contrast, anthropologists Ruth Benedict (1934) and Margaret Mead (1935, 1953, 1961) saw the impor-

Table 2–2 • Periodic Health Examination: Ages 11–24 Years

Interventions Considered and Recommended for the Periodic Health Examination	Leading Causes of Death
	Motor vehicle/other unintentional injuries
	Homicide
	Suicide
	Malignant neoplasms
	Heart diseases

Interventions for the General Population	
Screening	female barrier with spermicide*
Height and weight	Unintended pregnancy: contraception
Blood pressure[1]	Diet and Exercise
Papanicolaou (Pap) test[2] (females)	Limit fat and cholesterol; maintain caloric balance; emphasize grains, fruits, vegetables
Chlamydia screen[3] (females <20 yr)	Adequate calcium intake (females)
Rubella serology or vaccination hx[4] (females >12 yr)	Regular physical activity*
Assess for problem drinking	Dental Health
Counseling	Regular visits to dental care provider*
Injury Prevention	Floss, brush with fluoride toothpaste daily*
Lap/shoulder belts	**Immunizations**
Bicycle/motorcycle/ATV helmets*	Tetanus-diphtheria (Td) boosters (11–16 yr)
Smoke detector*	Hepatitis B[5]
Safe storage/removal of firearms*	MMR (11–12 yr)[6]
Substance Use	Varicella (11–12 yr)[7]
Avoid tobacco use	Rubella[4] (females >12 yr)
Avoid underage drinking and illicit drug use*	**Chemoprophylaxis**
Avoid alcohol/drug use while driving, swimming, boating, etc.*	Multivitamin with folic acid (females planning/capable of pregnancy)
Sexual Behavior	
STD prevention: abstinence*; avoid high-risk behavior*; condoms	

Continued

Table 2-2 • Periodic Health Examination: Ages 11-24 Years *Continued*

Interventions for High-Risk Populations

Population	Potential Interventions (see detailed high-risk definitions)
High-risk sexual behavior	RPR/VDRL (HR1); screen for gonorrhea (female) (HR2), HIV (HR3), chlamydia (female) (HR4); hepatitis A vaccine (HR5)
Injection or street drug use	RPR/VDRL (HR1); HIV screen (HR3); hepatitis A vaccine (HR5); PPD (HR6); advice to reduce infection risk (HR7)
TB contacts; immigrants; low income	PPD (HR6)
Native Americans/Alaska Natives	Hepatitis A vaccine (HR5); PPD (HR6); pneumococcal vaccine (HR8)
Travelers to developing countries	Hepatitis A vaccine (HR5)
Certain chronic medical conditions	PPD (HR6); pneumococcal vaccine (HR8); influenza vaccine (HR9)
Settings where adolescents and young adults congregate	Second MMR (HR10)
Susceptible to varicella, measles, mumps	Varicella vaccine (HR11); MMR (HR12)
Blood transfusion between 1978-1985	HIV screen (HR3)
Institutionalized persons; health care/lab workers	Hepatitis A vaccine (HR5); PPD (HR6); influenza vaccine (HR9)
Family h/o skin cancer; nevi; fair skin, eyes, hair	Avoid excess/midday sun, use protective clothing* (HR13)
Prior pregnancy with neural tube defect	Folic acid 4.0 mg (HR14)
Inadequate water fluoridation	Daily fluoride supplement (HR15)

HR1 = Persons who exchange sex for money or drugs, and their sex partners; persons with other STDs (including HIV); and sexual contacts of persons with active syphilis. Clinicians should also consider local epidemiology.

HR2 = Females who have: two or more sex partners in the last year; a sex partner with multiple sexual contacts; exchanged sex for money or drugs; or a history of repeated episodes of gonorrhea. Clinicians should also consider local epidemiology.

HR3 = Males who had sex with males after 1975; past or present injection drug use; persons who exchange sex for money or drugs, and their sex partners; injection drug-using, bisexual, or HIV-positive sex partner currently or in the past; blood transfusion during 1978-1985; persons seeking treatment for STDs. Clinicians should also consider local epidemiology.

HR4 = Sexually active females with multiple risk factors including: history of prior STD; new or multiple sex partners; age under 25; nonuse or inconsistent use of barrier contraceptives; cervical ectopy. Clinicians should consider local epidemiology of the disease in identifying other high-risk groups.

HR5 = Persons living in, traveling to, or working in areas where the disease is endemic and where periodic outbreaks occur (e.g., countries with high or intermediate endemicity; certain Alaska Native, Pacific Island, Native American, and religious communities); men who have sex with men; injection or street drug users. Vaccine may be considered for institutionalized persons and workers in these institutions, military personnel, and day-care, hospital, and laboratory workers. Clinicians should also consider local epidemiology.

HR6 = HIV positive, close contacts of persons with known or suspected TB, health care workers, persons with medical risk factors associated with TB, immigrants from countries with high TB prevalence, medically underserved low-income populations (including homeless), alcoholics, injection drug users, and residents of long-term care facilities. See appropriate text for indications for BCG vaccine.

HR7 = Persons who continue to inject drugs.

HR8 = Immunocompetent persons with certain medical conditions, including chronic cardiac or pulmonary disease, diabetes mellitus, and anatomic asplenia. Immunocompetent persons who live in high-risk environments or social settings (e.g., certain Native American and Alaska Native populations).

HR9 = Annual vaccination of: residents of chronic care facilities; persons with chronic cardiopulmonary disorders, metabolic diseases (including diabetes mellitus), hemoglobinopathies, immunosuppression, or renal dysfunction; and health care providers for high-risk patients. See appropriate text for indications for amantadine/rimantadine prophylaxis.

HR10 = Adolescents and young adults in settings where such individuals congregate (e.g., high schools and colleges), if they have not previously received a second dose.

HR11 = Healthy persons aged ≥13 yr without a history of chickenpox or previous immunization. Consider serologic testing for presumed susceptible persons aged ≥13 yr.

HR12 = Persons born after 1956 who lack evidence of immunity to measles or mumps (e.g., documented receipt of live vaccine on or after the first birthday, laboratory evidence of immunity, or a history of physician-diagnosed measles or mumps).

HR13 = Persons with a family or personal history of skin cancer, a large number of moles, atypical moles, poor tanning ability, or light skin, hair, and eye color.

HR14 = Women with prior pregnancy affected by neural tube defect who are planning pregnancy.

HR15 = Persons aged <17 yr living in areas with inadequate water fluoridation (<0.6 ppm).

---

[1]Periodic blood pressure for persons aged ≥21 yr. [2]If sexually active at present or in the past: q ≤3 yr. If sexual history is unreliable, begin Pap tests at age 18 yr. [3]If sexually active. [4]Serologic testing, documented vaccination history, and routine vaccination against rubella (preferably with MMR) are equally acceptable alternatives. [5]If not previously immunized: current visit, 1 and 6 mo later. [6]If no previous second dose of MMR. [7]If susceptible to chickenpox.
*The ability of clinician counseling to influence this behavior is unproven.
ATV = all-terrain vehicle; STD = sexually transmitted disease; MMR = measles-mumps-rubella; TB = tuberculosis; HIV = human immunodeficiency virus; RPR = rapid plasma reagin; VDRL = Venereal Disease Research Laboratories; PPD = purified protein derivative; BCG = bacille Calmette-Guérin.

tance of cultural influences on adolescence. They observed that in simpler societies in which the child had meaningful, responsible work to do and could see clearly the upcoming adult role, adolescence is smooth and serene.

Erikson believes the main conflict of the fifth stage in his theory to be **ego identity versus role diffusion.** The adolescent is preoccupied with how he or she looks to others, and how that image fits with his or her own view of the self. If this process is successful, a sense of ego identity emerges, culminating in what Erikson terms a career choice. If unsuccessful, if the teen is unsure of his or her skills, self-worth, or sexual identity, role confusion results. The adolescent feels cut adrift and experiences anxiety about being a social outcast.

Finding one's own identity is stressful. In the search for identity, teens often form cliques, wear fad clothing, and follow rock singers, movie stars, or charismatic heroes in an attempt to siphon identity from them. Falling in love also feeds the quest for personal identity; the teen projects his or her own ego qualities onto another person and tries to understand them as they are reflected by the loved one.

Cognitive Development

Adolescence corresponds to Piaget's fourth stage, in which the person focuses on **formal operations** and the ability to develop abstract thinking, deal with hypothetical situations, and make logical conclusions from reviewing evidence. Now, thinking is no longer confined to the concrete or the real but encompasses all that is possible. Abstract thinking is liberating. The adolescent is no longer limited to the present but can ponder the lessons of the past and the possibilities of the future. The adolescent now can analyze and use scientific reasoning. One can imagine hypotheses and then set up experiments to test them. One learns to use logic and solves problems by methodically eliminating each possibility, one by one. This opens the doors to new academic achievements such as mastering advanced mathematical concepts, chemistry, physics, or logic (Fig. 2–6).

This analytic thinking extends to values. Developing personal values is a part of the search for identity. The adolescent does not accept packaged values of parents or institutions but can reason through his or her inconsistencies and recognize injustices. The adolescent is sensitive to hypocrisy and notes when an adult professes a value (such as honesty) and then acts counter to it (such as cheating on income tax).

Behavioral Development

Socially, the adolescent is in limbo, because he or she rejects identity with the parents but is not yet sure of his or her own individual identity. The perfect solution to

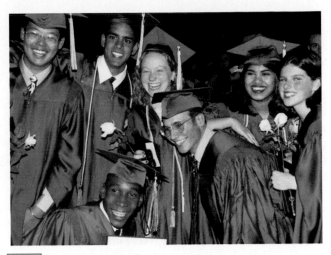

2–6

this dilemma is immersion in a peer group. Pressure to belong to a peer group intensifies at this age. The adolescent is influenced strongly by the group's norms for dress and behavior. By identifying with peers, the adolescent joins a sheltered workshop in which he or she feels safe and can experiment with various roles. Group members are allies in the universal goal of seeking freedom from parental domination.

Group identity means the adolescent spends more time away from home and the parents. Adolescents often feel ambivalent toward the parents. They desperately want to be independent from the parents but realize that economically, and even emotionally, this is impossible. Their stated desire to escape from parental dominance conceals their anxiety about leaving the safety of the family. The conflict is exacerbated when the parents try to maintain rigid control and use the protective stance that worked during earlier childhood. Often, things go smoother when the parents are not as strict, allow privacy, respect the adolescent's budding identity, and above all, take the adolescent seriously.

Developing close friendships is important to personal identity. In preadolescence, the experience of the relationship with the best friend is valuable in teaching intimacy, trust, and regard for another person. These lessons become a link in the new quest of developing close relationships with the opposite sex. Finding a girlfriend or boyfriend enables the adolescent to learn his or her own sex role identity. In many settings, group dating (youth groups, teen dances) is the norm at first. This decreases stress from paired dating. When adolescents do pair off, they usually have a monogamous relationship involving affection and fidelity.

Most adolescents worry that an occasional homosexual thought or act means that they are homosexual. These adolescent experiences are common and cannot turn a person into a gay or lesbian. Of course, some teenagers (about 3 to 6 percent) do discover that they have a homosexual orientation and that this lifestyle feels natural for them (Patterson, 1995).

The end of adolescence is more difficult to define. Some societies have recognized rites of passage, usually at puberty, when the young person earns a place in the adult world with its attendant responsibilities. But in complex Western societies, the adolescent remains dependent on the parents through the teen years and into the 20s for economic and educational reasons. This extends the period of adolescence. Consequently, the role is not well defined in our society, and this is a source of conflict.

Early Adulthood (20 to 40 Years)

The young adult is concerned with emancipation from his or her parents and building an independent lifestyle. The young adult has finished most formal schooling and is ready to embark on a chosen path (Fig. 2–7). The tasks of this era include

1. Growing independent from the parents' home and care
2. Establishing a career or vocation
3. Forming an intimate bond with another and choosing a mate
4. Learning to cooperate in a marriage relationship
5. Setting up and managing one's own household
6. Making friends and establishing a social group
7. Assuming civic responsibility and becoming a citizen in the community

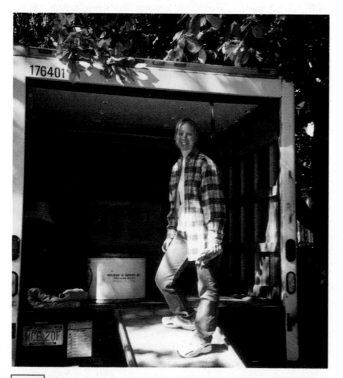

2–7

8. Beginning a parenting role
9. Forming a meaningful philosophy of life

Physical and cognitive developments now are steady and do not affect the young adult as much as they have before. Rather, sociocultural factors and values buffet the novice adult.

Physical Development

By early adulthood, the body reaches its maximum potential for growth and development. All body systems now operate at peak efficiency. The young adult enjoys maximum muscle tone and coordination, a high energy level, and optimum mental power. This person exudes freshness and vitality.

Since growth is finished, nutritional needs depend on maintenance and repair requirements and on activity levels. If activity decreases from its level during adolescence, calories must be reduced. Sensible nutrition is a major problem for many adults, and this is not confined to persons with low incomes. The diet should be high in fruits, vegetables, and grain but all too often is high in sugar, salt, and fat. A sedentary lifestyle adds further problems. However, more adults are learning that frequent steady exercise maintains weight, muscle strength, and joint flexibility; builds heart and lung capacity; and reduces stress. Table 2–2 lists these and other preventive counseling measures to address during health care visits.

Cognitive Development

During adolescence, cognitive functioning reached the new level of formal operations, or the capacity for abstract thinking. This level continues, but the young adult's thinking is different from the adolescent's. The young adult is less egocentric and operates in a more realistic and objective manner. Now, the young adult is close to maximum ability to acquire and use knowledge. The potential for sophisticated problem-solving and creative thinking is at a new height.

Education continues for many young adults, from formal courses in college to on-the-job training, military service, and continuing education classes. Usually, this education prepares the young adult to do some type of work. Work is an important factor in the young adult's life because it is tied closely with ego identity. A person with job satisfaction feels challenged, rewarded, and fulfilled. One who is frustrated with work feels bored and apathetic.

However, other young adults cannot find work. Those from dysfunctional families, from low-income households, and those who have recently immigrated to the United States lack the resources to obtain the education they need. Because the United States has become an increasingly technologic society, fewer jobs are available for people with little schooling. Unemployment has profound social implications, and one of them is a lack of money for health care. A frustrating clinical paradox arises for the health care provider. That is, nurses and physicians can assess a person, diagnose health problems, and treat or make appropriate referrals, but the individual may fail to comply when he or she does not have the money.

Psychosocial Development

Erikson's sixth stage covers the 1st years of early adulthood, from 20 to 24 years. He believes the major crisis to be resolved is that of **intimacy versus isolation.** Once self-identity is established after adolescence, it can be merged with another's in an intimate relationship. During the early 20s, the adult seeks the love, commitment, and intimacy of an intense lasting relationship. This mature relationship includes mutual trust, cooperation, sharing of feelings and goals, and complete acceptance of the other person. Although Erikson had a heterosexual union in mind, this intimacy could be satisfied through a homosexual relationship or through a bond with a cause or an institution.

Erikson believes that without a secure personal identity, a person cannot form a love relationship. The result is a person who is isolated, withdrawn, and lonely. This person may fill the void with numerous transient liaisons or promiscuity, but Erikson believes that these experiences will be found to be shallow and the person will feel remote and alone.

Daniel Levinson's (1986, 1996) time frame of early adulthood is much broader than Erikson's. It encompasses 22 to 40 years. Levinson believes that an adult's life alternates between periods of **structure building,** in which a lifestyle is fashioned, and periods of **transition,** in which this lifestyle is evaluated, appraised, and modified.

The era of Early Adulthood has two structure-building periods. In the 20s (about 22 to 28 years), the novice adult establishes the "entry structure," a first provisional lifestyle linking him or her to adult society. He or she is building a home base. The first set of important choices are made during this time concerning a mate, friends, an occupation, values, and lifestyle. In making these choices, the person must juggle the conflicting drives of (1) *exploring* many possibilities and keeping options open on the one hand and (2) securing some *stability* on the other hand (Levinson et al., 1986).

The Age Thirty Transition, age 28 to 33 years, is a time of self-reflection. Questions asked include "Where am I going?" and "Why am I doing these things?" This is the first major reassessment in life. A person ponders aspects that he or she wants to add, exclude, or modify in life. The person feels, "If there is anything I want to change I better start now, or it will be too late" (Levinson et al., 1986).

According to Levinson, the rest of the 30s (33 to 40 years) is characterized by settling down. A person takes the reforms or the reaffirmations established during the transitional period of the 30s and fashions a culminating life structure, one that realizes his or her youthful aspirations. During these years, the adult strives to establish a niche in society and to build a better life in all the choice points. This person is building a nest, using deliberation and seeking order and stability.

Sometimes, the reforms include having children. The addition of children brings a major readjustment to the couple's relationship. Roles are reshaped in the new family unit. For some couples, the father is more involved in child care than he was in past generations. The mother's role may include a choice between full-time parenting or a return to employment outside the home. More women are in the work force now. Although the opportunities are wider, the risk for stress exists because choices often must be made. The tension shifts from having no choice in a former traditional role to whether or not the right decision is being made now.

However, for many women, the luxury of having options does not exist. Single parents struggle to support themselves and their children. Often they have neither the time nor the financial resources to provide the basic needs for their children or for themselves.

Middle Adulthood (40 to 64 Years)

At some point around or after age 40, the realization dawns and grows that life is half over. No longer does the dream of young adulthood seem fully attainable. To some, it seems that there is more time to look back on than to see ahead. How the person deals with these feelings and builds a meaningful life structure is the task of middle adulthood. Its composite tasks include

1. Accepting and adjusting to the physical changes of middle age
2. Reviewing and redirecting career goals
3. Achieving desired performance in career
4. Developing hobby and leisure activities
5. Adjusting to aging parents
6. Helping adolescent children in their search for identity
7. Accepting and relating to the spouse as a person
8. Coping with an empty nest at home

Physical Development

A look in the mirror brings rueful recognition of the beginning of aging effects on the body. The skin loses its taut surface and forms wrinkles around the eyes, mouth, and forehead. Some notice pouches under the eyes and sagging jowls. The hair thins a little, starts to lose pigment, and turns gray, and in men the hairline often recedes. An abdominal paunch grows from increased fat deposits and decreased physical activity. Internally, most organ systems hold constant, with some small decrease in respiratory capacity and cardiac function. Sensory function remains intact except for some visual changes, e.g., decreased accommodation for near vision, or presbyopia.

In the late 40s and early 50s, females experience the **menopause,** the decreasing frequency and finally the cessation of menstruation. This involves a decrease in the female hormones, estrogen and progesterone, which brings attendant symptoms such as atrophy of reproductive organs, vasomotor disturbances, and mood swings (see Chapter 24). Although men do not have such an abrupt halt to reproductive ability, they experience a decrease in the production of testosterone, which causes decreased sperm and semen production and less-intense orgasms.

Middle-aged adults are suddenly aware of the occasional death of their peers. This is a rude reminder of their own mortality. The leading causes of death during middle adulthood are cancer, heart diseases, and injuries (Table 2–3). Morbidity also is increased, probably caused

Table 2–3 • Periodic Health Examination: Ages 25–64 Years

Interventions Considered and Recommended for the Periodic Health Examination	Leading Causes of Death
	Malignant neoplasms
	Heart diseases
	Motor vehicle and other unintentional injuries
	Human immunodeficiency virus (HIV) infection
	Suicide and homicide

Interventions for the General Population

Screening	**Injury Prevention**
Blood pressure	Lap/shoulder belts
Height and weight	Motorcycle/bicycle/ATV helmets*
Total blood cholesterol (men age 35–65, women age 45–65)	Smoke detector*
Papanicolaou (Pap) test (women)[1]	Safe storage/removal of firearms*
Fecal occult blood test[2] and/or sigmoidoscopy (≥50 yr)	**Sexual Behavior**
Mammogram ± clinical breast exam[3] (women 50–69 yr)	STD prevention: avoid high-risk behavior*; condoms/female barrier with spermicide*
Assess for problem drinking	Unintended pregnancy: contraception
Rubella serology or vaccination hx[4] (women of childbearing age)	**Dental Health**
Counseling	Regular visits to dental care provider*
Substance Use	Floss, brush with fluoride toothpaste daily*
Tobacco cessation	**Immunizations**
Avoid alcohol/drug use while driving, swimming, boating, etc.*	Tetanus-diphtheria (Td) boosters
Diet and Exercise	Rubella[4] (women of childbearing age)
Limit fat and cholesterol; maintain caloric balance; emphasize grains, fruits, vegetables	**Chemoprophylaxis**
Adequate calcium intake (women)	Multivitamin with folic acid (women planning or capable of pregnancy)
Regular physical activity*	Discuss hormone prophylaxis (peri- and postmenopausal women)

Interventions for High-Risk Populations

Population	Potential Interventions (see detailed high-risk definitions)
High-risk sexual behavior	RPR/VDRL (HR1); screen for gonorrhea (female) (HR2), HIV (HR3), chlamydia (female) (HR4); hepatitis B vaccine (HR5); hepatitis A vaccine (HR6)
Injection or street drug use	RPR/VDRL (HR1); HIV screen (HR3); hepatitis B vaccine (HR5); hepatitis A vaccine (HR6); PPD (HR7); advice to reduce infection risk (HR8)
Low income; TB contacts; immigrants; alcoholics	PPD (HR7)
Native Americans/Alaska Natives	Hepatitis A vaccine (HR6); PPD (HR7); pneumococcal vaccine (HR9)
Travelers to developing countries	Hepatitis B vaccine (HR5); hepatitis A vaccine (HR6)
Certain chronic medical conditions	PPD (HR7); pneumococcal vaccine (HR9); influenza vaccine (HR10)
Blood product recipients	HIV screen (HR3); hepatitis B vaccine (HR5)
Susceptible to measles, mumps, or varicella	MMR (HR11); varicella vaccine (HR12)
Institutionalized persons	Hepatitis A vaccine (HR6); PPD (HR7); pneumococcal vaccine (HR9); influenza vaccine (HR10)
Health care/lab workers	Hepatitis B vaccine (HR5); hepatitis A vaccine (HR6); PPD (HR7); influenza vaccine (HR10)
Family h/o skin cancer; fair skin, eyes, hair	Avoid excess/midday sun, use protective clothing* (HR13)
Previous pregnancy with neural tube defect	Folic acid 4.0 mg (HR14)

Table 2-3 • Periodic Health Examination: Ages 25-64 Years *Continued*

Interventions for High-Risk Populations

HR1 = Persons who exchange sex for money or drugs, and their sex partners; persons with other STDs (including HIV); and sexual contacts of persons with active syphilis. Clinicians should also consider local epidemiology.

HR2 = Women who exchange sex for money or drugs, or who have had repeated episodes of gonorrhea. Clinicians should also consider local epidemiology.

HR3 = Men who had sex with men after 1975; past or present injection drug use; persons who exchange sex for money or drugs, and their sex partners; injection drug-using, bisexual, or HIV-positive sex partner currently or in the past; blood transfusion during 1978-1985; persons seeking treatment for STDs. Clinicians should also consider local epidemiology.

HR4 = Sexually active women with multiple risk factors including: history of STD; new or multiple sex partners; nonuse or inconsistent use of barrier contraceptives; cervical ectopy. Clinicians should also consider local epidemiology.

HR5 = Blood product recipients (including hemodialysis patients), persons with frequent occupational exposure to blood or blood products, men who have sex with men, injection drug users and their sex partners, persons with multiple recent sex partners, persons with other STDs (including HIV), travelers to countries with endemic hepatitis B.

HR6 = Persons living in, traveling to, or working in areas where the disease is endemic and where periodic outbreaks occur (e.g., countries with high or intermediate endemicity; certain Alaska Native, Pacific Island, Native American, and religious communities); men who have sex with men; injection or street drug users. Consider for institutionalized persons and workers in these institutions, military personnel, and day-care, hospital, and laboratory workers. Clinicians should also consider local epidemiology.

HR7 = HIV positive, close contacts of persons with known or suspected TB, health care workers, persons with medical risk factors associated with TB, immigrants from countries with high TB prevalence, medically underserved low-income populations (including homeless), alcoholics, injection drug users, and residents of long-term care facilities.

HR8 = Persons who continue to inject drugs.

HR9 = Immunocompetent institutionalized persons aged ≥50 yr and immunocompetent persons with certain medical conditions, including chronic cardiac or pulmonary disease, diabetes mellitus, and anatomic asplenia. Immunocompetent persons who live in high-risk environments or social settings (e.g., certain Native American and Alaska Native populations).

HR10 = Annual vaccination of residents of chronic care facilities; persons with chronic cardiopulmonary disorders, metabolic diseases (including diabetes mellitus), hemoglobinopathies, immunosuppression, or renal dysfunction; and health care providers for high-risk patients.

HR11 = Persons born after 1956 who lack evidence of immunity to measles or mumps (e.g., documented receipt of live vaccine on or after the first birthday, laboratory evidence of immunity, or a history of physician-diagnosed measles or mumps).

HR12 = Healthy adults without a history of chickenpox or previous immunization. Consider serologic testing for presumed susceptible adults.

HR13 = Persons with a family or personal history of skin cancer, a large number of moles, atypical moles, poor tanning ability, or light skin, hair, and eye color.

HR14 = Women with previous pregnancy affected by neural tube defect who are planning pregnancy.

¹Women who are or have been sexually active and who have a cervix: q ≤ 3 yr. ²Annually. ³Mammogram q1-2 yr, or mammogram q1-2 yr with annual clinical breast examination. ⁴Serologic testing, documented vaccination history, and routine vaccination (preferably with MMR) are equally acceptable alternatives.

*The ability of clinician counseling to influence this behavior is unproven.

ATV = all-terrain vehicle; STD = sexually transmitted disease; TB = tuberculosis; RPR = rapid plasma reagin; VDRL = Venereal Disease Research Laboratories; HIV = human immunodeficiency virus; PPD = purified protein derivative; MMR = measles-mumps-rubella.

most often by obesity. Obesity is associated primarily with hypertension and also with cardiovascular disease, diabetes, and mobility dysfunction such as arthritis. Chronic smoking leads to health problems in middle adulthood.

Cognitive Development

Intelligence levels remain generally constant during middle adulthood. Intelligence is further enhanced by the knowledge that comes with life experience, self-confidence, a sense of humor, and flexibility. The middle-aged adult is interested in how new knowledge is applied, not just in learning for learning's sake. Continuing education courses meet the need to keep knowledge current in occupational and personal interest areas. Many middle-aged adults are seeking college degrees for the first time or are pursuing advanced degrees.

Psychosocial Development

Physical, personal, and social forces all interact during the era of middle adulthood. How a person reacts to the physical cues of aging affects his or her personality and self-perception. A success or disappointment in the career affects a person's self-image, stress level, and interpersonal relationships.

Erikson believed that the most important task for personality development is resolution of the crisis of **generativity versus stagnation.** Erikson believed that during the middle years adults have an urge to contribute to the next generation. This need can be fulfilled either by producing the next generation or by producing something to pass on to the next generation. Thus, middle-aged adults want to rear their own children or to engage in other creative, socially useful work. The motivation is to create and/or nurture those who will follow.

The middle-aged adult needs to be needed, to leave something behind, to leave his or her mark on the world. Generativity is sharing, giving, contributing to the growth of others. If this need is not fulfilled, the adult stagnates. Stagnation means experiencing boredom and a sense of emptiness in life, which leads to being inactive, self-absorbed, self-indulgent, a chronic complainer.

Levinson (1986) describes the era of middle adulthood as beginning with a mid-life transition. Roughly between 40 and 45 years, the person starts a major reassessment, "What have I done with my life?"

The rest of the 40s, according to Levinson, involves making choices and building a new life structure. The person confronts reality; some goals simply cannot be met. This must be accepted and goals adjusted. The person takes stock and emerges with a new perception of the self and the environment. For those who have come through the mid-life transition and have found inner meaning, life will be "less tyrannized by the ambitions, passions, and illusions of youth" (Levinson et al., 1986).

For women, the mid-life transition includes the issue that the biologic boundary of childbearing is now in sight. Women feel a time pinch that forces a survey of their life. Aging and biology force women to review options that were set aside and that will be closed off in the now-foreseeable future. Even those satisfied with the number of children that they have or those without children will face this review.

Whatever the central issue, all those in mid-life transition explore the meaning of their career, their family, and their personal identity. In terms of career, a person who spent the 30s searching for power and responsibility now may crave inner meaning (Levinson, 1986). Also, the middle-aged adult is aware of the time left until retirement. This may result in a reordering of career goals or in a new career path.

Career reassessment is intertwined with personal and family reassessment. New roles emerge as the middle-aged adult deals with growing children and aging parents. The adult often is caught in a "squeeze" between the simultaneously changing needs of adolescent children and aging parents.

Role realignment occurs in the individual's relationship with aging parents. Even if the parents are healthy and active, a role reversal occurs. The middle-aged adult gradually starts to take the parent's place as the one in charge. When one of the parents dies, the middle-aged adult is confronted with loss of the protective myth, "Death cannot happen to me or my loved ones" (Gould, 1979). The parent was a shield between the self and death. Once the parent dies, the middle-aged adult is more vulnerable and realizes the limited quantity of time left.

Another family task facing the middle-aged adult is to help the adolescent child in his or her search for identity. The parent must adjust to the adolescent's desire to be independent and less involved in the family activities and the need for increased responsibility. Some parents nurture the independence and delight in the budding individual. Others tend to be overprotective and controlling. They may feel that their adolescent is too immature. Or they do not want the adolescent to make the same mistakes that they did. The adolescent resents this attempt to relive the parent's life through his or her own. Also, some parents dread the empty nest.

Once the youngest child does leave home, the parent faces the empty nest. If the parent, often the mother, has focused only on the children, she may feel left with little to live for. Will she find something as important as the children to replace them? This dilemma is more poignant now than it was in the past when adult children stayed pretty close to home. With society's current mobility, the grown child often starts a new nuclear family at a faraway location.

The empty nest leaves parents alone as a couple again. They may face a relationship that is devoid of meaning apart from their children. They may find themselves dissatisfied, that they do not know each other, that they have drifted apart. Divorce may result and loom as a major crisis. Other couples find this a positive phase. Their marriage is happier with shared activities, increased freedom, and more time to travel. They look back on the shared memories of parenting with a satisfied smile.

Late Adulthood (65+ Years)

Although negative stereotypes exist for each age group, none is more prevalent than the one for aging adults. **Ageism** means discrimination based on age. It is a derogatory attitude that characterizes older adults as sick, senile, and useless and as a burden on the economy. It reveals our society's anxiety about aging. The attitude stems in part from our cultural emphasis on youth, beauty, and vigor. Other cultures respect and revere their aging members.

This ageist attitude is changing, partly because late adulthood now is the fastest-growing segment of our population and its members command attention. Older adults should be seen not as a homogeneous group with predictable reactions but as individuals with specific needs and widely divergent responses (Fig. 2–8).

Developmental tasks of this group include

1. Adjusting to changes in physical strength and health
2. Forming a new family role as an in-law and/or grandparent
3. Affiliating with one's age group
4. Adjusting to retirement and reduced income
5. Developing post-retirement activities that enhance self-worth and usefulness
6. Arranging satisfactory physical living quarters
7. Adjusting to the death of spouse, family members, and friends
8. Conducting a life review
9. Preparing for the inevitability of one's own death

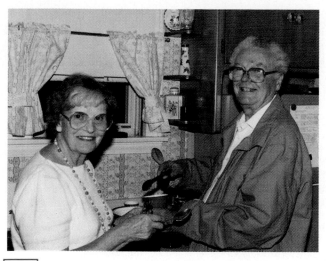

2-8

is known to be a lifelong process, its mechanism is not fully understood. An inevitable decline occurs in body functions that seems to be independent of stress, trauma, and disease. The degenerative effects of normal aging are described for each organ system in the corresponding chapter on physical examination.

Illness affects aging people more than those in other age groups. Incidence of chronic disease increases, resistance to illness decreases, and recuperative power decreases. That is, after an acute illness an aging person does not recover as quickly or as completely as a younger person. Everyday body aches and pains increase. Some older people become preoccupied with their physical discomfort, whereas others adjust to a few aches with equanimity. All these events mean that the aging person is increasingly dependent on the health care system for advice, health teaching, and physical care (Table 2-4).

Physical Development

Everyone does not age at the same rate. One person at 60 years can look older and feel weaker than another at 75 years. The widely divergent response depends on subjective attitude, physical activity, nutrition, personal habits, and the occurrence of physical illness. Although aging

Cognitive Development

Aging does not have a predictable effect on intelligence. Intellectual function depends on various factors, such as motivation, interest, sensory impairment, educational level, how far in the past that school learning occurred, deliberate caution, and a tendency to conserve time and emotional energy rather than acting assertively

Table 2-4 • Periodic Health Examination: Age 65 and Older

Interventions Considered and Recommended for the Periodic Health Examination	Leading Causes of Death
	Heart diseases
	Malignant neoplasms (lung, colorectal, breast)
	Cerebrovascular disease
	Chronic obstructive pulmonary disease
	Pneumonia and influenza

Interventions for the General Population

Screening	Injury Prevention
Blood pressure	Lap/shoulder belts
Height and weight	Motorcycle and bicycle helmets*
Fecal occult blood test[1] and/or sigmoidoscopy	Fall prevention*
Mammogram ± clinical breast exam[2] (women ≤69 yr)	Safe storage/removal of firearms*
Papanicolaou (Pap) test (women)[3]	Smoke detector*
Vision screening	Set hot water heater to <120–130°F*
Assess for hearing impairment	CPR training for household members
Assess for problem drinking	Dental Health
Counseling	Regular visits to dental care provider*
	Floss, brush with fluoride toothpaste daily*
Substance Use	Sexual Behavior
Tobacco cessation	STD prevention: avoid high-risk sexual behavior*; use condoms*
Avoid alcohol/drug use while driving, swimming, boating, etc.	**Immunizations**
Diet and Exercise	
Limit fat and cholesterol; maintain caloric balance; emphasize	Pneumococcal vaccine
grains, fruits, vegetables	Influenza[1]
Adequate calcium intake (women)	Tetanus-diphtheria (Td) boosters
Regular physical activity*	**Chemoprophylaxis**
	Discuss hormone prophylaxis (women)

Continued

Table 2–4 • Periodic Health Examination: Age 65 and Older *Continued*

Interventions for High-Risk Populations

Population	Potential Interventions (see detailed high-risk definitions)
Institutionalized persons	PPD (HR1); hepatitis A vaccine (HR2); amantadine/rimantadine (HR4)
Chronic medical conditions; TB contacts; low income; immigrants; alcoholics	PPD (HR1)
Persons ≥75 yr; or ≥70 yr with risk factors for falls	Fall prevention intervention (HR5)
Cardiovascular disease risk factors	Consider cholesterol screening (HR6)
Family h/o skin cancer; nevi; fair skin, eyes, hair	Avoid excess/midday sun, use protective clothing* (HR7)
Native Americans/Alaska Natives	PPD (HR1); hepatitis A vaccine (HR2)
Travelers to developing countries	Hepatitis A vaccine (HR2); hepatitis B vaccine (HR8)
Blood product recipients	HIV screen (HR3); hepatitis B vaccine (HR8)
High-risk sexual behavior	Hepatitis A vaccine (HR2); HIV screen (HR3); hepatitis B vaccine (HR8); RPR/VDRL (HR9)
Injection or street drug use	PPD (HR1); hepatitis A vaccine (HR2); HIV screen (HR3); hepatitis B vaccine (HR8); RPR/VDRL (HR9); advice to reduce infection risk (HR10)
Health care/lab workers	PPD (HR1); hepatitis A vaccine (HR2); amantadine/rimantadine (HR4); hepatitis B vaccine (HR8)
Persons susceptible to varicella	Varicella vaccine (HR11)

HR1 = HIV positive, close contacts of persons with known or suspected TB, health care workers, persons with medical risk factors associated with TB, immigrants from countries with high TB prevalence, medically underserved low-income populations (including homeless), alcoholics, injection drug users, and residents of long-term care facilities.

HR2 = Persons living in, traveling to, or working in areas where the disease is endemic and where periodic outbreaks occur (e.g., countries with high or intermediate endemicity; certain Alaska Native, Pacific Island, Native American, and religious communities); men who have sex with men; injection or street drug users. Consider for institutionalized persons and workers in these institutions, and day-care, hospital, and laboratory workers. Clinicians should also consider local epidemiology.

HR3 = Men who had sex with men after 1975; past or present injection drug use; persons who exchange sex for money or drugs, and their sex partners; injection drug-using, bisexual, or HIV-positive sex partner currently or in the past; blood transfusion during 1978–1985; persons seeking treatment for STDs. Clinicians should also consider local epidemiology.

HR4 = Consider for persons who have not received influenza vaccine or are vaccinated late; when the vaccine may be ineffective due to major antigenic changes in the virus; for unvaccinated persons who provide home care for high-risk persons; to supplement protection provided by vaccine in persons who are expected to have a poor antibody response; and for high-risk persons in whom the vaccine is contraindicated.

HR5 = Persons aged 75 years and older; or aged 70–74 with one or more additional risk factors including: use of certain psychoactive and cardiac medications (e.g., benzodiazepines, antihypertensives); use of ≥ four prescription medications; impaired cognition, strength, balance, or gait. Intensive individualized home-based multifactorial fall prevention intervention is recommended in settings where adequate resources are available to deliver such services.

HR6 = Although evidence is insufficient to recommend routine screening in elderly persons, clinicians should consider cholesterol screening on a case-by-case basis for persons ages 65–75 with additional risk factors (e.g., smoking, diabetes, or hypertension).

HR7 = Persons with a family or personal history of skin cancer, a large number of moles, atypical moles, poor tanning ability, or light skin, hair, and eye color.

HR8 = Blood product recipients (including hemodialysis patients), persons with frequent occupational exposure to blood or blood products, men who have sex with men, injection drug users and their sex partners, persons with multiple recent sex partners, persons with other STDs (including HIV), travelers to countries with endemic hepatitis B.

HR9 = Persons who exchange sex for money or drugs and their sex partners; persons with other STDs (including HIV); and sexual contacts of persons with active syphilis. Clinicians should also consider local epidemiology.

HR10 = Persons who continue to inject drugs.

HR11 = Healthy adults without a history of chickenpox or previous immunization. Consider serologic testing for presumed susceptible adults.

---

¹Annually. ²Mammogram q1–2 yr, or mammogram q1–2 yr with annual clinical breast exam. ³All women who are or have been sexually active and who have a cervix: q ≤ 3 yr. Consider discontinuation of testing after age 65 yr if previous regular screening with consistently normal results.

*The ability of clinician counseling to influence this behavior is unproven.

CPR = cardiopulmonary resuscitation; STD = sexually transmitted disease; TB = tuberculosis; PPD = purified protein derivative; HIV = human immunodeficiency virus; RPR = rapid plasma reagin; VDRL = Venereal Disease Research Laboratories.

(Murray and Zentner, 1993). Older adults do have a slower reaction time. They often have decreased ability for complex decision-making and decreased speed of performance, but no decrease in general knowledge occurs. Older adults experience little or no loss in verbal comprehension or in the application of experience. Memory declines are usually on short-term memory tasks that need deliberate processing, i.e., problems remembering names, where they placed their keys or other objects, appointments, or medication schedules (Berk, 1998).

Psychosocial Development

Levinson (1986) suggests a relationship between physical changes of the body and personality. By 60 years, most people are aware of some body decline. Although variations exist, most aging persons have at least one serious illness or limiting condition and are aware of the increasing frequency of death in peers. These issues, coupled with society's negative connotation of aging, lead to a fear that the person has lost all vestiges of youth, even those to which he or she had a tenuous hold during middle adulthood. The person fears ". . . that the youth within him is dying and that only the old man—an empty, dry structure devoid of energy, interests or inner resources—will survive for a brief and foolish old age" (Levinson et al., 1986). The task, then, is to look for a new form of youthfulness, a new force of inner growth to sustain the last era.

The era of late adulthood directs this inner youthfulness toward new creative endeavors. The older adult has stepped off center stage both in formal employment and in the family clan. This can be traumatic because it means a loss of recognition and authority. But now the person can direct energy inward. When financially and socially secure, the older adult can pursue whatever activity is important. One has paid one's dues to society and now can pursue whatever is pleasing. The person creates a new balance with society; he or she is less interested in society's extrinsic rewards and more interested in using inner resources.

Confronting Tasks. How an older adult responds to retirement depends largely on job satisfaction. If the job was rote and meaningless, the person may welcome the release provided by retirement. But if the job signified power and status, retirement may have a devastating effect. The retired person feels the loss of title and authority. A loss of professional associates who had common interests and were intellectually stimulating also occurs, and a social outlet is lost when co-workers had become a friendship group.

It is important to develop post-retirement activities that enhance self-worth and give a feeling of usefulness. These activities may include developing a new "semiretired" career, or a hobby, sport interest, or community service activity. The transition to retirement is eased if these activities are well in place before the last formal day on the job.

Having the retired person spend more time at home affects the marriage relationship. Traditionally, it was the husband who was suddenly at home and "under foot." Now more employed women exist who face the same retirement adjustment. Some couples do find that having one or both at home more means an invasion of previously held "turf," such as the kitchen, garden, or workshop. Other couples develop a more egalitarian relationship. They are now free of earlier sex role definitions and are able to share household tasks and leisure activities equally.

Family roles also are adjusted with the marriage of grown-up children and the addition of in-laws. How the sons- or daughters-in-law are absorbed into the family affects the older adult. This often involves a new role as grandparent. Being able to indulge and provide moral support to a grandchild is usually positive for all, unless the caretaking becomes a burden to the grandparent.

Retirement often involves financial adjustment. This may involve a reduced income, perhaps only social security and a small pension. This may be hard if the person is used to a higher standard of living. Even if the retired person owns his or her own home, the cost of maintaining it may exceed the income.

Establishing suitable living arrangements has both financial and family significance. In our culture, the extended family mostly has disappeared today. No longer do three generations live under one roof. In the past, the older adult contributed light household tasks that gave a sense of personal worth. Now, the contributions to the extended family that were made by the older family member have been replaced by advances in household mechanization, food processing, and day care centers.

Thus, most older adults choose to live independently, either as couples or alone. When it becomes difficult to manage self-care, they face the choice of moving in with grown children or moving into a retirement home or nursing home. All of these choices involve some disbursement of personal belongings and the relinquishing of some privacy.

Through the late adult years, each person is reminded of one's own limited time left by the increasing frequency of death and serious illness of friends, colleagues, siblings, or other family members, perhaps including the spouse.

The Life Review. One important task of late adulthood is performing a life review. Older adults have finished all or most of their life's work. Their contribution to society and to their own immortality are mostly completed (Levinson et al., 1986). The life review is a cataloging of life events, a considering of one's successes and failures with the perspective of age. The objective of the task is to gain a sense of integrity in reviewing one's life as a whole.

This period relates to Erikson's last ego stage, with its key polarity of **integrity versus despair.** A successful resolution to this final conflict occurs when the adult accepts "one's one and only life cycle as something that had to be and that, by necessity, permitted of no substitutions" (Erikson, 1963). The adult feels content with his or her one life on earth, satisfied that if it were possible to do it over again, he or she would live it the same way. The older adult reviews events, experiences, and relationships and realizes that these have been mostly good. There are cherished memories. The person has had a meaningful part in human history and can meet death with equanimity.

Failure to resolve this last crisis leaves the person with a sense of despair, resentment, futility, hopelessness, and a fear of death. However, a successful outcome completes a cycle. The contented older adult who does not fear death serves as a role model for younger adults that life can be trusted.

Levinson believes everyone has a sense of utter despair at some point during this time. To gain a sense of integrity, one has to confront the *lack* of integrity (Levinson et al., 1986). Some goals were not achieved, and what is worse, the damage is done and it is too late to set it right. The person realizes that whatever values were held, he or she cannot fully live up to them. This must be reconciled; it is an imperfect world. The task is to make peace with the self.

This final sense of what life is about is a close parallel to Erikson's last stage. Levinson likens the person's perspective at this time as a "view from the bridge" at the end of the life cycle (Levinson et al., 1986). One "must come finally to terms with the self—knowing it and loving it reasonably well, and being ready to give it up."

DEVELOPMENTAL SCREENING TESTS

The Denver II—Revision and Restandardization of the Denver Developmental Screening Test (DDST)

Age range: birth to 6 years
Time required: 10 to 25 minutes
Authors: W. Frankenburg, J. Dodds, P. Archer, B. Bresnick, H. Shapiro
Available from: Denver Developmental Materials, Inc.
P.O. Box 6919
Denver, CO 80206

This is a screening instrument designed to detect developmental delays in infants and preschoolers. It tests four functions: gross motor, language, fine motor-adaptive, and personal-social skills.

The Denver II is not an intelligence test; it does not predict current or future intellectual ability. It is not diagnostic; it does not suggest treatment regimens. What the Denver II does do is screen; it helps identify children who may be slow in development. This is important because early detection increases the opportunities for effective treatment.

The Denver II was revised in 1989 and restandardized for a sample including three ethnic groups, three residence categories (rural, suburban, and urban), and three

levels of maternal education (less than high school, high school, and more than high school). These norms should ameliorate the limitations of the earlier DDST concerning its relevance to various population groups (Frankenburg et al., 1981). The Denver II also appears to address the limitations experienced by Olade (1984) in using the earlier DDST in developing countries. Olade's study of African children in Nigeria suggested that language differences (naming certain colors, limited use of plurals and parents' last names) and unfamiliar interactive games (peek-a-boo) affected DDST results. These items are omitted or adjusted in the Denver II. However, the culture of developing countries still must be considered when using screening tests.

The Denver II easily is incorporated into the daily professional regimen of nurses, physicians, and teachers. The 125 items are arranged in chronologic order and are displayed in groupings corresponding to recommended ages for health maintenance visits (see Fig. 2–9). The clear pictorial charts aid in administering, scoring, and interpreting the test. It is reliable and economical. The materials are few in number, attractive to children, and easily maintained and replaced. The scoring avoids diagnostic labeling (such as mental retardation, language disorder, and cerebral palsy). Instead, the child's performance is scored either "normal," "abnormal," or "questionable," and includes an adjustment in scoring for premature infants.

Uses of the Denver II include (Frankenburg et al., 1981)

- Screening of infants, whose rapid rate of development makes it difficult to rely on professional opinion or on parent history alone
- Longitudinal following of a single child in health care or educational setting
- Follow-up in clinics, where a child may be seen briefly, infrequently, or by different examiners
- Prekindergarten screening

Adult Life Stress Measures

Some tools are available that attempt to quantify the impact of life change on a person's health. They are based on the assumption that a relationship exists between daily life stress and a person's susceptibility to physical and psychological problems. Many of the life change events are the developmental tasks discussed earlier in the chapter.

The Hassles and Uplifts Scale

Age range: adult
Author: DeLongis

This is a 53-item self-administered questionnaire whose purpose is to assess day-to-day stress (Table 2–5). Take

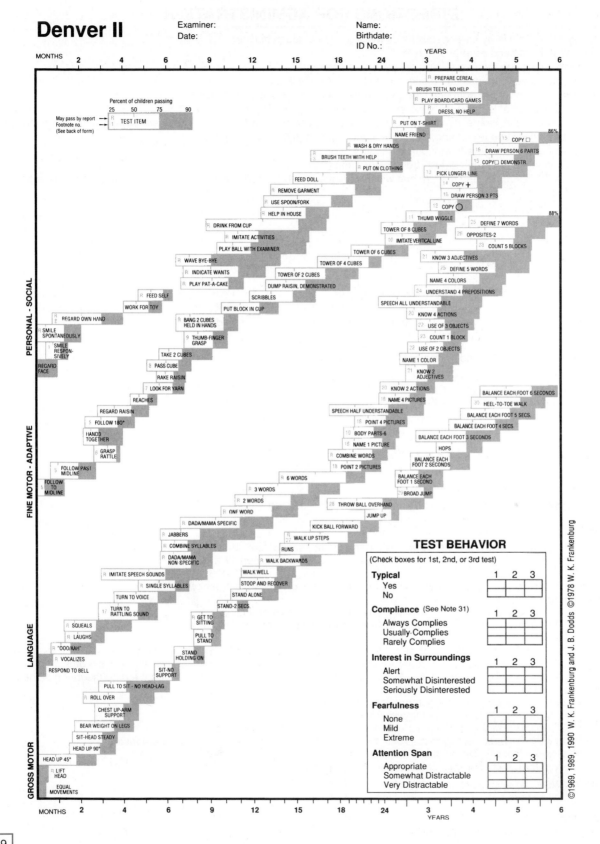

Continued on following page

DIRECTIONS FOR ADMINISTRATION

1. Try to get child to smile by smiling, talking or waving. Do not touch him/her.
2. Child must stare at hand several seconds.
3. Parent may help guide toothbrush and put toothpaste on brush.
4. Child does not have to be able to tie shoes or button/zip in the back.
5. Move yarn slowly in an arc from one side to the other, about 8" above child's face.
6. Pass if child grasps rattle when it is touched to the backs or tips of fingers.
7. Pass if child tries to see where yarn went. Yarn should be dropped quickly from sight from tester's hand without arm movement.
8. Child must transfer cube from hand to hand without help of body, mouth, or table.
9. Pass if child picks up raisin with any part of thumb and finger.
10. Line can vary only 30 degrees or less from tester's line. /
11. Make a fist with thumb pointing upward and wiggle only the thumb. Pass if child imitates and does not move any fingers other than the thumb.

  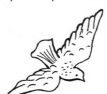 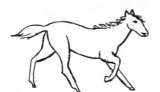 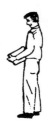

12. Pass any enclosed form. Fail continuous round motions.

13. Which line is longer? (Not bigger.) Turn paper upside down and repeat. (pass 3 of 3 or 5 of 6)

14. Pass any lines crossing near midpoint.

15. Have child copy first. If failed, demonstrate.

When giving items 12, 14, and 15, do not name the forms. Do not demonstrate 12 and 14.

16. When scoring, each pair (2 arms, 2 legs, etc.) counts as one part.
17. Place one cube in cup and shake gently near child's ear, but out of sight. Repeat for other ear.
18. Point to picture and have child name it. (No credit is given for sounds only.)
    If less than 4 pictures are named correctly, have child point to picture as each is named by tester.

      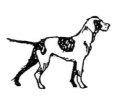 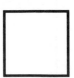

19. Using doll, tell child: Show me the nose, eyes, ears, mouth, hands, feet, tummy, hair. Pass 6 of 8.
20. Using pictures, ask child: Which one flies?... says meow?... talks?... barks?... gallops? Pass 2 of 5, 4 of 5.
21. Ask child: What do you do when you are cold?... tired?... hungry? Pass 2 of 3, 3 of 3.
22. Ask child: What do you do with a cup? What is a chair used for? What is a pencil used for? Action words must be included in answers.
23. Pass if child correctly places and says how many blocks are on paper. (1, 5).
24. Tell child: Put block **on** table; **under** table; **in front of** me, **behind** me. Pass 4 of 4. (Do not help child by pointing, moving head or eyes.)
25. Ask child: What is a ball?... lake?... desk?... house?... banana?... curtain?... fence?... ceiling? Pass if defined in terms of use, shape, what it is made of, or general category (such as banana is fruit, not just yellow). Pass 5 of 8, 7 of 8.
26. Ask child: If a horse is big, a mouse is __? If fire is hot, ice is __? If the sun shines during the day, the moon shines during the __? Pass 2 of 3.
27. Child may use wall or rail only, not person. May not crawl.
28. Child must throw ball overhand 3 feet to within arm's reach of tester.
29. Child must perform standing broad jump over width of test sheet (8 1/2 inches).
30. Tell child to walk forward, ∞∞∞∞→ heel within 1 inch of toe. Tester may demonstrate. Child must walk 4 consecutive steps.
31. In the second year, half of normal children are non-compliant.

OBSERVATIONS:

2–9 Continued

Table 2–5 • The Hassles and Uplifts Scale

HASSLES are irritants—things that annoy or bother you; they can make you upset or angry. UPLIFTS are events that make you feel good; they can make you joyful, glad, or satisfied. Some hassles and uplifts occur on a fairly regular basis and others are relatively rare. Some have only a slight effect, others have a strong effect.

This questionnaire lists things that can be hassles and uplifts in day-to-day life. You will find that during the course of a day some of these things will have been only a hassle for you and some will have been only an uplift. *Others will have been both a hassle AND an uplift.*

DIRECTIONS: Please think about how much of a hassle and how much of an uplift each item was for you today. Please indicate on the left-hand side of the page (under "HASSLES") how much of a hassle the item was by circling the appropriate number. Then indicate on the right-hand side of the page (under "UPLIFTS") how much of an uplift it was for you by circling the appropriate number.

Remember, circle one number on the left-hand side of the page *and* one number on the right-hand side of the page for *each* item.

PLEASE FILL OUT THIS QUESTIONNAIRE JUST BEFORE YOU GO TO BED.

HASSLES AND UPLIFTS SCALE

HOW MUCH OF A HASSLE WAS THIS ITEM FOR YOU TODAY?
HASSLES
0 = *None or not applicable*
1 = *Somewhat*
2 = *Quite a bit*
3 = *A great deal*

HOW MUCH OF AN UPLIFT WAS THIS ITEM FOR YOU TODAY?
UPLIFTS
0 = *None or not applicable*
1 = *Somewhat*
2 = *Quite a bit*
3 = *A great deal*

DIRECTIONS: Please circle one number on the left-hand side *and* one number on the right hand side for each item.

0 1 2 3	1. Your child(ren)	0 1 2 3
0 1 2 3	2. Your parents or parents-in-law	0 1 2 3
0 1 2 3	3. Other relative(s)	0 1 2 3
0 1 2 3	4. Your spouse	0 1 2 3
0 1 2 3	5. Time spent with family	0 1 2 3
0 1 2 3	6. Health or well-being of a family member	0 1 2 3
0 1 2 3	7. Sex	0 1 2 3
0 1 2 3	8. Intimacy	0 1 2 3
0 1 2 3	9. Family-related obligations	0 1 2 3
0 1 2 3	10. Your friend(s)	0 1 2 3
0 1 2 3	11. Fellow workers	0 1 2 3
0 1 2 3	12. Clients, customers, patients, etc.	0 1 2 3
0 1 2 3	13. Your supervisor or employer	0 1 2 3
0 1 2 3	14. The nature of your work	0 1 2 3
0 1 2 3	15. Your work load	0 1 2 3
0 1 2 3	16. Your job security	0 1 2 3
0 1 2 3	17. Meeting deadlines or goals on the job	0 1 2 3
0 1 2 3	18. Enough money for necessities (e.g., food, clothing, housing, health care, taxes, insurance)	0 1 2 3
0 1 2 3	19. Enough money for education	0 1 2 3
0 1 2 3	20. Enough money for emergencies	0 1 2 3
0 1 2 3	21. Enough money for extras (e.g., entertainment, recreation, vacations)	0 1 2 3
0 1 2 3	22. Financial care for someone who doesn't live with you	0 1 2 3
0 1 2 3	23. Investments	0 1 2 3
0 1 2 3	24. Your smoking	0 1 2 3
0 1 2 3	25. Your drinking	0 1 2 3
0 1 2 3	26. Mood-altering drugs	0 1 2 3
0 1 2 3	27. Your physical appearance	0 1 2 3
0 1 2 3	28. Contraception	0 1 2 3
0 1 2 3	29. Exercise(s)	0 1 2 3
0 1 2 3	30. Your medical care	0 1 2 3
0 1 2 3	31. Your health	0 1 2 3
0 1 2 3	32. Your physical abilities	0 1 2 3
0 1 2 3	33. The weather	0 1 2 3
0 1 2 3	34. News events	0 1 2 3
0 1 2 3	35. Your environment (e.g., quality of air, noise level, greenery)	0 1 2 3
0 1 2 3	36. Political or social issues	0 1 2 3
0 1 2 3	37. Your neighborhood (e.g., neighbors, setting)	0 1 2 3
0 1 2 3	38. Conserving (gas, electricity, water, gasoline, etc.)	0 1 2 3
0 1 2 3	39. Pets	0 1 2 3
0 1 2 3	40. Cooking	0 1 2 3
0 1 2 3	41. Housework	0 1 2 3
0 1 2 3	42. Home repairs	0 1 2 3
0 1 2 3	43. Yardwork	0 1 2 3
0 1 2 3	44. Car maintenance	0 1 2 3
0 1 2 3	45. Taking care of paperwork (e.g., paying bills, filling out forms)	0 1 2 3
0 1 2 3	46. Home entertainment (e.g., TV, music, reading)	0 1 2 3
0 1 2 3	47. Amount of free time	0 1 2 3
0 1 2 3	48. Recreation and entertainment outside the home (e.g., movies, sports, eating out, walking)	0 1 2 3
0 1 2 3	49. Eating (at home)	0 1 2 3
0 1 2 3	50. Church or community organizations	0 1 2 3
0 1 2 3	51. Legal matters	0 1 2 3
0 1 2 3	52. Being organized	0 1 2 3
0 1 2 3	53. Social commitments	0 1 2 3

Received March 21, 1986
Revision received July 20, 1987
Accepted August 4, 1987

From DeLongis A, Folkman S, Lazarus RS: The impact of daily stress on health and mood: Psychological and social resources as mediators. J Pers Soc Psychol 54(3):486–495, 1988. © 1988 by the American Psychological Association. Used with permission.

this test yourself just before you go to bed some day. Consider each item on the list, and circle a number on the left-hand side regarding how much of a hassle the item was for you that day. On the right-hand side, circle a number regarding how much of an uplift the same item was for you that day. Total scores are obtained by summing across ratings given to all items.

Relatively minor but frequently experienced stresses, termed Hassles in this tool, have been found to correlate strongly with negative health status (Weinberger, Hiner, and Tierney, 1987). DeLongis, Folkman, and Lazarus (1988) found a significant relationship between daily stress and concurrent or later occurrence of physical health problems, i.e., flu, sore throat, headaches, and backaches. There was great individual variation, however, with one third of the respondents reporting a somewhat improved health and mood with increased stress levels! Regarding daily stress and psychological disturbance, they found that individuals with unsupportive social relationships and low self-esteem had a greater risk of psychological and somatic health problems both on their stressful days and following their stressful days, than did individuals with positive social networks and high self-esteem (DeLongis, Folkman, and Lazarus, 1988).

Life Experiences Survey (LES)

Age range: adult
Authors: I.G. Sarason, J.H. Johnson, J.M. Siegel

This is a 47-item self-administered questionnaire that considers events that occurred over the past year. This test weighs the desirability or undesirability of life experiences. The assumption is that events considered *negative* by the respondent are more likely to be associated with stress. Also the respondent is allowed to rate the personal impact of the events experienced.

The respondent weighs the desirability or undesirability of each event on a 7-point scale, from extremely negative (-3) to extremely positive ($+3$) (Table 2–6). The negative and positive subscores are added to determine a total change score.

This test suggests a relationship between negative life changes and psychological problems. The effect of stress differs depending on individual characteristics, the degree of perceived control over the events, and the degree of psychosocial assets (Sarason et al., 1978).

Table 2–6 · Life Experiences Survey

Listed below are a number of events that sometimes bring about change in the lives of those who experience them and that necessitate social readjustment. *Please check those events that you have experienced in the recent past and indicate the time period during which you have experienced each event.* Be sure that all check marks are directly across from the items they correspond to.

Also, for each item checked below, *please indicate the extent to which you viewed the event as having either a positive or negative impact on your life* at the time the event occurred. That is, *indicate the type and extent of impact that the event had.* A rating of -3 would indicate an extremely negative impact. A rating of 0 suggests no impact either positive or negative. A rating of $+3$ would indicate an extremely positive impact.

	0–6 mo	7 mo to 1 yr	Extremely Negative	Moderately Negative	Somewhat Negative	No Impact	Slightly Positive	Moderately Positive	Extremely Positive
1. Marriage			-3	-2	-1	0	$+1$	$+2$	$+3$
2. Detention in jail or comparable institution			-3	-2	-1	0	$+1$	$+2$	$+3$
3. Death of spouse			-3	-2	-1	0	$+1$	$+2$	$+3$
4. Major change in sleeping habits (much more or much less sleep)			-3	-2	-1	0	$+1$	$+2$	$+3$
5. Death of close family member									
a. Mother			-3	-2	-1	0	$+1$	$+2$	$+3$
b. Father			-3	-2	-1	0	$+1$	$+2$	$+3$
c. Brother			-3	-2	-1	0	$+1$	$+2$	$+3$
d. Sister			-3	-2	-1	0	$+1$	$+2$	$+3$
e. Grandmother			-3	-2	-1	0	$+1$	$+2$	$+3$
f. Grandfather			-3	-2	-1	0	$+1$	$+2$	$+3$
g. Other (specify)			-3	-2	-1	0	$+1$	$+2$	$+3$
6. Major change in eating habits (much more or much less food intake)			-3	-2	-1	0	$+1$	$+2$	$+3$
7. Foreclosure on mortgage or loan			-3	-2	-1	0	$+1$	$+2$	$+3$
8. Death of close friend			-3	-2	-1	0	$+1$	$+2$	$+3$
9. Outstanding personal achievement			-3	-2	-1	0	$+1$	$+2$	$+3$
10. Minor law violations (traffic tickets, disturbing the peace, etc.)			-3	-2	-1	0	$+1$	$+2$	$+3$
11. *Male:* Wife/girlfriend's pregnancy			-3	-2	-1	0	$+1$	$+2$	$+3$
12. *Female:* pregnancy			-3	-2	-1	0	$+1$	$+2$	$+3$
13. Changed work situation (different work responsibility, major change in working conditions, working hours, etc.)			-3	-2	-1	0	$+1$	$+2$	$+3$

Table 2–6 • Life Experiences Survey *Continued*

	0–6 mo	7 mo to 1 yr	Extremely Negative	Moderately Negative	Somewhat Negative	No Impact	Slightly Positive	Moderately Positive	Extremely Positive
14. New job			−3	−2	−1	0	+1	+2	+3
15. Serious illness or injury of close family member									
a. Father			−3	−2	−1	0	+1	+2	+3
b. Mother			−3	−2	−1	0	+1	+2	+3
c. Sister			−3	−2	−1	0	+1	+2	+3
d. Brother			−3	−2	−1	0	+1	+2	+3
e. Grandfather			−3	−2	−1	0	+1	+2	+3
f. Grandmother			−3	−2	−1	0	+1	+2	+3
g. Spouse			−3	−2	−1	0	+1	+2	+3
h. Other (specify)			−3	−2	−1	0	+1	+2	+3
16. Sexual difficulties			−3	−2	−1	0	+1	+2	+3
17. Trouble with employer (in danger of losing job, being suspended, demoted, etc.)			−3	−2	−1	0	+1	+2	+3
18. Trouble with in-laws			−3	−2	−1	0	+1	+2	+3
19. Major change in financial status (a lot better off or a lot worse off)			−3	−2	−1	0	+1	+2	+3
20. Major change in closeness of family members (increased or decreased closeness)			−3	−2	−1	0	+1	+2	+3
21. Gaining a new family member (through birth, adoption, family member moving in, etc.)			−3	−2	−1	0	+1	+2	+3
22. Change in residence			−3	−2	−1	0	+1	+2	+3
23. Marital separation from mate (due to conflict)			−3	−2	−1	0	+1	+2	+3
24. Major change in church activities (increased or decreased attendance)			−3	−2	−1	0	+1	+2	+3
25. Marital reconciliation with mate			−3	−2	−1	0	+1	+2	+3
26. Major change in number of arguments with spouse (a lot more or a lot less arguments)			−3	−2	−1	0	+1	+2	+3
27. *Married male:* change in wife's work outside the home (beginning work, ceasing work, changing to a new job, etc.)			−3	−2	−1	0	+1	+2	+3
28. *Married female:* change in husband's work (loss of job, beginning new job, retirement, etc.)			−3	−2	−1	0	+1	+2	+3
29. Major change in usual type and/or amount of recreation			−3	−2	−1	0	+1	+2	+3
30. Borrowing more than $10,000 (buying home, business, etc.)			−3	−2	−1	0	+1	+2	+3
31. Borrowing less than $10,000 (buying car, TV, getting school loan, etc.)			−3	−2	−1	0	+1	+2	+3
32. Being fired from job			−3	−2	−1	0	+1	+2	+3
33. *Male:* wife/girlfriend having abortion			−3	−2	−1	0	+1	+2	+3
34. *Female:* having abortion			−3	−2	−1	0	+1	+2	+3
35. Major personal illness or injury			−3	−2	−1	0	+1	+2	+3
36. Major change in social activities, e.g., parties, movies, visiting (increased or decreased participation)			−3	−2	−1	0	+1	+2	+3
37. Major change in living conditions of family (building new home, remodeling, deterioration of home, neighborhood, etc.)			−3	−2	−1	0	+1	+2	+3
38. Divorce			−3	−2	−1	0	+1	+2	+3
39. Serious injury or illness of close friend			−3	−2	−1	0	+1	+2	+3
40. Retirement from work			−3	−2	−1	0	+1	+2	+3
41. Son or daughter leaving home (due to marriage, college, etc.)			−3	−2	−1	0	+1	+2	+3
42. Ending of formal schooling			−3	−2	−1	0	+1	+2	+3
43. Separation from spouse (due to work, travel)			−3	−2	−1	0	+1	+2	+3
44. Engagement			−3	−2	−1	0	+1	+2	+3
45. Breaking up with boyfriend/girlfriend			−3	−2	−1	0	+1	+2	+3
46. Leaving home for the first time			−3	−2	−1	0	+1	+2	+3
47. Reconciliation with boyfriend/girlfriend			−3	−2	−1	0	+1	+2	+3
Other recent experiences that have had an impact on your life. List and rate.									
48. _____ .			−3	−2	−1	0	+1	+2	+3
49. _____ .			−3	−2	−1	0	+1	+2	+3
50. _____ .			−3	−2	−1	0	+1	+2	+3

NURSING DIAGNOSES COMMONLY ASSOCIATED WITH
DEVELOPMENTAL DISORDERS

Diagnosis	Related Factors (Etiology)	Defining Characteristics (Symptoms and Signs)
CHILDHOOD		

Altered growth and development	Effects of physical disability
	Environmental and stimulation deficiencies
	Inadequate care-taking
	  Indifference
	  Inconsistent responsiveness
	  Multiple caretakers
	Prescribed dependence
	Separation from significant others
		Altered physical growth
		Decreased responses
		Delay or difficulty in performing skills that are typical of age group
		  Motor
		  Social
		  Expressive
		Flat affect
		Inability to perform self-care or self-control activities appropriate for age

ADOLESCENCE		
Decisional conflict	Unclear personal values/beliefs Peer pressure Lack of experience or interference with decision-making Support system deficit	Verbalized uncertainty about choices Verbalized undesired consequences of alternative actions being considered Vacillation among alternative choices Delayed decision-making
ADULTHOOD		
Ineffective family coping: compromised	Isolation of family members from one another Lack of support for family members Temporary family disorganization and role changes Effects of acute or chronic illness Incompatible or differing values, beliefs, or goals Unrealistic expectations	Ineffective responses to illness, disability, or situational crises Inability to demonstrate supportive behaviors Expressed concern about significant other's response to health problem Impaired intimacy or closeness Attempted assistive behaviors with less than satisfactory results
LATE ADULTHOOD		

Anticipatory grieving	Expected loss of
	  Friends
	  Occupation
	  Function
	  Home
	Mutiple crises
	Lack of social support system
		Expressed distress at potential loss
		Denial
		Guilt
		Sorrow
		Change in eating habits
		Change in sleep patterns
		Change in social patterns
		Decreased libido

Additional Related Nursing Diagnoses

ACTUAL	RISK/WELLNESS
Altered family processes	**Risk**
Altered role performance	Risk for caregiver role strain
Caregiver role strain	Risk for altered development
Parental role conflict	Risk for altered parenting
Personal identity disturbance	**Wellness**
Relocation stress syndrome	
Self-esteem disturbance	Health-seeking behavior
Social isolation	Potential for enhanced spiritual well-being

Bibliography

American Academy of Pediatrics Committee on Child Abuse and Neglect: Guidelines for distinguishing SIDS from child abuse fatalities. Pediatrics 94(1):124–126, 1994.

Appling SE: Wellness promotion and the elderly. Med Surg Nurs 6(1): 45–46, Feb 1997.

Barnard S, Edgar D: Pediatric Eye Care. Oxford, England, Blackwell Science, 1996.

Benedict R: Patterns of Culture. Boston, Houghton Mifflin, 1934.

Berk LE: Development Through the Lifespan. Boston: Allyn and Bacon, 1998.

Berk LE: Why children talk to themselves. Sci Am 271(5):60–65, Nov 1994.

Burns CM: Toward healthy people 2000: The role of the nurse practitioner and health promotion. J Am Acad Nurs Pract 6(1):29–35, 1994.

Burnside I, Haight B: Reminiscence and life review: Therapeutic interventions for older people. Nurse Pract 19(4):55–61, 1994.

Centers for Disease Control and Prevention: Guidelines for school and community programs to promote lifelong physical activity among young people. MMWR Morb Mortal Wkly Rep 46(RR6):1–36, Mar 7, 1997.

DeLongis A, Folkman S, Lazarus RS: The impact of daily stress on health and mood: Psychological and social resources as mediators. J Pers Soc Psychol 54(3):486–495, 1988.

Dwyer T, Ponsonby A, Blizzard L, et al: The contribution of changes in the prevalence of prone sleeping position to the decline in sudden infant death syndrome in Tasmania. JAMA 273(10):783–789, Mar 8, 1995.

Erikson EH: Childhood and Society. New York, WW Norton, 1963.

Erikson EH: Identity—Youth and Crisis. New York, WW Norton, 1968.

Finan SL: Promoting healthy sexuality: Guidelines for the school-age child and adolescent. Nurse Pract 22(11):62–72, Nov 1997.

Frankenburg WK, Fandal AW, Sciarillo W: The newly abbreviated and revised Denver Developmental Screening Test. J Pediatr 99(6): 995–999, 1981.

Gilbert-Barness E, Barness L: What we've learned about SIDS. Patient Care 30(5):98–118, Mar 15, 1996.

Gladwell M: Do parents matter? The New Yorker 74:54–64, Aug 17, 1998.

Gould RL: Transformations: Growth and Change in Adult Life. New York, Simon and Schuster, 1979.

Griffith H: Needed—a strong nursing position on preventive services. Image 25(4):272, 1993.

Griffith H: Resources to put more prevention into your practice. J Am Acad Nurse Pract 6(6):253–256, 1994.

Griffith HM, Rahman MI: Implementing the Put Prevention into Practice program. Nurse Pract 19(10):12–19, 1994.

Hall GS: Adolescence. New York, Appleton, 1916.

Healy LF: Adult periodic health assessment guides. Nurse Pract 22(2): 171–177, Feb 1997.

Hu H, Aro A, Payton M, et al: The relationship of bone and blood lead to hypertension. JAMA 275(15):1171–1176, April 17, 1996.

Landis BJ, Brykczynski KA: Employing prevention in practice. Am J Nurs 97(8):40–46, Aug 1997.

Levinson DJ: A conception of adult development. Am Psychol 41:3–13, 1986.

Levinson DJ: The seasons of a woman's life. New York, A.A. Knopf, 1996.

Levinson DJ, Darrow CN, Klein EB: The Seasons of a Man's Life, 2nd ed. New York, Ballantine, 1986.

Lockridge T: Now I lay me down to sleep: SIDS and infant sleep positions. Neonatal Network 16(7):25–31, Oct 1997.

Mead M: Coming of Age in Samoa. New York, Morrow, 1961.

Mead M: Growing Up in New Guinea. New York, Mentor, 1953.

Mead M: Sex and Temperament in Three Primitive Societies. New York, Morrow, 1935.

Murray RB, Zentner JP: Nursing Assessment and Health Promotion Strategies Through the Life Span, 5th ed. Englewood Cliffs, NJ, Prentice Hall, 1993.

Nay R: The 60 and better program: A primary health care program for the aged. Contemp Nurse 6(1):8–14, Mar 1997.

Olade RA: Evaluation of the Denver Developmental Screening Test as applied to African children. Nurs Res 33(4):204–207, 1984.

Padula CA: Development of the health-promotion activities of older adults measure. Public Health Nurs 14(2):123–128, Apr 1997.

Patterson CJ: Sexual orientation and human development: An overview. Dev Psych 31:3–11, 1995.

Piaget J: The Construction of Reality in the Child. New York, Balantine, 1975.

Piaget J: Judgment and Reasoning in the Child. Totowa, NJ, Littlefield, Adams, 1968.

Piomelli S: Childhood lead poisoning in the 90s. Pediatrics 93:508–510, 1994.

Reece SM: Community analysis for health planning: Strategies for primary care practitioners. Nurse Pract 23(10):46–59, Oct 1998.

Sarason EG, Johnson JH, Siegal JM: Assessing the impact of life changes—development of life experiences survey. J Consult Clin Psychol 45(5):932–946, 1978.

Singer L, Uphold CR, Graham MV, Hernandez B: Lead poisoning and associated risk factors among preschoolers enrolled in a head start program. Public Health Nurs 14(3):161–168, Jun 1997.

U.S. Preventive Services Task Force: Guide to Clinical Preventive Services, 2nd ed. Baltimore, MD, Williams & Wilkins, 1996.

U.S. Public Health Service: Counseling children and adolescents on safety. Nurse Pract 22(7):112–115, July 1997.

Weinberger M, Hiner SL, Tierney WM: In support of Hassles as a measure of stress in predicting health outcomes. J Behav Med 10(1):19–31, 1987.

Wong DL: Whaley and Wong's Nursing Care of Infants and Children, 6th ed. St. Louis, Mosby, 1999.

Woolf SH, Jonas S, Lawrence RS: Health Promotion and Disease Prevention in Clinical Practice. Baltimore, Williams & Wilkins, 1996.

CHAPTER THREE

Transcultural Considerations in Assessment

Cultural assessment refers to a systematic appraisal of an individual's beliefs, values, and practices conducted for the purpose of providing *culturally competent* health care. Derived from the Latin root *competere,* meaning "to strive together," *cultural competence* refers to the complex integration of knowledge, attitudes, and skills, which enhance cross-cultural communication, promote meaningful interactions with patients, and enable you to provide culturally appropriate, congruent and relevant health care. According to Campinha-Bacote et al. (1996), there are four components to developing cultural competence: cultural awareness, cultural knowledge, cultural skill, and cultural encounter. Because you may encounter people from literally hundreds of different cultures and subcultures in your professional career, it is virtually impossible to know about the culturally based, health-related beliefs and practices of them all. It is, however, possible to master the knowledge and skills associated with cultural assessment and learn about *some* of the cultural dimensions of care for individuals representing the groups you most frequently encounter.

One of the major challenges you will face in assessing people from culturally diverse backgrounds is overcoming your own *ethnocentrism.* Ethnocentrism is the tendency to view your own way of life as the most desirable, acceptable, or best, and to act in a superior manner toward another culture's lifeways. A related admonition is to beware of *cultural imposition,* the tendency to impose your beliefs, values, and patterns of behavior on individuals from another culture. These admonitions are more easily stated than lived.

Because health care providers deal with cultural values and belief systems, cultural assessments tend to be broad, comprehensive, and holistic. Cultural assessment consists of both *process* and *content. Process* refers to your approach to the patient and includes professional interactions, etiquette, perceptions of space/distance, and gender considerations. Cross-cultural communication is also an integral component of the assessment process, and these points are discussed in Chapter 4. The *content* of the cultural assessment, which follows below, consists of the actual data categories in which information about patients is gathered for the history and physical examination.

BASIC CHARACTERISTICS OF CULTURE

Culture has four basic characteristics. Culture is (1) *learned* from birth through the processes of language acquisition and socialization; (2) *shared* by all members of the same cultural group; (3) *adapted* to specific conditions related to environmental and technical factors and to the availability of natural resources; and (4) *dynamic* and ever changing.

Culture is a universal phenomenon, without which no person exists. Yet, the culture that develops in any given society is always specific and distinctive, encompassing all the knowledge, beliefs, customs, and skills acquired by members of the society. Within cultures, groups of individuals share different beliefs, values, and attitudes. Differences occur because of ethnicity, religion, education, occupation, age, and gender. When such groups function within a large culture, they are referred to as subcultural groups.

The term *subculture* is used for fairly large aggregates of people who have shared characteristics that are not common to all members of the culture and that enable them to be thought of as a distinguishable subgroup. Ethnicity, religion, occupation, health-related characteristics, age, and gender are frequently used to identify subcultural groups. Examples of subcultures based on *ethnicity* (those having common traits such as physical characteristics, language, or ancestry) include blacks, Hispanics, Native Americans, Korean-Americans, and Inuits; those based on *religion* include members of the more than 1200 recognized religions such as Catholics, Jews, Mormons, Muslims, and Buddhists; those based on *occupation* include individuals involved in health care professions, such as nursing or medicine, as well as the military; those based on a *health-related characteristic* include the blind, hearing impaired, or mentally retarded; those based on *age* include groups such as adolescents and older adults; and those based on *gender* or *sexual preference* include women, men, gay men, and lesbians.

When addressing the cultural dimensions of health care, some erroneously refer only to the federally defined ethnic minority groups, i.e., white, black, Hispanic, Asian/Pacific Islander, and Native American/Alaska Native. You should be mindful that hundreds of distinct cultural groups exist in the United States, not merely those identified by the U.S. government for statistical purposes. Furthermore, the federal classification system ignores unique characteristics of groups within the broad categories (e.g., more than 550 Native American tribes exist, each with specific beliefs and practices).

CULTURAL VALUES

According to Leininger (1995), the term *values* refers to a desirable or undesirable state of affairs. Values are a universal feature of all cultures, although the types and expressions of values differ widely. *Norms* are the rules by which human behavior is governed and result from the cultural values held by the group. All societies have rules or norms that specify appropriate and inappropriate behavior. Individuals are rewarded or punished as they conform to or deviate from the established norms. Values and norms are learned in childhood along with the acceptable and unacceptable behaviors associated with them.

Dominant Value Orientation

Every society has what is called a *dominant value orientation,* a basic value orientation that is shared by the majority of its members as a result of early common experiences. According to Kluckhohn (1990), there are a limited number of basic human problems for which all people must find some solution and five common human problems with respect to values and norms: 1) the innate human nature of people; 2) relationship to nature; 3) time dimension; 4) the purpose of existence; and 5) relationships with others.

Innate Human Nature. The innate human nature of people may be perceived as good, evil, or a combination. When conducting an interview, you may notice that some will indicate that human nature is unalterable or perfectible only with great discipline and effort, as people struggle to overcome a basically evil nature. For others, human nature is perceived to be fundamentally good, unalterable, and difficult or impossible to corrupt. The majority of people, however, are likely to view human nature in a mixed manner and may say, for example, "There are good people and bad people, good nurses and bad nurses. Every profession has its combination or mixture."

Relationship to Nature. In examining the ways in which our relationship to nature is perceived, there may be three perceptions: 1) *destiny,* in which the human person is subjugated to nature in a fatalistic, inevitable manner; 2) *harmony,* in which people and nature exist together as a single entity; and 3) *mastery,* in which it is believed that people are intended to overcome natural forces and put them to use for the benefit of humankind.

What does this values orientation have to do with health and illness? Let's examine three individuals who have been recently diagnosed with diabetes mellitus, each embracing one of the values orientations described. The person whose values orientation is destiny might say, "Why should I bother watching my diet? My diabetes is part of my genetic destiny and there is nothing I can do to change the outcome." The person whose values orientation embraces harmony might say, "If I follow the diet prescribed, I can achieve the balance and harmony necessary for health and wholeness by replacing what nature has failed to provide for me." Finally, the person whose values orientation leads to belief in active mastery might say, "I will overcome this diabetes no matter what. By eating the right foods and exercising, I will take charge of the situation and will ultimately be able to influence the course of my disease."

Time Dimension. Perhaps one of the major areas in which cultural conflicts between nurses and patients from culturally diverse backgrounds occur is the failure to understand each other's perception of *time.* According to Kluckhohn (1990), there are three major ways in which people can perceive time: (1) The focus may be on the *past,* with traditions and ancestors playing an important role in the person's life. For example, many Asians, Native Americans, East Indians, and Africans hold beliefs about ancestors and tend to value long-standing traditions. In times of crisis, such as illness, individuals with a value orientation emphasizing the past may consult with ancestors or ask for their guidance or protection during the illness. (2) The focus may be on the *present,* with little attention being paid to the past or the future. These individuals are concerned with "now," and the future is perceived as vague or unpredictable. You may have difficulty encouraging these individuals to prepare for the future, e.g., for discharge from the hospital, for future side effects or adverse reactions from the medication. In addition, they may fail to see the value of childhood immunizations or those aimed at preventing the flu, hepatitis, or other conditions afflicting adults. (3) For some people, the focus is on the *future,* with progress and change being highly valued. These individuals may express discontent with both the past and the present. In terms of health care, these individuals may inquire about the "latest treatment" and most modern equipment available for a particular problem and may express concern with nurses or physicians whom they perceive to be old-fashioned.

Purpose of Existence. In examining the purpose of humankind's existence, three major views are held by people from various cultures: 1) *being,* in which the emphasis is on the spontaneous expression of impulses and desires because they are viewed as an integral component of the personality (e.g., some members of Hispanic cultures); 2) *being-in-becoming,* in which inner control, meditation, and detachment are emphasized as ways to achieve self-realization (e.g., some members of Asian cultures); and 3) *doing,* in which active striving and accomplishment are paramount as the individual competes against externally applied standards of achievement (e.g., some members of Judeo-Christian religions in Western cultures, including the United States, Canada, and Australia).

Relationships With Others. Finally, let's consider the cultural values orientation concerning the relationships that exist with others. Relationships may be categorized in three ways: (1) *Lineal* relationships refer to those that exist by virtue of heredity and kinship ties. Lineal relationships follow an ordered succession and have continuity through time. (2) *Collateral* relationships focus primarily on group goals, and the family orientation is all-important. For example, some Asian-American people describe family honor and the importance of working together toward achievement of a group (versus personal) goal. (3) *Individual* relationships refer to personal autonomy and independence. Individual goals dominate, whereas group goals become secondary.

When making health-related decisions, people from culturally diverse backgrounds rely on relationships with others in various ways. If the cultural value orientation is lineal, the person may seek assistance from other members of the family and allow a relative (e.g., parent, grandparent, elder brother) to make decisions about important health-related matters. If collateral relationships are valued, decisions about the person may be interrelated with the impact of illness on the entire family or group. For example, among the Amish, the entire community is affected by the illness of a member because the community pays for health care from a common fund, members join together to meet the needs of both the person and his or her family throughout the illness, and the roles of dozens in the community are likely to be affected by the illness of a single member. Perhaps it is the value orientation toward *individual* relationships that is predominant among the majority of European Americans. Decision-making about health and illness is often an individual matter, with the person being the sole decider, although members of the nuclear family may participate to varying degrees.

Family

Despite the alarmingly high rate of divorce in the United States, the family remains the basic social unit. The essence of family consists of individuals living together as a unit. Although some social scientists argue that there are more than a dozen types of families, the following are commonly recognized types of families: (1) *nuclear* (husband, wife, and child[ren]); (2) *extended family* (nuclear plus blood relatives and even people who are not biologically related); (3) *blended* (husband, wife, and child[ren] from previous relationships); (4) *single parent* (either mother or father and at least one child); (5) *communal* (group of men, women, and children); (6) *cohabitation* (unmarried man and woman sharing a household with child[ren]); and (7) *gay/lesbian* (same-gender couple and child[ren]).

Each family modifies the culture of the larger group in ways that are uniquely its own. Some beliefs, practices, and customs are maintained, whereas others are altered or abandoned. You should also be aware that not all members of a cultural group behave according to the preconceived stereotype. For example, although many Chinese-American children behave in the manner congruent with the stereotype, showing respect for authority, polite social behavior, and moderate to soft voice, there are some who are disrespectful, impolite, and boisterous. Individual dif-ferences, changing norms over time, degree of acculturation, length of time the family has lived in the country, and other factors account for variation.

Relationships that may seem apparent sometimes warrant further exploration when interviewing people from culturally diverse backgrounds. For example, the dominant cultural group defines siblings as two persons with either the same mother, the same father, the same mother and father, or the same adoptive parents. In some Asian cultures, a sibling relationship is defined as one in which any infants are breast-fed by the same woman. In other cultures, certain kinship patterns, such as maternal first cousins, are defined as sibling relationships. In some African cultures, anyone from the same village or town may be called "brother" or "sister." Certain subcultures, such as members of the Roman Catholic or Orthodox religions (who may be further subdivided by ethnicity such as Italians, Polish, Spanish, Mexican, Greek, Russian, and so forth), recognize relationships such as *godmother* or *godfather* in which an individual who is not the biologic parent promises to assist with the moral and spiritual development of an infant and agrees to care for the child in the event of parental death. The godparent makes these promises during the religious ceremony of baptism.

When assessing families, it is important to identify key decision-makers and the primary provider of care because this individual may or may not be the biologic parent. Among some Hispanic groups, for example, female members of the nuclear or extended family such as sisters and aunts are primary providers of care. In some black families, the grandmother may be the decision-maker and primary caretaker of children. Remember that data about a person's family and social support network are useful in assessing the potential sources of psychosocial, emotional, physical, and financial support.

RELIGIOUS BELIEFS AND PRACTICES

As an integral component of the individual's culture, religious beliefs may influence the person's explanation of the cause(s) of illness, perception of its severity, and choice of healer(s). In times of crisis, such as serious illness and impending death, religion may be a source of consolation for the person and for his or her family. Religious dogma and spiritual leaders may exert considerable influence on the person's decision-making concerning acceptable medical and surgical treatment, choice of healer(s), and other aspects of the illness.

Religion and Spirituality

Religious concerns evolve from and respond to the mysteries of life and death, good and evil, and pain and suffering. In health care settings, you frequently encounter people who find themselves searching for a spiritual meaning to help explain their illness or disability. Some nurses find spiritual assessment difficult because of the abstract and personal nature of the topic, whereas others feel quite comfortable discussing spiritual matters. Comfort with your own spiritual beliefs is the foundation to effective assessment of spiritual needs in others.

An important distinction needs to be made between spirituality and religion. *Spirituality* is borne out of each person's unique life experience and his or her personal effort to find purpose and meaning in life. While the religions of the world offer various interpretations to many of life's mysteries, most people seek a personal understanding and interpretation at some time in their lives. Ultimately, this personal search becomes a pursuit to discover a supreme being (called by various names e.g., Allah, God, Yahweh, Jehovah, and so forth) or some unifying truth that will render meaning, purpose, and integrity to existence.

Religion refers to an organized system of beliefs concerning the cause, nature, and purpose of the universe, especially belief in or the worship of God or gods. There are more than 1500 religions in the United States. Eighty-five percent of Americans report religious affiliation with a Christian church. Among the Christian denominations, 66% are Protestant (Baptist, 21%; Methodist, 9%; Lutheran, 7%; Presbyterian, 5%; and Episcopalian, 2%), and 26% are Catholic. Those belonging to non-Christian religions total 6% of the population; the largest group, or 2%, are Jewish. Those reporting no religious affiliation account for 9% of the population (American Almanac, 1997).

 ## DEVELOPMENTAL CONSIDERATIONS

Illness during childhood may be an especially difficult clinical situation. Children as well as adults have spiritual needs that vary according to the child's developmental level and the religious climate that exists in the family. Parental perceptions about the illness of their child may be partially influenced by religious beliefs. For example, some parents may believe that a transgression against a religious law is responsible for a congenital anomaly in their offspring. Other parents may delay seeking medical care because they believe that prayer should be tried first. Certain types of treatment, e.g., administration of blood; medications containing caffeine, pork, or other prohibited substances; and selected procedures, may be perceived as *cultural taboos,* i.e., to be avoided (by both children and adults).

Values held by the dominant United States and Canadian culture, such as emphasis on independence, self-reliance, and productivity, influence aging members of society. North Americans define people as old at the chronologic age of 65 and then limit their work, in contrast to other cultures in which persons are first recog-

nized as being unable to work and then are identified as being old.

In adopting a cultural perspective in working with aging individuals from culturally diverse backgrounds, you should consider that the main task of these persons is to achieve a sense of integrity in accepting responsibility for their own lives and in gaining a sense of accomplishment. Individuals who achieve integrity see aging as a positive experience, make adjustments in their personal space and social relationships, maintain a sense of usefulness, and begin closure and life review.

Older persons may develop their own means of coping with illness through self-care, assistance from family members, and support from social groups. Some cultures have developed attitudes and specific behaviors for older adults that may include humanistic care and identification of family members as care providers. The older adults may have special family responsibilities, e.g., providing hospitality to visitors among Amish cultures and communicating to members of younger generations skills and accrued wisdom among Filipinos.

Older immigrants who have made major lifestyle adjustments in their move from their homeland to the United States or from a rural to an urban area (or vice versa) may not be aware of health care alternatives, preventive programs, health care benefits, and screening programs for which they are eligible. These individuals may also be in various stages of *culture shock,* a term used to describe the state of disorientation or inability to respond to the behavior of a different cultural group because of its sudden strangeness, unfamiliarity, and incompatibility to the stranger's perceptions and expectations.

HEALTH-RELATED BELIEFS AND PRACTICES

Before determining whether cultural practices are helpful, harmful, or neutral, you must first understand the logic of the belief system underlying the practice and then be certain that you fully grasp the nature and meaning of the practice from the person's cultural perspective.

Health and Culture

The first step in understanding the health care needs of others is to understand your own culturally based values, beliefs, attitudes, and practices. Sometimes this requires considerable introspection and may necessitate that you confront your own biases, preconceptions, and prejudices about specific racial, ethnic, religious, sexual, or socioeconomic groups.

Second, you need to identify the meaning of health to the patient, remembering that concepts are derived, in part, from the way in which members of their cultural group define health. Considerable research has been conducted on the various definitions of health that may be held by various groups. For example, Jamaicans may define health as having a good appetite, feeling strong and energetic, performing activities of daily living without difficulty, and being sexually active and fertile. For Italian women, health may mean the ability to interact socially and to perform routine tasks such as cooking, cleaning, and caring for self and others. On the other hand, some individuals of Mexican heritage believe that coughing, sweating, and diarrhea are a normal part of living, not symptoms of ill health—perhaps because of the high frequency of these conditions in the person's country of origin. Thus, individuals may define themselves or others in their group as healthy even though you identify them as having symptoms of disease.

Illness and Culture

For patients, symptom labeling and diagnosis depend on the degree of difference between the individual's behaviors and those the group has defined as normal, beliefs about the causation of illness, level of stigma attached to a particular set of symptoms, prevalence of the pathology, and the meaning of the illness to the individual and his or her family.

Throughout history, humankind has attempted to understand the cause of illness and disease. Theories of causation have been formulated based on religious beliefs, social circumstances, philosophical perspectives, and level of knowledge. You need to determine what the person believes has caused the illness.

Causes of Illness

Disease causation may be viewed in three major ways: from a biomedical or scientific, naturalistic or holistic, and magico-religious perspective.

Biomedical. The first, called the *biomedical* or *scientific* theory of illness causation, is based on the assumption that all events in life have a cause and effect, that the human body functions more or less mechanically (i.e., the functioning of the human body is analogous to the functioning of an automobile), that all life can be reduced or divided into smaller parts (e.g., the reduction of the human person into body, mind, and spirit), and that all of reality can be observed and measured (e.g., intelligence tests and psychometric measures of behavior). Among the biomedical explanations for disease is the germ theory, which posits that microscopic organisms such as bacteria and viruses are responsible for specific disease conditions. Most educational programs for physicians, nurses, and other health care providers embrace the biomedical or scientific theories that explain the causes of both physical and psychological illnesses.

Naturalistic. The second way in which people explain the cause of illness is from the *naturalistic* or *holistic*

perspective, a viewpoint that is found most frequently among Native Americans, Asians, and others who believe that human life is only one aspect of nature and a part of the general order of the cosmos. People from these groups believe that the forces of nature must be kept in natural balance or harmony.

Many Asians believe in the *yin/yang theory,* in which health is believed to exist when all aspects of the person are in perfect balance. Rooted in the ancient Chinese philosophy of *Tao,* the yin/yang theory states that all organisms and objects in the universe consist of yin and yang energy forces. The seat of the energy forces is within the autonomic nervous system where balance between the opposing forces is maintained during health. Yin energy represents the female and negative forces, such as emptiness, darkness, and cold; whereas yang forces are male and positive, emitting warmth and fullness. Foods are classified as hot and cold in this theory and are transformed into yin and yang energy when metabolized by the body. Yin foods are cold and yang foods are hot. Cold foods are eaten with a hot illness, and hot foods are eaten with a cold illness. The yin/yang theory is the basis for *Eastern* or *Chinese* medicine and is commonly embraced by Asian Americans.

The naturalistic perspective posits that the laws of nature create imbalances, chaos, and disease. Individuals embracing the naturalistic view use metaphors such as the healing power of nature, and they call the earth "Mother." From the perspective of the Chinese, for example, illness is not seen as an intruding agent but as a part of life's rhythmic course and as an outward sign of disharmony within.

Many Hispanic, Arab, black, and Asian groups embrace the *hot/cold theory* of health and illness, an explanatory model having its origins in the ancient Greek humoral theory. The four humors of the body—blood, phlegm, black bile, and yellow bile—regulate basic bodily functions and are described in terms of temperature, dryness, and moisture. The treatment of disease consists of adding or subtracting cold, heat, dryness, or wetness to restore the balance of the humors.

Beverages, foods, herbs, medicines, and diseases are classified as hot or cold according to their perceived effects on the body, not on their physical characteristics. Illnesses believed to be caused by cold entering the body include earache, chest cramps, paralysis, gastrointestinal discomfort, rheumatism, and tuberculosis. Among those illnesses believed to be caused by overheating are abscessed teeth, sore throats, rashes, and kidney disorders.

According to the hot/cold theory, the individual as a whole, not just a particular ailment, is significant. Those who embrace the hot/cold theory maintain that health consists of a positive state of total well-being, including physical, psychological, spiritual, and social aspects of the person. Paradoxically, the language used to describe this artificial dissection of the body into parts is itself a reflection of the biomedical/scientific perspective, not a naturalistic or holistic one.

Magico-Religious. The third major way in which people view the world and explain the causation of illness is from a *magico-religious* perspective. The basic premise of this explanatory model is that the world is seen as an arena in which supernatural forces dominate. The fate of the world and those in it depends on the action of supernatural forces for good or evil. Examples of magical causes of illness include belief in voodoo or witchcraft among some blacks and others from circum-Caribbean countries. *Faith healing* is based on religious beliefs and is most prevalent among certain Christian religions, including Christian Scientists, whereas various healing rituals may be found in many other religions such as Roman Catholicism, Mormonism (Church of Jesus Christ of Latter-Day Saints), and others.

Of course, it is possible to have a combination of world views, and many people are likely to offer more than one explanation for the cause of their illness. As a profession, nursing largely embraces the scientific/biomedical world view, but some other aspects have begun to gain popularity, including a wide variety of techniques for management of chronic pain such as acupuncture, herbs, hypnosis, therapeutic touch, and biofeedback. Belief in spiritual power is also held by many health care providers who may credit supernatural forces with various unexplained phenomena related to patients' health and illness states.

Healing and Culture

When self-treatment is unsuccessful, the individual may turn to the lay or folk healing systems, to spiritual or religious healing, or to scientific biomedicine. All cultures have their own preferred lay or popular healers, recognized symptoms of ill health, acceptable sick role behavior, and treatments. In addition to seeking help from you as a biomedical/scientific health care provider, patients may also seek help from folk or religious healers. Some people, such as those of Hispanic or Native American origins, may believe that the cure is incomplete unless healing of body, mind, and spirit are all carried out, although the division of the person into parts is itself a Western concept. For example, a Hispanic person with a respiratory infection may take the antibiotics prescribed by a physician or nurse practitioner and herbal teas recommended by a *curandero* and may say prayers for healing suggested by a Catholic priest.

The variety of healing beliefs and practices used by the many subcultural groups found in this country far exceeds the limitations of this chapter. It is important, however, that you be aware of the existence of alternative practices and recognize that, in addition to folk practices, many other alternative healing practices exist. Although it is dangerous to assume that all indigenous approaches to

healing are innocuous, the majority of practices are quite harmless, whether or not they are effective cures.

Folk Healers

Although numerous folk healers exist, you may find Hispanics turning to a *curandero(ra)*, *espiritualista* (spiritualist), *yerbo* (herbalist), or *sabedor* (healer who manipulates bones and muscles). Blacks may mention having received assistance from a *hougan* (a voodoo priest or priestess), *spiritualist,* or *"old lady"* (an older woman who has successfully raised a family and who specializes in child care and folk remedies). Native Americans may seek assistance from a *shaman* or *medicine (wo)man.* Asians may mention that they have visited *herbalists, acupuncturists,* or *bone setters.* Among the Amish the term *braucher* is used to refer to folk healers who use herbs and tonics in the home or community context. *Brauche,* a folk healing art, refers to sympathy curing, which is sometimes called *powwowing* in English. The treatments used by the braucher may be provided in conjunction with massage, foot treatments, acupressure, reflexology, or, less frequently, iridology (Andrews & Boyle, 1999; Wenger, 1995).

Each culture has its own healers, most of whom speak the person's native tongue, make house calls, and cost significantly less than healers practicing in the biomedical/scientific health care system. In addition to folk healers, many cultures have lay midwives (e.g., *parteras* for Hispanic women) or other health care provider available for meeting the needs of pregnant women (Finn, 1994).

In some religions, spiritual healers may be found among the ranks of the ordained and official religious hierarchy and may be known by a variety of names such as priest, bishop, elder, deacon, rabbi, brother, sister, and so forth. In other religions, a separate category of healer may be found, e.g., Christian Science "nurses" (not licensed by states) or practitioners.

TRANSCULTURAL EXPRESSION OF ILLNESS

Wide cultural variation exists in the manner in which certain symptoms and disease conditions are perceived, diagnosed, labeled, and treated. You should not assume that the perceived symptoms or complaints of patients are equivalent to the names of recognized diseases or syndromes familiar to nurses, physicians, and other health care professionals (Wenger, 1993). The same disease that is considered grounds for social ostracism in one culture may be reason for increased status in another. For example, epilepsy is seen as contagious and untreatable among Ugandans, as a cause for family shame among Greeks, as a reflection of a physical imbalance among Mexican-

Americans, and as a sign of having gained favor by enduring a trial by God among the Hutterites.

Bodily symptoms are also perceived and reported in a variety of ways. For example, people of Mediterranean descent tend to report common physical symptoms more often than persons of Northern European or Asian heritage. Among Chinese, no translation exists for the English word "sadness," yet all people experience the feeling of sadness at some time in life. To express emotion, Chinese patients somaticize their symptoms, or convert mental experiences or states into bodily symptoms, e.g., complain of cardiac symptoms because the center of emotion in the Chinese culture is the heart. You may collect in-depth data about the cardiovascular system only to learn subsequently that all diagnostic tests are negative. On further assessment, you may determine that the person has experienced a loss and is grieving, e.g., has experienced the death of a close friend or relative, or has been divorced or separated. Although some biomedical/scientific clinicians may refer to this as a psychosomatic illness, others recognize it as a culturally acceptable somatic expression of emotional disharmony (Wenger, 1993).

A discussion of pain follows to illustrate the cultural variability that may occur with a symptom of significant concern.

Transcultural Expression of Symptoms: Pain

To illustrate the manner in which symptom expression may reflect the person's cultural background, let's use an extensively studied symptom, pain. Pain is a universally recognized phenomenon and is an important aspect of assessment for people of various ages. Pain is a very private, subjective experience that is greatly influenced by cultural heritage. Expectations, manifestations, and management of pain are all embedded in a cultural context. The definition of pain, like that of health or illness, is culturally determined.

The term *pain* is derived from the Greek word for penalty, which helps explain the long association between pain and punishment in Judeo-Christian thought. The meaning of painful stimuli for individuals, the way people define their situation, and the impact of personal experience all help determine the experience of pain.

Much cross-cultural research has been conducted on pain. Pain has been found to be a highly personal experience, depending on cultural learning, the meaning of the situation, and other factors unique to the individual. Silent suffering has been identified as the most valued response to pain by health care professionals. The majority of nurses have been socialized to believe that in virtually any situation, self-control is better than open displays of strong feelings.

In research studies of nurses' attitudes toward pain, it

was discovered that the ethnic background of patients is important in the nurses' assessment of both physical and psychological pain. For example, nurses preconceive that Jewish and Spanish patients suffer the most and that Anglo-Saxon, German, and Asian patients suffer the least. In addition, nurses who infer relatively greater patient pain tended to report their own experiences as more painful. In general, nurses from Eastern and Southern European or African backgrounds tend to infer greater suffering than do nurses of Northern European backgrounds. Years of experience, current position, and area of clinical practice are unrelated to inferences of suffering (Ludwig-Beymer, 1999).

In addition to expecting variations in pain perception and tolerance, you should also expect variations in the expression of pain. It is a well-known fact that individuals turn to their social environment for validation and comparison. A first important comparison group is the family, which transmits cultural norms to its children.

Culture-Bound Syndromes

Some people may have a condition that is culturally defined, known as a *culture-bound syndrome*. Some of these conditions have no equivalent from a biomedical/scientific perspective, whereas others, such as anorexia nervosa and bulimia, are examples of the cultural aspects of illness among members of dominant group in the United States. Table 3–1 summarizes selected examples from among the more than 150 culture-bound syndromes that have been documented by medical anthropologists.

Culture and Treatment

After a symptom is identified, the first effort at treatment is often self-care. In the United States an estimated 70 to 90 percent of all illness episodes are treated first, or exclusively, through self-care, often with significant success (Lipson and Steiger, 1996). The availability of over-the-counter medications, relatively high literacy level of Americans, growing availability of herbal remedies and influence of the mass media in communicating health-related information to the general population have contributed to the high percentage of cases of self-treatment. Home treatments are attractive for their accessibility, especially when compared with the inconvenience associated with traveling to a physician, nurse practitioner, and pharmacist, particularly for people from rural or sparsely populated areas. Furthermore, home treatment may mobilize the person's social support network and provide the sick individual with a caring environment in which to convalesce. You should be aware, however, that not all home remedies are inexpensive. For example, urban black populations in the Southeast sometimes use medicinal po-

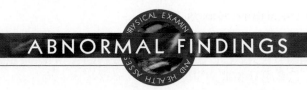
▼ Table 3–1   SELECTED CULTURE-BOUND SYNDROMES

Group	Disorder	Remarks
Blacks	Blackout	Collapse, dizziness, inability to move
	Low blood	Not enough blood or weakness of the blood, which is often treated with diet
	High blood	Blood that is too rich in certain nutrients due to ingestion of too much red meat or rich foods
	Thin blood	Occurs in women, children, and old people; renders the individual more susceptible to illness in general
	Diseases of hex, witchcraft, or conjuring	Sense of being doomed by spell; part of voodoo beliefs
Chinese/Southeast Asians	Koro	Intense anxiety that penis is retracting into body
Greeks	Hysteria	Bizarre complaints and behavior because the uterus leaves the pelvis for another part of the body
Hispanics	Empacho	Food forms into a ball and clings to the stomach or intestines causing pain and cramping
	Fatique	Asthmalike symptoms
	Mal ojo ("evil eye")	Fitful sleep, crying, diarrhea in children caused by a stranger's attention; sudden onset
	Pasmo	Paralysislike symptoms of face or limbs; prevented or relieved by massage
	Susto	Anxiety, trembling, phobias from sudden fright
Native Americans	Ghost	Terror, hallucinations, sense of danger
Indonesians	Latah	Hypersuggestibility, trancelike behavior
	Waswas	Excessive repetition of words or gestures
Japanese	Wagamama	Apathetic childish behavior with emotional outbursts
Koreans	Hwa-byung	Multiple somatic and psychological symptoms; "pushing up" sensation in the chest; palpitations; flushing; headache; sensation of a stomach mass; dysphoria, anxiety; irritability; and difficulty concentrating—highest incidence in married women
Whites	Anorexia nervosa	Excessive preoccupation with thinness; self-imposed starvation
	Bulimia	Gross overeating, then vomiting or fasting

Table 3–2 DISTRIBUTION OF SELECTED GENETIC TRAITS AND DISORDERS BY POPULATION OR ETHNIC GROUP

Ethnic or Population Group	Genetic or Multifactorial Disorder Present in Relatively High Frequency
Aland Islanders	Ocular albinism (Forsius-Eriksson type)
Amish	Limb-girdle muscular dystrophy (IN—Adams, Allen counties)
	Ellis-van Creveld syndrome (PA—Lancaster county)
	Pyruvate kinase deficiency (OH—Mifflin county)
	Hemophilia B (PA—Holmes county)
Armenians	Familial Mediterranean fever
	Familial paroxysmal polyserositis
Africans	Sickle-cell disease
	Hemoglobin C disease
	Hereditary persistence of hemoglobin F
	G6PD deficiency, African type
	Lactase deficiency, adult
	β-Thalassemia
Burmese	Hemoglobin E disease
Chinese	Alpha thalassemia
	G6PD deficiency, Chinese type
	Lactase deficiency, adult
Costa Ricans	Malignant osteopetrosis
Druze	Alkaptonuria
English	Cystic fibrosis
	Hereditary amyloidosis, type III
Inuit	Congenital adrenal hyperplasia
	Pseudocholinesterase deficiency
	Methemoglobinemia
French Canadians (Quebec)	Tyrosinemia
	Morquio syndrome
Finns	Congenital nephrosis
	Generalized amyloidosis syndrome, V
	Polycystic liver disease
	Retinoschisis
	Aspartylglycosaminuria
	Diastrophic dwarfism
Gypsies (Czech)	Congenital glaucoma
Hopi Indians	Tyrosinase positive albinism
Icelanders	Phenylketonuria
Irish	Phenylketonuria
	Neural tube defects
Japanese	Acatalasemia
	Cleft lip/palate
	Oguchi disease
Jews	Tay-Sachs disease (infantile)
Ashkenazi	Niemann-Pick disease (infantile)
	Gaucher disease (adult type)
	Familial dysautonomia (Riley-Day syndrome)
	Bloom syndrome
	Torsion dystonia
	Factor XI (PTA) deficiency

(Continued)

Table 3–2   DISTRIBUTION OF SELECTED GENETIC TRAITS AND DISORDERS BY POPULATION OR ETHNIC GROUP *Continued*

Ethnic or Population Group	Genetic or Multifactorial Disorder Present in Relatively High Frequency
Sephardi	Familial Mediterranean fever
	Ataxia-telangiectasia (Morocco)
	Cystinuria (Libya)
	Glycogen storage disease III (Morocco)
Oriental	Dubin-Johnson syndrome (Iran)
	Ichthyosis vulgaris (Iraq, India)
	Werdnig-Hoffmann disease (Karcite Jews)
	G6PD deficiency, Mediterranean type
	Phenylketonuria (Yemen)
	Metachromatic leukodystrophy (Habbanite Jews, Saudi Arabia)
Lapps	Congenital dislocation of hip
Lebanese	Dyggus-Melchior-Clausen syndrome
Mediterraneans (Italians, Greeks)	G6PD deficiency, Mediterranean type
	β-Thalassemia
	Familial Mediterranean fever
Navaho Indians	Ear anomalies
Polynesians	Clubfoot
Polish	Phenylketonuria
Portuguese	Joseph disease
Nova Scotia Acadians	Niemann-Pick disease, type D
Scandinavians (Norwegians, Swedes, Danes)	Cholestasis-lymphedema (Norwegians)
	Sjögren-Larsson syndrome (Swedes)
	Krabbe disease
	Phenylketonuria
Scots	Phenylketonuria
	Cystic fibrosis
	Hereditary amyloidosis, type III
Thai	Lactase deficiency, adult
	Hemoglobin E disease
Zuni Indians	Tyrosinase positive albinism

IN = Indiana; OH = Ohio; PA = Pennsylvania; PTA = plasma thromboplastin antecedent.
From Cohen FI: Clinical Genetics in Nursing Practice. Philadelphia, J.B. Lippincott Company, 1984.

tions that cost much more than the equivalent treatment with a biomedical intervention.

A wide variety of alternative or complementary interventions are gaining the recognition of health care professionals in the biomedical/scientific health care system. Acupuncture, acupressure, therapeutic touch, massage, therapeutic use of music, biofeedback, relaxation techniques, meditation, hypnosis, distraction, imagery, iridology, reflexology, herbal remedies, and others are interventions that people may use either alone or in combination with other treatments. Many pharmacies and grocery stores routinely carry herbal treatments for a wide variety of common illnesses.

CULTURE AND DISEASE PREVALENCE

For the past generation, the United States and Canada have enjoyed improvement in the health status of their people. Despite this fact, there continues to be disparity in deaths and illnesses experienced by racial and ethnic minority populations, and it is well known that diseases are not distributed equally among all segments of the population but rather tend to cluster around certain racial and ethnic subgroups. Abnormal biocultural variations may be genetic or acquired. Summarized in Table 3–2 is a list of selected genetic traits and disorders by population or ethnic group. This information is useful in assessing people from various subgroups because you are able to focus your assessment according to the increased statistical probability that a particular condition may occur. For example, if you are examining a black child with gastrointestinal symptoms, you may focus more on the possibility of lactose intolerance or sickle-cell anemia while considering cystic fibrosis, known primarily among white children, a much less likely source of the problem. Thus, in your assessment, you will want to be certain that you have gathered the appropriate data needed to support or to refute your suspicions.

In order to accurately assess individuals representing the hundreds of different subcultures found in North America, it is necessary to include cultural considerations during your assessment. Guidelines for gathering data from people of culturally diverse backgrounds have been suggested throughout this chapter and are interwoven throughout the remainder of the text. Awareness of cultural differences is foundational to understanding people's responses to health and illness because culture is all-pervasive and comprises the very fabric of the person's being.

Bibliography

American Almanac 1996–1997. Austin, TX, Hoover's Inc, 1997.

Andrews MM, Boyle JS: Competence in transcultural nursing care. Am J Nurs 97(8):16AAA–16DDD, Aug 1997.

Andrews MM, Boyle JS (Eds): Transcultural Concepts in Nursing Care, 3rd ed. Philadelphia, Lippincott-Raven Publishers, 1999.

Andrews MM, Hanson PA: Religion, culture and nursing. *In* Andrews MM, Boyle JS (Eds): Transcultural Concepts in Nursing Care, 3rd ed. Philadelphia, J.B. Lippincott Company, 1999, pp 378–443.

Campinha-Bacote J, Yahle T, Langenkamp M: The challenge of cultural diversity for nurse educators. J Con Educ Nur 27(2):59–64, 1996.

Eliason MJ: Cultural diversity in nursing care: The lesbian, gay or bisexual client. J Transcult Nur 5(1):14–20, 1993.

Finn JM: Culture care of Euro-American women during childbirth: Using Leininger's theory. J Transcult Nurs 5(2):25–37, 1994.

Gray M: Herbs: Multicultural folk medicines. Orthop Nurs 15(2):49–56, Mar–Apr 1996.

Grossman D: Cultural dimensions in home health nursing. Am J Nurs 96(7):33–36, July 1996.

Kluckhohn FR: Dominant and variant value orientations. *In* Brink PJ (Ed): Transcultural Nursing: A Book of Readings. Englewood Cliffs, NJ, Prentice Hall, 1990, pp 63–81.

Leininger MM: Transcultural Nursing: Concepts, Theories and Practices. New York, McGraw-Hill, Inc., 1995.

Leininger MM: Transcultural nursing research to transform nursing education and practice: 40 years. Image 29(4):341–347, 1997.

Lester N: Cultural competence: A nursing dialogue. Part 1. Am J Nurs 98(8):26–34, Aug 1998.

Lester N: Cultural competence: A nursing dialogue. Part 2. Am J Nurs 98(9):36–43, Sept 1998.

Lipson JG, Steiger NJ: Self-Care Nursing In a Multicultural Context. Thousand Oaks, MI, Sage Publications, 1996.

Ludwig-Beymer PA: Transcultural aspects of pain. *In* Andrews MM, Boyle JS (Eds): Transcultural Concepts in Nursing Care, 3rd ed. Philadelphia, J.B. Lippincott Company, 1999, pp 283–307.

U.S. Bureau of the Census: General Population Characteristics. Washington, DC, U.S. Government Printing Office, 1990.

Wenger AF. Cultural context, health, and health care decision making. J Transcult Nur 7(1):3–14, 1995.

Wenger AF: Cultural meaning of symptoms. Holistic Nurs Pract 7(2): 22–35, 1993.

Zatrick DF, Dimsdale JE: Cultural variations in response to painful stimuli. Psychosom Med 52:544–557, 1990.

CHAPTER FOUR

The Interview

The interview is a meeting between you and your patient. The meeting's goal is to record a complete health history. The health history is important in beginning to identify the person's health strengths and problems and as a bridge to the next step in data collection, the physical examination.

The interview is the first and really the most important part of data collection. It collects **subjective data**—what the person says about himself or herself. The interview is the first and the best chance a person has to tell you what *he or she* perceives the health state to be. Once people enter the health care system, they may relinquish some control. At the interview, however, the patient is still in charge. The individual knows everything about his or her own health state, and you know nothing. Your skill in interviewing will glean all the necessary information as well as build rapport for a successful working relationship.

When you have a successful interview, you

1. Gather complete and accurate data about the person's health state, including the description and chronology of any symptoms of illness.
2. Establish rapport and trust so the person feels accepted and thus free to share all relevant data.
3. Teach the person about the health state so that the person can participate in identifying problems.
4. Build rapport for a continuing therapeutic relationship; this rapport facilitates future diagnoses, planning, and treatment.
5. Begin teaching for health promotion and disease prevention.

Consider the interview as being similar to forming a contract between you and your patient. A contract consists of spoken or unspoken rules for behavior. In this case, the contract concerns what the person needs and expects from health care and what you, the health professional, have to offer. Your mutual goal is optimal health for the patient. The contract's terms include

● Time and place of the interview and succeeding physical examination
● Introduction of yourself and a brief explanation of your role
● The purpose of the interview
● How long it will take
● Expectation of participation for each person
● Presence of any other people, e.g., patient's family, other health professionals, students
● Confidentiality and to what extent it may be limited
● Any costs that the patient must pay

Although the patient already may know some of this information through telephone contact with receptionists or the admitting office, the remaining points need to be stated clearly at the outset. Any confusion could produce resentment and anger, rather than the openness and trust you need to facilitate the interview.

THE PROCESS OF COMMUNICATION

The vehicle that carries you and your patient through the interview is communication. Communication is exchanging information so that each person clearly understands the other. If you do not understand each other, if you have not *conveyed meaning,* no communication has occurred.

It is challenging to teach the skill of interviewing because initially most students think little needs to be learned. They assume that if they can talk and hear, they can communicate. But much more than talking and hearing is necessary. Communication is all behavior, conscious and unconscious, verbal and nonverbal. *All behavior has meaning.*

Sending

Likely, you are most aware of *verbal* communication—the words you speak, vocalizations, the tone of voice. *Nonverbal* communication also occurs—through posture, gestures, facial expression, eye contact, touch, even where you place your chair. Since nonverbal communication is under less conscious control than verbal communication, nonverbal communication probably is more reflective of your true feelings.

Receiving

Being aware of the messages you send is only part of the process. Your words and gestures must be interpreted in a *specific context* to have meaning. You have a specific context in mind when you send your words. The receiver puts his or her own interpretation on them. The receiver attaches meaning determined by his or her past experiences, culture, self-concept, as well as current physical and emotional state. Sometimes these contexts do not coincide. Remember how frustrating it may have been to try to communicate something to a friend, only to have your message totally misunderstood? Your message can be sabotaged by the listener's bias. It takes mutual understanding by the sender and receiver to have successful communication.

Even greater risk for misunderstanding exists in the health care setting than in a social setting. The patient usually has a health problem, and this factor emotionally charges your professional relationship. It *intensifies* the communication because the person feels dependent on you to get better.

Communication is a *basic skill* that can be learned and polished when you are a beginning practitioner. It is a tool, as basic to quality health care as the tools of inspection or palpation. To maximize your communicating skill, first you need to be aware of internal and external factors and their influence.

Internal Factors

Internal factors are those particular to the examiner, what you bring into the interview. Cultivate the three inner factors of liking others, empathy, and the ability to listen.

Liking Others. One essential factor for an examiner's "goodness of fit" into a helping profession is a genuine liking of other people. This means a generally optimistic view of people; an assumption of their strengths and a tolerance for their weaknesses (Benjamin, 1980). An atmosphere of warmth and caring is necessary. The patient must feel that he or she is accepted unconditionally.

The respect for other people extends to respect for their own control over their health. Your goal is *not* to make your patients dependent on you, but to help them to be increasingly responsible for themselves. You wish to promote their growth. You have the health care resources to offer patients. They must choose how to apply those resources to their own lives.

Empathy. Empathy means viewing the world from the other person's inner frame of reference while remaining yourself. Empathy means recognizing and accepting the other person's feelings without criticism. It is described as "feeling *with* the person rather than feeling *like* the person" (Bernstein and Bernstein, 1985). It does not mean you become lost in the other person at the expense of your own self. If this occurred you would cease to be helpful. Rather, it is to *understand with* the person how *he or she* perceives his or her world (Rogers, 1951).

The Ability to Listen. Listening is not a passive role in the communication process; it is active and demanding. Listening requires your complete attention. You cannot be preoccupied with your own needs or the needs of other patients, or you will miss something important with this one. For the time of this interview, no one is more important than this person. This person's needs are your sole concern.

Active listening is the route to understanding. You cannot be thinking of what you are going to say as soon as the person stops for breath. Listen to *what* the person says. The story may not come out in the order you would ask it, or will record it later. Let the person talk from his or her own outline; nearly everything that is said will be relevant. Listen to *the way* a person tells the story, such as difficulty with language, impaired memory, the tone of the person's voice, and even to what the person is leaving out.

CLINICAL ILLUSTRATION

Sandra B., 32 years of age, sought care for headaches she had during the last 3 months, which were unresponsive to aspirin and were interfering with her job. She was interviewed for 30 minutes. Through this time she never mentioned her husband, although they had been married only 5 months before. Finally the examiner asked, "I haven't heard you mention your husband. Tell me about him." It unfolded that Sandra's husband lost his job a few months after they were married because of alcohol-related work errors. Although Sandra related extreme personal stress and worry, she never thought that her headaches might be related to the stressful situation.

External Factors

Prepare the physical setting. The setting may be in a hospital room, an examination room in an office or clinic, or in the person's home (where you will have less control). In any location, optimal conditions are important to have a smooth interview.

Ensure Privacy. Aim for geographic privacy—a private room in the hospital, clinic, office, or home. This may involve asking an ambulatory roommate to step out for a while or finding an unoccupied room or an empty lounge. If geographic privacy is not available, "psychological privacy" by curtained partitions may suffice as long as the person feels sure no one can overhear the conversation or interrupt.

Refuse Interruptions. Most people resent interruptions except in cases of an emergency. Inform any support staff of your interview, and ask that they not interrupt you during this time. Discourage other health professionals from interrupting you with *their* need for access to the patient. You need to concentrate and to establish rapport. An interruption can destroy in seconds what you have spent many minutes building up.

Physical Environment
- Set the room temperature at a comfortable level.
- Provide sufficient lighting so that you can see each other clearly. Avoid facing the patient directly toward a strong light. The patient must squint into the full light, as if on stage.
- Reduce noise. Multiple stimuli are confusing. Turn off the television, radio, and any unnecessary equipment.
- Remove distracting objects or equipment. It is appropriate to leave some professional equipment (oto/ophthalmoscope, blood pressure manometer) in view. However, clutter, stacks of mail, files of other patients, or your lunch should not be seen. The room should advertise the professional nature of the interviewer.

- Place the distance between you and the patient at 4 to 5 feet (twice arm's length). If you place the patient any closer, you may invade his or her private space and you may create anxiety. If you place the patient farther away, you seem distant and aloof. (See the section on Transcultural Considerations for more information.)
- Arrange equal-status seating. Both you and the patient should be comfortably seated, at eye level. Avoid facing a patient across a desk or table because that feels like a barrier. Placing the chairs at 90 degrees is good because it allows the person either to face you or to look straight ahead from time to time (Fig. 4–1). Most important, avoid standing. Standing does two things: (1) it communicates your haste, and (2) it assumes superiority. Standing makes you loom over the patient as an authority figure. When you are sitting, the person feels some control in the setting.
- Arrange a face-to-face position when interviewing the hospitalized bedridden person. The person should not have to stare at the ceiling, because this causes him or her to lose the visual message of your communication.

Dress
- The patient should remain in street clothes except in the case of an emergency.
- Your appearance and clothing should be appropriate to the setting and should meet conventional professional standards: a uniform or lab coat over conservative clothing, a name tag, and neat hair. Avoid extremes.

Note-Taking. Some use of history forms and note-taking may be unavoidable. When you sit down later to record the interview, you cannot rely completely on memory to furnish details of previous hospitalizations or the review of body systems, for example. But be aware that note-taking during the interview has disadvantages:

- It breaks eye contact too often.
- It shifts your attention away from the person, diminishing his or her sense of importance.
- It can interrupt the patient's narrative flow. You may say "Please slow down, I'm not getting it all." Or, the patient sees you recording furiously, and in an effort to please you, adjusts his or her tempo to your writing. Either way, the patient's natural mode of expression is lost.
- It impedes your observation of the patient's nonverbal behavior.
- It is threatening to the patient during the discussion of sensitive issues, e.g., amount of alcohol and drug use, number of sexual partners, or incidence of physical abuse.

So keep note-taking to a minimum, and try to focus your attention on the person. Any recording you do should be secondary to the dialogue and should not interfere with the person's spontaneity. With experience, you will not rely on note-taking as much.

Tape and Video Recording. An audio tape documents a complete record of what was said during the interview. You cannot refer to it as easily as you can to your notes, but the tape is an excellent teaching tool to study objectively your performance as an interviewer. After listening, other students have said,

"I never realized how much I talked. I really dominated the patient."
"I have to watch my interrupting. I cut her off that time."
"There. That response really worked. She opened up. I want to be that effective more often."

Tapes demonstrate how you can improve your communication. And, as you gain experience, the tapes also document your advancing skills. This process is very rewarding.

A video recording takes the teaching-learning tool one step further because you can study both verbal and nonverbal communication at the same time. Initial anxiety is common among students who feel self-conscious and fear "making a fool" of themselves on camera, but the video can detect richer detail in nonverbal behavior.

"I must have crossed and uncrossed my legs 20 times! I never realized I did that. My fidgeting sure made Mr. J. look distracted."
"It was good that I leaned toward her when she paused that time. I think it helped her continue."
"I talked for five minutes nonstop about how to perform breast self examination, without ever letting Mrs. S. ask a question!"

If you use any tape recording, some ethical considerations are necessary. Explain to the person the purpose of

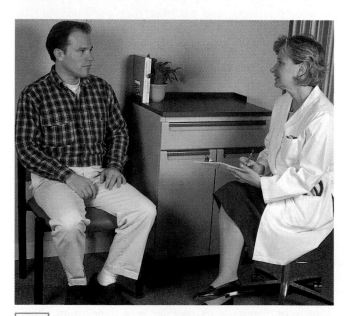

4–1

the recording (whether for teaching, supervision, research), exactly who will hear it (you, your supervisor), and that it will then be destroyed. Obtain consent before you start. Be thoroughly familiar with the equipment; fumbling with the controls is distracting. Arrange the microphone between you and the patient and place the rest of the recording equipment out of sight. It is likely that after a few moments, neither of you will be aware of the recording.

TECHNIQUES OF COMMUNICATION

Introducing the Interview

The patient is here and you are ready for the interview. If you are nervous about how to begin, remember to keep the beginning short. Probably, the patient is nervous, too, and is anxious to start. Address the person, using his or her surname, and shake hands if that seems comfortable. Introduce yourself and state your role in the agency (if you are a student, say so). If you are gathering a complete history, give the reason for this interview:

"Mrs. Sanchez, I would like to talk about your illness that caused you to come to the hospital."
"Ms. Taft, I want to ask you some questions about your health so that we can identify what is keeping you healthy and explore any problems."
"Mr. Craig, I want to ask you some questions about your health and your usual daily activities so that we can plan your care here in the hospital."

If the person is in the hospital, more than one health team member may be collecting a history. Patients are apt to feel exasperated because they believe they are repeating the same thing unless you give a reason for this interview.

After this brief introduction, ask an open-ended question (see the following section) and then let the person proceed. You do not need friendly small talk to build rapport. This is not a social visit; the person has some concern to talk about and wants to get on with it. You will build rapport best by letting him or her discuss the concern early.

The Working Phase

The working phase is the data-gathering phase. Verbal skills for this phase include your questions to the patient and your responses to what the patient has said. Two types of questions exist: open-ended and closed. Each type has a different place and function in the interview.

Open-Ended Questions

The **open-ended** question asks for narrative information. It states the topic to be discussed but only in general

terms. Use it to begin the interview, to introduce a new section of questions, and whenever the person introduces a new topic.

"Tell me how I can help you."
"What brings you to the hospital?"
"Tell me why you have come here today."
"How have you been getting along?"
"You mentioned shortness of breath. Tell me more about that."
"How have you been feeling since your last appointment?"

The open-ended question is unbiased; it leaves the person free to answer in any way. This question encourages the person to respond in paragraphs and to give a spontaneous account in any order chosen. It lets the person express herself or himself fully.

As the person answers, stop and *listen.* What usually happens is that the patient answers with a short phrase or sentence, pauses, and then looks at you expecting some direction of how to go on. What you do next is the key to the direction of the interview. If you pose new questions on other topics, you may lose much of the initial story. Instead, respond to the first statement with "Tell me about it," or "Anything else?" or merely look acutely interested. The person then will tell the story.

Closed or Direct Questions

Closed or **direct** questions ask for specific information. They elicit a short, one- or two-word answer, a yes or no, or a forced choice. Whereas the open-ended question allows the patient to have free rein, the direct question limits his or her answer (Table 4–1).

Table 4–1 • Comparison of Open-Ended and Closed Questions

Open-Ended	Direct, Closed
Use for narrative information	Use for specific information
Calls for long paragraph answers	Calls for short one- to two-word answers
Elicits feelings, opinions, ideas	Elicits cold facts
Builds and enhances rapport	Limits rapport and leaves interaction neutral

Use the direct questions after the person's opening narrative to fill in any details he or she left out. Also use direct questions when you need many specific facts, such as when asking about past health problems or during the review of systems. You need direct questions to speed up the interview. Asking all open-ended questions would be unwieldy and may take hours. But be careful not to overuse closed questions. Follow these guidelines:

1. Ask only one direct question at a time. Avoid bombarding the person with long lists: "Have you ever had

pain, double vision, watering or redness in the eyes?" Avoid double-barreled questions, such as "Do you exercise and follow a diet for your weight?" The person will not know which question to answer. And if the person answers "yes," you will not know which question the person has answered.

2. Choose language the person understands. You may need to use regional phrases or colloquial expressions. For example, "running off" means running away in standard English, but it means diarrhea to Appalachian mountain people.

Responses—Assisting the Narrative

You have asked the first open-ended question, and the patient answers. As the person talks, your role is to encourage free expression, but to not let the person wander off course. Your responses help the teller amplify the story.

Some people seek health care for short-term or relatively simple needs. Their history is direct and uncomplicated; for these people, two responses (facilitation and silence) may be all you need to get a complete picture. Other people have a complex story, a long history of a chronic condition, or accompanying emotions. Additional responses help you gather data without cutting them off.

There are nine types of verbal responses in all. The first five responses (facilitation, silence, reflection, empathy, clarification), involve your *reactions* to the facts or feelings the person has communicated. Your response focuses on the patient's frame of reference. Your own frame of reference does not enter into the response. In the last four responses (confrontation, interpretation, explanation, summary), you start to express your *own* thoughts and feelings. The frame of reference shifts from the patient's perspective to yours (Benjamin, 1980). In the first five responses, the patient leads; in the last four responses, you lead.

Facilitation. These responses encourage the patient to say more, to continue with the story ("mm-hmm, go on, continue, uh-huh"). Also called general leads, these responses show the person you are interested and will listen further. Simply maintaining eye contact, shifting forward in your seat with increased attention, nodding "Yes," or using your hand to gesture, "Yes, go on, I'm with you," encourage the person to continue talking.

Silence. Silence is golden after open-ended questions. Your silent attentiveness communicates that the patient has time to think, to organize what he or she wishes to say without interruption from you. This "thinking silence" is the one health professionals interrupt most often. The interruption destroys the person's train of thought. The patient is often interrupted because silence is uncomfortable to beginning examiners. They feel responsible for keeping the dialogue going and feel at fault if it stops.

But silence has advantages. One advantage is letting the person collect his or her thoughts. Also, silence gives you a chance to observe the person unobtrusively and to note nonverbal cues. Finally, silence gives you time to plan your next approach.

Reflection. This response echoes the patient's words. Reflection is repeating part of what the person has just said. In this example, it focuses further attention on a specific phrase and helps the person continue in his own way:

Patient: I'm here because of my water. It was cutting off.
Response: It was cutting off?
Patient: Yes, yesterday it took me 30 minutes to pass my water. Finally I got a tiny stream, but then it just closed off.

Reflection also can help express feeling behind a person's words. The feeling is already in the statement. You focus on it and encourage the person to elaborate:

Patient: It's so hard having to stay flat on my back in the hospital with this pregnancy. I have two more little ones at home. I'm so worried they are not getting the care they need.
Response: You feel worried and anxious about your children?

Think of yourself as a mirror reflecting the person's words or feelings. This helps the person to elaborate on the problem.

Empathy. A physical symptom, condition, or illness often has accompanying emotions. Many people have trouble expressing these feelings, perhaps because of confusion or embarrassment. In the reflecting example above, the person already had stated her feeling and you echoed it. But in the following example, he has not said it yet. An empathic response recognizes a feeling and puts it into words. It names the feeling and allows the expression of it. When the empathic response is used, the patient feels accepted and can deal with the feeling openly.

Patient: (sarcastically): This is just great. I have my own business, I direct 20 employees everyday, and now here I am having to call you for every little thing.
Response: It must be hard—one day having so much control, and now feeling dependent on someone else.

Your response does not cut off further communication as would happen by giving false reassurance ("Oh, you'll be back to work in no time"). Also, it does not deny the feeling and indicate that it is not justified ("Now I don't do *every*thing for you. Why, you are feeding yourself"). An empathic response recognizes the feeling, accepts it, and allows the person to express it without embarrassment. It strengthens rapport. The patient feels understood, which by itself is therapeutic, because it "bridges the isolation of illness" (Suchman et al., 1997). Other empathic responses are, "This must be very hard for you," "I understand," or just placing your hand on the person's arm.

Clarification. Use this when the person's word choice is ambiguous or confusing, e.g., "Tell me what you mean by 'tired blood.'" Clarification also is used to summarize the person's words, simplify the words to make them clearer, then ask if you are on the right track. You are asking for agreement, and the person can then confirm or deny your understanding.

Response: Now as I understand you, this heaviness in your chest comes when you shovel snow or climb stairs, and it goes away when you stop doing those things. Is that correct?
Patient: Yes, that's pretty much it.

Confrontation. Recall that in these last four responses, (confrontation, interpretation, explanation, summary), the frame of reference shifts from the patient's perspective to yours. These responses now include your own thoughts and feelings. Use the last four responses only when merited by the situation. If you use them too often, you take over at the patient's expense. In the case of confrontation, you have observed a certain action, feeling, or statement and you now focus the person's attention on it. You give your honest feedback about what you see or feel. This may focus on a discrepancy: "You say it doesn't hurt, but when I touch you here, you grimace." Or, it may focus on the person's affect: "You look sad" or "You sound angry." Or, you may confront the person when you notice parts of the story are inconsistent: "Earlier you said you were laying off alcohol and just now you said you had a few drinks after work."

Interpretation. This statement is not based on direct observation as is confrontation, but it is based on your inference or conclusion. It links events, makes associations, or implies cause: "It seems that every time you feel the stomach pain, you have had some kind of stress in your life." Interpretation also ascribes feelings and helps the person understand his or her own feelings in relation to the verbal message.

Patient: I have decided I don't want to take any more treatments. But I can't seem to tell my doctor that. Every time she comes in, I tighten up and can't say anything.
Response: Could it be that you're afraid of her reaction?

You do run a risk of making the wrong inference. If this is the case, the person will correct it. But even if the inference is corrected, interpretation helps to prompt further discussion of the topic.

Explanation. With these statements, you inform the person. You share factual and objective information. This may be for orientation to the agency setting: "Your din-

ner comes at 5:30 PM." Or, it may be to explain cause: "The reason you cannot eat or drink before your blood test is that the food will change the test results."

Summary. This is a final review of what you understand the person has said. It condenses the facts and presents a survey of how you perceive the health problem or need. It is a type of validation in that the person can agree with it or correct it. Both you and the patient should participate. When the summary occurs at the end of the interview, it signals that termination of the interview is imminent.

Ten Traps of Interviewing

The verbal skills discussed above are productive and enhance the interview. Now take time to consider nonproductive, defeating verbal messages, or traps. It is easy to fall into these traps because you are anxious to help. The danger is that they restrict the patient's response. The following traps are obstacles to obtaining complete data and to establishing rapport.

1. Providing False Assurance or Reassurance. A woman says, "Oh I just know this lump is going to turn out to be cancer." What happens inside you? The automatic response of many clinicians is to say, "Now don't worry. I'm sure you will be all right." This "courage builder" relieves *your* anxiety and gives you the false sense of having provided comfort. But for the woman it actually closes off communication. It trivializes her anxiety and effectively denies any further talk of it. (Also it promises something that may not happen, i.e., she may *not* be all right). Consider instead these responses:

"You are really worried about the lump, aren't you?"
"It must be hard to wait for the biopsy results."

These responses acknowledge the feeling and open the door for more communication.

A genuine, valid form of reassurance does exist. You *can* reassure patients that they are being listened to; that hope exists; that you understand what they say; and that you are providing good care (Bradley and Edinberg, 1990).

Patient: I feel so lost here since they transferred me to the medical center. No one comes to see me. No one here cares what happens to me.
Response: I care what happens to you. I am here today and I want you to know that I'll be here all week.

This type of reassurance makes a commitment to the patient, and it can have a powerful impact.

2. Giving Unwanted Advice. Know when to give advice and when to avoid giving it. Often, people seek health care because they want your professional advice and information on the management of a health problem: "My child has chickenpox. How should I take care of him?" This is a straightforward request for information that you have that the parent needs. You respond by giving a health prescription, a therapeutic plan based on your knowledge and experience.

In other situations, advice is different; it is based on a hunch or feeling. It is your personal opinion. Consider the woman who has just left a meeting with her consultant physician: "Dr. Kline just told me my only chance of getting pregnant is to have an operation. I just don't know. What would you do?" Does the woman really want your advice? If you answer, "If I were you, I'd . . ." then you would be making a mistake. You are not her. If you give your answer, you have shifted the accountability for decision-making from her to you. She has not worked out her own solution. She has learned nothing about herself.

Does the woman really want to know what you would do? Probably not. Instead, a better response is reflection:

Response: Have an operation?
Woman: Yes, and I'm terrified of being put to sleep.
   What if I don't wake up?

Now you know her *real* concern and can help her deal with it. She will have grown in the process and may be better equipped to meet her next decision.

When asked for advice, other preferred responses are,

"What are the pros and cons of _____ (this choice)
   for you?"
"What concerns do you have?"
"What is holding you back?"

Although it is quicker just to give advice, take the time to involve the patient in a problem-solving process. When a patient participates, he or she is more likely to learn and to change behavior.

3. Using Authority. "Your doctor/nurse knows best" is a response that promotes dependency and inferiority. The communication pathway looks something like this:

Interviewer: ↘

Patient: ↗

with your talk coming "down" and little from the patient going back "up" (Cornell, 1993). A better approach is to avoid using authority. Although you and the patient cannot have equality of professional skill and experience, you do have equally worthy roles in the health process, each respecting the other.

4. Using Avoidance Language. People use euphemisms such as "passed on" to avoid reality or to hide their feelings. They think if they just say the word "death," it might really happen. So to protect themselves, they evade the issue. Although it seems this will make comfortable potentially fearful topics, it does not. Not talking about the fear does not make it go away; it just

suppresses the fear and makes it even more frightening. Using direct language is the best way to deal with frightening topics.

5. Engaging in Distancing. This is the use of impersonal speech to put space between a threat and the self. "My friend has a problem. She is afraid she . . ." Or, "There is a lump in the left breast." By using "the" instead of "my," the woman can deny any association with her diseased breast and protect herself from it. Health professionals use distancing, too, to soften reality. This does not work because it communicates to the other person that you also are afraid of the procedure. The use of blunt specific terms actually is preferable to defuse anxiety.

6. Using Professional Jargon. What is called a myocardial infarction in the health profession is called a heart attack by most laypeople. Use of jargon sounds exclusionary and paternalistic. You need to adjust your vocabulary to the person, but avoid sounding condescending.

If a patient uses medical jargon, do not assume he or she always knows the correct meaning. For example, some people think "hypertensive" means that they are very tense. As a result, they take their medication only when feeling stressed and not when they feel relaxed. This misinformation must be corrected. They need to understand that hypertension is a chronic condition that needs consistent medication to avoid side effects. On the other hand, you do not need to feel that it is a moral imperative to correct all misstatements, e.g., when a patient says "prostrate" for prostate gland.

7. Using Leading or Biased Questions. Asking a man, "You don't smoke, do you?" implies that one answer is "better" than another. If the person wants to please you, either he is forced to answer in a way corresponding to your values or he feels guilty when he must admit the other answer. He risks your disapproval. And if he feels dependent on you for care, the last thing he wants to do is alienate you.

8. Talking Too Much. Some examiners positively associate helpfulness with verbal productivity. If the air has been thick with their oratory and advice, these examiners leave thinking they have met the patient's needs. Just the opposite is true. Anxious to please the examiner, the patient lets the professional talk at the expense of his or her need to express himself or herself. A good rule for every interviewer is to *listen more than you talk.*

9. Interrupting. Often, when you think you know what the person will say, you interrupt and cut the person off. This does not show you are clever. Rather, it signals you are impatient or bored with the interview.

A related trap is preoccupation with yourself by thinking of your next remark while the person is talking. The communication pathway looks like this: (Cornell, 1993)

Patient: ———➤   Interviewer ———➤

As the patient speaks, you are thinking about what to say next. Thus you cannot fully understand what the person says. You are so preoccupied with your own role as the interviewer that you are not really listening. Aim for a second of silence between the person's statement and your next response. Ideally, your communication pathway should look like this

◀——➤   ◀——➤

with two people talking, and two people listening (Cornell, 1993).

10. Using "Why" Questions. A young child asks, "Why does the moon look like the end of my fingernail?" The motive behind this question is an innocent search for information. This is quite different from that of an adult's "why" question, such as *Why* were you so late for your appointment?" The adult's use of why questions usually implies blame and condemnation; it puts the person on the defensive (Benjamin, 1980).

Consider your use of "why" questions in the health care setting. "Why did you take so much medication?" Or, let's say you ask a man who has just come to the emergency department, "Why did you wait so long before coming to the hospital?" The only possible answer to a "why" question is "because . . ." and the man may not know the answer. He may not have worked it out. You sound whining, accusatory, and judgmental. And the man now must produce an excuse to rationalize his own behavior. To avoid this trap say, "I see you started to have chest pains early in the day. What was happening between the time the pains started and the time you came to the emergency department?"

Nonverbal Skills

Learn to listen with your eyes as well as with your ears. Nonverbal modes of communication include physical appearance, posture, gestures, facial expression, eye contact, voice, and touch. Nonverbal messages are very important in establishing rapport and in conveying information, especially about feelings. Nonverbal messages provide clues to understanding feelings. When nonverbal and verbal messages are congruent, the verbal is reinforced. When they are incongruent, the nonverbal message tends to be the true one, because it is under less conscious control.

Physical Appearance. In his classic work, *The Stress of Life,* Hans Selye (1956) reports his interest in the body's total response to stress began as a student. Unbiased as yet by medical knowledge, he noted that some patients just "looked sick," even though they did not exhibit the specific characteristic signs that would lead to a precise medical diagnosis. Such people simply felt and looked ill or feverish. The same view can work for you.

Inattention to dressing or grooming suggests the person is too sick to maintain self-care or has an emotional dysfunction such as depression. Choice of clothing also sends a message, projecting such varied images as role (student, worker, or professional) or attitude (casual, suggestive, or rebellious).

Your own appearance sends a message to the patient. Professional dress varies among agencies and settings. Depending on the setting, the use of a professional uniform may create a positive stereotype (comfort, expertise, or ease of identification) or a negative stereotype (distance, authority, or formality). Whatever your personal choice in clothing or grooming, the aim should be to convey a competent, professional image.

Posture. Note the patient's position. An open position with extension of large muscle groups shows relaxation, physical comfort, and a willingness to share information. A closed position with arms and legs crossed looks defensive and anxious. Note any change in posture. If a person in a relaxed position suddenly tenses, it suggests discomfort with the new topic.

Your own calm, relaxed posture creates a feeling of warmth and trust and conveys an interest in the person. Standing and hastily filling out a history form with periodic peeks at your watch communicates you are busy with many more important things than interviewing this person. Even when your time is limited, appear calm and unhurried. Sit down, even if it is only for a few minutes, and look as if nothing else mattered except this person.

Gestures. Gestures send messages. For example, nodding or an open turning out of the hand shows acceptance, attention, or agreement. A wringing of the hands often indicates anxiety. Pointing a finger occurs with anger and vehemence. Also, hand gestures can reinforce a person's description of pain. When a crushing substernal chest pain is described, the person often holds the hand twisted into a fist in front of the sternum. Or, pain that is bright and sharply localized is shown by pointing one finger to the exact spot: "It hurts right here."

Facial Expression. The face reflects a wide variety of relevant emotions and conditions. The expression may look alert, relaxed, and interested or it may look anxious, angry, and suspicious. Physical conditions such as pain or shortness of breath also show in the expression.

Your own expression should reflect a professional who is attentive, sincere, and interested in the patient. Any expression of boredom, distraction, disgust, criticism, or disbelief is picked up by the other person, and rapport will dissolve.

Eye Contact. Lack of eye contact suggests that the person is shy, withdrawn, confused, bored, intimidated, apathetic, or depressed. This applies to examiners, too. You should aim to maintain eye contact, but do not "stare down" the person. Do not have a fixed, penetrating look but rather an easy gaze toward the person's eyes, with occasional glances away. One exception to this is when you are interviewing someone from a culture that avoids direct eye contact (see the section on Transcultural Considerations).

Voice. Beside the spoken words, meaning comes through the tone of voice, the intensity and rate of speech, the pitch, and any pauses. These are just as important as words in conveying meaning. For example, the tone of a person's voice may show sarcasm, disbelief, sympathy, or hostility. An anxious person often speaks in a loud, fast voice. A whining voice is similar; it has a high-pitched wavering quality and long, drawn-out syllables. A soft voice may indicate shyness or fear. A hearing-impaired person may use a loud voice.

Even the use of pauses conveys meaning. When your question is easy and straightforward, a patient's long unexpected pause indicates the person is taking time to think of an answer. This raises some doubt as to the honesty of the answer. Unusually frequent and long pauses, when combined with speech that is slow and monotonous and a weak breathy voice, indicate depression.

Touch. The meaning of physical touch is influenced by the person's age, sex, cultural background, past experience, and current setting. The meaning of touch is easily misinterpreted. In most Western cultures, physical touch is reserved for expressions of love and affection or for rigidly defined acts of greeting (see the section on Transcultural Considerations). Do not use touch during the interview unless you know the person well and are sure how it will be interpreted. When appropriate, touch communicates effectively, such as a touch of the hand or arm to signal empathy.

In sum, an examiner's nonverbal messages that are productive and enhancing to the relationship are those that show attentiveness and unconditional acceptance. Defeating, nonproductive nonverbal behaviors are those of inattentiveness, authority, and superiority (Table 4–2).

Closing the Interview

The session should end gracefully. An abrupt or awkward closing can destroy rapport and leave the person with a negative impression of the whole interview. To ease into the closing, ask the person,

"Is there anything else you would like to mention?"
"Are there any questions you would like to ask?"
"Are there any other areas I should have asked about?"

This gives the person the final opportunity for self-expression. Then, to indicate closing is imminent say, "Our interview is just about over." No new topic should be introduced now. This is a good time to give your summary or a recapitulation of what you have learned during

Table 4–2 • Nonverbal Behaviors of the Interviewer	
Positive	**Negative**
Appropriate professional appearance	Appearance objectionable to patient
Equal-status seating	Standing
Close proximity to patient	Sitting behind desk, far away, turned away
Relaxed open posture	Tense posture
Leaning slightly toward person	Slouched back
Occasional facilitating gestures	Critical or distracting gestures: pointing finger, clenched fist, finger-tapping, foot-swinging, looking at watch
Facial animation, interest	Bland expression, yawning, tight mouth
Appropriate smiling	Frowning, lip biting
Appropriate eye contact	Shifty, avoiding eye contact, focusing on notes
Moderate tone of voice	Strident, high-pitched tone
Moderate rate of speech	Rate too slow or too fast
Appropriate touch	Too frequent or inappropriate touch

the interview. The summary is a final statement of what you and the patient agree the health state to be. It should include positive health aspects, any health problems that have been identified, any plans for action, or an explanation of the following physical examination. As you part from patients, thank them for the time spent and for their cooperation.

 DEVELOPMENTAL CONSIDERATIONS

Interviewing The Parent

When your patient is a child, you must build rapport with two people—the child and the accompanying parent. Greet both by name, but with a younger child (1 to 6 years old), focus more on the parent. By ignoring the child temporarily, the child can size you up from a safe distance. The child can observe your interaction with the parent, see that the parent accepts and likes you, and relax (Fig. 4–2).

Begin by interviewing the parent and child together. If any sensitive topics arise (e.g., the parents' troubled relationship or the child's problems at school or with peers), explore them later when the parent is alone. Provide toys to occupy the child as you and the parent talk. This frees the parent to concentrate on the history. Also, it indicates the child's level of attention span or independent play. Through the interview, be alert to ways the parent and child interact.

For younger children, the parent will provide all or most of the history. Thus you are collecting the child's health data from the parent's frame of reference. Usually,

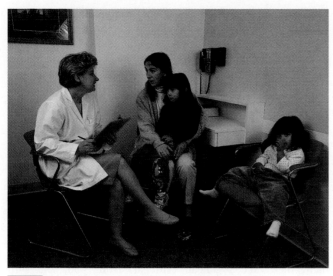

4-2

do?" Stoop down to meet the child at his or her eye level. Adult size can be overwhelming to young children and can emphasize their smallness.

Nonverbal communication is even more important to children than it is to adults. Children are quick to pick up feelings, anxiety, or comfort from nonverbal cues. Keep your physical appearance neat and clean, and avoid formal uniforms that distance you. Keep any gestures slow, deliberate, and close to your body. Children are frightened by quick or grandiose gestures. Do not try to maintain constant eye contact; this feels threatening to a small child. Use a quiet, measured voice, and choose simple words in your speech. Considering the child's level of language development is valuable in planning your communication.

The Infant

Nonverbal communication is the primary method. Most infants look calm and relaxed when all their needs are met, and they cry when they are frightened, hungry, tired, or uncomfortable. They respond best to firm, gentle handling and a quiet, calm voice. Your voice is comforting, even though they do not understand the words. Older infants have anxiety toward strangers. They are more cooperative when the parent is kept in view.

The Preschooler

A 2- to 6-year-old is egocentric. He or she sees the world mostly from his or her own point of view. Everything revolves around him or her. It may not work to cite the example of another child's behavior to get the child to cooperate. It has no meaning. Only the child's own experience is relevant.

Preschoolers' communication is direct, concrete, literal, and set in the present. Avoid expressions such as "climbing the walls," because they are easily misinterpreted by young children. Use short, simple sentences with a concrete explanation. Take time to give a short simple explanation for any unfamiliar equipment that will be used on the child. Preschoolers are *animistic;* they imagine inanimate objects can come alive and have human characteristics, e.g., they think that a blood pressure cuff can wake up and bite or pinch.

The School-Age Child

A child 7 to 12 years old can tolerate and understand others' viewpoints. This child is more objective and realistic. He or she wants to know functional aspects—how things work and why things are done.

Children of this age group have the verbal ability to add important data to the history. Interview the parent and child together, but when a presenting symptom or sign exists ask the child about it first, then gather data from the parent. For the well child seeking a checkup,

this viewpoint is reliable because most parents have the child's well-being as a priority and see cooperation with you as a way to enhance this well-being. But the possibility exists for parental bias. Bias can occur when parents are asked to describe the child's achievements, or whenever their own parenting ability seems called into question. For example, if you ask, "His fever was 103 and you did not bring him in?" you are implying a lack of parenting skill. This puts the parent on the defensive and increases anxiety. Instead, use open-ended questions that increase description and defuse threat, e.g., "What happened when the fever went up?"

A parent with more than one child has more than one set of data to remember. Be patient as the parent sorts through his or her memory to pull out facts of developmental milestones or past history. A comprehensive history may be lacking if the child is accompanied by a family friend or day care provider instead of the parent.

In collecting developmental data, avoid being judgmental about the age of achievement of certain milestones. Parents are understandably proud of their child's achievements and are sensitive to inferences that these milestones may occur late.

Refer to the child by name, not as "the baby." Refer to the parent by name, not the demeaning "Mother" or "Dad." Also, be clear when identifying the parents. The mother's present husband may not necessarily be the child's father. Instead of asking about "your husband's" health ask, "Is Joan's father in good health?"

Although most of your communication is with the parent, do not ignore the child completely. You need to make contact to ease into the physical examination later. Begin by asking about the toys the child is playing with or about a special doll or teddy bear brought from home: "Does your doll have a name?" or "What can your truck pose questions about school, friends, or activities directly to the child.

The Adolescent

Adolescents want to be adults, but they do not have the cognitive ability yet to achieve their goal. They are between two stages. Sometimes they are capable of mature actions, and other times they fall back on childhood response patterns, especially in times of stress. You cannot treat adolescents as children, yet you cannot overcompensate and assume that their communication style, learning ability, and motivation are consistently at an adult level.

Adolescents value their peers. They crave acceptance and sameness with their peers. Adolescents think no adult can understand them. Because of this, some act with aloof contempt, answering only in monosyllables. Others make eye contact and tell you what they think you want to hear, but inside they are thinking "You'll never know the full story about me."

This knowledge about adolescents is apt to paralyze you in communicating with them. However, successful communication is possible and rewarding. The guidelines are simple.

The first consideration is your attitude, which must be one of respect. Respect is the most important thing you can communicate to the adolescent. The adolescent needs to feel validated as a human being, accepted, and worthy.

Second, your communication must be totally honest. The adolescent's intuition is highly tuned and can detect phoniness or when information is withheld. Always give them the truth. Play it straight or you will lose them. They will cooperate if they understand your rationale.

Stay in character. Avoid using language that is absurd for your age or professional role. It is helpful to understand some of the jargon used by adolescents, but you cannot use those words yourself simply to try to bond with the adolescent. Do not try to be his or her peer. You are not, and they will not accept you as such.

Use icebreakers. Focus first on the adolescent, not on the problem. Although an adult just wants to get on with it and talk about the health concern immediately, the adolescent responds best when the focus is on him or her as a person. Show an interest in the adolescent. Ask open, friendly questions about school, activities, hobbies, friends. Refrain from asking questions about parents and family for now—these issues can be emotionally charged during adolescence.

Do not assume adolescents know *anything* about a health interview or a physical examination. Explain every step and give the rationale. They need direction. They will cooperate when they know the reason for the questions or actions. Encourage their questions. Adolescents are afraid they will sound "dumb" if they ask a question to which they assume everybody else knows the answer.

Keep your questions short and simple. "Why are you here?" sounds brazen to you, but it is effective with the adolescent. Be prepared for the adolescent who does *not* know why he or she is there. Some adolescents are pushed into coming to the examination by a parent.

The communication responses described for the adult need to be reconsidered when talking with the adolescent. Silent periods usually are best avoided. Giving adolescents a little time to collect their thoughts is acceptable, but a silence for other reasons is threatening. Also, avoid reflection. If you use reflection, the adolescent is likely to answer, "What?" They just do not have the cognitive skills to respond to that indirect mode of questioning. Also, adolescents are more sensitive to nonverbal communication than are adults. Be aware of your expressions and gestures. They are also more sensitive to any comment they take to mean criticism from you, and will withdraw.

Later in the interview, after you have developed rapport with the adolescent, you can address the topics that are emotionally charged, including alcohol and drug use, sexual behaviors, suicidal thoughts, and depression. Adolescents will assume that health professionals have similar values and standards of behavior as most of the other authority figures in their lives, and they may be reluctant to share this information. You can assure them that your questions are not intended to be curious or intrusive, but cover topics that are important for most teens and on which you have relevant health information to share.

If confidential material is uncovered during the interview, consider what can remain confidential and what you feel you must share for the well-being of the adolescent. State laws vary about confidentiality with minors, and in some states parents are not notified about, for example, birth control prescriptions or treatment for sexually transmitted diseases (STDs). However, if the adolescent talks about an abusive home situation, state that you must share this information with other health professionals for his or her own protection. Ask the adolescent, "Do you have a problem with that?" and then talk it through. Tell the adolescent, "You will have to trust that I will handle this information professionally and in your best interest."

Finally, take every opportunity for positive reinforcement. Praise every action regarding healthy lifestyle choices. "That's great that you don't smoke. You get lots of gold stars in my book for staying off the cigarettes. It's great for your heart, it will save you lots of money you can use on other things, and your skin won't be wrinkled when you get older."

The Older Adult

The aging adult has the developmental task of finding the meaning of life and the purpose of his or her own existence, and adjusting to the inevitability of death. Some people have developed comfortable and satisfying answers and greet you with a calm demeanor and self-assurance. Be alert for the occasional person who sounds hopeless and despairing about life at present and in the future. Symptoms of illness are even more frightening when they mean physical limitation or threaten independence.

Address the person always by the last name, e.g., "Hello, Mr. Choi." "Good morning, Mrs. Smith." Some older adults resent being called by their first name by younger persons, and almost all cringe at the ignominious "Grandma" or "Pop."

The interview usually takes longer with older adults because they have a longer story to tell. You may need to break up the interview into more than one visit, collecting the most important historical data first. Or certain portions of the data, such as past history or the review of systems, can be provided on a form that is filled out at home, as long as the person's vision and handwriting are adequate. Take time to review these parts with the person during the interview.

It is important to adjust the pace of the interview to the aging person. The older person has a great amount of background material to sort through, and this takes some time. Also, some aging persons need a greater amount of response time to interpret the question and process their answer. Avoid trying to hurry them along. This approach only affirms their stereotype of younger persons in general and health care providers in particular, i.e., people who are merely interested in numbers of patients and filling out forms. Any urge from you to get on with it

4–3

will surely make them retreat. You will lose valuable data, and their needs will not be met (Fig. 4–3).

Consider physical limitations when planning the interview. An aging person may fatigue earlier and may require that the interview be broken up into shorter segments. For the person with impaired hearing, face directly so that your mouth and face are fully visible. Do not shout; it does not help and actually distorts speech.

Touch is a nonverbal skill that is very important to older persons. Their other senses may be diminished, and touch grounds you in reality. Also, a hand on the arm or shoulder is an empathic message that communicates you empathize with the person and want to understand his or her problem (see section on Transcultural Considerations for exceptions).

INTERVIEWING PEOPLE WITH SPECIAL NEEDS

Hearing-Impaired People

Although many people will tell you in advance that they have a hearing deficit, others must be recognized by clues such as staring at your mouth and face, not attending unless looking at you, or speaking in a voice unusually loud or with guttural or garbled sounds. The deaf person may be familiar with some equipment in the hospital or office setting, or may have had previous experience with health care settings. But without full communication, the hearing-impaired person is sure to feel isolated and anxious. Ask the deaf person his or her preferred way to communicate—by signing, lip reading, or writing.

A complete health history requires a sign language interpreter. Since most health care professionals are not proficient in signing, try to find an interpreter through a social service agency or the person's own social network. You may use family members, but be aware that they sometimes edit for the person. Use the same guidelines as for the bilingual interpreter (see the section on Transcultural Considerations).

If the person prefers lip reading, be sure to face him or her squarely and have good lighting on your face. Examiners with a beard, moustache, or foreign accents are less effective. Do not exaggerate your lip movements because this distorts your words. Similarly, shouting distorts the reception of a hearing aid the person may wear. Speak slowly and supplement your voice with appropriate hand gestures or pantomime. Nonverbal cues are important adjuncts because the lip reader understands at best only 50 percent of your speech when relying solely on vision. Be sure the person understands your questions. Many hearing-impaired people nod "yes" just to be friendly and cooperative but really do not understand.

Written communication is efficient in sections such as past health history or review of systems. For the present history of illness, writing is very time consuming and laborious. The syntax of the person's written words will read normally if the hearing impairment occurred after speech patterns developed. If the deafness occurred before speech patterns developed, the written syntax follows that of signing, which is different from that of English.

Acutely Ill People

An emergency demands your prompt action. You must combine interviewing with physical examination skills to determine lifesaving actions. Although life support measures may be paramount, still try to interview the person as much as possible. Subjective data are crucial to determine the cause and course of the emergency. Abbreviate your questioning. Identify the main area of distress and question about that. Often family or friends can provide important data.

A hospitalized person with a critical or severe illness usually is too weak, too short of breath, or in too much pain to talk. First attend to the comfort of the person. Then establish a priority; find out immediately what parts of the history are the most relevant. Explore the first concern the person mentions. Begin to use closed, direct questions earlier. Finally, watch that your statements are very clear. When a person is very sick, he or she can misconstrue even the simplest sentence. The person will react according to preconceived ideas about what a serious illness means, so anything you say should be direct and precise.

People Under the Influence of Street Drugs or Alcohol

It is common for persons under the influence of alcohol or other mood-altering drugs to be admitted to a hospital; all of these drugs affect the central nervous system, putting the person at great risk for accidents and injuries. Also, chronic use creates complex medical problems that require increasing care.

Many substance abusers are poly-drug abusers. You may be faced with a wide range of patient behaviors due to current influence. Alcohol and the opioids (heroin, meperidine [Demerol], propoxyphene [Darvon]) are central nervous system depressants. Stimulants of the central nervous system (cocaine, amphetamine) can cause an intense high, agitation, and paranoid behavior. Hallucinogens cause bizarre, inappropriate, sometimes even violent, behavior accompanied by superhuman strength and insensitivity to pain.

When interviewing a person currently under the influence of alcohol or illicit drugs, ask simple and direct questions. Take care to make your manner and questions nonthreatening. Avoid confrontation at this point. Further, avoid any display of scolding or disgust, because this person may become belligerent. One priority is to find

out the time of the person's last drink and how much he or she drank at this episode as well as the name and amount of other drugs taken. This information will help assess any withdrawal patterns. For your own protection, be aware of hospital security or other personnel who could be called on for assistance.

Once he or she is sober, the hospitalized substance abuser should be assessed for the extent of the problem and the meaning of the problem for the person and family. Initially you will encounter denial and increased defensiveness; special interview techniques are needed.

Personal Questions

Occasionally, people will ask you questions about *your* personal life or opinions, such as "Are you married?" "Do you have children?" or "Do you smoke?" You do not need to answer every question. You may supply brief information when you feel it is appropriate, but be sensitive to the possibility that there may be a motive behind the personal questions such as loneliness or anxiety. Try directing your response back to the person's frame of reference. You might say, "No, I don't have children. I wonder if your question is related to how I can help you care for little Jamie?"

Sexually Aggressive People

On some occasions, personal questions extend to flirtatious compliments, seductive innuendo, or advances. Some people experience serious or chronic illness as a threat to their self-esteem and sexual adequacy. This creates anxiety that makes them act out in sexually aggressive ways.

Your response must make it clear that you are a health professional who can best care for the person by maintaining a professional relationship. At the same time, you should communicate that you accept the person and you understand the person's need to be self-assertive but that you cannot tolerate sexual advances. This may be difficult, considering that the person's words or gestures may have left you shocked, embarrassed, or angry. Your feelings are normal. A response that would open communication would be, "Your behavior makes me uncomfortable. I wonder if it relates to your illness or to being in the hospital?"

Crying

A beginning examiner usually feels horrified when the patient starts crying. But crying actually is a big relief to a person. Health problems come with powerful emotions. Worries about illness, death, or loss take a great amount of energy to keep bottled up inside. When you say something that "makes the person cry," do not think you have hurt the person. You have just hit on a topic that is important. Do not go on to a new topic. Just let the person cry and express his or her feelings fully. You can offer a tissue and wait until the crying subsides to talk. The person will regain control soon.

Sometimes your patient looks as if he or she is on the verge of tears but is trying hard to suppress them. Again instead of moving on to something new, acknowledge the expression ("You look sad"). Do not worry that you will open an uncontrollable floodgate. The person may cry but will be relieved, and you will have gained insight to a serious concern.

CLINICAL ILLUSTRATION

Alice P., a 49-year-old white divorced female with chronic alcoholism and skin yellow with jaundice has entered treatment for substance abuse. Today, she needs a pelvic examination and Pap smear.

Patient: I haven't had a pelvic exam in 5 years. I had a hysterectomy 18 years ago. They said I had "pre-invasive" cancer cells. (At this, Alice's lips fold in, her eyes squeeze shut, she puts hand to mouth, and breathes in audibly in jerks.)
Response: Alice, you look sad. (Puts hand on upper arm.)
Patient: (Crying freely now.) What if you find more cancer now? They can't operate on me with my liver so big. I'd never survive the anesthesia. And my father died of cancer. He had cirrhosis too, and they opened him up and he was full of cancer. He never woke up from surgery and he died 2 weeks later.
Response: I understand how worried you are. I think you have done the right thing to come in to treatment. That took courage. As for today, let's take one step at a time. Today we need to do the pelvic exam and Pap smear. There is no reason today to assume you need an operation. I'll do your exam today and I'll be here all week. We'll work together to help you get through this.
Alice: (Breathing deeply, sitting up straight, arms down and open at sides, making eye contact.) All right. I'm better now. Let's go ahead.

Anger

Occasionally you will try to interview a person who is already angry. Try not to personalize this anger; usually it does not relate to you. The person is showing aggression as a response to his or her own feelings of anxiety or helplessness. Do ask about the anger and hear the person out. Deal with the angry feelings before you ask anything else. An angry person cannot be an effective participant in a health interview.

Maybe because of an unrelated incident *you* are angry when you come into the interview. When you are angry, say so and tell the patient that you are angry at something or someone else. Otherwise the patient, unusually vulnerable and dependent on you, thinks you are angry at him or her.

Anxiety

Finally, take it for granted that nearly all sick people have some anxiety. This is a normal response to being sick. It makes some people aggressive and others dependent. Remember that the person is not reacting as typically as when he or she is healthy.

TRANSCULTURAL CONSIDERATIONS

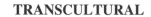

CROSS-CULTURAL COMMUNICATION

When two people come from different cultural backgrounds, the probability of miscommunication increases. Verbal and nonverbal communications are influenced by the cultural background of both the health care professional and the patient. *Cross-cultural* or *intercultural communication* refers to the communication process occurring between a health care professional and a patient, each with different cultural backgrounds, in which both attempt to understand the other's point of view from a cultural perspective.

Cultural Perspectives on Professional Interactions

Your professional interaction depends, to large extent, on the patient's cultural perception of health care providers and the degree of formality/informality that is considered appropriate. For example, some Southeast Asians expect those in authority, such as health care providers, to be authoritarian, directive, and detached. In seeking health care, some Asian Americans may expect the health care provider to intuitively know what is wrong with them, and you may actually lose some credibility by asking a fairly standard interview question such as, "What brings you here?" The Asian person may be thinking, "Don't you know why I'm here? You're supposed to be the one with all the answers."

The emphasis on social harmony among Asians and Native Americans may prevent the full expression of concerns or feelings during the interview. Such reserved behavior may leave you with the impression that the person agrees with or understands your explanation. Nodding or smiling by Asians may only reflect their cultural value for interpersonal harmony, not agreement with you. You may distinguish between socially compliant patient responses aimed at maintaining harmony and genuine concurrence by obtaining validation of your assumptions. You may accomplish this by inviting the person to respond frankly to your suggestions or by giving the person "permission" to disagree.

In contrast, Appalachians traditionally have close family interaction patterns, which often lead them to expect close personal relationships with health care providers. The Appalachian may evaluate your effectiveness on the basis of interpersonal skills rather than professional competencies. Appalachians are likely to be uncomfortable with the impersonal, bureaucratic orientation of most health care institutions. People of Latin American or Mediterranean origins often expect an even higher degree of intimacy and may attempt to involve you in their family system by expecting you to participate in personal activities and social functions. These individuals may come to expect personal favors that extend beyond the scope of your professional practice and may feel it is their privilege to contact you at home during any time of the day or night for care.

Etiquette

Etiquette refers to the conventional code of good manners that governs behavior and varies cross-culturally. Consider the cultural perceptions of some people from Hispanic, Middle Eastern, and African cultures who expect you to engage in conversation of a personal or social nature before they feel comfortable entering into the more personal and intimate aspects of the health history and physical examination. For these people, there is a high value placed on developing interpersonal relationships and getting to know about a person's family, personal concerns, and interests before they allow you to interact therapeutically. Recognizing that time constraints frequently affect the social interchange expected by individuals from some cultures, you should strive to incorporate the person's cultural needs with the health history data categories. For example, using a conversational tone of voice, you might begin the health history by inquiring about the patient's family members and their health.

You should be prepared for the converse, i.e., individuals from some cultures may want to interview *you*. They may ask questions about your family, marital status, salary, home address, telephone number, and so forth. Your own cultural beliefs will determine your level of comfort in responding to these questions. Remember that you aren't obligated to answer questions that you deem too personal and always have a right to protect your personal safety. For example, you are discouraged from providing your home telephone number. Rather, you should provide the patient with the hospital, clinic, or agency's business number. If you want the patient to be able to contact you while you're at home, you should ask a secretary or other third party at the heath care facility to call your home number. You may want to consider in advance which categories of questions you are willing to discuss and which ones you will politely avoid. If you refuse to answer certain questions about yourself, remember that the person may perceive your behavior as aloof and uncaring. Thus, the manner in which you reply to personal inquiries should be carefully worded, sensitive to the cultural needs of the patient, and congruent with your own cultural beliefs.

When meeting a patient for the first time, it is best to be formal, respectful, and polite. Unless a physical disability or handicap prevents you from doing so, you should be standing when you first greet the person and those accompanying him or her. Another aspect of etiquette concerns the use of *names* and *titles.* In order to ensure that a mutually respectful relationship is established, you should introduce yourself and indicate to the person how you prefer to be called, i.e., by first name, last name, and/or title. You should elicit the same information from the patient because this enables you to address the person in a manner that is culturally appropriate and could actually spare you considerable embarrassment. Everyone likes to be called by his or her correct name. You must be certain that you know your patients' names, pronounce them correctly, and follow cultural conventions concerning the use of titles. Avoid being unduly casual or familiar. For example, refrain from routinely using the person's first name before you have been invited to do so. The same guidelines should be followed when addressing the family members and other visitors.

Among Chinese, Vietnamese, and many other Asian groups, the family or surname is written and spoken first, followed by the first or given name. You will notice that this is exactly the opposite of most European-American cultures. Because politeness and formality frequently are valued by those from Asian cultures, you should address the person using the correct title (Mr., Mrs., Ms., Miss, Dr., and so forth) followed by the family or surname. Be aware that some Asians, particularly those who are members of Christian religions, also may have English names. Most Asian women do not use their husband's last name after marriage. You should be especially mindful of this when examining children in the presence of both parents. It is likely that you will need to refer to the husband and wife by different last names, e.g., Mr. Cai and Mrs. Li. In most Asian cultures, the child is given the father's last name. Depending on the degree of acculturation, some Asian Americans switch the order of their names in order to be consistent with the European-American custom. If you are in doubt, be sure to ask the patient or a significant other if the patient is unable to respond.

In traditional Chinese, Japanese, and other Asian cultures, when introduced to another, respect is shown by bowing. The more profound the bow, the deeper the respect. For example, it would be appropriate to bow very low to an older adult whose wisdom is highly regarded and less profoundly to an adolescent or a young adult. With Westernization, handshakes are now customary throughout most parts of Asia and among Asian Americans, but shaking someone's hand too firmly or vigorously is considered rude or intrusive. Most people of Asian descent will expect you to behave in a manner congruent with your cultural heritage. In other words, it is not necessary to bow when greeting Asian Americans but to greet them as you would other patients.

Because of the importance of family for people from Central and South America, two surnames are used, representing their father's and mother's last names. The paternal name is first, then the maternal name. For example, if the patient's name is Juan Diaz Hernandez, his father's last name is Diaz and his mother's last name is Hernandez. With immigration to the United States or Canada, some people with Spanish surnames drop their mother's name for the sake of brevity. Consider the number of spaces allowed for a person's name on a typical hospital admissions form, and it becomes evident why the name might be shortened. This is unfortunate because people lose part of their name, an important expression of their cultural identity.

Although there are dozens of Arab cultures and subcultures, customs pertaining to names are similar. Both males and females are given a first name as infants. The father's first name is used as the middle name and the last name is the family name. Some may prefer to be addressed as father (*abu*) or mother (*um*) of their oldest son, e.g., abu Walid or father of Walid. Because formality is emphasized in most Arab cultures, you should call patients Mr., Mrs., Ms., Miss, or Dr. followed by their last name unless invited to use more familiar first names or the abu/um form of the name. In most Arab cultures, etiquette requires either a gentle kiss on the cheeks or a handshake on arrival and departure for people of the same gender. When an Arab man is introduced to a woman, he usually waits for the woman to extend her hand first. This is done out of respect for the traditional beliefs about modesty in male-female relationships held by some Muslim women. When a handshake is not exchanged, the Muslim woman usually faces the man while bowing her head slightly and crossing her arms across her chest. In lieu of a handshake, this is a widely accepted, culturally appropriate gesture that is used when men and women are introduced in some Arab cultures.

With more than 550 federal and/or state-recognized Native American tribes, there is wide variation in the customs pertaining to names, titles, and etiquette. The majority tend to follow the dominant European-American cultural norms. In the Navajo culture, a health care provider may call an older adult grandfather or grandmother

as a sign of respect after getting to know him or her, but should be more formal during the initial introduction. Some Native American and Alaska natives have anglicized traditional names into surnames such as Running Deer, Flying Eagle, or Swift Bear, often reflecting the clan to which the person belongs. You should extend a gentle, nonaggressive handshake when introduced to a Native American patient.

Space and Distance

Both the patient's and your own sense of spatial distance are significant throughout the interview and physical examination, with culturally appropriate distance zones varying widely. For example, you may find yourself backing away from people of Hispanic, East Indian, or Middle Eastern origins who invade your personal space with regularity in an attempt to bring you closer into the space that is comfortable to them. Although you are uncomfortable with their close physical proximity, they are perplexed by your distancing behaviors and may perceive you as aloof and unfriendly. Summarized in Table 4–3 are the four distance zones identified for the functional use of space that are embraced by the dominant cultural group, including that of most health care professionals.

Table 4–3 · Functional Use of Space

Zone	Remarks
Intimate zone (0 to 1½ ft)	Visual distortion occurs
	Best for assessing breath and other body odors
Personal distance (1½ to 4 ft)	Perceived as an extension of the self similar to a bubble
	Voice is moderate
	Body odors inapparent
	No visual distortion
	Much of the physical assessment occurs at this distance
Social distance (4 to 12 ft)	Used for impersonal business transactions
	Perceptual information much less detailed
	Much of the interview occurs at this distance
Public distance (12+ ft)	Interaction with others impersonal
	Speaker's voice must be projected
	Subtle facial expressions imperceptible

From Hall E: Proxemics: The study of man's spatial relations. *In* Galdston I (Ed): Man's Image in Medicine and Anthropology. New York, International University Press, 1963, pp 109–120.

Cultural Considerations on Gender and Sexual Orientation

Violating cultural norms related to appropriate male-female relationships may jeopardize your professional relationship. Among Arab Americans, you may find that an adult male is never alone with a female (except his wife) and is generally accompanied by one or more other males when interacting with females. This behavior is culturally very significant, and failure to adhere to the *cultural code* (set of rules or norms of behavior used by a cultural group to guide their behavior and interpret situations) is viewed as a serious transgression, often one in which the lone male will be accused of sexual impropriety. The best way to ensure that cultural variables have been considered is to ask the person about culturally relevant aspects of male-female relationships, preferably at the beginning of the interview—before you have an opportunity to violate any culturally based practices. When you have determined that gender differences are important to the patient, you might try strategies such as offering to have a third person present when this is feasible. If a family member or friend has accompanied the patient, you might inquire whether the patient would like that person to be in the examination room during the history and/or physical examination.

The gender issue is further complicated by cultural beliefs about relationships with authority figures and cross-national perspectives on the status of various health care disciplines. For example, in many less developed nations, nursing is a low-status occupation. In some oil-rich Arab countries (e.g., Saudi Arabia, Kuwait), care for the sick is carried out by health care providers who are hired from abroad for the purpose of caring for the bodily needs of the sick, an activity that is considered undignified.

In approaching lesbian, gay, or bisexual individuals, you should be aware of heterosexist biases and the communication of these biases during the interview and physical examination. *Heterosexism* refers to the institutionalized belief that heterosexuality is the only natural choice and assumes it is the norm. For example, most health histories include a question concerning marital status. Although many same-sex couples are in committed, long-term monogamous relationships, seldom is there a category on the standard form that acknowledges this type of relationship. Although technically and legally the person may be single, this trivializes the relationship with his or her significant other. It also may have health-related implications if the person is diagnosed, for example, with a communicable disease, which may range in severity from a minor sore throat to a life-threatening condition such as HIV/AIDS. In extreme cases, lesbians have been subjected to unnecessary diagnostic procedures when the heterosexual assumption was made (Eliason, 1993).

OVERCOMING COMMUNICATION BARRIERS

Health care providers tend to have stereotypical expectations of the patient's behavior during the interview and physical examination. In general, we expect behavior to consist of undemanding compliance, an attitude of respect for the health care provider, and cooperation with requested behavior throughout the examination. Although patients may ask a few questions for the purpose of clarification, slight deference to recognized authority figures, i.e., health care providers, is expected. Individuals from culturally diverse backgrounds, however, may have significantly different perceptions about the appropriate role of the individual and his or her family when seeking health care. If you find yourself becoming annoyed that a patient is asking too many questions, assuming a defensive posture, or otherwise feeling uncomfortable, you might pause for a moment to examine the source of the conflict from a cross-cultural perspective.

During illness, culturally acceptable sick role behavior may range from aggressive, demanding behavior to silent passivity. According to Zatrick and Dimsdale (1990), complaining, demanding behavior during illness is often rewarded with attention among American Jewish and Italian groups, whereas Asians and Native Americans are likely to be quiet and compliant during illness. During the interview, Asians may provide you with the answers they think you want to hear, behavior consistent with the dominant cultural value for harmonious relationships with others. Thus, you should attempt to phrase questions or statements in a neutral manner that avoids foreshadowing an expected response. Appalachian people may reject an interviewer whom they perceive as prying or nosey owing to a cultural ethic of neutrality that mandates minding one's own business and avoiding assertive or argumentative behavior.

Working With (and Without) an Interpreter

Nearly 32 million people in the United States speak a language other than English at home (U.S. Bureau of the Census, 1990). Many also can read and write other languages. One of the greatest challenges in cross-cultural communication occurs when you and the patient speak different languages. After assessing the language skills of non–English-speaking people, you may find yourself in one of two situations: trying to communicate effectively through an interpreter or trying to communicate effectively when there is no interpreter.

Interviewing the non–English-speaking person requires a bilingual interpreter for full communication. Even the person from another culture or country who has a basic command of English (those for whom English is a second language) may need an interpreter when faced with the anxiety-provoking situation of entering a hospital, describing a strange symptom, or discussing sensitive topics such as those related to reproductive or urologic concerns.

It is tempting to ask a relative, friend, or even another patient to interpret because this person is readily available and probably would like to help. This is disadvantageous because it violates confidentiality for the patient, who may not want personal information shared with another. Furthermore, the friend or relative, although fluent in ordinary language usage, is likely to be unfamiliar with medical terminology, hospital or clinic procedures, and medical ethics.

Whenever possible, work with a bilingual team member or a trained medical interpreter. This person knows interpreting techniques, has a health care background, and understands patients' rights. The trained interpreter also is knowledgeable about cultural beliefs and health practices. This person can help you bridge the cultural gap and can advise you concerning the cultural appropriateness of your recommendations.

Although interpreters are trained to remain neutral, they can influence both the content of information exchanged and the nature of the interaction. Many trained medical interpreters are members of the linguistic community they serve. While this is largely beneficial, it has limitations. For example, interpreters often know patients and details of their circumstances before the interview begins. Although acceptance of a code of ethics governing confidentiality and conflicts of interest is part of the training interpreters receive, discord may arise when they relate information that the patient has not volunteered to the examiner.

It should be noted that being bilingual doesn't always mean the interpreter is culturally aware. The Hispanic or Latino cultures, for example, are so diverse that a Spanish-speaking interpreter from one country, class, race, and gender doesn't necessarily understand the cultural background of a Spanish-speaking person from another country and different circumstances. Even trained interpreters, who are often from urban areas and represent a higher socioeconomic class than the patients for whom they interpret, may be unaware of or embarrassed by rural attitudes and practices.

Although you will be in charge of the focus and flow of the interview, view yourself and the interpreter as a team. Ask the interpreter to meet the patient beforehand to establish rapport and to garner the patient's age, occupation, educational level, and attitude toward health care. This enables the interpreter to communicate on the patient's level.

Allow more time for this interview. With the third person repeating everything, it can take considerably longer than interviewing English-speaking people. You need to focus on priority data.

There are two styles of interpreting—line-by-line and summarizing. Translating line-by-line takes more time, but it ensures accuracy. Use this style for most of the interview. Both you and the patient should speak only a sentence or two, then allow the interpreter time. Use simple language yourself, not medical jargon that the interpreter must simplify before it can be translated. Summary translation progresses faster and is useful for teaching relatively simple health techniques with which the interpreter is already familiar. Be alert for nonverbal cues as the patient talks. These cues can give valuable data. A good interpreter also notes nonverbal messages and passes them on to you. Summarized in Table 4–4 are suggestions for the selection and use of an interpreter.

Although use of an interpreter is the ideal, you may find yourself in a situation with a non–English-speaking patient when no interpreter is available. Table 4–5 summarizes some suggestions for overcoming language barriers when no interpreter is present. Communicating with these patients may require that you combine verbal and nonverbal forms of communication.

Nonverbal Cross-Cultural Communication

Basically, there are five types of nonverbal behaviors that convey information about the person: 1) *vocal cues,* such as pitch, tone, and quality of voice, including moaning, crying, and groaning; 2) *action cues,* such as posture, facial expression, and gestures; 3) *object cues,* such as clothes, jewelry, and hair styles; 4) *use of personal and territorial space* in interpersonal transactions and care of belongings; and 5) *touch,* which involves the use of personal space and action (Lapierre and Padgett, 1991).

Unless you make an effort to understand the patient's nonverbal behavior, you may overlook important information such as that conveyed by facial expressions, silence, eye contact, touch, and other body language. Communication patterns vary widely transculturally even for such conventional social behaviors as smiling and handshaking. Among many Hispanic people, for example, smiling and handshaking are considered an integral part of sincere interactions and essential to establishing trust, whereas a Russian person might perceive the same behavior as insolent and frivolous.

Wide cultural variation exists when interpreting **silence.** Some individuals find silence extremely uncomfortable and make every effort to fill conversational lags with words. Conversely, many Native Americans consider silence essential to understanding and respecting the other person. A pause following your question signifies that what has been asked is important enough to be given thoughtful consideration. In traditional Chinese and Japanese cultures, silence may mean that the speaker wishes

Table 4–4 • Use of an Interpreter

Choosing an Interpreter
- Before locating an interpreter, identify the language the person speaks at home. Be aware that it may differ from the language spoken publicly (e.g., French is sometimes spoken by well-educated and upper-class members of certain Asian, African, or Middle Eastern cultures but it is not the language spoken in the home).
- Whenever possible, use a *trained* interpreter, preferably one who knows medical terminology.
- Avoid interpreters from a rival tribe, state, region, or nation (e.g., a Palestinian who knows Hebrew may not be the best interpreter for a Jewish person).
- Be aware of gender differences between interpreter and patient. In general, the same gender is preferred.
- Be aware of age differences between interpreter and patient. In general, an older, more mature interpreter is preferred to a younger, less experienced one.
- Be aware of socioeconomic differences between interpreter and patient.

Strategies for Effective Use of an Interpreter
- Plan what you want to say ahead of time. Meet privately with interpreter before the interview. Avoid confusing the interpreter by backing up, hesitating, or inserting a proviso.
- Ask the interpreter to provide a line-by-line verbatim account of the conversation. Ask for a detailed interpretation when provided with brief summaries of longer exchanges between interpreter and patient.
- Be patient. When using an interpreter, interviews often take two to three times longer.
- Longer-than-expected explanatory exchanges are often required to convey the meaning of words such as *stress, depression, allergy, preventive medicine,* and *physical therapy* because there may not be comparable terms in the language the patient understands.
- When discussing diagnostic tests such as mammograms, MRIs (magnetic resonance imaging), CT (computed tomography) scans, or those involving body fluids such as blood, urine, stool, spinal fluid, or saliva, be sure to clarify the nature of the test to the interpreter. Indicate the purpose of the test, exactly what will happen to the patient, approximately how long the test will take, whether the procedure is invasive or noninvasive, and what part(s) of the body will be tested.
- Be aware that the interpreter may modify or edit some aspects of the conversation, especially if he or she thinks you might not understand the cultural context of the patient's response (e.g., traditional or folk beliefs and practices related to healing).
- Avoid ambiguous statements and questions. Refrain from using conditional or indefinite phrasing such as "if," "would," and "could," especially for target languages, such as Khmer (Cambodia), that lack nuances of conditionality or distinctions of time other than simple past and present. Conditional statements may be mistaken for actual agreement or approval of a course of action.
- Avoid abstract expressions, idioms, similes, metaphors, and medical jargon.
- To ensure confidentiality and privacy, avoid using as interpreters children or strangers who may be visiting other patients.
- Be aware that an interpreter who is a nonrelative may seek compensation for services rendered. Be sure to negotiate fees ahead of time.

Recommendations for Institutions
- Maintain a current, computerized list of interpreters who may be contacted as needed.
- Network with area hospitals, colleges, universities, and other organizations that may serve as resources.
- Utilize over-the-telephone interpretation services provided by telephone companies. For example, since 1989 AT&T has operated the Language Line Services, which provides interpretation in more than 140 languages. Services are available around the clock every day of the year. Call (800) 628-8486 for further information on services and charges.

the listener to consider the content of what has been said before continuing. The English and Arabs may use silence out of respect for another's privacy, whereas the French, Spanish, and Russians may interpret it as a sign of agreement. Asian cultures often use silence to demonstrate respect for elders. Among some black communities, silence is used in response to what they perceive as a ridiculous question.

Eye contact is perhaps among the most culturally variable nonverbal behaviors. Although you probably have been taught to maintain eye contact when speaking with others, individuals from culturally diverse backgrounds may attribute other culturally based meanings to this behavior. Asian, Native American, Indochinese, Arab, and Appalachian people may consider direct eye contact impolite or aggressive, and they may avert their eyes when talking with you. Native Americans often stare at the floor during conversations, a culturally appropriate behavior indicating that the listener is paying close attention to the speaker. Some blacks may use *oculistics* (eye-rolling)

in response to what is perceived to be a ridiculous question. Among Hispanics, respect dictates appropriate deferential behavior in the form of downcast eyes toward others on the basis of age, sex, social position, economic status, and position of authority. Elders expect respect from younger individuals, adults from children, men from women, teachers from students, and employers from employees. By virtue of your authority status as a health care provider, with Hispanic people, your eye contact is expected but will not necessarily be reciprocated by the person.

In some cultures, including Arab, Hispanic, and black groups, *modesty for both women and men* is interrelated with eye contact. For Muslim-Arab women, modesty is, in part, achieved by avoiding eye contact with males (except for one's husband in private settings) and keeping the eyes downcast when encountering members of the opposite sex in public situations. In many cultures, the only woman who smiles and establishes eye contact with men in public is likely to be a prostitute. Hasidic Jewish

Table 4–5 • Overcoming Language Barriers: What to Do When No Interpreter is Available

1. Be polite and formal.
2. Pronounce name correctly. Use proper titles of respect, such as "Mr.," "Mrs.," "Ms.," "Dr." Greet the person using the last or complete name.
   Gesture to yourself and say your name.
   Offer a handshake or nod. Smile.
3. Proceed in an unhurried manner. Pay attention to any effort by the patient or family to communicate.
4. Speak in a low, moderate voice. Avoid talking loudly. Remember that there is a tendency to raise the volume and pitch of your voice when the listener appears not to understand. The listener may perceive that you are shouting and/or angry.
5. Use any words that you might know in the person's language. This indicates that you are aware of and respect his or her culture.
6. Use simple words, such as "pain" instead of "discomfort." Avoid medical jargon, idioms, and slang. Avoid using contractions, e.g., don't, can't, and won't. Use nouns repeatedly instead of pronouns.
   Example:
   Do not say: "He has been taking his medicine, hasn't he?"
   Do say:　"Does Juan take medicine?"
7. Pantomime words and simple actions while you verbalize them.
8. Give instructions in the proper sequence.
   Example:
   Do not say: "Before you rinse the bottle, sterilize it."
   Do say:　"First wash the bottle. Second, rinse the bottle."
9. Discuss one topic at a time. Avoid using conjunctions.
   Example:
   Do not say: "Are you cold and in pain?"
   Do say:　"Are you cold (while pantomiming)? Are you in pain?"
10. Validate if the person understands by having him or her repeat instructions, demonstrate the procedure, or act out the meaning.
11. Write out several short sentences in English and determine the person's ability to read them.
12. Try a third language. Many Indochinese speak French. Europeans often know two or more languages. Try Latin words or phrases.
13. Ask who among the person's family and friends could serve as an interpreter.
14. Obtain phrase books from a library or bookstore, make or purchase flash cards, contact hospitals for a list of interpreters, and use both a formal and an informal network to locate a suitable interpreter.

males also have culturally based norms concerning eye contact with females. You may observe the male avoiding direct eye contact and turning his head in the opposite direction when walking past or speaking to a woman. The preceding examples are intended to be illustrative, not exhaustive.

Touch

Without doubt, touching the patient is a necessary component of a comprehensive assessment. From a cultural perspective, however, you are urged to give careful consideration to issues concerning **touch.** While recognizing the benefits reported by many in establishing rapport with patients through touch, physical contact with patients conveys various meanings cross-culturally. In many cultures, such as Arab and Hispanic societies, male health care providers may be prohibited from touching or examining either all or certain parts of the female body. In many cultures, adolescent girls may prefer female health care providers or refuse to be examined by a male. You should be aware that the patient's significant others also may exert pressure on nurses by enforcing these culturally meaningful norms in the health care setting.

Touching children also may have associated meaning transculturally. For example, approximately 80 percent of the world's people believe in *mal ojo,* which literally translated means "evil of the eye." In this culture-bound syndrome, a child's illness may be attributed to excessive admiration by another person. Mal ojo is especially prevalent in Hispanic cultures. Many Asians believe that one's strength resides in the head and that touching the head is a sign of disrespect. The clinical significance of this is that you need to be aware that patting a child on the head or examining the fontanel of a Southeast Asian infant, for example, should be avoided or done only with parental permission. Whenever possible, you should explore alternative ways to express affection or to obtain information necessary for assessment of the patient's condition (e.g., hold the child on the lap, observe for other manifestations of increased intracranial pressure or signs of premature fontanel closure, or place one's hand over the mother's while asking for a description of what she feels).

In concluding this section, note this brief comment about same-sex relationships. In some cultures, it is considered an acceptable expression of friendship and affection to openly and publicly hold hands with or embrace members of the same sex without any sexual connotation being associated with the behavior. For example, you may notice that although a Nigerian American woman may not demonstrate overt affection for her husband or other male family members, she will hold hands with female relatives and friends while walking or talking with them. You may find that a patient displays similar behaviors and should feel free to discuss cultural differences and similarities openly with the person. The discussion should include how each person feels about the cultural practice and exploration of mutually acceptable—and unacceptable—avenues for communicating.

Bibliography

Arnold E, Boggs K: Interpersonal Relationships—Professional Communication Skills for Nurses, 2nd ed. Philadelphia, W.B. Saunders Company, 1995.
Andrews MM, Boyle JC: Transcultural Concepts in Nursing Care, 3rd ed. Philadelphia, Lippincott-Raven, 1998.
Benjamin A: The Helping Interview, 3rd ed. Boston, Houghton Mifflin, 1980.
Bernstein L, Bernstein RS: Interviewing—A Guide for Health Professionals, 4th ed. E. Norwalk, CT, Appleton & Lange, 1985.

Bradley JC, Edinberg MA: Communication in the Nursing Context, 3rd ed. E. Norwalk, CT, Appleton & Lange, 1990.

Cohen E, Mackenzie RG, Yates GL: HEADSS, a psychosocial risk assessment instrument: Implications for designing effective intervention programs for runaway youth. J Adolescent Health 12(7): 539–544, Nov 1991.

Cormier LS, et al: Interviewing & Helping Skills for Health Professionals, 2nd ed. Boston, MA, Jones & Bartlett, 1995.

Cornell D: Saying the words: Communication techniques. Nurs Management 24(3):42–44, 1993.

Earley T: The quare gene: What will happen to the secret language of the Appalachians? The New Yorker 73:80–85, Sep 21, 1998.

Edwards A, Tzelepis A, Klingbeil C, Melgar T, Speece M, Schubiner H, Burack R: Fifteen years of a videotape review program for internal medicine and medicine-pediatrics residents. Acad Med 71(7):744–748, July 1996.

Eliason MJ: Cultural diversity in nursing care: The lesbian, gay or bisexual client. J Transcul Nurs 5(1):14–20, 1993.

Enlow AJ, Forde DL, Brummel-Smith K: Interviewing and Patient Care, 4th ed. New York, Oxford University Press, 1996.

Forchuk C: Development of nurse-client relationships: What helps? J Am Psych Nurses Assoc 1(5):146–153, Oct 1995.

Lapierre ED, Padgett J: How can we become more aware of culturally specific body language and use this awareness therapeutically? J Psychosoc Nurs 29(11):38–41, 1991.

Lipkin M: Patient education and counseling in the context of modern patient-family communication. Patient Educ Counsel 27:5–11, 1996.

Lipkin M, Putnam S, Lazare A: The Medical Interview: Clinical Care, Education and Research. New York, Springer-Verlag, 1995.

Purtilo R: Health Professional and Patient Interaction, 5th ed. Philadelphia, W.B. Saunders Company, 1996.

Quirk M, Casey L: Primary care for women: The art of interviewing. J Nurse Midwifery 40(2):104–119, Mar–Apr 1995.

Roberts BL, Srour MI, Winkelman C: Videotaping: An important research strategy. Nurs Res 45(6):334–338, Nov/Dec 1996.

Rogers CR: Client-Centered Therapy, Boston, Houghton Mifflin, 1951.

Roye CF: Breaking through to the adolescent patient. Am J Nurs 95(12):19–23, Dec 1995.

Selye H: The Stress of Life. New York, McGraw-Hill, 1956.

Sharp PC, Pearce KA, Konen JC, Knudson MP: Using standardized patient instructors to teach health promotion interviewing skills. Fam Med 28(2):103–106, Feb 1996.

Suchman AL, Markakis K, Beckman HB, Frankel R: A model of empathic communication in the medical interview. JAMA 277(8):678–682, Feb 1997.

U.S. Bureau of the Census. 1990 Census of Population and Housing Data, Paper Listing (CPH.L. 133), and Summary Tape file 3C. Washington, DC: U.S. Government Printing Office.

Vannatta JB, Smith KR, Crandall S, Fischer PC, Williams K: Comparison of standardized patients and faculty in teaching medical interviewing. Acad Med 71(12):1360–1362, Dec 1996.

Zatrick DF, Dimsdale JE: Cultural variations in response to painful stimuli. Psychosom Med 52:544–557, 1990.

CHAPTER FIVE

The Complete Health History

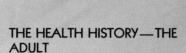

The purpose of the health history is to collect **subjective data,** what the person **says** about himself or herself. The history is combined with the **objective data** from the physical examination and laboratory studies to form the data base. The data base is used to make a judgment or a diagnosis about the health status of the individual.

The following health history provides a complete picture of the person's past and present health. It describes the individual as a whole and how the person interacts with the environment. It records health strengths and coping skills. The history should recognize and affirm what the person is doing right; what he or she is doing to help stay well. For the well person, the history is used to assess his or her lifestyle, including such factors as exercise, diet, risk reduction, and health promotion behaviors. For the ill person, it includes a detailed and chronologic record of the health problem. For all, the health history is a screening tool for abnormal symptoms, health problems, and concerns, and it records ways of responding to the health problems.

In many settings, the patient fills out a printed history form or checklist. This allows the person ample time to recall and consider such items as dates of health landmarks and relevant family history. The interview is then used to validate the written data and to collect more data on lifestyle management and current health problems.

Although history forms vary, most contain information in this sequence of categories:

1. Biographical data
2. Reason for seeking care
3. Present health or history of present illness
4. Past history
5. Family history
6. Review of systems
7. Functional assessment or activities of daily living (ADLs)

The health history discussed in the following section follows this format and presents a generic data base for all practitioners. Those in primary care settings may use all of it, whereas those in a hospital may focus primarily on the history of present illness and the functional, or patterns of living, data.

THE HEALTH HISTORY—THE ADULT

Biographical Data

Name, address and phone number, age and birthdate, birthplace, sex, marital status, race, ethnic origin, occupation, usual and present (an illness or disability may have prompted change in occupation).

Source of History

1. Record who furnishes the information—usually the person herself or himself—although the source may be a relative or friend.
2. Judge how reliable the informant seems and how willing he or she is to communicate. A reliable person always gives the same answers, even when questions are rephrased or are repeated later in the interview.
3. Note any special circumstances, such as the use of an interpreter. Sample statements include:

Patient herself, who seems reliable.
Patient's son, John Ramirez, who seems reliable.
Mrs. R. Fuentes, interpreter for Theresa Castillo who does not speak English.

Reason for Seeking Care*

This is a brief spontaneous statement in the person's own words that describes the reason for the visit. Think of it as the "title" for the story to follow. It states one (possibly two) symptoms or signs and their duration. A **symptom** is a subjective sensation that the person feels from the disorder. A **sign** is an objective abnormality that you as the examiner could detect on physical examination or in laboratory reports. Whatever the person says is the reason for seeking care is recorded, enclosed in quotation marks to indicate the person's exact words.

"Chest pain" for 2 hours.
"Earache and fussy all night."
"Need yearly physical for work."
"Want to start jogging and need checkup."

The reason for seeking care is not a diagnostic statement. Avoid translating it into the terms of a medical diagnosis. For example, Mr. J. Schmidt enters with shortness of breath, and you ponder writing "emphysema." Even if he is known to have emphysema from previous visits, it is not the chronic emphysema that prompted *this visit,* but rather the "increasing shortness of breath" for 4 hours.

Some people try to self-diagnose based on similar signs and symptoms in their relatives or friends, or based on conditions they know they have. Rather than record a woman's statement that she has "strep throat," ask her what symptoms she has that make her think this is true and record those symptoms.

Occasionally, a person may list *many* reasons for seeking care. The most important reason to the person may not necessarily be the one stated first. Try to focus on which is the most pressing concern by asking the person which one prompted him or her to seek help *now.*

Present Health or History of Present Illness

For the well person, this is a short statement about the general state of health.

For the ill person, this section is a chronologic record of the reason for seeking care, from the time the symptom first started until now. Isolate each reason for care identified by the person and say, for example, "Please tell me all about your headache, from the time it started, until the time you came to the hospital." If the concern started months or years ago, record what occurred during that time and find out why the person is seeking care *now.*

As the person talks, do not jump to conclusions and bias the story by adding your opinion. Collect *all* the data first. Although you want the person to respond in a narrative format without interruption from you, your final summary of any symptom the person has should include these *eight critical characteristics:*

1. **Location.** Be specific; ask the person to point to the location. If the problem is pain, note the precise site. "Head pain" is vague, whereas descriptions like "pain behind the eyes," "jaw pain," and "occipital pain" are more precise and are diagnostically significant. Is the pain localized to this site or radiating? Is the pain superficial or deep?
2. **Character** or **Quality.** This calls for specific descriptive terms such as burning, sharp, dull, aching, gnawing, throbbing, shooting, viselike. Use similes—Does blood in the stool look like sticky tar? Does blood in vomitus look like coffee grounds?
3. **Quantity** or **Severity.** Attempt to quantify the sign or symptom such as "profuse menstrual flow soaking five pads per hour." The symptom of pain is difficult to quantify because of individual interpretation. What one person may identify as

---

*In the past, this statement was called the "Chief Complaint" [CC]. This title is avoided now because it labels the person a "complainer," and more importantly, does not include wellness needs.

"terrible pain," another may describe as "not too bad." With pain, avoid adjectives and ask how it affects daily activities. Then the person might say, "I was so sick I was doubled up and couldn't move," or "I was able to go to work, but then I came home and went to bed."

4. **Timing** (Onset, Duration, Frequency). When did the symptom first appear? Give the specific date and time, or state specifically how long ago the symptom started prior to arrival (PTA). "The pain started yesterday" will not mean much when you return to read the record in the future. The report must include questions such as: How long did the symptom last (duration)? Was it steady (constant) or did it come and go during that time (intermittent)? Did it resolve completely and reappear days or weeks later (cycle of remission and exacerbation)?

5. **Setting.** Where was the person or what was the person doing when the symptom started? What brings it on? For example, "Did you notice the chest pain after shoveling snow, or did the pain start by itself?"

6. **Aggravating** or **Relieving Factors.** What makes the pain worse? Is it aggravated by weather, activity, food, medication, standing bent over, fatigue, time of day, season, and so on? What relieves it, e.g., rest, medication, or ice pack? What is the effect of any treatment? Ask, "What have you tried?" or, "What seems to help?"

7. **Associated Factors.** Is this primary symptom associated with any others, e.g., urinary frequency and burning associated with fever and chills? Review the body system related to this symptom now rather than wait for the review of systems.

8. **Patient's Perception.** Find out the meaning of the symptom by asking how it affects daily activities. Also ask directly, "What do you think it means?" This is crucial because it alerts you to potential anxiety if the person thinks the symptom may be ominous.

You may find it helpful to organize this same question sequence into the mnemonic **PQRST** to help remember all the points. Note that you still need to address the patient's perception of the problem.

P: Provocative or Palliative. What brings it on? What were you doing when you first noticed it? What makes it better? Worse?

Q: Quality or Quantity. How does it look, feel, sound? How intense/severe is it?

R: Region or Radiation. Where is it? Does it spread anywhere?

S: Severity Scale. How bad is it (on a scale of 1 to 10)? Is it getting better, worse, staying the same?

T: Timing. Onset—Exactly when did it first occur? Duration—How long did it last? Frequency—How often does it occur?

U: Understand Patient's Perception of the problem. What do you think it means?

Past Health

Past health events may have residual effects on the current health state. Also, the previous experience with illness may give clues as to how the person responds to illness and to the significance of illness for him or her.

Childhood Illnesses. Measles, mumps, rubella, chicken pox, pertussis, and strep throat. Avoid recording "usual childhood illnesses," because an illness common in the person's childhood may be unusual today, e.g., measles. Ask about serious illnesses that may have sequelae for the person in later years, e.g., rheumatic fever, scarlet fever, and poliomyelitis.

Accidents or Injuries. Auto accidents, fractures, penetrating wounds, head injuries (especially if associated with unconsciousness), and burns.

Serious or Chronic Illnesses. Diabetes, hypertension, heart disease, sickle-cell anemia, cancer, and seizure disorder.

Hospitalizations. Cause, name of hospital, how the condition was treated, how long the person was hospitalized, and name of the physician.

Operations. Type of surgery, date, name of the surgeon, name of hospital, and how the person recovered.

Obstetric History. Number of pregnancies (gravidity), number of deliveries in which the fetus reached full term (term), number of preterm pregnancies (preterm), number of incomplete pregnancies (abortions), and number of children living (living). This is recorded: Grav _____ Term _____ Preterm _____ Ab _____ Living _____. For each complete pregnancy, note the course of pregnancy; labor and delivery; sex, weight, and condition of each infant; and postpartum course. For any incomplete pregnancies, record the duration and whether the pregnancy resulted in spontaneous (S) or induced (I) abortion.

Immunizations. Measles-mumps-rubella, polio, diphtheria-pertussis-tetanus, hepatitis B, *Haemophilus influenzae* type b, pneumococcal vaccine. Note the date of the last tetanus immunization, last tuberculosis skin test, and last flu shot.

Last Examination Date. Physical, dental, vision, hearing, electrocardiogram, chest x-ray examinations.

Allergies. Note both the allergen (medication, food, or contact agent, such as fabric or environmental agent) and the reaction (rash, itching, runny nose, watery eyes, difficulty breathing). With a drug, this symptom should not be a side effect but a true allergic reaction.

Current Medications. Note all prescription and over-the-counter medications. Ask specifically about vitamins, birth control pills, aspirin, and antacids, because many people do not consider these to be medications. For each medication, note the name, dose, and schedule, and ask "How often do you take it each day?" "What is it for?" and "How long have you been taking it?"

Family History

Ask about the age and health or the age and cause of death of blood relatives, such as parents, grandparents, and siblings. These data may have genetic significance for the patient. Also ask about close family members, such as spouse and children. You need to know about the person's prolonged contact with any communicable disease or the effect of a family member's illness on this person.

Specifically ask for any family history of heart disease, high blood pressure, stroke, diabetes, blood disorders, cancer, sickle-cell anemia, arthritis, allergies, obesity, alcoholism, mental illness, seizure disorder, kidney disease, and tuberculosis. Construct a family tree, or genogram, to show this information clearly and concisely (Fig. 5–1).

Review of Systems

The purposes of this section are (1) to evaluate the past and present health state of each body system, (2) to double-check in case any significant data were omitted in the present illness section, and (3) to evaluate health promotion practices. The order of the examination of body systems is roughly head-to-toe. The items within each system are not inclusive, and only the most common symptoms are listed. If the present illness section covered one body system, you do not need to repeat all the data here. For example, if the reason for seeking care is earache, the present illness section describes most of the symptoms listed for the auditory system. Just ask now what was not asked in the present illness section. Medical terms are listed here, but they need to be translated for the patient. (Note that symptoms and health promotion activities are only listed here. These terms are repeated and expanded in each related physical examination chapter, along with suggested ways to pose questions and a rationale for each question.)

FAMILY TREE, or GENOGRAM

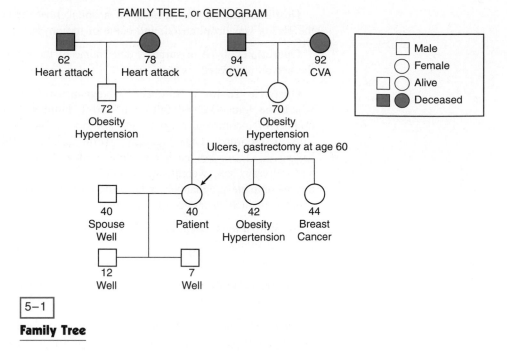

5–1

Family Tree

When recording information, avoid writing "negative" after the system heading. You need to record the *presence or absence* of all symptoms, otherwise the reader does not know about which factors you asked.

A common mistake made by beginning practitioners is to record some physical finding or objective data here, e.g., "skin warm and dry." Remember that the history should be limited to patient statements, or subjective data—factors that the person *says* were or were not present.

General Overall Health State. Present weight (gain or loss, period of time, by diet or other factors), fatigue, weakness or malaise, fever, chills, sweats or night sweats.

Skin. History of skin disease (eczema, psoriasis, hives), pigment or color change, change in mole, excessive dryness or moisture, pruritus, excessive bruising, rash or lesion.

Hair. Recent loss, change in texture. Nails: change in shape, color, or brittleness.

Health Promotion. Amount of sun exposure; method of self-care for skin and hair?

Head. Any unusually frequent or severe headache, any head injury, dizziness (syncope) or vertigo.

Eyes. Difficulty with vision (decreased acuity, blurring, blind spots), eye pain, diplopia (double vision), redness or swelling, watering or discharge, glaucoma or cataracts.

Health Promotion. Wears glasses or contacts; last vision check or glaucoma test; and how coping with loss of vision if any.

Ears. Earaches, infections, discharge and its characteristics, tinnitus or vertigo.

Health Promotion. Hearing loss, hearing aid use, how loss affects the daily life, any exposure to environmental noise, and method of cleaning ears.

Nose and Sinuses. Discharge and its characteristics, any unusually frequent or severe colds, sinus pain, nasal obstruction, nosebleeds, allergies or hay fever, or change in sense of smell.

Mouth and Throat. Mouth pain, frequent sore throat, bleeding gums, toothache, lesion in mouth or tongue, dysphagia, hoarseness or voice change, tonsillectomy, altered taste.

Health Promotion. Pattern of daily dental care, use of prostheses (dentures, bridge), and last dental checkup.

Neck. Pain, limitation of motion, lumps or swelling, enlarged or tender nodes, goiter.

Breast. Pain, lump, nipple discharge, rash, history of breast disease, any surgery on the breasts.

Health Promotion. Performs breast self-examination, including its frequency and method used, last mammogram.

Axilla. Tenderness, lump or swelling, rash.

Respiratory System. History of lung diseases (asthma, emphysema, bronchitis, pneumonia, tuberculosis), chest pain with breathing, wheezing or noisy breathing, shortness of breath, how much activity produces shortness of breath, cough, sputum (color, amount), hemoptysis, toxin or pollution exposure.

Health Promotion. Last chest x-ray study.

Cardiovascular. Precordial or retrosternal pain, palpitation, cyanosis, dyspnea on exertion (specify amount of exertion, e.g., walking one flight stairs, walking from chair to bath, or just talking), orthopnea, paroxysmal nocturnal dyspnea, nocturia, edema, history of heart murmur, hypertension, coronary artery disease, anemia.

Health Promotion. Date of last ECG or other heart tests.

Peripheral Vascular. Coldness, numbness and tingling, swelling of legs (time of day, activity), discoloration in hands or feet (bluish red, pallor, mottling, associated with position, especially around feet and ankles), varicose veins or complications, intermittent claudication, thrombophlebitis, ulcers.

Health Promotion. Does the work involve long-term sitting or standing? Avoid crossing legs at the knees? Wear support hose?

Gastrointestinal. Appetite, food intolerance, dysphagia, heartburn, indigestion, pain (associated with eating), other abdominal pain, pyrosis (esophageal and stomach burning sensation with sour eructation), nausea and vomiting (character), vomiting blood, history of abdominal disease (ulcer, liver or gallbladder, jaundice, appendicitis, colitis), flatulence, frequency of bowel movement, any recent change, stool characteristics, constipation or diarrhea, black stools, rectal bleeding, rectal conditions (hemorrhoids, fistula).

Health Promotion. Use of antacids or laxatives. (Alternatively, diet history and substance habits can be placed here.)

Urinary System. Frequency, urgency, nocturia (the number of times the person awakens at night to urinate, recent change), dysuria, polyuria or oliguria, hesitancy or straining, narrowed stream, urine color (cloudy or presence of hematuria), incontinence, history of urinary disease (kidney disease, kidney stones, urinary tract infections, prostate), pain in flank, groin, suprapubic region, or low back.

Health Promotion. Measures to avoid or treat urinary tract infections, use of Kegel exercises after childbirth.

Male Genital System. Penis or testicular pain, sores or lesions, penile discharge, lumps, hernia.

Health Promotion. Perform testicular self-examination? How frequently?

Female Genital System. Menstrual history (age at menarche, last menstrual period, cycle and duration, any amenorrhea or menorrhagia, premenstrual pain or dysmenorrhea, intermenstrual spotting), vaginal itching, discharge and its characteristics, age at menopause, menopausal signs or symptoms, postmenopausal bleeding.

Health Promotion. Last gynecologic checkup and last Papanicolaou smear.

Sexual Health. Presently in a relationship involving intercourse? Are the aspects of sex satisfactory to the patient and partner? Any dyspareunia (for female), any changes in erection or ejaculation (for male), and use of contraceptive? Is the contraceptive method satisfactory? Aware of contact with a partner who has any sexually transmitted disease (gonorrhea, herpes, chlamydia, venereal warts, acquired immunodeficiency syndrome [AIDS], or syphilis)?

Musculoskeletal System. History of arthritis or gout. In the joints: pain, stiffness, swelling (location, migratory nature), deformity, limitation of motion, noise with joint motion? In the muscles: any pain, cramps, weakness, gait problems or problems with coordinated activities? In the back: any pain (location and radiation to extremities), stiffness, limitation of motion, or history of back pain or disc disease?

Health Promotion. How much walking per day? What is the effect of limited range of motion on daily activities, such as on grooming, feeding, toileting, dressing? Are any mobility aids used?

Neurologic System. History of seizure disorder, stroke, fainting, blackouts. In motor function: weakness, tic or tremor, paralysis, or coordination problems. In sensory function: numbness and tingling (paresthesia). In cognitive function: memory disorder (recent or distant, disorientation). In mental status: any nervousness, mood change, depression, or any history of mental health dysfunction or hallucinations.

Health Promotion. Alternatively, data about interpersonal relationships, coping patterns placed here.

Hematologic System. Bleeding tendency of skin or mucous membranes, excessive bruising, lymph node swelling, exposure to toxic agents or radiation, blood transfusion and reactions.

Endocrine System. History of diabetes or diabetic symptoms (polyuria, polydipsia, polyphagia), history of thyroid disease, intolerance to heat and cold, change in skin pigmentation or texture, excessive sweating, relationship between appetite and weight, abnormal hair distribution, nervousness, tremors, and need for hormone therapy.

Functional Assessment (Including Activities of Daily Living)

Functional assessment measures a person's self-care ability in the areas of general physical health or absence of illness; ADLs, such as bathing, dressing, toileting, eating, walking; instrumental activities of daily living (IADLs), or those needed for independent living, such as housekeeping, shopping, cooking, doing laundry, using the telephone, managing finances; nutrition; social relationships and resources; self-concept and coping; and home environment.

Functional assessment may mean organizing the entire assessment around functional "pattern areas" (Gordon, 1994). Instruments that emphasize functional categories may help in leading to a nursing diagnosis.

Or, functional assessment may mean that the health history may be supplemented by a standardized instrument on functional assessment. These instruments objectively measure a person's present functional status and monitor any changes over time (Granger et al., 1979; Katz et al., 1963; Linn and Linn, 1982; Mahoney and Barthel, 1965; Pearlman, 1987).

Whether or not you use any of these formalized instruments, functional assessment questions such as those listed in the following section should be included in the standard health history. These questions provide data on the lifestyle and type of living environment to which the person is accustomed. Since some of the data may be judged private by the individual, the questions are best asked at this later point in the interview after you have had time to establish rapport.

Self-Esteem, Self-Concept. Education (last grade completed, other significant training), financial status (income adequate for lifestyle and/or health concerns), value-belief system (religious practices and perception of personal strengths).

Activity/Exercise. A daily profile reflecting usual daily activities: ask "Tell me how you spend a typical day." Note ability to perform ADLs: independent or needs assistance with feeding, bathing, hygiene, dressing, toileting, bed to chair transfer, walking, standing, or climbing stairs. Any use of wheelchair, prostheses, or mobility aids?

Record leisure activities enjoyed and exercise pattern (type, amount per day or week, method of warm-up session, method of monitoring the body's response to exercise).

Sleep/Rest. Sleep patterns, daytime naps, any sleep aids used.

Nutrition/Elimination. Record the diet by a recall of all food and beverages taken over the last 24 hours (see Chapter 7 for suggested method of inquiry). "Is that menu typical of most days?" Describe eating habits and current appetite. Ask "Who buys food and prepares food?" "Are your finances adequate for food?" "Who is present at mealtimes?" Indicate any food allergy or intolerance. Record daily intake of caffeine (coffee, tea, cola drinks).

Ask about usual pattern of bowel elimination and urinating, including problems with mobility or transfer in toileting, continence, use of laxatives.

Interpersonal Relationships/Resources. Social roles: "How would you describe your role in the family?" "How would you say you get along with family, friends, and co-workers?" Ask about support systems composed of family and significant others: "To whom could you go for support with a problem at work, with your health, or a personal problem?" Include contact with spouse, siblings, parents, children, friends, organizations, workplace: "Is time spent alone pleasurable and relaxing, or isolating?"

Coping and Stress Management. Kinds of stresses in life, especially in the last year, any change in lifestyle or any current stress, methods tried to relieve stress, and if these have been helpful.

Personal Habits. Tobacco, alcohol, street drugs: "Do you smoke cigarettes (pipe, use chewing tobacco)?" "At what age did you start?" "How many packs do you smoke per day?" "How many years have you smoked?" Record the number of packs smoked per day (PPD) and duration, e.g., 1 PPD × 5 years. Then ask, "Have you ever tried to quit?" and "How did it go?" to introduce plans about smoking cessation.

Alcohol. Health care professionals often fail to question about alcohol unless problems are obvious. However, alcohol interacts adversely with all medications, is a factor in many social problems such as assaults, rapes, and child abuse, contributes to half of all fatal traffic accidents, and accounts for 5% of all deaths in the United States. The later figure is actually an underestimate because alcohol-related conditions are underreported on death certificates (U.S. Department of Health and Human Services, 1993).

Be alert, then, to early signs of hazardous alcohol use. Ask whether the person drinks alcohol. If yes, ask specific questions about the amount and frequency of alcohol use: "When was your last drink of alcohol?" "How much did you drink that time?" "Out of the last 30 days, about how many days would you say that you drank alcohol?" "Have you ever had a drinking problem?"

You may wish to use a screening questionnaire to identify excessive or uncontrolled drinking, such as the Alcohol Use Disorder Identification Test (AUDIT) (Volk et al.,

1997), or the Cut Down, Annoyed, Guilty, and Eye-Opener Test (**CAGE**) (Ewing, 1984):

- Have you ever thought you should **C**ut down your drinking?
- Have you ever been **A**nnoyed by criticism of your drinking?
- Have you ever felt **G**uilty about your drinking?
- Do you drink in the morning? (i.e., an **E**ye opener?)

If the person answers "yes" to two or more CAGE questions, you should suspect alcohol abuse and continue with a more complete substance abuse assessment. If the person answers "no" to drinking alcohol, ask the reason for this decision (psychosocial, legal, health). Any history of alcohol treatment? Involvement in recovery activities? History of family member with problem drinking?

Street Drugs. Ask specifically about marijuana, cocaine, crack cocaine, amphetamines, barbiturates. Indicate frequency of use and how has usage affected work or family.

Environment/Hazards. Housing and neighborhood (living alone, knowledge of neighbors), safety of area, adequate heat and utilities, access to transportation, involvement in community services. Note environmental health, including hazards in workplace, hazards at home, use of seat belts, geographic or occupational exposures, travel or residence in other countries, including time spent abroad during military service.

Occupational Health. Ask the person to describe his or her job. Ever worked with any health hazard, such as asbestos, inhalants, chemicals, repetitive motion? Wear any protective equipment? Any work programs in place that monitor exposure? Aware of any health problems now that may be related to work exposure?

Note the timing of the reason for seeking care, and whether it may be related to work or home activities, job titles, or exposure history. Take a careful smoking history, which may contribute to occupational hazards. Finally, ask the person what he or she likes or dislikes about the job (Twining, 1995).

Perception of Health

Ask the person questions such as: "How do you define health?" "How do you view your situation now?" "What are your concerns?" "What do you think will happen in the future?" "What are your health goals?" "What do you expect from us as nurses, physicians, (or other health care providers)?"

 ## DEVELOPMENTAL CONSIDERATIONS

Children and Adolescents

The health history is adapted to include information specific for the age and developmental stage of the child, e.g., the mother's health during pregnancy, labor and delivery, and the perinatal period. Note that the developmental history and nutritional data are listed as separate sections because of their importance for current health.

Biographical Data

Include the child's name, nickname, address and phone number, parents' names and work numbers, child's age and birthdate, birthplace, sex, race, ethnic origin, and information on other children and family members at home.

Source of History

1. Person providing information and relation to child
2. Your impression of reliability of information
3. Any special circumstances, e.g., the use of an interpreter

Reason for Seeking Care

Record the parent's spontaneous statement. Because of the frequency of well child visits for routine health care, there will be more reasons such as "time for the child's checkup" or "she needs the next baby shot." Reasons for health problems may be initiated by the child, parent, or by a third party such as the classroom teacher.

Sometimes the reason stated may not be the real reason for the visit. A parent may have a "hidden agenda," such as the mother who brought her 4-year-old child in because "she looked pale." Further questioning revealed that the mother had heard recently from a former college friend whose own 4-year-old child had just been diagnosed with leukemia.

Present Health or History of Present Illness

If the parent or child seeks routine health care, include a statement about the usual health of the child and any common health problems or major health concerns.

Describe any presenting symptom or sign, using the same format as for the adult. Some additional considerations include

- Severity of pain: "How do you know the child is in pain," e.g., pulling at ears alerts parent to ear pain. Note effect of pain on usual behavior, e.g., does it stop child from playing?
- Associated factors, such as relation to activity, eating, and body position.
- The parent's intuitive sense of a problem. As the constant caregiver, this intuitive sense is often very accurate. Even if proved otherwise, this factor gives you an idea of parent's area of concern.
- Parent's coping ability and reaction of other family members to child's symptoms or illness.

Past Health

Prenatal Status. How was this pregnancy spaced? Was it planned? What was the mother's attitude toward the pregnancy? What was the father's attitude? Was there medical supervision for the mother? At what month was the supervision started? What was the mother's health during pregnancy? Were there any complications (bleeding, excessive nausea and vomiting, unusual weight gain, high blood pressure, swelling of hands and feet, infections—rubella or sexually transmitted diseases, falls)? During what month were diet and medications prescribed and/or taken during pregnancy (dose and duration)? Record the mother's use of alcohol, street drugs, or cigarettes and any x-ray studies taken during pregnancy.

Start with an open-ended question, "Tell me about your pregnancy." If she questions the relevancy of the statement, mention that these questions are important to gain a complete picture of the child's health.

Labor and Delivery. Parity of the mother, duration of the pregnancy, name of the hospital, course and duration of labor, use of anesthesia, type of delivery (vertex, breech, cesarean section), birth weight, Apgar scores, onset of breathing, any cyanosis, need for resuscitation, and use of special equipment or procedures.

Postnatal Status. Any problems in the nursery, length of hospital stay, neonatal jaundice, whether the baby was discharged with the mother, whether the baby was breast or bottle fed, weight gain, any feeding problems, "blue spells," colic, diarrhea, patterns of crying and sleeping, the mother's health postpartum, and the mother's reaction to the baby.

Childhood Illnesses. Age and any complications of measles, mumps, rubella, chickenpox, whooping cough, strep throat, and frequent ear infections. Also, any recent exposure to illness.

Serious Accidents or Injuries. Age of occurrence, extent of injury, how the child was treated, and complications of auto accidents, falls, head injuries, fractures, burns, and poisonings.

Serious or Chronic Illnesses. Age of onset, how the child was treated, and complications of meningitis or encephalitis; seizure disorders; asthma, pneumonia, and other chronic lung conditions; rheumatic fever; scarlet fever; diabetes; kidney problems; sickle-cell anemia; high blood pressure; and allergies.

Operations or Hospitalizations. Reason for care, age at admission, name of surgeon or primary care providers, name of hospital, duration of stay, how child reacted to hospitalization, and any complications. (If child reacted poorly, he or she may be afraid now and will need special preparation for the examination that is to follow.)

Immunizations. Age when administered, date administered, and any reactions following immunizations. Appendixes A–1 and A–2 list suggested immunization schedules. Because of recent outbreaks of measles across the United States, the American Academy of Pediatrics now is recommending two doses of the measles-mumps-rubella vaccine, one at 15 months and one at age 11 or 12 when the child enters middle school or junior high school (American Academy of Pediatrics, 1997).

Allergies. Any drugs, foods, contact agents, and environmental agents to which the child is allergic, and reaction to allergen. Note allergic reactions particularly common in childhood, such as allergic rhinitis, insect hypersensitivity, eczema, and urticaria.

Medications. Any prescription and over-the-counter medications (or vitamins) the child takes, including the dose, daily schedule, why the medication is given, and any problems.

Developmental History

Growth. Height and weight at birth and at 1, 2, 5, and 10 years, any periods of rapid gain or loss, and process of dentition (age of tooth eruption and pattern of loss).

Milestones. Age when child first held head erect, rolled over, sat alone, walked alone, cut his or her first tooth, said his or her first words with meaning, spoke in sentences, was toilet trained, tied shoes, dressed without help. Does the parent believe this development has been normal? How does this child's development compare with siblings or peers?

Current Development (Children 1 Month Through Preschool). Gross motor skills (rolls over, sits alone, walks alone, skips, climbs), fine motor skills (inspects hands, brings hands to mouth, pincer grasp, stacks blocks, feeds self, uses crayon to draw, uses scissors), language skills (vocalizes, first words with meaning, sentences, persistence of baby talk, speech problems), and personal-social skills (smiles, tracks movement with eyes to midline, past midline, attends to sound by turning head, recognizes own name). If the child is undergoing toilet training, indicate the method used, age of bladder/bowel control, parents' attitude toward toilet training, and terms used for toileting.

School-Age Child. Gross motor skills (runs, jumps, climbs, rides bicycle, general coordination), fine motor skills (ties shoelace, uses scissors, writes name and numbers, draws pictures), and language skills (vocabulary, verbal ability, able to tell time, reading level).

Nutritional History

The amount of nutritional information needed depends on the child's age; the younger the child, the more detailed and specific the data. For the infant, record whether breastfeeding or bottle-feeding is used. If the child is breast fed, record nursing frequency and duration, any supplements (vitamin, iron, fluoride, bottles), family support for nursing, and age and method of weaning. If the child is bottle fed, record type formula used, frequency and amount, any problems with feeding (spitting up, colic, diarrhea), supplements used, and any bottle propping. Record introduction of solid foods (age when the child began eating solids, which foods, whether foods are home or commercially made, amount given, child's reaction to new food, parent's reaction to feeding).

For preschool- and school-age children and adolescents, record the child's appetite, 24-hour diet recall (meals, snacks, amounts), vitamins taken, how much junk food is eaten, who eats with the child, food likes and dislikes, and parent's perception of child's nutrition.

A week-long diary of food intake may be more accurate than a spot 24-hour recall. Also, consider cultural practices in assessing child's diet (see Transcultural Considerations).

Family History

As with the adult, diagram a family tree for the child, including siblings, parents, grandparents. Give the age, health, or age and cause of death of each. Ask specifically for the family history of heart disease, high blood pressure, diabetes, blood disorders, cancer, sickle-cell anemia, arthritis, allergies, obesity, cystic fibrosis, alcoholism, mental illness, seizure disorder, kidney disease, mental retardation, learning disabilities, birth defects, and sudden infant death. (When interviewing the mother, ask about the "child's father," not "your husband," in case of the separation of child's biologic parents.)

Review of Systems

General. Significant gain or loss of weight, failure to gain weight appropriate for age, frequent colds, ear infections, illnesses, energy level, fatigue, overactivity, and behavior change (irritability, increased crying, nervousness).

Skin. Birthmarks, skin disease, pigment or color change, mottling, change in mole, pruritus, rash, lesion, acne, easy bruising or petechiae, easy bleeding, and changes in hair or nails.

Head. Headache, head injury, dizziness.

Eyes. Strabismus, diplopia, pain, redness, discharge, cataracts, vision changes, reading problems. Is the child able to see the board at school? Does the child sit too close to the television?

Health Promotion. Use of eyeglasses, date of last vision screening.

Ears. Earaches, frequency of ear infections, myringotomy tubes in ears, discharge (characteristics), cerumen, ringing or crackling, and whether parent perceives any hearing problems.

Health Promotion. How does the child clean his or her ears?

Nose and Sinuses. Discharge and its characteristics, frequency of colds, nasal stuffiness, nosebleeds, and allergies.

Mouth and Throat. History of cleft lip or palate, frequency of sore throats, toothache, caries, sores in mouth or tongue, tonsils present, mouth breathing, difficulty chewing, difficulty swallowing, and hoarseness or voice change.

Health Promotion. Child's pattern of brushing teeth and last dental checkup.

Neck. Swollen or tender glands, limitation of movement, or stiffness.

Breast. For preadolescent and adolescent girls, when did they notice that their breasts were changing? What is the girl's self-perception of development? For older adolescents, does the girl perform breast self-examination? (See Chapter 15 for suggested phrasing of questions.)

Respiratory System. Croup or asthma, wheezing or noisy breathing, shortness of breath, chronic cough.

Cardiovascular System. Congenital heart problems, history of murmur, and cyanosis (what prompts this condition). Is there any limitation of activity, or can the child keep up with peers? Is there any dyspnea on exertion, palpitations, high blood pressure, or coldness in the extremities?

Gastrointestinal System. Abdominal pain, nausea and vomiting, history of ulcer, frequency of bowel movements, stool color and characteristics, diarrhea, constipation or stool-holding, rectal bleeding, anal itching, history of pinworms, and use of laxatives.

Urinary System. Painful urination, polyuria/oliguria, narrowed stream, urine color (cloudy, dark), history of urinary tract infection, whether toilet trained, when toilet training was planned, any problems, bed wetting (when the child started, frequency, associated with stress, how child feels about it).

Male Genital System. Penis or testicular pain, whether told if testes are descended, any sores or lesions, discharge, hernia or hydrocele, or swelling in scrotum during crying. For the preadolescent and adolescent boy, has he noticed any change in the penis and scrotum? Is the boy familiar with normal growth patterns, nocturnal emissions, and sex education? Screen for sexual abuse. (See Chapter 22 for suggested phrasing of questions.)

Female Genital System. Has the girl noted any genital itching, rash, vaginal discharge? For the preadolescent and adolescent girl, when did menstruation start? Was she prepared? Screen for sexual abuse. (See Chapter 24 for suggested phrasing of questions.)

Sexual Health. What is the child's attitude toward the opposite sex? Who provides sex education? How does the family deal with sex education, masturbation, dating patterns? Is the adolescent in a relationship involving intercourse? Does he or she have information on birth control and sexually transmitted diseases? (See Chapters 22 and 24 for suggested phrasing of questions.)

Musculoskeletal System. In bones and joints: arthritis, joint pain, stiffness, swelling, limitation of movement, gait strength and coordination. In muscles: pain, cramps, and weakness. In the back: pain, posture, spinal curvature, and any treatment.

Neurologic System. Numbness and tingling. (Behavior and cognitive issues are covered in the sections on development and interpersonal relationships.)

Hematologic Systems. Excessive bruising, lymph node swelling, and exposure to toxic agents or radiation.

Endocrine System. History of diabetes or thyroid disease; excessive hunger, thirst, or urinating; abnormal hair distribution; and precocious or delayed puberty.

Functional Assessment (Including Activities of Daily Living)

Interpersonal Relationships. Within the family constellation, record the child's position in family; whether the child is adopted; who lives with the child; who is the primary caretaker; who is the caretaker if both parents work outside of the home; any support from relatives, neighbors, or friends; and the ethnic or cultural milieu.

Indicate family cohesion. Does the family enjoy activities as a unit? Has there been a recent family change or crisis (death, divorce, move)? Record information on child's self-image and level of independence. Does the child use a security blanket or toy? Is there any repetitive behavior (bed-rocking, head-banging), pica, thumb-sucking, or nail-biting? Note method of discipline used. Indicate type used at home. How effective is it? Who disciplines the child? Is there any occurrence of negativism, temper tantrums, withdrawal, or aggressive behavior?

Provide information on the child's friends: whether the child makes friends easily. How does the child get along with friends? Does he or she play with same-age or older or younger children?

Activity and Rest. Record the child's play activities. Indicate amount of active and quiet play, outdoor play, time watching television, and special hobbies or activities. Record sleep and rest. Indicate pattern and number of hours at night and during the day and the child's routine at bedtime. Is the child a sound sleeper, or is he or she wakeful? Does the child have nightmares, night terrors, or somnambulation? How does the parent respond? Does the child have naps during the day?

Record school attendance. Has the child had any experience with day care or nursery school? In what grade is the child in school? Has the child ever skipped a grade or been held back? Does the child seem to like school? What is his or her school performance? Are the parent and child satisfied with the performance? Were days missed in school? Provide a reason for the absence. (These questions give an important index to child's functioning outside the home.)

Economic Status. Ask about the mother's occupation and father's occupation. Indicate the number of hours each parent is away from home. Do parents perceive their income as adequate? What is the effect of illness on financial status?

Home Environment. Where does family live (house, apartment)? Is the size of the home adequate? Is there access to an outdoor play area? Does the child share a room, have his or her own bed, and have toys appropriate for his or her age?

Environmental Hazards. Inquire about home safety (precautions for poisons, medications, household products, presence of gates for stairways, and safe yard equipment). Provide information on the child's residence (adequate heating, ventilation, bathroom facilities), neighborhood (residential or industrial, age of neighbors, safe play areas, playmates available, distance to school, amount of traffic, is area remote or congested and overcrowded, is crime a problem, presence of air or water pollution), and automobile (child safety seat, seat belts).

Coping/Stress Management. Does the child have the ability to adapt to new situations? Record recent stressful experiences (death, divorce, move, loss of special friend). How does the child cope with stress? Has there been any recent change in behavior or mood? Has counseling ever been sought?

Habits. Has the child ever tried cigarette smoking? How much did he or she smoke? Has the child ever tried alcohol? How much alcohol did he or she drink weekly or daily? Has the child ever tried other drugs (marijuana, cocaine, amphetamines, barbiturates)?

Health Promotion. Who is the primary health care provider? When was the child's last checkup? Who is the dental care provider, and when was the last dental checkup? Provide date and result of screening for vision, hearing, urinalysis, phenylketonuria, hematocrit, tuberculosis skin test, sickle-cell trait, blood lead, and other tests specific for high-risk population.

The Older Adult

This health history includes the same format as that described for the younger adult, as well as some additional questions. These questions address ways in which the ADLs may have been affected by normal aging processes or by the effects of chronic illness or disability. There is no specific age at which to ask these additional questions. Use them when it seems appropriate.

It is important for you to recognize positive health measures; what the person has been doing to help himself or herself stay well and to live to an older age. Older people have spent a lifetime with a traditional health care system that searches only for pathology and what is wrong with their health. It may be a pleasant surprise to have a health professional affirm the things that they are "doing right" and to note health strengths.

As you study the following, keep in mind the format for the "younger" adult. **Only** *additional* **questions or a varying focus are addressed here.**

Reason for Seeking Care

It may take time to figure out the reason that the older person has come in for an examination. An aging person may shrug off a symptom as evidence of growing old and may be unsure whether it is "worth mentioning." Also, some older people have a conservative philosophy toward their health status: "If it isn't broken, don't fix it." These people come for care only when something is blatantly wrong.

Another older person may have many chronic problems, such as diabetes, hypertension, or constipation. It is challenging to filter out what brought the person in this time. The final statement should be the *person's* reason for seeking care, not your assumption of what the problem is.

Past Health

General Health. Health state in the last 5 years.

Accidents or Injuries, Serious or Chronic Illnesses, Hospitalizations, Operations. These areas may produce lengthy responses, and the person probably will not relate them in chronologic order. Let the person talk freely; you can reorder the events later when you do the write-up. The amount of data included here can indicate the amount of stress the person has faced during his or her lifetime. This section of the history can be filled out at home or before the interview if the person's vision and writing ability are adequate. Then you can concentrate remaining time of the interview on reviewing pertinent data and on the present health of the person.

Last Examination. Most recent mammography, proctoscopy, and tonometry.

Obstetric Status. It is *not* necessary to collect a detailed account of each pregnancy and delivery if the woman has passed menopause and has no gynecologic symptoms. Merely record the number of pregnancies and the health of each newborn.

Current Medications. For each medication, record the name, purpose, and daily schedule. Does the person have a system to remember to take the medicine? Does medicine seem to work? Are there any side effects? If so, does the person feel like skipping medicine because of them? Also consider the following issues:

- Some older persons take a large number of drugs, prescribed by different physicians.
- The person may not know drug name or purpose. When this occurs, ask the person to bring in the drug to be identified.
- Is cost a problem? When the person is unable to afford a drug, he or she may decrease the dosage, take one pill instead of two, or not refill the empty bottle immediately.

- Is traveling to the pharmacy to refill a prescription a problem?
- Is the person taking any over-the-counter medications? Some people use local pharmacist for self-treatment.
- Has the person ever shared medications with neighbors or friends? Some establish "lay referral" networks by comparing symptoms and thus medications.

Family History

This is not as useful in predicting which familial diseases the person may contract, because most of those will have occurred at an earlier age. But these data are useful to assess which diseases or causes of death of relatives the person has experienced. Also it describes the person's existing social network.

Review of Systems

Remember, these are *additional* items to question for the older adult. Refer to the history for the younger adult for the basic list.

General. Present weight and what the person would like to weigh (gives idea of body image).

Skin. Change in sensation to pain, heat, or cold.

Eyes. Use of bifocal glasses, any trouble adjusting to far vision (problems with stairs).

Ears. Increased sensitivity to background noise and whether conversation sounds garbled or distorted.

Mouth. Use of dentures, when the person wears them (always, all day, only at meals, only at social occasions, or never), method of cleaning, any difficulty wearing the dentures (loose, pain, makes whistling or clicking noise), cracks at corners of the mouth.

Respiratory System. Shortness of breath and level of activity that produces it. Shortness of breath often is an early sign of cardiac dysfunction, but many older people dismiss it as "a cold" or getting "winded" because of old age.

Cardiovascular System. If chest pain occurs, the person may not feel it as intensely as a younger person. Instead, the older adult may feel dyspnea on exertion.

Peripheral Vascular System. Wears constrictive clothing, garters, or rolls stockings at knees. Any color change at feet or ankles.

Urinary System. Urinary retention, incomplete emptying, straining to urinate, change in force of stream. If a weakened stream occurs, men may note the need to stand closer to toilet. Women may note incontinence when coughing, laughing, or sneezing.

Sexual Health. Ask about any changes in sexual relationship the person has experienced. Note for men it is normal for an erection to develop slowly. (See Chapter 22.) Note for women any vaginal dryness or pain with intercourse. Note for all whether aspects of sex are satisfactory and whether adequate privacy exists for sexual relationship.

Musculoskeletal System. Gait change (balance, weakness, difficulty with steps, fear of falling), use of any assistive device (cane, walker). Any joint stiffness? During what part of the day does the stiffness occur? Does pain or stiffness occur with activity or rest?

Neurologic System. Any problem with memory (recent or remote) or disorientation (time of day, in what settings).

Functional Assessment (Including Activities of Daily Living)

Functional assessment measures how a person manages day-to-day activities. For older people, the meaning of health becomes those activities that they can or cannot do. The *impact* of a disease on their daily activities and over-all quality of life (called the *disease burden*) is more important to older people than the actual disease diagnosis or pathology (Bernstein, 1992). Thus, the functional assessment—because it emphasizes function—is very important in assessing older people.

Many functional assessment instruments are available that objectively measure a person's present functional status and monitor any changes over time. Most instruments measure the performance of specific tasks such as the ADLs and IADLs. The Comprehensive Older Person's Evaluation (Table 5–1) is particularly useful because it contains the basic ADL/IADL functional assessment as well as physical, social, psychological, demographic, financial, and legal issues.

Whether or not a standardized instrument is used, the following functional assessment questions are important additions to the older adult's health history.

Self-Concept, Self-Esteem. When the aging person was an adolescent, educational opportunities were not as available as they are today, nor were they equally available for women. The aging person may be sensitive about having achieved the level of only elementary school education or less.

Occupation. Past positions, volunteer activities, and community activities. Many people continue to work past the age of 65; they grew up with a strong work ethic and are proud to continue. If the person is retired, how has he or she adjusted to the change in role? It may mean loss of social role or social status, loss of personal relationships formed at work, and reduced income.

Activity and Exercise. How does the person spend a typical day in work, hobbies, and leisure activities? Is there any day this routine changes, e.g., Sunday visits from family? Note that the person suffering from chronic illness or disability may have a self-care deficit, musculoskeletal changes such as arthritis, and mental confusion.

List significant leisure activities, hobbies, sports, community activities. Is there a community senior citizen center available for nutrition, social network, and screening of health status?

What is the type, amount, and frequency of the exercise? Is a warm-up included? How does the body respond?

Sleep and Rest. Usual sleep pattern, feel rested during day? Is energy sufficient to carry out daily activities? Need naps? Is there a problem with night wakenings (nocturia, shortness of breath, light sleep, insomnia [difficulty falling asleep, awakening during night, early morning wakening])? If no routine, tend to nap all afternoon? Does insomnia worsen with lack of a daily schedule?

Nutrition/Elimination. Record a 24-hour recall. Is this typical of most days? (Nutrition may vary greatly. Ask the person to keep a weekly log to bring in.) What are the meal patterns? Are there three full meals or five to six smaller meals per day? How many convenience foods and soft foods are used? Who prepares meals? Eat alone? Who shops for food? How are groceries transported home? Is the income adequate for groceries? Is there a problem preparing meals (adequate vision, motor deficit, adequate energy)? Are the appliances and water and utilities adequate for meal preparation? Is there any difficulty chewing or swallowing? What are the food preferences (aging persons often eat high amounts of carbohydrates because these foods are cheaper, easier to make, and easier to chew).

Interpersonal Relationships/Resources. Who else is at home with you? Live alone? Is this satisfactory? Have a pet? How close are family or friends? How often see family or friends? If infrequent, experience this as a loss?

Table 5-1 • Comprehensive Older Person's Evaluation

Name (print): _____ Date of visit: _____

Chief complaint: _____

Today I will ask you about your overall health and function and will be using a questionnaire to help me obtain this information. The first few questions are to check your memory.

Preliminary Cognition Questionnaire: *Record if answer is correct with (+); if answer is incorrect, with (−). Record total number of errors.*

	(+, −)
1) What is the date today?	_____
2) What day of the week is it?	_____
3) What is the name of this place?	_____
4) What is your telephone number or room number? (*record answer:* _____) *If subject does not have phone, ask:* What is your street address?	_____
5) How old are you? (*record answer:* _____)	_____
6) When were you born? (*record answer from records if patient cannot answer:* _____)	_____
7) Who is the president of the United States now?	_____
8) Who was the president just before him?	_____
9) What was your mother's maiden name?	_____
10) Subtract 3 from 20 and keep subtracting from each new number you get, all the way down.	_____
Total errors	_____

If more than 4 errors, ask #11. If more than 6 errors, complete questionnaire from informant.

11) Do you think you would benefit from a legal guardian, someone who would be responsible for your legal and financial matters? Do you have a living will? Would you like one?
   a) No
   b) Has functioning legal guardian for sole purpose of managing money
      (*describe:* _____)
   c) Has legal guardian
   d) Yes

Demographic Section
1) Patient's race or ethnic background (*record:* _____)
2) Patient's gender (*circle*)   Male   Female
3) How far did you go in school?
   a) Postgraduate education
   b) Four-year degree
   c) College or technical school
   d) High school complete
   e) High school incomplete
   f) 0–8 years

Social Support Section: Now there are a few questions about your family and friends.
4) Are you married, widowed, separated, divorced, or have you never been married?
   a) Now married
   b) Widowed
   c) Separated
   d) Divorced
   e) Never married
5) Who lives with you? (*circle all responses*)
   a) Spouse
   b) Other relative or friend (*specify:* _____)
   c) Group living situation (non-health)
   d) Lives alone
   e) Nursing home, number of years _____

6) Have you talked to any friends or relatives by phone during the last week?
   a) Yes
   b) No
7) Are you satisfied by seeing your relatives and friends as often as you want to, or are you somewhat dissatisfied about how little you see them?
   a) Satisfied (*skip to* #8)
   b) No (*ask* A)
      A) Do you feel you would like to be involved in a Senior Citizens Center for social events, or perhaps meals?
         1) No
         2) Is involved (*describe:* _____)
         3) Yes
8) Is there someone who would take care of you for as long as you needed if you were sick or disabled?
   a) Yes (*skip to* C)
   b) No (*ask* A)
      A) Is there someone who would take care of you for a short time?
         1) Yes (*skip to* C)
         2) No (*ask* B)
      B) Is there someone who could help you now and then?
         1) Yes (*ask* C)
         2) No (*ask* C)
      C) Whom would we call in case of an emergency? (*record name and telephone:* _____)
      _____)

Financial Section
9) Do you own, or are you buying, your own home?
   a) Yes (*skip to* #10)
   b) No (*ask* A)
      A) Do you feel you need assistance with housing?
         1) No
         2) Has subsidized or other housing assistance
         3) Yes (*describe:* _____)
      B) What type of housing did you have prior to coming here?
10) Are you covered by private medical insurance, Medicare, Medicaid, or some disability plan? (*circle all that apply*)
   a) Private insurance (*specify and skip to* #11: _____)
   b) Medicare
   c) Medicaid
   d) Disability (*specify and ask* A: _____)
   e) None
   f) Other (*specify:* _____)
      A) Do you feel you need additional assistance with your medical bills?
         1) No
         2) Yes
11) Which of these statements best describes your financial situation?
   a) My bills are no problem to me (*skip to* #12)
   b) My expenses make it difficult to meet my bills (*ask* A)
   c) My expenses are so heavy that I cannot meet my bills (*ask* A)
      A) Do you feel that you need financial assistance such as: (*circle all that apply*)
         1) Food stamps
         2) Social Security or disability payments
         3) Assistance in paying your heating or electrical bills
         4) Other financial assistance? (*describe:* _____)

Continued

Table 5–1 • Comprehensive Older Person's Evaluation *Continued*

Psychological Health Section: The next few questions are about how you feel about your life in general. There are no right or wrong answers, only what best applies to you. Please answer yes or no to each question.

	Yes	No

12) Is your daily life full of things that keep you interested?

13) Have you, at times, very much wanted to leave home?

14) Does it seem that no one understands you?

15) Are you happy most of the time?

16) Do you feel weak all over much of the time?

17) Is your sleep fitful and disturbed?

18) Taking everything into consideration, how would you describe your satisfaction with your life in general at the present time— good, fair, or poor?
   a) Good
   b) Fair
   c) Poor

19) Do you feel you now need help with your mental health; for example, a counselor or psychiatrist?
   a) No
   b) Has (*specify:* _____)
   c) Yes

Physical Health Section: The next few questions are about your health.

20) During the past month (30 days), how many days were you so sick that you couldn't do your usual activities, such as working around the house or visiting with friends? _____

21) Relative to other people your age, how would you rate your overall health at the present time: excellent, good, fair, poor, or very poor?
   a) Excellent (*skip to #22*)
   b) Very good (*skip to #22*)
   c) Good (*ask A*)
   d) Fair (*ask A*)
   e) Poor (*ask A*)
      A) Do you feel you need additional medical services such as a doctor, nurse, visiting nurse or physical therapist? *circle all that apply)*
         1) Doctor
         2) Nurse
         3) Visiting nurse
         4) Physical therapist
         5) None

22) Do you use an aid for walking, such as a wheelchair, walker, cane, or anything else? (*circle aid usually used*)
   a) Wheelchair
   b) Other (*specify:* _____)
   c) Visiting nurse
   d) Walker
   e) None

23) How much do your health troubles stand in the way of your doing things you want to do: not at all, a little, or a great deal?
   a) Not at all (*skip to #24*)
   b) A little (*ask A*)
   c) A great deal (*ask A*)
      A) Do you think you need assistance to do your daily activities; for example, do you need a live-in aide or choreworker?
         1) Live-in aide

      2) Choreworker
      3) Has aide, choreworker, or other assistance (*describe:* _____)
      4) None needed

24) Have you had, or do you currently have, any of the following health problems? *If yes, place an "X" in appropriate box and describe; medical record information may be used to help complete this section.)*

	HX	CURRENT	DESCRIBE
a) Arthritis or rheumatism?			
b) Lung or breathing problem?			
c) Hypertension?			
d) Heart trouble?			
e) Phlebitis or poor circulation problems in arms or legs?			
f) Diabetes or low blood sugar?			
g) Digestive ulcers?			
h) Other digestive problem?			
i) Cancer?			
j) Anemia?			
k) Effects of stroke?			
l) Other neurological problem? (*specify:* _____)			
m) Thyroid or other glandular problem? (*specify:* _____)			
n) Skin disorders such as pressure sores, leg ulcers, burns?			
o) Speech problem?			
p) Hearing problem?			
q) Vision or eye problem?			
r) Kidney or bladder problems, or incontinence?			
s) A problem of falls?			
t) Problem with eating or your weight? (*specify:* _____)			
u) Problem with depression or your nerves? (*specify:* _____)			
v) Problem with your behavior (*specify:* _____)			
w) Problem with your sexual activity?			
x) Problem with alcohol?			
y) Problem with pain?			
z) Other health problems? (*specify:* _____)			

Immunizations: _____

25) What medications are you currently taking, or have been taking, in the last month? (May I see your medication bottles?) *(If patient cannot list, ask categories a–r and note dosage and schedule, or obtain information from medical or pharmacy records and verify accuracy with the patient.)*

Continued

Table 5–1 • Comprehensive Older Person's Evaluation *Continued*

Allergies:	Rx (DOSAGE AND SCHEDULE)		YES	NO	DESCRIBE (INCLUDE NEEDS)
a) Arthritis medication		a) Use the telephone?			
b) Pain medication		b) Get to places out of walking distance (using transportation)?			
c) Blood pressure medication					
d) Water pills or pills for fluid		c) Shop for clothes and food?			
e) Medication for your heart		d) Do your housework?			
f) Medication for your lungs		e) Handle your money?			
g) Blood thinners		f) Feed yourself?			
h) Medication for your circulation		g) Dress and undress yourself?			
i) Insulin or diabetes medication		h) Take care of your appearance?			
j) Seizure medication		i) Get in and out of bed?			
k) Thyroid pills		j) Take a bath or shower?			
l) Steroids		k) Prepare your meals?			
m) Hormones		l) Do you have any problem getting to the bathroom on time?			
n) Antibiotics					
o) Medicine for nerves or depression					
p) Prescription sleeping pills					
q) Other prescription drugs					
r) Other nonprescription drugs					

26) Many people have problems remembering to take their medications, especially ones they need to take on a regular basis. How often do you forget to take your medications? Would you say you forget often, sometimes, rarely, or never?
a) Never
b) Rarely
c) Sometimes
d) Often

Activities of Daily Living: The next set of questions asks whether you need help with any of the following activities of daily living.
27) I would like to know whether you can do these activities without any help at all, or if you need assistance to do them. Do you need help to: (*If yes, describe, including patient needs.*)

28) During the past 6 months, have you had any help with such things as shopping, housework, bathing, dressing and getting around?
a) Yes (*specify:* _____)
b) No
Signature of person completing the form:
_____

(Reprinted with permission from Pearlman R: Development of a functional assessment questionnaire for geriatric patients: COPE. J Chronic Dis 40:85S–94S, 1987. With permission from Elsevier Science.)

Live with family, such as a spouse, children, or a sibling? Is this a satisfactory arrangement? What is the role in family for preparation of meals, housework, and other activities? Are there any conflicts?

On whom depend for emotional support? For help with problems? Who meets affection needs?

Coping and Stress Management. Has there been a recent change in lifestyle, such as loss of occupation, spouse, friends, move from home, illness of self or family member, or has income been decreased? How dealing with stress? If a loved one has died, how responding to the loss? "How do you feel about being 'alone' and having to take on unfamiliar responsibilities now?"

Environment/Hazards. Home safety: one floor or are there stairs, state of repair, is money adequate to maintain home, exits for fire, heating and utilities adequate, how long in the present home? Transportation: own auto, last driver's test, consider self a safe driver, income adequate for maintenance, public transportation access, receive

Table 5–2 • Cultural Assessment*

Brief History of the Cultural Group With Which the Person Identifies

- With what cultural group(s) does the person affiliate (e.g., Hispanic, Polish, Navajo, or combination)? To what degree does the person identify with the cultural group (e.g., "we" concept of solidarity or a fringe member)?
- What is the person's reported racial affiliation (e.g., black, Native American, Asian, and so on)?
- Where was the person born?
- Where has the person lived (country, city) and when (during what years)? Note: If a recent relocation to the United States, knowledge of prevalent diseases in country of origin may be helpful.

Values Orientation

- What are the person's attitudes, values, and beliefs about birth, death, health, illness, health care providers?
- How does the person view work, leisure, education?
- How does the person perceive change?

Cultural Sanctions and Restrictions

- How does the persons's cultural group regard expression of emotion and feelings, spirituality, and religious beliefs? How are dying, death, and grieving expressed in a culturally appropriate manner?
- How is modesty expressed by men and women? Are there culturally defined expectations about male-female relationships, including the health care relationship?
- Does the person have any restrictions related to sexuality, exposure of body parts, certain types of surgery (e.g., amputation, vasectomy, hysterectomy)?
- Are there any restrictions against discussion of dead relatives or fears related to the unknown?

Communication

- What language does the person speak at home? What other languages does the person speak or read? In what language would the person prefer to communicate with you?
- Does the person need an interpreter? If so, is there a relative or friend whom he or she would like to interpret? Is there anyone whom the person would prefer did not interpret (e.g., member of the opposite sex, a person younger/older than the person, member of a rival tribe or nation)?
- How does the person feel about health care providers who are not of the same cultural background (e.g., black, middle-class nurse and Hispanic of a different social class)? Does the person prefer to receive care from a nurse or doctor of the same cultural background, gender, and/or age?

Health-Related Beliefs and Practices

- To what cause(s) does the person attribute illness and disease (e.g., divine wrath, imbalance in hot/cold or yin/yang, punishment for moral transgressions, hex, soul loss)?
- What does the person believe promotes health (eating certain foods, wearing amulets to bring good luck, exercise, prayer, rituals to ancestors, saints, or intermediate deities)?
- What is the person's religious affiliation (e.g., Judaism, Islam, Pentecostalism, West African voodooism, Seventh-Day Adventism, Catholicism, Mormonism)?
- Does the person rely on cultural healers (e.g., curandero, shaman, spiritualist, priest, minister, monk?) Who determines when the person is sick and when he or she is healthy? Who determines the type of healer and treatment that should be sought?

- In what types of cultural healing practices does the person engage (use of herbal remedies, potions, massage, wearing of talismans or charms to discourage evil spirits, healing rituals, incantations, prayers)?
- How are biomedical/scientific health care providers perceived? How does the person and his or her family perceive nurses or physicians? What are the expectations of nurses and nursing care?
- What is appropriate "sick role" behavior? Who determines what symptoms constitute disease/illness? Who decides when the person is no longer sick? Who cares for the person at home?
- How does the person's cultural group view mental disorders? Are there differences in acceptable behaviors for physical versus psychological illnesses?

Nutrition

- What is the meaning of food and eating to the person? With whom does the person usually eat? What types of foods are eaten? What does the person define as food? What does the person believe composes a "healthy" versus an "unhealthy" diet?
- How are foods prepared at home (type of food preparation, cooking oil(s) used, length of time foods are cooked, especially vegetables, amount and type of seasoning added to various foods during preparation)?
- Do religious beliefs and practices influence the person's diet (e.g., amount, type, preparation or delineation of acceptable food combinations, such as kosher diets)? Does the person abstain from certain foods at regular intervals, on specific dates determined by the religious calendar, or at other times?
- If the person's religion mandates or encourages fasting, what does the term "fast" mean (e.g., refraining from certain types or quantities of foods, eating only during certain times of the day)? For what period of time is the person expected to fast?
- During fasting, does the person refrain from liquids/beverages? Does the religion allow exemption from fasting during illness? If so, does the person believe that an exemption applies to him or her?

Socioeconomic Considerations

- Who composes the person's social network (family, peers, and cultural healers)? How do they influence the person's health or illness status?
- How do members of the person's social support network define caring (e.g., being continuously present, doing things for the person, looking after the person's family)? What are the roles of various family members during health and illness?
- How does the person's family participate in the nursing care (e.g., bathing, feeding, touching, being present)?
- Does the cultural family structure influence the person's response to health or illness (e.g., beliefs, strengths, weaknesses, and social class)? Is there a key family member whose role is significant in health-related decisions (e.g., grandmother in many black families, eldest adult son in Asian families)?
- Who is the principal wage earner in the person's family? What is the total annual income? (Note: This is a potentially sensitive question that should be asked only if necessary.) Is there more than one wage earner? Are there other sources of financial support (extended family, investments)?
- What impact does economic status have on lifestyle, place of residence, living conditions, ability to obtain health care, discharge planning?

Continued

Table 5–2 • Cultural Assessment *Continued*

Organizations Providing Cultural Support

• What influence do ethnic/cultural organizations have on the person's receiving health care (e.g., Organization of Migrant Workers, National Association for the Advancement of Colored People (NAACP), Black Political Caucus, churches, schools, Urban League, community-based health care programs and clinics)?

Educational Background

• What is the person's highest educational level obtained?
• Can the person read and write English, or is another language preferred? If English is the second language, are materials available in the primary language?
• What learning style is most comfortable/familiar? Does the person prefer to learn through written materials, oral explanation, or demonstration?

Religious Affiliation

• What is the role of religious beliefs and practices during health and illness?
• Are there healing rituals or practices that the person believes can promote wellbeing or hasten recovery from illness? If so, who performs these?

• What is the role of significant religious representatives during health and illness? Are there recognized healers (e.g., Islamic imams, Christian Scientist practitioners or nurses, Catholic priests, Mormon elders, Buddhist monks)?

Spiritual Considerations

• Does the person have religious objects in the environment?
• Does the person wear outer- or undergarments having religious significance?
• Are get-well greeting cards religious in nature or from a religious representative?
• Does the person appear to pray at certain times of the day or before meals?
• Does the person make special dietary requests (e.g., Kosher diet; vegetarian diet; diet free from caffeine, pork, shellfish, or other specific food items)?
• Does the person read religious magazines or books?
• Does the person mention God (Allah, Buddha, Yahweh, or a synonym), prayer, faith, or other religious topics?
• Is a request made for a visit by a member of the clergy or other religious representative?
• Is there an expression of anxiety or fear about pain, suffering, death?
• Does the person prefer to interact with others or to remain alone?

Data for spiritual considerations from Andrews MM, Hanson PA: Religion, culture, and nursing. *In* Andrews MM, Boyle JS (Eds): Transcultural Concepts in Nursing Care, 2nd ed. Philadelphia, J.B. Lippincott Company, 1995.

*Cultural Assessment is reprinted in a format intended for direct use with patients in Jarvis CM: *Student Laboratory Manual for Physical Examination and Health Assessment,* 3rd ed. (Philadelphia, W.B. Saunders Company, 2000.

drives from community resources, friends? Neighborhood: secure in personal safety at day or night; danger of loss of possessions; amount of noise and pollution; access to family and friends, grocery store, drug store, laundry, church, temple, mosque, health care facilities?

TRANSCULTURAL **CONSIDERATIONS**

Cultural Assessment

One aspect of a comprehensive health history concerns the collection of data related to culturally based beliefs and practices about health and illness. A *cultural assessment* refers to a systematic appraisal or examination of individuals, groups, and communities in relation to their cultural beliefs, values, and practices to determine explicit nursing needs and intervention practices within the cultural context of the people being evaluated (Leininger, 1991). Cultural assessments tend to be broad and comprehensive because they deal with cultural values, belief systems, and ways of living now and in the recent past. However, you can learn to appraise segments of these larger areas, such as a particular cultural value, and then relate this finding to other aspects such as cultural practices. Table 5–2 summarizes major data categories pertaining to culture and offers suggested questions that you might ask the person to elicit the information.

Bibliography

American Academy of Pediatrics: *1997 Red Book*. Report of the Committee on Infectious Diseases, 24th ed. Elk Grove Village, IL. American Academy of Pediatrics, 1997.

Andersen SJ, Johnson MA: Caring for patients on the edge of decline. Am J Nurs 96(12):16B–16D, Dec 1996.

Andrews MM, Boyle JS (Eds): Transcultural Concepts in Nursing Care, 2nd ed. Philadelphia, J.B. Lippincott Company, 1995.

Bernstein LH: A public health approach to functional assessment. Caring 11 (12):32–38, 1992.

Byrnes K: Conducting the pediatric health history: A guide. Pediatr Nurs 22(2):135–137, Mar–Apr 1996.

Campbell LA, Thompson BL: Evaluating elderly patients: A critique of comprehensive functional assessment tools. Nurse Pract 15(8):11–18, 1990.

Caulker-Burnett I: Primary care screening for substance abuse. Nurs Pract 19(6):42–48, 1994.

Ewing JA: Detecting alcoholism: The CAGE questionnaire. JAMA 252: 1905–1907, 1984.

Fleming KC et al: Practical functional assessment of elderly persons: A primary care approach. Mayo Clin Proc 70:890–910, Sept 1995.

Gordon M: Nursing Diagnosis: Process and Application. St. Louis, Mosby-Year Book, 1994.

Granger CV, Albrecht GL, Hamilton BB: Outcome of comprehensive medical rehabilitation: Measures of PULSES profile and the Barthel index. Arch Phys Med Rehabil 60:145–154, 1979.

Granger CV, Ottenbacher KJ, Baker JG, Sehgal A: Reliability of a brief outpatient functional outcome assessment measure. Am J Phys Med Rehabil 74(6):469–475, Nov–Dec 1995.

Jackson PL: Age-specific well child charting forms. Nurs Pract 19(3): 14–18, 1994.

Katz S, Ford AB, Moskowitz RS, et al: Studies of illness in the aged. The Index of ADL: A standardized measure of biological and psychosocial function. JAMA 185:94–98, 1963.

Kempen GIJ, Steverink N, Ormel J, Deeg DJH: The assessment of ADL among frail elderly in an interview survey: Self-report versus performance-based tests and determinants of discrepancies. J Gerontol 51B(5):254–260, 1996.

Leininger M: Culture care diversity and universality: A theory of nursing. New York, National League for Nursing, 1991.

Lekan-Rutledge D: Functional assessment. *In* Matteson M, McConnell ES (Eds): Gerontological Nursing, 2nd ed. Philadelphia, W.B. Saunders Company, 1996.

Linn MW, Linn BS: The rapid disability rating scale—2. J Am Geriatr Soc 30(6):378–382, 1982.

Mahon SM: Identification and education of persons with a hereditary predisposition to malignancy. Nurs Pract 22(6):18–31, June 1997.

Mahoney FI, Barthel DW: Functional evaluation: The Barthel Index. Md State Med J 14:61–65, 1965.

Pearlman R: Development of a functional assessment questionnaire for geriatric patients: The comprehensive older persons' evaluation (COPE). J Chronic Dis 40:85S–94S, 1987.

Staab AM: Adult immunization: Recommendations for optimal protection. Clin Rev 8(10):55–77, Oct 1998.

Stone AT, Wyman JF, Salisbury SS (Eds): Clinical Gerontological Nursing: A Guide to Advanced Practice, 2nd ed. Philadelphia, W.B. Saunders Company, 1998.

Twining S: The occupational and environmental health history: Guidelines for the primary care nurse practitioner. Nurse Pract Forum 6(2):64–71, June 1995.

U.S. Department of Health and Human Services: Alcohol and Health (Publication No. ADM-281-91-0003). Alexandria, VA, National Institutes of Health, National Institute on Alcohol Abuse and Alcoholism, 1993.

Volk RJ, Steinbauer JR, Cantor SB, Holzer CE: The Alcohol Use Disorders Identification Test (AUDIT) as a screen for at-risk drinking in primary care patients of different racial/ethnic backgrounds. Addiction 92(2):197–206, 1997.

Williams GD: Preoperative assessment and health history interview. Nurs Clin North Am 32(2):395–416, June 1997.

CHAPTER SIX

Mental Status Assessment

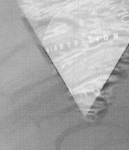

Function

DEFINING MENTAL STATUS

DEVELOPMENTAL CONSIDERATIONS

Infants and Children

The Aging Adult

COMPONENTS OF THE MENTAL STATUS EXAMINATION

Objective Data

APPEARANCE

BEHAVIOR

COGNITIVE FUNCTIONS

Judgment

THOUGHT PROCESSES AND PERCEPTIONS

SUPPLEMENTAL MENTAL STATUS EXAMINATION

DEVELOPMENTAL CONSIDERATIONS

Infants and Children

The Aging Adult

Behavior

Cognitive Functions

Supplemental Mental Status Examination

Application & Critical Thinking

NURSING DIAGNOSES

Abnormal Findings

LEVELS OF CONSCIOUSNESS

SPEECH DISORDERS

ABNORMALITIES OF MOOD AND AFFECT

ABNORMALITIES OF THOUGHT PROCESS

ABNORMALITIES OF THOUGHT CONTENT

ABNORMALITIES OF PERCEPTION

DELIRIUM, DEMENTIA, AND AMNESTIC DISORDERS

SUBSTANCE USE DISORDERS

SCHIZOPHRENIA

MOOD DISORDERS

ANXIETY DISORDERS

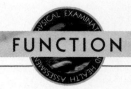
DEFINING MENTAL STATUS

Mental status is a person's emotional and cognitive functioning. Optimal functioning aims toward simultaneous life satisfaction in work, in caring relationships, and within the self. Mental health is relative and ongoing. Everyone has "good" and "bad" days. Usually, mental status strikes a balance, allowing the person to function socially and occupationally.

The stress surrounding a traumatic life event (death of a loved one, serious illness) tips the balance, causing transient dysfunction. This is an expected response to a trauma. Mental status assessment at this time can identify remaining strengths and can help the individual mobilize resources and use coping skills.

A **mental disorder** is apparent when a person's response is much greater than the expected reaction to a traumatic life event. A mental disorder is defined as a significant behavioral or psychological *pattern* that is associated with distress (a painful symptom) or disability (impaired functioning) and has a significant risk of pain, disability, or death, or a loss of freedom (American Psychiatric Association, 1994). Mental disorders include **organic disorders** (due to brain disease of *known* specific organic cause, e.g., delirium, dementia, intoxication, and withdrawal), and **psychiatric mental illness** (in which organic etiology has not yet been established, e.g., anxiety disorder or schizophrenia). Mental status assessment documents a dysfunction and determines how that dysfunction affects self-care in everyday life.

Mental status cannot be scrutinized directly like the characteristics of skin or heart sounds. Its functioning is *inferred* through assessment of an individual's behaviors:

Consciousness: being aware of one's own existence, feelings, and thoughts and aware of the environment. This is the most elementary of mental status functions.

Language: using the voice to communicate one's thoughts and feelings. This is a basic tool of humans, and its loss has a heavy social impact on the individual.

Mood and affect: both of these elements deal with the prevailing feelings; **affect** is a temporary expression of feelings or state of mind, and **mood** is more durable, a prolonged display of feelings that color the whole emotional life.

Orientation: the awareness of the objective world in relation to the self.

Attention: the power of concentration, the ability to focus on one specific thing without being distracted by many environmental stimuli.

Memory: the ability to lay down and store experiences and perceptions for later recall. *Recent* memory evokes day-to-day events; *remote* memory brings up years' worth of experiences.

Abstract reasoning: pondering a deeper meaning beyond the concrete and literal.

Thought process: the *way* a person thinks, the logical train of thought.

Thought content: *what* the person thinks—specific ideas, beliefs, the use of words.

Perceptions: an awareness of objects through any of the five senses.

DEVELOPMENTAL CONSIDERATIONS

Infants and Children

The maturation of emotional and cognitive functioning is described in detail in Chapter 2. It is difficult to separate and trace the development of just one aspect of mental status. All aspects are interdependent. For example, consciousness is rudimentary at birth because the cerebral cortex is not yet developed; the infant cannot distinguish the self from the mother's body. Consciousness gradually develops along with language, so that by 18 to 24 months the child learns that he or she is separate from objects in the environment and has words to express this. We also can trace language development: from the differentiated crying at 4 weeks, the cooing at 6 weeks, through one-word sentences at 1 year to multiword sentences at 2 years. Yet the concept of language as a social tool of communication occurs around 4 to 5 years of age, coincident with the child's readiness to cooperatively play with other children.

Attention gradually increases in span through preschool years so that, by school age, most children are able to sit and concentrate on their work for a period of time. Some children are late in developing concentration. School readiness coincides with the development of the thought process; around age 7, thinking becomes more logical and systematic, and the child is able to reason and understand. Abstract thinking, the ability to consider a hypothetical situation, usually develops between ages 12 and 15, although a few adolescents never achieve it.

The Aging Adult

The aging process leaves the parameters of mental status mostly intact. There is no decrease in general knowledge and little or no loss in vocabulary. Response time is slower than in youth; it takes a bit longer for the brain to process information and react to it. Thus, performance on timed intelligence tests may be lower for the aging person, not because intelligence has declined, but because it takes longer to respond to the questions. The slower response time affects new learning; if a new presentation is rapidly paced, the older person does not have time to respond to it (Birren and Schaie, 1996).

Recent memory, which requires some processing (e.g., medication instructions, 24-hour diet recall, names of new acquaintances), is somewhat decreased with aging. Remote memory is not affected.

Age-related changes in sensory perception can affect mental status. For example, vision loss (as detailed in Chapter 12) may result in apathy, social isolation, and depression. Hearing changes are common in older adults (see the discussion of presbycusis in Chapter 13). Age-related hearing loss involves high sound frequencies. Consonants are high-frequency sounds, so older people who have difficulty hearing them have problems with normal conversation. This problem produces frustration, suspicion, and social isolation, and also makes the person look confused.

The era of older adulthood contains more potential for loss than do earlier eras, such as loss of loved ones, loss of job status and prestige, loss of income, and the loss of an energetic and resilient body. The grief and despair surrounding these losses can affect mental status. These losses can result in disorientation, disability, or depression.

COMPONENTS OF THE MENTAL STATUS EXAMINATION

The full mental status examination is a systematic check of emotional and cognitive functioning. The steps described here, though, rarely need to be taken in their entirety. Usually, you can assess mental status through the context of the health history interview. During that time, keep in mind the four main headings of mental status assessment:

appearance, behavior, cognition,
and thought processes, or
A, B, C, T

Integrating the mental status examination into the health history interview is sufficient for most people. You will collect ample data to be able to assess mental health strengths and coping skills, and to screen for any dysfunction.

It is necessary to perform a full mental status examination when you discover any abnormality in affect or behavior, and in the following situations:

- Family members concerned about a person's behavioral changes, e.g., memory loss, inappropriate social interaction.
- Brain lesions (trauma, tumor, brain attack [formerly known as cerebrovascular accident or stroke]). A mental status assessment documents any emotional or cognitive change associated with the lesion. Not recognizing these changes hinders care planning and creates problems with social readjustment.
- Aphasia (the impairment of language secondary to brain damage). A mental status examination assesses language dysfunction as well as any emotional problems associated with it, such as depression or agitation.
- Symptoms of psychiatric mental illness, especially with acute onset.

In every mental status examination, note these factors from the health history that could affect your interpretation of the findings:

- Any known illnesses or health problems, such as alcoholism or chronic renal disease
- Current medications whose side effects may cause confusion or depression
- The usual educational and behavioral level—note that factor as the normal baseline, and do not expect performance on the mental status examination to exceed it
- Responses to personal history questions, indicating current stress, social interaction patterns, sleep habits, drug and alcohol use

In the following examination, the sequence of steps forms a *hierarchy* in which the most basic functions (consciousness, language) are assessed first. The first steps must be accurately assessed to ensure validity for the steps to follow. That is, if consciousness is clouded, then the person cannot be expected to have full attention and to cooperate with new learning. Or, if language is impaired, subsequent assessment of new learning or abstract reasoning (anything that requires language functioning) can give erroneous conclusions.

Normal Range of Findings	Abnormal Findings

APPEARANCE

Posture. *Posture* is erect and *position* is relaxed.

Body movements. *Body movements* are voluntary, deliberate, coordinated, and smooth and even.

Dress. *Dress* is appropriate for setting, season, age, gender, and social group. Clothing fits and is put on appropriately.

Grooming and hygiene. The person is clean and well groomed, hair is neat and clean, women have moderate or no make-up, men are shaved or beard or moustache are well groomed. Nails are clean (though some jobs leave nails chronically dirty). Note: A disheveled appearance in a previously well-groomed person is significant. Use care in interpreting clothing that is disheveled, bizarre, or in poor repair, because these sometimes reflect the person's economic status or a deliberate fashion trend.

Abnormal Findings

Sitting on edge of chair or curled in bed, tense muscles, frowning, darting watchful eyes, restless pacing occur with anxiety and with hyperthyroidism. Sitting slumped in chair, slow walk, dragging feet occur with depression and some organic brain diseases.

Restless, fidgety movements, or hyperkinetic appearance occur with anxiety.
Apathy and psychomotor slowing occur with depression and organic brain disease.
Abnormal posturing and bizarre gestures occur with schizophrenia.
Facial grimaces.

Inappropriate dress can occur with organic brain syndrome.
Eccentric dress combination and bizarre make-up occur with schizophrenia or manic syndrome.

Unilateral neglect (total inattention to one side of body) occurs following some cerebrovascular accidents.
Inappropriate dress, poor hygiene, and lack of concern with appearance occur with depression and severe Alzheimer's disease. Meticulously dressed and groomed appearance and fastidious manner may occur with obsessive-compulsive disorders.

Normal Range of Findings	Abnormal Findings

BEHAVIOR

Level of Consciousness. The person is awake, alert, aware of stimuli from the environment and within the self, and responds appropriately to stimuli.

Facial Expression. The look is appropriate to the situation and changes appropriately with the topic. There is comfortable eye contact unless precluded by cultural norm, e.g., Native American.

Speech. Judge the quality of speech by noting that the person makes laryngeal sounds effortlessly and shares conversation appropriately.

The pace of the conversation is moderate, and stream of talking is fluent.

Articulation (ability to form words) is clear and understandable.

Word choice is effortless and appropriate to educational level. The person completes sentences, occasionally pausing to think.

Mood and Affect. Judge this by body language and facial expression, and by asking directly, "How do you feel today," or "How do you usually feel?" The mood should be appropriate to the person's place and condition and change appropriately with topics. The person is willing to cooperate with you.

COGNITIVE FUNCTIONS

Orientation. You can discern orientation through the course of the interview, or ask for it directly, using tact. "Some people have trouble keeping up with the dates while in the hospital. Do you know today's date?" Assess:

Time: day of week, date, year, season
Place: where person lives, present location, type of building, name of city and
  state
Person: own name, age, who examiner is, type of worker

Many hospitalized people normally have trouble with the exact date but are fully oriented on the remaining items.

Abnormal Findings column:

Lethargic, obtunded. See Table 6–3, Levels of Consciousness.

Flat, masklike expression occurs with parkinsonism and depression.

Dysphonia is abnormal volume, pitch, see Table 6–4.
Monopolizes interview. Silent, secretive, or uncommunicative.
Slow, monotonous speech with parkinsonism, depression. Rapid-fire, pressured, and loud talking occur with manic syndrome.
Dysarthria is distorted speech, see Table 6–4. Misuse of words; omits letters, syllables, or words; transposes words; occurs with aphasia. Circumlocution, or repetitious abnormal patterns: neologism, echolalia, see Table 6–6.
Unduly long word-finding or failure in word search occurs with aphasia.

See Table 6–5, Abnormalities of Mood and Affect. Wide mood swings occur with manic syndrome. Bizarre mood is apparent in schizophrenia.

Disorientation occurs with organic brain disorders, such as delirium and dementia. Orientation is usually lost in this order—first to time, then to place, and rarely to person.

Attention Span. Check the person's ability to concentrate by noting whether he or she completes a thought without wandering. Note any distractibility or difficulty attending to you. Or, give a series of directions to follow and note the correct sequence of behaviors, e.g., "Please take this glass of water with your left hand, drink from it, shift it to your right hand, and set it on the table." Note that attention span commonly is impaired in people who are anxious, fatigued, or drug intoxicated.

Digression from initial thought. Irrelevant replies to questions. Easily distracted; "stimulus bound," i.e., any new stimulus quickly draws attention. Confusion, negativism.

Recent Memory. Assess recent memory in the context of the interview by the 24-hour diet recall or by asking the time the person arrived at the agency. Ask questions you can corroborate. This screens for the occasional person who confabulates or makes up answers to fill in the gaps of memory loss.

Recent memory deficit occurs with organic disorders, e.g., delirium, dementia, amnestic syndrome, or Korsakoff's syndrome in chronic alcoholism.

Remote Memory. In the context of the interview, ask the person verifiable past events, e.g., describe past health, the first job, birthday and anniversary dates, and historical events that are relevant for that person.

Remote memory is lost when cortical storage area for that memory is damaged, such as in Alzheimer's dementia or any disease that damages the cerebral cortex.

New Learning—The Four Unrelated Words Test. This tests the person's ability to lay down new memories. It is a highly sensitive and valid memory test. It requires more effort than does the recall of personal or historic events. It also avoids the danger of unverifiable material.

To the person, say, "I am going to say four words. I want you to remember them. In a few minutes I will ask you to recall them." To be sure the person has understood, have the words repeated. Pick four words with semantic and phonetic diversity:

1. brown
2. honesty
3. tulip
4. eyedropper

1. fun
2. carrot
3. ankle
4. loyalty

After 5 minutes, ask for the recall of the four words. To test the duration of memory, ask for a recall at 10 minutes and at 30 minutes. The normal response for persons under 60 years is an accurate three- or four-word recall after a 5-, 10-, and 30-minute delay (Strub and Black, 1993).

People with Alzheimer's dementia score a zero- or one-word recall. Impaired new learning ability also occurs with anxiety (due to inattention and distractibility) and depression (due to lack of effort mobilized to remember).

Additional Testing for Persons with Aphasia

Word Comprehension. Point to articles in the room, parts of the body, articles from pockets, and ask the person to name them.

Reading. Ask the person to read available print. Be aware that reading is related to educational level. Use caution that you are not just testing literacy.

Writing. Ask the person to make up and write a sentence. Note coherence, spelling, and parts of speech (the sentence should have a subject and verb).

Aphasia is the loss of the ability to speak or write coherently, or to understand speech or writing, due to a brain attack (cerebral vascular accident or CVA). See Table 6–4, Speech Disorders. This functioning is important in planning health teaching and rehabilitation.

Normal Range of Findings	Abnormal Findings

Higher Intellectual Function

These tests measure problem-solving and reasoning abilities. Results are closely related to the person's general intelligence and must be assessed considering educational and cultural background. Tests of higher intellectual functioning have been used to discriminate between organic brain disease and psychiatric disorders; errors on the tests indicate organic dysfunction.

Although they have been widely used, there is little evidence that most of these tests are valid in detecting organic brain disease (Keller and Manschreck, 1981). Furthermore, most of these tests have little relevance for daily clinical care. Thus, many time-honored, standard tests of higher intellectual function are not discussed here, such as fund of general knowledge, digit span repetition, calculation, proverb interpretation and similarities to test abstract reasoning, or hypothetical situations to test judgment.

Judgment

A person exercises judgment when he or she can compare and evaluate the alternatives in a situation and reach an appropriate course of action. Rather than testing the person's response to a hypothetical situation (e.g., "What would you do if you found a stamped, addressed envelope lying on the sidewalk?"), you should be more interested in the person's judgment about daily or long-term life goals, the likelihood of acting in response to delusions or hallucinations, and the capacity for violent or suicidal behavior.

To assess judgment in the context of the interview, note what the person says about job plans, social or family obligations, and plans for the future. Job and future plans should be realistic, considering the person's health situation. Also, ask the person to describe the rationale for personal health care, and how he or she decided about whether or not to comply with prescribed health regimens. The person's actions and decisions should be realistic.

Impaired judgment (unrealistic or impulsive decisions, wish fulfillment), occurs with mental retardation, emotional dysfunction, schizophrenia, and organic brain disease.

THOUGHT PROCESSES AND PERCEPTIONS

Thought Processes. Ask yourself, "Does this person make sense? Can I follow what the person is saying?" The *way* a person thinks should be logical, goal directed, coherent, and relevant. The person should complete a thought.

Illogical, unrealistic thought processes. Digression from initial thought. Ideas run together. Evidence of blocking (person stops in middle of thought). See Table 6–6, Abnormalities of Thought Process.

Thought Content. *What* the person says should be consistent and logical.

Obsessions, compulsions. See Table 6–7, Abnormalities of Thought Content.

Perceptions. The person should be consistently aware of reality. The perceptions should be congruent with yours. Ask the following questions:

● How do people treat you?
● Do other people talk about you?
● Do you feel like you are being watched, followed, or controlled?
● Is your imagination very active?
● Have you heard your name when alone?

Illusions, hallucinations. See Table 6–8, Abnormalities of Perception. Auditory and visual hallucinations occur with psychiatric and organic brain disease and with psychedelic drugs. Tactile hallucinations occur with alcohol withdrawal.

|

Screen for Suicidal Thoughts. When the person expresses feelings of sadness, hopelessness, despair or grief, it is important to assess any possible risk of physical harm to himself or herself. Begin with more general questions. If you hear affirmative answers, continue with more specific questions:

- Have you ever felt so blue you thought of hurting yourself?
- Do you feel like hurting yourself now?
- Do you have a plan to hurt yourself?
- What would happen if you were dead?
- How would other people react if you were dead?

It is very difficult to question people about possible suicidal wishes, especially for beginning examiners. Examiners fear invading privacy and may have their own normal denial of death and suicide. However, the risk is far greater if you skip these questions when you have the slightest clue that they are appropriate. You may be the only health professional to pick up clues of suicide risk. You are responsible for encouraging the person to talk about suicidal thoughts. Sometimes you cannot prevent a suicide when someone really wishes to kill himself or herself. However, for the people who are ambivalent, and they are the majority, you can buy time so the person can be helped to find an alternate route to the situation.

A precise suicide plan to take place in the next 24 to 48 hours using a lethal method constitutes high risk. Important clues and warning signs of suicide:

Prior suicide attempts
Depression, hopelessness
Social withdrawal, running away
Self-mutilation
Hypersomnia or insomnia
Slowed psychomotor activity
Anorexia
Verbal suicide messages (defeat, failure, worthlessness, loss, giving up, desire to kill self)
Death themes in art, jokes, writing, behaviors
Saying goodbye (giving away prized possessions)

Additional content on mental disorders is listed in Table 6–9, Delirium, Dementia, and Amnestic Disorders; Table 6–10, Substance Use Disorders; Table 6–11, Schizophrenia; Table 6–12, Mood Disorders; and Table 6–13, Anxiety Disorders.

SUPPLEMENTAL MENTAL STATUS EXAMINATION

The Mini-Mental State is a simplified scored form of the cognitive functions of the mental status examination (Folstein et al., 1975; replicated by Depaulo and Folstein, 1978; Table 6–1). It is quick and easy, includes a standard set of only 11 questions, and requires only 5 to 10 minutes to administer. It is useful for both initial and serial measurement, so you can demonstrate worsening or improvement of cognition over time and with treatment. It concentrates only on cognitive functioning, not on mood or thought processes. It is a valid detector of organic disease; thus, it is a good screening tool to detect dementia and delirium and to differentiate these from psychiatric mental illness.

The maximum score on the test is 30; people with normal mental status average 27. Scores between 24 and 30 indicate no cognitive impairment.

Scores that occur with dementia and delirium are classified as follows: 18–23 = mild cognitive impairment; 0–7 = severe cognitive impairment.

Table 6-1 • Mini-Mental State Examination

Patient _____ Examiner _____ Date _____

Maximum Score	Score	
		Orientation
5	( )	What is the (year) (season) (date) (day) (month)?
5	( )	Where are we: (state) (county) (town) (hospital) (floor)
		Registration
3	( )	Name three objects: (Apple, Penny, Table) 1 second to say each. Then ask the patient all three after you have said them. Give 1 point for each correct answer. Then repeat them until he or she learns all three. Count trials and record. Trials _____
		Attention and Calculation
5	( )	Serial 7's. 1 point for each correct. Stop after five answers. Alternatively spell "world" backwards.
		Recall
3	( )	Ask for the three objects repeated above. Give 1 point for each correct.
		Language
9	( )	Name a pencil, and watch (2 points)

Repeat the following "No ifs, ands, or buts." (1 point)
Follow a three-stage command:
   "Take a paper in your right hand, fold it in half, and put it on the floor." (3 points)
Read and obey the following:
   CLOSE YOUR EYES (1 point)
Write a sentence (1 point)
Copy design (overlapping pentagons) (1 point)

Overlapping pentagons

Total Score _____
ASSESS level of consciousness along a continuum _____
Alert   Drowsy   Stupor   Coma

Instructions for Administration of Mini-Mental State Examination

Orientation

(1) Ask for the date. Then ask specifically for parts omitted, e.g., "Can you also tell me what season it is?" One point for each correct.
(2) Ask in turn "Can you tell me the name of this hospital?" (town, country, etc.). One point for each correct.

Registration

Ask the patient if you may test his or her memory. Then say the names of three unrelated objects, clearly and slowly, about 1 second for each. After you have said all three, ask him or her to repeat them. This first repetition determines his or her score (0–3), but keep saying them until he or she can repeat all three, up to six trials. If he or she does not eventually learn all three, recall cannot be meaningfully tested.

Attention and Calculation

Ask the patient to begin with 100 and count backwards by 7. Stop after five subtractions (93, 86, 79, 72, 65). Score the total number of correct answers.
If the patient cannot or will not perform this task, ask him or her to spell the word "world" backwards. The score is the number of letters in correct order, e.g., dlrow = 5, dlorw = 3.

Recall

Ask the patient if he or she can recall the three words you previously asked him or her to remember. Score 0–3.

Language

Naming: Show the patient a wrist watch and ask him or her what it is. Repeat for pencil. Score 0–2.
Repetition: Ask the patient to repeat the sentence after you. Allow only one trial. Score 0 or 1.
Three-stage command: Give the patient a piece of plain blank paper and repeat the command. Score 1 point for each part correctly executed.
Reading: On a blank piece of paper print the sentence "Close your eyes," in letters large enough for the patient to see clearly. Ask him or her to read it and do what it says. Score 1 point only if he or she actually closes his or her eyes.
Writing: Give the patient a blank piece of paper and ask him or her to write a sentence for you. Do not dictate a sentence, it is to be written spontaneously. It must contain a subject and verb and be sensible. Correct grammar and punctuation are not necessary.
Copying: On a clean piece of paper, draw intersecting pentagons, each side about 1 inch, and ask him or her to copy it exactly as it is. All 10 angles must be present, and 2 must intersect to score 1 point. Tremor and rotation are ignored.
Estimate the patient's level of sensorium along a continuum, from alert on the left to coma on the right.

From Folstein MF, Folstein SE, McHugh PR: Mini-mental state. J Psychiatric Res 12:189–198, 1975. Reprinted with permission. © 1975, 1998 Mini-Mental LLC.

DEVELOPMENTAL CONSIDERATIONS

Infants and Children

The mental status assessment of infants and children covers behavioral, cognitive, and psychosocial development, and examines how the child is coping with his or her environment. Essentially, you will follow the same A-B-C-T guidelines as for the adult, with special consideration for developmental milestones. Your best examination "technique" arises from thorough knowledge of developmental milestones as described in Chapter 2. Abnormalities are often problems of *omission;* the child does not achieve a milestone you would expect.

The parent's health history, especially the sections on the developmental history and personal history, yields most of the mental status data.

In addition, the Denver II screening test (see Chapter 2) gives you a chance to interact directly with the young child to assess mental status. For the child from birth to 6 years of age, the Denver II helps identify those who may be slow in development in behavioral, language, cognitive, and psychosocial areas. An additional language test is the Denver Articulation Screening Exam.

For school-age children, ages 7 to 11, who have grown beyond the age when developmental milestones are very useful, the "Behavioral Checklist" (Table 6–2) is an additional tool that can be given to the parent along with the history. It covers five major areas: mood, play, school, friends, and family relations. It is easy to administer and lasts about 5 minutes.

For the adolescent, follow the same A-B-C-T guidelines as described for the adult.

Table 6–2 • Behavioral Checklist

1. Prefers to play alone
2. Gets hurt in major accidents
3. Does he/she ever play with fire?
4. Has difficulties with teachers
5. Gets poor grades in school
6. Is absent from school
7. Becomes angry easily
8. Daydreams
9. Feels unhappy
10. Acts younger than other children his/her age
11. Does not listen to parents
12. Does not tell the truth
13. Unsure of himself/herself
14. Has trouble sleeping
15. Seems afraid of someone or something
16. Is nervous and jumpy
17. Has a nervous habit
18. Does not show feelings
19. Fights with other children
20. Is understanding of other people's feelings
21. Refuses to share
22. Shows jealousy
23. Takes things that are not his/hers
24. Blames others for his/her troubles
25. Prefers to play with children not his/her age
26. Gets along well with grown-ups
27. Teases others

Scoring is a point system: 0—never; 1—sometimes; 2—often.
Scoring is reversed for items 20 and 26.

From Jellinek M, Evans N, Knight R: Use of a behavior checklist on a pediatric inpatient unit. J Pediatr 94:156–158, 1979.

Scores between 15 and 22 indicate closer following; scores above 22 warrant psychiatric evaluation.

Normal Range of Findings	Abnormal Findings

The Aging Adult

It is important to conduct even a brief examination of all older people admitted to the hospital. Confusion is common in aging people and is easily misdiagnosed. Between one-third and one-half of older adults admitted to acute-care medical and surgical services show varying degrees of confusion. In the community, about 5% of adults over 65 and almost 20% of those over 75 have some degree of clinically detectable impaired cognitive function (Kane et al., 1994).

Check sensory status before assessing any aspect of mental status. Vision and hearing changes due to aging may alter alertness and leave the person looking confused. When older people cannot hear your questions, they may test worse than they actually are. One group of 21 older people with psychiatric mental illness tested significantly better when they wore hearing aids (Kreeger et al., 1995).

Follow the same A-B-C-T guidelines as described for the younger adult with these *additional* considerations:

Behavior

Level of Consciousness. In a hospital or extended care setting, the Glasgow Coma Scale (see Chapter 21) is a quantitative tool that is useful in testing consciousness in aging persons in whom confusion is common. It gives a numerical value to the person's response in eye-opening, best verbal response, and best motor response. This system avoids ambiguity when numerous examiners care for the same person.

Cognitive Functions

Orientation. Many aging persons experience social isolation, loss of structure without a job, a change in residence, or some short-term memory loss. These factors affect orientation, and this person may not provide the precise date or complete name of agency. You may consider aging persons oriented if they know *generally* where they are and the present period. That is, consider them oriented to time if the year and month are correctly stated. Orientation to place is accepted with the correct identification of the type of setting (e.g., the hospital) and the name of the town.

New Learning. In people of normal cognitive function, an age-related decline occurs in performance in the Four Unrelated Words Test described on p. 108 (Strub and Black, 1993). Persons in the eighth decade average two of four words recalled over 5 minutes. They will improve their performance at 10 and 30 minutes after being reminded by verbal cues, e.g., "one word was a color; a common flower in Holland is _____."

People with Alzheimer's dementia do not improve their performance on subsequent trials.

Supplemental Mental Status Examination

Set Test. The Set Test was developed specifically for use with an aging population. The original study tested people 65 to 85 years of age. It is a quantifiable test, designed to screen for dementia (Isaacs and Kennie, 1973). The test is easy to administer and takes less than 5 minutes. Ask the person to name 10 items in each of four categories or sets: fruits, animals, colors, and towns (FACT). Do not coach, prompt, or hurry the person. Each correct answer is one point. The maximum total score is 40. No one with a score over 25 has been found to have dementia. (Note: Since this is a verbal test, do not use it with persons with hearing impairments or aphasia.)

Set Test scores of less than 15 indicate dementia. Scores between 15 and 24 show less association with dementia and should be evaluated carefully.

The Set Test is a more holistic approach to testing cognitive function. It assesses mental function as a whole instead of examining individual parts of cognitive function. That is, by asking the person to categorize, name, remember, and count the items in the test, you are really assessing this person's alertness, motivation, concentration, short-term memory, and problem-solving ability.

 SUMMARY CHECKLIST: Mental Status Assessment

1: Appearance
Posture
Body movements
Dress
Grooming and hygiene

2: Behavior
Level of consciousness
Facial expression
Speech (quality, pace, articulation, word choice)
Mood and affect

3: Cognitive functions
Orientation
Attention span
Recent and remote memory
New learning—the Four Unrelated Words test
Judgment

4: Thought processes
Thought processes
Thought content
Perceptions
Screen for suicidal thoughts (when indicated)

5: Perform the Mini-Mental State Examination

APPLICATION AND CRITICAL THINKING

SAMPLE CHARTING

Appearance: Person's posture is erect, with no involuntary body movements. Dress and grooming are appropriate for season and setting.

Behavior: Person is alert, with appropriate facial expression and fluent, understandable speech. Affect and verbal responses are appropriate.

Cognitive functions: Oriented to time, person, place. Able to attend cooperatively with examiner. Recent and remote memory intact. Can recall four unrelated words at 5-, 10-, and 30-minute testing intervals. Future plans include returning to home and to local university once individual therapy is established and medication is adjusted.

Thought processes: Perceptions and thought processes are logical and coherent. No suicide ideation.

Score on Mini-Mental State examination is 28.

CLINICAL CASE STUDY

Lola P. is a 79-year-old white married woman, with a recent hospitalization for evaluation of increasing memory loss, confusion, and socially inappropriate behavior. Her family reports that Mrs. P's hygiene and grooming have decreased, she eats very little and has lost weight, does not sleep through the night, has angry emotional outbursts that are unlike her former demeanor, and does not recognize her younger grandchildren. Her husband reports that she has drifted away from the stove while cooking, allowing food to burn on the stovetop. He has found her wandering through the house in the middle of the night, unsure of where she was. She used to "talk on the phone for hours" but now he has to push her into conversations. During this hospitalization, Mrs. P. has undergone a series of medical tests, including a negative lumbar puncture test, normal electroencephalogram (EEG), and a benign head computed tomography (CT) scan. Her physician now suggests a diagnosis of senile dementia of the Alzheimer's type (SDAT).

Appearance: Sitting quietly, somewhat slumped, picking on loose threads on her dress. Hooded, zippered sweatshirt top worn over dress. Hair is gathered in loose ponytail with stray wisps. No make-up.

Behavior: Awake and gazing at hands and lap. Expression is flat and vacant. Will make eye contact when called by name, although gaze quickly shifts back to lap. Speech is a bit slow but articulate; some trouble with word choice.

Cognitive functions: Oriented to person and place. Can state the season, but not the day of the week or the year. Is not able to repeat the correct sequence of complex directions involving lifting and shifting glass of water to other hand. Scores a one-word recall on the Four Unrelated Words test. Cannot tell examiner how she would plan a grocery shopping trip.

Thought processes: Experiences blocking in train of thought. Thought content is logical. Acts cranky and suspicious with family members. No suicide ideation.

Mini-Mental State examination score is 17, and shows poor recall ability and marked difficulty with serial 7s.

 ASSESSMENT

Chronic confusion
Impaired social interaction
Impaired memory

NURSING DIAGNOSES COMMONLY ASSOCIATED WITH MENTAL HEALTH DISORDERS

Diagnosis	Related Factors (Etiology)	Defining Characteristics (Symptoms and Signs)

Altered thought processes	Psychological conflicts
	Social isolation
	Side effects of sedatives, narcotics, or anesthetics
	Sleep deprivation
	Sensory overload or deprivation
	Stress
	Anxiety
	Depression
	Effects of aging
	Emotional trauma
	Exposure to unfamiliar environment
	Fear of the unknown
	Impaired judgment
	Limited attention span
	Loss of memory
	Negative reactions from others
	Actual loss of:
	   Control
	   Familiar objects
	   Routine surroundings
	   Significant other
		Agitation or depressed behavior
		Altered sleep patterns
		Inappropriate affect or social behavior
		Cognitive dissonance
		Confabulations
		Delusions or hallucinations
		Disorientation to time, place, person
		Distractibility
		Egocentricity
		Fabrication
		Hyper/hypovigilance
		Impaired ability to make decisions, solve problems, reason, abstract, conceptualize, calculate
		Inaccurate interpretation of environment
		Inability to perceive and/or repeat message clearly
		Memory deficits
		Non-reality-based thinking
		Nonsensical speech
		Obsessions

Continued

Diagnosis	Related Factors (Etiology)	Defining Characteristics (Symptoms and Signs)
Powerlessness	Immobility Difficulty in performing self-care Low self-esteem Cultural role Communication barriers Loss of financial independence Lifestyle of helplessness Lack of knowledge or skills Health care environment Illness-related regimen	Anger Violent behavior Anxiety Resentment Guilt Apathy Devalues own feelings or opinions Reluctance to express true feelings, fearing alienation from caregiver Verbal expressions of having no control over situation, outcome, or self-care Expressions of doubt about self-worth or role performance
Risk for violence (self-directed or directed at others)	Substance abuse or withdrawal Toxic reaction to medication Explosive, impulsive, immature personality Paranoia Panic state Rage reaction Manic excitement Loneliness Perceived threat to self-esteem Response to catastrophic event Suicidal behavior Change in mental or physical health status Feelings of alienation Physical, sexual, or psychological abuse Manipulative behavior Developmental crisis Lack of support systems Actual or potential loss of significant other Significant change in lifestyle	Rage Overt and aggressive acts Self-destructive behavior Aggression Increased motor activity Hostile, threatening verbalizations Body language: clenched fists, facial expressions, rigid posture, tautness Provocative behavior Increasing anxiety level Depression Paranoid ideation Expresses intent to harm self or others Possession of destructive means: gun, knife, or other weapon Hallucinations, delusions
Spiritual distress	Loss of significant others Challenged belief and value system Beliefs opposed by family, peers, or health care providers Disruption in usual religious activity Effects of personal and family disasters or major life changes	Feeling separated or alienated from deity Feelings of helplessness or hopelessness Expresses concerns about meaning of life and death and/or belief system Verbalizes inner conflict about beliefs Inability to participate in usual religious practices Regards illness as punishment

Other Related Nursing Diagnoses

ACTUAL	RISK/WELLNESS
Anxiety (see Chapter 16) Confusion, acute Confusion, chronic Family processes: Alcoholism, altered Impaired adjustment Impaired social interaction Ineffective individual coping Memory, impaired Personal identity disturbance Self-esteem disturbance Social isolation	**Risk** Risk for caregiver role strain **Wellness** Spiritual well-being, potential for enhanced

Table 6–3 LEVELS OF CONSCIOUSNESS

These terms are commonly used in clinical practice. They spread over a continuum from full alertness to deep coma. The terms are qualitative and therefore are not always reliable. (A *quantitative* tool that serves the same purpose and eliminates ambiguity is the Glasgow Coma Scale in Chapter 21.) These terms are widely accepted, however, and are useful as long as all co-workers agree on definitions and are consistent in their application. To increase clarity when using these terms, record also:

1. The level of stimulus used, ranging progressively from
   a. Name called in normal tone of voice
   b. Name called in loud voice
   c. Light touch on person's arm
   d. Vigorous shake of shoulder
   e. Pain applied

2. The person's response
   a. Amount and quality of movement
   b. Presence and coherence of speech
   c. Opening of eyes and making of eye contact
3. What the person does on cessation of your stimulus

(1) Alert

Awake or readily aroused, oriented, fully aware of external and internal stimuli and responds appropriately, conducts meaningful interpersonal interactions.

(2) Lethargic (or Somnolent)

Not fully alert, drifts off to sleep when not stimulated, can be aroused to name when called in normal voice but looks drowsy, responds appropriately to questions or commands but thinking seems slow and fuzzy, inattentive, loses train of thought, spontaneous movements are decreased.

(3) Obtunded

(Transitional state between lethargy and stupor; some sources omit this level.)

Sleeps most of time, difficult to arouse—needs loud shout or vigorous shake, acts confused when is aroused, converses in monosyllables, speech may be mumbled and incoherent, requires constant stimulation for even marginal cooperation.

(4) Stupor or Semi-Coma

Spontaneously unconscious, responds only to persistent and vigorous shake or pain; has appropriate motor response (i.e., withdraws hand to avoid pain); otherwise can only groan, mumble, or move restlessly; reflex activity persists.

(5) Coma

Completely unconscious, no response to pain or to any external or internal stimuli (e.g., when suctioned, does not try to push the catheter away), light coma has some reflex activity but no purposeful movement, deep coma has no motor response.

Acute Confusional State (Delirium)

Clouding of consciousness (dulled cognition, impaired alertness); inattentive; incoherent conversation; impaired recent memory and confabulatory for recent events; often agitated and having visual hallucinations; disoriented, with confusion worse at night when environmental stimuli are decreased.

Adapted from Strub RL, Black, FW: The Mental Status Examination in Neurology, 3rd ed. Philadelphia, F.A. Davis, 1993, with permission.

Table 6–4 SPEECH DISORDERS

Condition	Disorder of	Description
Dysphonia	Voice	Difficulty or discomfort in talking, with abnormal pitch or volume, due to laryngeal disease. Voice sounds hoarse or whispered, but articulation and language are intact.
Dysarthria	Articulation	Distorted speech sounds; speech may sound unintelligible; basic language (word choice, grammar, comprehension) intact.
Aphasia	Language comprehension and production secondary to brain damage	True language disturbance, defect in word choice and grammar or defect in comprehension; defect is in *higher* integrative language processing.

Types of Aphasia

An earlier dichotomy classified aphasias as expressive (difficulty producing language) or receptive (difficulty understanding language). Since all people with aphasia have some difficulty with expression, beginning examiners tend to classify them all as expressive. The following system is more descriptive.

Condition	Description
Global aphasia	The most common and severe form. Spontaneous speech is absent or reduced to a few stereotyped words or sounds. Comprehension is absent or reduced to only the person's own name and a few select words. Repetition, reading, and writing are severely impaired. Prognosis for language recovery is poor. Caused by a large lesion that damages most of combined anterior and posterior language areas.
Broca's aphasia	Expressive aphasia. The person can understand language but cannot express him- or herself using language. This is characterized by nonfluent, dysarthric, and effortful speech. The speech is mostly nouns and verbs (high-content words) with few grammatic fillers, termed "agrammatic" or "telegraphic" speech. Repetition and reading aloud are severely impaired. Auditory and reading comprehensions are surprisingly intact. Lesion is in anterior language area called the *motor speech cortex* or *Broca's area.*
Wernicke's aphasia	Receptive aphasia. The linguistic opposite of Broca's aphasia. The person can hear sounds and words but cannot relate them to previous experiences. Speech is fluent, effortless, and well articulated but has many paraphasias (word substitutions that are malformed or wrong) and neologisms (made up words) and often lacks substantive words. Speech can be totally incomprehensible. Often, there is a great urge to speak. Repetition, reading, and writing also are impaired. Lesion is in posterior language area called the *Association auditory cortex* or *Wernicke's area.*

(For a discussion of other types of aphasia [e.g., conduction, anomic, transcortical, and so on], please consult a neurology text.)

Table 6–5   ABNORMALITIES OF MOOD AND AFFECT

Type of Mood or Affect	Definition	Clinical Example
Flat affect (blunted affect)	Lack of emotional response; no expression of feelings; voice monotonous and face immobile	Topic varies, expression does not
Depression	Sad, gloomy, dejected; symptoms may occur with rainy weather, after a holiday, or with an illness; if the situation is temporary, symptoms fade quickly	"I've got the blues."
Depersonalization (lack of ego boundaries)	Loss of identity, feels estranged, perplexed about own identity and meaning of existence	"I don't feel real." "I feel like I'm not really here."
Elation	Joy and optimism, overconfidence, increased motor activity, not necessarily pathologic	"I'm feeling very happy."
Euphoria	Excessive well-being, unusually cheerful or elated, which is inappropriate considering physical and mental condition, implies a pathologic mood	"I am high." "I feel like I'm flying." "I feel on top of the world."
Anxiety	Worried, uneasy, apprehensive from the anticipation of a danger whose source is unknown	"I feel nervous and high strung." "I worry all the time." "I can't seem to make up my mind."
Fear	Worried, uneasy, apprehensive, external danger is known and identified	Fear of flying in airplanes
Irritability	Annoyed, easily provoked, impatient	Person internalizes a feeling of tension, and a seemingly mild stimulus "sets him (or her) off"
Rage	Furious, loss of control	Person has expressed violent behavior toward self or others
Ambivalence	The existence of opposing emotions toward an idea, object, person	A person feels love and hate toward another at the same time
Lability	Rapid shift of emotions	Person expresses euphoric, tearful, angry feelings in rapid succession
Inappropriate affect	Affect clearly discordant with the content of the person's speech	Laughs while discussing admission for liver biopsy

Table 6–6 ABNORMALITIES OF THOUGHT PROCESS

Type of Process	Definition	Clinical Example
Blocking	Sudden interruption in train of thought, unable to complete sentence, seems related to strong emotion	"Forgot what I was going to say."
Confabulation	Fabricates events to fill in memory gaps	Gives detailed description of his long walk around the hospital although you know Mr. J. remained in his room all afternoon.
Neologism	Coining a new word, invented word has no real meaning except for the person, may condense several words	"I'll have to turn on my thinkilator."
Circumlocution	Round-about expression, substituting a phrase when cannot think of name of object	Says "the thing you open the door with" instead of "key."
Circumstantiality	Talks with excessive and unnecessary detail, delays reaching point; sentences have a meaningful connection but are irrelevant (this occurs normally in some people)	"When was my surgery? Well I was 28, I was living with my aunt, she's the one with psoriasis, she had it bad that year because of the heat, the heat was worse then than it was the summer of '82, . . ."
Loosening associations	Shifting from one topic to an unrelated topic; person seems unaware that topics are unconnected	"My boss is angry with me and it wasn't even my fault. (pause) I saw that movie too, Lassie. I felt really bad about it. But she kept trying to land the airplane and she never knew what was going on."
Flight of ideas	Abrupt change, rapid skipping from topic to topic, practically continuous flow of accelerated speech; topics usually have recognizable associations or are plays on words	"Take this pill? The pill is blue. I feel blue. (sings) She wore blue velvet."
Word salad	Incoherent mixture of words, phrases, and sentences; illogical, disconnected, includes neologisms	"Beauty, red based five, pigeon, the street corner, sort-of."
Perseveration	Persistent repeating of verbal or motor response, even with varied stimuli	"I'm going to lock the door, lock the door. I walk every day and I lock the door. I usually take the dog and I lock the door."
Echolalia	Imitation, repeats others' words or phrases, often with a mumbling, mocking, or mechanical tone	Nurse: "I want you to take your pill." Patient (mocking): "Take your pill. Take your pill."
Clanging	Word choice based on sound, not meaning, includes nonsense rhymes and puns	"My feet are cold. Cold, bold, told. The bell tolled for me."

Table 6-7 ABNORMALITIES OF THOUGHT CONTENT

Type of Content	Definition	Clinical Example
Phobia	Strong, persistent, irrational fear of an object or situation, feels driven to avoid it	Cats, dogs, heights, enclosed spaces
Hypochondriasis	Morbid worrying about his or her own health, feels sick with no actual basis for that assumption	Preoccupied with the fear of having cancer; any symptom or physical sign means cancer
Obsession	Unwanted, persistent thoughts or impulses; logic will not purge them from consciousness; experienced as intrusive and senseless	Violence (parent having repeated impulse to kill a loved child); contamination (becoming infected by shaking hands)
Compulsion	Unwanted repetitive, purposeful act; driven to do it; behavior thought to neutralize or prevent discomfort or some dreaded event	Hand-washing, counting, checking and rechecking, touching
Delusions	Firm, fixed, false beliefs; irrational; person clings to delusion despite objective evidence to contrary	Grandiose—person believes he or she is God, famous historical, or sports figure, or other well-known person. Persecution—"They are out to get me."

Table 6-8 ABNORMALITIES OF PERCEPTION

Type of Perception	Definition	Clinical Example
Hallucination	Sensory perceptions for which there are no external stimuli; may strike any sense: visual, auditory, tactile, olfactory, gustatory	Visual: seeing an image (ghost) of a person who is not there; auditory: hearing voices or music
Illusion	*Mis*perception of an actual existing stimulus, by any sense	Folds of bedsheets appear to be animated

Table 6-9   DELIRIUM, DEMENTIA, AND AMNESTIC DISORDERS*

Delirium

A. **Disturbance of consciousness** (i.e., reduced clarity of awareness of the environment) with reduced ability to focus, sustain, or shift attention

B. A **change in cognition** (such as memory deficit, disorientation, language disturbance) or the development of a perceptual disturbance

C. The disturbance **develops over a short period of time** (usually hours to days) and tends to fluctuate during the course of the day

Delirium may be due to a **general medical condition:** systemic infections, metabolic disorders (e.g., hypoxia, hypercarbia, hypoglycemia), fluid or electrolyte imbalances, liver or kidney disease, thiamine deficiency, postoperative states, hypertensive encephalopathy, or following seizures or head trauma.

Delirium also may be **substance-induced** (i.e., due to a drug of abuse, a medication, or toxin exposure).

Dementia

A. The development of multiple cognitive deficits manifested by both
   1. **Memory impairment** (impaired ability to learn new information or to recall previously learned information)
   2. One (or more) of the following **cognitive disturbances:**
      a. Aphasia (language disturbance)
      b. Apraxia (impaired ability to carry out motor activities despite intact motor function)
      c. Agnosia (failure to recognize or identify objects despite intact sensory function)
      d. Disturbance in executive functioning (i.e., planning, organizing, sequencing, abstracting)

B. The cognitive deficits must be sufficiently severe to cause **impairment in occupational or social functioning** and must represent a decline from a previously higher level of functioning

Dementias have a common symptom presentation but are differentiated based on etiology, e.g., senile dementia of the Alzheimer's type or SDAT (course is characterized by gradual onset and continuing cognitive decline); dementia due to cerebrovascular disease (characterized by focal neurological signs and symptoms, e.g., exaggeration of deep tendon reflexes, extensor plantar response, gait abnormalities, weakness of an extremity); human immunodeficiency virus disease; head trauma; Parkinson's disease, and others.

Amnestic Disorder

A. The development of **memory impairment** (inability to learn new information or to recall previously learned information) in the absence of other significant cognitive impairments

B. The memory disturbance causes significant **impairment in social or occupational functioning** and represents a significant decline from a previous level of functioning

This may be due to pathology (closed head trauma, penetrating missile wounds, surgical intervention, hypoxia, infarction of the posterior cerebral artery, herpes simplex encephalitis), or it may be substance-induced, e.g., alcohol-induced amnestic disorder due to thiamine deficiency associated with prolonged, heavy ingestion of alcohol.

---

*The terms *organic mental disorder* and *organic brain syndrome* are no longer used for these disorders. These diagnostic categories are meant to be illustrative, not inclusive. Please refer to the original source for additional details and for further categories.

Adapted from the American Psychiatric Association: Diagnostic and Statistical Manual of Mental Disorders, 4th ed. Washington, DC, American Psychiatric Association, 1994. Reprinted with permission from the Diagnostic and Statistical Manual of Mental Disorders, 4th ed. © 1994 American Psychiatric Association.

Table 6–10 SUBSTANCE USE DISORDERS

"Substances" refer to those agents taken nonmedically to alter mood or behavior

Intoxication: ingestion of substance produces maladaptive behavior changes due to effects on the central nervous system

Abuse: daily use needed to function, inability to stop, impaired social and occupational functioning, recurrent use when it is physically hazardous, substance-related legal problems

Dependence: physiologic dependence on substance

Tolerance: requires increased amount of substance to produce same effect

Withdrawal: cessation of substance produces a syndrome of physiologic symptoms

Substance	Intoxication	Withdrawal
Alcohol	**Appearance.** Unsteady gait, incoordination, nystagmus, flushed face **Behavior.** Sedation, relief of anxiety, dulled concentration, impaired judgment, expansive, uninhibited behavior, talkativeness, slurred speech, impaired memory, irritability, depression, emotional lability	**Uncomplicated.** (Shortly after cessation of drinking, lasts 5 to 7 days.) Coarse tremor of hands, tongue, eyelids; anorexia; nausea and vomiting; malaise; autonomic hyperactivity (tachycardia, sweating, elevated blood pressure); headache; insomnia; anxiety; depression or irritability; transient hallucinations or illusions **Withdrawal delirium, "delirium tremens."** (Much less common than uncomplicated, occurs within 1 week of cessation.) Coarse, irregular tremor; marked autonomic hyperactivity (tachycardia, sweating); vivid hallucinations; delusions; agitated behavior; fever
Sedatives, hypnotics	Similar to alcohol **Appearance.** Unsteady gait, incoordination **Behavior.** Talkativeness, slurred speech, inattention, impaired memory, irritability, emotional lability, sexual aggressiveness, impaired judgment, impaired social or occupational functioning	Anxiety or irritability; nausea or vomiting; malaise; autonomic hyperactivity (tachycardia, sweating); orthostatic hypotension; coarse tremor of hands, tongue, and eyelids; marked insomnia; grand mal seizures
Nicotine	**Appearance.** Alerting, increased systolic blood pressure, increased heart rate, vasoconstriction **Behavior.** Nausea, vomiting, indigestion (first use); loss of appetite, head rush, dizziness, jittery feeling, mild stimulant	Vasodilation, headaches; anger, irritability, frustration, anxiety, nervousness, awakening at night, difficulty concentrating, depression, hunger, impatience or restlessness, desire to smoke
Cannabis (marijuana)	**Appearance.** Injected (reddened) conjunctivae, tachycardia, dry mouth, increased appetite, especially for "junk" food **Behavior.** Euphoria, anxiety, slowed time perception, increased perceptions, impaired judgment, social withdrawal, suspiciousness or paranoid ideation	
Cocaine	**Appearance.** Pupillary dilation, tachycardia or bradycardia, elevated or lowered blood pressure, sweating, chills, nausea, vomiting, weight loss **Behavior.** Euphoria, talkativeness, hypervigilance, pacing, psychomotor agitation, impaired social or occupational functioning, fighting, grandiosity, visual or tactile hallucinations	Dysphoric mood (anxiety, depression, irritability), fatigue, insomnia or hypersomnia, psychomotor agitation

Continued

Table 6–10   SUBSTANCE USE DISORDERS *Continued*

Substance	Intoxication	Withdrawal
Amphetamines	Similar to cocaine **Appearance.** Pupillary dilation, tachycardia, or bradycardia, elevated or lowered blood pressure, sweating or chills, nausea and vomiting, weight loss. **Behavior.** Elation, talkativeness, hypervigilance, psychomotor agitation, fighting, grandiosity, impaired judgment, impaired social and occupational functioning	Dysphoric mood (anxiety, depression, irritability), fatigue, insomnia or hypersomnia, psychomotor agitation
Opiates (morphine, heroin, meperidine)	**Appearance.** Pinpoint pupils, decreased blood pressure, pulse, respirations, and temperature **Behavior.** Lethargy; somnolence; slurred speech; initial euphoria followed by apathy, dysphoria, and psychomotor retardation; inattention; impaired memory; impaired judgment; impaired social or occupational functioning	Dilated pupils, lacrimation, runny nose, tachycardia, fever, elevated blood pressure, piloerection, sweating, diarrhea, yawning, insomnia, restlessness, irritability, depression, nausea, vomiting, malaise, tremor, muscle and joint pains; symptoms are remarkably similar to clinical picture of influenza

Table 6–11   SCHIZOPHRENIA*

A. Characteristic Symptoms

Two (or more) of the following, each present for a significant part of a 1-month period:

1. Delusions, i.e., involving a phenomenon that the person's culture would regard as totally implausible, such as thought broadcasting, being controlled by a dead person
2. Hallucinations (auditory are most common), e.g., voices speaking directly to the person or commenting on his or her ongoing behavior
3. Disorganized speech, e.g., frequent derailment or incoherence
4. Grossly disorganized or catatonic behavior
5. Negative symptoms, i.e., affective flattening, alogia (inability to speak), or avolition

B. Social/Occupational Dysfunction

One or more major areas of functioning such as work, interpersonal relations, or self-care are markedly below the level achieved prior to onset of the disturbance

C. Duration

Continuous signs persist for at least 6 months, including at least 1 month of symptoms from Criterion A (i.e., active phase) and may include periods of prodromal or residual symptoms

---

*These diagnostic categories are meant to be illustrative, not inclusive. The reader is referred to the original source or a psychiatry textbook for further categories and schizophrenia subtypes, such as Paranoid Type, Catatonic Type, Disorganized Type.

Adapted from American Psychiatric Association: Diagnostic and Statistical Manual of Mental Disorders, 4th ed. Washington, DC, American Psychiatric Association, 1994. Reprinted with permission from the Diagnostic and Statistical Manual of Mental Disorders, 4th ed. © 1994 American Psychiatric Association.

Table 6-12   MOOD DISORDERS*

Major Depressive Episode

Characteristics

A. Five (or more) of the following symptoms present during the same 2-week period and represent a change from previous functioning; at least one of the symptoms is either 1. depressed mood or 2. loss of interest or pleasure

Note: Do not include symptoms that are clearly caused by a general medical condition, or delusions, or hallucinations

1. **Depressed mood** most of the day nearly every day, as indicated by either subjective report (e.g., feels sad or empty) or by observation by others (e.g., appears tearful)
   Note: In children and adolescents, can be irritable mood
2. Markedly **diminished interest or pleasure** in all, or almost all, activities most of the day nearly every day
3. Significant **weight loss** when not dieting, weight gain (e.g., a change of >5% body weight in a month), or decrease or increase in appetite nearly every day.
   Note: In children, consider failure to make expected weight gains
4. **Insomnia** or hypersomnia nearly every day
5. **Psychomotor agitation** or retardation nearly every day
6. **Fatigue** or loss of energy nearly every day
7. Feelings of **worthlessness** or excessive or inappropriate guilt nearly every day
8. **Diminished ability to think** or concentrate, or indecisiveness, nearly every day
9. Recurrent **thoughts of death** (not just fear of dying), recurrent suicidal ideation without a specific plan, or a suicide attempt or a specific plan for committing suicide

B. The symptoms cause clinically significant distress or impairment in social, occupational, or other important areas of functioning

C. The symptoms are not due to the direct physiological effects of a substance (e.g., drug of abuse, a medication) or a general medical condition (e.g., hypothyroidism) and are not better accounted for by bereavement, i.e., loss of a loved one (unless persist for longer than 2 months or are characterized by functional impairment, morbid preoccupation with worthlessness, suicidal ideation, psychotic symptoms, or psychomotor retardation)

Manic Episode

Characteristics

A. A distinct period of abnormally and **persistently elevated, expansive, or irritable mood,** lasting at least 1 week (or any duration if hospitalization is necessary)

B. During the period of mood disturbance, three (or more) of the following symptoms have persisted (four if the mood is only irritable):

1. Inflated self-esteem or grandiosity
2. Decreased need for sleep (e.g., feels rested after only 3 hours of sleep)
3. More talkative than usual or pressure to keep talking
4. Flight of ideas or subjective experience that thoughts are racing
5. Distractibility (i.e., attention too easily drawn to unimportant or irrelevant external stimuli)
6. Increase in goal-directed activity (either socially, at work or school, or sexually) or psychomotor agitation
7. Excessive involvement in pleasurable activities that have a high potential for painful consequences (e.g., engaging in unrestrained buying sprees, sexual indiscretions, or foolish business investments)

C. The mood disturbance is sufficiently severe to cause marked impairment in occupational functioning or in usual social activities or relationships with others, or to necessitate hospitalization to prevent harm to self or others, or there are psychotic features

D. The symptoms are not due to the direct physiological effects of a substance (e.g., a drug of abuse, a medication) or a general medical condition (e.g., hyperthyroidism)

Continued

Table 6–12   MOOD DISORDERS* *Continued*

Major depressive disorder is characterized by one or more major depressive episodes (i.e., at least 2 weeks of depressed mood or loss of interest accompanied by at least four additional symptoms of depression); **dysthymic disorder** is characterized by at least 2 years of depressed mood for more days than not, accompanied by additional depressive symptoms; **bipolar disorder** is characterized by one or more manic episodes usually accompanied by major depressive episodes.

---

*These diagnostic categories are meant to be illustrative, not inclusive. The reader is referred to the original source or a psychiatry textbook for further categories, such as personality disorders or somatiform disorders.

Adapted from American Psychiatric Association: Diagnostic and Statistical Manual of Mental Disorders, 4th ed. Washington, DC, American Psychiatric Association, 1994. Reprinted with permission from the Diagnostic and Statistical Manual of Mental Disorders, 4th ed. © 1994 American Psychiatric Association.

Table 6–13   ANXIETY DISORDERS*

Panic Attack

A discrete period of **intense fear or discomfort,** in which four (or more) of the following symptoms developed abruptly and reached a peak within 10 minutes:

1. Palpitations, pounding heart, or accelerated heart rate
2. Sweating
3. Trembling or shaking
4. Sensations of shortness of breath or smothering
5. Feeling of choking
6. Chest pain or discomfort
7. Nausea or abdominal distress
8. Feeling dizzy, unsteady, lightheaded, or faint
9. Derealization (feelings of unreality) or depersonalization (being detached from oneself)
10. Fear of losing control or going crazy
11. Fear of dying
12. Paresthesias (numbness or tingling sensations)
13. Chills or hot flashes

Agoraphobia

A. Anxiety about being in places or situations from which escape might be difficult (or embarrassing) or in which help may not be available in the event of having a panic attack or paniclike symptoms—agoraphobic fears typically involve being outside the home alone; being in a crowd or standing in a line; being on a bridge; and traveling in a bus, train, or automobile

B. The situations are avoided (e.g., travel is restricted), are endured with marked distress or with anxiety about having a panic attack or paniclike symptoms, or require the presence of a companion

Panic Disorder

A. Both 1. and 2. occur:

1. Recurrent unexpected panic attacks (see above)
2. At least one of the attacks has been followed by 1 month (or more) of one (or more) of the following:
   a. Persistent concern about having additional attacks
   b. Worry about the implications of the attack or its consequences (e.g., losing control, having a heart attack, "going crazy")
   c. A significant change in behavior related to the attacks

B. Agoraphobia may be present or absent

Table 6–13 ANXIETY DISORDERS* Continued

Specific Phobia

A. Marked and persistent fear that is excessive or unreasonable, cued by a specific object or situation (e.g., flying, heights, animals, receiving an injection, seeing blood)

B. Exposure to the phobic stimulus almost invariably provokes an immediate anxiety response, which may be a panic attack.
Note: In children, the anxiety may be expressed by crying, tantrums, freezing, or clinging

C. The person recognizes that the fear is excessive or unreasonable

D. The phobic situation is avoided or is endured with intense anxiety or distress

E. This interferes significantly with the person's normal routine, occupational (or academic) functioning, or social activities or relationships

Social Phobia

A. A marked and persistent fear of one or more social or performance situations in which the person is exposed to unfamiliar people or to possible scrutiny by others; the individual fears that he or she will act in a way (or show anxiety symptoms) that will be humiliating or embarrassing

B.–E.: The same as in specific phobia (above).

Obsessive-Compulsive Disorder

A. Person has either **obsessions:**

1. Recurrent and persistent thoughts, impulses, or images that are experienced as intrusive and inappropriate and that cause marked anxiety or distress
2. The thoughts, impulses, or images are not simply excessive worries about real-life problems
3. The person attempts to ignore or suppress such thoughts, impulses, or images, or to neutralize them with some other thought or action
4. The person recognizes that the obsessional thoughts are a product of his or her own mind (not imposed from without)

or **compulsions:**

1. Repetitive behaviors (e.g., hand-washing, ordering, checking) or mental acts (e.g., praying, counting, repeating words silently) that the person feels driven to perform in response to an obsession, or according to rules that must be applied rigidly
2. The behaviors or mental acts are aimed at preventing or reducing distress or at preventing some dreaded event or situation

B. At some point, the person has recognized that the obsessions or compulsions are excessive or unreasonable

C. The obsessions or compulsions cause marked distress, are time consuming, or significantly interfere with the person's normal routine, occupational (or academic) functioning, or usual social activities or relationships

Posttraumatic Stress Disorder

A. The person has been exposed to a traumatic event in which

1. The person experienced, witnessed, or was confronted with the actual or threatened death or serious injury of self or others
2. The person's response involved intense fear, helplessness, or horror

B. The traumatic event is persistently reexperienced by:
1. Recurrent and intrusive distressing recollections of the event, including images, thoughts, or perceptions
2. Recurrent distressing dreams of the event
3. Acting or feeling as if the traumatic event were recurring

Continued

Table 6–13   ANXIETY DISORDERS* Continued

C. Persistent avoidance of stimuli associated with the trauma and numbing of general responsiveness (e.g., feeling of detachment or estrangement from others, unable to have loving feelings, sense of a foreshortened future)

D. Persistent symptoms of increased arousal:

1. Difficulty falling or staying asleep
2. Irritability or outbursts of anger
3. Difficulty concentrating

4. Hypervigilance
5. Exaggerated startle response

Generalized Anxiety Disorder

A. Excessive anxiety and worry occurring more days than not for at least 6 months about a number of events or activities (such as work or school performance)

B. The person finds it difficult to control the worry

C. The anxiety and worry are associated with three (or more) of the following:

1. Restlessness or feeling keyed up or on edge
2. Being easily fatigued
3. Difficulty concentrating or mind going blank

4. Irritability
5. Muscle tension
6. Sleep disturbance

*These diagnostic categories are meant to be illustrative, not inclusive. The reader is referred to the original source or a psychiatry textbook for further details and categories of anxiety disorders.

Adapted from American Psychiatric Association: Diagnostic and Statistical Manual of Mental Disorders, 4th ed. Washington, DC, American Psychiatric Association, 1994. Reprinted with permission from the Diagnostic and Statistical Manual of Mental Disorders, 4th ed. © 1994 American Psychiatric Association.

Bibliography

American Psychiatric Association: Diagnostic and Statistical Manual of Mental Disorders, 4th ed. Washington, DC, American Psychiatric Association, 1994.

Birren JE, Schaie KW (Eds): Handbook of the Psychology of Aging, 4th ed. San Diego, CA, Academic Press, Inc., 1996.

Callahan CM, Hendrie HC, Tierney WM: Documentation and evaluation of cognitive impairment in elderly primary care patients. Ann Intern Med 122(6):422–428, Mar 15, 1995.

Clark CC: Posttraumatic stress disorder: How to support healing. Am J Nurs 97(8):27–32, Aug 1997.

Depaulo JR Jr, Folstein MF: Psychiatric disturbances in neurological patients: Detection, recognition and hospital course. Ann Neurol 4:225–228, 1978.

Dolamore MJ, Libow LS, Mulvihill MN, et al: Mental status guide: FROMAJE for use with frail elders. J Gerontol Nurs 20(6):29–35, June 1994.

Dubin S: The Mini-Mental State Exam. Am J Nurs 98(11):16D, Nov 1998.

Eden BM, Foreman MD: Problems associated with underrecognition of delirium in critical care: A case study. Heart Lung 25(5):388–400, Sept–Oct 1996.

Farrell KR, Ganzini L: Misdiagnosing delirium as depression in medically ill elderly patients. Arch Intern Med 155:2459–2464, Dec 1995.

Ferrera PC, Chan L: Initial management of the patient with altered mental status. Am Fam Phys 55(5):1773–1780, Apr 1997.

Fleming KC, Evans JM, Weber DC, Chutka DS: Practical functional assessment of elderly persons: A primary-care approach. Mayo Clin Proc 70:890–910, 1995.

Folstein MF, Folstein SE, McHugh PR: "Mini-mental state": A practical method for grading the cognitive state of patients for the clinician. J Psychiatr Res 12:189–198, 1975.

Foreman MD, Zane D: Nursing strategies for acute confusion in elders. Am J Nurs 96(4):44–52, Apr 1996.

Isaacs A: Depression and your patient. Am J Nurs 98(7):26–31, July 1998.

Isaacs B, Kennie A: The set test as an aid to the detection of dementia in old people. Br J Psychiatry 123:467–470, 1973.

Kane RL, Ouslander JG, Abrass IB: Essentials of Clinical Geriatrics, 3rd ed. New York, McGraw-Hill, Inc., 1994.

Keller MB, Manschreck TC: The bedside mental status examination-reliability and validity. Compr Psychiatry 22(5):500–511, 1981.

Kennedy CW, Polivka BJ, Steel JS: Psychiatric symptoms in a community-based medically ill population. Home Healthcare Nurs 15(6):431–440, 1997.

Krach P: Assessment of depressed older persons living in a home setting. Home Healthcare Nurs 13(3):61–64, 1995.

Kreeger JL, Raulin ML, Grace J, Priest BL: Effect of hearing enhancement on mental status ratings in geriatric psychiatric patients. Am J Psychiatry 152(4):629–631, Apr 1995.

Mangino M, Middlemiss C: Alzheimer's disease: Preventing and recognizing a misdiagnosis. Nurs Pract 22(10):58–75, 1997.

McConnell EA: Assessing altered mental status. Nursing 27(4):32d–32h, Apr 1997.

Mezey M, Mitty E, Ramsey G: Assessment of decision-making capacity: Nursing's role. J Gerontol Nurs 23(3)28–35, Mar 1997.

Roy-Byrne P, Dagadakis C, Ries R, et al: A psychiatrist-rated battery of measures for assessing the clinical status of psychiatric inpatients. Psychiatr Serv 46(4):347–352, Apr 1995.

Strub RL, Black FW: The Mental Status Examination in Neurology, 3rd ed. Philadelphia, F.A. Davis, 1993.

Sullivan-Marx EM: Delirium and physical restraint in the hospitalized elderly. Image 26(4):295–300, 1994.

Tombaugh TN, McIntyre, NJ: The Mini-Mental State Examination: A comprehensive review. J Am Geriatr Soc 40(9):922–935, 1992.

Tully MW, Matrakas KL, Muir J, Musallam K: The Eating Behavior Scale: A simple method of assessing functional ability in patients with Alzheimer's disease. J Gerontol Nurs 23(7):9–15, July 1997.

Unger JB: Sedentary lifestyle as a risk factor for self-reported poor physical and mental health. Am J Health Promot 10(1):15–17, Sept–Oct 1995.

U.S. Public Health Service: Adult screening for depression. Nurs Pract 21(5):82–86, May 1996.

Valente SM: Evaluating suicide risk in the medically ill patient. Nurse Pract 18(9):41–50, 1993.

Valente SM: Recognizing depression in elderly patients. Am J Nurs 94(12):18–25, Dec 1994.

Vermeersch PEH, Henly SJ: Validation of the structure for the "Clinical Assessment of Confusion-A." Nurs Res 46(4):208–213, July–Aug 1997.

Walker C: Homeless people and mental health. Am J Nurs 98(11):26–33, Nov 1998.

CHAPTER SEVEN

Nutritional Assessment

DEFINING NUTRITIONAL STATUS

Nutritional status refers to the degree of balance between nutrient intake and nutrient requirements. This balance is affected by many factors, including physiologic, psychosocial, developmental, cultural, and economic.

Optimal nutritional status is achieved when sufficient nutrients are consumed to support day-to-day body needs and any increased metabolic demands due to growth, pregnancy, or illness. Persons having optimal nutritional status are more active, have fewer physical illnesses, and live longer than persons who are malnourished.

Undernutrition occurs when nutritional reserves are depleted and/or when nutrient intake is inadequate to meet day-to-day needs or added metabolic demands. Vulnerable groups—infants, children, pregnant women, recent immigrants, persons with low incomes, hospitalized people, and aging adults—are at risk for impaired growth and development, lowered resistance to infection and disease, delayed wound healing, longer hospital stays, and higher health care costs.

Overnutrition is caused by the consumption of nutrients—especially calories, sodium, and fat—in excess of body needs. A major nutritional problem today, overnutrition can lead to obesity and related diseases (e.g., diabetes, hypertension). Nearly 14 percent of children, 12 percent of adolescents, and 33 percent of adults are estimated to be overweight. Among African-American and Mexican-American women, the rate is approximately 50 percent. Overweight during childhood and adolescence is associated with overweight during adulthood, and the prevalence of overweight in all age categories continues to increase (Anonymous, MMWR, 1997).

 DEVELOPMENTAL CONSIDERATIONS

Infants and Children

The time from birth to 4 months of age is the most rapid period of growth in the life cycle. Although infants lose weight during the first few days of life, birth weight is usually regained by the 7th to 10th day after birth. Thereafter, infants double their birth weight by 4 months and triple it by 1 year of age. Breastfeeding is recommended for full-term infants for the 1st year of life because breast milk is ideally formulated to promote normal infant growth and development and natural immunity. Although relatively few contraindications to breastfeeding

exist, women who are human immunodeficiency virus (HIV) positive should not breastfeed, since HIV can be transmitted through breast milk. The number of pounds gained during the second year approximates the birth weight.

Infants increase their length by 50 percent during the first year of life and double it by 4 years of age. Brain size also increases very rapidly during infancy and childhood. By age 2 years, the brain has reached 50 percent of its adult size; by age 4, 75 percent; and by age 8, 100 percent. For this reason, infants and children younger than 2 should not drink skim or low-fat milk or be placed on low-fat diets—fat (calories and essential fatty acids) is required for proper growth and central nervous system development.

The Recommended Dietary Allowances (RDAs) for infants and children are illustrated in Appendix B.

Adolescence

Following a period of slow growth in late childhood, adolescence is characterized by rapid physical growth and endocrine and hormonal changes. Caloric and protein requirements increase to meet this demand, and because of bone growth and increasing muscle mass (and, in girls, the onset of menarche), calcium and iron requirements also increase. Typically, these increased requirements cannot be met by three meals per day; therefore, nutritious snacks play an important role in achieving adequate nutrient intake. The recommended ranges of caloric and protein intakes for adolescents are shown in Appendix B.

In general, boys grow taller and have less body fat than girls. The percent of body fat increases in females to about 25 percent and decreases in males (replaced by muscle mass) to about 12 percent. Typically, girls double their body weight between the ages of 8 and 14; boys double their body weight between the ages of 10 and 17 years.

Pregnancy and Lactation

To support the synthesis of maternal and fetal tissues, sufficient calories, protein, vitamins, and minerals must be consumed. The National Academy of Sciences (NAS) recommends a weight gain of 25 to 35 lb for women of normal weight, 28 to 40 lb for underweight women, and 15 to 25 lb for overweight women. See Appendix B for increased requirements of pregnancy and lactation. Appendix C gives recommended weight gain guidelines based on body mass index, and illustrates curves of desirable weight gain during pregnancy, as recommended by the Subcommittee on Nutritional Status and Weight Gain During Pregnancy (National Academy of Sciences, 1990).

Adulthood

During adulthood, growth and nutrient needs stabilize. Most adults are in relatively good health. However, unhealthy habits such as cigarette smoking, stressful lifestyles, lack of exercise, excessive alcohol intake, and diets high in saturated fat, cholesterol, salt, and sugar and low in fiber can be factors in the development of hypertension, obesity, atherosclerosis, cancer, osteoporosis, and diabetes mellitus. The adult years, therefore, are an important time for education, to preserve health and to prevent or delay the onset of chronic disease. The RDAs for this group (persons aged 23 to 50 years) for protein, energy, vitamin, and mineral intakes are shown in Appendix B.

The Aging Adult

As people age, a number of changes occur that make them prone to undernutrition or overnutrition. Poor physical or mental health, social isolation, alcoholism, limited functional ability, poverty, and polypharmacy are the major risk factors for malnutrition in older adults (Dwyer, 1991). Normal physiologic changes in aging adults that directly affect nutritional status include poor dentition, decreased visual acuity, decreased saliva production, slowed gastrointestinal motility, decreased gastrointestinal absorption, and diminished olfactory and taste sensitivity.

Socioeconomic conditions frequently have a significant effect on the nutritional status of the aging adult. Decline of extended families and increased mobility of families reduce available support systems. Facilities for meal preparation and eating, transportation to grocery stores, physical limitations, income, and social isolation are frequent problems and can obviously interfere with the acquisition of a balanced diet. Medications must also be considered, because aging adults frequently take multiple medications that have a potential for interaction with nutrients and with one another.

The most important nutritional feature of the older years is the decrease in energy requirements due to loss of lean body mass, the most metabolically active tissue. Between the ages of 51 and 75, energy needs decrease by approximately 200 kcal/day in both men and women. After age 75, energy needs decrease by 500 kcal and 400 kcal/day in males and females, respectively. The protein requirement of 0.8 g/kg/day for younger adults is appropriate for the healthy older person. In both men and women, height decreases slowly beginning during the early 30s, leading to an average lifetime height loss of 2.9 cm in men and 4.9 cm in women (Bowman and Rosenberg, 1982).

TRANSCULTURAL CONSIDERATIONS

Because foods and eating customs are culturally distinct, each person has a unique cultural heritage that may affect nutritional status. Immigrants commonly maintain traditional eating customs long after the language and manner of dress of an adopted country become routine (especially for holidays and observance of religious customs). Occupation, class, religion, gender, and health awareness also have a great bearing on eating customs. Within the last decade, hundreds of thousands of Southeast Asians, Mexicans, and Cubans have immigrated to the United States. Not only do their food habits change to accommodate their new cultures, but their food habits have influence on their adoptive country. The popularity of tofu, stir-fried vegetables, tortillas, and rice and beans is just one example of these influences on American eating habits.

Newly arriving immigrants may be at nutritional risk for a variety of reasons. They frequently come from countries with limited food supplies caused by poverty, poor sanitation, war, or political strife. General undernutrition, hypertension, diarrhea, lactose intolerance, osteomalacia (soft bones), scurvy, and dental caries are among the more common nutrition-related problems of new immigrants from developing countries.

When immigrants arrive in the United States, other factors contribute to their nutritional problems: They are in a new country with a completely new language, culture, and society. They are faced with unfamiliar foods, food storage, food preparation, and food-buying habits. Many familiar foods are difficult or impossible to obtain. Low income may also limit their access to familiar foods. When traditional food habits are disrupted by a new culture, borderline deficiencies or adverse nutritional consequences may result. As an example, Japanese immigrants to the United States have increased risk of colon and breast cancer as they adapt to a diet in the United States that is higher in saturated fats and cholesterol (Hunter and Willett, 1996; Potter, 1996).

Cultural heritage also plays a role in nutrient needs. For example, studies have shown that black women have lower hemoglobin levels than white women independent of iron intake, and that their risk for osteoporosis is significantly less despite lower overall calcium intake. Or, cultural values may conflict with optimum nutrition (e.g., many cultures worldwide consider obesity an indication of beauty, affluence, and well-being).

Because rapid changes in eating patterns and customs are occurring in all countries, what are considered customs today may not be considered traditional in a few years. The best way to learn about the eating patterns of a people is to talk with them, eat with them, and ask about their dietary customs. It is important to keep in mind that recent immigrant groups, such as the Southeast

Asians, are often shorter and weigh less than their Western counterparts, so American standard tables of weight for age, height for age, and weight for height may not be appropriate to evaluate growth and development of immigrant children. At present no reliable standards to evaluate every immigrant group exist.

The cultural factors that must be considered are the cultural definition of food, frequency and number of meals eaten away from home, form and content of ceremonial meals, amount and types of foods eaten, and regularity of food consumption. Because inaccuracies may occur, the 24-hour dietary recalls or 3-day food records used traditionally for assessment may be inadequate when dealing with people from culturally diverse backgrounds. Standard dietary handbooks may fail to provide culture-specific diet information because nutritional content and exchange tables are generally based on Western diets (Pennington, 1998). Another source of error may originate from cultural patterns of eating. For example, many low-income ethnic groups eat sparingly or moderately during the week (i.e., simple rice or bean dishes), while weekend meals are markedly more elaborate (i.e., meats, fruits, vegetables, and sweets are added).

Although you may assume that the term "food" is a universal concept, you should have the person clarify what is meant by the term. For example, certain Latin American groups do not consider chili peppers—an important source of vitamins A and C—to be food and thus fail to list them as vegetables on daily food records. Among Vietnamese refugees, the dietary intake of calcium may appear inadequate, particularly with the low consumption of dairy products common among members of this group. Daily soups prepared by soaking bones in acidified broth or pickled or sweet and sour meats such as pork ribs (vinegar leaches calcium from the bones and makes it available to the body) are, however, commonly consumed, thus providing adequate quantities of calcium to meet daily requirements. Tofu is also a good source of calcium if calcium salts are used to precipitate the curd. For Mexican Americans, tortillas prepared from corn treated with lime water significantly increase dietary calcium. In Middle Eastern countries, yogurt and feta cheese are the major dietary sources of calcium since milk is not commonly consumed by adults.

Food itself is only one part of eating. In some cultures, social contacts during meals are restricted to members of the immediate or extended family. For example, in some Middle Eastern cultures, men and women eat meals separately, or women may be permitted to eat with their husbands, but not with other males. Among some Hispanic groups, the male breadwinner is served first, then women and children. Etiquette during meals, the use of hands, type of eating utensils (e.g., chopsticks, special flatware), and protocols governing the order in which food is consumed during a meal all vary cross-culturally.

Dietary Practices of Selected Cultural Groups

It is necessary to avoid *cultural stereotyping*, the tendency to view individuals of common cultural backgrounds similarly and according to a preconceived notion of how they "ought" to behave. For example, despite widely held stereotypes, we know that there are Chinese who do not like rice, Italians who despise spaghetti, Irish who dislike corned beef and cabbage, and so forth. Aggregate dietary preferences among people from certain cultural groups, however, can be described (e.g., characteristic ethnic dishes, methods of food preparation). Refer to nutrition texts on the topic for detailed information about culture-specific diets and the nutritional value of ethnic foods.

Cultural food preferences are often interrelated with religious dietary beliefs and practices. Many religions use foods as symbols in celebrations and rituals. Knowing the person's religious practices related to food enables you to suggest improvements or modifications that do not conflict with dietary laws. Table 7-1 summarizes dietary practices for selected religious groups.

Other issues are fasting and other religious observations that may limit a person's food or liquid intake during specified times (e.g., many Catholics fast and abstain from meat on Ash Wednesday and the Fridays of Lent. Muslims fast from dawn to sunset during the month of Ramadan in the Islamic calendar and eat only twice a day—before dawn and after sunset; Jews observe a 24-hour fast on Yom Kippur).

PURPOSES AND COMPONENTS OF NUTRITIONAL ASSESSMENT

Nutritional status can be determined by the application of nutritional assessment techniques. In general, these techniques are noninvasive, inexpensive, and easy to perform.

The purposes of nutritional assessment are to (1) identify individuals who are malnourished or are at risk of developing malnutrition; (2) provide data for designing a nutrition plan of care that will prevent or minimize the development of malnutrition; and (3) establish baseline data for evaluating the efficacy of nutritional care.

Nutrition screening, the first step in assessing nutritional status, may be completed in any setting (e.g., clinic, home, hospital, long-term care). Based on easily

Table 7–1 • Religious Dietary Practices

Religious Group	Food Restrictions
Church of Jesus Christ of Latter-Day Saints (Mormonism)	No alcoholic beverages No stimulants (caffeinated beverages such as coffee, tea, sodas) Observant Mormons fast (refrain from food and liquids) on the first Sunday of each month.

Judaism
 	
   Orthodox—strict observance
 	
   Conservative—nominal observance
 	
   Reform—less ceremonial emphasis and minimum observance of dietary laws
	The *laws of kashrut* dictate which foods are permissible under religious law:
	
	1. Only meat from cloven-hoofed animals that chew cud (cattle, sheep, goat, ox, or deer) is allowed. These animals must be slaughtered ritually in a manner that results in minimal pain to the animal and maximal blood drainage. There are two methods used to prepare *kosher* (meaning "properly preserved" or "fit for eating") meats: (a) The meat is soaked in cold water for 30 minutes, salted, and drained to deplete blood content. It is then washed under cold water and drained again before cooking *or* (b) the meat is first prepared by quickly searing or cooking over an open flame, which permits liver to be eaten.
	
	2. Meat and dairy products cannot be served at the same meal, nor can they be cooked or served in the same set of dishes or eaten with the same utensils. Fish, eggs, vegetables, and fruits are considered *parve* or neutral and may be eaten with dairy products or meat meals.
	
	3. Fish with fins and scales are allowed. No shellfish (crab, lobster, shrimp, clam, oyster) or scavenger fish (catfish, shark, porpoise) may be eaten. Crocodile, frog, snail, snake, and tortoise also are prohibited.
	
	Additional dietary laws are followed during the week of Passover. No bread or product with yeast may be eaten; instead *matzah* or unleavened bread is eaten. Products that are fermented or can cause fermenting or souring may not be eaten.

Islam	Pork, pork products, animal shortening, and alcohol are strictly prohibited. The slaughter of poultry, beef, and lamb must be done ritually by a Muslim to ensure that it is *halal*. Fasting is common. During the month of Ramadan, no foods or beverages are consumed until after sunset.
Roman Catholicism	Abstinence from meat and meat products (gravy, soups) and fasting on Ash Wednesday and the Fridays during a 40-day period of religious observance called Lent. Rules of fasting apply to those between the ages of 12 and 65.
Seventh-Day Adventism	Fermented or alcoholic beverages are prohibited. Optional vegetarianism may take three forms: (a) strict vegetarians (syn. *vegans*)—people who include no animal-derived products in their diet; (b) ovolactovegetarians—people who use milk, milk products, and eggs but no meats in their diet; and (c) semivegetarians—Adventists who refrain from pork or pork products, shellfish, and blood. Snacking between meals is discouraged.

obtained data, nutrition screening is a quick and easy way to identify individuals at nutrition risk. Parameters used for nutrition screening typically include weight and weight history, conditions associated with increased nutritional risk, diet information, and routine laboratory data. A variety of valid tools are available for screening different populations. For example, the Nutrition Screening Initiative form (see Figure 7–1) was designed and validated in the outpatient, geriatric population (Dwyer, 1991) and the Admission Nutrition Screening Tool (Kovacevich et al., 1997) was validated for use by nurses in hospitalized patients (Table 7–2).

The warning signs of poor nutritional health are often overlooked. Use this checklist to find out if you or someone you know is at nutritional risk.

Read the statements below. Circle the number in the yes column for those that apply to you or someone you know. For each yes answer, score the number in the box. Total your nutritional score.

DETERMINE YOUR NUTRITIONAL HEALTH

	YES
I have an illness or condition that made me change the kind and/or amount of food I eat.	2
I eat fewer than 2 meals per day.	3
I eat few fruits or vegetables, or milk products.	2
I have 3 or more drinks of beer, liquor or wine almost every day.	2
I have tooth or mouth problems that make it hard for me to eat.	2
I don't always have enough money to buy the food I need.	4
I eat alone most of the time.	1
I take 3 or more different prescribed or over-the-counter drugs a day.	1
Without wanting to, I have lost or gained 10 pounds in the last 6 months.	2
I am not always physically able to shop, cook and/or feed myself.	2
	TOTAL

Total Your Nutritional Score. If it's —

0-2   **Good!** Recheck your nutritional score in 6 months.

3-5   **You are at moderate nutritional risk.** See what can be done to improve your eating habits and lifestyle. Your office on aging, senior nutrition program, senior citizens center or health department can help. Recheck your nutritional score in 3 months.

6 or more   **You are at high nutritional risk.** Bring this checklist the next time you see your doctor, dietitian or other qualified health or social service professional. Talk with them about any problems you may have. Ask for help to improve your nutritional health.

These materials developed and distributed by the Nutrition Screening Initiative, a project of:

 AMERICAN ACADEMY OF FAMILY PHYSICIANS

 THE AMERICAN DIETETIC ASSOCIATION

 NATIONAL COUNCIL ON THE AGING, INC.

* Remember that warning signs suggest risk, but do not represent diagnosis of any condition.

7–1

Table 7–2 · Admission Nutrition Screening Tool

A. Diagnosis

If the patient has at least ONE of the following diagnoses, circle and proceed to section E to consider the patient AT NUTRITIONAL RISK and stop here.

- Anorexia nervosa/bulimia nervosa
- Malabsorption (celiac sprue, ulcerative colitis, Crohn's disease, short bowel syndrome)
- Multiple trauma (closed head injury, penetrating trauma, multiple fractures)
- Decubitus ulcers
- Major gastrointestinal surgery within the past year
- Cachexia (temporal wasting, muscle wasting, cancer, cardiac)
- Coma
- Diabetes
- End-stage liver disease
- End-stage renal disease
- Nonhealing wounds

B. Nutrition Intake History

If the patient has at least ONE of the following symptoms, circle and proceed to section E to consider the patient AT NUTRITIONAL RISK and stop here.

- Diarrhea (>500 ml × 2 days)
- Vomiting (>5 days)
- Reduced intake (<½ normal intake for >5 days)

C. Ideal Body Weight Standards

Compare the patient's current weight for height to the ideal body weight chart.
If at <80% of ideal body weight, proceed to section E to consider the patient AT NUTRITIONAL RISK and stop here.

D. Weight History

Any recent unplanned weight loss? No ___ Yes ___ Amount (lbs or kg) ___
  If yes, within the past _____ weeks or _____ months
  Current weight (lbs or kg) _____
  Usual weight (lbs or kg) _____
  Height (ft, in, or cm) _____
Find percentage of weight loss:

$$\frac{\text{usual wt} - \text{current wt}}{\text{usual wt}} \times 100 = \underline{\hspace{1cm}} \% \text{ wt loss}$$

Compare the % wt loss with the chart values and circle appropriate value

Length of Time	Significant (%)	Severe (%)
1 week	1–2	>2
2–3 weeks	2–3	>3
1 month	4–5	>5
3 months	7–8	>8
5+ months	10	>10

If the patient has experienced a significant or severe weight loss, proceed to section E and consider the patient AT NUTRITIONAL RISK

E. Nurse Assessment

Using the above criteria, what is this patient's nutritional risk? (circle one)

    LOW NUTRITIONAL RISK   AT NUTRITIONAL RISK

Source: Adapted from Kovacevich DS, Boney AR, Braunschweig CL, Perez A, Stevens M: Nutrition risk classification: A valid and reproducible tool for nurses. Nutr Clin Practice 12:20–25, 1997. Used with permission.

Individuals identified at nutritional risk during screening should undergo a **comprehensive nutritional assessment,** which includes dietary history and intake information, physical examination for clinical signs, anthropometric measures, and laboratory tests. The skills needed to collect the dietary history and to perform the physical examination are described in the Subjective Data and Objective Data sections that follow. Table 7–3 is an example of a form for compiling comprehensive nutritional assessment data.

Various methods for collecting current dietary intake information are available—24-hour recall, food frequency questionnaire, and food diary. During hospitalization, documentation of nutritional intake can best be achieved through calorie counts of nutrients consumed and/or infused.

The easiest and most popular method for obtaining information about dietary intake is the **24-hour recall.** The individual or family member completes a questionnaire or is interviewed and asked to recall everything eaten within the last 24 hours. However, several significant sources of error may occur when this method is used: (1) The individual or family member may not be able to recall the type or amount of food eaten; (2) intake within the last 24 hours may be atypical of usual intake; (3) the individual or family member may alter the truth for a variety of reasons; and (4) snack items and use of gravies, sauces, and condiments may be underreported.

To counter some of the difficulties inherent in the 24-hour recall method, a **food frequency questionnaire** may also be completed. With this tool, information is collected on how many times per day, week, or month the individual eats particular foods. Drawbacks to the use of the food frequency questionnaire are (1) it does not quantify amount of intake, and (2) like the 24-hour recall, it relies on the individual's or family member's memory for how often a food was eaten.

Food diaries or records require asking the individual or family member to write down everything consumed for a certain period of time. Three days—two weekdays and one weekend day—are customarily used. A food diary is most complete and accurate if the individual is instructed to record information immediately after eating. Potential problems with the food diary include (1) noncompliance, (2) inaccurate recording, (3) atypical intake on the recording days, and (4) conscious alteration of diet during the recording period.

Direct observation of the feeding and eating process can lead to detection of problems not readily identified through standard nutrition interviews. For example, observing the typical feeding techniques used by a parent or caregiver and the interaction between the individual and caregiver can be of value when assessing failure to thrive in children or unintentional weight loss in older adults.

Table 7–3 • Comprehensive Nutritional Assessment Form

Scored
PG-SGA*

Institutional Code:_____ Patient Code: _____
Setting: Inpt   Outpt Clinic/Office   Homecare   Hospice
Patient Name: _____
Medical Record # (optional): _____
Sex: Male   Female   Age: _____

History

---

1. Weight   *See Table A*

In summary of my current and recent weight:

I currently weigh about _____ pounds

I am about _____ feet _____ inches tall

Six months ago I weighed about _____ pounds

One month ago I weighed about _____ pounds

During the past two weeks, my weight has

☐ decreased (1)   ☐ not changed (0)   ☐ increased (0)

---

2. Food Intake

As compared to my normal, I would rate my food intake during the past month as either:

☐ unchanged (0)

☐ more than usual (1)

☐ less than usual (1)

I am now taking: ☐ little solid food (2)

☐ only liquids (3)

☐ only nutritional supplements (3)

☐ very little of anything (4)

---

3. Symptoms During the past two weeks, I have had the following problems that kept me from eating enough (check all that apply):

☐ no problems eating (0)

☐ no appetite, just did not feel like eating (3)

☐ nausea (1)   ☐ vomiting (3)

☐ constipation (1)   ☐ diarrhea (3)

☐ mouth sores (2)   ☐ dry mouth (1)

☐ pain: (where?) (3) _____

☐ things taste funny or have no taste (1)

☐ smells bother me (1)

☐ other** (1) _____

---

4. Functional Capacity

Over the past month, I would rate my activity as generally:

☐ normal with no limitations (0)

☐ not my normal self, but able to be up and about with fairly normal activities (1)

☐ not feeling up to most things, but in bed less than half the day (2)

☐ able to do little activity and spend most of the day in bed or chair (3)

☐ pretty much bedridden, rarely out of bed (3)

Patient Signature _____

**Depression, money, dental problems, etc.

THE REMAINDER OF THIS FORM WILL BE COMPLETED BY YOUR DOCTOR, NURSE, OR THERAPIST. THANK YOU.

5. Disease and Its Relationship to Nutritional Requirements   *See Table B*

Primary diagnoses (specify) _____

Stage, if known _____

Metabolic demand: *See Table C* ☐ no stress ☐ low stress ☐ moderate stress ☐ high stress

Physical

For each trait specify: 0 = normal 1 = mild 2 = moderate 3 = severe   *See Table D*

___ loss of subcutaneous ___ muscle wasting ___ ankle edema ___sacral edema ___ ascites
fat (triceps, chest)   (quadriceps, deltoids)

SGA Rating
Select One *See Table E*

☐ A: well nourished   ☐ B: moderately (or suspected) malnourished   ☐ C: severely malnourished

Clinician Signature _____ RD RN PA MD DO Other: _____ Date _____

Table A. Criteria for Scoring Weight Loss

Weight loss in 6 months	Points	Weight loss in 1 month	Points
20% or greater	4	10% or greater	4
10–19.9%	3	5–9.9%	3
6–9.9%	2	3–4.9%	2
2–5.9%	1	2–2.9%	1
0–1.9%	0	0–1.9%	0

Table 7–3 • Comprehensive Nutritional Assessment Form *Continued*

Table B. Scoring Criteria for Diseases or Conditions

Category	Points
Cancer	1
AIDS	1
Pulmonary or cardiac cachexia	1
Presence of decubitus, open wound, or fistula	1
Presence of trauma	1
Age greater than 65 years	1

Table C. Scoring of Metabolic Stressors

Stressor	None (0)	Low (1)	Moderate (2)	High (3)
Fever (°F)*	No fever	>99 and <101	≥101 and <102	≥102
Fever duration	No fever	<72 hr		Lasting >72 hr
Steroids	No steroids	Low-dose steroids (<10 mg prednisone equivalents/day)	Moderate steroids (≥10, <30 mg prednisone equivalents/day)	High-dose steroids (≥30 mg prednisone equivalents/day)

Table D. Components of Quick Physical Examination (none to +++)

Fat Status	Muscle Status	Fluid Status
Eyes	Temples	Skin and skin turgor
Triceps fat pinch	Shoulders	Eyes
Anterior lower ribs	Clavicle	Ankles
	Scapula	Sacrum
	Thumb/index press	Abdomen for ascites
	Thigh and calf	

Table E. PG-SGA Staging Guide

Variable	Stage A: Well Nourished	Stage B: Moderately Malnourished or Suspected of Being Malnourished	Stage C: Severely Malnourished
Weight	No weight loss or recent nonfluid weight gain	a. Approximately 5% weight loss within 1 month (or 10% in 6 months) b. No weight stabilization or weight (i.e., continued loss)	a. >5% loss in one month (or >10% loss in 6 months) b. No weight stabilization or weight gain
Intake	No deficit or significant recent improvement	Definite decrease in intake	Severe deficit in intake
Nutrition impact symptoms	None or significant recent improvement allowing adequate intake	Presence of nutrition impact symptoms (Box 3 of PG-SGA)	Presence of nutrition impact symptoms (Box 3 of PG-SGA)
Functionality	No deficit or significant recent improvement	Moderate functional deficit or recent functional deterioration	Severe functional deficit or recent significant functional deterioration
Physical exam	No deficit or chronic deficit in the face of recent improvement in all history categories listed above	Evidence of mild to moderate loss of ● Subcutaneous fat and/or ● Muscle mass and/or ● Muscle tone on palpation	Obvious signs of malnutrition (e.g., severe loss of subcutaneous tissues, possible edema)

The PG-SGA scoring is based on the points found in parentheses on the PG-SGA form. Where a point score is not included on the form, Tables A–E are used for scoring.

Table F. Triaging Nutritional Intervention

Additive scores are used to define specific nutritional intervention pathways including education and/or symptom management, aggressive oral nutrition, enteral/parenteral triage.

An *additive score of 0 to 1* indicates that no intervention is required at this time. Although these examples include only the patient section of the form, the total additive scores include addition of both the patient and clinician scores.

An *additive score of 2 to 3* is an indication for patient education by a dietitian or nurse, with pharmacologic triage by the nurse or physician as indicated by the symptom survey.

An *additive score of 4 to 8* requires the intervention of the dietitian, working in conjunction with the nurse or physician as indicated by the symptom check-off for pharmacologic management.

An *additive score of ≥9* indicates a critical need for symptom management and/or nutritional intervention. These patients require an interdisciplinary discussion to address all the aspects that have an impact on the nutritional status as well as to address the potential need for nonoral nutritional options, including enteral or parenteral. This decision should be dictated by the presence or absence GI function.

© Ottery 1997

*PG-SGA = Patient-Generated Subjective Global Assessment. © Ottery 1997
For additional information concerning the PG-SGA, contact F. Ottery, MD, PhD. at (215) 351-4050 or e-mail noatpres@mem.po.com

Table 7–4 • Recommended Number of Servings

Food Group	Child (2–5 yrs)	Child (≥6 yrs)/Teen	Adult	Pregnant	Lactating
Milk	3	3	2	3	3
Meat/protein	1–1.5	2	2	3	3
	1–1.5	2	2	2	2
Vegetable	2	3	3	3	3
Bread/cereal	4	6	6	6	6
Fats/sweets	—	—	—	—	—

The Food Guide Pyramid (Figure 7–2), recommended number of servings (Table 7–4), dietary guidelines (Table 7–5), and the RDAs (Appendix B) are most often used as a basis for determining nutritional adequacy of diet. One shortcoming of the RDAs is that they are not meant to be applied to sick individuals, whose nutrient requirements may be very different from those of healthy individuals. Specific nutrient values of foods can be obtained from several publications (e.g., *Bowes and Church's Food Values of Portions Commonly Used,* Pennington, 1998) and from nutrition labels and food manufacturers' information.

Table 7–5 • Summary of Major Dietary Guidelines

1. Reduce overall fat consumption to about 30% of total calorie intake
2. Increase complex carbohydrate intake (fruits, vegetables, grains) to about 60% of total calorie intake; reduce intake of refined and processed sugars to about 10% of total calorie intake
3. Limit protein consumption to about 10% of total calorie intake
4. Reduce cholesterol consumption to about 300 mg/d
5. Limit intake of sodium to about 3–5 g/d
6. Increase fiber intake to 25–35 g/d
7. Eat a variety of foods in each of the major food groups and maintain a healthy weight

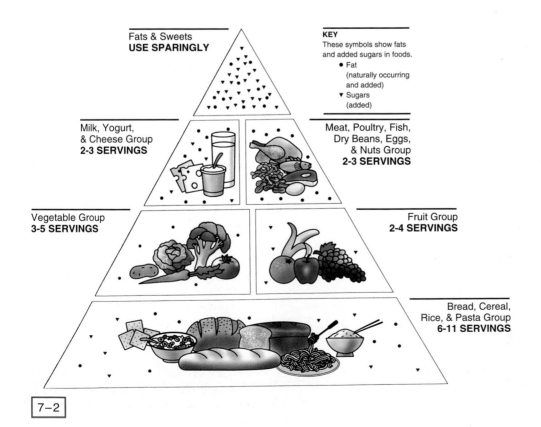

7–2

1. Eating patterns
2. Usual weight
3. Changes in appetite, taste, smell, chewing, swallowing
4. Recent surgery, trauma, burns, infection
5. Chronic illnesses
6. Vomiting, diarrhea, constipation

7. Food allergies or intolerances
8. Medications and/or nutritional supplements
9. Self-care behaviors
10. Alcohol or illegal drug use
11. Exercise and activity patterns
12. Family history

Examiner Asks	Rationale
❶ Eating patterns. • Number of meals/snacks per day? • Kind and amount of food eaten? • Fad or special diets? • Where is food eaten? • Food preferences and dislikes? • Religious or cultural restrictions? • Able to feed self?	Most individuals are knowledgeable about, or interested in, the foods they consume. If misconceptions are present, begin gradual instruction to correct them. Ethnic/religious beliefs or feeding difficulties may affect intake of certain foods.
❷ Usual weight. What is your usual weight? • 20% below or above desirable weight? • Recent weight change? • How much lost or gained? • Over what time period? • Reason for loss or gain?	Persons who have had a recent, unintentional weight loss or who are obese are at nutritional risk. Underweight individuals are vulnerable because their fuel reserves may be depleted. Excess weight is associated with a number of health problems, ranging from hypertension to cancer. Protein and calorie needs are often overlooked in acutely ill obese persons.
❸ Changes in appetite, taste, smell, chewing, swallowing. • Type of change? • When did change occur?	Poor appetite, taste and smell alterations, as well as chewing and swallowing difficulties interfere with adequate nutrient intake and increase the likelihood of nutritional risk.
❹ Recent surgery, trauma, burns, infection. • When? • Type? • How treated? • Conditions that increase nutrient loss (e.g., draining wounds, effusions, blood loss, dialysis)?	Persons who have had recent surgery, trauma, sepsis, or conditions causing nutrient losses may have caloric and nutrient needs that are two or three times greater than normal.
❺ Chronic illnesses. • Type? • When diagnosed?	Individuals with chronic illnesses that affect nutrient use (e.g., diabetes mellitus, pancreatitis, or malabsorption) or

Examiner Asks	Rationale
• How treated? • Dietary modifications? • Recent cancer chemotherapy or radiation therapy?	those receiving cancer treatment are twice as likely to have nutritional deficits.
6 Vomiting, diarrhea, constipation. Any problems? • Due to? • How long?	Gastrointestinal symptoms such as vomiting, diarrhea, or constipation may interfere with nutrient intake or absorption.
7 Food allergies or intolerances. • Any problematic foods? • Type of reaction? • How long?	Food allergies and intolerances may exacerbate adverse symptoms and result in nutrient deficiencies (e.g., diarrhea after milk ingestion).
8 Medications and/or nutritional supplements. • Prescription medications? • Nonprescription? • Use over a 24-hour period? • Type of vitamin/mineral, herbal, or alternative supplement? • Amount? • Duration of use?	Analgesics, antacids, anticonvulsants, antibiotics, diuretics, laxatives, antineoplastic drugs, steroids, and oral contraceptives are among the drugs that can interact with nutrients, impairing their digestion, absorption, metabolism, or utilization. Nutritional supplements may cause harmful side effects if taken in large amounts.
9 Self-care behaviors. • Meal preparation facilities? • Transportation for travel to market? • Adequate income for food purchase? • Who prepares meals and does shopping? • Environment during mealtimes?	Socioeconomic factors may interfere with ingestion of adequate amounts of food or usual diet.
10 Alcohol or illegal drug use. • When was last drink of alcohol? • Amount taken that episode? • Amount alcohol each day? Each week? • Duration of use? • (Repeat questions for each drug used.)	These agents are often substituted for nutritious foods and may increase requirements for some nutrients. Also, pregnant women who smoke, drink alcohol, or use illegal drugs give birth to a disproportionate number of infants with low birth weights, failure to thrive, and other complications.
11 Exercise and activity patterns. • Amount? • Type?	Caloric and nutrient needs increase with increased activity and exercise, especially competitive sports and manual labor. Inactive or sedentary lifestyles often lead to excess weight gain.
12 Family history. Family or personal history of heart disease, osteoporosis, cancer, gout, GI disorders, obesity, or diabetes? • Effect of each on eating patterns? • Effect on activity patterns?	Long-term nutritional deficiencies or excesses may first become manifest as disease, such as these common examples during the adult years. Early identification of nutritional alterations permits dietary and activity modifications to occur promptly—at a time when the body can recover more fully.

Examiner Asks	Rationale

ADDITIONAL HISTORY FOR INFANTS AND CHILDREN

Dietary histories of infants and children are generally obtained from the child's parents, guardian, baby sitter, or day care center. Usually, the person responsible for food preparation is able to provide a fairly accurate dietary history. Having the caregivers keep a thorough daily food diary and occasionally requesting 24-hour recalls during clinic visits are the most commonly employed techniques for this population group.

1 Gestational nutrition.
- Maternal history of alcohol or illegal drug use?
- Any diet-related complications during gestation?
- Infant's birth weight?
- Any evidence of delayed physical or mental growth?

Low birth weight (<2500 g) is a major factor in infant morbidity and mortality. Poor gestational nutrition, low maternal weight gain, and maternal alcohol and drug use—all factors in low birth weight—can lead to birth defects and delayed growth and development.

2 Infant breast or bottle fed.
- Type, frequency, amount, and duration of feeding?
- Any difficulties encountered?
- Timing and method of weaning?

Well-nourished infants experience appropriate physical and social growth and development. Inexperienced mothers may encounter problems with either breastfeeding or bottle-feeding or have questions about whether the infant is receiving adequate amounts of food.

3 Child willing to eat what you prepare.
- Any special likes or dislikes?
- How much will child eat?
- How do you control non-nutritious snack foods?
- How do you avoid food aspiration?

The preschool period is one of increasing growth for the child. Lifelong food habits are forming. Use of small portions, finger foods, simple meals, and nutritious snacks are strategies to improve dietary intake. Foods likely to be aspirated should be avoided (e.g., hot dogs, nuts, grapes, round candies, popcorn).

ADDITIONAL HISTORY FOR THE ADOLESCENT

1 Your present weight.
- What would you like to weigh?
- How do you feel about your present weight?
- On any special diet to lose weight?
- On other diets to lose weight? If so, were they successful?
- Constantly think about "feeling fat?"
- Intentionally vomit or use laxatives or diuretics after eating?

Obesity, particularly in girls, may precipitate fad dieting and malnutrition. Also, because of adolescents' increased body awareness and self-consciousness, they are prone to develop eating disorders such as anorexia nervosa or bulimia, conditions in which the real or perceived body image does not compare favorably to an ideal image—that found in advertisements or pictures of fashion models.

2 Use of anabolic steroids or other agents to increase muscle size and physical performance?
- When?

Once confined to male professional athletes, the use of anabolic steroids and other performance-enhancing agents

Examiner Asks	Rationale

- How much?
- Any problems?

now extends to junior high, high school, and college males and females. Adverse effects include personality disorders, aggressiveness, and liver and other organ damage.

3 **What snacks or fast foods do you like to eat?**
- When?
- How much?

An accurate dietary history may be difficult to obtain from the adolescent because of the frequency of between-meal snacks and meals eaten on the run. These often are omitted or forgotten during the interview or in a food diary.

4 **Age first started menstruating.**
- What is your menstrual flow like?

Menarche is usually delayed if malnutrition is present. Likewise, amenorrhea or scant menstrual flow is associated with nutritional deficiency.

ADDITIONAL HISTORY FOR THE PREGNANT FEMALE

1 **How many times have you been pregnant?**
- When?
- Any problems encountered during previous pregnancies?
- Problems this pregnancy?

If the mother is multiparous, with pregnancies occurring less than 1 year apart, there is a greatly increased chance that her nutritional reserves are depleted. Note previous complications of pregnancy such as excessive vomiting, anemia, or gestational diabetes. Slower gastrointestinal motility and pressure from the fetus may cause constipation, hemorrhoids, and indigestion. A past history of giving birth to a low-birth-weight infant suggests past nutritional problems. Giving birth to an infant with a birth weight of 4.5 kg (10 lbs) or more may signal the presence of *latent* diabetes in the mother.

2 **What foods do you prefer when pregnant?**
- What foods do you avoid?
- Crave any particular foods?

The expectant mother may be extremely vulnerable to familial, cultural, and traditional influences for food choices. Cravings for or aversions to particular foods are common, frequently psychological in origin, and should be evaluated for their potential contribution to, or interference with, dietary intake.

ADDITIONAL HISTORY FOR THE AGING ADULT

1 **How does your diet differ from when you were in your 40s and 50s?**
- Why?
- What factors affect the way you eat?

Note any physiologic changes of aging or socioeconomic changes that affect nutritional status.

Examiner Asks	Rationale
❷ Review the "Determine Your Nutritional Health" checklist (Figure 7–1).	The Nutritional Screening Initiative (White et al., 1991) is a three-step approach for nutrition screening of the elderly. The nutrition checklist in Figure 7–1 is completed by the older person or caregiver and identifies major risk factors and indicators of poor nutritional status. Persons identified at risk should undergo Level 1 and/or Level 2 screening depending on whether they are at moderate or high risk of poor nutritional status. (See sample forms in Jarvis C: *Laboratory Manual for Physical Examination and Health Assessment.*)

OBJECTIVE DATA

▶ **Equipment Needed**

Lange or Harpenden skinfold calipers

Ross Insertion Tape or other measurement tape

Anthropometer

Pen or pencil

Nutritional assessment data form

CLINICAL SIGNS

Observation of an individual's general appearance—obese, cachectic (fat and muscle wasting), or edematous—can provide clues to overall nutritional status. More specific clinical signs and symptoms suggestive of nutritional deficiencies can be detected through a physical examination. Because clinical signs are late manifestations of malnutrition, only in areas in which rapid turnover of epithelial tissue occurs—skin, hair, mouth, lips, and eyes—are the nutritional deficiencies readily detectable. These signs may also be non-nutritional in origin. Therefore, laboratory testing is required to make an accurate diagnosis. Laboratory tests for assessment of nutritional status are reviewed later in this chapter. Clinical signs of various nutritional deficiencies are summarized in Table 7–6 and are depicted in the section on abnormalities at the end of this chapter (See Table 7–8).

Table 7–6 · Clinical Signs of Malnutrition

Area of Examination	Normal Appearance	Signs Associated With Malnutrition	Nutrient Deficiency
Skin	Smooth, no signs of rashes, bruises, flaking	Dry, flaking, scaly	Vitamin A, vitamin B-complex, linoleic acid
		Petechiae/ecchymoses	Vitamins C and K
		Follicular hyperkeratosis (dry, bumpy skin)	Vitamin A, linoleic acid
		Cracks in skin, lesions on the hands, legs, face, or neck	Niacin, tryptophan
		Pellagrous dermatosis (hyperpigmentation of skin exposed to sunlight)	Niacin
		Nasolabial seborrhea	Riboflavin, vitamin B_6
		Acneiform forehead rash	Vitamin B_6
		Eczema	Linoleic acid
		Xanthomas (excessive deposits of cholesterol)	Excessive serum levels of LDLs or VLDLs
Hair	Shiny, firm, does not fall out easily, healthy scalp	Dull, dry, sparse	Protein, zinc, linoleic acid
		Color changes	Copper or protein
		Corkscrew hair	Copper
Eyes	Corneas are clear, shiny; membranes are pink and moist; no sores at corners of eyelids	Foamy plaques (Bitot's spots)	Vitamin A
		Dryness (xerophthalmia)	Vitamin A
		Softening (keratomalacia)	Vitamin A
		Pale conjunctivae	Iron, vitamins B_6, B_{12}
		Red conjunctivae	Riboflavin
		Blepharitis	B-complex, biotin
Lips	Smooth, not chapped or swollen	Cheilosis (vertical cracks in lips)	Riboflavin, niacin
		Angular stomatitis (red cracks at sides of mouth)	Riboflavin, niacin, iron, vitamin B_6
Tongue	Red in appearance; not swollen or smooth, no lesions	Glossitis (beefy red)	Vitamin B-complex
		Pale	Iron
		Papillary atrophy	Niacin
		Papillary hypertrophy	Multiple nutrients
		Magenta/purplish colored	Riboflavin
Gums	Reddish-pink, firm, no swelling or bleeding	Bleeding	Vitamin C
Nails	Smooth, pink	Brittle, ridged, or spoon shaped (koilonychia)	Iron
		Splinter hemorrhages	Vitamin C
Musculoskeletal	Erect posture, no malformations, good muscle tone, can walk or run without pain	Pain in calves, thighs	Thiamine
		Osteomalacia	Vitamin D, calcium
		Rickets	Vitamin D, calcium
		Joint pain	Vitamin C
		Muscle wasting	Protein, carbohydrate, fat
Neurologic	Normal reflexes, appropriate affect	Peripheral neuropathy	Thiamine, vitamin B_6
		Hyporeflexia	Thiamine
		Disorientation or irritability	Vitamin B_{12}

▶ **Normal Range of Findings**   **Abnormal Findings**

ANTHROPOMETRIC MEASURES

Anthropometry is the measurement and evaluation of growth, development, and body composition. The most commonly used anthropometric measures are height, weight, triceps skinfold thickness, elbow breadth, and arm and head circumferences. Measurement of height, weight, and head circumference is described in Chapter 9.

Derived Weight Measures

Three derived weight measures are used to depict changes in body weight.
Body weight as a percentage of ideal body weight is calculated using the following formula:

► Normal Range of Findings	Abnormal Findings

$$\text{Percent Ideal Body Weight} = \frac{\text{Current Weight}}{\text{Ideal Weight}} \times 100$$

(Ideal weight is based on the Metropolitan Life Insurance Tables, 1983; cited in Chapter 9.)

The **percent usual body weight** is calculated as follows:

$$\text{Percent Usual Body Weight} = \frac{\text{Current Weight}}{\text{Usual Weight}} \times 100$$

Recent weight change is calculated using the following formula:

$$\frac{\text{Usual Weight} - \text{Current Weight}}{\text{Usual Weight}} \times 100$$

Skinfold Thickness

Skinfold thickness measurements provide an estimate of body fat stores or the extent of obesity or undernutrition. Although other sites can be used (biceps, subcapsular, or suprailiac skinfolds), the triceps skinfold (TSF) is most commonly selected because of its easy accessibility and because standards and techniques are most developed for this site. To measure TSF thickness:

1. Have the ambulatory person stand with arms hanging freely at the sides and back to the examiner. (Nonambulatory persons should lie on one side. The uppermost arm should be fully extended, with the palm of the hand resting on the thigh.)
2. Using the thumb and forefinger of your left hand, gently grasp a fold of skin and fat on the posterior aspect of the person's left upper arm, midway between the acromion process of the scapula and the olecranon process (the tip of the elbow). Gently pull the skinfold away from the underlying muscle (Fig. 7–3).

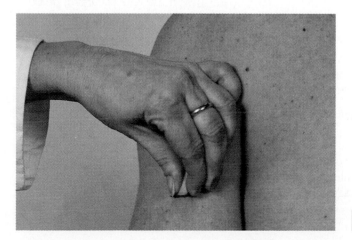

7–3

Abnormal Findings column:

A current weight of 80 to 90 percent of ideal weight is suggestive of mild malnutrition; 70 to 80 percent, of moderate malnutrition; and less than 70 percent, of severe malnutrition.

Obesity is defined as >120 percent ideal body weight.

A current weight of 85 to 95 percent of usual body weight is an indication of mild malnutrition; 75 to 84 percent, of moderate malnutrition; and less than 75 percent, of severe malnutrition.

An unintentional loss of >5 percent of body weight over 1 month, >7.5 percent of body weight over 3 months, or >10 percent of body weight over 6 months is considered clinically significant.

▶ Normal Range of Findings	Abnormal Findings

3. While grasping the skinfold, pick up the calipers with your right hand and depress the spring-loaded lever. Apply caliper jaws horizontally to the fat fold. Release the lever of the calipers while holding the skinfold. Wait 3 seconds, then take a reading. Repeat three times and average the three skinfold measurements (Fig. 7–4).

TSF values that are 10 percent below or above standard are suggestive of undernutrition and overnutrition, respectively.

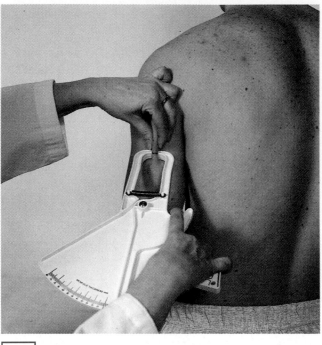

7–4

4. Record measurements to the nearest 5 mm (0.5 cm) on the nutritional assessment data form. Compare the person's measurements with standards by age, sex, and body frame size (see Appendixes D and E).

Conditions such as edema or subcutaneous emphysema may produce falsely high readings. Nonreproducible readings may be due to instrument malfunctions, use of plastic calipers (which are less accurate), or examiner error.

Mid-Upper Arm Circumference

Mid-upper arm circumference (MAC) estimates skeletal muscle mass and fat stores.

1. Have the person stand or sit with arm hanging fully extended and relaxed by the side of the body.
2. Loop the insertion tape or measuring tape around the arm at the midpoint of the upper arm (midway between the acromion and olecranon processes).
3. Position the tape horizontally at the midpoint, then tighten it firmly around the arm, but not so tightly as to cause skin contour indentation or pinching (Fig. 7–5).

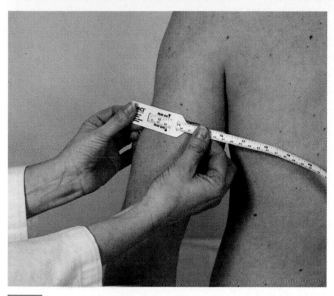

7-5

4. Note and record the measurement (in centimeters) on the appropriate form. Compare with norms (Appendix F).

For example, a normal mid-upper arm circumference for a 20-year-old female ranges from 23 to 34.5 cm; for a 20-year-old male, the normal range is 27.2 to 37.2 cm. Remember that accurate MAC and TSF measurements are difficult to obtain and interpret in older adults because of sagging skin, changes in fat distribution, and declining muscle mass.

Individuals whose measurements fall below the 10th percentile or above the 95th percentile warrant further medical and nutritional evaluation. Very high or very low readings may be due to examiner error.

Derived Anthropometric Measures

Although the MAC is of little value in and of itself, when combined with the TSF measurement, it is possible to indirectly determine the arm muscle *circumference* and arm muscle *area*.

Mid-upper arm muscle circumference (MAMC) estimates skeletal muscle reserves or the amount of lean body mass and is derived from the TSF and MAC measures using the following formula:

$$MAMC = MAC - (\pi \times TSF)$$

where

$$\pi = 3.14$$
$$MAC = \text{mid-upper arm circumference (in cm)}$$
$$TSF = \text{triceps skinfold (in mm)}$$
$$MAMC = \text{mid-upper arm muscle circumference (in cm)}$$

Record calculation on data forms. Compare with norms (Appendix F).

MAMC is dependent on accurate measurement of the MAC and TSF. In general, a MAMC that is 90 percent of standard is suggestive of mild malnutrition, 60 to 90 percent suggests moderate malnutrition; and less than 60 percent is indicative of severe malnutrition.

▶ **Normal Range of Findings**   **Abnormal Findings**

Mid-arm muscle area (MAMA) is a good indicator of lean body mass and thus skeletal protein reserves. These reserves are important in growing children and are especially valuable in evaluating persons who may be malnourished because of chronic illness, multiple surgeries, or inadequate dietary intake.

The equation for calculating MAMA is:

$$MAMA = \frac{(MAC - MAMC)^2}{4\pi}$$

where

$$MAMA = \text{mid-arm muscle area (in cm}^2)$$
$$MAC = \text{mid-upper arm circumference (in cm)}$$
$$MAMC = \text{mid-upper arm muscle circumference (in cm)}$$
$$4\pi = 4 \times 3.14 = 12.56$$

Record calculation on data forms. Compare with norms (Appendices D and E).

A newer technique to measure body composition is **bioelectrical impedance analysis (BIA).** Gaining more widespread use, the procedure resembles an electrocardiogram. An imperceptibly small electrical current passes through electrodes attached to the extremities of an individual yielding values which are used to calculate body muscle mass and fat stores ("Bioelectrical Impedance Analysis," 1996).

MAMA is considered to be a more sensitive measure of long-standing malnutrition than MAMC. A MAMA of 90 percent of standard reflects mild malnutrition; 60 to 90 percent, moderate malnutrition; and less than 60 percent, severe malnutrition.

Arm Span or Total Arm Length

Measurement of arm span is useful for those situations in which height is difficult to measure, such as in children with cerebral palsy or scoliosis or in aging persons with spinal curvature. Arm span, which is nearly equivalent to height, is sometimes used clinically instead of height (Mitchell and Lipschitz, 1982). Ask the person to hold the arms straight out from the sides of the body. Measure the distance from the tip of the middle finger on one hand to that on the other hand.

Frame Size

Frame size is calculated to determine appropriate range of ideal body weight. Most weight standards, such as the Metropolitan Life Insurance Tables of ideal weight for height, contain classifications of weight by frame size. Elbow breadth, a measure of skeletal breadth, is the most accurate method to determine frame size (Frisancho and Flegel, 1983). To measure it, you must be familiar with the use of flat-blade sliding calipers or a broad-blade anthropometer.

1. Instruct the person to extend the right arm forward, perpendicular to the body. Bend the elbow to a 90-degree angle, with the palm of the hand turned laterally (Fig. 7–6).
2. Facing the person, place the calipers on the condyles of the humerus (a broad-blade anthropometer may be needed if the calipers do not extend to the breadth of the elbow).
3. Read the distance between the condyles; record measurement (in centimeters) on the appropriate form. Assess whether small, medium, or large frame size using the norms (Appendix G).

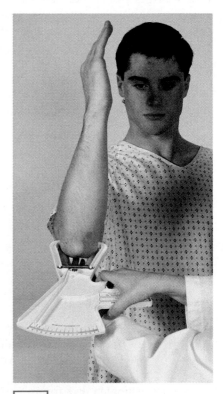

7–6

▶ Normal Range of Findings	Abnormal Findings

Body Mass Index

Body mass index is a simple indicator of total body fat or obesity. In children, adolescent girls, and older adults, it provides an especially useful estimate of obesity.

$$\text{Body Mass Index} = \frac{\text{Weight (in kilograms)}}{\text{Height (in meters)}^2} \quad or \quad \frac{\text{Weight (in pounds)}}{\text{Height (in inches)}^2 \times 704.5}$$

A body mass index of 27 or greater indicates obesity.

Waist-to-Hip Ratio

The waist-to-hip ratio assesses body fat distribution as an indicator of health risk (Folsom et al., 1993). Obese persons with a greater proportion of fat in the upper body, especially in the abdomen, have android obesity; obese persons with most of their fat in the hips and thighs have gynoid obesity.

$$\text{Waist-to-Hip Ratio} = \frac{\text{Waist Circumference}}{\text{Hip Circumference}}$$

where waist circumference is measured in inches at the smallest circumference below the rib cage and above the umbilicus, and hip circumference is measured in inches at the largest circumference of the buttocks.

A waist-to-hip ratio of 1.0 or greater in men or 0.8 or greater in women is indicative of android (upper body obesity) and increasing risk for obesity-related diseases and early mortality.

 DEVELOPMENTAL CONSIDERATIONS

Infants, Children, and Adolescents

Weight. During infancy, childhood, and adolescence, height and weight should be measured at regular intervals, because longitudinal growth is one of the best indices of nutritional status over time. See Chapter 9 for techniques.

Skinfold Thickness. Determination of skinfold thickness and/or body mass index may be useful in evaluating childhood and teenage overnutrition.

An estimated 15 percent or more of children and teenagers in the United States are obese.

The Pregnant Female

Weight. Measure weight monthly up to 30 weeks gestation, then every 2 weeks until the last month of pregnancy, when weight should be measured weekly. Appendix C illustrates approximate weight gain considered normal for each week of pregnancy.

The expectant mother should be considered at nutritional risk if her weight is 10 percent or more below ideal or 20 percent or more above the norm for her height and age group.

The Aging Adult

Height. With age, height declines in both men and women very slowly from the early 30s, leading to an average 2.9-cm loss in men and 4.9-cm loss in women (Bowman and Rosenberg, 1982). Height measures may not be accurate in individuals confined to a bed or wheelchair or those over 60 years of age (because of osteoporotic changes). Therefore, arm span, which is correlated with height, may be a better measure for the elderly.

|

Other Measurements. MAC and TSF measures may not be accurate and are difficult to obtain in older adults (because of sagging skin, changes in fat distribution, and declining muscle mass). (See Frisancho [1984] for data on weight and TSF thickness by height in U.S. men and women age 55 to 74 years.) Body mass index and waist-to-hip ratio are better indicators of obesity in this age group.

LABORATORY STUDIES

Routine laboratory tests are of particular value in nutritional assessment because they are objective, can detect preclinical nutritional deficiencies, and can be used to confirm subjective findings. Use caution, however, when interpreting test results that may be outside normal ranges, because they do not always reflect a nutritional problem and because standards for aging adults have not yet been firmly established.

The best routinely performed laboratory indicators of nutritional status are hemoglobin, hematocrit, cholesterol, triglycerides, total lymphocyte count, and serum albumin. Glucose, low- and high-density lipoproteins, prealbumin, transferrin, and total protein levels also provide meaningful information.

Hemoglobin

The hemoglobin determination is used to detect iron deficiency anemia. Normal values are as follows: **Infants,** 1 to 3 days—14.5 to 22.5 g/dl; 2 months—9.0 to 14.0 g/dl; **Children,** 6 to 12 years—11.5 to 15.5 g/dl; **Adults, males**—14 to 18 g/dl, females—12 to 16 g/dl.

Increased hemoglobin levels are suggestive of hemoconcentration due to polycythemia vera or dehydration.

Decreased hemoglobin levels may indicate anemia, recent hemorrhage, or hemodilution caused by fluid retention.

Hematocrit

Hematocrit, a measure of cell volume, is also an indicator of iron status. Normal values are as follows: **Infants,** 1 to 3 days—44 to 72 percent; 2 months—28 to 42 percent; **Children,** 6 to 12 years—35 to 45 percent; **Adults, males**—37 to 49 percent, females—36 to 46 percent.

A low value indicates insufficient hemoglobin formation, and for this reason, hematocrit and hemoglobin values should be interpreted together.

Cholesterol

Total cholesterol is measured to evaluate fat metabolism and to assess the risk of cardiovascular disease. Normal cholesterol concentrations vary with age and gender and may range from 120 mg/dl to 200 mg/dl.

Coronary heart disease risk steadily increases as serum cholesterol rises. Serum cholesterol levels of 200 to 239 mg/dl (borderline high) are associated with moderate risk and 240 mg/dl or more (high) with high risk of coronary heart disease, including myocardial infarction, stroke, and peripheral vascular disease.

|

Triglycerides

Serum triglycerides are used to screen for hyperlipidemia and to determine the risk of coronary artery disease. Triglyceride values are age related. Some controversy exists over the most appropriate normal ranges, but the following are fairly widely accepted: **ages 0 to 19,** 10 to 100 mg/dl; **ages 20 to 65,** 40 to 200 mg/dl.

Serum triglyceride levels are also associated with coronary heart disease. Serum triglycerides are categorized as: borderline, 250 to 500 mg/dl, or high, more than 500 mg/dl.

Total Lymphocyte Count

The most commonly used tests of immune function are total lymphocyte count (TLC) and skin testing, also called delayed cutaneous hypersensitivity testing. TLC is an important indicator of visceral protein status, and therefore, of cellular immune function.

The TLC is derived from the white blood cell count (WBC) and the differential count:

$$TLC = WBC \times \frac{\text{Number of Lymphocytes in Differential}}{100 \text{ cells}}$$

where TLC is calculated in cells per cubic millimeter.

Normal values for all age categories are between 1800 and 3000 cells/mm^3.

Non-nutritional factors that affect TLC include hypoalbuminemia, metabolic stress (e.g., major surgery, trauma, sepsis), infection, cancer, and chronic diseases.

Total lymphocyte counts of 1500 to 1800 indicate mild lymphocyte depletion; 900 to 1500, moderate depletion; and less than 900, severe depletion.

Skin Testing

Adequate immunity can also be demonstrated by a positive reaction to multiple skin test antigens. In these tests of immune function, at least six antigens are injected intradermally in the forearm area, and the response (redness and/or induration) is noted at 24 and 48 hours. A 5-mm or greater response to more than one antigen is generally considered to be a positive reaction (i.e., indicative of adequate immunity).

Commonly used antigens include *Candida,* tetanus toxoid, diphtheria toxoid, streptococcus, old tuberculin, proteus, trichophyton.

A response of less than 5 mm indicates anergy or immunoincompetence. Anergy occurs with malnutrition, hepatic failure, infection, and immunosuppressive drugs (e.g., chemotherapy agents, steroids).

Lymphopenia and the lack of a positive response to skin test antigens place the person at increased risk of infection, sepsis, and other complications.

Serum Proteins

Serum albumin is another common measurement of visceral protein status. Because of its relatively long half-life (17 to 20 days) and large body pool (4.0 to 5.0 g/kg), albumin is not an early indicator of protein malnutrition.

Normal serum albumin concentration in infants and children older than 6 months and adults ranges from 3.5 to 5.5 g/dl.

Low serum albumin levels may be caused by reasons other than protein-calorie malnutrition—for example, altered hydration status and decreased liver function.

▶ | Normal Range of Findings | Abnormal Findings

Levels of **serum transferrin,** an iron-transport protein, can be measured directly or by an indirect measurement of total iron-binding capacity. Serum transferrin, with a half-life of 8 to 10 days, may be a more sensitive indicator of visceral protein status than albumin.

The most widely used formula for computing serum transferrin is

$$\text{Serum Transferrin} = (0.8 \times \text{Total Iron-Binding Capacity}) - 43$$

The normal values for serum transferrin are 170 to 250 mg/dl.

Prealbumin, or thyroxine-binding prealbumin, serves as a transport protein for thyroxine (T_4) and retinol-binding protein. With a shorter half-life (48 hours) than either albumin or transferrin, prealbumin is sensitive to acute changes in protein status and sudden demands on protein synthesis. Normal prealbumin levels range from 15 to 25 mg/dl.

Nitrogen Balance

Nitrogen balance is also used as an index of protein nutritional status. Nitrogen is released with the catabolism of amino acids and is excreted in the urine as urea. Nitrogen balance therefore indicates whether the person is anabolic (positive nitrogen balance) or catabolic (negative nitrogen balance).

Nitrogen balance is estimated by a formula based on urine urea nitrogen (UUN) excreted during the previous 24 hours:

$$\text{Nitrogen} = \text{Nitrogen Intake} - \text{Nitrogen Excretion}$$
$$= \text{Protein Intake}/6.25 - (\text{24-hour UUN} + 4)$$

where

Nitrogen balance is determined in grams
24-hour UUN = urinary urea nitrogen, measured in grams
4 = nonurea nitrogen losses via feces, skin, sweat, and lungs, measured in grams

Creatinine-Height Index

The creatinine-height index (CHI) is a method of estimating the amount of skeletal muscle mass. Creatinine is derived from the breakdown of creatine, an energy-containing complex found in muscle. Creatinine is excreted unchanged in the urine at a constant rate in proportion to the amount of body muscle.

Abnormal Findings

In general, a serum albumin level of 2.8 to 3.5 g/dl represents moderate visceral protein depletion, and less than 2.8 g/dl denotes severe depletion (Wallach, 1996).

Levels of 150 to 170 mg/dl, are considered evidence of mild deficiency; 100 to 150 mg/dl, moderate deficiency; and levels less than 100 mg/dl, severe deficiency. (Lee and Nieman, 1996). Because a variety of clinical conditions can alter serum albumin and transferrin levels, consider the person's history in conjunction with these values for accurate interpretation.

Prealbumin levels are elevated in renal disease and reduced by surgery, trauma, burns, and infection. Prealbumin levels of 10 to 15 mg/dl indicate mild depletion; 5 to 10 mg/dl, moderate depletion; and less than 5 mg/dl, severe depletion.

In response to stress and increased protein demand, the body rapidly mobilizes its protein compartments, which results in increased production of urea and excretion of urea in the urine. With infection, an estimated loss of 9 to 11 g/day of UUN can be expected. In patients with major burns, 12 to 18 g/day of urea nitrogen may be expected in the urine (Blackburn et al., 1977).

Creatinine height index is calculated by first measuring urinary creatinine using a carefully collected 24-hour urine specimen. This value is then compared with ideal urinary creatinine levels from a creatinine for height standard table, by means of the following equation:

$$\text{CHI} = \frac{\text{Actual 24-hour Urine Creatinine}}{\text{Ideal 24-hour Urine Creatinine for Height}} \times 100$$

The person's CHI is then compared with a CHI standard table to determine the degree of skeletal muscle depletion.

DEVELOPMENTAL CONSIDERATIONS

In infancy and childhood, laboratory tests are performed only when undernutrition is suspected or if the child has acute or chronic illnesses that affect nutritional status.

During adolescence, unless overt disease is suspected, laboratory evaluation of hemoglobin and hematocrit levels and urinalysis for glucose and protein levels are adequate.

In pregnancy, hemoglobin and hematocrit values can be used to detect deficiencies of protein, folacin, vitamin B_{12}, and iron. Urine is frequently tested for glucose and protein (albumin), which can signal diabetes, preeclampsia, and renal disease.

In older adulthood, all serum and urine data must be interpreted with an understanding of declining renal efficiency and a tendency for aging adults to be overhydrated or underhydrated.

TRANSCULTURAL CONSIDERATIONS

Biocultural Variations in Laboratory Studies

Biocultural variations occur with some laboratory tests, such as *hemoglobin/ hematocrit, serum cholesterol, and serum transferrin*. The normal *hemoglobin level* for blacks is 1 g lower than for other groups, a factor that should be considered in the treatment of anemia. Data indicate that Native Americans, Hispanics, Asian Americans, and whites do not differ in this factor.

The difference between blacks and whites with respect to *serum cholesterol* is quite interesting. At birth, blacks and whites have similar serum cholesterol levels, but during childhood blacks have higher serum cholesterol levels than whites (5 mg/100 ml). These differences reverse during adulthood when black adults have lower serum cholesterol levels than white adults. The Pima Indians

The validities of CHI and nitrogen balance studies are dependent on the accuracy of the 24-hour urine collection. Failure to obtain an accurate sample, abnormal renal function, and certain other conditions can result in underestimation of creatinine and nitrogen losses.

Assuming an accurate 24-hour urine specimen has been collected, a CHI of 60 to 80 percent of standard indicates a moderate deficit in body mass. A value of less than 60 percent indicates a severe deficit of body muscle mass (Blackburn et al., 1977). Stress, fever, and trauma can increase urinary creatinine excretion.

|

have considerably lower serum cholesterol levels than whites, both during childhood (20 to 30 mg/100 ml lower) and adulthood (50 to 60 mg/100 ml lower).

In a study of children 1 to 3½ years of age, *serum transferrin* levels were found to differ between white and black children. The mean value for white children was 200 to 400 mg/100 ml, whereas the mean for black children was 341.4. The higher serum transferrin levels in black children may be due to their lowered hemoglobin/hematocrit levels. Transferrin levels increase in the presence of anemia. If the hemoglobin and hematocrit levels are normally lower in blacks, then higher transferrin levels should be considered normal (Jackson, 1990).

SERIAL ASSESSMENT

To monitor nutritional status in malnourished individuals or in individuals at risk for malnutrition, serial measurements of nutritional assessment parameters are made at routine intervals. At a minimum, weight and dietary intake should be evaluated weekly. Because the other nutritional assessment parameters change more slowly, data on these indicators may be collected biweekly or monthly.

Based on the findings of the nutritional assessment, the type of malnutrition can be diagnosed. The four major types of malnutrition are obesity, marasmus, kwashiorkor, and marasmus-kwashiorkor mix (Table 7–7). Each type of malnutrition has characteristic clinical and laboratory findings and a distinct cause.

 SUMMARY CHECKLIST: Nutritional Assessment

1: Obtain a health history relevant to nutritional status

2: Elicit dietary history, if indicated

3: Inspect skin, hair, eyes, oral cavity, nails, and musculoskeletal and neurologic systems for clinical signs and symptoms suggestive of nutritional deficiencies

4: Measure height, weight, and other anthropometric parameters, as indicated

5: Review relevant laboratory tests

APPLICATION AND CRITICAL THINKING

SAMPLE CHARTING

 Subjective

No history of diseases or surgery that would alter intake/requirements; no recent weight changes; no appetite changes; socioeconomic history is noncontributory. Does not smoke, drink alcohol, or use illegal, prescription, or over-the-counter drugs; no food allergies. Sedentary lifestyle; plays golf once per week.

Continued

▶ **Objective**

Dietary intake is adequate to meet protein and energy needs. No clinical signs of nutrient deficiencies. Height, weight, and screening laboratory tests within normal ranges.

CLINICAL CASE STUDY 1

R.G. is a single, 33-year-old white male high school teacher with a primary diagnosis of HIV infection.

▶ **Subjective**

6 months prior to admission (PTA)—no appetite changes; no anorexia or nausea; no weight loss; occasional "flulike symptoms" (fever and chills).

1 day PTA—symptoms include intractable diarrhea (1 to 2 L/day); fever; anorexia; pain with swallowing; weight loss of 17 kg; and depression. States that he feels helpless and that friends and family are avoiding him. "I would rather just get it over with." Daily caloric intake averages 1000 kcal (usual intake is 2000 kcal).

▶ **Objective**

Avoids eye contact and answers questions with short responses during history.

Inspection. Slightly raised patches resembling milk curds present in mouth and throat. General appearance is pale and cachectic.

Anthropometric. Height is 166.4 cm (65.5 inches). Current weight is 50.9 kg (112 lb); usual and ideal body weight is 68 kg (150 lb). TSF measures 8.5 mm (normal value is 12.5).

Laboratory. Serum albumin (1.86 g/dl) and total lymphocyte count (1000/mm³) are well below normal ranges. Stool is of watery consistency; stool analysis reveals *Cryptosporidium* infection.

▶ ASSESSMENT

- Altered nutrition: less than body requirements R/T anorexia, fever, diarrhea, and oral *Candida albicans*
- Malnutrition (marasmus)
- Reactive depression related to diagnosis and future

CLINICAL CASE STUDY 2

E.F. is an 87-year-old widow who lives alone in her own home. She has enjoyed good health all of her life.

▶ **Subjective**

During the past year, she has experienced declining memory and no longer cooks or drives. Relies on children to take her grocery shopping and prepare occasional meals. Income adequate. Describes her appetite as excellent. Spends her days watching television and reading. Experiences occasional constipation. Eats a well-balanced diet and enjoys high-carbohydrate foods such as cookies, candy, and doughnuts because they are easy to chew. Caloric intake is 1800 kcal/day.

▶ **Objective**

Inspection. No clinical signs of nutrient deficiencies.

Anthropometric. Height is 160 cm (63 inches). Current weight is 56.8 kg (125 lb); usual weight is 56.8 kg (125 lb), and ideal weight is 56.4 kg (124 lb).

Laboratory. Hemoglobin, hematocrit, and albumin values within normal limits.

▶ ASSESSMENT

- Normal nutriture
- Constipation related to inactivity and diet high in refined carbohydrates

NURSING DIAGNOSES COMMONLY ASSOCIATED WITH NUTRITIONAL DISORDERS

Diagnosis	Related Factors (Etiology)	Defining Characteristics (Symptoms and Signs)

Altered nutrition: less than body requirements	Increased energy and nutrient needs:
	  Periods of rapid growth and development
	  Pregnancy
	  Draining wounds
	  Infection
	  Surgery
	Inadequate nutrient intake:
	  Anorexia
	  Nausea and vomiting
	  Fatigue
	  Socioeconomic factors
	  Substance abuse
	Maldigestion or malabsorption (short bowel syndrome, pancreatitis)
	Drug-nutrient interactions
	Alteration in taste or smell
	Dysphagia
	Inability to chew
	Decreased level of consciousness
	Stress
	Decreased salivation
	Effects of hypercatabolic states (cancer, burns, infection)
	Effects of aging—decreased sense of taste
		Loss of body weight with adequate food intake
		Body weight 20% or more under ideal weight for height
		Aversion to eating
		Diarrhea and/or steatorrhea
		Inadequate food intake
		Triceps skinfold (TSF) <60% of standard measurement
		Midarm circumference (MAC <60% of standard measurement
		Abdominal pain or cramping
		Sore, inflamed buccal cavity
		Pale conjunctival and mucous membranes
		Poor muscle tone or skin turgor
		Loss of hair
		Decreased serum albumin or total protein
		Decreased serum transferrin or iron binding capacity
		Metabolic demands in excess of intake
		Anemia
		Lack of interest in food
		Reported or evidence of lack of food

Altered nutrition: more than body requirements	Lack of physical exercise/decreased activity pattern
	Eating in response to stress or emotional trauma
	Eating as a comfort measure/substitute gratification
	Learned eating behaviors
	Decreased metabolic need
	Lack of knowledge regarding nutritional needs
	Perceived lack of control
	Ethnic and cultural values
	Lack of social support for weight loss
	Decreased self-esteem
	Negative body image
		Weight 10%–20% over ideal for height and frame
		Reported and observed dysfunctional eating patterns:
		  Pairing food with other activities
		  Concentrating food intake at end of day
		  Eating in response to external cues such as time of day
		  Eating in response to internal cues other than hunger, e.g., anxiety
		Sedentary activity level
		Body mass index >27
		TSF > 15 mm for men and >25 mm for women
		Serum cholesterol ≥200 mg/dl
		Serum triglycerides >250 mg/dl

Other Related Nursing Diagnoses

ACTUAL	RISK/WELLNESS
Altered oral mucous membrane (See Chapter 14) Body image disturbance (See Chapter 11) Impaired skin integrity (See Chapter 10) Fluid volume deficit (See Chapter 10) Fluid volume excess (See Chapter 16) Ineffective breast feeding Constipation Diarrhea Knowledge deficit: nutrition Impaired swallowing Self-care deficit: feeding/eating	**Risk** Risk for constipation Risk for fluid volume deficit Risk for fluid volume imbalance **Wellness** Compliance with prescribed diet Increasing knowledge about adequate nutrition Improving nutritional intake

Table 7–7   CLASSIFICATION OF MALNUTRITION

Type/Etiology	Clinical Features	Anthropometric Measures	Laboratory Findings
Obesity due to caloric excess, refers to weights more than 20% above ideal body weight. Persons who are 100% or more above ideal body weight are categorized as morbidly obese. The causes of over-weight and obese conditions are complex and multifaceted; genetic, social, cultural, patho-logic, psychological, and physiologic factors have all been implicated. Regardless of its cause, the underlying prob-lem is usually an imbalance of caloric intake and caloric expenditure. In most cases, a small caloric surplus over a long period of time results in the extra pounds. Although visceral protein levels and im-munocompetence are gener-ally normal in the obese indi-vidual, anthropometric measures are above normal.	Obese appearance	Weight >120% standard for height Body mass index >27 Triceps skinfold (TSF) >10% standard Waist-to-hip ratio >1.0 (men) or >0.8 (women)	Serum cholesterol ≥200 mg/dl Serum triglycerides >250 mg/dl
Marasmus (protein-calorie malnutrition) is due to inade-quate intake of protein and calories or prolonged starva-tion. Anorexia, bowel obstruc-tion, cancer cachexia, and chronic illness are among the clinical conditions leading to marasmus. Marasmus is char-acterized by decreased anthro-pometric measures — weight loss and subcutaneous fat and muscle wasting. Visceral pro-tein levels may remain within normal ranges.	Starved appearance 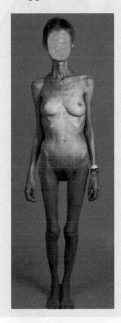	Weight ≤80% standard for height TSF < 90% standard Midarm muscle circum-ference (MAMC) ≤90% standard	Creatinine-height index < 80% standard

Continued

Table 7-7 CLASSIFICATION OF MALNUTRITION *Continued*

Type/Etiology	Clinical Features	Anthropometric Measures	Laboratory Findings
Kwashiorkor (protein malnutrition) is due to diets that may be high in calories but that contain little or no protein, e.g., low-protein liquid diets, fad diets, and long-term use of dextrose-containing intravenous fluids. Individuals with kwashiorkor, in contrast to those with marasmus, have decreased visceral protein levels and depressed immune function, but generally they have adequate anthropometric measures. These individuals may, therefore, appear well nourished or even obese.	Well-nourished appearance Edematous	Weight $\geq$ 100% standard for height TSF $\geq$ 100% standard	Serum albumin $<$ 3.5 g/dl Serum transferrin $<$ 150 mg/dl Lymphocytes $<$ 1,500 mm^3 Anergy
Marasmus/kwashiorkor mix is due to prolonged inadequate intake of protein and calories (e.g., severe starvation, severe catabolic states). This mix combines elements of both marasmus and kwashiorkor. Nutritional assessment findings include muscle, fat, and visceral protein wasting, along with immune incompetence. Individuals with marasmus-kwashiorkor mix are usually those who have undergone acute catabolic stress, such as major surgery, trauma, or burns in combination with prolonged starvation. Without nutritional support, this type of malnutrition is associated with the highest risk of morbidity and mortality.	Emaciated appearance	Weight $\leq$ 70% standard TSF $\leq$ 80% standard MAMC $\leq$ 60% standard	Serum albumin $<$ 2.8 g/dl Serum transferrin $<$ 100 mg/dl Lymphocytes $<$ 900 mm^3 Anergy Creatinine-height index $\leq$ 60% standard

▼ **Table 7–8   ABNORMALITIES DUE TO NUTRITIONAL DEFICIENCES**

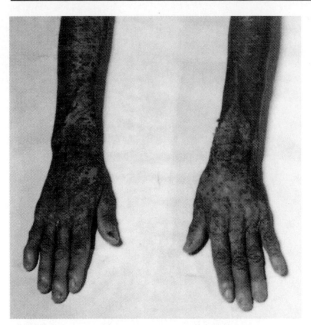

Pellagra

Pigmented keratotic scaling lesions resulting from a deficiency of niacin. These lesions are especially prominent in areas exposed to the sun, such as hands, forearms, neck, and legs.

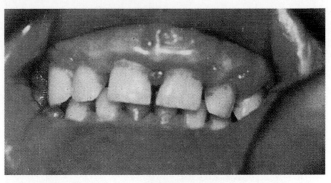

Scorbutic Gums

Deficiency of vitamin C. Gums are swollen, ulcerated, and bleeding due to vitamin C-induced defects in oral epithelial basement membrane and periodontal collagen fiber synthesis.

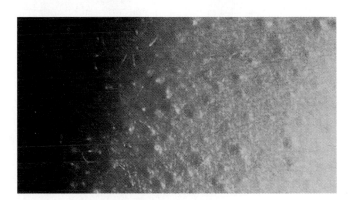

Follicular Hyperkeratosis

Dry, bumpy skin associated with vitamin A and/or linoleic acid (essential fatty acid) deficiency. Linoleic acid deficiency may also result in eczematous skin, especially in infants.

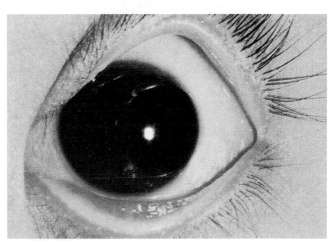

Bitot's Spots

Foamy plaques of the cornea that are a sign of vitamin A deficiency. Severe depletion may result in conjunctival xerosis (drying) and progress to corneal ulceration, and finally destruction of the eye (keratomalacia).

Continued

Table 7–8 ABNORMALITIES DUE TO NUTRITIONAL DEFICIENCIES *Continued*

ABNORMAL FINDINGS

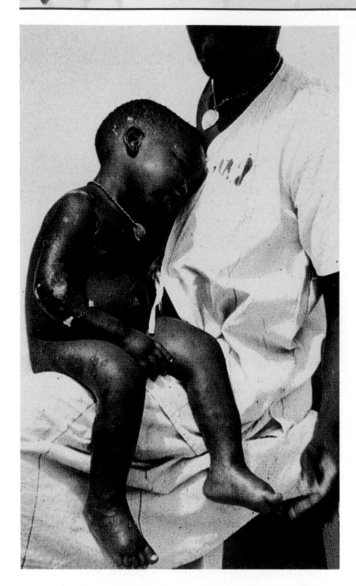

Kwashiorkor

Occurs in children and adults whose diets contain mostly carbohydrate and little or no protein and are under stress (growth, parasitic or viral infections, major surgery, trauma, or burns).

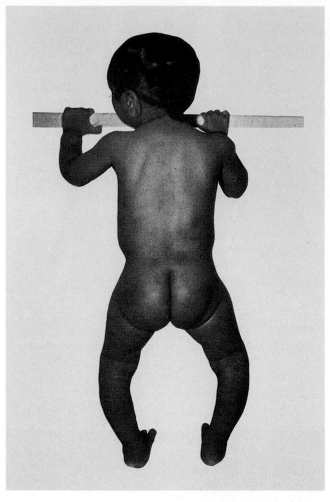

Rickets

Sign of vitamin D and calcium deficiencies in children (disorders of cartilage cell growth, enlargement of epiphyseal growth plates) and adults (osteomalacia).

Magenta Tongue ▶

"Magenta tongue" is a sign of riboflavin deficiency. In contrast, a pale tongue is probably attributable to iron deficiency; a beefy red–colored tongue is caused by vitamin B-complex deficiency.

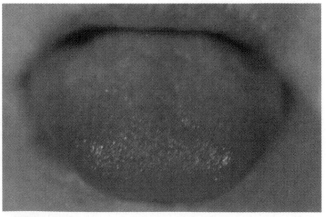

Continued

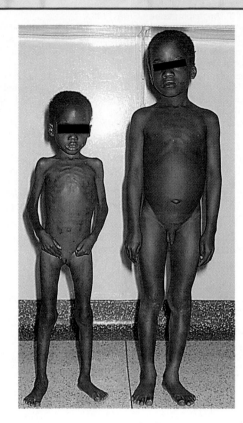

◄ **HIV Infection Discordant twins**

An HIV-infected 4½-year-old girl with her uninfected twin brother. The girl has been sickly since shortly after birth and suffers from HIV-associated malnutrition.

Bibliography

Anonymous: Position of the American Dietetic Association: Child and adolescent food and nutrition programs. J Am Diet Assoc 96(9), 913–917, 1996.

Anonymous: Update: Prevalence of overweight among children, adolescents, and adults—United States, 1988–1994. MMWR Morb Mortal Wkly Rep 46(9): 198–202, 1997.

Battaglia FC, Thureen PJ: Nutrition of the fetus and premature infant. Nutrition 13(10):903–906, 1997.

Bioelectrical impedance analysis in body composition measurement: National Institutes of Health Technology Assessment Conference Statement. Am J Clin Nutr 64(Suppl. 3): 524S–532S, 1996.

Blackburn GL, Bistrian BR, Maini BS, et al: Nutritional and metabolic assessment of the hospitalized patient. J Parenteral Enter Nutr 1(1): 11–22, 1977.

Bowman BB, Rosenberg IH: Assessment of nutritional status of the elderly. Am J Clin Nutr 35:1142–1151, 1982.

Bronner YL, Paige DM: Current concepts in infant nutrition. J Nurse Midwifery 37:43S–58S, 1992.

Charney P: Nutrition assessment in the 1990s: Where are we now? Nutr Clin Pract 10:131–139, 1995.

Curtas S: Nutrition assessment of the adult. *In* Hennessy K, Orr M (Eds): Nutrition Support Nursing: Core Curriculum. Silver Spring, MD, American Society for Parenteral and Enteral Nutrition, 1996.

Detsky AS, Smalley PS, Chang J: Is this patient malnourished? JAMA 271(1):54–58, 1994.

Dwyer JT: Screening Older Americans' Nutritional Health: Current Practices and Future Possibilities [Monograph]. Washington, DC, Nutrition Screening Initiative, 1991.

Evans-Stoner E: Nutrition assessment: A practical approach. Nurs Clin North Am 32(4):637–650, 1997.

Folsom AR, Kaye SA, Sellers TA, et al: Body fat distribution and 5-year risk of death in older women. JAMA 269(4):483–487, 1993.

Frisancho AR: Anthropometric Standards for the Assessment of Growth and Nutritional Status. Ann Arbor, MI, University of Michigan Press, 1990.

Frisancho AR: New standards of weight and body composition by frame size and height for assessment of nutritional status of adults and the elderly. Am J Clin Nutr 40:808–819, 1984.

Frisancho AR, Flegel PN: Elbow breadth as a measure of frame size for U.S. males and females. Am J Clin Nutr 31:311–314, 1983.

Giotta MP: Nutrition during pregnancy: Reducing obstetric risk. J Perinat Neonat Nurs 6(4):1–12, 1993.

Grindel CG, Costello, MC: Nutrition screening: An essential assessment parameter. MedSurg Nurs 5(3):145–156, 1996.

Hammond K: Physical assessment: A nutritional perspective. Nurs Clin North America 32(4):779–790, 1997.

Hunter J, Willett WC: Nutrition and breast cancer. Cancer Causes Control 7(1):56–58, 1996.

Jackson RT: Separate hemoglobin standards for blacks and whites: A critical review of the case for separate and unequal hemoglobin standards. Med Hypotheses 32:181–189, 1990.

Keithley JK, Keller A, Vazquez J: Promoting good nutrition: Using the food guide pyramid in clinical practice. MedSurg Nurs 5(6):397–403, 1996.

Kolasa KM, Weismiller DG: Nutrition during pregnancy. Am Fam Phys 56(1):205–212, 1997.

Kovacevich DS, Boney AR, Braunschweig CL, Perez A, Stevens M: Nutrition risk classification: A valid and reproducible tool for nurses. Nutr Clin Prac 12:20–25, 1997.

Lee RD, Nieman D: Nutritional Assessment, 2nd ed. St. Louis, Mosby-Yearbook, 1996.

Mahan KL, Escott-Stump S: Krauses's Food, Nutrition, and Diet Therapy, 9th ed. Philadelphia, W.B. Saunders, 1996.

Mitchell CO, Lipschitz DA: Arm length measurement as an alternative to height in nutritional assessment of the elderly. J Parenteral Enter Nutr 6:226–229, 1982.

Muscari ME: Screening for anorexia and bulimia. Am J Nurs 98(11): 22–24, Nov 1998.

National Academy of Sciences: Nutrition During Lactation. Washington, DC, National Academy Press, 1991.

National Academy of Sciences: Nutrition During Pregnancy. Washington, DC, National Academy Press, 1990.

National Cholesterol Education Program: Report of the Expert Panel on Population Strategies for Blood Cholesterol Reduction. Bethesda, MD, U.S. Department of Health and Human Services, Public Health Service, National Institutes of Health, National Heart, Lung, Blood Institute, 1990.

North American Diagnosis Association: Classification of nursing diagnosis. Proceedings of the Ninth National Conference, Philadelphia, J.B. Lippincott Company, 1991.

Ottery FD: Definition of standardized nutritional assessment and interventional pathways in oncology. Nutrition 12(Suppl. 1): S15–S19, 1996.

Pennington JAT: Bowes and Church's Food Values of Portions Commonly Used, 17th ed. Philadelphia, J.B. Lippincott Company, 1998.

Phaneuf C: Screening elders for nutritional deficits. Am J Nurs 96(3): 58–60, Mar 1996.

Posthauer ME, Dorse B, Foiles RA, Escott-Stump S, Lysen L, Balogun L: Identifying patients at risk: ADA's definitions for nutrition screening and nutrition assessment. J Am Diet Assoc 94(8):838–839, 1994.

Potter JD: Nutrition and colorectal cancer. Cancer Causes Control 7(1): 127–146, 1996.

Recommended Daily Dietary Allowances, 10th ed. Washington, DC, National Academy of Sciences, National Research Council Food and Nutrition Board, 1989.

Spector RE: Cultural Diversity in Health and Illness, 4th ed. Norwalk, CT, Appleton-Century-Crofts, 1996.

Subcommittee on Nutritional Status and Weight Gain During Pregnancy, Food and Nutrition Board, National Academy of Sciences: Nutrition During Pregnancy, Parts I and II. Washington, DC, National Academy Press, 1990.

Sucher KP, Kittler PG: Food and Culture in America: A Nutrition Handbook, 2nd ed. New York, Van Nostrand Reinhold, 1997.

Wallach J: Interpretation of Diagnostic Tests, 6th ed. Boston, Little, Brown & Company, 1996.

Whitaker RC, Wright JA, Pepe MS, et al: Predicting obesity in young adulthood from childhood and parental obesity. N Engl J Med 337(13):869–873, Sept 1997.

White JV, Dwyer JT, Possner BM, et al: Nutrition screening initiative: Development and implementation of the public awareness checklist and screening tools. J Am Diet Assoc 92:163–167, 1992.

White JV, Ham RJ, Lipschitz DA: Nutrition Screening Initiative: Toward a Common View [Monograph]. Washington, DC, Nutrition Screening Initiative, 1991.

Nutrition-Related Internet Sites

U.S. Food and Nutrition Information Center http://www.nal.usda.gov/fnic/etext/fnic.html

National Nutrition Program http://www.dcpc.nci.nih.gov/5aday/

Weight Management Program http://www.obesity.com/

FDA Center for Food Safety and Nutrition http://vm.cfsan.fda.gov/index/html

American Dietetic Association http://www.eatright.org

Child/Adolescent Nutrition and Health http://ificinfo.health.org/index3.htm

UNIT 2

Physical Examination

CHAPTER EIGHT

Assessment Techniques and Approach to the Clinical Setting

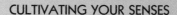

The health history described in the preceding chapters provides **subjective** data for health assessment, the individual's *own* perception of the health state. Unit 2 presents **objective** data, the signs perceived by the examiner through the physical examination.

The physical examination requires that the examiner develop technical skills and a knowledge base. The technical skills are the tools to gather data. You will relate those data to your knowledge base and to your previous experience. A sturdy knowledge base enables you to look *for,* rather than merely look *at.* Consider a statement by the eighteenth century German poet Goethe, "We see only what we know." To recognize a significant finding, you need to know what to look for.

CULTIVATING YOUR SENSES

You will use your senses—sight, smell, touch, and hearing—to gather data during the physical examination. You always have perceived the world through your senses, but now they will be focused in a new way. Applying your senses to assess each individual's health state may seem awkward at first, but this will be polished with repetition and tutored practice. The skills requisite for the physical examination are **inspection, palpation, percussion,** and **auscultation.** The skills are performed one at a time and in this order.

Inspection

Inspection is concentrated watching. It is close, careful scrutiny, first of the individual as a whole and then of each body system. Inspection begins the moment you first meet the individual and develop a "general survey." (Specific data to consider for the general survey are presented in the following chapter.) Then as you proceed through the examination, start the assessment of each body system with inspection.

Inspection always comes first. Initially, you may feel embarrassed "staring" at the person without also "doing something." But do not be too eager to touch the person. A focused inspection takes time and yields a surprising amount of data. Train yourself not to rush through inspection by placing your hands in your pockets or holding them behind your back.

Learn to use each person as his or her own control and compare the right and left sides of the body. The two sides are nearly symmetric. Inspection requires good lighting, adequate exposure, and occasional use of certain instruments (otoscope, ophthalmoscope, penlight, nasal and vaginal specula) to enlarge your view.

Palpation

Palpation follows and often confirms points you noted during inspection. Palpation applies your sense of touch to assess these factors: texture, temperature, moisture, or-

gan location and size, as well as any swelling, vibration or pulsation, rigidity or spasticity, crepitation, presence of lumps or masses, and presence of tenderness or pain. Different parts of the hands are best suited for assessing different factors:

- Fingertips—best for fine tactile discrimination, such as skin texture, swelling, pulsation, and determining presence of lumps
- A grasping action of the fingers and thumb—to detect the position, shape, and consistency of an organ or mass
- The dorsa (backs) of hands and fingers—best for determining temperature because the skin here is thinner than on the palms
- Base of fingers (metacarpophalangeal joints) or ulnar surface of the hand—best for vibration.

Your palpation technique should be slow and systematic. A person stiffens when touched suddenly, making it difficult for you to feel very much. Use a calm, gentle approach. Warm your hands by kneading them together or holding them under warm water. Identify any tender areas, and palpate them last.

Start with light palpation to detect surface characteristics and to accustom the person to being touched. Then perform deeper palpation, perhaps by helping the person use relaxation techniques such as imagery or deep breathing. Your sense of touch becomes blunted with heavy or continuous pressure. When deep palpation is needed (as for abdominal contents), intermittent pressure is better than one long continuous palpation. Avoid any situation in which deep palpation could cause internal injury or pain.

Bimanual palpation requires the use of both of your hands to envelop or capture certain body parts or organs, such as the kidneys, uterus, or adnexa, for more precise delimitation (see Chapters 19 and 24).

Percussion

Percussion is tapping the person's skin with short, sharp strokes to assess underlying structures. The strokes yield a palpable vibration and a characteristic sound that depicts the location, size, and density of the underlying organ. Why learn percussion when an x-ray study is so much more accurate? Because your percussing hands are always available, are easily portable, give instant feedback, and have no radiative side effects. Percussion has the following uses:

- Mapping out the *location* and *size* of an organ by exploring where the percussion note changes between the borders of an organ and its neighbors
- Signaling the *density* (air, fluid, or solid) of a structure by a characteristic note
- Detecting an abnormal mass if it is fairly superficial; the percussion vibrations penetrate about 5 cm deep— a deeper mass would give no change in percussion

- Eliciting pain if the underlying structure is inflamed, as with sinus areas or over the kidney
- Eliciting a deep tendon reflex using the percussion hammer.

Two methods of percussion can be used—*direct* (sometimes called immediate) and *indirect* (or mediate). In direct percussion, the striking hand directly contacts the body wall. This produces a sound and is used in percussing the infant's thorax or the adult's sinus areas. *Indirect* percussion is used more often, and involves both hands. The striking hand contacts the stationary hand fixed on the person's skin. This yields a sound and a subtle vibration. The procedure is:

The Stationary Hand. Hyperextend the middle finger (sometimes called the pleximeter) and place its distal portion, the phalanx and distal interphalangeal joint, *firmly* against the person's skin. Avoid the person's ribs and scapulae. Percussing over a bone yields no data because it always sounds "dull." Lift the rest of the stationary hand up off the person's skin (Fig. 8–1). Otherwise the resting hand will dampen off the produced vibrations, just as a drummer uses the hand to halt a drum roll.

The Striking Hand. Use the middle finger of your dominant hand as the *striking-finger* (sometimes called the plexor) (Fig. 8–2). Hold your forearm close to the skin surface, with your upper arm and shoulder steady. Scan your muscles to make sure they are steady but not rigid. The action is all in the wrist, and it *must* be relaxed. Spread your fingers, swish your wrist, and bounce your middle finger off the stationary one. Aim for just behind the nail bed or at the distal interphalangeal joint; the goal is to hit the portion of the finger that is pushing the hardest into the skin surface. Flex the striking finger so that its tip, not the finger pad, makes contact. It hits directly at right angles to the stationary finger.

Percuss two times in this location using even, staccato blows. Lift the striking finger off quickly; a resting finger damps off vibrations. Then move to a new body location and repeat, keeping your technique even. The force of the blow determines the loudness of the note. You do not need a very loud sound; use just enough force to achieve a clear note. The thickness of the person's body wall will be a factor. You will need a stronger percussion stroke for persons with obese or very muscular body walls.

Percussion can be an awkward technique for beginning examiners. You may feel surprised and embarrassed if your striking finger misses your stationary hand completely. You may wince if the fingernail of your striking finger is too long and painfully gouges your stationary finger. As with all new skills, refinement follows practice. After a few weeks your hand placement becomes precise and feels natural, and your ears learn to perceive the subtle difference in percussion notes.

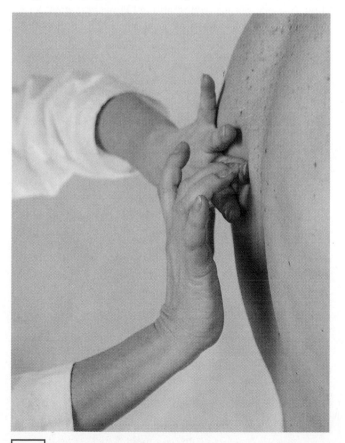

8–1

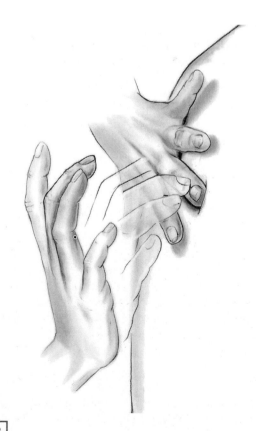

8–2

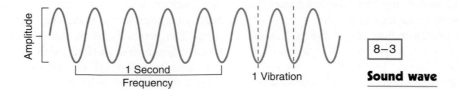

8–3

Sound wave

Production of Sound. All sound results from vibration of some structure (Fig. 8–3). Percussing over a body structure causes vibrations that produce characteristic waves and are heard as "notes" (Table 8–1). Each of the five percussion notes is differentiated by the following components:

1. **Amplitude** (or intensity), a loud or soft sound. The louder the sound, the greater the amplitude. Loudness depends on the force of the blow and the structure's ability to vibrate.
2. **Pitch** (or frequency), the number of vibrations per second, written as "cps," or cycles per second. More rapid vibrations produce a high-pitched tone; slower vibrations yield a low-pitched tone.
3. **Quality** (timbre), a subjective difference due to a sound's distinctive overtones. A pure tone is a sound of one frequency. Variations within a sound wave produce overtones. Overtones allow you to distinguish a C on a piano from a C on a violin.
4. **Duration,** the length of time the note lingers.

A basic principle is that a structure with relatively more air (such as the lungs) produces a louder, deeper, and longer sound because it vibrates freely, while a denser, more solid structure (such as the liver) gives a softer, higher, shorter sound because it does not vibrate as easily. Although Table 8–1 describes five "normal" percussion notes, variations occur in clinical practice. The "note" you hear depends on the nature of the underlying structure, as well as the thickness of the body wall and your correct technique. Do not learn these various notes just from written description. Practice on a willing partner.

Auscultation

Auscultation is listening to sounds produced by the body, such as the heart and blood vessels and the lungs and abdomen. Likely you already have heard certain body sounds with your ear alone, for example, the harsh gurgling of very congested breathing. However, most body

Table 8–1 • Characteristics of Percussion Notes

	Amplitude	Pitch	Quality	Duration	Sample Location
Resonant	Medium-loud	Low	Clear, hollow	Moderate	Over normal lung tissue
Hyperresonant	Louder	Lower	Booming	Longer	Normal over child's lung Abnormal in the adult, over lungs with increased amount of air, as in emphysema
Tympany	Loud	High	Musical and drumlike (like the kettle drum)	Sustained longest	Over air-filled viscus, e.g., the stomach, the intestine
Dull	Soft	High	Muffled thud	Short	Relatively dense organ, as liver or spleen
Flat	Very soft	High	A dead stop of sound, absolute dullness	Very short	When no air is present, over thigh muscles, bone, or over tumor

sounds are very soft and must be channeled through a **stethoscope** for you to evaluate them. The stethoscope does not magnify sound, but does block out extraneous room sounds. Of all the equipment you will use, the stethoscope quickly becomes a very personal instrument. Take time to learn its features and to fit one individually to yourself.

The fit and quality of the stethoscope are important. You cannot assess what you cannot hear through a poor instrument. The slope of the earpieces should point forward toward your nose. This matches the natural slope of your ear canal and efficiently blocks out environmental sound. If necessary, use pliers to parallel the slope of the earpieces with that of your ear canals. The earpieces should fit snugly, but if they hurt, they are inserted too far. Adjust the tension and experiment with different rubber or plastic earplugs to achieve the most comfort. The tubing should be of thick material, with an internal diameter of 4 mm (⅛ in), and about 30 to 36 cm (12 to 14 in) long. Longer tubing may distort the sound.

Choose a stethoscope with two endpieces—a diaphragm and a bell (Fig. 8–4). You will use the **diaphragm** most often because its flat edge is best for high-pitched sounds—breath, bowel, and normal heart sounds. (Since your stethoscope touches many people, clean the endpieces with an alcohol swab to eliminate a possible vector of infection.) Hold the diaphragm firmly against the person's skin, firm enough to leave a slight ring afterward. The **bell** endpiece has a deep, hollow cuplike shape. It is best for soft, low-pitched sounds such as extra

heart sounds or murmurs. Hold it lightly against the person's skin, just enough that it forms a perfect seal. Any harder causes the person's skin to act as a diaphragm, obliterating the low-pitched sounds.

Before you can evaluate body sounds, you must eliminate any confusing artifacts:

• Any extra room noise can produce a "roaring" in your stethoscope, so the room must be quiet.
• Keep the examination room warm. If the person starts shivering, the involuntary muscle contractions could drown out other sounds.
• Warm the stethoscope endpiece by rubbing it in your palm. This avoids the "chandelier sign" elicited when placing a cold endpiece on a warm chest!
• The friction on the endpiece from a male's hairy chest causes a crackling sound that mimics an abnormal breath sound called *crackles* or *rales*. To minimize this problem, wet the hair before auscultating the area.
• Never listen through a gown. Reach under a gown to listen, but take care that no clothing rubs on the stethoscope.
• Finally, avoid your own "artifact," such as breathing on the tubing, or the "thump" from bumping the tubing together.

Auscultation is a skill that beginning examiners are eager to learn, but one that is difficult to master. First, you must learn the wide range of normal sounds. Once you can recognize normal sounds, you can distinguish the abnormal sounds and "extra" sounds. Be aware that in some body locations you may hear more than one sound; this can be confusing. You will need to listen selectively, to only one thing at a time. As you listen, ask yourself: What am I *actually hearing?* . . . What *should* I be hearing at this spot?

SETTING

The examination room should be warm and comfortable, quiet, private, and well lit. When possible, stop any distracting noises, such as humming machinery, radio or television, or people talking, that could make it difficult to hear body sounds. Your time with the individual should be secure from interruptions from other health care personnel. Lighting with natural daylight is best, although it is often not available; artificial light from two sources will suffice and will prevent shadows. A wall-mounted or gooseneck stand lamp is needed for high-intensity lighting.

Position the examination table so that both sides of the person are easily accessible (Fig. 8–5). The table should be at a height at which you can stand without stooping and should be equipped to raise the person's head up to 45 degrees. A roll-up stool is used for the sections of the examination for which you must be sitting. A bedside stand or table is needed to lay out all your equipment.

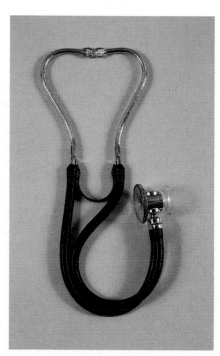

8–4

Stethoscope diaphragm (left) and bell (right)

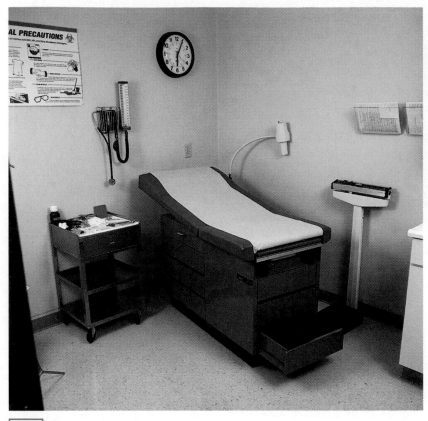

8-5

EQUIPMENT

During the examination, you do not want to be searching for equipment or to have to leave the room to find an item. Have all your equipment at easy reach and laid out in an organized fashion (Fig. 8–6). The following items are usually needed for a screening physical examination:

- Platform scale with height attachment
- Skinfold calipers
- Sphygmomanometer
- Stethoscope with bell and diaphragm endpieces
- Thermometer
- Flashlight or penlight
- Otoscope/ophthalmoscope
- Tuning fork
- Nasal speculum (if a short, broad speculum is not included with the otoscope)
- Tongue depressor
- Pocket vision screener
- Skin-marking pen
- Flexible tape measure and ruler marked in centimeters
- Reflex hammer
- Sharp object (sterile needle or split tongue blade)
- Cotton balls
- Bivalve vaginal speculum

- Clean gloves
- Materials for cytologic study
- Lubricant
- Fecal occult blood test materials

Most of the equipment is described as it comes into use throughout the text. However, consider these introductory comments on the otoscope and ophthalmoscope.

The **otoscope** funnels light into the ear canal and onto the tympanic membrane. The base serves both as the power source by holding a battery and as the handle. To attach the head, press it down onto the male adaptor end of the base and turn clockwise until you feel a stop. To turn the light on, press the red button rheostat down and clockwise. (Always turn it off after use to increase the life of the bulb and battery.) Five different-sized specula are available to attach to the head (Fig. 8–7). (The short broad speculum is for viewing the nares.) Choose the largest one that will fit comfortably into the person's ear canal. See Chapter 13 for technique on use of the otoscope.

The **ophthalmoscope** illuminates the internal eye structures. Its system of lenses and mirrors enables you to look through the pupil at the fundus (background) of the eye, much like looking through a keyhole at a room beyond. The ophthalmoscope head attaches to the base male adaptor just as the otoscope head does (Fig. 8–8).

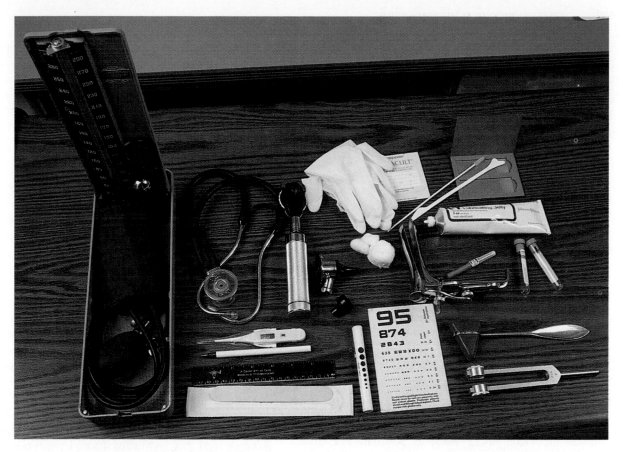

8-6

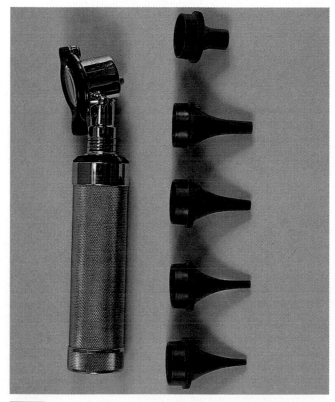

8-7

Otoscope

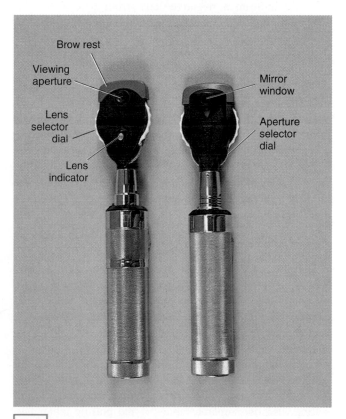

8-8

Brow rest

Viewing aperture

Lens selector dial

Lens indicator

Mirror window

Aperture selector dial

Ophthalmoscope

The head has five different parts:

1. Viewing aperture, with five different apertures
2. Aperture selector dial on the front
3. Mirror window on the front
4. Lens selector dial
5. Lens indicator

Select the aperture to be used (Fig. 8–9).

○ Large (full spot) for dilated pupils

○ Small for undilated pupils

● Red-free filter — a green beam, used to examine the optic disc for hemorrhage (which looks black) and melanin deposits (which look gray)

⊞ Grid — to determine fixation pattern and to assess size and location of lesions on the fundus

▯ Slit — to examine the anterior portion of the eye and to assess elevation or depression of lesions on the fundus

8–9

Rotating the lens selector dial brings the object into focus. The lens indicator shows a number, or *diopter,* that indicates the value of the lens in position. The black numbers indicate a positive lens, from 0 to +40. The red numbers indicate a negative lens, from 0 to −20. The ophthalmoscope can compensate for myopia (nearsightedness) or hyperopia (farsightedness) but will not correct for astigmatism. See Chapter 12 for details on how to hold the instrument and what to inspect.

The following equipment occasionally will be used, depending on the individual's needs: goniometer to measure joint range of motion, Doppler to augment pulse or blood pressure measurement, fetoscope for auscultating fetal heart tones, and pelvimeter to measure pelvic width.

For a child you also will need appropriate pediatric-sized endpieces for stethoscope and otoscope specula, materials for developmental assessment, appropriate-age toys, and a nipple or pacifier for an infant.

A Clean Field

Do not let your stethoscope become a *staph*-oscope! Stethoscopes and other equipment that are frequently used on many patients can become a common vehicle for transmission of infection. Cleaning with an alcohol swab between patients is an effective control.

Designate a "clean" versus a "used" area for handling of your equipment. In a hospital setting, you may use the bedside stand for your clean surface and the overbed table for the used equipment surface. Or, in a clinic setting, use two separate areas of the pull-up table. Distinguish the clean area by one or two disposable paper towels. On the towels, place all the new, newly cleaned, or newly alcohol-swabbed equipment that you will use on

this patient. Use alcohol swabs to clean all equipment that you carry from patient to patient, e.g., your stethoscope endpieces, the reflex hammer, ruler. As you proceed through the examination, pick up each piece of equipment from the clean area, and after use on the patient, relegate it to the used area, or (as in the case of tongue blades, gloves) throw it directly in the trash.

A SAFER ENVIRONMENT

In addition to monitoring the cleanliness of your equipment, take all steps to avoid any possible transmission of infection between patients or between patient and examiner. A *nosocomial* infection (an infection acquired during hospitalization) is a hazard because hospitals have sites that are possible reservoirs for virulent microorganisms. Some of these microorganisms have become resistant to antibiotics, such as methicillin-resistant *Staphylococcus aureus* (MRSA), vancomycin-resistant *Enterococcus* (VRE), or multidrug-resistant tuberculosis. Other microorganisms include those for which there is currently no known cure, such as HIV.

The single most important step to decrease risk of microorganism transmission is to wash your hands promptly and thoroughly for 10 to 15 seconds (or longer if hands appear visibly soiled). Wash hands (1) before and after physical contact with each patient, (2) after inadvertent contact with blood, body fluids, secretions, excretions, (3) after contact with any equipment contaminated with body fluids, and (4) after removing gloves.

Wear gloves when the potential exists for contact with any body fluids (e.g., blood, mucous membranes, body fluids, drainage, open skin lesions). Wearing gloves is *not* a protective substitute to washing hands, however, because gloves may have undetectable holes or may become torn during use, or hands may become contaminated as gloves are removed. Wear a gown, mask, and protective eye wear when the potential exists for any blood or body fluid spattering (e.g., suctioning, arterial puncture).

The Centers for Disease Control and Prevention (CDC) guidelines include the latest epidemiologic information for decreasing transmission of blood-borne and other infections in hospitals (Garner, 1996). The guidelines include two tiers of precautions. **Standard Precautions** (Table 8–2) are intended for use with *all* patients regardless of their risk or presumed infection status. Standard Precautions are designed to reduce the risk of transmission of microorganisms from both recognized and unrecognized sources, and they apply to (1) blood; (2) all body fluids, secretions, and excretions *except sweat,* whether or not they contain visible blood; (3) nonintact skin; and (4) mucous membranes (Garner, 1996).

The second tier is **Transmission-Based Precautions,** intended for use with patients with documented or suspected transmissible infections. They are designed *in ad-*

Table 8–2 • Standard Precautions for Use With All Patients

A. **Wash hands** after touching blood, body fluids, secretions, excretions, and contaminated items, whether or not wearing gloves. Wash hands immediately after gloves are removed and between patient contacts. May need to wash hands between procedures on the same patient to prevent cross-contamination of different body sites.

B. **Wear clean gloves** when touching blood, body fluids, secretions, excretions, items contaminated with these, mucous membranes, and nonintact skin. Change gloves between tasks and procedures on the same patient after contact with material that may contain a high concentration of microorganisms. Remove gloves promptly after use, before touching noncontaminated items, and before going to another patient, and wash hands immediately.

C. **Wear a mask and eye protection** to protect mucous membranes during procedures and patient care activities that are likely to generate splashes of blood, body fluids, secretions, and excretions.

D. **Wear a gown** (clean, nonsterile, appropriate to activity) to protect skin and prevent soiling of clothing during procedures and patient care activities that are likely to generate splashes of blood, body fluids, secretions, or excretions. Remove a soiled gown promptly and wash hands.

E. **Take care with used patient care equipment** soiled with blood, body fluids, secretions, and excretions; handle it in a manner that prevents skin and mucous membrane exposure, contamination of clothing, and transfer of microorganisms to other patients and environments. Do not use the reusable equipment on another patient until it has been cleaned and reprocessed appropriately. Discard single-use items appropriately.

F. **Design and follow adequate hospital or clinic procedures** for the routine care, cleaning, and disinfection of environmental surfaces, beds, bed rails, bedside equipment, and other frequently touched surfaces.

G. **Take care with used linen** soiled with blood, body fluids, secretions, and excretions; handle, transport, and process this linen in a manner that prevents skin and mucous membrane exposure and contamination of clothing, and that avoids transfer of microorganisms to other patients and environments.

H. **Prevent injuries due to bloodborne pathogens** when using or handling needles, scalpels, and other sharp instruments. Never recap used needles, manipulate them using both hands, or direct the point of a needle toward any part of the body; rather, use either a one-handed "scoop" technique or an appropriate mechanical device. Do not remove used needles from disposable syringes by hand or otherwise bend, break, or manipulate used needles by hand. Place used disposable syringes, needles, scalpel blades, and other sharp items in appropriate puncture-resistant containers.

Use mouthpieces, resuscitation bags, or other ventilation devices instead of mouth-to-mouth resuscitation methods in areas where the need for resuscitation is predictable.

I. **Place in a private room** any patient who contaminates the environment or who does not or cannot assist in appropriate hygiene or environmental control.

Adapted from Garner JS: Guidelines for Isolation Precautions in Hospitals. Atlanta, GA, Public Health Service, U.S. Department of Health and Human Services, Centers for Disease Control and Prevention, 1996.

dition to Standard Precautions to interrupt transmission in hospitals. There are three types of transmission-based precautions: airborne, droplet, and contact. They may be combined for diseases that have multiple routes of transmission, e.g., varicella (chickenpox) (Appendices A and H).

APPROACH TO THE CLINICAL SETTING

General Approach

Consider your emotional state and that of the person being examined. The patient is usually anxious, owing to the anticipation of being examined by a stranger and the unknown outcome of the examination. If anxiety can be reduced, the person will feel more comfortable and the data gathered will more closely describe the person's natural state. Anxiety can be reduced by an examiner who is confident and self-assured, as well as considerate and unhurried.

Usually, a beginning examiner feels anything *but* self-assured! Most worry about their technical skill, about missing something significant, or about forgetting a step. Many are embarrassed themselves about encountering a partially dressed individual. All these fears are natural and common. The best way to minimize them is with a lot of tutored practice on a healthy willing subject, usually a fellow student. You have to feel comfortable with your motor skills before you can absorb what you are actually seeing or hearing in a "real" patient. This comes with practice under the guidance of an experienced tutor, in an atmosphere in which it is acceptable to make mistakes and to ask questions. Your subject should "act like a patient" so that you can deal with the "real" situation while still in a safe setting. After you feel comfortable with the laboratory setting, accompany your tutor as he or she examines an actual patient so that you can observe an experienced examiner.

Hands On

With this preparation, it is possible to interact with your own patient in a confident manner. Begin by measuring the person's height, weight, blood pressure, temperature, pulse, and respirations (see Chapter 9). If needed, measure visual acuity at this time using the Snellen eye chart. All of these are familiar, relatively nonthreatening actions; they will gradually accustom the person to the examination. Then ask the person to change into an examining gown, leaving his or her underpants on. This will feel more comfortable, and the underpants easily can be removed just before the genital examination. Unless your assistance is needed, leave the room as the person undresses.

As you reenter the room, wash your hands in the person's presence. This indicates you are protective of this person and are starting fresh for him or her. Explain each step in the examination and how the person can cooperate. Encourage the person to ask questions. Keep your own movements slow, methodical, and deliberate.

Begin by touching the person's hands, checking skin color, nail beds, and metacarpophalangeal joints (Fig. 8–

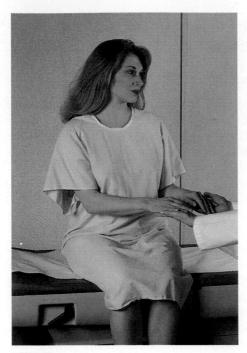

8–10

10; see Chapters 10 and 20). Again, this is a less threatening way to ease a person into being touched. Most people are used to having relative strangers touch their hands.

As you proceed through the examination, avoid distractions and concentrate on one step at a time. The sequence of the steps may differ depending on the age of the person and your own preference. However, you should establish a system that works for you and stick to it to avoid omissions. Organize the steps so the person does not change positions too often. Although proper exposure is necessary, use additional drapes to maintain the person's privacy and to prevent chilling.

Do not hesitate to write out the examination sequence and refer to it as you proceed. The patient will accept this as quite natural if you explain you are making brief notations to ensure accuracy. Many agencies use a printed form. You will find that you will glance at the form less and less as you gain experience. Even with a form, you sometimes may forget a step in the examination. When you realize this, perform the maneuver in the next logical place in the sequence. (See Chapter 26 for the sequence of steps in the complete physical examination.)

As you proceed through the examination, occasionally offer some brief teaching about the person's body. For example, you might say, "This tapping on your back (percussion) is a little like playing different drums. The different notes I hear tell me where each organ starts and stops. You probably can hear the difference yourself from within your body." Or, "Everyone has two sounds for each heartbeat, something like this—lub-dup. Your own beats sound normal." Do not do this with every single

step, or you will be hard pressed to make a comment when you do come across an abnormality. But some sharing of information builds rapport and increases the person's confidence in you as an examiner. It also gives the person a little more control in a situation in which it is easy to feel completely helpless.

At some point, you will want to linger in one location to concentrate on some complicated findings. To avoid anxiety, tell the person, "I always listen to heart sounds on a number of places on the chest. Just because I am listening a long time does not necessarily mean anything is wrong with you." And it follows that sometimes you will discover a finding that may be abnormal and you want another examiner to double check. You need to give the person some information, yet you should not alarm the person unnecessarily. Say something like, "I do not have a complete assessment of your heart sounds. I want Ms. Wright to listen to you too."

At the end of the examination, summarize your findings and share the necessary information with the person. Thank the person for the time spent. In a hospital setting, apprise the person of what is scheduled next. Before you leave a hospitalized person, lower the bed, make the person comfortable and safe, and return the bedside table, television, or any equipment to the way it was originally.

 DEVELOPMENTAL CONSIDERATIONS

Children are different from adults. Their difference in size is obvious. Their bodies grow in a predictable pattern that is assessed during the physical examination. However, their behavior also is different. Behavior grows and develops through predictable stages, just as the body does. Each examiner needs to know the expected emotional and cognitive features of these stages and to perform the physical examination based on developmental principles (Erikson, 1963; Wong, 1999).

With all children, the goal is to increase their comfort in the setting. This approach reveals their natural state as much as possible and will give them a more positive memory of health care providers. Remember that a "routine" examination is anything but routine to the child. You can increase their comfort by attending to the following developmental principles and approaches. The *order* of the developmental stages is more meaningful than the exact chronologic age. Each child is an individual and will not fit exactly into one category. For example, if your efforts to "play games" with the preschooler are rebuffed, modify your approach to the security measures used with the toddler.

The Infant

Erikson defines the major task of infancy as establishing trust. An infant is completely dependent on the parent for his or her basic needs. If these needs are met

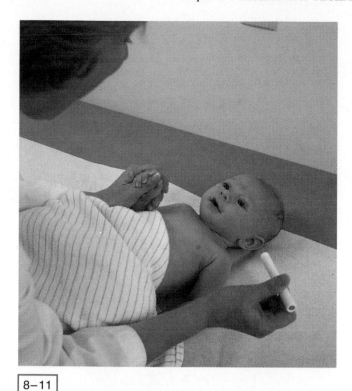

8–11

- Use a soft, crooning voice during the examination; the baby responds more to the feeling in the tone of the voice than to what is actually said.
- An infant likes eye contact; lock eyes from time to time.
- Smile; a baby prefers a smiling face to a frowning one. (Often beginning examiners are so absorbed in their technique that they look serious or stern.) Take time to play.
- Keep movements smooth and deliberate, not jerky.
- Use a pacifier for crying or during invasive steps.
- Offer brightly colored toys for a distraction when the infant is fussy.
- Let an older baby touch the stethoscope or tongue blade.

Sequence

- Seize the opportunity with a sleeping baby to listen to heart, lung, and abdomen sounds first.
- Perform least distressing steps first. (See the sequence in Chapter 26.) Save the invasive steps of examination of the eye, ear, nose, and throat until last.
- Elicit the Moro or "startle" reflex at the end of the examination because it may cause the baby to cry.

The Toddler

This is Erikson's stage of developing autonomy. However, the need to explore the world and be independent is in conflict with the basic dependency on the parent. This often results in frustration and negativism. The toddler may be difficult to examine; do not take this personally. Since he or she is acutely aware of the new environment, the toddler may be frightened and cling to the parent. Also, the toddler has fear of invasive procedures and dislikes being restrained (Fig. 8–12).

promptly and consistently, the infant feels secure and learns to trust others.

Position

- The parent always should be present to understand normal growth and development and for the child's feeling of security.
- Place the neonate or young infant flat on a padded examination table (Fig. 8–11). The infant also may be held against the parent's chest for some steps.
- Once the baby can sit without support (around 6 months), as much of the examination as possible should be performed while the infant is in the parent's lap.
- By 9 to 12 months, the infant is acutely aware of the surroundings. Anything outside the infant's range of vision is "lost," so the parent must be in full view.

Preparation

- Timing should be 1 to 2 hours after feeding, when the baby is not too drowsy or too hungry.
- Maintain a warm environment. A neonate may require an overhead radiant heater.
- An infant will not object to being nude. Have the parent remove outer clothing, but leave a diaper on a boy.
- An infant does not mind being touched, but make sure your hands and stethoscope endpiece are warm.

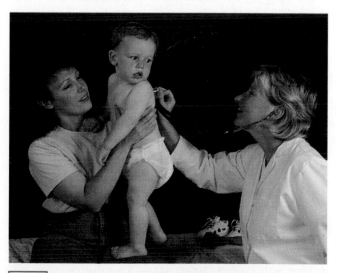

8–12

Position

- The toddler should be sitting up on the parent's lap for all of the examination. When the toddler must be supine (as in the abdominal examination), move chairs to sit knee-to-knee with parent. Have the toddler lie in the parent's lap with the toddler's legs in your lap.
- Enlist the aid of a cooperative parent to help position the toddler during invasive procedures. The child's legs can be captured between the parent's. An arm of the parent can encircle the child's head, holding it against the chest and the other arm can hold the child's arms. (See Figure 14–22.)

Preparation

- Children of 1 or 2 years of age can understand symbols, so a security object, such as a special blanket or teddy bear, is helpful.
- Begin by greeting the child and the accompanying parent by name, but with a child 1 to 6 years old, focus more on the parent. By essentially "ignoring" the child at first, you allow the child to adjust gradually and to size you up from a safe distance. Then turn your attention gradually to the child, at first to a toy or object the child is holding, or perhaps to compliment a dress, the hair, or what a big girl or boy the child is. If the child is ready, you will note these signals: eye contact with you, smiling, talking with you, or accepting a toy or a piece of equipment.
- A 2-year-old child does not like to take off his or her clothes; have the parent undress the child one part at a time.
- Children 1 or 2 years of age like to say "No." Do not offer a choice when there really is none. Avoid saying, "May I listen to your heart now?" When the 1- or 2-year-old child says "No," and you go ahead and do it anyway, you lose trust. Instead, use clear firm instructions, in a tone that expects cooperation, "Now it is time for you to lie down so I can check your tummy."
- Also, 1- or 2-year-old children like to make choices. When possible, enhance autonomy by offering the *limited option,* "Shall I listen to your heart next, or your tummy?"
- Demonstrate the procedures on the parent (see Fig. 13–14).
- Praise the child when he or she is cooperative.

Sequence

- Collect some objective data during the history, which is a less stressful time. While you are focusing on the parent, note the child's gross motor and fine motor skills and gait.
- Begin with "games," the Denver II test, or cranial nerve testing.
- Start with nonthreatening areas. Save distressing procedures, such as examination of the head, ear, nose, or throat, for last.

The Preschool Child

The child at this stage displays developing initiative. The preschooler takes on tasks independently and plans the task and sees it through. A child of this age is often cooperative, helpful, and easy to involve. However, children of this age have fantasies and may see illness as punishment for being "bad." The concept of body image is limited. The child fears any body injury or mutilation, so he or she will recoil from invasive procedures, e.g., tongue blade, rectal temperature, injection, and venipuncture.

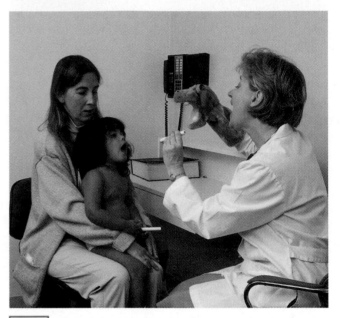

8–13

Position

- With a 3-year-old child, the parent should be present and may hold the child on his or her lap (Fig. 8–13).
- A 4- or 5-year-old child usually feels comfortable on the examining table, with the parent present.

Preparation

- A preschooler can talk. Verbal communication becomes helpful now, but remember that the child's understanding is still limited. Use short, simple explanations.
- The preschooler is usually willing to undress. Leave underpants on until the genital examination.
- Talk to the child and explain the steps in the examination exactly.
- Do not allow a choice when there is none.
- As with the toddler, enhance the autonomy of the preschooler by offering choice when possible.
- Allow the child to play with equipment to reduce fears (Fig. 8–14).

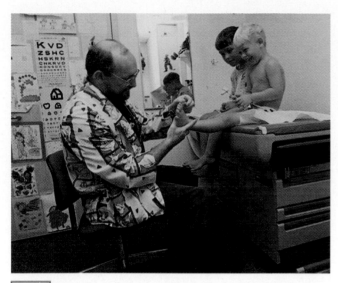

8–14 Courtesy of *The Pantagraph*, Bloomington, Illinois, August 10, 1998.

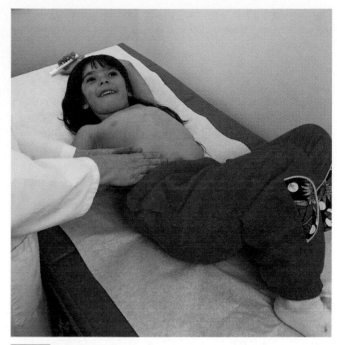

8–15

- A preschooler likes to help; have the child hold the stethoscope for you.
- Use games. Have the child "blow out" the light on the penlight as you listen to the breath sounds. Or, pretend to listen to the heart sounds of the child's teddy bear first. One technique that is absorbing to a preschooler is to trace their shape on the examining table paper (Wong, 1999). You can comment on how big the child is, then fill in the outline with a heart or stomach and listen to the paper doll first. After the examination, the child can take the paper doll home as a souvenir.
- Use a slow, patient, deliberate approach. Do not rush.
- During the examination give the preschooler needed feedback and reassurance: "Your tummy feels just fine."
- Compliment the child on his or her cooperation.

Sequence

- Examine the thorax, abdomen, extremities, and genitalia first. Though the preschooler is usually cooperative, continue to assess head, eye, ear, nose, and throat last.

The School-Age Child

During the school-age period, the major task of the child is developing industry. The child is developing basic competency in school and in social networks and desires the approval of parents and teachers. When successful, the child has a feeling of accomplishment. During the examination, the child is cooperative and is interested in learning about the body. Language is more sophisticated now, but do not overestimate and treat the school-age child as a small adult. The child's level of understanding does not match that of his or her speech.

Position

- The school-age child should be sitting on the examination table.
- A 5-year-old child has a sense of modesty. To maintain privacy, let the older child (an 11- or 12-year-old child) decide whether parents or siblings should be present.

Preparation

- Break the ice with small talk about family, school, friends, music, or sports.
- The child should undress himself or herself, leave underpants on, and use a gown and drape.
- Demonstrate equipment—a school-aged child is curious to know how equipment works.
- Comment on the body and how it works (Fig. 8–15). An 8- or 9-year-old child has some understanding of the body and is interested to learn more. It is rewarding to see the child's eyes light up when he or she hears the heart sounds.

Sequence

- As with the adult, progress from head to toes.

The Adolescent

The major task of adolescence is developing a self-identity. This takes shape from various sets of values and different social roles (son or daughter, sibling, and student). In the end, each person needs to feel satisfied and comfortable with who he or she is. In the process, the adolescent is increasingly self-conscious and introspective. Peer group values and acceptance are important.

Position

- The adolescent should be sitting on the examination table.
- Examine the adolescent alone, without parent or sibling present.

Preparation

- The body is changing rapidly. During the examination, the adolescent needs feedback that his or her own body is healthy and developing normally.
- The adolescent has keen awareness of body image, often comparing himself or herself to peers. Apprise the adolescent of the wide variation among teenagers on the rate of growth and development (see Sex Maturity Rating, Chapters 15, 22, and 24).
- Communicate with some care. Do not treat the teenager like a child, but do not overestimate and treat him or her like an adult either.
- Since the person is idealistic at this age, the adolescent is ripe for health teaching. Positive attitudes developed now may last through adult life. Focus your teaching on ways the adolescent can promote wellness.

Sequence

- As with the adult, a head-to-toe approach is appropriate. Examine genitalia last, and do it quickly.

The Aging Adult

During later years, the tasks are developing the meaning of life and one's own existence and adjusting to changes in physical strength and health.

Position

- The older adult should be sitting on the examination table.
- Arrange the sequence to allow as few position changes as possible.
- Allow rest periods when needed.

Preparation

- Adjust examination pace to meet possible slowed pace of the aging person. It is better to break the complete examination into a few visits than to rush through the examination and turn off the person.
- Use physical touch (unless there is a cultural contrain-

dication). This is especially important with the aging person because other senses, such as vision and hearing, may be diminished.
- Do not mistake diminished vision or hearing for confusion. Confusion of sudden onset may signify a disease state. It is noted by short-term memory loss, diminished thought process, diminished attention span, and labile emotions (see Mental Status Assessment, Chapter 6).
- Be aware that aging years contain more of life's stress. Loss is inevitable, including changes in physical appearance of the face and body, declining energy level, loss of job through retirement, loss of financial security, loss of long-time home, and death of friends or spouse. How the person adapts to these losses significantly affects health assessment.

Sequence

- Use the head-to-toe approach as in the younger adult.

The Ill Person

For the person in some distress, alter the position during the examination. For example, a person with shortness of breath or ear pain may want to sit up, whereas a person with faintness or overwhelming fatigue may want to be supine. Initially, it may be necessary just to examine the body areas appropriate to the problem, collecting a *mini data base*. You may return to finish a complete assessment after the initial distress is resolved.

Bibliography

Berk LE: Infants, Children, and Adolescents, 3rd ed. Boston, Allyn and Bacon, 1999.
Breathnach AS, Jenkins DR, Pedler SJ: Stethoscopes as possible vectors of infection by staphylococci. BMJ 305:1573–1574, Dec 19–26, 1992.
Calkins E, Ford AB, Katz PR: Practice of Geriatrics, 2nd ed. Philadelphia, W.B. Saunders Company, 1992.
Erikson EH: Childhood and Society. New York, W.W. Norton, 1963.
Faria SH, Glidden C: Assessment of the child: What's different? Home Care Provider 2(6):282–286, Dec 1997.
Garner JS, Hospital Infection Control Practices Advisory Committee: Guideline for Isolation Precautions in Hospitals. Atlanta, GA, Public Health Service, U.S. Department of Health and Human Services, Centers for Disease Control and Prevention, 1996.
Goldberg EA: Physical assessment of children ages 1 to 10 years. ANNA J 24(2):209–217, 1997.
Moser R: Preventing pedianosis: The illnesses we get from kids. Adv Nurse Pract 3(12):31–34, Dec 1995.
Ricchini W: Sound advice about stethoscopes. Adv Nurse Pract 6(5):65–66, May 1998.
Stone AT, Wyman JF, Salisbury SS: Clinical Gerontological Nursing, 2nd ed. Philadelphia, W.B. Saunders Company, 1997.
Thomas DO: Assessing children—It's different. RN 19:38–45, Apr 1996.
Wong DL: Whaley and Wong's Nursing Care of Infants and Children, 6th ed. St. Louis, Mosby, 1999.

CHAPTER NINE

General Survey, Measurement, Vital Signs

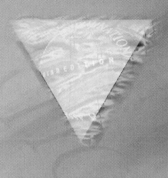

The general survey is a study of the whole person, covering the general health state and any obvious physical characteristics. It is an introduction for the physical examination that will follow; it should give an overall impression, a "gestalt," of the person (see Sample Charting). Objective parameters are used to form the general survey, but these apply to the whole person, not just to one body system.

Launch a general survey at the moment you first encounter the person. What leaves an immediate impression? Does the person stand promptly as his or her name is called and walk easily to meet you? Or does the person look sick, rising slowly or with effort, with shoulders slumped and eyes without luster or downcast? Is the hospitalized person conversing with visitors, involved in reading or television, or lying perfectly still? Even as you introduce yourself and shake hands, you collect data. Does the person fully extend the arm, shake your hand firmly, make eye contact, or smile? Are the palms dry or wet and clammy? As you proceed through the health history, the measurements, and the vital signs, note the following points that will add up to the general survey. Consider these four areas: **physical appearance, body structure, mobility,** and **behavior.**

▶ Normal Range of Findings	Abnormal Findings

THE GENERAL SURVEY

Physical Appearance

Age—The person appears his or her stated age.

Appears older than stated age, as with chronic illness, chronic alcoholism.

Sex—Sexual development is appropriate for gender and age.

Delayed or precocious puberty.

Level of consciousness—The person is alert and oriented, attends to your questions and responds appropriately.

Confused, drowsy, lethargic (see Table 6–3, Levels of Consciousness).

Skin color—Color tone is even, pigmentation varying with genetic background, skin is intact with no obvious lesions.

Pallor, cyanosis, jaundice, erythema, any lesions (see Chapter 10).

Facial features—Facial features are symmetric with movement.

Immobile, masklike, asymmetric, drooping (see Table 11–5, Abnormal Facial Appearances with Chronic Illness).

No signs of acute distress are present.

Respiratory signs—shortness of breath, wheezing.

Pain, indicated by facial grimace, holding body part.

► Normal Range of Findings	Abnormal Findings

Body Structure

Stature—The height appears within normal range for age, genetic heritage (see Measurement, p. 194).

Excessively short or tall (see Table 9–6, Abnormalities in Body Height and Proportion).

Nutrition—The weight appears within normal range for height and body build; body fat distribution is even.

Cachectic, emaciated.

Simple obesity, with even fat distribution.

Centripetal (truncal) obesity—fat concentrated in face, neck, trunk, with thin extremities, as in Cushing's syndrome (hyperadrenalism) (see Table 9–6).

Symmetry—Body parts look equal bilaterally and are in relative proportion to each other.

Unilateral atrophy or hypertrophy.

Asymmetric location of a body part.

Posture—The person stands comfortably erect as appropriate for age. Note the normal "plumb line" through anterior ear, shoulder, hip, patella, ankle. Exceptions are the standing toddler who has a normally protuberant abdomen ("toddler lordosis") and the aging person who may be stooped with kyphosis.

Rigid spine and neck; moves as one unit, e.g., arthritis.

Stiff and tense, ready to spring from chair, fidgety movements.

Shoulders slumped; looks deflated, e.g., depression.

Position—The person sits comfortably in a chair or on the bed or examination table, arms relaxed at sides, head turned to examiner.

Tripod—leaning forward with arms braced on chair arms, occurs with chronic pulmonary disease.

Sitting straight up and resists lying down, e.g., congestive heart failure.

Curled up in fetal position, e.g., acute abdominal pain.

Body build, contour—proportions are

1. Arm span (fingertip to fingertip) equals height.
2. Body length from crown to pubis roughly equal to length from pubis to sole.

Elongated arm span, arm span greater than height, e.g., Marfan's syndrome hypogonadism (see Table 9–6).

Missing extremities or digits; webbed digits; shortened limb.

Obvious physical deformities—Note any congenital or acquired defects.

Mobility

Gait—Normally, the base is as wide as the shoulder width; foot placement is accurate; the walk is smooth, even, and well-balanced; and associated movements, such as symmetric arm swing, are present.

Exceptionally wide base. Staggered, stumbling.

Shuffling, dragging, nonfunctional leg.

Limping with injury.

Propulsion—difficulty stopping (see Table 21–6, Abnormal Gaits).

Range of motion—Note full mobility for each joint, and that movement is deliberate, accurate, smooth, and coordinated. (See Chapter 20 for information on more detailed testing of joint range of motion.)

No involuntary movement.

> Limited joint range of motion.
> Paralysis—absent movement.
> Movement jerky, uncoordinated.
> Tics, tremors, seizures (see Table 21–5, Abnormalities in Muscle Movement).

Behavior

Facial expression—The person maintains eye contact (unless a cultural taboo exists), expressions are appropriate to the situation, e.g., thoughtful, serious, or smiling. (Note expressions both while the face is at rest and while the person is talking.)

> Flat, depressed, angry, sad, anxious. However, note that anxiety is common in ill people. Also, some people smile when they are anxious.

Mood and affect—The person is comfortable and cooperative with the examiner and interacts pleasantly.

> Hostile, distrustful, suspicious, crying.

Speech—Articulation (the ability to form words) is clear and understandable.

> Dysarthria and dysphagia. Speech defect, monotone, garbled speech.

The stream of talking is fluent, with an even pace.
The person conveys ideas clearly.
Word choice is appropriate to culture and education.
The person communicates in prevailing language easily by himself or herself or with an interpreter.

> Extremes of few words or constant talking.

Dress—Clothing is appropriate to the climate, looks clean and fits the body, and is appropriate to the person's culture and age group, e.g., normally, Amish women wear clothing from the nineteenth century, Indian women wear saris, Arab men wear long robes. Culturally determined dress should not be labeled as bizarre by Western standards.

> Trousers too large and held up by belt suggest weight loss, as does the addition of new holes in belt. If the belt is moved to a looser fit, it may indicate obesity or ascites.
> Consistent wear of certain clothing may provide clues: neck scarves may conceal thyroidectomy scar; long sleeves may conceal needle marks of drug abuse; broad-brimmed hats may reveal sun intolerance of lupus erythematosus; Velcro fasteners instead of buttons may indicate chronic motor dysfunction.

Personal hygiene—The person appears clean and groomed appropriately for his or her age, occupation, and socioeconomic group. (Note that a wide variation of dress and hygiene is "normal." Many cultures do not include use of deodorant or women shaving legs.)

Hair is groomed, brushed. Women's make-up is appropriate for age and culture.

> In a previously carefully groomed woman, unkempt hair and absent make-up may indicate malaise or illness.

| ► Normal Range of Findings | Abnormal Findings |

MEASUREMENT

Weight

Use a standardized *balance* scale. Instruct the person to remove his or her shoes and heavy outer clothing before standing on the scale. When a sequence of repeated weights is necessary, aim for approximately the same time of day and the same type of clothing worn each time. Record the weight in kilograms and in pounds.

Show the person how his or her own weight matches up to the recommended range for height (Table 9–1). Compare the person's current weight with that from the previous health visit. A recent weight loss may be explained by successful dieting. A weight gain usually reflects overabundant caloric intake, unhealthy eating habits, and sedentary lifestyle.

An unexplained weight loss may be a sign of a short-term illness (e.g., fever, infection, disease of the mouth or throat) or a chronic illness (endocrine disease, malignancy, mental health dysfunction).

Obesity is >120 percent ideal body weight and occasionally may be due to endocrine disorders, drug therapy (e.g., corticosteroids), or mental depression.

Table 9–1 • Height and Weight Tables for Men and Women According to Frame, Ages 25–59

Height*		Weight†		
Feet	*Inches*	*Small Frame*	*Medium Frame*	*Large Frame*
Men				
5	2	128–134	131–134	138–150
5	3	130–136	133–143	140–153
5	4	132–138	135–145	142–156
5	5	134–140	137–148	144–160
5	6	136–142	139–151	146–164
5	7	138–145	142–154	149–168
5	8	140–148	145–157	152–172
5	9	142–151	148–160	155–176
5	10	144–154	151–163	158–180
5	11	146–157	154–166	161–184
6	0	149–160	157–170	164–188
6	1	152–164	160–174	168–192
6	2	155–168	164–178	172–197
6	3	158–172	167–182	176–202
6	4	162–176	171–187	181–207
Women				
4	10	102–111	109–121	118–131
4	11	103–113	111–123	120–134
5	0	104–115	113–126	122–137
5	1	106–118	115–129	125–140
5	2	108–121	118–132	128–143
5	3	111–124	121–135	131–147
5	4	114–127	124–138	134–151
5	5	117–130	127–141	137–155
5	6	120–133	130–144	140–159
5	7	123–136	133–147	143–163
5	8	126–139	136–150	146–167
5	9	129–142	139–153	149–170
5	10	132–145	142–156	152–173
5	11	135–148	145–159	155–176
6	0	138–151	148–162	158–179

*Shoes with 1-inch heels.
†Weight in pounds. Men: allow 5 lb of clothing. Women: allow 3 lb of clothing.
Courtesy of Metropolitan Life Insurance Company, 1983.

|

Height

Use the measuring pole on the balance scale. Align the extended headpiece with the top of the head. The person should be shoeless, standing straight, and looking straight ahead.

Note that measurement of skinfold thickness is described in Chapter 7.

VITAL SIGNS

Temperature

Cellular metabolism requires a stable core, or "deep body," temperature of a mean of 37.2° C (99° F). The body maintains a steady temperature through a thermostat, or feedback mechanism, regulated in the hypothalamus of the brain. The thermostat balances heat production (from metabolism, exercise, food digestion, external factors) with heat loss (through radiation, evaporation of sweat, convection, conduction).

The various routes of temperature measurement reflect the body's core temperature. The normal oral temperature in a resting person is 37° C (98.6° F), with a range of 35.8 to 37.3° C (96.4 to 99.1° F). The rectal temperature measures 0.4 to 0.5° C (0.7 to 1° F) higher. The normal temperature is influenced by

- A diurnal cycle of 1 to 1.5° F, with the trough occurring in the early morning hours and the peak occurring in late afternoon to early evening.
- The menstruation cycle in women. Progesterone secretion, occurring with ovulation at midcycle, causes a 0.5 to 1.0° F rise in temperature that continues until menses.
- Exercise. Moderate to hard exercise increases body temperature.
- Age. Wider normal variations occur in the infant and young child due to less effective heat control mechanisms. In older adults, temperature is usually lower than in other age groups, with a mean of 36.2° C (97.2° F).

The **oral** temperature is accurate and convenient. The oral sublingual site has a rich blood supply from the carotid arteries that quickly responds to changes in inner core temperature. Shake the *mercury-in-glass* thermometer down to 35.5° C (96° F) and place it at the base of the tongue in either of the posterior sublingual pockets, *not* in front of the tongue. Instruct the person to keep his or her lips closed. Leave in place 3 to 4 minutes if the person is afebrile (Baker et al., 1984), and up to 8 minutes if febrile (Nichols and Kucha, 1972). (Take other vital signs during this time.) Wait 15 minutes if the person has just taken hot or iced liquids (Cole, 1993) and 2 minutes if he or she has just smoked.

The **electronic thermometer** has the advantages of swift and accurate measurement (usually in 20 to 30 seconds) as well as safe, unbreakable, disposable probe covers. The instrument must be fully charged and correctly calibrated. Most children enjoy watching their temperature numbers advance on the box.

The **axillary** temperature is safe and accurate for infants and young children when the environment is reasonably controlled (see Developmental Considerations, p. 194).

Take a **rectal** temperature only when the other routes are not practical, e.g., for comatose or confused persons, for persons in shock, or for those who cannot close the mouth because of breathing or oxygen tubes, wired mandible, or other facial dysfunction or if no tympanic membrane thermometer equipment is available. Wear gloves and insert a lubricated rectal thermometer (with a short, blunt tip) only 2 to 3 cm (1 in) into the adult rectum, directed toward the umbilicus,

The thermostatic function of the hypothalamus may become scrambled during illness or central nervous system disorders.

Hyperthermia, or fever, is caused by pyrogens secreted by toxic bacteria during infections or from tissue breakdown such as that following myocardial infarction, trauma, surgery, or malignancy. Neurologic disorders (e.g., a cerebral vascular accident, cerebral edema, brain trauma, tumor, or surgery) also can reset the brain's thermostat at a higher level, resulting in heat production and conservation.

Hypothermia is usually due to accidental, prolonged exposure to cold. It also may be purposefully induced to lower the body's oxygen requirements during heart or peripheral vascular surgery, neurosurgery, amputation, or gastrointestinal hemorrhage.

and leave in place for 2½ minutes. Disadvantages to the rectal route are patient discomfort, time-consuming and disruptive activity, and risk of cross-contamination.

The **tympanic membrane thermometer (TMT)** is the newest development in temperature monitoring. It senses the infrared emissions of the tympanic membrane (eardrum). The tympanic membrane shares the same vascular supply that perfuses the hypothalamus (the internal carotid artery), thus it is an accurate measurement of core temperature (Henker and Coyne, 1995).

The tympanic membrane thermometer is a noninvasive, nontraumatic device that is extremely quick and efficient. The probe tip has the shape of an otoscope, the instrument used to inspect the ear. Gently place the covered probe tip in the person's ear canal (see Fig. 9–14 on p. 199). Do not force it and do not occlude the canal. Activate the device and you can read the temperature in 2 to 3 seconds.

There is minimal chance of cross-contamination using the tympanic thermometer because the ear canal is lined with skin and not mucous membrane. This thermometer is very successful in use with unconscious patients or with those who are unable or unwilling to cooperate with traditional techniques (i.e., those in critical care units, emergency departments, recovery areas, labor and delivery units, and pediatric care settings). Nurses and patients, including parents and children, all favor the use of the tympanic thermometer over the usual rectal and oral thermometers because of its speed, convenience, safety, reduced risk of injury and infection, and noninvasiveness.

Report the temperature in degrees Celsius unless your agency uses the Fahrenheit scale. Use this conversion:

$$\text{degrees C} = \tfrac{5}{9}\,(\text{F} - 32)$$
$$\text{degrees F} = (\tfrac{9}{5} \cdot \text{C}) + 32$$

Familiarize yourself with both scales. Note that it is far easier to learn to *think* in the centigrade scale than to take the time for paper-and-pencil conversions. Begin by memorizing these convenient equivalents:

$$104.0° \text{ F} = 40.0° \text{ C}; \quad 98.6° \text{ F} = 37.0° \text{ C}; \quad 95.0° \text{ F} = 35.0°\text{C}.$$

Pulse

With every beat, the heart pumps an amount of blood—the **stroke volume**—into the aorta. This is about 70 ml in the adult. The force flares the arterial walls and generates a pressure wave, which is felt in the periphery as the **pulse.** Palpating the peripheral pulse gives the rate and rhythm of the heartbeat, as well as local data on the condition of the artery. The *radial* pulse is usually palpated while vital signs are measured.

Using the pads of your first three fingers, palpate the radial pulse at the flexor aspect of the wrist laterally along the radius bone (Fig. 9–1). Push until you feel the strongest pulsation. If the rhythm is regular, count the number of beats in 30 seconds and multiply by 2. Although the 15-second interval is frequently practiced, any one-beat error in counting results in a recorded error of four beats per minute. The 30-second interval is the most accurate and efficient when heart rates are normal or rapid and when rhythms are regular (Hollerbach and Sneed, 1990). However, if the rhythm is irregular, count for a full minute. As you begin the counting interval, start your count with "zero" for the first pulse felt. The second pulse felt is "one," and so on. Assess the pulse, including (1) rate, (2) rhythm, (3) force, and (4) elasticity.

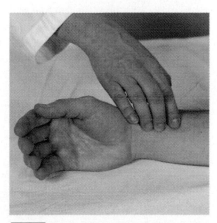

9–1

Rate. In the resting adult, the normal heart rate range is 60 to 100 beats per minute (bpm). The rate normally varies with age, being more rapid in infancy and childhood and more moderate during adult and older years. The rate also varies with gender; after puberty, females have a slightly faster rate than males (Table 9–2).

Table 9–2 • Normal Resting Pulse Rates Across Age Groups

Age	Average (Beats Per Minute)	Normal Limits
Newborn	120	70–190
1 yr	120	80–160
2 yr	110	80–130
4 yr	100	80–120
6 yr	100	75–115
8 yr	90	70–110
10 yr	90	70–110
12 yr		
Female	90	70–110
Male	85	65–105
14 yr		
Female	85	65–105
Male	80	60–100
16 yr		
Female	80	60–100
Male	75	55–95
18 yr		
Female	75	55–95
Male	70	50–90
Well-conditioned athlete	May be 50–60	50–100
Adult	74–76	60–100
Aging	74–76	60–100

In the adult, a heart rate less than 60 bpm is called **bradycardia.** This occurs normally in the well-trained athlete whose heart muscle develops along with the skeletal muscles. The stronger, more efficient heart muscle pushes out a larger stroke volume with each beat, thus requiring fewer beats per minute to maintain a stable cardiac output. (Review the equation $CO = SV \times R$, or Cardiac Output = Stroke Volume $\times$ Rate, in Chapter 17.) A more rapid heart rate, over 100 bpm, is **tachycardia.** It occurs normally with anxiety or with increased exercise to match the body's demand for increased metabolism.

Some researchers propose that the range of normal resting heart rate for adults should be shifted down to new limits of 50 to 90 bpm, rather than the traditional 60 to 100 bpm (Spodick, 1993; Wood, 1994). Revising the limits down would account for the physically fit individuals who have resting heart rates well below 60 and often 50 bpm. Also, lowering the tachycardia threshold would agree with studies that show heart rates over 90 bpm do occur with conditions of sepsis and following myocardial infarction.

Rhythm. The rhythm of the pulse normally has an even tempo. However, one irregularity that is commonly found in children and young adults is **sinus arrhythmia.** Here the heart rate varies with the respiratory cycle, speeding up at the peak of inspiration and slowing to normal with expiration. Inspiration momentarily causes a decreased stroke volume from the left side of the heart; to

For descriptions of abnormal rates and rhythms, see Table 18–1, Variations in Arterial Pulse.

compensate, the heart rate increases. (See Chapter 17 for a full discussion on sinus arrhythmia.) If any other irregularities are felt, auscultate heart sounds for a more complete assessment (see Chapter 17).

Force. The force of the pulse shows the strength of the heart's stroke volume. A "weak, thready" pulse reflects a decreased stroke volume, e.g., as occurs with hemorrhagic shock. A "full, bounding" pulse denotes an increased stroke volume, as with anxiety, exercise, and some abnormal conditions. The pulse force is recorded using a three-point scale:

3+ —full, bounding
2+ —normal
1+ —weak, thready
0—absent

Some agencies use a four-point scale; make sure your system is consistent with that used by the rest of your staff. Either scale is somewhat subjective. Experience will increase your clinical judgment.

Elasticity. With normal elasticity, the artery feels springy, straight, resilient.

Chapter 17 presents assessment of the precordium, including listening to the heart rate and rhythm as well as the quality of heart sounds. Chapter 18, on peripheral vascular assessment, presents further data on other pulse sites.

Respirations

Normally, a person's breathing is relaxed, regular, automatic, and silent. Since most people are unaware of their breathing, do not mention that you will be counting the respirations, because sudden awareness may alter the normal pattern. Instead, maintain your position of counting the radial pulse and unobtrusively count the respirations. Count for 30 seconds or for a full minute if you suspect an abnormality. Avoid the 15-second interval. The result can vary by a factor of + or −4, which is significant with such a small number.

Note that respiratory rates presented in Table 9−3 normally are more rapid in infants and children. Also, a fairly constant ratio of pulse rate to respiratory rate exists, which is about 4:1. Normally, both pulse and respiratory rates rise as a response to exercise or anxiety. More detailed assessment on respiratory status is presented in Chapter 16.

Table 9–3 • Normal Respiratory Rates

Age	Breaths Per Minute
Neonate	30–40
1 yr	20–40
2 yr	25–32
4 yr	23–30
6 yr	21–26
8 yr	20–26
10 yr	20–26
12 yr	18–22
14 yr	18–22
16 yr	16–20
18 yr	12–20
Adult	10–20

Blood Pressure

Blood pressure (BP) is the force of the blood pushing against the side of its container, the vessel wall. The strength of the push changes with the event in the cardiac cycle. The **systolic** pressure is the maximum pressure felt on the artery during left ventricular contraction, or systole. The **diastolic** pressure is the elastic recoil, or resting, pressure that the blood exerts constantly between each contraction. The **pulse pressure** is the difference between the systolic and diastolic and reflects the stroke volume (Fig. 9–2). The **mean arterial pressure (MAP)** is the pressure forcing blood into the tissues, averaged over the cardiac cycle. This is not an arithmetic average of systolic and diastolic pressures because diastole lasts longer. Rather, it is a value closer to diastolic pressure plus one-third the pulse pressure.

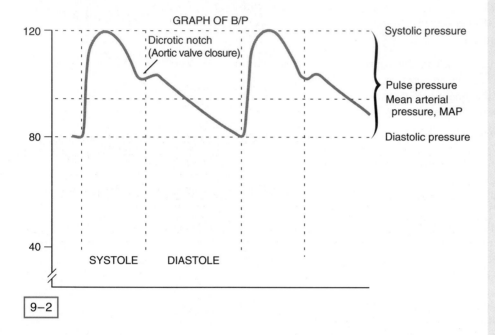

9–2

The average BP in the young adult is 120/80 mm Hg, although this varies normally with many factors, such as

- **Age.** Normally, a gradual rise occurs through childhood and into adult years (see Fig. 9–17).
- **Sex.** Before puberty, no difference exists between males and females. After puberty, females usually show a lower BP reading than male counterparts. After menopause, BP in females is higher than in male counterparts.
- **Race.** In the United States, a black adult's BP is usually higher than that of a white person of the same age. The incidence of hypertension is twice as high in blacks as in whites. The reasons for this difference are not understood fully but appear to be due to genetic heritage and environmental factors.
- **Diurnal rhythm.** A daily cycle of a peak and a trough occurs: the BP climbs to a high in late afternoon or early evening, and then declines to an early morning low.
- **Weight.** BP is higher in obese persons than in persons of normal weight of the same age (including adolescents).
- **Exercise.** Increasing activity yields a proportionate increase in BP. Within 5 minutes of terminating the exercise, the BP normally returns to baseline.

Normal Range of Findings	Abnormal Findings

- **Emotions.** The BP momentarily rises with fear, anger, and pain as a result of stimulation of the sympathetic nervous system.
- **Stress.** The BP is elevated in persons experiencing continual tension because of their lifestyle, occupational stress, or life problems.

FACTORS CONTROLLING BLOOD PRESSURE

FACTOR	CONDITION		RESULT
Cardiac output	↑	with heavy exercise to meet body demand for increased metabolism	↑ B/P
	↓	with pump failure (weak pumping action after myocardial infarction, or in shock)	↓ B/P
Vascular resistance	↑	resistance (vasoconstriction)	↑ B/P
	↓	resistance (vasodilatation)	↓ B/P
Volume	↓	volume (hemorrhage)	↓ B/P
	↑	volume (increased sodium and water retention, intravenous fluid overload)	↑ B/P
Viscosity	↑	viscosity (increased hematocrit in polycythemia)	↑ B/P
Elasticity of arterial walls	↑	rigidity, hardening as in arteriosclerosis (heart pumping against greater resistance)	↑ B/P

9–3

The level of **BP** is determined by five factors:

1. **Cardiac output.** If the heart pumps more blood into the container (i.e., the blood vessels), the pressure on the container walls increases (Fig. 9–3).
2. **Peripheral vascular resistance.** This is the opposition to blood flow through the arteries. When the container becomes smaller (e.g., such as with constricted vessels), the pressure needed to push the contents becomes greater.
3. **Volume of circulating blood.** This is how tightly the blood is packed into the arteries. Increasing the contents in the container increases the pressure.
4. **Viscosity.** The "thickness" of blood is determined by its formed elements, the blood cells. When the contents are thicker, the pressure increases.
5. **Elasticity of vessel walls.** When the container walls are stiff and rigid, the pressure needed to push the contents increases.

Blood pressure is measured using a stethoscope and a *sphygmomanometer* of either the mercury or the aneroid type. The mercury type is accurate and reliable but not as portable as the aneroid. However, the aneroid gauge is subject to drift, and must be recalibrated at least once each year against a reliable mercury manometer.

The cuff consists of an inflatable rubber bladder inside a cloth cover. The width of the rubber bladder should equal 40 percent of the circumference of the person's arm. The length of the bladder should equal 80 percent of this circumference.

The cuff size is important; using a cuff that is too narrow yields a falsely high BP because it takes extra pressure to compress the artery.

Available cuffs include six sizes that fit newborns to the extra-large adult, as well as tapered cuffs for the cone-shaped obese arm, and thigh cuffs. Match the appropriate size cuff to the person's arm size and shape and not to the person's age (Fig. 9–4).

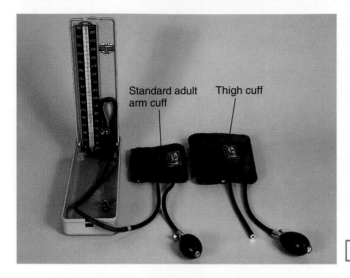

Standard adult arm cuff   Thigh cuff

9–4

Arm Pressure. A comfortable, relaxed person yields a valid blood pressure. Many people are anxious at the beginning of an examination; allow at least a 5-minute rest before measuring the BP. Then take two or more BP measurements separated by two minutes.

For each person, verify BP in both arms once, either on admission or for the first complete physical examination. It is not necessary to continue to check both arms for screening or monitoring. Occasionally a 5- to 10-mm Hg difference may occur in BP in the two arms (if values are different, use the higher value).

The person may be sitting or lying, with the bare arm supported at heart level. Place the mercury manometer so that it is vertical and at your eye level.

Palpate the brachial artery, which is located just above the antecubital fossa, medial to the biceps tendon. With the cuff deflated, center it about 2.5 cm (1 in) above the brachial artery and wrap it evenly.

Now palpate the brachial or the radial artery (Fig. 9–5). Inflate the cuff until the artery pulsation is obliterated and then 20 to 30 mm Hg beyond. This

A difference in the two arms of more than 10 to 15 mm Hg may indicate arterial obstruction on the side with the lower reading.

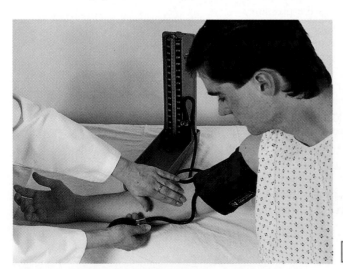

9–5

▶ Normal Range of Findings	Abnormal Findings

will avoid missing an **auscultatory gap,** which is a period when Korotkoff's sounds disappear during auscultation (Table 9–4).

Deflate the cuff quickly and completely; then wait 15 to 30 seconds before reinflating so that the blood trapped in the veins can dissipate.

Place the bell of the stethoscope over the site of the brachial artery, making a light but airtight seal (Fig. 9–6). The diaphragm endpiece is usually adequate, but the bell is designed to pick up low-pitched sounds such as the sounds of a blood pressure reading. So if you have a bell, use it.

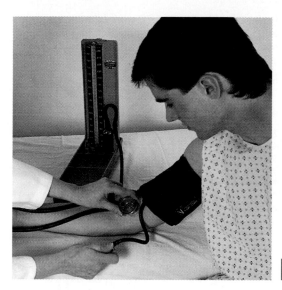

9–6

Rapidly inflate the cuff to the maximal inflation level you determined. Then deflate the cuff slowly and evenly, about 2 mm Hg per heartbeat. Note the points at which you hear the first appearance of sound, the muffling of sound, and the final disappearance of sound. These are phases I, IV, and V of **Korotkoff's sounds,** which are the components of a BP reading first described by a Russian surgeon in 1905 (Table 9–4).

For all age groups, the fifth Korotkoff phase is now used to define diastolic pressure (Joint National Committee–VI[JNC-VI], 1997). However, when a variance greater than 10 to 12 mm Hg exists between phases IV and V, record *both* phases along with the systolic reading, e.g., 142/98/80. Clear communication is important because the results significantly affect diagnosis and planning of care. See Table 9–5 for a list of common errors in blood pressure measurement.

Orthostatic (or Postural) Vital Signs. Take serial measurements of pulse and blood pressure when: you suspect volume depletion; the person is known to have hypertension or is taking antihypertensive medications; or the person reports fainting or syncope. Have the person rest supine for 2 or 3 minutes, take baseline readings of pulse and BP, and then repeat the measurements with the person sitting and then standing. For the person who is too weak or dizzy to stand, assess supine and then sitting with legs dangling. When the position is changed from supine to standing, normally a slight decrease (less than 10 mm Hg) in systolic pressure may occur.

Record the BP using even numbers. Also record the person's position, arm used, and cuff size if different from the standard adult cuff. Record the pulse rate and rhythm, noting whether the pulse is regular.

An auscultatory gap occurs in about 5 percent of people, most often in hypertension due to a noncompliant arterial system.

Hypotension, abnormally low BP; **hypertension,** abnormally high BP (see parameters in Table 9–8, Abnormalities in Blood Pressure).

Orthostatic hypotension, a drop in systolic pressure of more than 20 mm Hg, and/or orthostatic pulse increases of 20 bpm or more, occurs with a quick change to a standing position. These changes are due to abrupt peripheral vasodilatation without a compensatory increase in cardiac output. Orthostatic changes also occur with prolonged bedrest, older age, hypovolemia, and some drugs.

Table 9–4 • Korotkoff Sounds

Phase	Quality	Description	Rationale
Cuff correctly inflated	No sound		Cuff inflation compresses brachial artery. Cuff pressure exceeds heart's systolic pressure, occluding brachial artery blood flow.
I	Tapping	Soft, clear tapping, increasing in intensity	The SYSTOLIC pressure. As the cuff pressure lowers to reach intraluminal systolic pressure, the artery opens, and blood first spurts into the brachial artery. Blood is at very high velocity because of small opening of artery and large pressure difference across opening. This creates turbulent flow, which is audible.
Auscultatory gap*	No sound	Silence for 30–40 mm Hg	Sounds temporarily disappear during end of phase I, then reappear in phase II. Common with hypertension. If undetected, results in falsely low systolic or falsely high diastolic reading.
II	Swooshing	Softer murmur follows tapping	Turbulent blood flow through still partially occluded artery.
III	Knocking	Crisp, high-pitched sounds	Longer duration of blood flow through artery. Artery closes just briefly during late diastole.
IV	Abrupt muffling	Sound mutes to a low-pitched, cushioned murmur; blowing quality	Artery no longer closes in any part of cardiac cycle. Change in quality, not intensity.
V	Silence		Decreased velocity of blood flow. Streamlined blood flow is silent. The last audible sound (marking the disappearance of sounds) is DIASTOLIC pressure. The fifth Korotkoff is now used to define diastolic pressure in all age groups (JNC-VI, 1997).

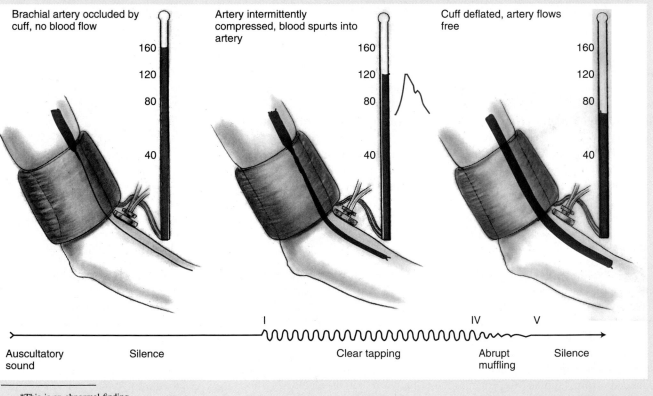

*This is an abnormal finding.

Normal Range of Findings   **Abnormal Findings**

Table 9-5 • Common Errors in Blood Pressure Measurement

Factor	Result	Rationale
Taking blood pressure reading when person is anxious or angry or has just been active	Falsely high	Sympathetic nervous system stimulation
Faulty arm position		
Above level of heart	Falsely low	Eliminates effect of hydrostatic pressure
Below level of heart	Falsely high	Additional force of gravity added to brachial artery pressure
Person supports own arm	Falsely high diastolic	Sustained isometric muscular contraction
Examiner's eyes are not level with meniscus of mercury column		
Looking up at meniscus	Falsely high	Parallax
Looking down on meniscus	Falsely low	
Inaccurate cuff size*		
Cuff too narrow for extremity	Falsely high	Needs excessive pressure to occlude brachial artery
Cuff wrap is too loose or uneven, or bladder balloons out of wrap	Falsely high	Needs excessive pressure to occlude brachial artery
Failure to palpate radial artery while inflating		
Inflating not high enough	Falsely low systolic	Miss initial systolic tapping or may tune in during *auscultatory gap* (tapping sounds disappear for 10 to 40 mm Hg and then return; common with hypertension)
Inflating cuff too high	Pain	
Pushing stethoscope too hard on brachial artery	Falsely low diastolic	Excessive pressure distorts artery and the sounds continue
Deflating cuff		
Too quickly	Falsely low systolic and/or falsely high diastolic	Insufficient time to hear tapping
Too slowly	Falsely high diastolic	Venous congestion in forearm makes sounds less audible
Halting during descent and reinflating cuff to recheck systolic	Falsely high diastolic	Venous congestion in forearm
Failure to wait 1–2 min before repeating entire reading	Falsely high diastolic	Venous congestion in forearm
Any observer error		
Examiner's "subconscious bias"; a preconceived idea of what blood pressure reading *should* be owing to person's age, race, sex, weight, history, or condition	Error anywhere	
Examiner's haste	Error anywhere	
Faulty technique		
Examiner's digit preference, "hears" more results that end in zero than would occur by chance alone, e.g., 130/80		
Diminished hearing acuity		
Defective or inaccurately calibrated equipment		

*This is the most common error.

Thigh Pressure. When BP measured at the arm is excessively high, particularly in adolescents and young adults, compare it with the thigh pressure to check for **coarctation** of the aorta (a congenital form of narrowing). Normally, the *thigh pressure is higher* than that in the arm. If possible, turn the person into the prone position on the abdomen. (If the person must remain in the supine position, bend the knee slightly.) Wrap a large cuff, 18 to 20 cm, around the lower third of the thigh, centered over the popliteal artery on the back of the

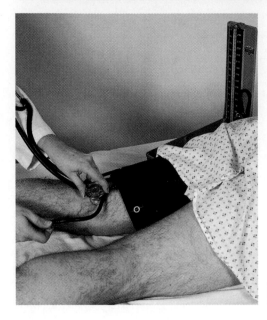

9–7

knee. Auscultate the popliteal artery for the reading (Fig. 9–7). Normally, the systolic value is 10 to 40 mm Hg higher in the thigh than in the arm, and the diastolic pressure is the same.

 DEVELOPMENTAL CONSIDERATIONS

Infants and Children

General Survey

Physical appearance, body structure, mobility—Note the same basic elements as with the adult, with consideration to age and development.

Behavior—note the response to stimuli and level of alertness appropriate for age.

Parental bonding—note the child's interactions with parents, that parent and child show a mutual response and are warm and affectionate, appropriate to the child's condition. The parent provides appropriate physical care of child and promotes new learning.

Measurement

Weight. Weigh an infant on a platform-type balance scale (Fig. 9–8). To check calibration, set the weight at zero and observe the beam balance. Guard the baby so that he or she does not fall. Weigh to the nearest 10 g (½ oz) for infants and 100 g (¼ lb) for toddlers.

With **coarctation of the aorta,** arm pressures are high. Thigh pressure is *lower* because the blood supply to the thigh is below the constriction.

Some signs of child abuse are that the child avoids eye contact; the child exhibits no separation anxiety when you would expect it for age; the parent is disgusted by child's odor, sounds, drooling, or stools.

Deprivation of physical or emotional care.

Signs of physical abuse (see Chapter 10).

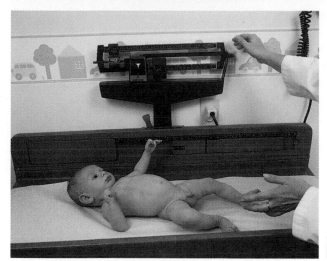

9-8

By age 2 or 3 years, use the upright scale. Leave underpants on the child. Some young children are fearful of the rickety standing platform and may prefer sitting on the infant scale. Use the upright scale with preschoolers and school-age children, maintaining modesty with light clothing (Fig. 9–9).

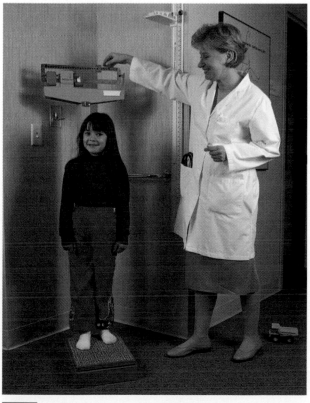

9-9

▶

Length. Until age 2 years, measure the infant's body length supine using a horizontal measuring board (Fig. 9–10). Hold the head in the midline. Because the infant normally has flexed legs, extend them momentarily by holding the knees together and pushing them down until the legs are flat on the table. Avoid using a tape measure along the infant's length because this is inaccurate.

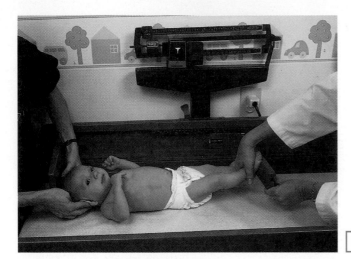

9–10

By age 2 or 3 years, measure the child's height by standing the child against the pole on the platform scale or back against a flat ruler taped to the wall (Fig. 9–11). (Sometimes a child will stand more erect against the solid wall than against the narrow measuring pole on the scale.) Encourage the child to stand straight and tall and to look straight ahead without tilting the head. The shoulders, buttocks, and heels should touch the wall. Hold a book or flat board on the child's head at a right angle to the wall. Mark just under the book, noting the measure to the nearest 1 mm (⅛ in).

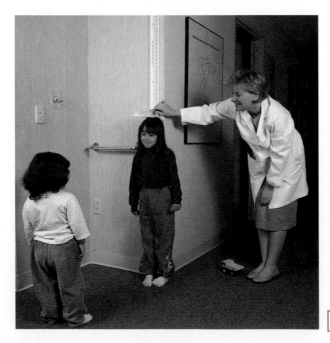

9–11

▶ Normal Range of Findings

Abnormal Findings

Physical growth is perhaps the best index of a child's general health. The child's height and weight are recorded at every health care visit to determine normal growth patterns. The results are plotted on growth charts based on data from the National Center for Health Statistics (NCHS). (See Appendix I for samples of the two groups of charts: one group for weight and height charts from birth to 36 months for girls and boys, and the second group from 2 to 18 years for males and females.)

Healthy childhood growth is continuous but uneven, with rapid growth spurts occurring during infancy and adolescence. Results are more reliable when comparing numerous growth measures over a long time. These charts also compare the individual child's measurements against the general population. Normal limits range from the 5th to the 95th percentile on the standardized charts.

Use your judgment and consider the genetic background of the small-for-age child. Explore the growth patterns of the parents and siblings. Be aware that the statistical averages for the United States charts are based on norms for white children and may not necessarily generalize to other ethnic groups. Studies indicate that black children weigh less than white children during the first 2 years of life, but afterward black children tend to be taller and heavier than white children of the same age. Asian children (particularly girls) are found to be shorter and lighter than white counterparts (Barr et al., 1972; Robson et al., 1975). Race-specific standards are needed before making judgments on growth of infants and children. Otherwise an excessive number of black infants or Asian children may be judged to be below normal when they actually may be normal for their own population group (see Transcultural Considerations, p. 205).

Further explore any growth measure that:

- Falls below the 5th or above the 95th percentile with no genetic explanation
- Shows a wide percentile difference between height and weight e.g., a 10th percentile height with a 95th percentile weight
- Shows that growth has suddenly stopped when it had been steady
- Fails to show normal growth spurts during infancy and adolescence

Head Circumference. Measure the infant's head circumference at birth and at each well child visit up to age 2 years, then yearly up to age 6 years (Fig. 9–12). Circle the tape around the head at the prominent frontal and occipital bones; the widest span is correct. Plot the measurement on standardized growth charts. Compare the infant's head size with that expected for age. A series of measurements is more valuable than a single figure to show the *rate* of head growth.

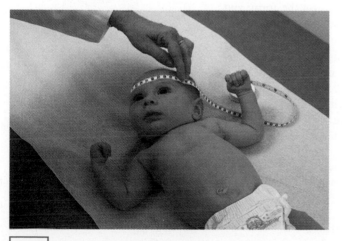

9–12

Normal Range of Findings	Abnormal Findings

The newborn's head measures about 32 to 38 cm (average around 34 cm) and is about 2 cm larger than the chest circumference. The chest grows at a faster rate than the cranium; at some time between 6 months and 2 years, both measurements are about the same, and after age 2, the chest circumference is greater than the head circumference.

Measurement of the chest circumference is valuable in a comparison with the head circumference but not necessarily by itself. Encircle the tape around the chest at the nipple line. It should be snug, but not so tight that it leaves a mark (Fig. 9–13).

Enlarged head circumference occurs with increased intracranial pressure (see Chapter 11, Head and Neck).

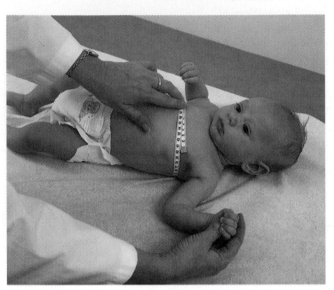

9–13

Assessment of Gestational Age. Occasionally, you will need to compare birth weight with a newborn's gestational age (GA) to assess maturity. Fetal maturity is the ability of the infant's organ systems to adapt to extrauterine life and is closely related to GA. GA is the number of weeks from the first day of the mother's last menstrual period (LMP) to the newborn's date of birth. Normal GA for a full-term newborn is 38 to 42 weeks.

The most commonly used method of assessing GA is the New Ballard Score (Ballard et al., 1991). Examine the newborn regarding the six neuromuscular maturity signs and the six physical maturity signs described on the form, and record the scores in each adjacent box (Appendix J). Scores range from 0 to 4 or 5, with the new addition of −1 scores that reflect signs of extreme prematurity. Add the two maturity scores to determine the maturity rating, and compare this maturity rating with the corresponding week of GA. Then enter the newborn's weight, length, and head circumference on the three grids at the vertical axis for the newborn's GA (Appendix J). Plotted scores that fall within the 10th to the 90th percentile show that a newborn is AGA, or appropriate for gestational age. That indicates this newborn grew at a normal rate during fetal life, regardless of being born at term, preterm, or postterm.

At the 50th percentile, a baby of average GA (40 weeks) measures an average weight of 3200 g (7 lb, 1 oz), an average length of 49 cm (19.3 in), and an average head circumference of 34 cm (13.5 in).

Preterm—less than 38 weeks
Postterm—more than 42 weeks

SGA, or small for gestational age, occurs with scores below the 10th percentile, indicating the infant grew at a retarded rate during fetal life. LGA, or large for gestational age, occurs with scores above the 90th percentile, indicating this infant grew at an accelerated rate during fetal life.

▶ Normal Range of Findings	Abnormal Findings

Vital Signs

Measure vital signs with the same purpose and frequency as you would in an adult. With an *infant,* reverse the order of vital sign measurement to respiration, pulse, and temperature. Taking a rectal temperature may cause the infant to cry, which will increase the respiratory and pulse rate, thus masking the normal resting values. A *preschooler's* normal fear of body mutilation is increased with any invasive procedure. Whenever possible, avoid the rectal route and take a tympanic, inguinal, or axillary temperature. When this is not feasible, use the reverse order and measure the rectal temperature last. Promote the cooperation of the *school-age child* by explaining the procedure completely and encouraging the child to handle the equipment. Your approach to measuring vital signs with the *adolescent* is much the same as with the adult.

Temperature

Tympanic. If you have TMT equipment available, use it for any age child (Fig. 9–14). The TMT is quite useful with toddlers who squirm at the restraint needed for the rectal route, and it is useful with preschoolers who are not yet able to cooperate for an oral temperature yet fear the disrobing and invasion of a rectal temperature. The TMT measurement is so rapid that it is usually over before the child realizes it.

The TMT use with newborns has remained questionable (Bliss-Holtz, 1995). Cusson, Madonia, and Taekman (1997) found that the temperature of the environment has a significant effect on temperature measurements. The superheated environment of the radiant warmer and particularly the incubator resulted in a significant elevation of tympanic membrane temperature over rectal, inguinal, or axillary measurement—a difference that could influence clinical management. They recommended the inguinal route. However, for infants in room-air bassinets, the TMT thermometers are the recommended screening tool because the differences between tympanic and rectal or axillary measurements were much less (Cusson et al., 1997).

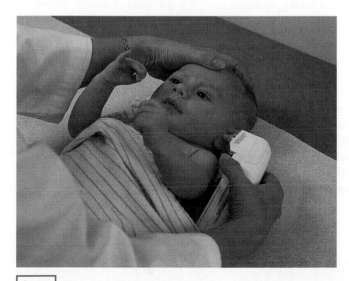

9–14

Inguinal. The inguinal route is safer than the rectal site. Its results may be closer to core temperature than the axillary site because the inguinal area has a rich supply of blood vessels, it lacks the brown fat tissue that interferes with axillary temperatures, and you can form a tight skin-to-skin seal (Bliss-Holtz, 1995; Cusson et al., 1997). Abduct the infant's leg and locate the femoral pulse. Place the bulb of the thermometer lateral to the pulse site, and adduct the leg to create a seal. A stable temperature will register in 3 to 5 minutes (Bliss-Holtz, 1995).

Axillary. The axillary route is safer and more accessible than the rectal route; however, its accuracy and reliability have been questioned (Bliss-Holtz, 1995; Cusson et al., 1997). When cold receptors are stimulated, brown fat tissue in the area releases heat through chemical energy, which artificially raises skin temperature. Studies on preterm infants show only small differences between axillary and rectal temperature measurement, which may be because brown fat is not present until 34 weeks gestation (Bliss-Holtz, 1995). When the axillary route is used, place the tip well into the axilla, and hold the child's arm close to the body. A stable axillary temperature will register by 5½ minutes (Bliss-Holtz, 1995).

Oral. When the TMT is not available, use the oral route when the child is old enough to keep the mouth closed and does not bite on the glass thermometer. This is usually at age 5 or 6, although some 4-year-old children can cooperate. When available, use an electronic thermometer because it is unbreakable and it registers quickly.

Rectal. Use this route with infants or with other age groups when the TMT is not available and other routes are not feasible, such as with the child who is unable to cooperate, agitated, unconscious, critically ill, or seizure prone. An infant may be supine or side lying, with the examiner's hand flexing the knees up onto the abdomen. (When supine, cover the boy's penis with a diaper.) An infant also may lie prone across the adult's lap. Separate the buttocks with one hand, and insert the lubricated stubby-tipped thermometer *no farther than* 2.5 cm (1 in). Any deeper insertion risks rectal perforation because the colon curves posteriorly at 3 cm (1¼ in). The temperature will register by 3 minutes.

Normally, rectal temperatures measure higher in infants and young children than in adults, with an average of 37.8°C (100° F) at 18 months. Also, the temperature normally may be elevated in the late afternoon, after vigorous playing or after eating.

Up to ages 6 to 8, children have higher fevers with illness than adults do. Even with minor infections, fevers may elevate to 39.5 to 40.5° C (103 to 105° F).

Pulse

Palpate or auscultate an apical rate with infants and toddlers. (See Chapter 17 for location of apex and technique.) In children older than 2 years, use the radial site. Count the pulse for a full minute to take into account normal irregularities, such as sinus arrhythmia. The heart rate normally fluctuates more with infants and children than with adults in response to exercise, emotion, and illness.

Respirations

Watch the infant's abdomen for movement, because the infant's respirations are normally more diaphragmatic than thoracic (Fig. 9–15). Count a full minute, because the pattern varies significantly from rapid breaths to short periods of apnea. Note the normal rate in Table 9–4.

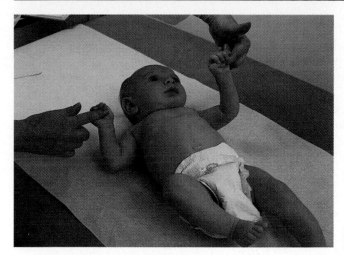

9–15

Blood Pressure

In children age 3 and older, and in younger children at risk, measure a routine BP at least annually. For accurate measurement in children, make some adjustment in the choice of equipment and technique. The most common error is to use the incorrect size cuff. The cuff width must cover two-thirds of the upper arm, and the cuff bladder must completely encircle it.

Use a pediatric-sized endpiece on the stethoscope to locate the sounds. If possible, allow a crying infant to become quiet for 5 to 10 minutes before measuring the BP; crying may elevate the systolic pressure by 30 to 50 mm Hg. New guidelines state that the disappearance of sound (phase V Korotkoff) can now be used for the diastolic reading in children as well as adults (JNC-VI, 1997; NHBPEP, 1996). Note the new guidelines for normal BP values by age groups *based on the child's height* (Appendix K). In children, height is more strongly correlated with BP than is age. The new charts avoid the misclassification as normotensive or hypertensive of children who are at the extremes of normal growth (NHBPEP, 1996). That is, for children of the same age, BP classified as 90th and 95th percentiles are lower for very short children, while tall children are given a higher normal range.

Children under 3 years of age have such small arm vessels that it is difficult to hear Korotkoff's sounds using a stethoscope. Instead, use an electronic BP device that uses *oscillometry,* such as Dinamap, and gives a digital readout for systolic, diastolic, and MAP and pulse. Or, use a *Doppler* ultrasound device to amplify the sounds. This instrument is easy to use and can be used by one examiner. (Note the technique for using the Doppler on p. 203).

Further explore any blood pressure that is greater than the 95th percentile and refer for diagnostic evaluation. For the child whose BP falls in the 90 to 95th percentile and whose high BP cannot be explained by height or weight, monitor the BP every 6 months (Purath, 1995).

The Aging Adult

General Survey

Physical appearance—By the eighth and ninth decades, body contour is sharper, with more angular facial features, and body proportions are redistributed. (See measuring weight and height, p. 183.)

Posture—A general flexion occurs by the eighth or ninth decade.

Gait—Older adults often use a wider base to compensate for diminished balance, arms may be held out to help balance, and steps may be shorter or uneven.

Measurement

Weight. The aging person appears sharper in contour with more prominent bony landmarks than the younger adult. Body weight decreases during the 80s and 90s. This factor is more evident in males, perhaps because of greater muscle shrinkage. The distribution of fat also changes during the 80s and 90s. Even with good nutrition, subcutaneous fat is lost from the face and periphery (especially the forearms), whereas additional fat is deposited on the abdomen and hips (Fig. 9–16).

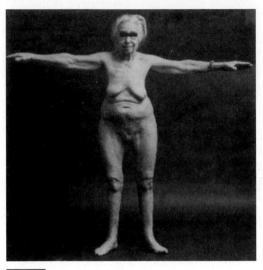

9–16

Height. By the 80s and 90s, many people are shorter than they were in their 70s. This results from shortening in the spinal column due to thinning of the vertebral discs and shortening of the individual vertebrae as well as the postural changes of kyphosis and slight flexion in the knees and hips. Since long bones do not shorten with age, the overall body proportion looks different; a shorter trunk with relatively long extremities (Fig 9–16).

Vital Signs

Temperature. Changes in the body's temperature regulatory mechanism leave the aging person less likely to develop fever but at a greater risk of developing hypothermia. Thus, the temperature is a less reliable index of the older person's true health state. Sweat gland activity is also diminished.

Pulse. The normal range of heart rate is 60 to 100 bpm, but the rhythm may be slightly irregular. The radial artery may feel stiff, rigid, and tortuous in an older person, although this condition does not necessarily imply vascular disease in the heart or brain. The increasingly rigid arterial wall needs a faster upstroke of blood, so the pulse is actually easier to palpate.

Respirations. Aging causes a decrease in vital capacity and a decreased inspiratory reserve volume. You may note a shallower inspiratory phase and an increased respiratory rate.

Blood Pressure. The aorta and major arteries tend to harden with age. As the heart pumps against a stiffer aorta, the systolic pressure increases, leading to a widened pulse pressure (see Fig. 9–17 for mean BP readings in apparently healthy persons from birth to old age). With many older people, both the systolic and diastolic pressures increase, making it difficult to distinguish normal aging values from abnormal hypertension.

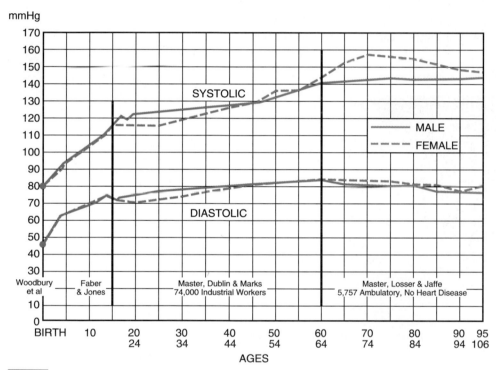

9–17

Mean blood pressure readings in apparently healthy people, birth to old age

ADDITIONAL TECHNIQUES

The Doppler Technique

In many situations, pulse and BP measurement are enhanced using an electronic device, the *Doppler ultrasonic flowmeter*. The Doppler technique works by a principle discovered in the nineteenth century by an Austrian physicist, Johannes Doppler. Sound varies in pitch in relation to the distance between the sound source and the listener; the pitch is higher when the distance is small, and the pitch lowers as the distance increases. Think of a railroad train speeding toward you; its train whistle sounds higher the closer it gets, and the pitch of the whistle lowers as the train fades away.

Here, the sound source is the blood pumping through the artery in a rhythmic manner. A handheld transducer picks up changes in sound frequency as the blood flows and ebbs and it amplifies them. The listener hears a whooshing pulsatile beat.

The Doppler technique is used to locate the peripheral pulse sites (see Chapter 18 for further discussion of this technique). For BP measurement, the Doppler technique will augment Korotkoff's sounds (Fig. 9–18). Through this technique, you can evaluate sounds that are hard to hear with a stethoscope, such as those in critically ill individuals with a low BP, in infants with small arms, and in obese persons in whom the sounds are muffled by layers of fat. Also, proper cuff placement is difficult on the obese person's cone-shaped upper arm. In this situation, you can place the cuff on the more even forearm and hold the Doppler probe over the radial artery. For either location, use this procedure:

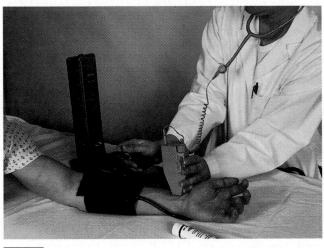

9–18

- Apply coupling gel to the transducer probe.
- Turn Doppler on.
- Touch the probe to the skin, holding the probe perpendicular to the artery.
- A pulsatile whooshing sound indicates location of the artery. You may need to rotate the probe, but maintain contact with the skin. Do not push the probe too hard or you will wipe out the pulse.
- Inflate the cuff until the sounds disappear, then proceed another 20 to 30 mm Hg beyond that point.
- Slowly deflate the cuff, noting the point at which the first whooshing sounds appear. This is the systolic pressure.
- It is difficult to hear the muffling of sounds or a reliable disappearance of sounds indicating the diastolic pressure (phases IV and V of Korotkoff's sounds). However, the systolic pressure alone gives valuable data on the level of tissue perfusion and on blood flow through patent vessels.

▶ | Normal Range of Findings | Abnormal Findings |

PROMOTING HEALTH AND SELF-CARE

As you measure height and weight and collect vital signs, it is a good time to begin a teaching plan to help the client keep these physical signs within normal limits. The 1997 Joint National Committee on Detection, Evaluation, and Treatment of High Blood Pressure considers the following **lifestyle modifications** to be the foundation of hypertension control. Even if your patient is normotensive and has body weight in normal limits, the following lifestyle modifications will help keep blood pressure under control (JNC-VI, 1997).

- Lose weight, if you are more than 10 percent above ideal weight.
- Limit alcohol intake to no more than 1 oz of ethanol (i.e., 24 oz [720 ml] of beer, 10 oz [300 ml] of wine, or 2 oz [60 ml] of 100-proof whiskey) per day or 0.5 oz (15 ml) of ethanol per day for women and lighter-weight people.
- Get regular aerobic exercise (e.g., a 30- to 45-minute brisk walk) most days of the week.
- Cut sodium intake from the average 150 mmol/L (150 mEq/L) to less than 100 mmol/L (100 mEq/L) per day (less than 2.3 g of sodium or 6 g of sodium chloride).
- Include the recommended daily allowances of potassium, calcium, and magnesium in your diet.
- Stop smoking.
- Reduce dietary saturated fat and cholesterol.

TRANSCULTURAL CONSIDERATIONS

General Appearance

Cultural differences are found in the body proportions of individuals. In general, white males are 1.27 cm (0.5 in) taller than black males, whereas white and black women are, on the average, the same height. Sitting-to-standing height ratios reveal that blacks of both sexes have longer legs and shorter trunks than whites. Because proportionately most of the weight is in the trunk, white men appear more obese than black men. Asians are markedly shorter, weigh less, and have smaller body frames.

Despite their longer legs, black women are consistently heavier than white women at every age, with black women carrying an average of 9.1 kg (20 lb) more than white women between the ages of 35 and 64 years (Overfield, 1995).

Bone length, as revealed by stature, shows definite biocultural differences, with blacks having longer legs and arms than whites. Asians and Native Americans have, on the average, longer trunks and shorter limbs than whites. Blacks tend to be wide shouldered and narrow hipped, whereas Asians tend to be wide hipped and narrow shouldered. Shoulder width is largely produced by the clavicle. Because the clavicle is a long bone, this explains why taller people have wide shoulders, whereas shorter people have narrower shoulders.

Although not all groups have been studied, research on selected populations reveals that children of some immigrant groups to the United States are taller than their peers in the country of origin. For example, Japanese Americans residing in Hawaii are taller than those Japanese living in Japan. Although the sitting-to-standing height ratio is the same, Italians in California are 3.8 cm (1.5 in) taller than those of the same age living in Italy (Hulse, 1968; Overfield, 1995). This indicates that the increase in height occurs in both the long bones and the spine (Brues, 1977).

The height increase in migrants is theorized to be the result of two factors: (1) better nutrition provided in the United States and (2) decreased interference with growth from infectious diseases during the formative years. Furthermore, the overall height of Americans increased 1.8 cm (0.7 in) for men and 1.3 cm (0.5 in) for women during the 10-year period studied (Abraham et al., 1976).

Biocultural differences also exist in the amount of body fat and the distribution of fat throughout the body. In general, individuals from lower socioeconomic groups are more obese than those from middle socioeconomic groups, who are more obese than members from upper socioeconomic groups. In addition to socioeconomic considerations, blacks tend to have smaller (1 mm) skinfold thicknesses in their arms than whites, but the distribution of fat on the trunk is similar.

SAMPLE CHARTING

A.J. is a 47-year-old black female high school principal, well nourished, well developed, appears stated age. She is alert, oriented, cooperative, with no signs of acute distress. Ht 163 cm (5′4″), Wt 57 kg (126 lbs), TPR 37° C—76—14, B/P 146/84 right arm, sitting.

CLINICAL CASE STUDY*

Mrs. Grazia Sanchez is a 76-year-old Hispanic female, retired secretary, in previous good health, who is brought to the emergency department by her 83-year-old husband. They have both been ill during the night with nausea, vomiting, abdominal pain, and diarrhea, which they attribute to eating "bad food" at a buffet-style restaurant the night before. Mr. Sanchez's condition has improved during the next day, but Mrs. Sanchez is worse, with severe vomiting, diarrhea, weakness, dizziness, and abdominal pain.

 Subjective

Extreme fatigue. Weakness and dizziness occur whenever tries to sit or stand up, "Feels like I'm going to black out." Severe nausea and vomiting, thirsty but cannot keep anything down; even sips of water result in "dry heaves." Abdominal pain is moderate aching, intermittent. Diarrhea is watery brown stool, profuse during the night, somewhat diminished now.

 Objective

Vital signs: temp 99°F, BP (supine) 102/64, pulse (supine) 70, regular rhythm, respirations 18.

Helped to seated, leg dangling position, vitals: BP 74/52, pulse 138, regular rhythm, respirations 20. Skin pale and moist (diaphoretic).

Reports lightheaded and dizzy in seated position. Returned to supine.

Respiratory: breath sounds clear in all fields, no adventitious sounds.

Cardiovascular: regular rate (70 bpm) and rhythm when supine, S_1 and S_2 are not accentuated or diminished, no extra sounds. All pulses present, 2+ and equal bilaterally. Carotids 2+ with no carotid bruit.

Abdomen: bowel sounds hyperactive, skin pale and moist, abdomen soft and mildly tender to palpation. No enlargement of liver or spleen.

Neuro: level of consciousness alert and oriented; pupils equal, round, react to light and accommodation. Sensory status normal. Mild weakness in arms and legs. Gait and standing leg strength not tested due to inability to stand. Deep tendon reflexes 2+ and equal bilaterally. Down-going toes.

 ASSESSMENT

Orthostatic hypotension, orthostatic pulse increase, and syncopal symptoms, R/T hypovolemia

Diarrhea, possibly R/T ingestion of contaminated food

Risk for hyperthermia, R/T dehydration and aging

Fluid volume deficit

*Please note that space does not allow a detailed plan for each clinical case study in this text. Please consult the appropriate text for current treatment plan.

Continued

NURSING DIAGNOSES COMMONLY ASSOCIATED WITH MEASUREMENT OR VITAL SIGN DISORDERS

Diagnosis	Related Factors (Etiology)	Defining Characteristics (Symptoms and Signs)

Hyperthermia	Dehydration
	Effects of
	    Illness or trauma involving temperature regulation
	    Medications/anesthesia
	    Aging
	Exposure to hot environment
	Inability to perspire
	Inability to regulate environmental temperature
	    No air conditioning
	    Isolette temperature for infants
	Increased metabolic rate
	Vigorous activity
		Increase in body temperature above normal range
		Skin flushed or warm to the touch
		Increased respiratory rate
		Tachycardia
		Seizures/convulsions
		Shivering
		Weakness, faintness
		Perspiration
		Verbal reports of feeling hot

Other Related Nursing Diagnoses

ACTUAL	RISK/WELLNESS
Bathing/hygiene self-care deficit Dressing/grooming self-care deficit Hypothermia Nutrition: more than body requirements, altered Nutrition: less than body requirements, altered Thermoregulation, ineffective	**Risk** Risk for altered body temperature Risk for fluid volume deficit **Wellness** Enhanced health-seeking behavior related to request for hypertension management by diet and exercise

Table 9–6   ABNORMALITIES IN BODY HEIGHT AND PROPORTION

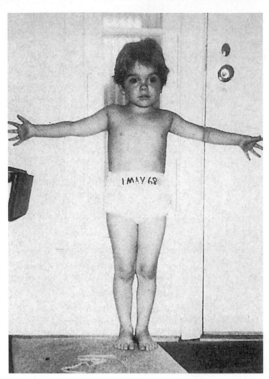

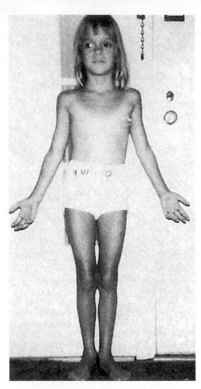

Hypopituitary Dwarfism

Deficiency in growth hormone in childhood results in retardation of growth and delayed puberty. The 6-year-old girl at left appears much younger than her chronologic age, with infantile facial features and chubbiness. The same girl at right 15 months later after treatment with growth hormone shows increased height, more mature facies, and loss of infantile fat.

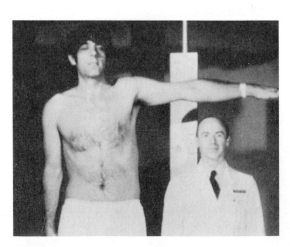

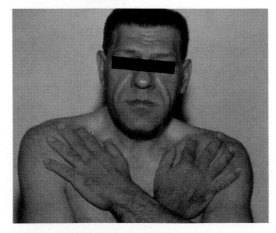

Gigantism

Excessive secretion of growth hormone by the anterior pituitary. When this occurs during childhood, before closure of bone epiphyses in puberty, it causes increased height and weight and delayed sexual development.

Acromegaly (Hyperpituitarism)

Excessive secretion of growth hormone in adulthood, after normal completion of body growth, causes overgrowth of bone in the face, head, hands, and feet, but no change in height. Internal organs also enlarge (e.g., cardiomegaly).*

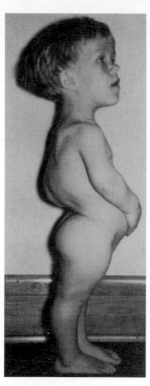

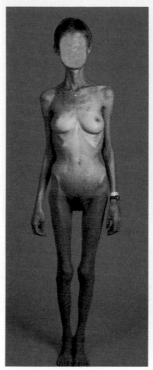

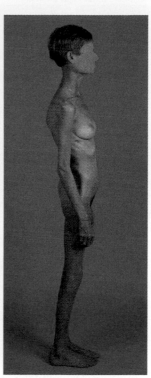

Achondroplastic Dwarfism

Congenital skeletal malformation due to genetic disorder characterized by relatively large head, short stature, short limbs, thoracic kyphosis, prominent lumbar lordosis, and abdominal protrusion. The mean adult height in men is about 131.5 cm (51.8 in) and in women about 125 cm (49.2 in).

Anorexia Nervosa

A serious psychological disorder characterized by severe and debilitating weight loss and amenorrhea in an otherwise healthy adolescent or young woman. Behavior is characterized by fanatic concern about weight, distorted body image (perceives self as fat despite skeletal appearance), starvation diets, frenetic exercise patterns, and striving for perfection.

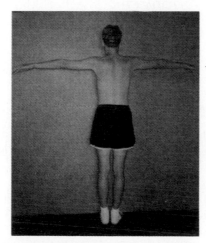

◄ Marfan's Syndrome

Abraham Lincoln, Paganini, and Rachmaninoff are thought to have had this inherited connective tissue disorder, characterized by tall, thin stature (greater than 95th percentile), arachnodactyly (long, thin fingers), hyperextensible joints, arm span greater than height, pubis-to-sole measurement exceeding crown-to-pubis measurement, sternal deformity, high-arched narrow palate, and pes planus. Early morbidity and mortality occur due to cardiovascular complications such as mitral regurgitation and aortic dissection.

Table continued on following page

Table 9–6 ABNORMALITIES IN BODY HEIGHT AND PROPORTION *Continued*

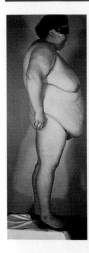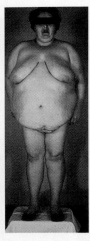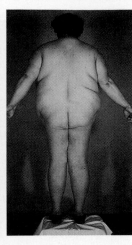

◀ **Endogenous Obesity—Cushing's Syndrome**

Either administration of adrenocorticotropic hormone (ACTH) or excessive production of ACTH by the pituitary will stimulate the adrenal cortex to secrete excess cortisol. This causes Cushing's syndrome, characterized by weight gain and edema with central trunk and cervical obesity (buffalo hump) and round plethoric face (moon face). Excessive catabolism causes muscle wasting, weakness, thin arms and legs, reduced height, and thin, fragile skin with purple abdominal striae, bruising, and acne. Note the obesity here is markedly different from *exogenous obesity* due to excessive caloric intake, in which body fat is evenly distributed and muscle strength is intact.

Table 9–7 RISK STRATIFICATION AND TREATMENT

Cardiovascular Risk Stratification in Patients With Hypertension

Major Risk Factors	*Target Organ Damage/Clinical Cardiovascular Disease*
Smoking	Heart diseases
Dyslipidemia	Left ventricular hypertrophy
Diabetes mellitus	Angina or prior myocardial infarction
Age >60 y	Prior coronary revascularization
Sex (men and postmenopausal women)	Heart failure
Family history of cardiovascular disease: women <65 y or men <55 y	Stroke or transient ischemic attack
	Nephropathy
	Peripheral arterial disease
	Retinopathy

Risk Stratification and Treatment

Blood Pressure Stages (mm Hg)	*Risk Group A (No Risk Factors; No TOD/ CCD)*	*Risk Group B (At Least 1 Risk Factor, Not Including Diabetes; No TOD/CCD)*	*Risk Group C (TOD/ CCD and/or Diabetes, With or Without Other Risk Factors)*
High-normal (130–139/85–89)	Lifestyle modification	Lifestyle modification	Drug therapy
Stage 1 (140–159/90–99)	Lifestyle modification (up to 12 mo)	Lifestyle modification (up to 6 mo)	Drug therapy
Stages 2 and 3 (≥160/≥100)	Drug therapy	Drug therapy	Drug therapy

Lifestyle Modifications for Hypertension Prevention and Management

- Lose weight if overweight
- Limit alcohol intake to no more than 1 oz (30 ml) of ethanol (e.g., 24 oz [720 ml] of beer, 10 oz [300 ml] of wine, or 2 oz [60 ml] of 100-proof whiskey) per day or 0.5 oz (15 ml) of ethanol per day for women and lighter-weight people
- Increase aerobic physical activity (30–45 min most days of the week)
- Reduce sodium intake to no more than 100 mmol/d (2.4 g of sodium or 6 g of sodium chloride)
- Maintain adequate intake of dietary potassium (approximately 90 mmol/d)
- Maintain adequate intake of dietary calcium and magnesium for general health
- Stop smoking and reduce intake of dietary saturated fat and cholesterol for overall cardiovascular health

From Joint National Committee on Prevention, Detection, Evaluation and Treatment of High Blood Pressure–VI: The Sixth Report of the Joint National Committee on Prevention, Detection, Evaluation, and Treatment of High Blood Pressure. Arch Intern Med 157(21):2389–2528, Nov 24, 1997.

Table 9-8 ABNORMALITIES IN BLOOD PRESSURE

Hypotension

In normotensive adults: < 95/60
In hypertensive adults: < the person's average reading, but > 95/60
In children: < expected value for age

Occurs with	Rationale
Acute myocardial infarction	Decreased cardiac output
Shock	Decreased cardiac output
Hemorrhage	Decrease in total blood volume
Vasodilatation	Decrease in peripheral vascular resistance
Addison's disease (hypofunction of adrenal glands)	

Associated Symptoms and Signs

In conditions of decreased cardiac output, a low BP is accompanied by an increased pulse, dizziness, diaphoresis, confusion, and blurred vision. The skin feels cool and clammy because the superficial blood vessels constrict to shunt blood to the vital organs. An individual having an acute MI (myocardial infarction) may also complain of crushing substernal chest pain, high epigastric pain, and shoulder or jaw pain.

Hypertension

Essential or Primary Hypertension

This occurs from no known cause but is responsible for about 95% of cases of hypertension in adults.

Classification and Follow-Up of Blood Pressure for Adults Age 18 and Older*

Category	Systolic		Diastolic	Follow-up Recommended§
Optimal†	< 120	and	< 80	
Normal	< 130	and	< 85	Recheck in 2 y
High-normal	130–139	or	85–89	Recheck in 1 y‡
Hypertension‡				
Stage 1	140–159	or	90–99	Confirm within 2 mo‡
Stage 2	160–179	or	100–109	Evaluate or refer to source of care within 1 mo
Stage 3	≥ 180	or	N ≥ 110	Evaluate or refer to source of care immediately or within 1 wk depending on clinical situation

*Not taking antihypertensive drugs and not acutely ill. When systolic and diastolic blood pressures fall into different categories, the higher category should be selected to classify the individual's blood pressure status. For example, 160/92 mm Hg should be classified as stage 2 hypertension, and 174/120 mm Hg should be classified as stage 3 hypertension. Isolated systolic hypertension is defined as systolic blood pressure 140 mm Hg or greater and diastolic blood pressure less than 90 mm Hg and staged appropriately (e.g., 170/82 mm Hg is defined as stage 2 isolated systolic hypertension). In addition to classifying stages of hypertension on the basis of average blood pressure levels, clinicians should specify presence or absence of target organ disease and additional risk factors. This specificity is important for risk classification and treatment. If systolic and diastolic categories are different, follow recommendations for shorter follow-up. 160/86 mm Hg should be evaluated or referred to source of care within 1 month.

†Optimal blood pressure with respect to cardiovascular risk is less than 120/80 mm Hg. However, unusually low readings should be evaluated for clinical significance.

‡Based on the average of 2 or more readings taken at each of 2 or more visits after an initial screening.

§Modify the scheduling of follow-up according to reliable information about past blood pressure measurements, other cardiovascular risk factors, or target organ disease.

‡Provide advice about lifestyle modifications (see p. 205 in text).

Data on classification of hypertension in adults adapted from the Sixth Report of the Joint National Committee on Prevention, Detection, Evaluation and Treatment of High Blood Pressure (JNC-VI), reprinted in Arch Intern Med 157(21):2389–2528, Nov 24, 1997.

Bibliography

Abraham SJ, Clifford L, Najjar MF: Height and weight of adults 18–74 years of age in the United States. Advancedata 3:1–8, 1976.

Baker NC, Cerone SB, Gaze N, Knapp TR: The effect of type of thermometer and length of time inserted on oral temperature measurements of afebrile subjects. Nurs Res 33:109–111, 1984.

Ballard JL, Khoury JC, Wedig K, et al: New Ballard score, expanded to extremely premature infants. J Pediatr 119:417–423, 1991.

Barr GD, Allen CM, Shinefield HR: Height and weight of 7,500 children of three skin colors. Am J Dis Child 124:866–872, 1972.

Bartlett EM: Temperature measurement: Why and how in intensive care. Intensive Crit Care Nurs 12(1):50–54, 1996.

Bayne CG: Vital signs: Are we monitoring the right parameters? Nurs Manage 28(5):74–77, May 1997.

Bhatia T: The fifth vital sign. RT: J Respir Care Pract 9(1):55–60, 1996.

Bliss-Holtz J: Methods of newborn infant temperature monitoring: A research review. Issues Compr Pediatr Nurs 18(4):287–298, Oct–Dec 1995.

Brown JK, Knapp TR, Radke KJ: Sex, age, height, and weight as predictors of selected physiologic outcomes. Nurs Res 46(2):101–104, Mar–Apr 1997.

Brown KA: Malignant hyperthermia. Am J Nurs 97(10):33, Oct 1997.

Brues AM: People and Races. New York, Macmillan, 1977.

Burton M: Pheochromocytoma. Am J Nurs 97(11):57, Nov 1997.

Carroll P: Using pulse oximetry in the home. Home Healthcare Nurse 15(2):88–97, Feb 1997.

Clayton LH, Dilley KB: Cushing's syndrome. Am J Nurs 98(7):40–41, July 1998.

Cole FL: Temporal variation in the effects of iced water on oral temperature. Res Nurs Health 16(2): 107–111, 1993.

Cornell S: Rethinking hypertension in children: New guide offers standards for diagnosis. Adv Nurs Pract 5(1):39–42, Jan 1977.

Cusson RM, Madonia JA, Taekmen JB: The effect of environment on body site temperatures in full-term neonates. Nurs Res 46(4):202–207, July–Aug 1997.

Girard N: Preoperative assessment. Nurse Pract Forum 8(4):140–146, Dec 1997.

Goldberg EA: Physical assessment of children ages 1 to 10 years. ANNA J 24(2):209–217, Apr 1997.

Goldy D: Circulatory overload secondary to blood transfusion. Am J Nurs 98(7):33, July 1998.

Helgeson DM, Berg CL, Juhl N: Blood pressure comparison in a selected Native American and white population. Public Health Nurs 10(1):36–41, 1993.

Henker R, Coyne C: Comparison of peripheral temperature measurements with core temperature. AACN Clin Issues 6(1):21–30, Feb 1995.

Hollerbach AD, Sneed NV: Accuracy of radial pulse assessment by length of counting interval. Heart Lung 19(33):258–264, 1990.

Hulse FS: The breakdown of isolates and hybrid vigor among the Italian Swiss. Proceedings of the 12th International Congress on Genetics 2:177, 1968.

Hurley ML: New hypertension guidelines. RN 61(3):25–28, Mar 1998.

Joint National Committee VI: The sixth report of the Joint National Committee on the Prevention, Detection, Evaluation, and Treatment of High Blood Pressure. Arch Intern Med 157(21):2389–2528, Nov 24, 1997.

Kaiser DK: Patient assessment pitfalls. Emergency 28(10):26–31, Oct 1996.

Keddington RK: A triage vital sign policy for a children's hospital emergency department. J Emerg Nurs 24(2):189–192, 1998.

Kohl J: Heat stroke. Am J Nurs 96(7):51, July 96.

Moody LY: Pediatric cardiovascular assessment and referral in the primary care setting. Nurse Pract 22(1):120–134, Jan 1997.

Murphy L, Linn L: Managing vital signs monitoring problems. Nursing 26(11):32gg–jj, 1996.

National High Blood Pressure Education Program (NHBPEP): Update on the 1987 task force report on high blood pressure in children and adolescents. Pediatrics 98(4):649–667, 1996.

Nichols GA, Kucha D: Oral measurements. Am J Nurs 72:1091–1093, 1972.

O'Hanlon-Nichols T: Basic assessment series: The adult cardiovascular system. Am J Nurs 97(12):34–40, Dec 1997.

Overfield T: Biologic Variation in Health and Illness: Race, Age and Sex Differences. Menlo Park, CA, Addison Wesley, 1995.

Purath J: Pediatric hypertension: Assessment and management. Pediatr Nurs 21(2):173–177, Mar–Apr 1995.

Robson JR, Larkin FH, Bursick JH, Peri KP: Growth standards for infants and children: A cross-sectional study. Pediatrics 56:1014–1020, 1975.

Roper M: Assessing orthostatic vital signs. Am J Nurs 96(8):43–46, Aug 1996.

Spodick DH: Redefinition of normal sinus heart rate. Chest 104(3):939–941, 1993.

Tallon RW: Oximetry: State of the art. Nurs Manage 27(11):43–44, Nov 1996.

Thomas DO: Assessing children—It's different. RN 59(4):38–45, Apr 1996.

U.S. Public Health Service: Adult blood pressure screening. Nurse Pract 21(2):112–116, 19 Feb 1996.

Vermette E: Malignant hyperthermia. Am J Nurs 98(4):45, Apr 1998.

Wong DL: Nursing Care of Infants and Children, 6th ed. St. Louis, CV Mosby, 1999.

Wood K: Commentary on redefinition of normal sinus heart rate. AACN Nursing Scan Crit Care 4(2):28, 1994.

Zaiser DK: Patient assessment pitfalls. Emergency 28(10):26–31, Oct 1996.

CHAPTER TEN

Skin, Hair, and Nails

Think of the skin as the body's largest organ system—it covers 20 square feet of surface area in the average adult. The skin is the sentry that guards the body from environmental stresses (e.g., trauma, pathogens, dirt) and adapts it to other environmental influences (e.g., heat, cold).

SKIN

The skin has two layers—the outer highly differentiated *epidermis* and the inner supportive *dermis* (Fig. 10–1). Beneath these layers is a third layer, the *subcutaneous* layer of adipose tissue.

Epidermis. The *epidermis* is thin but tough. Its cells are bound tightly together into sheets that form a rugged protective barrier. It is stratified into several zones. The inner **stratum germinativum,** or basal cell layer, forms new skin cells. Their major ingredient is the tough, fibrous protein *keratin.* The melanocytes interspersed along this layer produce the pigment *melanin,* which gives brown tones to the skin and hair. All people have the same number of melanocytes; however, the amount of melanin they produce varies with genetic, hormonal, and environmental influences.

From the basal layer, the new cells migrate up and flatten into the **stratum corneum.** This outer horny cell layer consists of dead keratinized cells that are interwoven and closely packed. The cells are constantly being shed, or desquamated, and are replaced with new cells from below. The epidermis is completely replaced every 4 weeks. In fact, each person sheds about 1 lb of skin each year.

The epidermis is uniformly thin except on the surfaces that are exposed to friction, such as the palms and the soles. On these surfaces, skin is thicker because of work and weight-bearing. The epidermis is avascular; it is nourished by blood vessels in the dermis below.

Skin color is derived from three sources: (1) mainly from the brown pigment melanin, (2) also from the yellow-orange tones of the pigment carotene, and (3) from

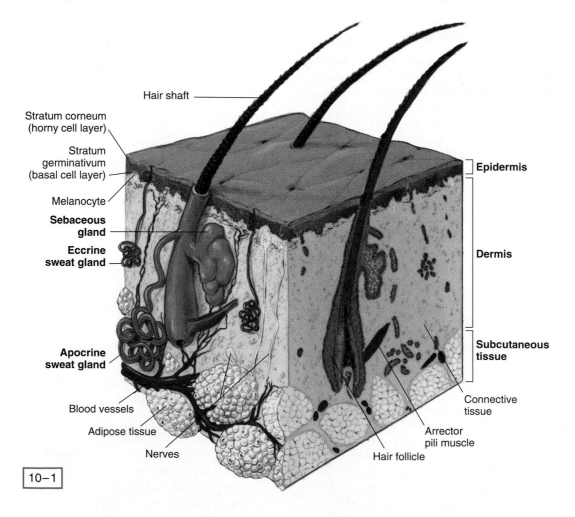

Hair shaft

Stratum corneum (horny cell layer)

Stratum germinativum (basal cell layer)

Melanocyte

Sebaceous gland

Eccrine sweat gland

Apocrine sweat gland

Blood vessels

Adipose tissue

Nerves

Epidermis

Dermis

Subcutaneous tissue

Connective tissue

Arrector pili muscle

Hair follicle

10–1

the red-purple tones in the underlying vascular bed. All people have skin of varying shades of brown, yellow, and red; the relative proportion of these shades affects the prevailing color. Skin color is further modified by the thickness of the skin and by the presence of edema.

Dermis. The *dermis* is the inner supportive layer consisting mostly of connective tissue, or *collagen*. This is the tough, fibrous protein that enables the skin to resist tearing. The dermis also has resilient elastic tissue that allows the skin to stretch with body movements. The nerves, sensory receptors, blood vessels, and lymphatics lie in the dermis. Also, appendages from the epidermis, such as the hair follicles, sebaceous glands, and sweat glands, are embedded in the dermis.

Subcutaneous Layer. The *subcutaneous layer* is adipose tissue, which is made up of lobules of fat cells. The subcutaneous tissue stores fat for energy, provides insulation for temperature control, and aids in protection by its soft cushioning effect. Also, the loose subcutaneous layer gives skin its increased mobility over structures underneath.

EPIDERMAL APPENDAGES

These structures are formed by a tubular invagination of the epidermis down into the underlying dermis.

Hair. Hair is *vestigial* for humans; it no longer is needed for protection from cold or trauma. However, hair is highly significant in most cultures for its cosmetic and psychological meaning (see Transcultural Considerations).

Hairs are threads of keratin. The hair *shaft* is the visible projecting part, and the *root* is below the surface embedded in the follicle. At the root, the *bulb matrix* is the expanded area where new cells are produced at a high rate. Hair growth is cyclical with active and resting phases. Each follicle functions independently so that while some hairs are resting, others are growing. Around the hair follicle are the muscular *arrector pili,* which contract and elevate the hair so that it resembles "goose flesh" when the skin is exposed to cold or in emotional states.

People have two types of hair. Fine, faint **vellus hair** covers most of the body (except the palms and soles, the dorsa of the distal parts of the fingers, the umbilicus, the glans penis, and inside the labia). The other type is **terminal hair,** the darker thicker hair that grows on the scalp and eyebrows and, after puberty, on the axillae, pubic area, and the face and chest in the male.

Sebaceous Glands. These glands produce a protective lipid substance, *sebum,* which is secreted through the hair follicles. Sebum oils and lubricates the skin and hair and forms an emulsion with water that retards water loss from the skin. (Dry skin results from loss of water, not directly from loss of oil.) Sebaceous glands are everywhere except on the palms and soles. They are most abundant in the scalp, forehead, face, and chin.

Sweat Glands. There are two types. The **eccrine** glands are coiled tubules that open directly onto the skin surface and produce a dilute saline solution called sweat. The evaporation of sweat reduces body temperature. Eccrine glands are widely distributed through the body and are mature in the 2-month-old infant.

The **apocrine** glands produce a thick, milky secretion and open into the hair follicles. They are located mainly in the axillae, anogenital area, nipples, and navel and are vestigial in humans. They become active during puberty, and secretion occurs with emotional and sexual stimulation. Bacterial flora residing on the skin surface react with apocrine sweat to produce characteristic musky body odor. The functioning of apocrine glands decreases in the aging adult.

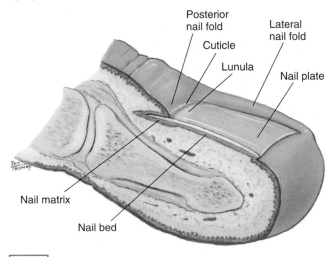

10-2

Nails. The nails are hard plates of keratin on the dorsal edges of the fingers and toes (Fig. 10–2). The nail plate is clear with fine longitudinal ridges that become prominent in aging. Nails take their pink color from the underlying nail bed of highly vascular epithelial cells. The lunula is the white opaque semilunar area at the proximal end of the nail. It lies over the nail matrix where new keratinized cells are formed. The nail folds overlap the posterior and lateral borders. The cuticle works like a gasket to cover and protect the nail matrix.

FUNCTION OF THE SKIN

The skin is a waterproof, almost indestructible covering that has protective and adaptive properties:

- **Protection.** Skin minimizes injury from physical, chemical, thermal, and light wave sources.
- **Prevents penetration.** Skin is a barrier that stops invasion of microorganisms and loss of water and electrolytes from within the body.
- **Perception.** Skin is a vast sensory surface holding the

neurosensory end-organs for touch, pain, temperature, and pressure.

- **Temperature regulation.** Skin allows heat dissipation through sweat glands and heat storage through subcutaneous insulation.
- **Identification.** People identify one another by unique combinations of facial characteristics, hair, skin color, and even fingerprints. Self-image is often enhanced or deterred by the way society's standards of beauty measure up to each person's perceived characteristics.
- **Communication.** Emotions are expressed in the sign language of the face and in the body posture. Vascular mechanisms such as blushing or blanching also signal emotional states.
- **Wound repair.** Skin allows cell replacement of surface wounds.
- **Absorption and excretion.** Skin allows limited excretion of some metabolic wastes, by-products of cellular decomposition such as minerals, sugars, amino acids, cholesterol, uric acid, and urea.
- **Production of vitamin D.** The skin is the surface on which ultraviolet light converts cholesterol into vitamin D.

 ## DEVELOPMENTAL CONSIDERATIONS

Infants and Children

The hair follicles develop in the fetus at 3 months' gestation; by midgestation most of the skin is covered with **lanugo,** the fine downy hair of the newborn. In the first few months after birth, this is replaced by fine vellus hair. Terminal hair on the scalp, if present at birth, tends to be soft and to suffer a patchy loss, especially at the temples and occiput. Also present at birth is **vernix caseosa,** the thick, cheesy substance made up of sebum and shed epithelial cells.

The newborn's skin is similar in structure to the adult's, but many of its functions are not fully developed. The newborn's skin is thin, smooth, and elastic and is relatively more permeable than that of the adult, so the infant is at greater risk for fluid loss. Sebum, which holds water in the skin, is present for the first few weeks of life, producing milia and cradle cap in some babies. Then sebaceous glands decrease in size and production and do not resume functioning until puberty. Temperature regulation is ineffective. Eccrine sweat glands do not secrete in response to heat until the first few months of life and then only minimally throughout childhood. The skin cannot protect much against cold because it cannot contract and shiver and because the subcutaneous layer is inefficient. Also, the pigment system is inefficient at birth.

As the child grows, the epidermis thickens, toughens, and darkens and the skin becomes better lubricated. Hair growth accelerates. At puberty, secretion from apocrine sweat glands increases in response to heat and emotional stimuli, producing body odor. Sebaceous glands become more active—the skin looks oily, and acne develops. Subcutaneous fat deposits increase, especially in females.

Secondary sex characteristics that appear during adolescence are evident in the integument (i.e., skin). In the female, the diameter of the areola enlarges and darkens, and breast tissue develops. Coarse pubic hair develops in males and females, then axillary hair, and then coarse facial hair in males.

The Pregnant Female

The change in hormone levels results in increased pigment in the areolae and nipples, vulva, and sometimes in the midline of the abdomen (**linea nigra**) or in the face (**chloasma**). Hyperestrogenemia probably also causes the common vascular spiders and palmar erythema. Connective tissue develops increased fragility, resulting in **striae gravidarum,** which may develop in the skin of the abdomen, breasts, or thighs. Metabolism is increased in pregnancy; as a way to dissipate heat, the peripheral vasculature dilates, and the sweat and sebaceous glands increase secretion. Fat deposits are laid down, particularly in the buttocks and hips, as maternal reserves for the nursing baby.

The Aging Adult

The skin is a mirror that reflects aging changes that proceed in *all* our organ systems; it just happens to be the one organ we can view directly. The aging process carries a slow atrophy of skin structures. The aging skin loses its elasticity; it folds and sags. By the 70s to 80s, it looks parchment thin, lax, dry, and wrinkled.

The epidermis's outer layer, *stratum corneum,* thins and flattens. This allows chemicals easier access into the body. Wrinkling occurs because the underlying dermis thins and flattens. A loss of elastin, collagen, and subcutaneous fat occurs as well as a reduction in muscle tone. The loss of collagen increases the risk for shearing, tearing injuries.

Sweat glands and sebaceous glands decrease in number and function, leaving dry skin. Decreased response of the sweat glands to thermoregulatory demand also puts the aging person at greater risk for heat stroke. The vascularity of the skin diminishes, while the vascular fragility increases; a minor trauma may produce dark red discolored areas, or **senile purpura.**

Sun exposure and, to a somewhat lesser extent, cigarette smoking further accentuate aging changes in the skin. Coarse wrinkling, decreased elasticity, atrophy, speckled and uneven coloring, more pigment changes, and a yellowed leathery texture occur. Chronic sun damage is even more prominent in pale or light-skinned persons.

An accumulation of factors place the aging person at risk for skin disease and breakdown: the thinning of the skin, the decrease in vascularity and nutrients, the loss of protective cushioning of the subcutaneous layer, a lifetime of environmental trauma to skin, the social changes of aging (e.g., less nutrition, limited financial resources), the increasingly sedentary lifestyle, and the chance of immobility. When skin breakdown does occur, subsequent cell replacement is slower, and wound healing is delayed.

In the aging hair matrix, the number of functioning melanocytes decreases so the hair looks gray or white and feels thin and fine. A person's genetic script determines the onset of graying and the number of gray hairs. Hair distribution changes. Males may have a symmetric W-shaped balding in the frontal areas. Some testosterone is present in both males and females; as it decreases with age, axillary and pubic hair decrease. As the female's estrogen also decreases, testosterone is unopposed and the female may develop some bristly facial hairs. Nails grow more slowly. Their surface is lusterless and is characterized by longitudinal ridges due to local trauma at the nail matrix.

Because the aging changes in the skin and hair can be viewed directly, they carry profound psychological impact. For many people, self-esteem is linked to a youthful appearance. This view is compounded by media advertising in Western society. Although sagging and wrinkling skin and graying and thinning hair are normal processes of aging, they prompt a loss of self-esteem for many adults.

TRANSCULTURAL CONSIDERATIONS

Awareness of normal biocultural differences and the ability to recognize the unique clinical manifestations of disease are especially important for darkly pigmented people. As described earlier, melanin is responsible for the various colors and tones of skin observed among people from culturally diverse backgrounds. Melanin protects the skin against harmful ultraviolet rays, a genetic advantage accounting for the lower incidence of skin cancer among darkly pigmented blacks and Native Americans. Areas of the skin affected by hormones and, in some cases, differing for culturally diverse people, are the sexual skin areas, such as the nipples, areola, scrotum, and labia majora. In general, these areas are darker than other parts of the skin in both adults and children, especially among blacks and Asians.

The apocrine and eccrine sweat glands are important for fluid balance and for thermoregulation. When apocrine gland secretions are contaminated by normal skin flora, odor results. Most Asians and Native Americans have a mild body odor or none at all, whereas whites and blacks tend to have strong body odor.

Inuits have made an interesting environmental adaptation, whereby they sweat less than whites on their trunks and extremities but more on their faces. This adaptation allows for temperature regulation without causing perspiration and dampness of their clothes, which would decrease their ability to insulate against severe cold weather and would pose a serious threat to their survival.

The amount of chloride excreted by sweat glands varies widely, and blacks have lower salt concentrations in their sweat than whites do. A study of Ashkenazic Jews (Jews of European descent) and Sephardic Jews (Jews of Northern African and Middle Eastern descent) revealed that those of European origins had a lower percentage of sweat chlorides.

Perhaps one of the most obvious and widely variable racial differences occurs with the hair. The hair of blacks varies widely in texture. It is very fragile and ranges from long and straight to short, spiraled, thick, and kinky. The hair and scalp have a natural tendency to be dry and require daily combing, gentle brushing, and the application of oil. In comparison, people of Asian backgrounds generally have straight, silky hair.

Hair condition is significant in diagnosing and treating certain disease states. For example, hair texture becomes dry, brittle, and lusterless with inadequate nutrition. The hair of black children with severe malnutrition (e.g., marasmus) frequently changes not only in texture but in color. The child's hair often becomes less kinky and assumes a copper-red color.

SUBJECTIVE DATA

1. Previous history of skin disease (allergies, hives, psoriasis, eczema)
2. Change in pigmentation
3. Change in mole (size or color)
4. Excessive dryness or moisture
5. Pruritus
6. Excessive bruising
7. Rash or lesion
8. Medications
9. Hair loss
10. Change in nails
11. Environmental or occupational hazards
12. Self-care behaviors

Examiner Asks	Rationale
1 **Previous history of skin disease.** Any **previous skin disease** or problem?	
● How was this treated?	
● Any family history of allergies or allergic skin problem?	Significant familial predisposition: allergies, hay fever, psoriasis, atopic dermatitis (eczema), acne.
● Any known allergies to drugs, plants, animals?	Identify offending allergen.
● Any birthmarks, tattoos?	Use of nonsterile equipment to apply tattoos increases risk of hepatitis.
2 **Change in pigmentation.** Any **change in skin color** or **pigmentation?**	Localized change: hypopigmentation—loss of pigmentation; hyperpigmentation—increase in color.
● A generalized color change (all over), or localized?	Generalized change suggests systemic illness: pallor, jaundice, cyanosis.
3 **Change in mole.** Any **change in a mole:** color, size, shape, sudden appearance of tenderness, bleeding, itching?	Signs suggest neoplasm in pigmented nevus. Person may be unaware of change in nevus on back or buttock that he or she cannot see.
● Any "sores" that do not heal?	
4 **Excessive dryness or moisture.** Any change in the feel of your skin: temperature, **moisture,** texture?	Seborrhea—oily.
● Any excess **dryness?** Is this seasonal or constant?	Xerosis—dry.
5 **Pruritus.** Any skin itching? Is this mild (prickling, tingling) or intense (intolerable)?	Pruritus is the most common of skin symptoms; occurs with dry skin, aging, drug reactions, allergy, obstructive jaundice, uremia, lice.
● Does it awaken you from sleep?	
● Where is the itching? When did it start?	Presence or absence of pruritus may be significant for diagnosis. Scratching may cause excoriation of primary lesion.
● Any other skin pain or soreness? Where?	
6 **Excessive bruising.** Any excess **bruising?** Where on the body?	Multiple cuts and bruises, bruises in various stages of healing, bruises above knees and elbows, and illogical explanation—consider the possibility of abuse. Frequent falls may be due to dizziness of neurologic or cardiovascular origin. Also, frequent minor trauma may be a side effect of alcoholism or other drug abuse.
● How did this happen?	
● How long have you had it?	
7 **Rash or lesion.** Any skin **rash or lesion?**	Rashes are a common cause of seeking health care. A careful history is important; it may be an accurate predictor of the type of lesion you will see in the examination and its cause.
● Onset. When did you first notice it?	
● Location. Where did it start?	Identify the primary site—it may give clue to cause.
● Where did it spread?	Migration pattern, evolution.
● Character or quality. Describe the color.	
● Is it raised or flat? Any crust, odor? Does it feel tender, warm?	
● Duration. How long have you had it?	
● Setting. Anyone at home or work with a similar rash? Have you been camping, acquired a new pet, tried a new food, drug? Does the rash seem to come with stress?	Identify new or relevant exposure. Identify any household or social contacts with similar symptoms.

Examiner Asks	Rationale
• Alleviating and aggravating factors. What home care have you tried? Bath, lotions, heat? Do they help, or make it worse? • Associated symptoms. Any itching, fever?	Myriad over-the-counter remedies are available. Many people have tried them and seek professional help only when they do not see improvement.
• What do you think rash/lesion means?	Assess person's perception of cause. May need to deal with fear of cancer, tick-borne illnesses, or sexually transmitted diseases.
• Coping strategies. How has rash/lesion affected your self-care, hygiene, ability to function at work/home/socially?	Assess effectiveness of coping strategies. Chronic skin diseases may increase risk of loss of self-esteem, social isolation, and anxiety.
• Any new or increased stress in your life?	Stress can exacerbate chronic skin illness.
8 Medications. What **medications** do you take? • Prescription and over-the-counter? • Recent change?	Drugs may produce allergic skin eruption: aspirin, antibiotics, barbiturates, some tonics. Drugs may increase sunlight sensitivity and give burn response: sulfonamides, thiazide diuretics, oral hypoglycemic agents, and tetracycline. Drugs can cause hyperpigmentation: antimalarials, antineoplastic agents, hormones, metals, tetracycline.
• How long on medication?	Even after a long time on medication, a person may develop sensitivity.
9 Hair loss. Any recent **hair loss?** • A gradual or sudden onset? Symmetric? Associated with fever, illness, increased stress?	Alopecia is a significant loss. A full head of hair equates with vitality in many cultures. If this is treated as a trivial problem, the person may seek alternative, unproven methods of treatment.
• Any unusual hair growth? • Any recent change in texture, appearance?	Hirsutism.
10 Change in nails. Any **change in nails:** shape, color, brittleness? Do you tend to bite or chew nails?	
11 Environmental or occupational hazards. Any **environmental** or **occupational hazards?** • Any hazard-related problems with your occupation, e.g., dyes, toxic chemicals, radiation? • How about hobbies? Do you perform any household or furniture repair work? • How much sun exposure do you get from outdoor work, leisure activities, sunbathing, tanning salons?	Majority of skin neoplasms result from occupational or environmental agents. People at risk include coal workers; farmers who are exposed to the sun, sailors, outdoor workers; also creosote workers, roofers. Unprotected sun exposure accelerates aging and produces lesions. At more risk: light-skinned people, those over 40, and those regularly in sun.
• Recently been bitten by insect: bee, tick, mosquito?	Identify contactants that produce lesions or contact dermatitis.
• Any recent exposure to plants, animals in yard work, camping?	For people with chronic recurrent urticaria (hives), tell them to keep diary of meals and environment to identify precipitating factors.

Examiner Asks	Rationale

⓬ Self-care behaviors. What do you do to care for your skin, hair, nails? What cosmetics, soaps, chemicals do you use?
- Clip cuticles on nails, use adhesive for false fingernails?

Assess **self-care** and influence on self-concept—may be important with this society's media stress on high norms of beauty. Many over-the-counter remedies are costly and exacerbate skin problems.

- If you have allergies, how do you control your environment to minimize exposure?
- Do you perform a skin self-examination?

ADDITIONAL HISTORY FOR INFANTS AND CHILDREN

❶ Does the child have any birthmarks?

❷ Was there any change in skin color as a newborn?
- Any jaundice? Which day after birth?
- Any cyanosis? What were the circumstances?

❸ Have you noted any rash or sores? What seems to bring it on?
- Have you introduced a new food or formula? When? Does your child eat chocolate, cow's milk, eggs?

Generalized rash—consider allergic reaction to new food.
Irritability and general fussiness may indicate the presence of pruritus.

❹ Does the child have any diaper rash? How do you care for this? How do you wash diapers? Do you use rubber pants? How do you clean skin?

Occlusive diapers or infrequent changing may cause rash. Infant may be allergic to certain detergent or to disposable wipes.

❺ Does the child have any burns or bruises?
- Where?
- How did it happen?

A careful history is important to distinguish expected childhood bumps and bruises from any lesion that may indicate child abuse or neglect: cigarette burns; excessive bruising, especially above knees or elbows; linear whip marks. With abuse, the history often will not coincide with the physical appearance and location of lesion.

❻ Has the child had any exposure to contagious skin conditions: scabies, impetigo, lice? Or to communicable diseases: measles, chickenpox, scarlet fever? Or to toxic plants: poison ivy?
- Are the child's vaccinations up to date?

❼ Does the child have any habits or habitual movements, e.g., nail-biting, twisting hair, rubbing head on mattress?

❽ What steps are taken to protect the child from sun exposure? What about sunscreens and sunblocks? How do you treat a sunburn?

Between 60 and 80 percent of a person's lifetime sun exposure occurs before 18 years of age. One or more severe sunburns during childhood double the risk of malignant melanoma in later life (Heffernan and O'Sullivan, 1998).

Examiner Asks	Rationale

ADDITIONAL HISTORY FOR THE ADOLESCENT

1 Have you noticed any skin problems such as pimples, blackheads?
 ● How long have you had them?
 ● How do you treat this?
 ● How do you feel about it?

About 70 percent of teens will have acne, and the psychological effect often is more significant than the physical effect. Self-treatment is common. Many myths surround the cause of acne, which you may need to clear up. Cause is unknown; acne is not caused by poor diet, oily complexion, or contagion, and has no relation to sexual practices.

ADDITIONAL HISTORY FOR THE AGING ADULT

1 What changes have you noticed in your skin in the last few years?

Assess impact of aging on self-concept. For some, normal aging changes may cause distress.

Note that many changes attributed to aging are due to chronic sun damage. Aging people are at greater risk of sun damage.

2 Any delay in wound healing?
 ● Any skin itching?

Pruritus is very common with aging. Consider side effects of medicine or systemic disease (e.g., liver or kidney disease, cancer, lymphoma), but senile pruritus is usually due to dry skin (xerosis). Exacerbated by too-frequent bathing or use of soap. Scratching with dirty, jagged fingernails produces excoriations.

3 Any other skin pain?

Some diseases produce more intense sensations of pain, itching in aging people, e.g., herpes zoster (shingles). Other diseases may reduce pain sensation in extremities, e.g., diabetes. Also, some aging people tolerate chronic pain as "part of growing old," and hesitate to "complain."

4 Any change in feet, toenails? Any bunions? Is it possible to wear shoes?

Some aging people cannot reach down to their feet to give self-care.

5 Do you experience frequent falls?

Multiple bruises, trauma from falls.

6 Any history of diabetes, peripheral vascular disease?

Increased risk for skin lesions in feet or ankles.

7 What do you do to care for your skin?

The application of bland lotions is important to retain moisture in aging skin.

Examiner Asks	Rationale
	But dermatitis may ensue from certain cosmetics, creams, ointments, and dyes applied to achieve a youthful appearance. Aging skin has a delayed inflammatory response when exposed to irritants. If the person is not alerted by warning signs (e.g., pruritus, redness), exposure may continue and dermatitis may ensue.

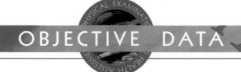

OBJECTIVE DATA

PREPARATION

Try to control external variables that may influence skin color and confuse your findings, both in light-skinned and in dark-skinned persons (Table 10–1).

Learn to consciously attend to skin characteristics. The danger is one of omission. You grow so accustomed to seeing the skin that you are likely to ignore it as you assess the organ systems underneath. Yet the skin holds information about the body's circulation, nutritional status, and signs of systemic diseases as well as topical data on the integument itself.

Know the person's normal skin coloring. Baseline knowledge is important to assess color or pigment changes. If this is the first time you are examining the person, ask about his or her usual skin color and about any self-monitoring practices.

The Complete Physical Examination. Although it is presented alone in this chapter, skin assessment is *integrated* throughout the complete examination; it is not a separate step. At the beginning of the examination, assessing the person's hands and fingernails is a nonthreatening way to accustom him or her to your touch. Most people are used to having relative strangers shake their hand or touch their arm. As you move through the examination, scrutinize the outer skin surface first before you concentrate on the underlying structures. Separate intertriginous areas (areas with skinfolds) such as under large breasts, obese abdomen, and the groin and inspect them thoroughly. These areas are dark, warm, and moist and provide the perfect conditions for irritation or infection. Last, always remove the person's socks and inspect the feet, toenails, and the area between the toes.

The Regional Examination. At times, an individual seeks health care because of a skin change and your assessment will be focused on the skin alone. Ask the person to remove his or her clothing and assess the skin as one entity. Stand back at first to get an overall impression; this helps reveal distribution

► Equipment Needed

Strong direct lighting (natural daylight is ideal to evaluate skin characteristics but is usually not available in the clinical area)

Small centimeter ruler

Penlight

Gloves

Needed for special procedures:

Wood's light (filtered ultraviolet light)

Magnifying glass, for minute lesions

Materials for laboratory tests: potassium hydroxide (KOH), glass slide

Table 10–1 • External Variables Influencing Skin Color

Variable		Causes		Misleading Outcome
Emotions				
Fear, anger	⟶	Peripheral vasoconstriction	⟶	False pallor
Embarrassment	⟶	Flushing in face and neck	⟶	False erythema
Environment				
Hot room	⟶	Vasodilatation	⟶	False erythema
Chilly or air-conditioned room, mist tents	⟶	Vasoconstriction	⟶	False pallor, coolness
Cigarette smoking	⟶	Vasoconstriction	⟶	False pallor
Physical				
Prolonged elevation	⟶	Decreased arterial perfusion	⟶	Pallor, coolness
Dependent position	⟶	Venous pooling	⟶	Redness, warmth, distended veins
Immobilization, prolonged inactivity	⟶	Slowed circulation	⟶	Pallor, coolness, nail beds pale, prolonged capillary filling time

Data from Roach L. Dark skins: Recognizing and interpreting color changes. Crit Care Update 5–15, 1977.

patterns. Then inspect lesions carefully. With a skin rash, check all areas of the body because there are some locations the person cannot see. You cannot rely on the history alone that the rash is limited to one location. Inspect mucous membranes, too, because some disorders have characteristic lesions here.

The skills used are inspection and palpation because some skin changes have accompanying signs that can be felt.

▶ Normal Range of Findings	Abnormal Findings

SKIN

Inspect and palpate

Color

General Pigmentation

Observe the skin tone. Normally, it is consistent with genetic background and varies from pinkish tan to ruddy dark tan or from light to dark brown and may have yellow or olive overtones. Dark-skinned people normally have areas of lighter pigmentation on the palms, nail beds, and lips (Fig. 10–3A).

An acquired condition is **vitiligo**, the complete absence of melanin pigment in patchy areas of white or light skin on the face, neck, hands, feet, body folds, and around orifices (Fig. 10–3B). Vitiligo can occur in all races, although dark-skinned people are more severely affected and potentially suffer a greater threat to their body image.

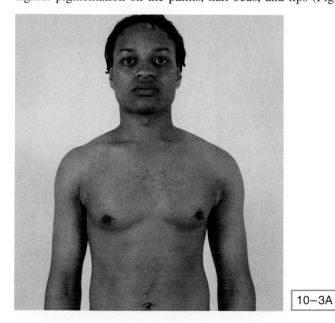

10–3A

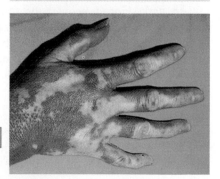

10–3B

Vitiligo

223

Normal Range of Findings	Abnormal Findings

General pigmentation is darker in sun-exposed areas. Common (benign) pigmented areas also occur:

- **Freckles** (ephelides)—small, flat macules of brown melanin pigment that occur on sun-exposed skin (Fig. 10–4A).

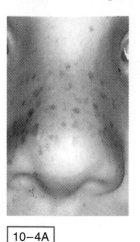

10–4A

Freckles

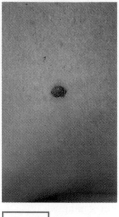

10–4B

Junctional nevus

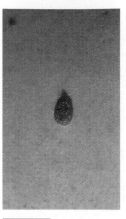

10–4C

Compound nevus

- **Mole** (nevus)—a proliferation of melanocytes, tan to brown color, flat or raised. Acquired nevi are characterized by their symmetry, small size (6 mm or less), smooth borders, and single uniform pigmentation. The **junctional nevus** (Fig. 10–4B) is macular only and occurs in children and adolescents. It progresses to the **compound nevi** in young adults (Fig. 10–4C) that are macular and papular. The intradermal nevus (mainly in older age) has nevus cells in only the dermis.
- **Birthmarks**—may be tan to brown in color.

Widespread Color Change

Note any color change over the entire body skin, such as pallor (white), erythema (red), cyanosis (blue), and jaundice (yellow). Note whether the color change is transient and expected or if it is due to pathology.

In dark-skinned people, the amount of normal pigment may mask color changes. Lips and nail beds show some color change, but they vary with the person's skin color and may not always be accurate signs. The more reliable sites are those with the least pigmentation, such as under the tongue, the buccal mucosa, the palpebral conjunctiva, and the sclera. See Table 10–2 for specific clues to assessment.

Pallor. When the red-pink tones from the oxygenated hemoglobin in the blood are lost, the skin takes on the color of connective tissue (collagen), which is mostly white. Pallor is common in acute high-stress states such as anxiety or fear, due to the powerful peripheral vasoconstriction from sympathetic nervous

Danger signs: abnormal characteristics of pigmented lesions are summarized in the mnemonic **ABCDE**:

Asymmetry of a pigmented lesion (one that is *not* regularly round or oval)

Border irregularity (notching, scalloping, ragged edges or poorly defined margins)

Color variation (areas of brown, tan, black, blue, red, white, or combination thereof)

Diameter greater than 6 mm; i.e., the size of a pencil eraser (although early melanomas may be diagnosed at a smaller size) (NIH, 1992)

Elevation and **E**nlargement

Additionally, individuals may report change in mole's size, a new pigmented lesion, and development of itching, burning or bleeding in a mole. Any of these signs should raise suspicion of malignant melanoma and warrant referral.

Ashen gray color in dark skin or marked pallor in whites occurs with anemia, shock, arterial insufficiency (see Table 10–2).

system stimulation. The skin also looks pale with vasoconstriction from exposure to cold and cigarette smoking and in the presence of edema.

Look for pallor in dark-skinned people by the absence of the underlying red tones that normally give brown or black skin its luster. The brown-skinned individual demonstrates pallor with a more yellowish-brown color, and the black-skinned person will appear ashen or gray. Generalized pallor can be observed in the mucous membranes, lips, and nail beds. The palpebral conjunctiva and nail beds are preferred sites for assessing the pallor of anemia. When inspecting the conjunctiva, lower the lid sufficiently to visualize the conjunctiva near the *outer* canthus as well as the inner canthus. The coloration is often lighter near the inner canthus.

The pallor of impending shock is accompanied by other subtle manifestations, such as increasing pulse rate, oliguria, apprehension, and restlessness.

Anemias, particularly chronic iron deficiency anemia, may become manifest by "spoon" nails, which have a concave shape. A lemon yellow tint of the face and slightly yellow sclera accompany pernicious anemia, which is also indicated by neurologic deficits and a red, painful tongue. Fatigue, exertional dyspnea, rapid pulse, dizziness, and impaired mental function accompany most severe anemias.

Erythema. This is an intense redness of the skin due to excess blood (hyperemia) in the dilated superficial capillaries. This sign is *expected* with fever, local inflammation, or with emotional reactions, e.g., blushing in vascular flush areas (cheeks, neck, and upper chest).

When erythema is associated with fever or localized inflammation, it is characterized by increased skin temperature due to the increased rate of blood flow through the blood vessels. Since you cannot see inflammation in dark-skinned persons, it is often necessary to palpate the skin for increased warmth, taut or tightly pulled surfaces that may be indicative of edema, and hardening of deep tissues or blood vessels.

Erythema occurs with polycythemia, venous stasis, carbon monoxide poisoning, and the extravascular presence of red blood cells (petechiae, ecchymosis, hematoma) (see Tables 10–2 and 10–7).

Cyanosis. This is a bluish mottled color that signifies decreased perfusion; the tissues are not adequately perfused with oxygenated blood. Be aware that cyanosis can be a nonspecific sign. A person who is anemic could have hypoxemia without ever looking blue because not enough hemoglobin is present (either oxygenated or reduced) to color the skin. On the other hand, a person with polycythemia (an increase in the number of red blood cells) looks ruddy blue at all times and may not necessarily be hypoxemic. This person just is unable to fully oxygenate the massive numbers of red blood cells. Lastly, do not confuse cyanosis with the common and normal bluish tone on the lips of dark-skinned persons of Mediterranean origin.

Cyanosis is difficult to observe in darkly pigmented persons (see Table 10–2). Given that most conditions causing cyanosis also cause decreased oxygenation of the brain, other clinical signs, such as changes in level of consciousness and signs of respiratory distress, will be evident.

Cyanosis indicates hypoxemia and occurs with shock, heart failure, chronic bronchitis, and congenital heart disease.

Jaundice. Jaundice is exhibited by a yellow color, indicating rising amounts of bilirubin in the blood. Except for physiologic jaundice in the newborn (p. 236), jaundice does not occur normally. Jaundice is *first* noted in the junction of the hard and soft palate in the mouth and in the sclera. But do not confuse scleral jaundice with the normal yellow subconjunctival fatty deposits that are common in the outer sclera of dark-skinned persons. The scleral yellow of jaundice extends up to the edge of the iris.

Jaundice occurs with hepatitis, cirrhosis, sickle-cell disease, transfusion reaction, and hemolytic disease of the newborn.

As levels of serum bilirubin rise, jaundice is evident in the skin over the rest of the body. This is best assessed in direct natural daylight. Common calluses on palms and soles often look yellow—do not interpret these as jaundice.

Light or clay-colored stools and dark golden urine often accompany jaundice in both light- and dark-skinned people.

Temperature

Note the temperature of your own hands. Then use the backs (dorsa) of your hands to palpate the person and check bilaterally. The skin should be warm, and the temperature should be equal bilaterally; warmth suggests normal circulatory status. Hands and feet may be slightly cooler in a cool environment.

Hypothermia. Generalized coolness may be induced, such as in hypothermia used for surgery or high fever. Localized coolness is expected with an immobilized extremity, as when a limb is in a cast or with an intravenous infusion.

General hypothermia accompanies central circulatory disturbance, such as in shock.

Localized hypothermia occurs in peripheral arterial insufficiency and Raynaud's disease.

Hyperthermia. Generalized hyperthermia occurs with an increased metabolic rate, such as in fever, or after heavy exercise. A localized area feels hyperthermic with trauma, infection, or sunburn.

Hyperthyroidism has an increased metabolic rate, causing warm, moist skin.

Moisture

Perspiration appears normally on the face, hands, axilla, and skinfolds in response to activity, a warm environment, or anxiety. **Diaphoresis,** or profuse perspiration, accompanies an increased metabolic rate, such as occurs in heavy activity or fever.

Look for **dehydration** in the oral mucous membranes. Normally there is none, and the mucous membranes look smooth and moist. Be aware that dark skin may normally look dry and flaky, but this does not necessarily indicate systemic dehydration.

Diaphoresis occurs with thyrotoxicosis and with stimulation of the nervous system with anxiety or pain.

With dehydration, mucous membranes look dry and the lips look parched and cracked. With extreme dryness the skin is fissured, resembling cracks in a dry lake bed.

Texture

Normal skin feels smooth and firm, with an even surface.

Hyperthyroidism—skin feels smoother and softer, like velvet.

Hypothyroidism—skin feels rough, dry, and flaky.

Thickness

The epidermis is uniformly thin over most of the body, although thickened callus areas are normal on palms and soles. A callus is a circumscribed overgrowth of epidermis and is an adaptation to excessive pressure. On the palms and soles, calluses develop from the friction of work and weight-bearing.

Very thin, shiny skin (atrophic) occurs with arterial insufficiency.

▶

Edema

Edema is fluid accumulating in the intercellular spaces and is not present normally. To check for edema, imprint your thumbs firmly against the ankle malleolus or the tibia. Normally the skin surface stays smooth. If your pressure leaves a dent in the skin, "pitting" edema is present. Its presence is graded on a 4-point scale:

1 + Mild pitting, slight indentation, no perceptible swelling of the leg
2 + Moderate pitting, indentation subsides rapidly
3 + Deep pitting, indentation remains for a short time, leg looks swollen
4 + Very deep pitting, indentation lasts a long time, leg is very swollen

This scale is somewhat subjective; outcomes vary among examiners (see further content on grading scale in Chapter 18).

Edema masks normal skin color as well as obscures pathologic conditions such as jaundice or cyanosis because the fluid lies between the surface and the pigmented and vascular layers. It makes dark skin look lighter.

Mobility and Turgor

Pinch up a large fold of skin on the anterior chest under the clavicle (Fig. 10–5). Mobility is the skin's ease of rising, and turgor is its ability to return to place promptly when released. This reflects the elasticity of the skin.

Edema is most evident in dependent parts of the body (feet, ankles, and sacral areas), where the skin looks puffy and tight. Edema makes the hair follicles more prominent, so you note a pig-skin or orange-peel look (called *peau d'orange*).

Unilateral edema—consider a local or peripheral cause.

Bilateral edema or edema that is generalized over the whole body (anasarca)—consider a central problem such as congestive heart failure, kidney failure.

Mobility is decreased when edema is present.

Poor turgor is evident in severe dehydration or extreme weight loss; the pinched skin recedes slowly or "tents" and stands by itself.

Scleroderma, literally "hard skin," is a chronic connective tissue disorder associated with decreased mobility (see Table 11–5).

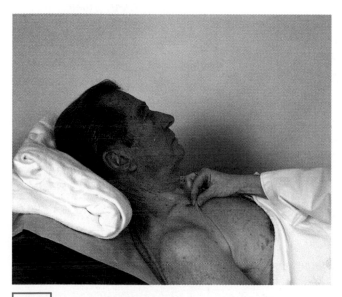

10–5

Normal Range of Findings	Abnormal Findings

Vascularity or Bruising

Cherry (senile) angiomas are small (1 to 5 mm), smooth, slightly raised bright red dots that commonly appear on the trunk in all adults over 30 (Fig. 10–6). They normally increase in size and number with aging and are not significant.

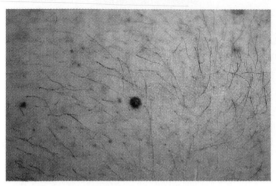

10–6

Cherry angioma

Any bruising (ecchymosis) should be consistent with the expected trauma of life. There are normally no venous dilatations or varicosities.

Document the presence of any tattoos (a permanent skin design from indelible pigment) on the person's chart. Advise the person that the use of tattoo needles and tattoo parlor equipment of doubtful sterility increases the risk of hepatitis.

Lesions

If any lesions are present, note their:

1. Color.
2. Elevation: flat, raised, or pedunculated.
3. Pattern or shape: the grouping or distinctness of each lesion, for example, annular, grouped, confluent, linear. The pattern may be characteristic of a certain disease.
4. Size, in centimeters: Use a ruler to measure. Avoid household descriptions such as "quarter size" or "pea size."
5. Location and distribution on body: Is it generalized or localized to area of a specific irritant; around jewelry, watchband, around eyes?
6. Any exudate. Note its color and/or odor.

Multiple bruises at different stages of healing and excessive bruises above knees or elbows should raise concern about physical abuse (see Table 10–6).

Needle marks or tracks from intravenous injection of street drugs may be visible on the antecubital fossae or forearms or on any available vein.

Lesions are traumatic or pathologic changes in previously normal structures. When a lesion develops on previously unaltered skin, it is **primary**. However, when a lesion changes over time or changes because of a factor such as scratching or infection, it is **secondary**. Study Table 10–3 for the shapes and Tables 10–4 and 10–5 for the characteristics of primary and secondary skin lesions. The terms used (macule, papule, and so forth) are helpful to describe any lesion you encounter.

▶ Normal Range of Findings	Abnormal Findings

Palpate lesions. Wear a glove if you anticipate contact with blood, mucosa, any body fluid, or skin lesion. Roll a nodule between the thumb and index finger to assess depth. Gently scrape a scale to see if it comes off. Note the nature of its base or if it bleeds when the scale comes off. Note the surrounding skin temperature. However, the erythema associated with rashes is not always accompanied by noticeable increases in skin temperature.

Does the lesion blanch with pressure or stretch? Stretching the area of skin between your thumb and index finger decreases (blanches) the normal underlying red tones, thus providing more contrast and brightening the macules. Red macules from dilated blood vessels *will* blanch momentarily, whereas those from extravasated blood (petechiae) do not. Blanching also helps identify a macular rash in dark-skinned people.

Use a magnifier and light for closer inspection of the lesion (Fig. 10–7). Use a Wood's light, i.e., an ultraviolet light filtered through a special glass, to detect fluorescing lesions. With the room darkened, shine the Wood's light on the area.

Note the pattern and characteristics of common skin lesions (see Table 10–8) and malignant skin lesions (Table 10–9), and lesions associated with AIDS (Table 10–10).

Lesions with blue-green fluorescence indicate fungal infection, e.g., tinea capitis (scalp ringworm).

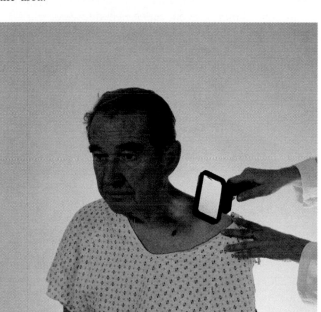

10–7

Potassium Hydroxide (KOH) Preparation. Microscopic examination of skin scrapings helps diagnose superficial fungal infections. Use a sharp sterile blade and lightly scrape the scale from the edge of a scaling lesion. Place on a clean slide. Add a drop of 10 to 20 percent potassium hydroxide (KOH) to dissolve nonfungal skin debris and send to the lab.

HAIR

Inspect and palpate

Color

Hair color comes from melanin production and may vary from pale blonde to total black. Graying begins as early as the third decade of life because of reduced melanin production in the follicles. Genetic factors affect the age of onset of graying.

| Normal Range of Findings | Abnormal Findings |

Texture

Scalp hair may be fine or thick and may look straight, curly, or kinky. It should look shiny, although this characteristic may be lost with the use of some beauty products such as dyes, rinses, or permanents.

Note dull, coarse, or brittle scalp hair.

Gray, scaly, well-defined areas with broken hairs accompany tinea capitis, a ringworm infection found mostly in school-age children (see Table 10–11).

Distribution

Fine vellus hair coats the body, whereas coarser terminal hairs grow at the eyebrows, eyelashes, and scalp. During puberty, distribution conforms to normal male and female patterns. At first, coarse curly hairs develop in the pubic area, then in the axillae, and last in the facial area in boys. In the genital area, the female pattern is an inverted triangle; the male pattern is an upright triangle with pubic hair extending up to the umbilicus. In Asians, body hair may be diminished.

Genital hair absent or with abnormal configuration suggests endocrine abnormalities.

Hirsutism—excess body hair. In females, this forms a male pattern of hair distribution on the face and chest and indicates the presence of endocrine abnormalities (see Table 10–11).

Lesions

Separate the hair into sections and lift it, observing the scalp. With a history of itching, inspect the hair behind the ears and in the occipital area as well. All areas should be clean and free of any lesions or pest inhabitants. Many people normally have seborrhea (dandruff), which is indicated by loose white flakes.

Head or pubic lice. Distinguish dandruff from nits (eggs) of lice, which are oval, adherent to hair shaft, and cause intense itching (see Table 10–11).

NAILS

Inspect and palpate

Shape and Contour

The nail surface is normally slightly curved or flat, and the posterior and lateral nail folds are smooth and rounded. Nail edges are smooth, rounded, and clean, suggesting adequate self-care.

Spoon nails (see Table 10–12). Jagged nails, bitten to the quick, or traumatized nail folds from chronic nervous picking suggest nervous habits.

Chronically dirty nails suggest poor self-care or some occupations in which it is impossible to keep them clean.

Normal Range of Findings	Abnormal Findings

The Profile Sign. View the index finger at its profile and note the angle of the nail base; it should be about 160 degrees (Fig. 10–8). The nail base is firm to palpation. Curved nails are a variation of normal with a convex profile. They may look like clubbed nails, but notice that the angle between nail base and nail is normal, i.e., 160 degrees or less.

Clubbing of nails occurs with congenital chronic cyanotic heart disease and with emphysema and chronic bronchitis.

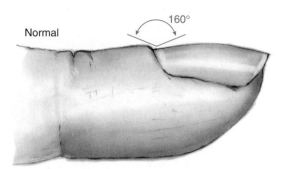

Normal

160°

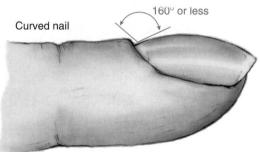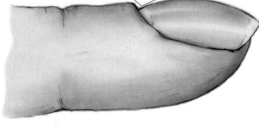

Curved nail

160° or less

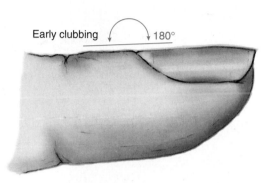

Early clubbing   180°

10–8

In early clubbing, the angle straightens out to 180 degrees, and the nail base feels spongy to palpation.

Consistency

The surface is smooth and regular, not brittle or splitting.

Pits, transverse grooves, or lines may indicate a nutrient deficiency or may accompany acute illness in which nail growth is disturbed (see Table 10–12).

Nail thickness is uniform.

Nails are thickened and ridged with arterial insufficiency.

The nail is firmly adherent to the nail bed, and the nail base is firm to palpation.

A spongy nail base accompanies clubbing.

Normal Range of Findings	Abnormal Findings

Color

The translucent nail plate is a window to the even, pink nail bed underneath.

Dark-skinned people may have brown-black pigmented areas or linear bands or streaks along the nail edge (Fig. 10–9). All people normally may have white hairline linear markings from trauma or picking at the cuticle (Fig. 10–10). Note any abnormal marking in the nail beds.

Cyanosis or marked pallor.

Brown linear streaks (especially sudden appearance) are abnormal in light-skinned people and may indicate melanoma.

Splinter hemorrhages, transverse ridges, or Beau's lines (see Table 10–12).

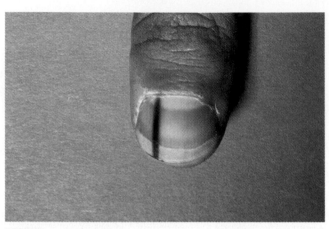

10–9

Linear pigmentation

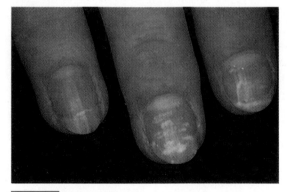

10–10

Leukonychia striata

Capillary refill. Depress the nail edge to blanch and then release, noting the return of color. Normally, color return is instant, or at least within a few seconds in a cold environment. This indicates the status of the peripheral circulation. A sluggish color return takes longer than 1 or 2 seconds.

Inspect the toenails. Separate the toes and note the smooth skin in between.

Cyanotic nail beds or sluggish color return, consider cardiovascular or respiratory dysfunction.

PROMOTING HEALTH AND SELF-CARE
Teach Skin Self-Examination

Teach all adults to examine their skin once a month, using the ABCDE rule (see p. 224) to raise warning signals of any suspicious lesions. Use a well-lighted room that has a full-length mirror. It helps to have a small handheld mirror. Ask a relative to search skin areas difficult to see (e.g., behind ears, back of neck, back). Follow the sequence outlined in Figure 10–11 and report any suspicious lesions promptly to a physician or nurse.

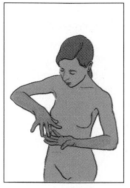

1. Undress completely. Check forearms, palms, space between fingers. Turn over hands and study the backs.

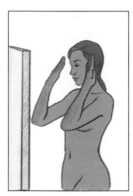

2. Face mirror; bend arms at elbow. Study arms in mirror.

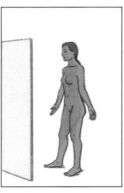

3. Face mirror and study entire front of body. Start at face, neck, torso, working down to lower legs.

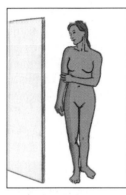

4. Pivot to right side facing mirror. Study sides of upper arms, working down to ankles. Repeat with left side.

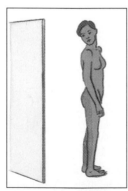

5. With back to mirror, study buttocks, thighs, lower legs.

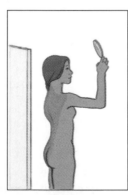

6. Use the hand-held mirror to study upper back.

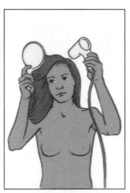

7. Use the hand-held mirror to study scalp, lifting the hair. A blow-dryer on a cool setting helps to lift hair.

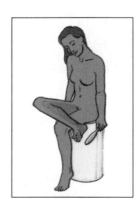

8. Sit on chair or bed. Study insides of each leg and soles of feet. Use the small mirror to help.

10–11

Skin self-examination

DEVELOPMENTAL CONSIDERATIONS

Use the same examination as described in the previous sections for the adult. Common variations follow.

Infants

Skin Color—General Pigmentation. Black newborns initially have lighter-toned skin than their parents because of a pigment function that is not yet in full production. Their full melanotic color is evident in the nail beds and scrotal folds. The **mongolian spot** is a common variation of hyperpigmentation in black, Asian, Native American, and Hispanic newborns (Fig. 10–12). It is a blue-black to purple macular area at the sacrum or buttocks, but sometimes it occurs on the abdomen, thighs, shoulders, or arms. It is due to deep dermal melanocytes. It gradually fades during the first year. By adulthood these spots are lighter but are frequently still visible. Mongolian spots are present in 90 percent of blacks, 80 percent of Asians and Native Americans, and 9 percent of whites. If you are unfamiliar with mongolian spots, be careful not to confuse them with bruises. Recognition of this normal variation is particularly important when dealing with children who might be erroneously identified as victims of child abuse.

Bruising is a common soft tissue injury that follows a rapid, traumatic, or breech birth.

Multiple bruises in various stages of healing, or pattern injury, suggest child abuse (see Table 10–6).

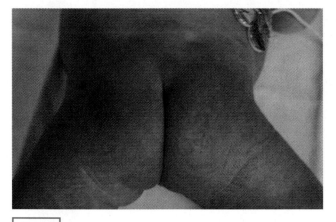

10–12

Mongolian spot

The **café au lait spot** is a large round or oval patch of light brown pigmentation (hence, the name "coffee with milk"), which is usually present at birth (Fig. 10–13). Most often these patches are normal.

Six or more café au lait macules, each more than 1.5 cm in diameter, are diagnostic of neurofibromatosis, an inherited neurocutaneous disease.

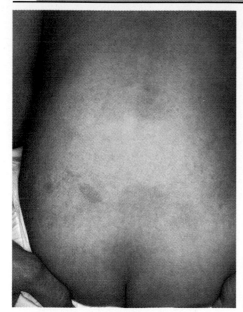

10-13

Café au lait spot

Skin Color Change. Three erythematous states are common variations in the neonate. (1) The newborn's skin has a beefy red flush for the first 24 hours because of vasomotor instability; then the color fades to its normal color. (2) Another finding, the **Harlequin color change,** occurs when the baby is in a side-lying position. The lower half of the body turns red and the upper half blanches with a distinct demarcation line down the midline. The cause is unknown, and its occurrence is transient. (3) Finally, **erythema toxicum** is a common rash that appears in the first 3 to 4 days of life. Sometimes called the "flea bite" rash or newborn rash, it consists of tiny, punctate, red macules and papules on the cheeks, trunk, chest, back, and buttocks (Fig. 10–14). The cause is unknown; no treatment is needed.

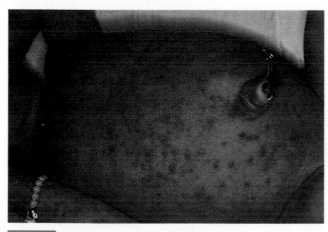

10-14

Erythema toxicum

▶ Normal Range of Findings | Abnormal Findings

Two temporary cyanotic conditions may occur. (1) A newborn may have **acrocyanosis,** a bluish color around the lips, hands and fingernails, and feet and toenails. This may last for a few hours and disappear with warming. (2) **Cutis marmorata** is a transient mottling in the trunk and extremities in response to cooler room temperatures (Fig. 10–15). It forms a reticulated red or blue pattern over the skin.

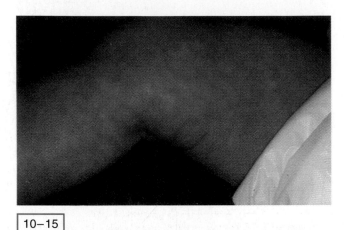

10–15

Cutis marmorata

Persistent generalized cyanosis indicates distress, possibly cyanotic congenital heart disease.

Persistent or pronounced cutis marmorata occurs with Down syndrome or prematurity.

Green-brown discoloration of the skin, nails, and cord occurs with passing of meconium in utero, indicating fetal distress.

Physiologic jaundice is a common variation in about half of all newborns. A yellowing of the skin, sclera, and mucous membranes develops after the 3rd or 4th day of life because of the increased numbers of red blood cells that hemolyze following birth. The hemoglobin in the red blood cells is metabolized by the liver and spleen; its pigment is converted into bilirubin.

Carotenemia also produces a yellow-orange color in light-skinned persons but no yellowing in the sclera or mucous membranes. It comes from ingesting large amounts of foods containing carotene, a vitamin A precursor. Carotene-rich foods are popular as prepared infant foods, and the absorption of carotene is enhanced by mashing, pureeing, and cooking. The color is best seen on the palms and soles, the forehead, tip of the nose and nasolabial folds, the chin, behind the ears, and over the knuckles; it fades to normal color within 2 to 6 weeks of withdrawing carotene-rich foods from the diet.

Moisture. The vernix caseosa is the moist, white, cream-cheese–like substance that covers part of the skin in all newborns. Perspiration is present after 1 month of age.

Texture. A common variation occurring in the infant is **milia** (Fig. 10–16). Milia are tiny white papules on the cheeks, forehead, and across the nose and chin due to sebum that occludes the opening of the follicles. Tell parents not to squeeze the lesions; milia resolve spontaneously within a few weeks.

Jaundice on the first day of life may indicate hemolytic disease. Jaundice after 2 weeks of age may indicate biliary tract obstruction.

Green-tinged vernix occurs with meconium staining.

In children, excessive sweating may accompany hypoglycemia, heart disease, or hyperthyroidism.

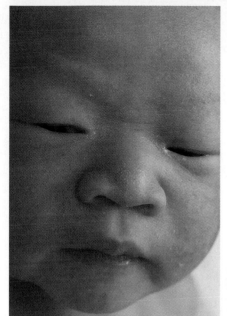

10–16

Milia

Thickness. In the neonate, the epidermis is normally thin but you will also note well-defined areas of subcutaneous fat. The baby's skin dimples over joints, but there is no break in the skin. Check for any defect or break in the skin, especially over the length of the spine.

Lack of subcutaneous fat occurs in prematurity and malnutrition.

A red sacrococcygeal dimple occurs with a pilonidal cyst or sinus (see Table 23–1).

Mobility and Turgor. Test mobility and turgor over the abdomen in an infant.

Poor turgor, or "tenting," indicates dehydration or malnutrition.

Vascularity or Bruising. Some vascular markings are common birthmarks in the newborn. A **storkbite** (salmon patch) is a flat, irregularly shaped red or pink patch found on the forehead, eyelid, or upper lip, but most commonly at the back of the neck (nuchal area) (Fig. 10–17). It is present at birth and usually fades during the first year.

Port-wine stain, strawberry mark (immature hemangioma), cavernous hemangioma (see Table 10–6).

Bruising may suggest abuse (see Table 10–7).

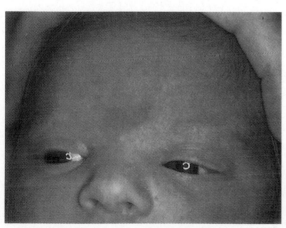

10–17

Storkbite

Hair. A newborn's skin is covered with fine downy lanugo (Fig. 10–18), especially in a preterm infant. Dark-skinned newborns have more lanugo than lighter-skinned newborns. Scalp hair may be lost in the few weeks following birth, especially at the temples and occiput. It grows back slowly.

Scaly crusted scalp occurs with seborrheic dermatitis (craddle cap (see Table 10–10).

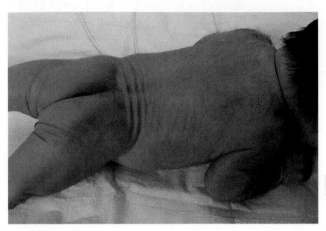

10–18

Lanugo

Nails. A newborn's nail beds may be blue (cyanotic) for the first few hours of life; then they turn pink.

Adolescents

The increase in sebaceous gland activity creates increased oiliness and **acne** (Fig. 10–19). Acne is the most common skin problem of adolescence. Almost all teens have some acne, even if it is the milder form of open comedones (blackheads) and closed comedones (whiteheads). Severe acne includes papules, pustules, and nodules. Acne lesions usually appear on the face and sometimes on the chest, back, and shoulders. Acne may appear in children as early as 7 to 8 years of age; then the lesions increase in number and severity and peak at 14 to 16 years in girls and at 16 to 19 years in boys.

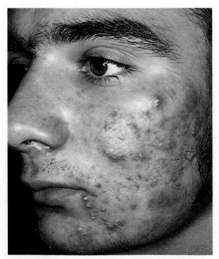

10–19

Acne

The Pregnant Female

Striae are jagged linear "stretch marks" of silver to pink color that appear during the second trimester on the abdomen, breasts, and sometimes thighs. They occur in one-half of all pregnancies. They fade after delivery but do not disappear. Another skin change on the abdomen is the **linea nigra,** a brownish black line down the midline (see Fig. 25–3). **Chloasma** is an irregular brown patch of hyperpigmentation on the face. It may occur with pregnancy or in women taking oral contraceptive pills. Chloasma disappears after delivery or stopping the pills. **Vascular spiders** occur in two-thirds of pregnancies in white women and less often in blacks. These lesions have tiny red centers with radiating branches and occur on the face, neck, upper chest, and arms.

The Aging Adult

Skin Color and Pigmentation. The lesions discussed in the following sections are common variations of hyperpigmentation:

Senile Lentigines. These lesions are commonly called liver spots and are small, flat, brown macules (Fig. 10–20). These circumscribed areas are clusters of melanocytes that appear following extensive sun exposure. They appear on the forearms and dorsa of the hands. They are not malignant and require no treatment.

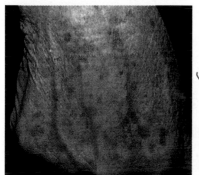

10–20
Lentigines

Keratoses. These lesions are raised, thickened areas of pigmentation that look crusted, scaly, and warty. One type, **seborrheic keratoses,** looks dark, greasy, and "stuck on" (Fig. 10–21). They develop mostly on the trunk but also on the face and hands and on unexposed as well as on sun-exposed areas. They do not become cancerous.

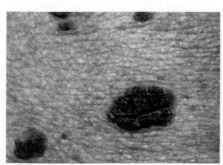

10–21
Seborrheic keratosis

Another type, **actinic (senile or solar) keratoses,** are less common (Fig. 10–22). These lesions are red-tan scaly plaques that increase over the years to become raised and roughened. They may have a silvery white scale adherent to the plaque. They occur on sun-exposed surfaces and are directly related to sun exposure. They are premalignant and may develop into squamous cell carcinoma.

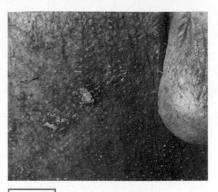

10–22 **Actinic keratosis**

Moisture. Dry skin (xerosis) is common in the aging person because of a decline in the size, number, and output of the sweat glands and sebaceous glands. The skin itches and looks flaky and loose.

Texture. Common variations occurring in the aging adult are **acrochordons,** or "skin tags," which are overgrowths of normal skin that form a stalk and are polyplike (Fig. 10–23). They occur frequently on eyelids, cheeks and neck, and axillae and trunk.

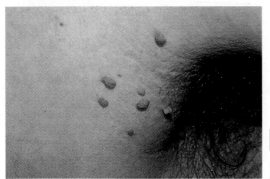

10–23

Skin tags

Sebaceous hyperplasia consists of raised yellow papules with a central depression. They are more common in men, occurring over the forehead, nose, or cheeks. They have a pebbly look (Fig. 10–24).

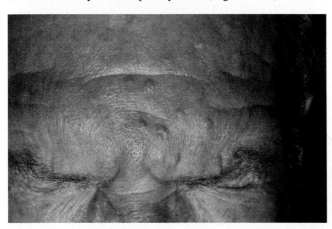

10–24

Sebaceous hyperplasia

Thickness. With aging, the skin looks as thin as parchment and the subcutaneous fat diminishes. Thinner skin is evident over the dorsa of the hands, forearms, lower legs, dorsa of feet, and over bony prominences. The skin may feel thicker over the abdomen and chest.

Normal Range of Findings	Abnormal Findings

Mobility and Turgor. The turgor is decreased (less elasticity), and the skin recedes slowly or "tents" and stands by itself (Fig. 10–25).

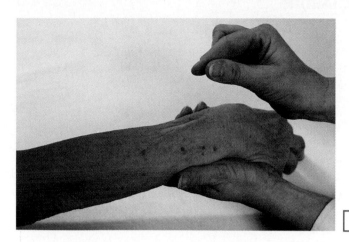

10–25

Hair. With aging, the hair growth decreases, and the amount decreases in the axillae and pubic areas. After menopause, white women may develop bristly hairs on the chin or upper lip resulting from unopposed androgens. In men, coarse terminal hairs develop in the ears, nose, and eyebrows, although the beard is unchanged. Male-pattern balding, or alopecia, is a genetic trait. It is usually a gradual receding of the anterior hairline in a symmetric W shape. In men and women, scalp hair gradually turns gray because of the decrease in melanocyte function.

Nails. With aging, the nail growth rate decreases, and local injuries in the nail matrix may produce longitudinal ridges. The surface may be brittle or peeling and sometimes yellowed. Toenails also are thickened and may grow misshapen, almost grotesque. The thickening may be a process of aging or it may be due to chronic peripheral vascular disease.

Fungal infections are common in aging, with thickened crumbling toenails and erythematous scaling on contiguous skin surfaces.

SUMMARY CHECKLIST: Skin, Hair, and Nails Exam

1: Inspect the skin:
Color
General pigmentation
Areas of hypopigmentation
  or hyperpigmentation
Abnormal color changes

2: Palpate the skin:
Temperature
Moisture
Texture
Thickness
Edema
Mobility and turgor
Hygiene
Vascularity or bruising

3: Note any lesions:
Color
Shape and configuration
Size
Location and distribution on
  body

4: Inspect and palpate the hair:
Texture
Distribution
Any scalp lesions

5: Inspect and palpate the nails:
Shape and contour
Consistency
Color

6: Teach skin self-examination

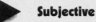

SAMPLE CHARTING

▶ **Subjective**

No history of skin disease; no present change in pigmentation or in nevi; no pruritus, bruising, rash, or lesions. On no medications. No work-related skin hazards. Uses sun block cream when outdoors.

▶ **Objective**

Skin: color tan-pink, even pigmentation, with no nevi. Warm to touch, dry, smooth, and even. Turgor good, no lesions.
Hair: even distribution, thick texture, no lesions or pest inhabitants.
Nails: no clubbing or deformities. Nail beds pink with prompt capillary refill.

CLINICAL CASE STUDY 1*

Ethan E. is a 3-year-old white male presenting with his mother, who seeks health care because of Ethan's fever, fatigue, and rash of 3 days duration.

▶ **Subjective**

2 weeks PTA (prior to arrival)—Ethan was playing with child who was subsequently diagnosed as having chickenpox.
3 days PTA—mother reports fever 100° to 101° F and fatigue, irritability. That evening noted "tiny blisters" on chest and back.
1 day PTA—blisters on chest changed to white with scab on top. New eruption of blisters on shoulders, thighs, face. Intense itching and scratching.

▶ **Objective**

Temp 38.0° C (100.4° F), P 110, R 24
Skin: generalized vesiculopustular rash covering face, trunk, upper arms, and thighs. Small vesicles on face, pustules and red-honey–colored crusts on trunk. Otherwise skin is warm and dry, turgor good.
Ears: tympanic membranes pearl-gray with landmarks intact. No discharge.
Mouth and throat: mucosa dark pink, no lesions. Tonsils 1 +, no exudate. No lymphadenopathy.
Heart: S$_1$, S$_2$ normal, not accentuated or diminished, no murmurs or extra sounds.
Lungs: hyperresonant to percussion. Breath sounds clear, no adventitious sounds.

▶ ASSESSMENT

Varicella
Impaired skin integrity R/T infection and scratching

---

*Please note that space does not allow a detailed plan for each sample clinical problem in this text. Please consult the appropriate text for current treatment plans.

CLINICAL CASE STUDY 2

Myra G. is a 79-year-old widowed, retired college professor, in good health up until recent hospitalization following a fall.

Problem List   1   Fractured right hip—hip pinning   11/24

11/27

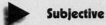

Subjective

Aching pain in left hip (nonoperative side).

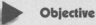

Objective

Erosion 2 × 2 cm with surrounding erythema covering L ischium. Erosion is moist, no active bleeding. Area very warm and tender to touch.

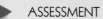

ASSESSMENT

Pressure sore, L hip
Impaired skin integrity R/T immobility and pressure
Pain, acute

NURSING DIAGNOSES COMMONLY ASSOCIATED WITH SKIN, HAIR, AND NAIL DISORDERS

Diagnosis	Related Factors (Etiology)	Defining Characteristics (Symptoms and Signs)

Impaired skin integrity	Altered
	   Nutritional state
	   Oxygen transport
	   Sensation
	Autoimmune dysfunction
	Decreased circulation
	Edema
	Effects of aging, medication
	Infection
	Skeletal prominence
	Excretions/secretions
	Allergy (drugs, foods)
	Chemical substances on skin
	Immobility
	Insect/animal bites
	Pressure
	Radiation
	Restraint
	Stress
	Surgery
		Blisters
		Bruising
		Callus
		Chafing
		Cyanosis
		Disruption of
		   Skin surface
		   Skin layers
		Dryness
		Erythema
		Induration
		Lesions
		Necrosis
		Pallor
		Pruritus

Continued

NURSING DIAGNOSES COMMONLY ASSOCIATED WITH SKIN, HAIR, AND NAIL DISORDERS *Continued*

Diagnosis	Related Factors (Etiology)	Defining Characteristics (Symptoms and Signs)

Self-care deficit: bathing/hygiene	Effects of
	  Aging
	  Trauma
	  Surgery
	  Chronic illness
	Muscular weakness
	Fatigue
	Pain
	Immobility
	Presence of external devices—intravenous lines, casts, traction
	Visual impairment
	Stiffness
	Depression
	Knowledge deficit
	Lack of motivation
	Perceptual or cognitive impairment
	Confusion
	Grieving
		Dirt or stains on body
		Requests help in bathing
		Body odor
		Halitosis
		Inability to wash body or body parts

Fluid volume deficit	Loss of body fluids or electrolytes
	Diaphoresis
	Diarrhea
	Increased insensible water loss
	Nausea and/or vomiting
	Excessive drainage through artificial orifices or lumens, wounds, or drainage tubes
	Diuretic therapy
	Exposure to extreme heat
	Excessive use of alcohol, enemas, or laxatives
		Concentrated urine, blood
		Decreased
		  Blood pressure
		  Skin turgor
		  Urine output
		Dry skin
		Dry mucous membranes
		Increased
		  Body temperature
		  Pulse rate
		Thirst
		Sudden weight loss

Other Related Nursing Diagnoses

ACTUAL	RISK/WELLNESS
Body image disturbance Ineffective thermoregulation Knowledge deficit Pain Self-esteem disturbance	**Risk** Risk for infection Risk for impaired skin integrity Risk for trauma **Wellness** Enhanced health-seeking behavior R/T request for information on skin self-exam

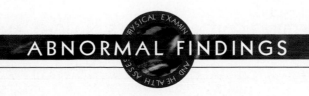

ABNORMAL FINDINGS

Table 10–2 DETECTING COLOR CHANGES IN LIGHT AND DARK SKIN

Etiology	Note Appearance	
	Light Skin	Dark Skin
Pallor		
Anemia—decreased hematocrit Shock—decreased perfusion, vasoconstriction	Generalized pallor	Brown skin appears yellow-brown, dull; black skin appears ashen gray, dull; skin loses its healthy glow—check areas with least pigmentation, such as conjunctivae, mucous membranes
Local arterial insufficiency	Marked localized pallor, e.g., lower extremities, especially when elevated	Ashen gray, dull; cool to palpation
Albinism—total absence of pigment melanin throughout the integument	Whitish pink	Tan, cream, white
Vitiligo—patchy depigmentation from destruction of melanocytes	Patchy milky white spots, often symmetric bilaterally	Same
Cyanosis		
Increased amount of unoxygenated hemoglobin Central—chronic heart and lung disease cause arterial desaturation Peripheral—exposure to cold, anxiety	Dusky blue Nail beds dusky	Dark but dull, lifeless; only severe cyanosis is apparent in skin—check conjunctiva, oral mucosa, nail beds
Erythema		
Hyperemia—increased blood flow through engorged arterioles, such as in inflammation, fever, alcohol intake, blushing	Red, bright pink	Purplish tinge, but difficult to see; palpate for increased warmth with inflammation, taut skin, and hardening of deep tissues
Polycythemia—increased red blood cells, capillary stasis	Ruddy blue in face, oral mucosa, conjunctiva, hands and feet	Well concealed by pigment—check for redness in lips

Continued

Table 10–2 DETECTING COLOR CHANGES IN LIGHT AND DARK SKIN *Continued*

	Note Appearance	
Etiology	**Light Skin**	**Dark Skin**
Erythema *Continued*		
Carbon monoxide poisoning	Bright cherry red in face and upper torso	Cherry red color in nail beds, lips, and oral mucosa
Venous stasis—decreased blood flow from area, engorged venules	Dusky rubor of dependent extremities; a prelude to necrosis with pressure sore	Easily masked; use palpation for warmth or edema
Jaundice		
Increased serum bilirubin, over 2 to 3 mg/100 ml due to liver inflammation or hemolytic disease such as after severe burns, some infections	Yellow in sclera, hard palate, mucous membranes, then over skin	Check sclera for yellow near limbus; do not mistake normal yellowish fatty deposits in the periphery under the eyelids for jaundice—jaundice best noted in junction of hard and soft palate and also palms
Carotenemia—increased serum carotene from ingestion of large amounts of carotene-rich foods	Yellow-orange in forehead, palms and soles, nasolabial folds, but no yellowing in sclera or mucous membranes	Yellow-orange tinge in palms and soles
Uremia—renal failure causes retained uro-chrome pigments in the blood	Orange-green or gray overlying pallor of anemia; may also have ecchymoses and purpura	Easily masked; rely on laboratory and clinical findings
Brown-Tan		
Addison's disease—cortisol deficiency stimulates increased melanin production	Bronzed appearance, an "eternal tan," most apparent around nipples, perineum, genitalia, and pressure points (inner thighs, buttocks, elbow, axillae)	Easily masked; rely on lab and clinical findings
Café au lait spots—due to increased melanin pigment in basal cell layer	Tan to light brown, irregularly shaped, oval patch with well-defined borders	

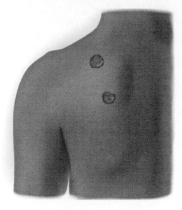

ANNULAR, or circular, begins in center and spreads to periphery, e.g., tinea corporis or ringworm, tinea versicolor, pityriasis rosea.

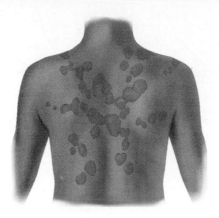

CONFLUENT, lesions run together, e.g., urticaria (hives).

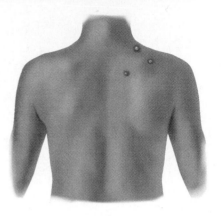

DISCRETE, distinct, individual lesions that remain separate, e.g., molluscum.

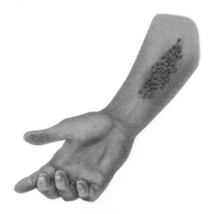

GROUPED, clusters of lesions, e.g., vesicles of contact dermatitis.

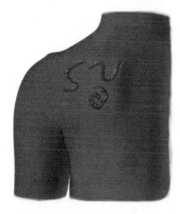

GYRATE, twisted, coiled spiral, snakelike.

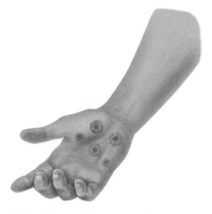

TARGET, or iris, resembles iris of eye, concentric rings of color in the lesions, e.g., erythema multiforme.

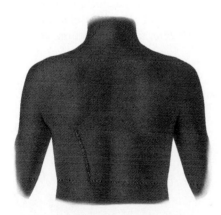

LINEAR, a scratch, streak, line, or stripe.

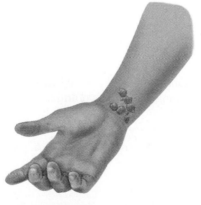

POLYCYCLIC, annular lesions grow together, e.g., lichen planus, psoriasis.

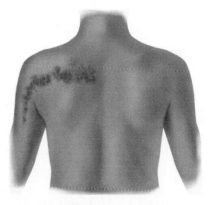

ZOSTERIFORM, linear arrangement along a nerve route, e.g., herpes zoster.

▼ Table 10–4   PRIMARY SKIN LESIONS*

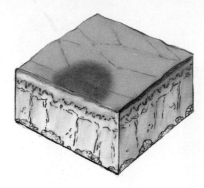

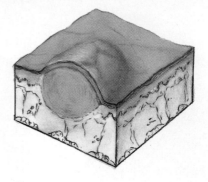

Macule

Solely a color change, flat and circumscribed, of less than 1 cm. Examples: freckles, flat nevi, hypopigmentation, petechiae, measles, scarlet fever.

Patch

Macules that are larger than 1 cm. Examples: mongolian spot, vitiligo, café au lait spot, chloasma, measles rash.

Papule

Something you can feel, i.e., solid, elevated, circumscribed, less than 1 cm diameter, due to superficial thickening in the epidermis. Examples: elevated nevus (mole), lichen planus, molluscum, wart (verruca).

Plaque

Papules coalesce to form surface elevation wider than 1 cm. A plateaulike, disc-shaped lesion. Examples: psoriasis, lichen planus.

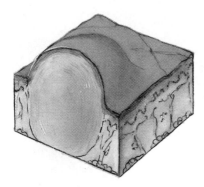

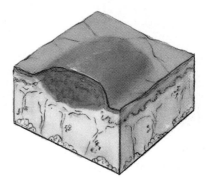

Nodule

Solid, elevated, hard or soft, larger than 1 cm. May extend deeper into dermis than papule. Examples: xanthoma, fibroma, intradermal nevi.

Tumor

Larger than a few centimeters in diameter, firm or soft, deeper into dermis; may be benign or malignant, although "tumor" implies "cancer" to most people. Examples: lipoma, hemangioma.

Wheal

Superficial, raised, transient, and erythematous; slightly irregular shape due to edema (fluid held diffusely in the tissues). Examples: mosquito bite, allergic reaction, dermographism.

Urticaria (Hives)

Wheals coalesce to form extensive reaction, intensely pruritic.

*The immediate result of a specific causative factor; primary lesions develop on previously unaltered skin.

Table 10—4   PRIMARY SKIN LESIONS* Continued

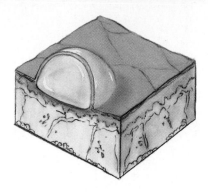

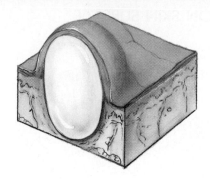

Vesicle

Elevated cavity containing free fluid, up to 1 cm. Clear serum flows if wall is ruptured. Examples: herpes simplex, early varicella (chickenpox), herpes zoster (shingles), contact dermatitis.

Cyst

Encapsulated, fluid-filled cavity in dermis or subcutaneous layer, tensely elevating skin. Examples: sebaceous cyst, wen.

Bulla

Larger than 1 cm diameter; usually single chambered (unilocular); superficial in epidermis; it is thin walled, so it ruptures easily. Examples: friction blister, pemphigus, burns, contact dermatitis.

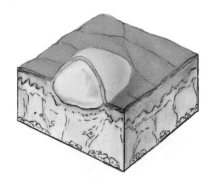

Pustule

Turbid fluid (pus) in the cavity. Circumscribed and elevated. Examples: impetigo, acne.

▼ Table 10–5   SECONDARY SKIN LESIONS*

DEBRIS ON SKIN SURFACE

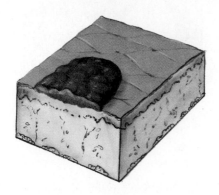

Crust

The thickened, dried-out exudate left when vesicles/pustules burst or dry up. Color can be red-brown, honey, or yellow, depending on the fluid's ingredients (blood, serum, pus). Examples: impetigo (dry, honey-colored), weeping eczematous dermatitis, scab following abrasion.

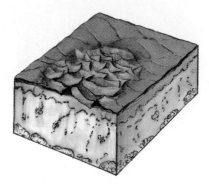

Scale

Compact, desiccated flakes of skin, dry or greasy, silvery or white, from shedding of dead excess keratin cells. Examples: following scarlet fever or drug reaction (laminated sheets), psoriasis (silver, micalike), seborrheic dermatitis (yellow, greasy), eczema, ichthyosis (large, adherent, laminated), dry skin.

BREAK IN CONTINUITY OF SURFACE

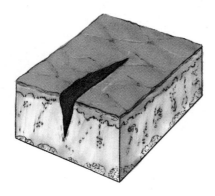

Fissure

Linear crack with abrupt edges, extends into dermis, dry or moist. Examples: cheilosis—at corners of mouth due to excess moisture; athlete's foot.

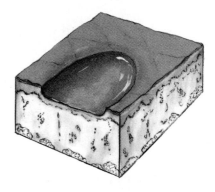

Erosion

Scooped out but shallow depression. Superficial; epidermis lost; moist but no bleeding; heals without scar because erosion does not extend into dermis.

---

*Resulting from a change in a primary lesion due to the passage of time; an evolutionary change.

Note: Combinations of primary and secondary lesions may coexist in the same person. Such combined designations may be termed papulosquamous, maculopapular, vesiculopustular, or papulovesicular.

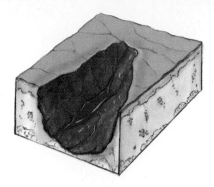

Ulcer

Deeper depression extending into dermis, irregular shape; may bleed; leaves scar when heals. Examples: stasis ulcer, pressure sore, chancre.

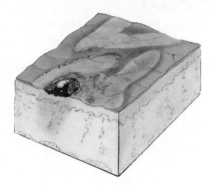

Excoriation

Self-inflicted abrasion; superficial; sometimes crusted; scratches from intense itching. Examples: insect bites, scabies, dermatitis, varicella.

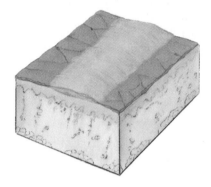

Scar

After a skin lesion is repaired, normal tissue is lost and replaced with connective tissue (collagen). This is a permanent fibrotic change. Examples: healed area of surgery or injury, acne.

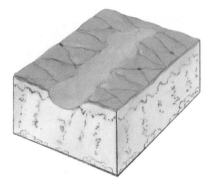

Atrophic Scar

Resulting skin level depressed with loss of tissue; a thinning of the epidermis. Example: striae.

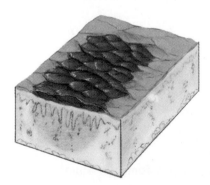

Lichenification

Prolonged intense scratching eventually thickens the skin and produces tightly packed sets of papules; looks like surface of moss (or lichen).

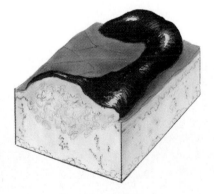

Keloid

A hypertrophic scar. The resulting skin level is elevated by excess scar tissue, which is invasive beyond the site of original injury. May increase long after healing occurs. Looks smooth, rubbery, "clawlike," and has a higher incidence among blacks.

▼ Table 10–6 VASCULAR LESIONS

HEMANGIOMAS

Due to a benign proliferation of blood vessels in the dermis.

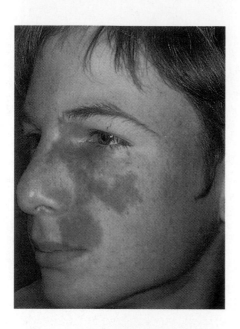

◀ **Port-Wine Stain (Nevus Flammeus)**

A large, flat macular patch covering the scalp or face, frequently along the distribution of cranial nerve V. The color is dark red, bluish, or purplish and intensifies with crying, exertion, or exposure to heat or cold. The marking consists of mature capillaries. It is present at birth and usually does not fade. The use of yellow light lasers now makes photoablation of the lesion possible, with minimal adverse effects.

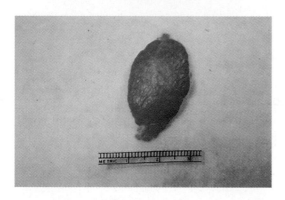

◀ **Strawberry Mark (Immature Hemangioma)**

A raised bright red area with well-defined borders about 2 to 3 cm in diameter. It does not blanch with pressure. It consists of immature capillaries, is present at birth or develops in the first few months, and usually disappears by age 5 to 7. Requires no treatment, although parental and peer pressure may prompt treatment.

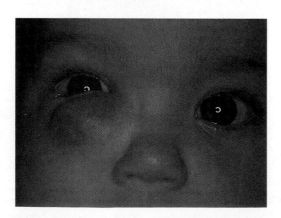

◀ **Cavernous Hemangioma (Mature)**

A reddish-blue, irregularly shaped, solid and spongy mass of blood vessels. It may be present at birth, may enlarge during the first 10 to 15 months, and will not involute spontaneously.

TELANGIECTASES

Due to vascular dilatation; permanently enlarged and dilated blood vessels that are visible on the skin surface. Examples are

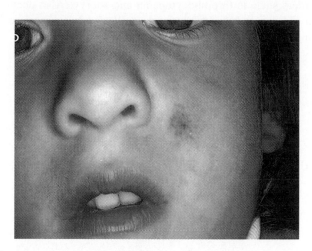

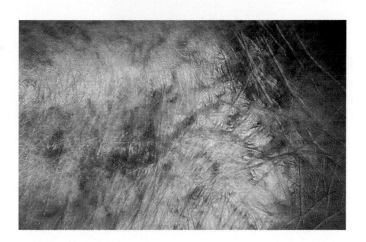

Spider or Star Angioma

A fiery red, star-shaped marking with a solid circular center. Capillary radiations extend from the central arterial body. With pressure, note a central pulsating body and blanching of extended legs. Develops on face, neck, or chest; may be associated with pregnancy, chronic liver disease, or estrogen therapy, or may be normal.

Venous Lake

A blue-purple dilatation of venules and capillaries in a star-shaped, linear, or flaring pattern. Pressure causes them to empty or disappear. Located on the legs near varicose veins and also on the face, lips, ears, and chest.

PURPURIC LESIONS

Due to blood flowing out of breaks in the vessels. Red blood cells and blood pigments are deposited in the tissues (extravascular). Difficult to see in dark-skinned people.

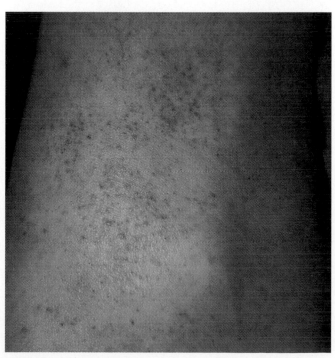

◀ Petechiae

Tiny punctate hemorrhages, less than 2 mm, round and discrete, dark red, purple, or brown in color. Due to bleeding from superficial capillaries; will not blanch. May indicate abnormal clotting factors. In dark-skinned people petechiae are best visualized in the areas of lighter melanization, such as the abdomen, buttocks, and volar surface of the forearm. When the skin is black or very dark brown, petechiae cannot be seen in the skin. Most of the diseases that cause bleeding and microembolism formation, such as thrombocytopenia, subacute bacterial endocarditis, and other septicemias, are characterized by the presence of petechiae in the mucous membranes as well as on the skin. Thus, you should inspect for petechiae in the mouth, particularly the buccal mucosa, and in the conjunctiva.

Table continued on following page

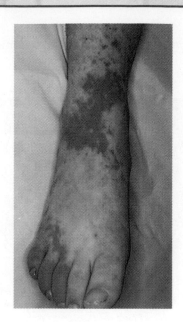

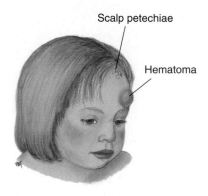

Purpura

Confluent and extensive patch of petechiae and ecchymoses, flat macular hemorrhage. Seen in generalized disorders such as thrombocytopenia and scurvy. Also occurs in old age as blood leaks from capillaries in response to minor trauma and diffuses through dermis.

Scalp petechiae

Hematoma

LESIONS DUE TO TRAUMA OR ABUSE

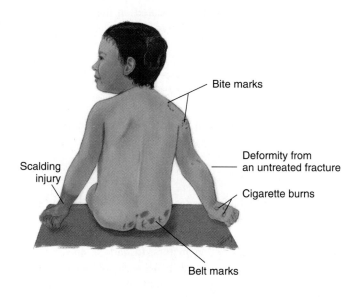

Bite marks

Deformity from
an untreated fracture

Cigarette burns

Scalding
injury

Belt marks

Hematoma

A hematoma is a bruise you can feel. It elevates the skin and is seen as swelling. Multiple petechiae and purpura may occur on the face when prolonged vigorous crying or coughing raises venous pressure.

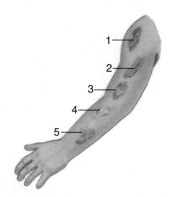

1
2
3
4
5

Pattern Injury

Pattern injury is a bruise or wound whose shape suggests the instrument or weapon that caused it, e.g., belt buckle, broomstick, burning cigarette, pinch marks, bite marks, or scalding hot liquid. Inflicted scalding-water immersion burns usually have a clear border, like a glove or sock, indicating body part was held under water intentionally. Deformity results from an untreated fracture because the bone heals out of alignment.

These physical signs suggest child abuse, together with a history that does not match the severity or type of injury, and indicates impaired or dysfunctional parent-child relationship.

Ecchymosis (Bruise)

A large patch of capillary bleeding into tissues. Color in light-skinned person is first 1—red-blue or purple immediately after or within 24 hours of trauma, 2—blue to purple (1 to 5 days), 3—green (5 to 7 days), 4—yellow (7 to 10 days), 5—brown to disappearing (10 to 14 days). A recent bruise in dark-skinned person is deep dark purple. Pressure on a bruise will *not* cause it to blanch. A bruise usually occurs from trauma; also from bleeding disorders and liver dysfunction.

Table 10–7 COMMON SKIN LESIONS IN CHILDREN

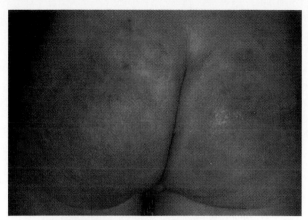

Diaper Dermatitis

Red, moist maculopapular patch with poorly defined borders in diaper area, extending along inguinal and gluteal folds. History of infrequent diaper changes or occlusive coverings. Inflammatory disease due to skin irritation from ammonia, heat, moisture, occlusive diapers.

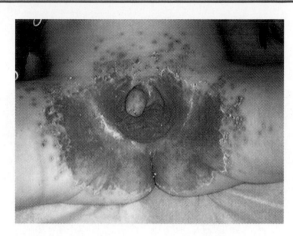

Intertrigo (Candidiasis)

Scalding red, moist patches with sharply demarcated borders, some loose scales. Usually in genital area extending along inguinal and gluteal folds. Aggravated by urine, feces, heat, moisture, the *Candida* fungus infects the superficial skin layers.

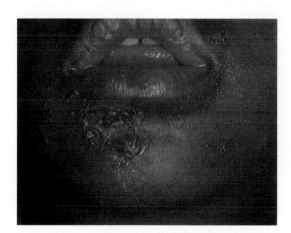

Impetigo

Moist, thin-roofed vesicles with thin erythematous base. Rupture to form thick honey-colored crusts. Contagious bacterial infection of skin; most common in infants and children.

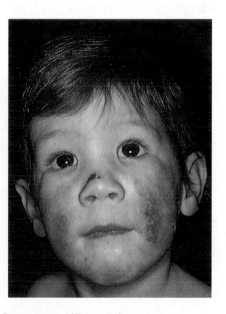

Atopic Dermatitis (Eczema)

Erythematous papules and vesicles, with weeping, oozing, and crusts. Lesions usually on scalp, forehead, cheeks, forearms and wrists, elbows, backs of knees. Paroxysmal and severe pruritus. Family history of allergies.

Table continued on following page

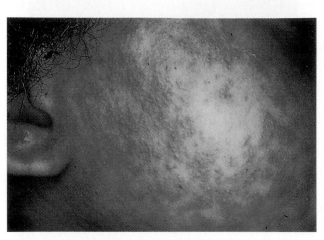

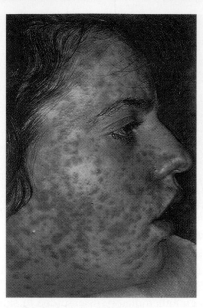

Measles (Rubeola) in Dark Skin

Measles (Rubeola) in Light Skin

Red-purple maculopapular blotchy rash in dark skin (on left) and in light skin (on right) appears on 3rd or 4th day of illness. Rash appears first behind ears and spreads over face, then over neck, trunk, arms, and legs; looks "coppery" and does not blanch. Also characterized by Koplik's spots in mouth—bluish white, red-based elevations of 1 to 3 mm.

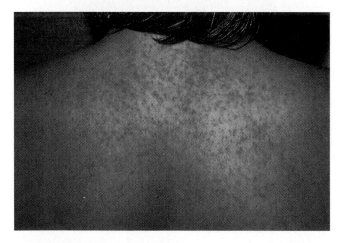

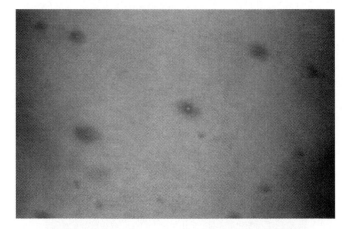

German Measles (Rubella)

Pink papular rash (similar to measles but paler) first appears on face, then spreads. Distinguished from measles by presence of neck lymphadenopathy and absence of Koplik's spots.

Chickenpox (Varicella)

Small tight vesicles first appear on trunk, then spread to face, arms, and legs (not palms or soles). Shiny vesicles on an erythematous base are commonly described as the "dewdrop on a rose petal." Vesicles erupt in succeeding crops over several days, then become pustules, and then crusts. Intensely pruritic.

Table 10-8 COMMON SKIN LESIONS

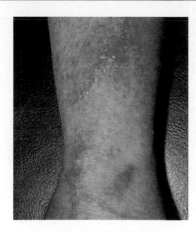

Primary Contact Dermatitis

Local inflammatory reaction to an irritant in the environment or an allergy. Characteristic location of lesions often gives clue. Often erythema shows first, followed by swelling, wheals (or urticaria), or maculopapular vesicles, scales. Frequently accompanied by intense pruritus. Example here: poison ivy.

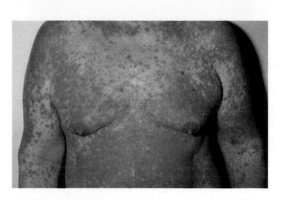

Allergic Drug Reaction

Erythematous and symmetric rash, usually generalized. Some drugs produce urticarial rash or vesicles and bullae. History of drug ingestion.

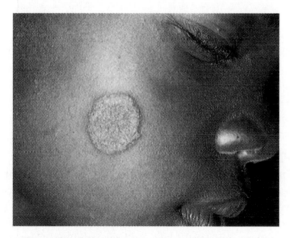

Tinea Corporis (Ringworm of the Body)

Scales—hyperpigmented in whites, depigmented in dark-skinned persons—on chest, abdomen, back of arms, forming multiple circular lesions with clear centers.

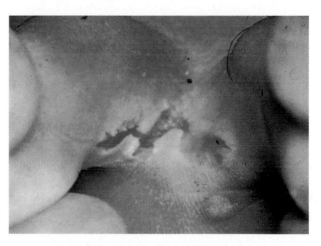

Tinea Pedis (Ringworm of the Foot)

"Athlete's foot," a fungal infection, first appears as small vesicles between toes, sides of feet, soles. Then grows scaly and hard. Found in chronically warm moist feet: children after gymnasium activities, athletes, aging adults who cannot dry their feet well.

Table continued on following page

Table 10–8   COMMON SKIN LESIONS *Continued*

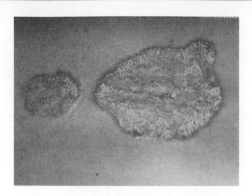

Psoriasis

Scaly erythematous patch, with silvery scales on top. Usually on scalp, outside of elbows and knees, low back, and anogenital area.

Tinea Versicolor

Fine, scaling, round patches of pink, tan, or white (hence the name), which do not tan in sunlight, due to a superficial fungal infection. Usual distribution is on neck, trunk, and upper arms—a short-sleeved turtleneck sweater area. Most common in otherwise healthy young adults.

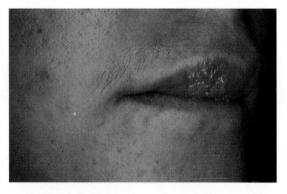

Labial Herpes Simplex (Cold Sores)

Herpes simplex virus (HSV) infection has a prodrome of skin tingling and sensitivity. Then, lesion erupts with tight vesicles followed by pustules, and then produces acute gingivostomatitis with many shallow, painful ulcers. Common location is upper lip, also in oral mucosa and tongue.

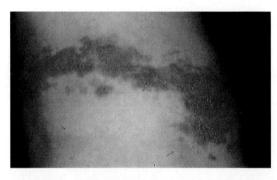

Herpes Zoster (Shingles)

Small grouped vesicles emerge along route of cutaneous sensory nerve, then pustules, then crusts. Caused by the varicella zoster virus (VZV), a reactivation of the dormant virus of chickenpox. Acute appearance, practically always unilateral, does not cross midline. Commonly on trunk, can be anywhere. If on ophthalmic branch of cranial nerve V, it poses risk to eye. Most common in adults over 50. Pain is often severe and long lasting in aging adults, called postherpetic neuralgia.

Table 10–9 MALIGNANT SKIN LESIONS

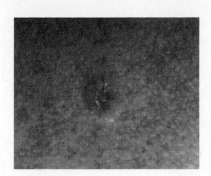

Basal Cell Carcinoma

Usually starts as a skin-colored papule (may be deeply pigmented) with a translucent top and overlying telangiectasia. Then develops rounded pearly borders with central red ulcer, or looks like large open pore with central yellowing. Most common form of skin cancer; slow but inexorable growth.

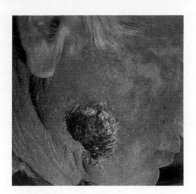

Squamous Cell Carcinoma

Erythematous scaly patch with sharp margins, 1 cm or more. Develops central ulcer and surrounding erythema. Usually on hands or head, areas exposed to solar radiation. Less common than basal cell carcinoma but grows rapidly.

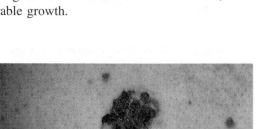

Malignant Melanoma

Half of these lesions arise from pre-existing nevi. Usually brown, can be tan, black, pink-red, purple, or mixed pigmentation. Often irregular or notched borders. May have scaling, flaking, oozing texture. Common locations are on the trunk and back in men and women, on the legs in women, and on the palms, soles of feet, and the nails in blacks.

Table 10–10   SKIN LESIONS ASSOCIATED WITH AIDS

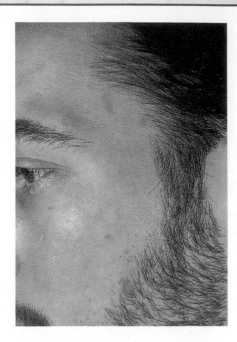

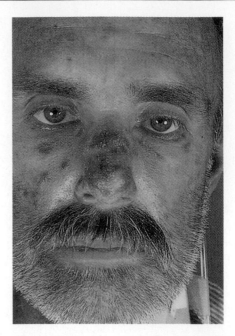

Epidemic Kaposi's Sarcoma. Patch Stage.

An aggressive form of Kaposi's sarcoma is one of the diseases that characterize the epidemic AIDS. Here, multiple patch-stage early lesions are faint pink on the temple and beard area. They easily could be mistaken for bruises or nevi and be ignored.

Epidemic Kaposi's Sarcoma. Advanced Disease.

Advanced stage, widely disseminated lesions involving skin, mucous membranes, and visceral organs. Here, violet-colored tumors cover the nose and face, and a tiny cherry-red tumor nodule is on the inner canthus of the right eye.

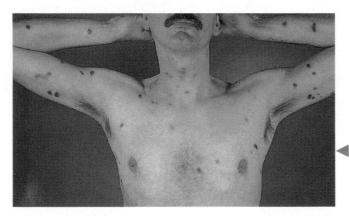

◀ Epidemic Kaposi's Sarcoma. Plaque Stage.

Evolving lesions develop into raised papules or thickened plaques. These are oval in shape and vary in color from red to brown.

ABNORMAL FINDINGS

Table 10–11   ABNORMAL CONDITIONS OF HAIR

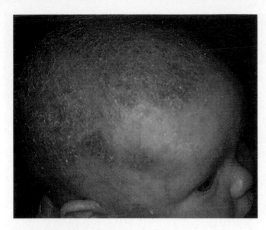

Seborrheic Dermatitis (Cradle Cap)

Thick, yellow to white, greasy, adherent scales with mild erythema on scalp and forehead; very common in early infancy. Resembles eczema lesions except cradle cap is distinguished by absence of pruritus, "greasy" yellow-pink lesions, and negative family history of allergy.

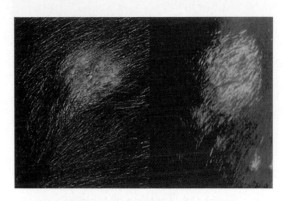

Tinea Capitis (Scalp Ringworm)

Rounded patchy hair loss on scalp, leaving broken-off hairs, pustules, and scales on skin. Due to fungal infection; lesions may fluoresce blue-green under Wood's light. Usually seen in children and farmers; highly contagious, may be transmitted by another person, by domestic animals, or from soil.

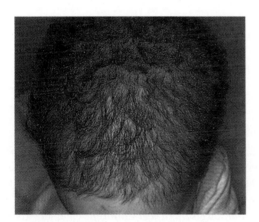

Toxic Alopecia

Patchy, asymmetric balding that accompanies severe illness or use of chemotherapy where growing hairs are lost and resting hairs are spared. Regrowth occurs after illness or discontinuation of toxin.

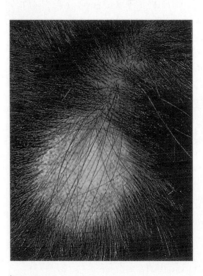

Alopecia Areata

Sudden appearance of a sharply circumscribed, round or oval balding patch, usually with smooth, soft, hairless skin underneath. Unknown cause; when limited to a few patches, person usually has complete regrowth.

Table continued on following page

Table 10–11 ABNORMAL CONDITIONS OF HAIR *Continued*

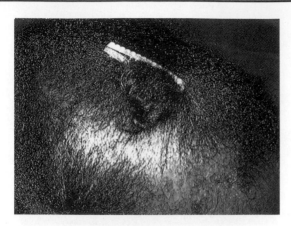

Traumatic Alopecia: Traction Alopecia

Linear or oval patch of hair loss along hair line, a part, or scattered distribution; due to trauma from hair rollers, tight braiding, tight pony tail, barrettes.

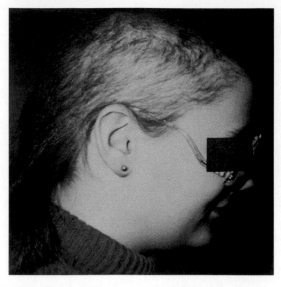

Trichotillomania

Traumatic self-induced hair loss usually due to compulsive twisting or plucking. Forms irregularly shaped patch, with broken-off, stublike hairs of varying lengths; person is never completely bald. Occurs as child rubs or twirls area absently while falling asleep, reading, or watching television. In adults it can be a serious problem and is usually a sign of a personality disorder.

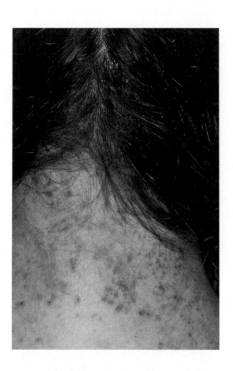

◄ Pediculosis Capitis (Head Lice)

History includes intense itching of the scalp, especially the occiput. The nits (eggs) of lice are easier to see in the occipital area and around the ears, appearing as 2- to 3-mm oval translucent bodies, adherent to the hair shafts. Common among school-age children. Over-the-counter pediculicide shampoos are available; however, nit removal by daily combing of wet hair with a fine-tooth metal comb is especially important.

Table 10–11 ABNORMAL CONDITIONS OF HAIR *Continued*

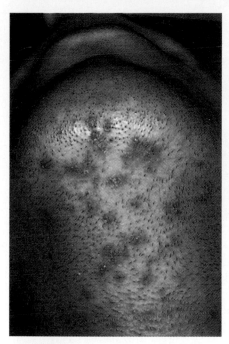

Folliculitis

Superficial infection of hair follicles. Multiple pustules, "whiteheads," with hair visible at center and erythematous base. Usually on arms, legs, face, and buttocks.

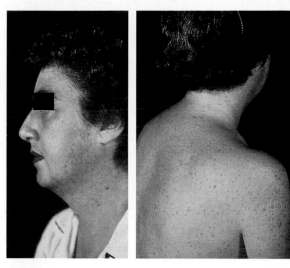

Hirsutism

Excess body hair in females forming a male sexual pattern (upper lip, face, chest, abdomen, arms, legs), due to endocrine or metabolic dysfunction, or occasionally idiopathic.

Furuncle and Abscess ▶

Red, swollen, hard, tender, pus-filled lesion due to acute localized bacterial (usually staphylococcal) infection; usually on back of neck, buttocks, occasionally on wrists or ankles. Furuncles are due to infected hair follicles, whereas abscesses are due to traumatic introduction of bacteria into the skin. Abscesses are usually larger and deeper than furuncles.

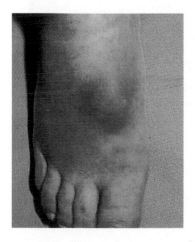

Table 10–12   ABNORMAL CONDITIONS OF THE NAILS

ABNORMAL FINDINGS

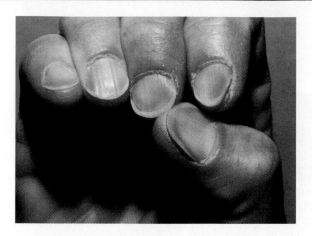

Koilonychia (Spoon Nails)

Thin depressed nails with lateral edges tilted up, forming a concave profile. May be congenital or a hereditary trait, occasionally due to hypochromic anemia.

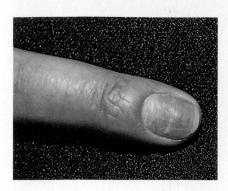

Paronychia

Red, swollen, tender inflammation of the nail folds. Acute paronychia is usually a bacterial infection; chronic paronychia is most often a fungal infection from a break in the cuticle in those who perform "wet" work.

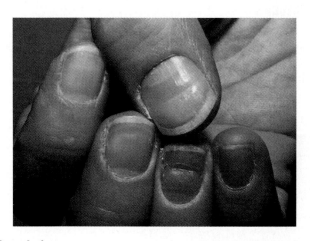

Beau's Line

Transverse furrow or groove. A depression across the nail that extends down to the nail bed. Occurs with any trauma that temporarily impairs nail formation, such as acute illness, toxic reaction, or local trauma. Dent appears first at the cuticle and moves forward as nail grows.

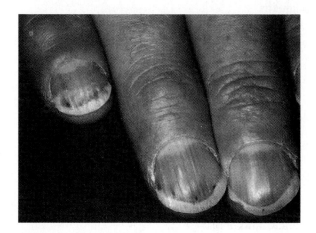

Splinter Hemorrhages

Red-brown linear streaks, embolic lesions, occur with subacute bacterial endocarditis; also may occur with minor trauma.

Table 10–12   ABNORMAL CONDITIONS OF THE NAILS *Continued*

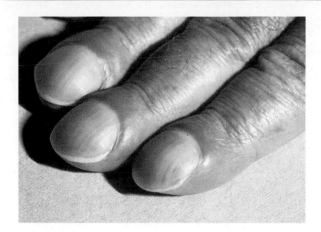

Late Clubbing

Proximal edge of nail elevates, angle is greater than 180 degrees. Distal phalanx looks rounder and wider. Seen with chronic obstructive pulmonary disease and congenital heart disease with cyanosis. Occurs first in thumb and index finger.

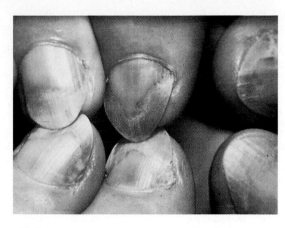

Onycholysis

Loosening of the nail plate, usually beginning at the distal edge and progressing proximally.

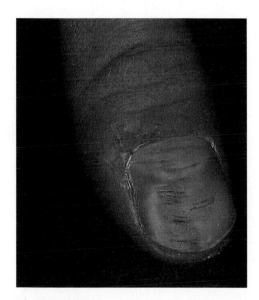

Habit-Tic Dystrophy

Depression down middle of nail or multiple horizontal ridges, due to continuous picking of cuticle by another finger of same hand, which causes injury to nail base and nail matrix.

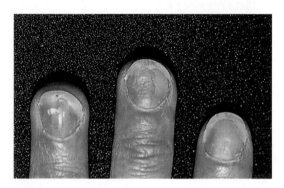

Pitting

Pitting, crumbling of the nails with distal detachment often occurs with psoriasis.

Bibliography

Bjorgen S: Herpes zoster. Am J Nurs 98(2):46–47, Feb 1998.

Chalmers DA: Rosacea: Recognition and management for the primary care provider. Nurs Pract 22(1):18–30, Oct 1997.

Devlin BK, Reynolds E: Child abuse: How to recognize it, how to intervene. Am J Nurs 94(3):26–32, 1994.

Friedman-Kien AE: Color Atlas of AIDS, 2nd ed. Philadelphia, W.B. Saunders Company, 1996.

Galen BA: Acne vulgaris. Primary Care Pract 1(1):88–92, Mar–Apr 1997.

Gallagher J: Management of cutaneous symptoms. Semin Oncol Nurs 11(4):239–247, Nov 1995.

Harkins L: Contact dermatitis. Primary Care Pract 1(1):97–99, Mar–Apr 1997.

Heffernan AE, O'Sullivan A: Pediatric sun exposure. Nurse Pract 23(7):67–86, July 1998.

Hurwitz S: Clinical Pediatric Dermatology, 2nd ed. Philadelphia, W.B. Saunders Company, 1993.

Kosko DA: Dermatologic manifestations of human immunodeficiency virus disease. Primary Care Pract 1(1):50–61, Mar–Apr 1997.

Lawton S: Assessing the skin. Professional Nurse 13(4):S5–S7, 1998.

Levin S: Effect of age, ethnic background and disease on sweat chloride. Isr J Med Sci 2(3):333–337, 1966.

Lobato MN, Vugia DJ, Friedman IJ: Tinea capitis in California children: A population-based study of a growing epidemic. Pediatrics 99(4):551–554, Apr 1997.

Lookingbill DP, Marks JG: Principles of Dermatology, 2nd ed. Philadelphia, W.B. Saunders Company, 1993.

Moore AV: Stopping the spread of scabies. Am J Nurs 97(10):68–69, Oct 1997.

NIH Consensus Development Panel on Melanoma: Diagnosis and treatment of early melanoma. JAMA 268:1314–1319, 1992.

Nowazek V, Neeley MA: Health assessment of the older patient. Crit Care Nurs 19(2):1–6, 1996.

Phillips LP, Caruso ES, Paine LL: Primary care for women: Comprehensive dermatologic assessment. J Nurse Midwifery 40(2):172–186, Mar–Apr 1995.

Pigott KG: Lice and scabies. Primary Care Pract 1(1):93–96, Mar–Apr 1997.

Polednak A: Connective tissue responses in negroes in relation to disease. Am J Physical Anthropol 41:49–55, 1974.

Reifsnider E: Common adult infectious skin conditions. Nurs Pract 22(11):17–33, Nov 1997.

Resnick B: Dermatologic problems in the elderly. Primary Care Pract 1(1):14–31, Mar–Apr 1997.

Schaefer O: Regional sweating in Eskimos compared with Caucasians. Can J Physiol Pharmacol 52(5):960–965, 1974.

Scott CB, Moloney MF: Physical urticaria: A common misdiagnosis. Nurse Pract 21(11):42–61, Nov 1996.

Singleton JK: Pediatric dermatoses: Three common skin disruptions in infancy. Nurse Pract 22(6):32–50, June 1997.

Sinni-McKeehen B: Scaling skin disorders. Primary Care Pract 1(1):3–13, Mar–Apr 1997.

Swinyer T: Recognizing and managing rosacea. Am J Nurs 97(12):16AAA–16DDD, Dec 1997.

Taffe AS: Acne treatment: A comprehensive review of pharmacotherapy. Primary Care Pract 1(1):70–87, Mar–Apr 1997.

Talbot L, Curtis L: The challenges of assessing skin indicators in people of color. Home Healthcare Nurse 14(3):167–171, 1996.

Webb JA, Friedman LC, Bruce SB, Weinberg AD, Cooper P: Demographic, psychosocial, and objective risk factors related to perceived risk of skin cancer. J Cancer Educ 11(3):174–177, 1996.

Weyer D: Skin: A window to the immune system—Recognizing and treating HIV-related lesions. Adv Nurs Pract 5(10):23–31, Oct 1997.

Wysocki AB: A review of the skin and its appendages. Adv Wound Care 8(2):53–70, Mar–Apr 1995.

CHAPTER ELEVEN

Head and Neck, Including Regional Lymphatics

THE HEAD

The **skull** is a rigid bony box that protects the brain and special sense organs, and it includes the bones of the cranium and the face (Fig. 11–1). Note the location of these **cranial bones:** frontal, parietal, occipital, and temporal. Use these names to describe any of your findings in the corresponding areas.

The adjacent cranial bones unite at meshed immovable joints called the **sutures.** The bones are not firmly joined at birth; this allows for the mobility and change in shape needed for the birth process. The sutures gradually ossify during early childhood. The **coronal** suture *crowns* the head from ear to ear at the union of the frontal and parietal bones. The **sagittal** suture *separates* the head lengthwise between the two parietal bones. The **lambdoid** suture separates the parietal bones crosswise from the occipital bone.

The 14 **facial bones** also articulate at sutures (note the nasal bone, zygomatic bone, and maxilla), except for the mandible (the lower jaw). It moves up, down, and sideways from the temporomandibular joint, which is anterior to each ear.

The cranium is supported by the cervical vertebrae: C1, the "atlas"; C2, the "axis"; and down to C7. The C7 vertebra has a long spinous process that is palpable when the head is flexed. Feel this useful landmark, the **vertebra prominens,** on your own neck.

The human **face** has myriad appearances and a large array of facial expressions that reflect mood. The expressions are formed by the facial muscles (Fig. 11–2), which are mediated by cranial nerve VII, the facial nerve. Facial muscle function is symmetric bilaterally, except for an occasional quirk or wry expression.

Facial structures also are symmetric; the eyebrows, eyes, ears, nose, and mouth appear about the same on both sides. The palpebral fissures, the openings between the eyelids, are equal bilaterally. Also, the nasolabial folds, the creases extending from the nose to each corner of the mouth, should look symmetric. Facial sensations of pain or touch are mediated by the three sensory branches of cranial nerve V, the trigeminal nerve. (Testing for

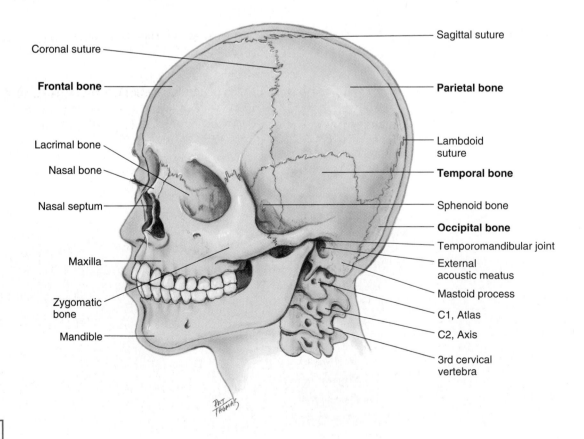

Coronal suture

Frontal bone

Lacrimal bone

Nasal bone

Nasal septum

Maxilla

Zygomatic bone

Mandible

Sagittal suture

Parietal bone

Lambdoid suture

Temporal bone

Sphenoid bone

Occipital bone

Temporomandibular joint

External acoustic meatus

Mastoid process

C1, Atlas

C2, Axis

3rd cervical vertebra

11–1

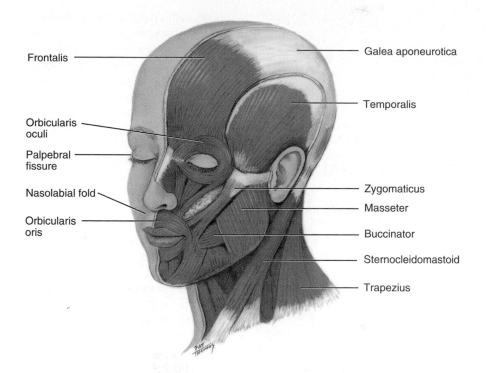

Frontalis

Galea aponeurotica

Temporalis

Orbicularis oculi

Palpebral fissure

Nasolabial fold

Orbicularis oris

Zygomaticus

Masseter

Buccinator

Sternocleidomastoid

Trapezius

11-2

Facial muscles

sensory function is described in Chapter 21, Neurologic System.)

Two pairs of **salivary glands** are accessible to examination on the face (Fig. 11-3). The **parotid** glands are in the cheeks over the mandible, anterior to and below the ear. They are the largest of the salivary glands but are not normally palpable. The **submandibular** glands are beneath the mandible at the angle of the jaw. A third pair, the **sublingual** glands, lie in the floor of the mouth. (Salivary gland function follows in Chapter 14.) The **temporal artery** lies superior to the temporalis muscle, and its pulsation is palpable anterior to the ear.

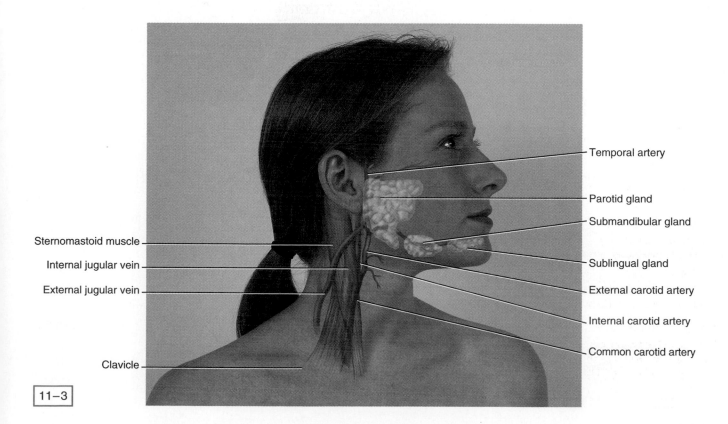

Temporal artery

Parotid gland

Submandibular gland

Sublingual gland

External carotid artery

Internal carotid artery

Common carotid artery

Sternomastoid muscle

Internal jugular vein

External jugular vein

Clavicle

11-3

THE NECK

The **neck** is delimited by the base of the skull and inferior border of the mandible above, and by the manubrium sterni, the clavicle, the first rib, and the first thoracic vertebra below. Think of the neck as a *conduit* for the passage of many structures, which are lying in close proximity: vessels, muscles, nerves, lymphatics, and viscera of the respiratory and digestive systems. Blood vessels include the common and internal carotid arteries and their associated veins. The internal carotid branches off the common carotid, and runs inward and upward to supply the brain; the external carotid supplies the face, salivary glands, and superficial temporal area. The carotid artery and internal jugular vein lie beneath the sternomastoid muscle. The external jugular vein runs diagonally across the sternomastoid muscle. (Assessment of the neck vessels is discussed in Chapter 17.)

The major **neck muscles** are the **sternomastoid** and the **trapezius** (Fig. 11–4); they are innervated by cranial nerve XI, the spinal accessory. The sternomastoid muscle arises from the sternum and the medial part of the clavicle and extends diagonally across the neck to the mastoid process behind the ear. It accomplishes head rotation and head flexion. The two trapezius muscles form a trapezoid shape on the upper back. Each arises from the occipital bone and the vertebrae and extends fanning out to the scapula and clavicle. The trapezius muscles move the shoulders and extend and turn the head.

The sternomastoid muscle divides each side of the neck into two triangles. In front of the sternomastoid, the **anterior triangle** lies between the sternomastoid and the midline of the body, with its base up along the lower border of the mandible and its apex down at the suprasternal notch. The **posterior triangle** is behind the sternomastoid muscle, with the trapezius muscle on the other side and with its base along the clavicle below. It contains the posterior belly of the omohyoid muscle. These triangles are helpful guidelines when describing findings in the neck.

The **thyroid gland** is an important endocrine gland with a rich blood supply. It straddles the trachea in the middle of the neck (Fig. 11–5). This highly vascular endocrine gland synthesizes and secretes thyroxine (T_4) and triiodothyronine (T_3), hormones that stimulate the rate of cellular metabolism. The gland has two lobes, both conical in shape, each curving posteriorly between the trachea and the sternomastoid muscle. The lobes are connected in the middle by a thin isthmus lying over the second and third tracheal rings. (Sometimes a third lobe, the pyramidal lobe, is present. It is cone shaped, usually on the left, and extends up toward the hyoid bone from the isthmus or from the neighboring lobe.)

Just above the thyroid isthmus, within about 1 cm, is the **cricoid** cartilage or upper tracheal ring. The **thyroid** cartilage is above that, with a small palpable notch in its upper edge. This is the prominent "Adam's apple" in males. And the highest is the **hyoid** bone, palpated high in the neck at the level of the floor of the mouth.

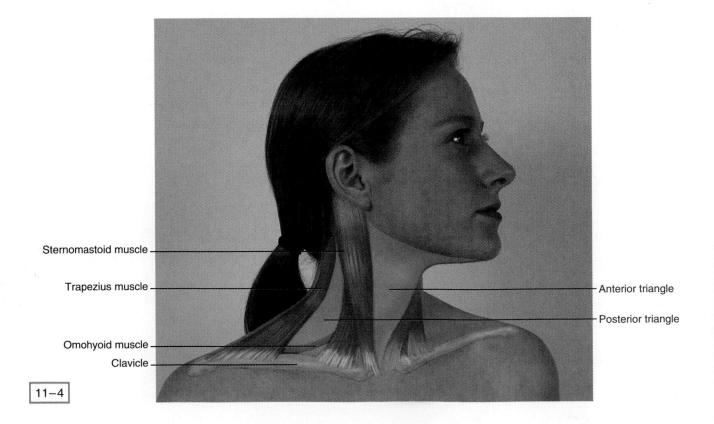

Sternomastoid muscle

Trapezius muscle

Omohyoid muscle

Clavicle

Anterior triangle

Posterior triangle

11–4

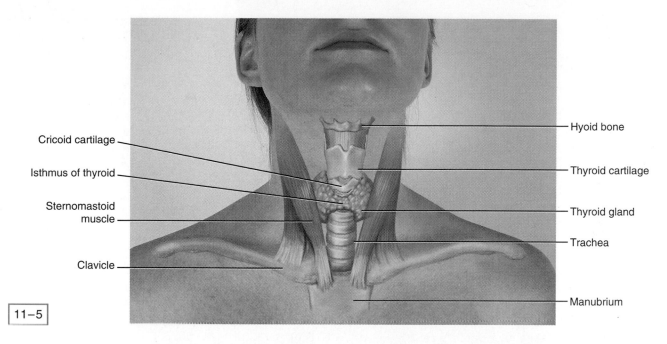

Cricoid cartilage

Isthmus of thyroid

Sternomastoid muscle

Clavicle

Hyoid bone

Thyroid cartilage

Thyroid gland

Trachea

Manubrium

11–5

LYMPHATICS

The head and neck have a rich supply of **lymph nodes** (Fig. 11–6). Although sources differ as to their nomenclature, one commonly used system is given here. Note that their labels correspond to adjacent structures.

- Preauricular, in front of the ear
- Posterior auricular (mastoid), superficial to the mastoid process

- Occipital, at the base of the skull
- Submental, midline, behind the tip of the mandible
- Submandibular, halfway between the angle and the tip of the mandible
- Jugulodigastric, under the angle of the mandible
- Superficial cervical, overlying the sternomastoid muscle
- Deep cervical, deep under the sternomastoid muscle
- Posterior cervical, in the posterior triangle along the edge of the trapezius muscle
- Supraclavicular, just above and behind the clavicle, at the sternomastoid muscle

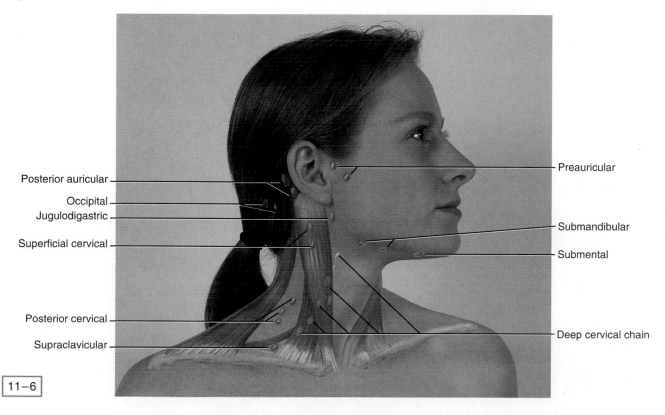

Posterior auricular

Occipital

Jugulodigastric

Superficial cervical

Posterior cervical

Supraclavicular

Preauricular

Submandibular

Submental

Deep cervical chain

11–6

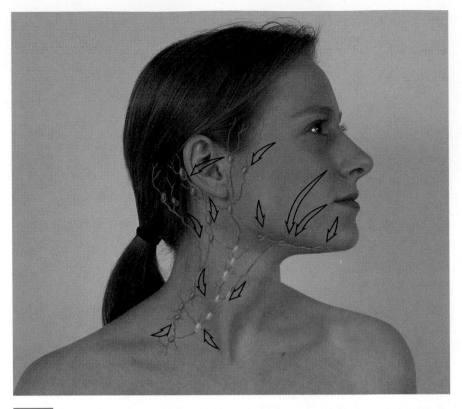

11-7

You also should be familiar with the direction of the drainage patterns of the lymph nodes (Fig. 11–7). When nodes are abnormal, check the area they drain for the source of the problem. Explore the area proximal (upstream) to the location of the abnormal node.

The lymphatic system is an extensive vessel system, which is separate from the cardiovascular system and is phylogenetically older. It is described in full in Chapter 18. The lymphatics are a major part of the immune system, whose job it is to detect and eliminate foreign substances from the body. The vessels allow the flow of clear, watery fluid (lymph) from the tissue spaces into the circulation. Lymph nodes are set at intervals along the lymph vessels like beads on a string. The nodes are small

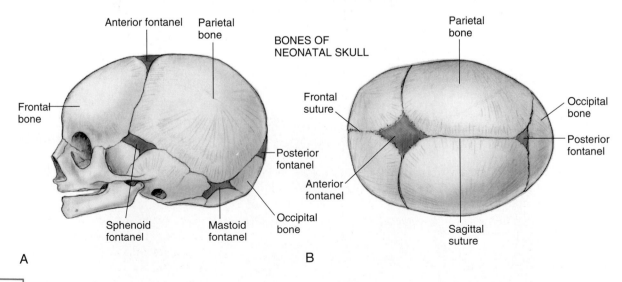

11-8

oval clusters of lymphatic tissue. They filter the lymph and engulf pathogens, preventing potentially harmful substances from entering the circulation. Nodes are located throughout the body but are accessible to examination only in four areas: head and neck, arms, axillae, and inguinal region. The greatest supply is in the head and neck.

DEVELOPMENTAL CONSIDERATIONS

Infants and Children

The bones of the neonatal skull are separated by sutures and by **fontanels,** the spaces where the sutures intersect (Fig. 11–8). These membrane-covered "soft spots" allow for growth of the brain during the 1st year. They gradually ossify; the triangle-shaped posterior fontanel is closed by 1 to 2 months, and the diamond-shaped anterior fontanel closes between 9 months and 2 years.

During the fetal period, head growth predominates. Head size is greater than chest circumference at birth. The head size grows during childhood, reaching 90 percent of its final size when the child is 6 years old. But during infancy, trunk growth predominates so that head size changes in proportion to body height. Facial bones grow at varying rates, especially nasal and jaw bones. In the toddler, the mandible and maxilla are small and the

nasal bridge is low, so that the whole face seems small compared with the skull.

Lymphoid tissue is well developed at birth and grows to adult size when the child is 6 years old. The child's lymphatic tissue continues to grow rapidly until age 10 or 11, actually exceeding its adult size before puberty. Then the lymphatic tissue slowly atrophies.

The appearance of acne in adolescence was discussed in the previous chapter. Facial hair also appears on boys at this time—first on the upper lip, then on cheeks and lower lip, last on the chin. A noticeable enlargement of the thyroid cartilage occurs and with it, the voice deepens.

The Pregnant Female

The thyroid gland enlarges slightly during pregnancy owing to hyperplasia of the tissue and increased vascularity.

The Aging Adult

The facial bones and orbits appear more prominent, and the facial skin sags owing to decreased elasticity, decreased subcutaneous fat, and decreased moisture in the skin. The lower face may look smaller if teeth have been lost.

SUBJECTIVE DATA

1. Headache
2. Head injury
3. Dizziness

4. Neck pain, limitation of motion
5. Lumps or swelling
6. History of head or neck surgery

Examiner Asks	Rationale
1 Headache. Any *unusually frequent* or *unusually severe* **headaches?** • Onset. When did *this kind* of headache start? • Gradual, over hours, or a day? • Or, suddenly, over minutes, or less than 1 hour? • Ever had *this kind* of headache before?	This is a more meaningful question than "Do you ever have headaches?" because most people have had at least one headache. Since many conditions have a headache as a symptom, a detailed history is important. A red flag is a severe headache in an adult or child who has never had it before.

Examiner Asks	Rationale
• Location. Where do you feel it: frontal, temporal, behind your eyes, like a band around the head, in the sinus area, or in the occipital area?	Tension headaches tend to be occipital or frontal or with bandlike tightness; migraines (vascular) tend to be supraorbital, retroorbital, or frontotemporal; cluster headaches (vascular) produce pain around the eye, temple, forehead, and cheek.
• Is pain localized on one side, or all over?	Unilateral or bilateral, e.g., with cluster headaches pain is always unilateral and always on the same side of the head.
• Character. Throbbing (pounding, shooting) or aching (viselike, constant pressure, dull)?	Character is typically viselike with tension headache, throbbing with migraine or temporal arteritis.
• Is it mild, moderate, or severe?	Quantity is often severe with migraine, or excruciating with cluster headache.
• Course and duration. What time of day do the headaches occur: morning, evening, awaken you from sleep? How long do they last? Hours, days? Have you noted any daily headaches, or several within a time period?	Migraines occur about two per month, each lasting 1 to 3 days; one to two cluster headaches occur per day, each lasting ½ to 2 hours for 1 or 2 months, then complete remission may last for months or years.
• Precipitating factors. What brings it on: activity or exercise, work environment, emotional upset, anxiety, alcohol? (Also note signs of depression.)	Alcohol ingestion and daytime napping typically precipitate cluster headaches, whereas alcohol, letdown after stress, menstruation, and eating chocolate or cheese precipitate migraines.
• Associated factors. Any relation to other symptoms: any nausea and vomiting? (Note which came first, headache or nausea.) Any vision changes, pain with bright lights, neck pain or stiffness, fever, weakness, moodiness, stomach problems?	Nausea, vomiting, and visual disturbances are associated with migraines; eye reddening and tearing, eyelid drooping, rhinorrhea, and nasal congestion are associated with cluster headaches; anxiety and stress are associated with tension headaches; nuchal rigidity and fever are associated with the headache of meningitis or encephalitis.
• Do you have any other illness?	Hypertension, fever, hypothyroidism, and vasculitis produce headaches.
• Do you take any medications?	Oral contraceptives, bronchodilators, alcohol, nitrates, as well as carbon monoxide inhalation, produce headaches.
• What makes it worse: movement, coughing, straining, exercise? • Pattern. Any family history of headache? What is the frequency of your headaches: once a week? Are your headaches occurring closer together? Are they getting worse? Or are they getting better? (For females) When do they occur in relation to your menstrual periods?	Migraines are associated with family history of migraine.
• Effort to treat. What seems to help: going to sleep, medications, positions, rubbing the area?	With migraines, people lie down to feel better, whereas with cluster headaches they need to move—even to pace the floor—to feel better.
• Coping strategies. How have these headaches affected your self-care, or your ability to function at work, home, and socially?	

Examiner Asks	Rationale

2 **Head injury.** Any **head injury** or blow to your head?
- Onset. When? Please describe exactly what happened.
- Setting: any hazardous conditions? Were you wearing a helmet or hard hat?
- How about yourself just before injury: dizzy, lightheaded, had a blackout, had a seizure?
  Lose consciousness and then fall? (Note which came first.)
  Knocked unconscious? Or did you fall and lose consciousness a few minutes later?

Loss of consciousness *before* a fall may have a cardiovascular cause, e.g., heart block.

- Any history of illness, e.g., heart trouble, diabetes, epilepsy?
- Location. Exactly where did you hit your head?
- Duration. How long were you unconscious?
  Any symptoms afterward—headache, vomiting, projectile vomiting?
  Any change in level of consciousness since injury: dazed or sleepy?

A change in the level of consciousness is of prime importance in evaluating a neurologic deficit.

- Associated symptoms. Any pain in the head or the neck, vision change, discharge from ear or nose—is it bloody or watery? Are you able to move all extremities? Any tremors, staggered walk, numbness and tingling?
- Pattern. Symptoms become worse, better, unchanged since injury?
- Effort to treat. Emergency department or hospitalized? Any medications?

3 **Dizziness.** Experienced any **dizziness?**
   (Determine exactly what the person means by dizziness.) Was it a feeling of lightheadedness or of falling? Or was it a spinning sensation?

Dizziness is a lightheaded, swimming sensation or a feeling of falling. True *vertigo* is true rotational spinning owing to neurologic dysfunction (labyrinthine-vestibular apparatus, vestibular nuclei in brain stem).
   When vertigo is *objective,* the perception is that the room spins. When vertigo is *subjective,* the perception is that the person spins.

- Onset. Abrupt or gradual? After a change in position, such as sudden standing?
- Associated factors. Any nausea and vomiting, pallor, immobility, decreased hearing acuity, or tinnitus along with the dizziness?

4 **Neck pain.** Any **neck pain?**
- Onset. How did the pain start: injury, automobile accident, after lifting, from a fall? Or with fever? Or did it have a gradual onset?

Acute onset of stiffness along with headache and fever occurs with meningeal inflammation.

- Location. Does pain radiate? To the shoulders, arms?
- Associated symptoms. Any **limitations to range of motion,** numbness or tingling in shoulders, arms, or hands?
- Precipitating factors. What movements cause pain? Do you need to lift or bend at work or home?
  Does stress seem to bring it on?

Pain creates a vicious circle. Tension increases pain and disability, which produces more anxiety.

- Coping strategies. Able to do your work, to sleep?

Examiner Asks	Rationale

⑤ Lumps or swelling. Any **lumps or swelling** in the neck? Any recent infection? Any tenderness?

Tenderness usually indicates acute infection.

For a lump that persists, how long have you had it? Has it changed in size?

A persistent lump should arouse suspicion of malignancy. For persons over 40 years, suspect malignancy until proven otherwise.

● Any history of prior irradiation of head, neck, upper chest?

Increased risk for salivary and thyroid tumors.

● Any difficulty swallowing?

Dysphagia.

● Do you smoke? For how long? How many packs a day? Do you chew tobacco?

Smoking and chewing tobacco increase risk of oral and respiratory cancer.

● When was your last alcohol drink? How much alcohol do you drink a day?

Smoking and large alcohol consumption together increase the risk of cancer.

● Ever had a thyroid problem? Overfunctioning or underfunctioning? How was it treated: surgery, irradiation, any medication?

⑥ History of head or neck surgery. Ever had surgery of the head or neck? For what condition? When did the surgery occur? How do you feel about results?

Surgery for head and neck cancer often is disfiguring and increases risk of body image disturbance.

ADDITIONAL HISTORY FOR INFANTS AND CHILDREN

① Did the mother use alcohol or street drugs during pregnancy? How often? How much was used per episode?

Alcohol increases the risk of fetal alcohol syndrome, which has distinctive facial features (see Table 11–3). Cocaine use causes neurologic, developmental, and emotional problems.

② Was delivery vaginal or by cesarean section? Any difficulty? Use of forceps?

Forceps may increase the risk of caput succedaneum, cephalhematoma, and Bell's palsy.

③ What were you told about the baby's growth? Was it on schedule? Did the head seem to grow and fontanels close on schedule? At what age (in months) did the baby achieve head control?

ADDITIONAL HISTORY FOR THE AGING ADULT

① If dizziness is a problem, how does this affect your daily activities? Are you able to drive safely, maneuver about the house safely?

Assess self-care. Assess potential for injury.

② If neck pain is a problem, how does this affect your daily activities? Are you able to drive, perform at work, do housework, sleep, look down when using stairs?

THE HEAD

Inspect and palpate the skull
Size and Shape

Note the general size and shape. *Normocephalic* is the term that denotes a round symmetric skull that is appropriately related to body size. Be aware that "normal" includes a wide range of sizes.

To assess shape, place your fingers in the person's hair and palpate the scalp. The skull normally feels symmetric and smooth. The cranial bones that have normal protrusions are the forehead, the lateral edge of each parietal bone, the occipital bone, and the mastoid process behind each ear. There is no tenderness to palpation.

Temporal Area

Palpate the temporal artery above the zygomatic (cheek) bone between the eye and top of the ear.

The temporomandibular joint is just below the temporal artery and anterior to the tragus. Palpate the joint as the person opens the mouth, and note normally smooth movement with no limitation or tenderness.

Inspect the face
Facial Structures

Inspect the face, noting the facial expression and its appropriateness to behavior or reported mood. Anxiety is common in the hospitalized or ill person.

Although the shape of facial structures may vary somewhat among races, they always should be symmetric. Note symmetry of eyebrows, palpebral fissures, nasolabial folds, and sides of the mouth.

Note any abnormal facial structures (coarse facial features, exophthalmos, changes in skin color or pigmentation), or any abnormal swelling. Also note any involuntary movements (tics) in the facial muscles. Normally none occur.

Abnormal Findings column:

Deformities include microcephaly, abnormally small head; macrocephaly, abnormally large head, e.g., hydrocephaly; and acromegaly, Paget's disease, see Table 11–1, p. 290.

Note lumps, depressions, or abnormal protrusions.

The artery looks more tortuous and feels hardened and tender with temporal arteritis.

Crepitation, limited range of motion, or tenderness.

Hostility or embarrassment.
Tense, rigid muscles may indicate anxiety or pain; a flat affect may indicate depression; excessive smiling may be inappropriate.

Marked asymmetry with central brain lesion (e.g., brain attack or cerebrovascular accident) or with peripheral cranial nerve VII damage (Bell's palsy). See Table 11–5.

Edema in the face is noted first around the eyes (periorbital) and the cheeks where the subcutaneous tissue is relatively loose.
Note grinding of jaws, tics, fasciculations, or excessive blinking.

Normal Range of Findings   **Abnormal Findings**

THE NECK

Inspect and palpate the neck
Symmetry

Head position is centered in the midline, and the accessory neck muscles should be symmetric. The head should be held erect and still.

> Head tilt occurs with muscle spasm.
> Rigid head and neck occur with arthritis.

Range of Motion (ROM)

Note any limitation of movement during active motion. Ask the person to touch the chin to the chest, turn the head to the right and left, try to touch each ear to the shoulder (without elevating shoulders), and to extend the head backward. When the neck is supple, motion is smooth and controlled.

> Note pain at any particular movement.
> Note ratchety movement or limitation of movement that may be due to cervical arthritis or inflammation of neck muscles. With arthritis, the neck is rigid and the person turns at the shoulders rather than the neck.

Test muscle strength and the status of cranial nerve XI by trying to resist the person's movements with your hands as the person shrugs the shoulders and turns the head to each side.

As the person moves the head, note enlargement of the salivary glands and lymph glands. Normally no enlargement is present. Note a swollen parotid gland when the head is extended; look for swelling below the angle of the jaw. Also, note thyroid gland enlargement. Normally none is present.

> Thyroid enlargement may be a unilateral lump, or it may be diffuse and look like a doughnut lying across the lower neck (see Table 11–2).

Also note any obvious pulsations. The carotid artery runs medial to the sternomastoid muscle, and it creates a brisk localized pulsation just below the angle of the jaw. Normally, there are no other pulsations while the person is in the sitting position (see Chapter 17, Heart and Neck Vessels).

Lymph Nodes

Using a gentle circular motion of your fingerpads, palpate the lymph nodes (Fig. 11–9). (Normally, the salivary glands are not palpable. When symptoms warrant, check for parotid tenderness by palpating in a line from the outer corner of the eye to the lobule of the ear.) Beginning with the preauricular lymph nodes in front of the ear, palpate the 10 groups of lymph nodes in a routine order. Many nodes are closely packed, so you must be systematic and thorough in your examination. Once you establish your sequence, do not vary or you may miss some small nodes.

> The parotid is swollen with mumps (see Table 11–2).
> Parotid enlargement has been found with AIDS.

▶ Normal Range of Findings   Abnormal Findings

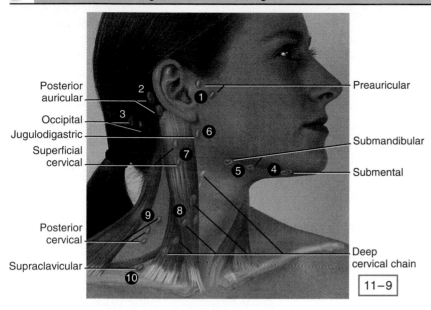

Posterior auricular
Occipital
Jugulodigastric
Superficial cervical
Posterior cervical
Supraclavicular

Preauricular
Submandibular
Submental
Deep cervical chain

11–9

Use gentle pressure because strong pressure could push the nodes into the neck muscles. It is usually most efficient to palpate with both hands, comparing the two sides symmetrically. However, the submental gland under the tip of the chin is easier to explore with one hand. When you palpate with one hand, use your other hand to position the person's head. For the deep cervical chain, tip the person's head toward the side being examined to relax the ipsilateral muscle (Fig. 11–10). Then you can press your fingers under the muscle. Search for the supraclavicular node by having the person hunch the shoulders and elbows forward (Fig. 11–11); this relaxes the skin. The inferior belly of the omohyoid muscle crosses the posterior triangle here; do not mistake it for a lymph node.

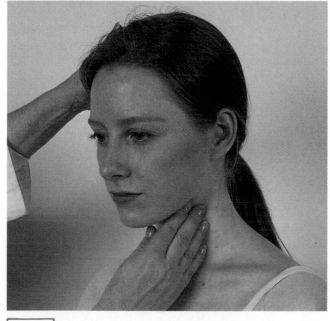

11–10

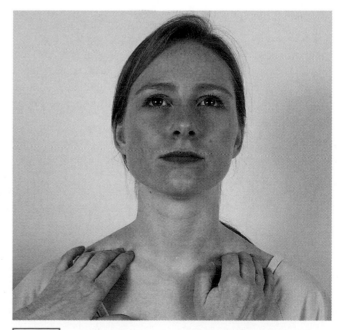

11–11

▶

If any nodes are palpable, note their location, size, shape, delimitation (discrete or matted together), mobility, consistency, and tenderness. Cervical nodes often are palpable in healthy persons, although this palpability decreases with age (Fig. 11–12). Normal nodes feel movable, discrete, soft, and nontender.

Lymphadenopathy is enlargement of the lymph nodes (> 1 cm) due to infection, allergy, or neoplasm.

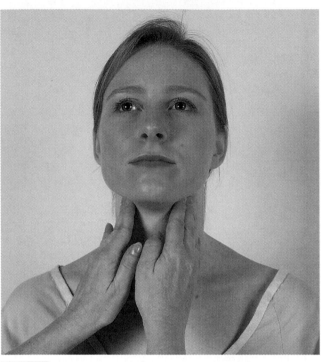

11–12

If nodes are enlarged or tender, check the area they drain for the source of the problem. For example, those in the upper cervical or submandibular area often relate to inflammation or a neoplasm in the head and neck. Follow up on or refer your findings. An enlarged lymph node, particularly when you cannot find the source of the problem, deserves prompt attention.

The following criteria are common clues but are not definitive in all circumstances.

- Acute infection—nodes are bilateral, enlarged, warm, tender, and firm but freely movable.
- Chronic inflammation, e.g., in tuberculosis the nodes are clumped.
- Cancerous nodes are hard, unilateral, nontender, and fixed.
- Nodes with HIV infection are enlarged, firm, nontender, and mobile. Occipital node enlargement is common with HIV infection.

▶ | Normal Range of Findings | Abnormal Findings |

- A single, enlarged, nontender, hard, left supraclavicular node (Virchow's node) may indicate a neoplasm in the thorax or abdomen.
- Painless, rubbery, discrete nodes that gradually appear occur with Hodgkin's lymphoma.

Trachea

Normally, the trachea is midline; palpate for any tracheal shift. Place your index finger on the trachea in the sternal notch, and slip it off to each side (Fig. 11–13). The space should be symmetric on both sides. Note any deviation from the midline.

Conditions of tracheal shift:

- The trachea is *pushed to the unaffected* (or healthy) side with an aortic aneurysm, a tumor, unilateral thyroid lobe enlargement, and pneumothorax.
- The trachea is *pulled toward the affected* (diseased) side with large atelectasis, pleural adhesions, or fibrosis.
- Tracheal tug is a rhythmic downward pull that is synchronous with systole and that occurs with aortic arch aneurysm.

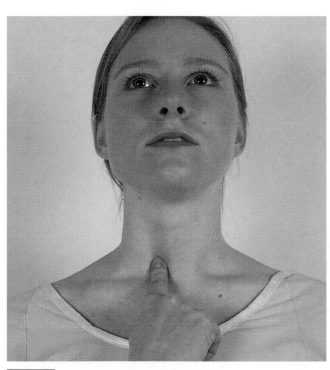

11–13

Thyroid Gland

The thyroid gland is difficult to palpate; arrange your setting to maximize your likelihood of success. Position a standing lamp to shine tangentially across the neck to highlight any possible swelling. Supply the person with a glass of water, and first inspect the neck as the person takes a sip and swallows. Thyroid tissue moves up with a swallow.

Look for diffuse enlargement or a nodular lump.

Posterior Approach. To palpate, move behind the person (Fig. 11–14). Ask the person to sit up very straight and then to bend the head slightly forward and to the right. This will relax the neck muscles. Use the fingers of your left hand to push the trachea slightly to the right.

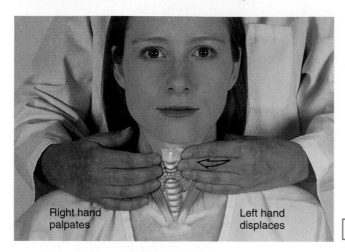

Right hand palpates   Left hand displaces   11–14

Then curve your right fingers between the trachea and the sternomastoid muscle, retracting it slightly, and ask the person to take a sip of water. The thyroid moves up under your fingers with the trachea and larynx as the person swallows. Reverse the procedure for the left side.

Usually you cannot palpate the normal adult thyroid. If the person has a long, thin neck, you sometimes will feel the isthmus over the tracheal rings. The lateral lobes usually are not palpable; check them for enlargement, consistency, symmetry, and the presence of nodules.

Abnormalities include enlarged lobes that are easily palpated before swallowing, or are tender to palpation, or the presence of nodules or lumps. See Table 11–2.

Anterior Approach. This is an alternate method of palpating the thyroid, but it is more awkward to perform, especially for a beginning examiner. Stand facing the person. Ask him or her to tip the head forward and to the right. Use your right thumb to displace the trachea slightly to the person's right. Hook your left thumb and fingers around the sternomastoid muscle. Feel for lobe enlargement as the person swallows (Fig. 11–15).

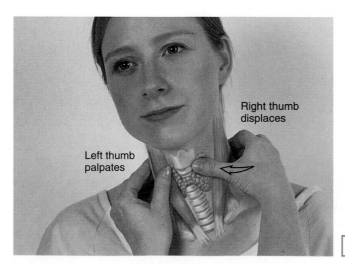

Left thumb palpates   Right thumb displaces   11–15

| Normal Range of Findings | Abnormal Findings

Auscultate the Thyroid

If the thyroid gland is enlarged, auscultate it for the presence of a **bruit.** This is a soft, pulsatile, whooshing, blowing sound heard best with the bell of the stethoscope. The bruit is not present normally.

 DEVELOPMENTAL CONSIDERATIONS

Infants and Children

Skull

Measure an infant's **head size** with measuring tape at each visit up to age 2, then yearly up to age 6. (Measurement of head circumference is presented in detail in Chapter 9.)

The newborn's head measures about 32 to 38 cm (average around 34 cm), and is 2 cm larger than chest circumference. At age 2, both measurements are the same. During childhood, the chest circumference grows to exceed head circumference by 5 to 7 cm.

Observe the infant's head from all angles, not just the front. The contour should be symmetric. Some racial variation occurs in normal head shapes; Nordic children tend to have long heads, and Asian children have broad heads.

Two common variations in the newborn cause the shape of the skull to look markedly asymmetric: A **caput succedaneum** is edematous swelling and ecchymosis of the presenting part of the head due to birth trauma (Fig. 11–16). It feels soft, and it may extend across suture lines. It gradually resolves during the first few days of life and needs no treatment.

Abnormal Findings

A bruit occurs with accelerated or turbulent blood flow, indicating hyperplasia of the thyroid, e.g., hyperthyroidism.

Note an abnormal increase in head size or failure to grow.

Microcephalic—head circumference below norms for age.

Macrocephalic—an enlarged head for age, or rapidly increasing in size. This may be due to hydrocephalus (increased cerebrospinal fluid).

Frontal bulges, or "bossing," occur with prematurity, rickets, or congenital syphilis.

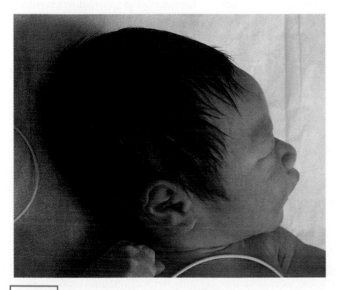

11–16

Caput succedaneum

A **cephalhematoma** is a subperiosteal hemorrhage, which is also a result of birth trauma (Fig. 11–17). It is soft, fluctuant, and well defined over one cranial bone because the periosteum (i.e., the covering over each bone) holds the bleeding in place. It appears several hours after birth and gradually increases in size. No discoloration is present, but it looks bizarre, so parents need reassurance that it will be reabsorbed during the first few weeks of life without treatment. Rarely, a large hematoma may persist to 3 months.

An infant with cephalhematoma is at greater risk for jaundice as the red blood cells within the hematoma are broken down and reabsorbed.

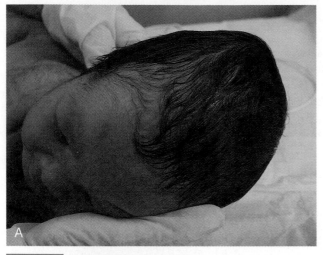

11–17A   **Cephalhematoma**

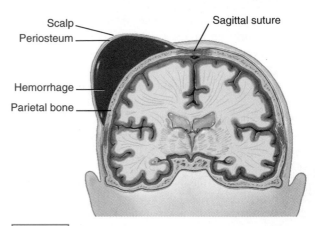

Scalp
Periosteum
Sagittal suture
Hemorrhage
Parietal bone

11–17B

As you palpate the newborn's head, the suture lines feel like ridges. By 5 to 6 months, they are smooth and not palpable.

A newborn's head may feel asymmetric and the involved ridges more prominent due to *molding* of the cranial bones during engagement and passage through the birth canal. Molding is overriding of the cranial bones; usually, the parietal bone overrides the frontal or occipital bone. Reassure parents that this lasts only a few days or a week. Babies delivered by cesarean section are noted for their evenly round heads. Also, some asymmetry may occur if an infant continually sleeps in one position; this is a flattening of the dependent cranial bone, usually the occiput.

Gently palpate the skull and **fontanels** while the infant is calm and somewhat in a sitting position (crying, lying down, or vomiting may cause the anterior fontanel to look full and bulging). The skull should feel smooth and fused except at the fontanels. The fontanels feel firm, slightly concave, and well defined against the edges of the cranial bones. You may see slight arterial pulsations in the anterior fontanel.

The posterior fontanel may not be palpable at birth. If it is, it measures 1 cm and closes by 1 to 2 months. The anterior fontanel may be small at birth and enlarge to 2.5 cm by 2.5 cm. A large diameter of 4 to 5 cm occasionally may be normal under 6 months. A small fontanel usually is normal. The anterior fontanel closes between 9 months and 2 years. Early closure may be insignificant if head growth proceeds normally.

Sutures palpable when the child is older than 6 months.

Marked asymmetry, as in *craniosynostosis,* a severe deformity due to premature closure of the sutures, is abnormal. See Table 11–1.

Flattening also occurs with rickets or mental retardation.

A true tense or bulging fontanel occurs with acute increased intracranial pressure.
Depressed and sunken fontanels occur with dehydration or malnutrition.
Marked pulsations occur with increased intracranial pressure.

Delayed closure or larger-than-normal fontanel size occurs with hydrocephalus, Down syndrome, hypothyroidism, or rickets.

Normal Range of Findings	Abnormal Findings

<table>
<tr><td>

Note the infant's **head posture** and **head control.** The infant can turn the head side to side by 2 weeks and shows the **tonic neck reflex** when supine and the head is turned to one side (extension of same arm and leg, flexion of opposite arm and leg). The tonic neck reflex disappears between 3 and 4 months, and then the head is maintained in the midline. Head control is achieved by 4 months, when the baby can hold the head erect and steady when pulled to a vertical position. (See Chapter 20, Musculoskeletal System, and Chapter 21, Neurologic System, for further details.)

</td><td>

A small fontanel is a sign of microcephaly, as is early closure.

Tonic neck reflex lasting longer than 5 months indicates brain damage.

In children, head tilt occurs with habit spasm, poor vision, and brain tumor.

Head lag after 4 months is significant; it may indicate mental or motor retardation.

</td></tr>
</table>

Face

Check **facial features** for symmetry, appearance, and presence of swelling. Note symmetry of wrinkling when the infant cries or smiles, e.g., both sides of the lips rise and both sides of forehead wrinkle. Children love to comply when you ask them to "make a face." Normally, no swelling is evident. Parotid gland enlargement is seen best when the child sits and looks up at the ceiling; the swelling appears below the angle of the jaw.

Unilateral immobility indicates nerve damage (central or peripheral), e.g., note angle of mouth droop on paralyzed side.

Some facies are characteristic of congenital abnormalities or of chronic allergy. See Tables 11–3 and 11–4.

Neck

An infant's neck looks short; it lengthens during the first 3 to 4 years. You can see the neck better by supporting the infant's shoulders and tilting the head back a little. This positioning also enhances palpation of the trachea, which is buried deep in the neck. Feel for the row of cartilaginous rings in the midline or just slightly to the right of midline.

Assess muscle development with gentle passive ROM. Cradle the infant's head with your hands and turn it side to side and test forward flexion, extension, and rotation. Note any resistance to movement, especially flexion. Ask a child to actively move through the ROM, as you would an adult.

A short neck or webbing (loose fanlike folds) may indicate a congenital abnormality, such as Down or Turner syndrome, or it may occur alone.

Head tilt and limited ROM occur with torticollis (wryneck), or from sternomastoid muscle injury during birth or a congenital defect.

Resistance to flexion (nuchal rigidity) and pain on flexion indicate meningeal irritation or meningitis.

During infancy, cervical lymph nodes are not palpable normally. But a child's lymph nodes are—they feel more prominent than an adult's until after puberty when lymphoid tissue begins to atrophy. Palpable nodes less than 3 mm are normal. They may be up to 1 cm in size in the cervical and inguinal areas but are discrete, move easily, and are nontender. Children have a higher incidence of infection, so you will expect a greater incidence of inflammatory adenopathy. No other mass should occur in the neck.

Cervical nodes larger than 1 cm are considered enlarged.

Thyroglossal duct cyst—cystic lump high up in midline, freely movable, and rises up when swallowing.

Supraclavicular nodes enlarge with Hodgkin's disease.

The thyroid gland is difficult to palpate in an infant due to the short, thick neck. The child's thyroid may be palpable normally.

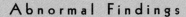

▶ | Normal Range of Findings | Abnormal Findings

Special Procedures

Palpation. *Craniotabes* is a softening of the skull's outer layer. With a newborn, pressure along the suture of the parietal and occipital bones above the ear produces a snapping sensation due to the pliable skull bone. It is like indenting a ping pong ball and feeling it snap back. Do not attempt this unless craniotabes is suspected because of other abnormal findings, and even then avoid excessive pressure. Craniotabes may be normal, especially with premature infants.

Craniotabes may occur with rickets, hydrocephaly, or congenital syphilis.

Percussion. With an infant, you may directly percuss with your plexor finger against the head surface. This yields a resonant or "cracked pot" sound, which is normal before closure of the fontanels.

The sound occurs with hydrocephalus due to separation of cranial sutures (Macewen's sign).

Auscultation. Bruits are common in the skull in children under 4 or 5 years of age or in children with anemia. They are systolic or continuous and are heard over the temporal area.

After 5 years of age, bruits indicate increased intracranial pressure, aneurysm, or arteriovenous shunt.

Transillumination. Use this procedure if you suspect an abnormal head size or an intracranial lesion. In a completely darkened room, hold a rubber-collared flashlight firmly against the infant's skull. You need a tight fit against the head. Explore all regions of the head: frontal, both sides, occiput (Fig. 11–18). A small ring of light around the flashlight is normal (less than 2 cm in the frontal area, less than 1 cm in the occipital area). But you should not see a larger halo around the rubber collar.

Presence of a halo of light through the skull indicates a loss or thinning of cerebral cortex. If the cortex is absent, the entire cranium lights up (Fig. 11–19).

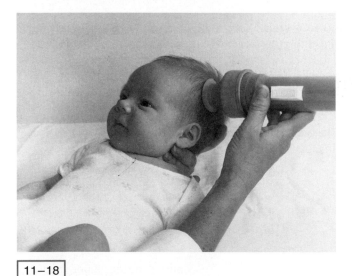

11–18

11–19

Hydranencephaly

The Pregnant Female

During the second trimester, chloasma may show on the face. This is a blotchy, hyperpigmented area over the cheeks and forehead that fades after delivery. The thyroid gland may be palpable normally during pregnancy.

Normal Range of Findings	Abnormal Findings

The Aging Adult

The temporal arteries may look twisted and prominent. In some aging adults, a mild rhythmic tremor of the head may be normal. *Senile tremors* are benign and include head nodding (as if saying yes or no) and tongue protrusion. If some teeth have been lost, the lower face looks unusually small, with the mouth sunken in.

The neck may show an increased cervical concave curve when the head and jaw are extended forward to compensate for kyphosis of the spine. During the examination, direct the aging person to perform ROM slowly; he or she may experience dizziness with side movements. An aging person may have prolapse of the submandibular glands, which could be mistaken for a tumor. But drooping submandibular glands will feel soft and be present bilaterally.

SUMMARY CHECKLIST: Head and Neck, Including Regional Lymphatics Exam

1: Inspect and palpate the skull
General size and contour
Note any deformities, lumps, tenderness
Palpate temporal artery, temporomandibular joint

2: Inspect the face
Facial expression
Symmetry of movement (cranial nerve VII)
Any involuntary movements, edema, lesions

3: Inspect and palpate the neck
Active ROM
Enlargement of salivary glands, lymph nodes, thyroid gland
Position of the trachea
4: Auscultate the thyroid (if enlarged) for bruit

APPLICATION AND CRITICAL THINKING

SAMPLE CHARTING

Subjective
Denies any unusually frequent or severe headache; no history of head injury, dizziness, or syncope; no neck pain, limitation of motion, lumps, or swelling.

Objective
Head. Normocephalic, no lumps, no lesions, no tenderness.
Face. Symmetric, no drooping, no weakness, no involuntary movements.
Neck. Supple with full ROM, no pain. Symmetric, no lymphadenopathy or masses. Trachea midline, thyroid not palpable. No bruits.

Continued

CLINICAL CASE STUDY 1

Frank V. is a 57-year-old insurance executive who is in his 4th postoperative day after a transurethral resection of the prostate gland. He also has chronic hypertension, managed by oral hydrochlorothiazide, exercise, and a low-salt diet.

 Subjective

Complaining of dizziness, a lightheaded feeling that occurred on standing and cleared on sitting. No previous episodes of dizziness. Denies palpitations, nausea, or vomiting. States urine pink tinged as it was yesterday with no red blood. No pain meds today. On 2nd day of same antihypertensive medication he took before surgery.

 Objective

BP 142/88 RA sitting, 94/58 RA standing. Pulse 94 sitting and standing, regular rhythm, no skipped beats. Temp 37° C. Color tannish-pink, no pallor, skin warm and dry. Neuro: alert and oriented to person, place, and time. Speech clear and fluent. Moving all extremities, no weakness. No nystagmus, no ataxia, past pointing normal. Romberg's sign negative (normal). Intake/output in balance. Urine faint pink tinged, no clots.

Lab: Hct 45, serum chemistries normal.

 ASSESSMENT

Orthostatic hypotension
Risk for injury R/T orthostatic hypotension

CLINICAL CASE STUDY 2

Mara is a 19-year-old single white female college student with a past history of good health and no chronic illnesses, who enters the outpatient clinic today stating, "I think I've had a stroke!"

 Subjective

One day PTA: first noticed at dinner at college cafeteria when joking with friends, started to stick out tongue and roll tongue and could not do it, right side of tongue was not working. Mara left room to look in mirror and became scared; when smiled, noticed right side was not working. Tried to pucker lips, could not. Could not whistle, could not raise eyebrow, "I looked like a Vulcan." No other movement disorder below neck. Mild pain behind right ear with buzzing in ear. Able to sleep last night, but roommate said Mara's right eyelid did not close completely during sleep.

Today: still no movement on complete right side of face. Feeling self-conscious in class and during conversations with friends. Now has taste aversion, fluids with high water content taste especially bitter. No hearing loss.

Objective

T 37° C, P 64, R 14, B/P 108/78.

Forehead appears smooth and immobile on right, unable to wrinkle right side. Unable to close right eye, Bell's phenomenon present when attempts to close (right eyeball rolls upward), right palpebral fissure appears wider. No corneal reflex on right. Unable to whistle or puff right cheek. Absent nasolabial fold on right. Mouth droops on right, sags on right when tries to smile. Slight drooling. Left side of face responds appropriately to all these movements. Superficial sensation intact.

Rest of musculoskeletal system intact: able to hold balance while standing, able to walk, walk heel-to-toe, do knee bend on each knee. Arm strength and range of motion intact.

ASSESSMENT

Right-sided facial paralysis, consistent with Bell's palsy
Body image disturbance R/T effects of loss of facial function
Risk for fluid volume deficit R/T taste aversion and dietary alteration
Risk for sensory deficit, visual impairment, R/T effects of neurologic impairment

NURSING DIAGNOSES COMMONLY ASSOCIATED WITH HEAD AND NECK DISORDERS

Diagnosis	Related Factors (Etiology)	Defining Characteristics (Symptoms and Signs)

Body image disturbance	Effects of loss of body part(s)
	 Effects of loss of body function
		Verbal or nonverbal response to actual or perceived change in structure and/or function
		 Verbalization of
		   Fear of rejection or of reaction by others
		   Negative feelings about body
		 Not looking at and/or touching body part
		 Preoccupation with loss or change
		 Refusal to verify actual change or loss
		 Hiding or overexposing body part
		 Change in social involvement
		 Depersonalization of part or loss by use of impersonal pronouns

Impaired swallowing	Neuromuscular impairment
	   Decreased/absent gag reflex
	   Facial paralysis
	   Decreased strength or excursion of muscles of mastication
	 Mechanical obstruction
	   Edema
	   Tracheostomy tube
	   Tumor
	 Limited awareness
	 Excessive/inadequate salivation
	 Fatigue
	 Reddened, irritated oropharyngeal cavity
		Observed evidence of difficulty swallowing
		 Evidence of aspiration
		 Reported pain on swallowing
		 Dehydration
		 Weight loss

Other Related Nursing Diagnoses

ACTUAL	RISK
Pain (see Chapter 14) Sensory/perceptual alteration	Risk for fluid volume deficit Risk for infection Risk for ineffective airway clearance

 ## ASSESSMENT VIDEO CRITICAL THINKING QUESTIONS

The Saunders *Physical Examination and Health Assessment* Video Series—HEAD, EYES, AND EARS—AND NOSE, MOUTH, THROAT, AND NECK—will direct you to consider the following:
1. How do examination techniques and findings differ when palpating the head of an adult and the head of an infant?
2. Describe characteristics of normal and abnormal cervical lymph nodes.

ABNORMAL FINDINGS

ABNORMAL FINDINGS

▼ Table 11–1   ABNORMALITIES IN HEAD SIZE AND CONTOUR

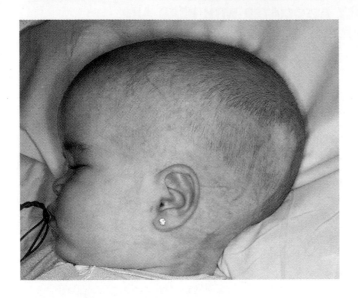

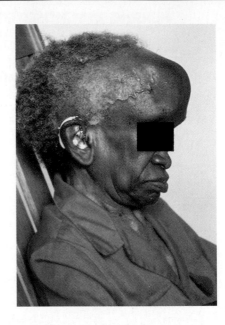

Hydrocephalus

Obstruction of drainage of cerebrospinal fluid results in excessive accumulation, increasing intracranial pressure, and enlargement of the head. The face looks small compared with the enlarged cranium. The increasing pressure also produces dilated scalp veins, frontal bossing, and downcast or "setting sun" eyes (sclera visible above iris). The cranial bones thin, sutures separate, and percussion yields a "cracked pot" sound (Macewen's sign).

Paget's Disease of Bone (Osteitis Deformans)

A localized bone disease of unknown etiology that softens, thickens, and deforms bone. It affects 3 percent of adults over age 40 and 10 percent over age 80 and occurs more often in males. The disease is characterized by bowed long bones, sudden fractures, frontal bossing, and enlarging skull bones which form an acorn-shaped cranium. Enlarging skull bones press on cranial nerves, causing symptoms of headache, vertigo, tinnitus, progressive deafness, as well as optic atrophy and compression of the spinal cord.

Reprinted from the Clinical Slide Collection on the Rheumatic Diseases. © 1991, 1995, 1997. Used by permission of the American College of Rheumatology.

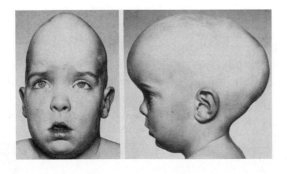

◀ Craniosynostosis

Premature closure of one or more sutures while brain growth continues. Skull growth stops at right angles to closed suture. Deformity depends on involved sutures; closure of the sagittal suture results in a long, narrow head, and closure of the coronal suture involves the head, the face, and the orbits. Also note exophthalmos and drooping eyelids.

Table 11–1   ABNORMALITIES IN HEAD SIZE AND CONTOUR *Continued*

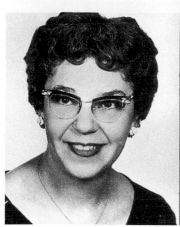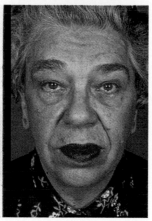

◄ **Acromegaly**

Excessive secretion of growth hormone from the pituitary, after puberty, creates an enlarged skull and thickened cranial bones. Note the elongated head, massive face, prominent nose and lower jaw, heavy eyebrow ridge, and coarse facial features, especially when compared with the same woman's face on the left pictured several years before she had a pituitary tumor.

▼ **Table 11–2   SWELLINGS ON THE HEAD OR NECK**

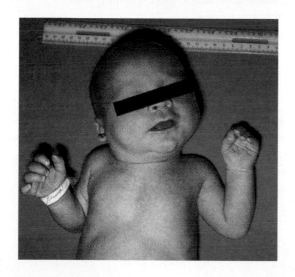

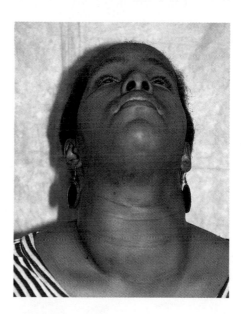

Torticollis (Wryneck)

A hematoma in one sternomastoid muscle, probably injured by intrauterine malposition, results in head tilt to one side and limited neck ROM to the opposite side. You will feel a firm, discrete, nontender mass in mid-muscle on the involved side. This requires treatment, or the muscle becomes fibrotic and permanently shortened with permanent limitation of ROM, asymmetry of head and face, and visual problems from a nonhorizontal position of the eyes.

Thyroid—Multiple Nodules

Multiple nodules usually indicate inflammation or a multinodular goiter rather than a neoplasm. However, suspect any rapidly enlarging or firm nodule.

Thyroid—Single Nodule (not illustrated)

Most solitary nodules are benign, although a solitary nodule poses a greater risk of malignancy than do multiple nodules and poses a greater risk in a young person. Suspect any painless, rapidly growing nodule, especially the appearance of a single nodule in a young person. Cancerous nodules tend to be hard and are fixed to surrounding structures.

Table continued on following page

Table 11–2 SWELLINGS ON THE HEAD OR NECK *Continued*

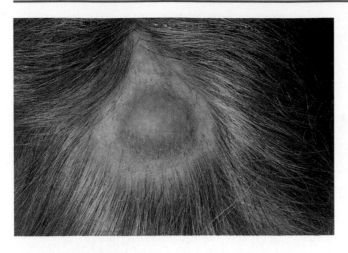

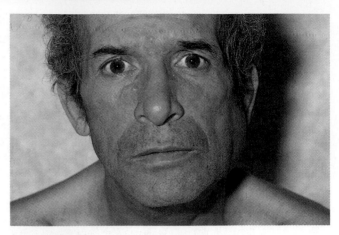

Pilar Cyst (Wen)

Smooth, firm, fluctuant swelling on the scalp. Tense pressure of the contents causes overlying skin to be shiny and taut. It is a benign growth.

Parotid Gland Enlargement

Rapid painful inflammation of the parotid occurs with mumps. Parotid swelling also occurs with blockage of a duct, abscess, or tumor. Note swelling anterior to lower ear lobe.

 Table 11–3 PEDIATRIC FACIAL ABNORMALITIES

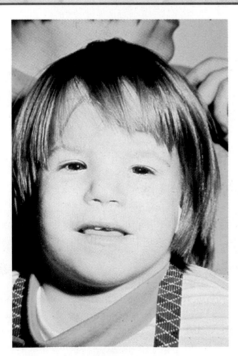

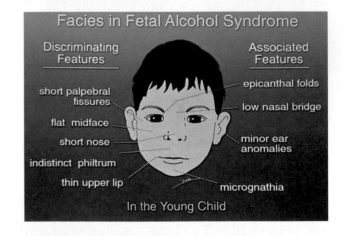

Fetal Alcohol Syndrome

A pregnant woman who abuses alcohol is at great risk of producing a baby with a wide range of growth and developmental abnormalities. Facial malformations may be recognizable at birth. Characteristic facies include narrow palpebral fissures, epicanthal folds, and midfacial hypoplasia.

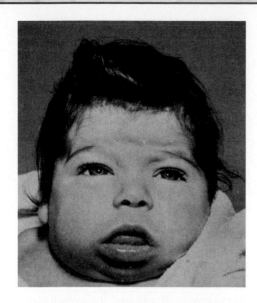

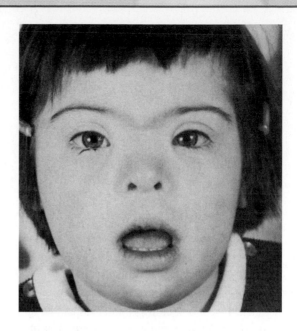

Cretinism—Congenital Hypothyroidism

Thyroid deficiency at an early age produces impaired growth and neurologic deficit. Characteristic facies include low hairline, hirsute forehead, swollen eyelids, narrow palpebral fissures, widely spaced eyes, depressed nasal bridge, puffy face, thick tongue protruding through an open mouth, and a dull expression. Head size is normal, but the anterior and posterior fontanels are wide open.

Down Syndrome

Chromosomal aberration (trisomy 21). Head and face characteristics may include slanted eyes with inner epicanthal folds, flat nasal bridge, small broad flat nose, protruding thick tongue, ear dysplasia, and short broad neck with webbing.

▼ Table 11–4   FACIAL FEATURES WITH CHRONIC ALLERGIES

 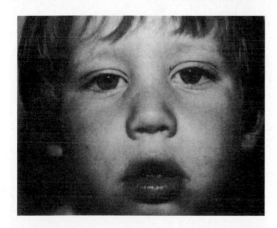

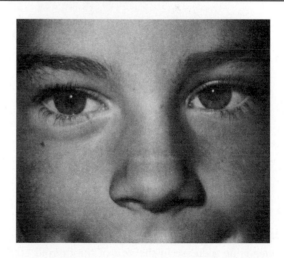

Atopic (Allergic) Facies

Children with chronic allergies such as atopic dermatitis often develop characteristic facial features. These include exhausted face, blue shadows below the eyes ("allergic shiners") from sluggish venous return, a double or single crease on the lower eyelids (Morgan's lines), central facial pallor, and open-mouth breathing (allergic gaping). The open mouth breathing can lead to malocclusion of the teeth and malformed jaw because the child's bones are still forming.

Allergic Crease

The transverse line on the nose is also a feature of chronic allergies. It is formed when the child chronically uses the hand to push the nose up and back (the "allergic salute") to relieve itching and to free swollen turbinates, which allows air passage.

▼ **Table 11–5   ABNORMAL FACIAL APPEARANCES WITH CHRONIC ILLNESSES**

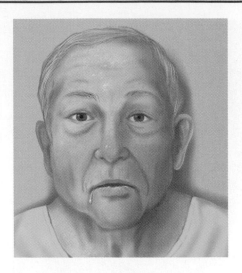

Parkinson's Syndrome

A deficiency of the neurotransmitter dopamine and degeneration of the basal ganglia in the brain. The immobility of features produces a face that is flat and expressionless, "masklike," with elevated eyebrows, staring gaze, oily skin, and drooling.

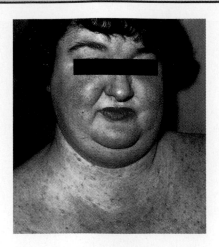

Cushing's Syndrome

With excessive secretion of corticotropin hormone (ACTH) and chronic steroid use, the person develops a plethoric, rounded, "moonlike" face, prominent jowls, red cheeks, hirsutism on the upper lip, lower cheeks, and chin, and acneiform rash on the chest.

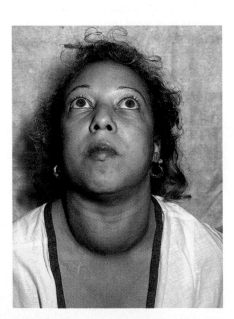

Hyperthyroidism

Goiter is an increase in the size of the thyroid gland and occurs with hyperthyroidism, Hashimoto's thyroiditis, and hypothyroidism. Graves' disease (shown here) is the most common cause of hyperthyroidism, manifested by goiter and exophthalmos (bulging eyeballs). Symptoms include nervousness, fatigue, weight loss, muscle cramps, and heat intolerance; signs include tachycardia, shortness of breath, excessive sweating, fine muscle tremor, thin silky hair and skin, infrequent blinking, and a staring appearance.

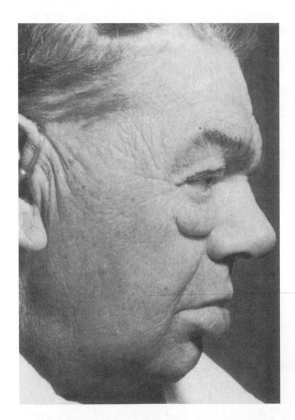

Myxedema (Hypothyroidism)

A deficiency of thyroid hormone, when severe, causes a nonpitting edema or myxedema. Note puffy edematous face, especially around eyes (periorbital edema), coarse facial features, dry skin, and dry coarse hair and eyebrows.

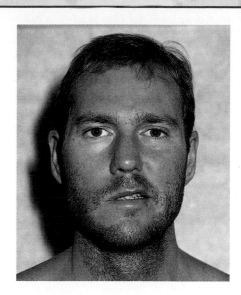

Bell's Palsy (Right Side)

A **lower motor neuron** lesion **(peripheral),** producing cranial nerve VII paralysis, which is almost always unilateral. It has a rapid onset, and its cause is currently thought to be herpes simplex virus (HSV). Note complete paralysis of one-half of the face; person cannot wrinkle forehead, raise eyebrow, close eye, whistle, or show teeth on the right side. Usually presents with smooth forehead, wide palpebral fissure, flat nasolabial fold, drooling, and pain behind the ear.

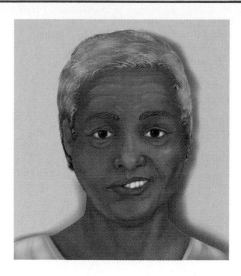

Brain Attack or Cerebrovascular Accident

An **upper motor neuron** lesion **(central).** A "stroke" is an acute neurologic deficit due to an obstruction of a cerebral vessel, as in atherosclerosis, or a rupture in a cerebral vessel. Note paralysis of lower facial muscles, but also note that the upper half of face is not affected owing to the intact nerve from the unaffected hemisphere. The person is still able to wrinkle the forehead and to close the eyes.

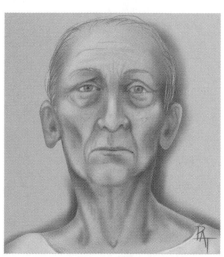

Cachectic Appearance

Accompanies chronic wasting diseases such as cancer, dehydration, and starvation. Features include sunken eyes, hollow cheeks, and exhausted defeated expression.

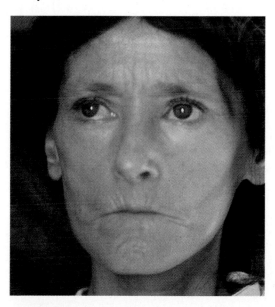

Scleroderma

Literally, "hard skin," this collagen disease is characterized by chronic hardening and shrinking of connective tissue. This can occur in any body organ (skin, heart, esophagus, kidney, lung). Characteristic facies: hard, shiny skin on forehead and cheeks; thin, pursed lips with radial furrowing; absent skinfolds; muscle atrophy on face and neck; absence of expression.

Bibliography

Allen TG: Evaluating and treating headaches. Am J Nurs 94(4):16B–16H, 1994.

Baker JT: Adrenal disorders: A primary care approach. Primary Care Pract 1(5):527–536, Nov–Dec 1997.

Barett E: Primary care for women: Assessment and management of headache. J Nurse Midwifery 41(2):117–124, Mar–Apr 1996.

Berman GD: Chronic headache: Management strategies that make sense. Patient Care 30(2):54–66, Jan 30, 1996.

Bierman CW, Pearlman DS: Allergic Diseases from Infancy to Adulthood, 3rd ed. Philadelphia, W.B. Saunders Company, 1996.

Billue JS: Bell's palsy: An update on idiopathic facial paralysis. Nurse Pract 22(8):88–107, Aug 1997.

Chabon SL: Identification and evaluation of thyroid nodules. Primary Care Pract 1(5):499–506, Nov–Dec 1997.

Childs SG: Syncope: Categories and considerations for practice. J Emerg Nurs 21:125–134, Apr 1995.

Costa M: Trigeminal neuralgia. Am J Nurs 98(6):42–43, June 1998.

Dowd TR: Primary care approach to lymphadenopathy. Nurs Pract 19(12):36–43, Dec 1994.

Galen BA: Rhinitis. Primary Care Pract 1(2):129–141, May–June 1997.

Gilkison CR: Thyrotoxicosis: Recognition and management. Primary Care Pract 1(5):485–498, Nov–Dec 1997.

Heitman B, Irizarry A: Hypothyroidism: Common complaints, perplexing diagnosis. Nurse Pract 20(3):54–60, 1995.

Karmel-Ross K, Lepp M: Assessment and treatment of children with congenital muscular torticollis. Phys Occup Ther Pediatr 17(2):21–67, 1997.

Kingston L, Reynolds D, Phillips LP: Primary care for women: Comprehensive assessment of the head and neck. J Nurse Midwifery 40(2):187–201, Mar–Apr 1995.

Longo DL, Arun B: Cervical adenopathy: A clinical approach to diagnosis. Consultant 36(11):2345–2352, Nov 1996.

McMorrow ME: Myxedema coma. Am J Nurs 96(10):55, Oct 1996.

Phillips LP, Campbell LR, Barger MK: Primary care for women: Management of common problems of the head and neck. J Nurse Midwifery 41(2):101–116, Mar–Apr 1996.

Schilling JS: Hyperthyroidism: Diagnosis and management of Graves' disease. Nurse Pract 22(6):72–97, June 1997.

Skelly AH, Elasy TA: Endocrine disorders. Primary Care Pract 1(5):459–473, Nov–Dec 1997.

Smith R: Diagnosing headache. Hosp Med 33(7):26–34, July 1997.

U.S. Public Health Service: Adult screening for cancer detection: Thyroid examination and function. Nurs Pract 20(5):64–67, May 1995.

Webster J: Vasovagal syncope. Am J Nurs 98(2):16CCC–16DDD, Feb 1998.

CHAPTER TWELVE

Eyes

EXTERNAL ANATOMY

The eye is the sensory organ of vision. Humans are very visual beings. Over half of the neocortex is involved with processing visual information (Wehenmeyer and Gallman, 1997).

Because this sense is so important to humans, the eye is well protected by the bony orbital cavity, which is surrounded with a cushion of fat. The **eyelids** are like two movable shades that further protect the eye from injury, strong light, and dust. The upper eyelid is the larger and more mobile one. The eyelashes are short hairs in double or triple rows that curve outward from the lid margins, filtering out dust and dirt.

The **palpebral fissure** is the elliptical open space between the eyelids (Fig. 12–1). When closed, the lid margins approximate completely. When open, the upper lid covers part of the iris. The lower lid margin is just at the **limbus,** the border between the cornea and sclera. The **canthus** is the corner of the eye, the angle where the lids meet. At the inner canthus, the **caruncle** is a small fleshy mass containing sebaceous glands.

Within the upper lid, **tarsal plates** are strips of connective tissue that give it shape (Fig. 12–2). The tarsal plates contain the **meibomian glands,** modified sebaceous glands that secrete an oily lubricating material onto the lids. This stops the tears from overflowing and helps to form an airtight seal when the lids are closed.

The exposed part of the eye has a transparent protective covering, the **conjunctiva.** The conjunctiva is a thin mucous membrane folded like an envelope between the eyelids and the eyeball. The *palpebral* conjunctiva lines the lids and is clear, with many small blood vessels. It forms a deep recess and then folds back over the eye. The *bulbar* conjunctiva overlays the eyeball, with the white sclera showing through. At the limbus, the conjunctiva merges with the cornea. The cornea covers and protects the iris and pupil.

The **lacrimal apparatus** provides constant irrigation to keep the conjunctiva and cornea moist and lubricated (Fig. 12–3). The lacrimal gland, in the upper outer corner over the eye, secretes tears. The tears wash across the eye and are drawn up evenly as the lid blinks. The tears drain into the **puncta,** visible on the upper and lower lids at the inner canthus. The tears then drain into the nasolacrimal sac, through the one-half-inch long nasolacrimal duct, and empty into the inferior meatus inside the nose. A tiny fold of mucous membrane prevents air from being forced up the nasolacrimal duct when the nose is blown.

Extraocular Muscles. Six muscles attach the eyeball to its orbit (Fig. 12–4) and serve to direct the eye to points of interest. These extraocular muscles give the eye both straight and rotary movement. The four straight, or *rectus,* muscles are the superior, inferior, lateral, and medial rectus muscles. The two slanting, or *oblique,* muscles are the superior and inferior muscles.

Each muscle is coordinated, or yoked, with one in the other eye. This ensures that when the two eyes move, their axes always remain parallel (called *conjugate movement*). Parallel axes are important because the human

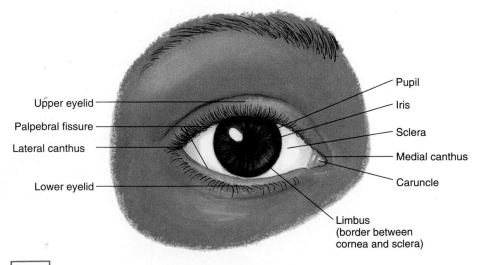

Upper eyelid

Palpebral fissure

Lateral canthus

Lower eyelid

Pupil

Iris

Sclera

Medial canthus

Caruncle

Limbus
(border between
cornea and sclera)

12–1

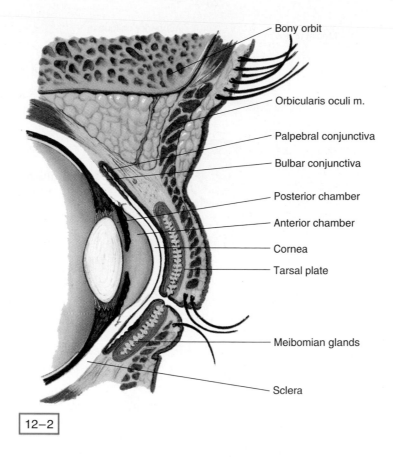

Bony orbit

Orbicularis oculi m.

Palpebral conjunctiva

Bulbar conjunctiva

Posterior chamber

Anterior chamber

Cornea

Tarsal plate

Meibomian glands

Sclera

12–2

brain can tolerate seeing only one image. Although some animals can perceive two different pictures through each eye, human beings have a binocular, single-image visual system. This occurs because our eyes move as a pair. For example, the two yoked muscles that allow looking to the far right are the right lateral rectus and the left medial rectus.

Movement of the extraocular muscles is stimulated by three cranial nerves. Cranial nerve VI, the abducens nerve, innervates the lateral rectus muscle (which abducts the eye); cranial nerve IV, the trochlear nerve, innervates the superior oblique muscle; and cranial nerve III, the oculomotor nerve, innervates all the rest—the superior, inferior, and medial rectus and the inferior oblique muscles.

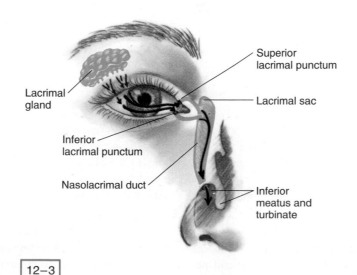

Lacrimal gland

Superior lacrimal punctum

Lacrimal sac

Inferior lacrimal punctum

Nasolacrimal duct

Inferior meatus and turbinate

12–3

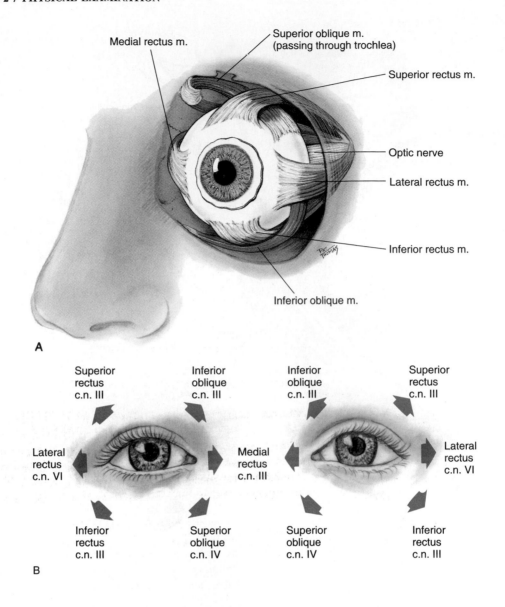

A

Medial rectus m.

Superior oblique m.
(passing through trochlea)

Superior rectus m.

Optic nerve

Lateral rectus m.

Inferior rectus m.

Inferior oblique m.

B

| Superior rectus c.n. III | Inferior oblique c.n. III | | Inferior oblique c.n. III | Superior rectus c.n. III |

Lateral rectus c.n. VI

Medial rectus c.n. III

Lateral rectus c.n. VI

| Inferior rectus c.n. III | Superior oblique c.n. IV | | Superior oblique c.n. IV | Inferior rectus c.n. III |

12–4

Muscle attachments (A) and direction of movement (B)

INTERNAL ANATOMY

The eye is a sphere composed of three concentric coats: (1) the outer fibrous **sclera,** (2) the middle vascular **choroid,** and (3) the inner nervous **retina** (Fig. 12–5). Inside the retina is the transparent vitreous body. The only parts accessible to examination are the sclera anteriorly and the retina through the ophthalmoscope.

The Outer Layer. The **sclera** is a tough, protective, white covering. It is continuous anteriorly with the smooth, transparent cornea, which covers the iris and pupil. The cornea is part of the refracting media of the eye,

bending incoming light rays so they will be focused on the inner retina.

The **cornea** is very sensitive to touch; contact with a wisp of cotton stimulates a blink in both eyes, called the *corneal reflex.* The trigeminal nerve (cranial nerve V) carries the afferent sensation into the brain, and the facial nerve (cranial nerve VII) carries the efferent message that stimulates the blink.

The Middle Layer. The **choroid** has dark pigmentation to prevent light from reflecting internally, and is heavily vascularized to deliver blood to the retina. Anteriorly, the choroid is continuous with the ciliary body and the iris. The muscles of the ciliary body control the thick-

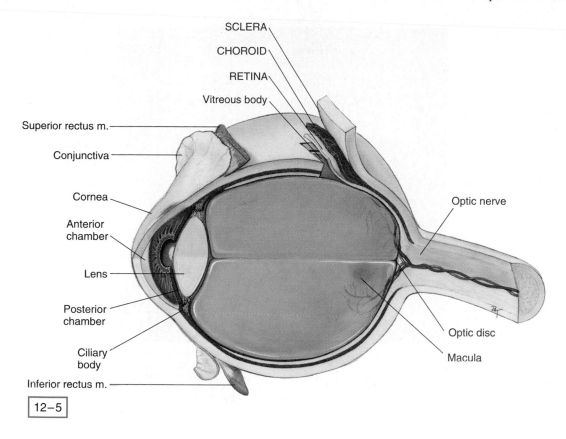

SCLERA
CHOROID
RETINA
Vitreous body
Superior rectus m.
Conjunctiva
Cornea
Anterior chamber
Lens
Posterior chamber
Ciliary body
Inferior rectus m.
Optic nerve
Optic disc
Macula

12–5

ness of the lens. The iris functions as a diaphragm, varying the opening at its center, the pupil. This controls the amount of light admitted into the retina. The muscle fibers of the iris contract the pupil in bright light and to accommodate for near vision, and dilate the pupil when the light is dim and for far vision. The color of the iris varies from person to person.

The **pupil** is round and regular. Its size is determined by a balance between the parasympathetic and sympathetic chains of the autonomic nervous system. Stimulation of the parasympathetic branch, through cranial nerve III, causes constriction of the pupil. Stimulation of the sympathetic branch dilates the pupil and elevates the eyelid. As mentioned earlier, the pupil size also reacts to the amount of ambient light and to accommodation, or focusing an object on the retina.

The **lens** is a biconvex disc located just posterior to the pupil. The transparent lens serves as a refracting medium, keeping a viewed object in continual focus on the retina. Its thickness is controlled by the ciliary body; the lens bulges for focusing on near objects, and flattens for far objects.

The **anterior chamber** is posterior to the cornea and in front of the iris and lens. It contains the aqueous humor that is produced continually by the ciliary body. The continuous flow of fluid serves to deliver nutrients to the surrounding tissues and to drain metabolic wastes. Intraocular pressure is determined by a balance between the amount of aqueous produced and resistance to its outflow at the angle of the anterior chamber.

The Inner Layer. The **retina** is the visual receptive layer of the eye in which light waves are changed into nerve impulses. The retinal structures viewed through the ophthalmoscope are the optic disc, the retinal vessels, the general background, and the macula (Fig. 12–6).

The **optic disc** (or optic papilla) is the area in which fibers from the retina converge to form the optic nerve. Located toward the nasal side of the retina, it has these characteristics: a color that varies from creamy yellow-orange to pink; a round or oval shape; margins that are distinct and sharply demarcated, especially on the temporal side; and a physiologic cup, the smaller circular area inside the disc where the blood vessels exit and enter.

The **retinal vessels** normally include a paired artery and vein extending to each quadrant, growing progressively smaller in caliber as they reach the periphery. The arteries appear brighter red and narrower than the veins, and the arteries have a thin sliver of light on them (the arterial light reflex). The general background of the fundus varies in color, depending on the person's skin color. The **macula** is located on the temporal side of the fundus. It is a slightly darker pigmented region surrounding the **fovea centralis,** the area of sharpest and keenest vision. The macula receives and transduces light from the center of the visual field.

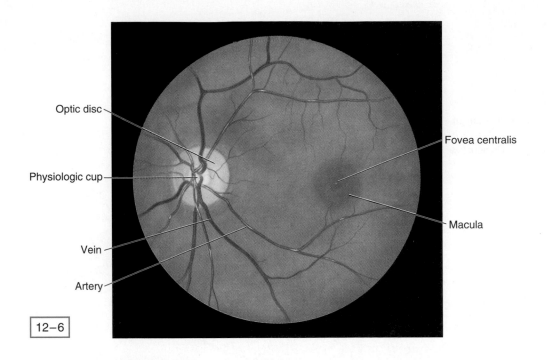

Optic disc

Physiologic cup

Vein

Artery

Fovea centralis

Macula

12–6

VISUAL PATHWAYS AND VISUAL FIELDS

Objects reflect light. The light rays are refracted through the transparent media (cornea, aqueous humor, lens, and vitreous body) and strike the retina. The retina transforms the light stimulus into nerve impulses that are conducted through the optic nerve and the optic tract to the visual cortex of the occipital lobe.

The image formed on the retina is upside down and reversed from its actual appearance in the outside world (Fig. 12–7). That is, an object in the upper temporal visual field of the right eye reflects its image onto the lower nasal area of the retina. All retinal fibers collect to form the optic nerve, but they maintain this same spatial arrangement, with nasal fibers running medially and temporal fibers running laterally.

At the optic chiasm, nasal fibers (from both temporal visual fields) cross over. The left optic tract now has fibers from the left half of each retina, and the right optic tract contains fibers only from the right. Thus, the right side of the brain looks at the left side of the world.

VISUAL REFLEXES

Pupillary Light Reflex. The pupillary light reflex is the normal constriction of the pupils when bright light shines on the retina (Fig. 12–8). It is a subcortical reflex arc (i.e., a person has no conscious control over it); the afferent link is cranial nerve II, the optic nerve, and the efferent path is cranial III, the oculomotor nerve. When one eye is exposed to bright light, a *direct light reflex*

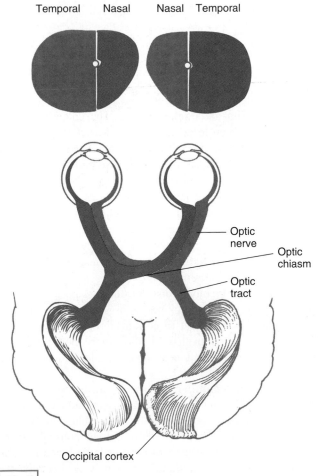

LEFT VISUAL FIELD   RIGHT VISUAL FIELD

Temporal   Nasal   Nasal   Temporal

Optic nerve

Optic chiasm

Optic tract

Occipital cortex

12–7

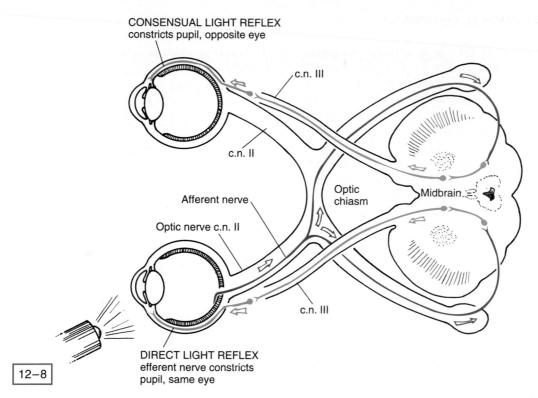

CONSENSUAL LIGHT REFLEX
constricts pupil, opposite eye

c.n. III

c.n. II

Optic
chiasm

Midbrain

Afferent nerve

Optic nerve c.n. II

c.n. III

DIRECT LIGHT REFLEX
efferent nerve constricts
pupil, same eye

12–8

occurs (constriction of that pupil) as well as a *consensual light reflex* (simultaneous constriction of the other pupil). This happens because the optic nerve carries the sensory afferent message in and then synapses with both sides of the brain. For example, consider the light reflex in a person who is blind in one eye. Stimulation of the normal eye produces both a direct and a consensual light reflex. Stimulation of the blind eye causes no response because the sensory afferent in cranial nerve II is destroyed.

Fixation. This is a reflex direction of the eye toward an object attracting a person's attention. The image is fixed in the center of the visual field, the fovea centralis. This consists of very rapid ocular movements to put the target back on the fovea, and somewhat slower (smooth pursuit) movements to track the target and keep its image on the fovea. These ocular movements are impaired by drugs, alcohol, fatigue, and inattention.

Accommodation. This is adaptation of the eye for near vision. It is accomplished by increasing the curvature of the lens through movement of the ciliary muscles. Although the lens cannot be observed directly, the components of accommodation that can be observed are convergence (motion toward) of the axes of the eyeballs and pupillary constriction.

 DEVELOPMENTAL CONSIDERATIONS

Infants and Children

At birth, eye function is limited but it matures fully during the early years. Peripheral vision is intact in the newborn. The macula, the area of keenest vision, is ab-

sent at birth but is developing by 4 months and is mature by 8 months. Eye movements may be poorly coordinated at birth. By 3 to 4 months of age, the infant establishes binocularity and can fixate on a single image with both eyes simultaneously. Most neonates (80 percent) are born farsighted; this gradually decreases after age 7 to 8 years.

In structure, the eyeball reaches adult size by 8 years. At birth, the iris shows little pigment, and the pupils are small. The lens is nearly spherical at birth, growing flatter throughout life. Its consistency changes from that of soft plastic at birth to rigid glass in old age.

The Aging Adult

Changes in eye structure contribute greatly to the distinct facial changes of the aging person. The skin loses its elasticity, causing wrinkling and drooping; fat tissues and muscles atrophy; and the external eye structures appear as on p. 327. Lacrimal glands involute, causing decreased tear production and a feeling of dryness and burning.

On the globe itself, the cornea may show an infiltration of degenerative lipid material around the limbus (see discussion of *arcus senilis,* p. 328). Pupil size decreases. The lens loses elasticity, becoming hard and glasslike. This glasslike quality decreases its ability to change shape in order to accommodate for near vision, and this condition is termed **presbyopia.** The average age at which people experience presbyopia is 40 years (Friedman, Pineda, and Kaiser, 1998). By age 70 years, the normally transparent fibers of the lens begin to thicken and yellow. This is nuclear sclerosis, or the beginning of a senile cataract.

Inside the globe, floaters appear in the vitreous due to debris that can accumulate because the vitreous is not continuously renewed as the aqueous humor is. Retinal structures are described on p. 328.

Visual acuity may diminish gradually after age 50 years, and even more so after age 70 years. Near vision is commonly affected owing to the decreased power of accommodation in the lens (presbyopia). As early as the fourth decade, a person may have blurred vision and difficulty reading. Also, the aging person needs more light to see because of a decreased adaptation to darkness, and this condition may affect the function of night driving.

In the aging population, the most common causes of decreased visual functioning are:

1. Cataract formation, or lens opacity. Some cataract formation should be expected by age 70. Studies indicate that 46 percent of people aged 75 to 85 have developed cataracts (Kane, Ouslander, and Abrass, 1994).
2. Glaucoma, or increased ocular pressure. The incidence increases with age to 7.2 percent at ages 75 to 85, affecting men at higher rates than women (Kane et al., 1994). Chronic, open-angle glaucoma is the most common type and involves a gradual loss of peripheral vision.
3. Macular degeneration. Loss of central vision, the area of clearest vision, is the most common cause of blindness. It affects 28 percent of those aged 75 to 85, with women affected more often than men (Kane et al., 1994). With this, the person is unable to read fine print, sew, or do fine work and may have difficulty distinguishing faces. Depending on how much the lifestyle is oriented around activities requiring close work, loss of central vision may cause great distress. Peripheral vision is not affected, so the per-

son can manage self-care and will not become completely disabled.

TRANSCULTURAL CONSIDERATIONS

Racial differences are evident in the palpebral fissures. Persons of Asian origins are often identified by their characteristic eyes, whereas the presence of narrowed palpebral fissures in non-Asian individuals may be diagnostic of a serious congenital anomaly, *Down syndrome.*

Culturally based variability exists in the color of the iris and in retinal pigmentation, with darker irides having darker retinas behind them. Individuals with light retinas generally have better night vision but can suffer pain in an environment that has too much light.

Racial Variations in Disease. Primary open-angle glaucoma affects blacks three to six times more often than whites, and is six times more likely to cause blindness in blacks than in whites (Friedman et al., 1998). Reasons for this are not known. What is even more surprising are the results from a 1998 study showing that the efficacy of treatment approach to glaucoma is different for blacks and whites (Gaasterland et al., 1998). For blacks, the best outcomes were when the regimen started with argon laser treatments and then followed, if necessary, by a trabeculectomy (surgery to create a tunnel between the anterior chamber in the eye and the subconjunctival space, thereby helping the drainage of aqueous humor). For whites, outcomes were better when the regimen started with the trabeculectomy, and then later included the laser treatments if needed. It is not known why racial groups respond differently to treatment.

SUBJECTIVE DATA

1. Vision difficulty (decreased acuity, blurring, blind spots)
2. Pain
3. Strabismus, diplopia
4. Redness, swelling
5. Watering, discharge
6. Past history of ocular problems
7. Glaucoma
8. Use of glasses or contact lenses
9. Self-care behaviors

Examiner Asks	Rationale

1 **Vision difficulty (decreased acuity, blurring, blind spots).** Any **difficulty seeing** or any blurring? Come on suddenly, or progress slowly? In one eye or both?
• Constant, or does it come and go?

- Do objects appear out of focus, or does it feel like a clouding over objects? Does it feel like "grayness" of vision?
- Do spots move in front of your eyes? One or many? In one or both eyes?

Floaters are common with myopia or after middle age owing to condensed vitreous fibers. Usually they are not significant. Acute onset of floaters ("shade" or "cobwebs") may occur with retinal detachment.

- Any halos/rainbows around objects? Or rings around lights?

Halos around lights occur with acute narrow-angle glaucoma.

- Any blind spot? Does it move as you shift your gaze? Any loss of peripheral vision?

Scotoma is a blind spot in the visual field surrounded by an area of normal or decreased vision. This occurs with glaucoma and with optic nerve and visual pathway disorders.

- Any night blindness?

Night blindness occurs with optic atrophy, glaucoma, or vitamin A deficiency.

2 **Pain.** Any **eye pain?** Please describe.
- Come on suddenly?

Note: Consider *sudden onset* of eye symptoms or vision change (pain, floaters, blind spot, loss of peripheral vision) as a possible emergency. Refer immediately.

- Quality—a burning or itching?

Quality may be valuable diagnostic indicator.

- Or sharp, stabbing pain or pain with bright light?

Photophobia is the inability to tolerate light.

- A foreign body sensation? Or deep aching? Or headache in brow area?

(Note: some common eye diseases cause no pain, e.g., refractive errors, cataract, glaucoma.)

3 **Strabismus, diplopia.** Any history of crossed eyes? Now or in the past? Does this occur with eye fatigue?
- Ever see double? Constant, or does it come and go? In one eye or both?

Strabismus is a deviation in the anteroposterior axis of the eye.
Diplopia is the perception of two images of a single object.

4 **Redness, swelling.** Any **redness** or **swelling** in the eyes?
- Any infections? Now or in the past?
- When do these occur? In a particular time of year? Are they seasonal?

5 **Watering, discharge.** Any **watering,** or excessive tearing?

Lacrimation (tearing) and epiphora (excessive tearing) are due to irritants or obstruction in drainage of tears.

- Any **discharge?** Any matter in the eyes? Is it hard to open your eyes in the morning? What color is the discharge?
- How do you remove matter from eyes?

Purulent discharge is thick and yellow colored. Crusts form at night. Assess hygiene practices and knowledge of cross-contamination.

6 **Past history of ocular problems.** Any **past history** of injury or surgery to eye? Or any history of allergies?

Allergens may cause irritation of conjunctiva or cornea, e.g., make-up, contact lens solution.

7 **Glaucoma.** Ever been tested for **glaucoma?** Results?
- Any family history of glaucoma?

Glaucoma is an eye disease characterized by increased intraocular pressure.

8 **Use of glasses or contact lenses.** Do you wear **glasses** or **contact lenses?** How do they work for you?

- Last time your prescription was checked? Was it changed?
- If you wear contact lenses, are there any problems such as pain, photophobia, watering, or swelling?
- How do you care for contacts? How long do you wear them? How do you clean them? Do you remove them for certain activities?

Assess self-care behaviors.

9 Self-care behaviors. Last vision test? Who tested it?
- Ever tested for color vision?
- Any environmental conditions at home or at work that may affect your eyes? For example, flying sparks, metal bits, smoke, dust, chemical fumes? If so, do you wear goggles to protect your eyes?

Self-care behaviors for eyes and vision.

Ocular diseases or injuries may be work related, e.g., an auto mechanic with a foreign body from metal working.

10 What medications are you taking? Systemic or topical? Do you take any medication specifically for the eyes?

Some medications have ocular side effects, e.g., prednisone may cause cataracts or increased intraocular pressure.

11 If you have experienced a vision loss, how do you cope? Do you have books with large print, books on audio tape, Braille?
- Do you maintain living environment the same?
- Do you sometimes fear complete loss of vision?

A constant spatial layout eases navigation through the home.

ADDITIONAL HISTORY FOR INFANTS AND CHILDREN

1 Any vaginal infections in the mother at time of delivery?

Certain forms of vaginitis (gonorrhea, genital herpes) have ocular sequelae for the newborn.

2 Considering age of child, which developmental milestones of vision have you (parent) noted?

Studies indicate the parent is most often the one to detect vision problems.

3 Does the child have routine vision testing at school?

4 Are you (parent) aware of safety measures to protect child's eyes from trauma? Do you inspect toys?
- Have you taught the child safe care of sharp objects, and how to carry and how to use them?

ADDITIONAL HISTORY FOR THE AGING ADULT

1 Have you noticed any visual difficulty with climbing stairs or driving?

Any loss of depth perception.

2 When was the last time you were tested for glaucoma?
- Any aching pain around eyes? Any loss of peripheral vision?
- If you have glaucoma, how do you manage your eyedrops?

Assess compliance; it may be a problem if symptoms are absent. Assess ability to administer eyedrops.

3 Do you have any problem with night vision?

4 Is there a history of cataracts? Any loss or progressive blurring of vision?

5 Do your eyes ever feel dry? burning? What do you do for this?

Decreased tear production may occur with aging.

6 Any decrease in usual activities, such as reading or sewing?

Macular degeneration causes a loss in central visual acuity.

Preparation

Position the person sitting up with the head at your eye level.

Equipment Needed

Snellen eye chart
Handheld visual screener
Opaque card or occluder
Penlight
Applicator stick
Ophthalmoscope

Normal Range of Findings	Abnormal Findings

CENTRAL VISUAL ACUITY

Test visual acuity
Snellen Eye Chart

The Snellen alphabet chart is the most commonly used and accurate measure of visual acuity. It has lines of letters arranged in decreasing size.

Place the Snellen chart in a well-lit spot at eye level. Position the person on a mark exactly 20 feet from the chart. Hand the person an opaque card with which to shield one eye at a time during the test; inadvertent peeking may result when shielding the eye with the person's own fingers (Fig. 12–9). If the person wears glasses or contact lenses, leave them on. Remove only reading glasses because they will blur distance vision. Ask the person to read through the chart to the smallest line of letters possible. Encourage the person to try the next smallest line also. (Note: Use a Snellen "E" chart for people who cannot read letters. See p. 323.)

Hesitancy, squinting, leaning forward, misreading letters.

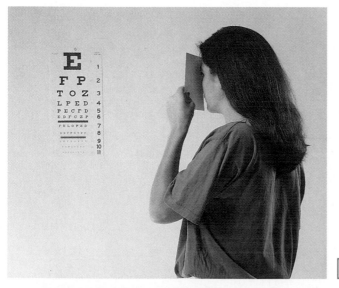

12–9

Record the result using the numeric fraction at the end of the last successful line read. Indicate whether or not the person missed any letters or if corrective lenses were worn, e.g., "O.D.* 20/30 − 1, with glasses."

---

*O.D., oculus dexter, or right eye.

▶ Normal Range of Findings | Abnormal Findings

Normal visual acuity is 20/20. Contrary to some people's impression, the numeric fraction is *not* a percentage of normal vision. Instead, the top number (numerator) indicates the distance the person is standing from the chart, while the denominator gives the distance at which a normal eye could have read that particular line. Thus "20/20" means, "You can read at 20 feet what the normal eye could have read at 20 feet."

The larger the denominator, the poorer the vision. If vision is poorer than 20/30, refer the person to an ophthalmologist or optometrist. Impaired vision may be due to refractive error, opacity in the media (cornea, lens, vitreous), or disorder in the retina or optic pathway.

If the person is unable to see even the largest letters, shorten the distance to the chart until it is seen and record that distance, e.g., "10/200." If visual acuity is even lower, assess whether the person can count your fingers when they are spread in front of the eyes or distinguish light perception using your penlight.

Near Vision

For people over 40 years of age or for those who report increasing difficulty reading, test near vision using a handheld vision screener with various sizes of print (e.g., a Jaeger card) (Fig. 12–10). Hold the card in good light about 35 cm (14 inches) from the eye—this distance equals the print size on the 20-ft chart. Test each eye separately, with glasses on. A normal result is "14/14" in each eye, read without hesitancy and without moving the card closer or farther away. When no vision screening card is available, ask the person to read from a magazine or newspaper.

Presbyopia, the decrease in power of accommodation with aging, is suggested when the person moves the card farther away.

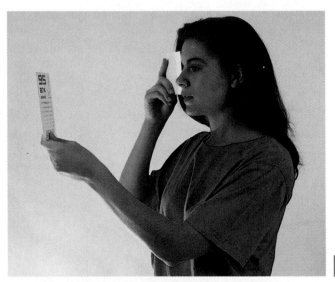

12–10

VISUAL FIELDS

Test visual fields
Confrontation Test

This is a gross measure of peripheral vision. It compares the person's peripheral vision with your own, assuming yours is normal (Fig. 12–11). Position yourself at eye level with the person, about 2 ft away. Direct the person to cover one eye with an opaque card, and with the other eye to look straight at you. Cover your own eye opposite to the person's covered one. Hold a pencil or your flicking finger as a target midline between you and the other person, and slowly advance it in from the periphery in several directions.

▶ Normal Range of Findings	Abnormal Findings

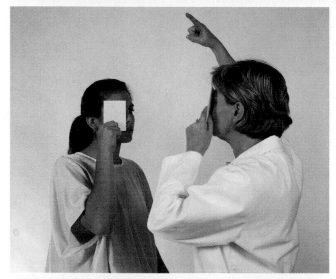

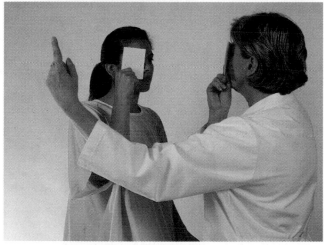

12–11

Ask the person to say "now" as the target is first seen; this should be just as you see the object also. (This works with all but the temporal visual field, with which you would need a 6-ft arm to avoid being seen initially! With the temporal direction, start the object somewhat behind the person.) Estimate the angle between the anteroposterior axis of the eye and the peripheral axis where the object is first seen. Normal results are about 50 degrees upward, 90 degrees temporal, 70 degrees down, and 60 degrees nasal (Fig. 12–12).

If the person is unable to see the object as examiner does, the test suggests peripheral field loss. Refer the person to an optometrist for more precise testing using a tangent screen (see Table 12–1 on p. 333).

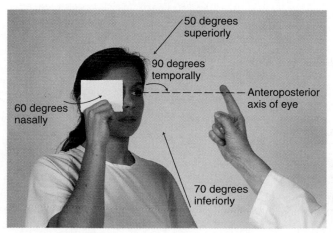

50 degrees
superiorly

90 degrees
temporally

Anteroposterior
axis of eye

60 degrees
nasally

70 degrees
inferiorly

12–12

Range of peripheral motion

EXTRAOCULAR MUSCLE FUNCTION

Inspect extraocular muscle function
Corneal Light Reflex (The Hirschberg Test)

Assess the parallel alignment of the eye axes by shining a light toward the person's eyes. Direct the person to stare straight ahead as you hold the light about 30 cm (12 inches) away. Note the reflection of the light on the corneas; it should be in exactly the same spot on each eye. See Figure 12–33 for symmetry of the corneal light reflex.

Cover Test

This test detects small degrees of deviated alignment by interrupting the fusion reflex that normally keeps the two eyes parallel. Ask the person to stare straight ahead at your nose even though the gaze may be interrupted. With an opaque card, cover one eye. As it is covered, note the uncovered eye. A normal response is a steady fixed gaze (Fig. 12–13A).

Asymmetry of the light reflex indicates deviation in alignment due to eye muscle weakness or paralysis. If you see this, perform the cover test.

If the eye jumps to fixate on the designated point, it was out of alignment before.

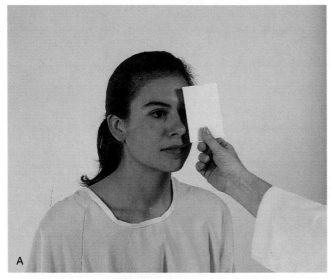

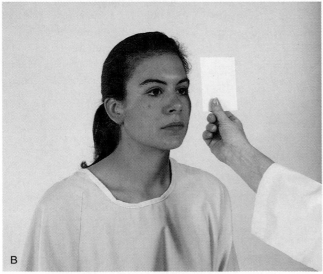

12–13

|

Meanwhile, the macular image has been suppressed on the covered eye. If muscle weakness exists, the covered eye will drift into a relaxed position. Now uncover the eye and observe it for movement. It should stare straight ahead (Fig. 12–13*B*). If it jumps to re-establish fixation, eye muscle weakness exists. Repeat with the other eye.

Diagnostic Positions Test

Leading the eyes through the six cardinal positions of gaze will elicit any muscle weakness during movement (Fig. 12–14). Ask the person to hold the head steady and to follow the movement of your finger, pen, or penlight only with the eyes. Hold the target back about 12 inches so the person can focus on it comfortably, and move it to each of the six positions, hold it momentarily, then back to center. Progress clockwise. A normal response is parallel tracking of the object with both eyes.

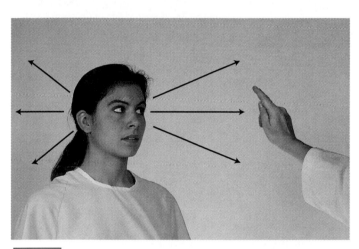

12–14

In addition to parallel movement, note any **nystagmus,** a fine oscillating movement best seen around the iris. Mild nystagmus at extreme lateral gaze is normal; nystagmus at any other position is not.

Finally, note that the upper eyelid continues to overlap the superior part of the iris, even during downward movement. You should not see a white rim of sclera between the lid and the iris. If noted, this is termed "lid lag."

EXTERNAL OCULAR STRUCTURES

Inspect external eye structures
Begin with the most external points, and logically work your way inward.

General

Already you will have noted the person's ability to move around the room, with vision functioning well enough to avoid obstacles, and to respond to your directions. Also note the facial expression; a relaxed expression accompanies adequate vision.

A **phoria** is a mild weakness noted only when fusion is blocked. **Tropia** is more severe, a constant malalignment of the eyes (see Table 12–2).

Eye movement is not parallel. Failure to follow in a certain direction indicates weakness of an extraocular muscle (EOM) or dysfunction of cranial nerve innervating it.

Nystagmus occurs with disease of the semicircular canals in the ears, a paretic eye muscle, multiple sclerosis, or brain lesions.

Lid lag occurs with hyperthyroidism.

Groping with hands.
Squinting or craning forward.

► Normal Range of Findings

Abnormal Findings

Eyebrows

Normally the eyebrows are present bilaterally, move symmetrically as the facial expression changes, and have no scaling or lesions.

Absent lateral third of hair with hypothyroidism.

Unequal or absent movement with nerve damage.

Scaling with seborrhea.

Eyelids and Lashes

The upper lids normally overlap the superior part of the iris, and approximate completely with the lower lids when closed. The skin is intact without redness, swelling, discharge, or lesions.

The palpebral fissures are horizontal in non-Asians, whereas Asians normally have an upward slant.

Note that the eyelashes are evenly distributed along the lid margins, and curve outward.

Lid lag with hyperthyroidism.

Incomplete closure creates risk for corneal damage.

Ptosis, drooping of upper lid.

Periorbital edema, lesions (see Tables 12–3 and 12–4).

Ectropion and entropion (see Table 12–3).

Eyeballs

The eyeballs are aligned normally in their sockets with no protrusion or sunken appearance. Blacks normally may have a slight protrusion of the eyeball beyond the supraorbital ridge.

Exophthalmos, protruding eyes, and enophthalmos, sunken eyes (see Table 12–3).

Conjunctiva and Sclera

Ask the person to look up. Using your thumbs, slide the lower lids down along the bony orbital rim. Take care not to push against the eyeball. Inspect the exposed area (Fig. 12–15). The eyeball looks moist and glossy. Numerous small blood vessels normally show through the transparent conjunctiva. Otherwise, the

General reddening (see Table 12–5).

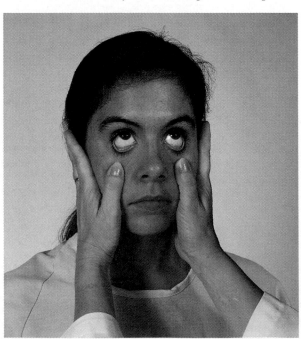

12–15

Normal Range of Findings	Abnormal Findings

conjunctivae are clear and show the normal color of the structure below—pink over the lower lids, and white over the sclera. Note any color change, swelling, or lesions.

The sclera is china white, although blacks occasionally have a gray-blue or "muddy" color to the sclera. Also in dark-skinned people, you normally may see small brown macules (like freckles) on the sclera, which should not be confused with foreign bodies or petechiae. Lastly, blacks may have yellowish fatty deposits beneath the lids away from the cornea. Do not confuse these yellow spots with the overall scleral yellowing that accompanies jaundice.

Eversion of the Upper Lid

This maneuver is not part of the normal examination, but it is useful when you must inspect the conjunctiva of the upper lid, as with eye pain or suspicion of a foreign body. Most people are apprehensive of any eye manipulation. Enhance their cooperation by using a calm and gentle, yet deliberate, approach.

1. Ask the person to keep both eyes open and look down. This relaxes the eyelid, whereas closing it would tense the orbicularis muscle.
2. Slide the upper lid up along the bony orbit to lift up the eyelashes.
3. Grasp the lashes between your thumb and forefinger and gently pull down and outward.
4. With your other hand, place the tip of an applicator stick on the upper lid above the level of the internal tarsal plates (Fig. 12–16).

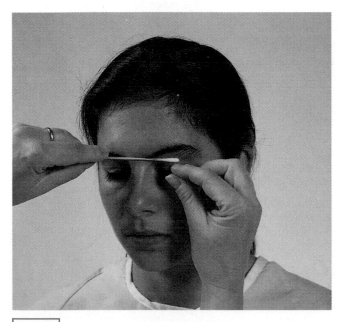

12–16

5. Gently push down with the stick as you lift the lashes up. This uses the edge of the tarsal plate as a fulcrum and flips the lid inside out. Take special care not to push in on the eyeball.

Abnormal Findings column:

Cyanosis of the lower lids.

Pallor near the outer canthus of the lower lid may indicate anemia (the inner canthus normally contains less pigment).

Scleral icterus is an even yellowing of the sclera extending up to the cornea, indicating jaundice.

Tenderness, foreign body, discharge, or lesions.

6. Secure the everted position by holding the lashes against the bony orbital rim (Fig. 12–17).

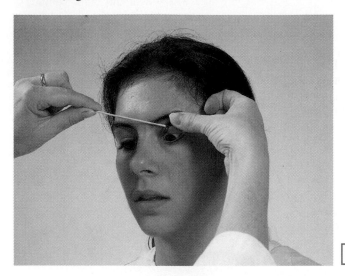

12–17

7. Inspect for any color change, swelling, lesion, or foreign body.
8. To return to normal position, gently pull the lashes outward as the person looks up.

Lacrimal Apparatus

Ask the person to look down. With your thumbs, slide the outer part of the upper lid up along the bony orbit. Inspect for any redness or swelling.

Normally, the puncta drain the tears into the lacrimal sac. Presence of excessive tearing may indicate blockage of the nasolacrimal duct. Check this by pressing the index finger against the sac, just inside the lower orbital rim, not against the side of the nose (Fig. 12–18). Pressure will slightly evert the lower lid, but there should be no other response to pressure.

Swelling of the lacrimal gland may show as a visible bulge in the outer part of the upper lid.

Puncta red, swollen, tender to pressure.

Watch for any regurgitation of fluid out of the puncta, which confirms duct blockage.

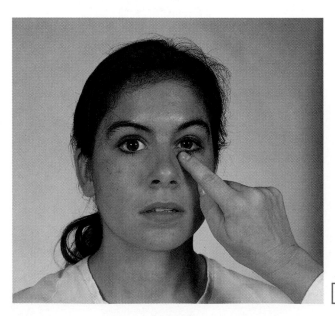

12–18

| ▶ N o r m a l   R a n g e   o f   F i n d i n g s | A b n o r m a l   F i n d i n g s |

ANTERIOR EYEBALL STRUCTURES

Inspect anterior eyeball structures

Cornea and Lens

Shine a light from the side across the cornea, and check for smoothness and clarity. This oblique view highlights any abnormal irregularities in the corneal surface. There should be no opacities (cloudiness) in the cornea, the anterior chamber, or the lens behind the pupil. Do not confuse an **arcus senilis** with an opacity. The arcus senilis is a normal finding in aging persons and is illustrated on p. 328.

A corneal abrasion causes irregular ridges in reflected light, producing a shattered look to light rays (see Table 12–6).

Iris and Pupil

The iris normally appears flat, with a round regular shape and even coloration. Note the size, shape, and equality of the pupils. Normally the pupils appear round, regular, and of equal size in both eyes. In the adult, resting size is from 3 to 5 mm. A small number of people (5 percent) normally have pupils of two different sizes, termed **anisocoria.**

Irregular shape.

Although they may be normal, all unequally sized pupils call for a consideration of central nervous system injury.

To test the **pupillary light reflex,** darken the room and ask the person to gaze into the distance. (This dilates the pupils.) Advance a light in from the side* and note the response. Normally you will see (1) constriction of the same-sided pupil (a *direct light reflex*) and (2) simultaneous constriction of the other pupil (a *consensual light reflex*).

Dilated pupils.

Dilated and fixed pupils.

Constricted pupils.

Unequal or no response to light (see Table 12–7).

In the acute care setting, gauge the pupil size in millimeters, both before and after the light reflex. Recording the pupil size in millimeters is more accurate when many nurses and physicians care for the same person, or when small changes may be significant signs of increasing intracranial pressure. Normally, the resting size is 3, 4, or 5 mm, and decreases equally in response to light. A normal response is designated by

$$R \frac{3}{1} = \frac{3}{1} L.$$

This indicates that both pupils measure 3 mm in the resting state and that both constrict to 1 mm in response to light. A graduated scale printed on a handheld vision screener or taped onto a tongue blade facilitates your measurement (see Fig. 21–58 in Chapter 21).

---

*Always advance the light in from the *side* to test the light reflex. If you advance from the front, the pupils will constrict to accommodate for near vision. Thus you do not know what the pure response to the light would have been.

Test for **accommodation** by asking the person to focus on a distant object (Fig. 12–19). This process dilates the pupils. Then have the person shift the gaze to a near object, such as your finger held about 7 to 8 cm (3 inches) from the nose. A normal response includes (1) pupillary constriction and (2) convergence of the axes of the eyes.

Absence of constriction or convergence.

Asymmetric response.

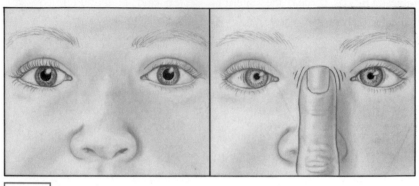

12–19

Far vision—pupils dilate   **Near vision—pupils constrict**

Record the normal response to all these maneuvers as PERRLA, or **P**upils **E**qual, **R**ound, **R**eact to **L**ight and **A**ccommodation.

THE OCULAR FUNDUS

Inspect the ocular fundus

The ophthalmoscope enlarges your view of the eye so that you can inspect the **media** (anterior chamber, lens, vitreous) and the **ocular fundus** (the internal surface of the retina). It accomplishes this by directing a beam of light through the pupil to illuminate the inner structures. Thus, using the ophthalmoscope is like peering through a keyhole (the pupil) into an interesting room beyond.

The ophthalmoscope should function as an appendage of your own eye. This takes some practice. Practice holding the instrument and focusing at objects around the room before you approach a "real" person. Hold the ophthalmoscope right up to your eye, braced firmly against the cheek and brow. Extend your index finger onto the lens selector dial so that you can refocus as needed during the procedure without taking your head away from the ophthalmoscope to look. Now, look about the room, moving your head and the instrument together, as one unit. Keep both your eyes open; just view the field through the ophthalmoscope.

Recall that the ophthalmoscope contains a set of lenses that control the focus (Fig. 12–20). The unit of strength of each lens is the *diopter*. The black numbers indicate a positive diopter; they focus on objects nearer in space to the ophthalmoscope. The red numbers show a negative diopter and are for focusing on objects farther away.

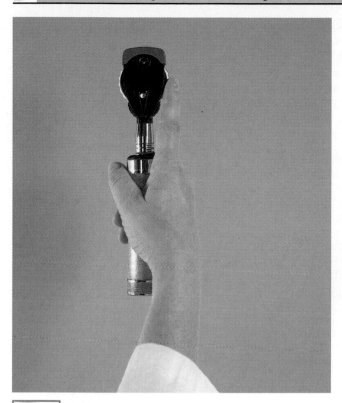

12–20

To examine a person, darken the room to help dilate the pupils. (Dilating eyedrops are not needed during a screening examination. When indicated, they dilate the pupils for a wider look at the fundus background and macular area. Eyedrops are used only when glaucoma can be completely ruled out, because dilating the pupils in the presence of glaucoma can precipitate an acute episode.) Remove eyeglasses from yourself or the other person; they obstruct close movement and you can compensate for their correction by using the diopter setting. Contact lenses may be left in; they pose no problem as long as they are clean.

Select the large round aperture with the white light for the routine examination. If the pupils are small, use the smaller white light. (Although the instrument has other shape and colored apertures, these are rarely used in a screening examination.) The light must have maximum brightness; replace old or dim batteries.

Tell the person, "Please keep looking at that light switch (or mark) on the wall across the room, even though my head will get in the way." Staring at a distant fixed object helps to dilate the pupils and to hold the retinal structures still.

Match sides with the person. That is, hold the ophthalmoscope in your *right* hand up to your *right* eye to view the person's *right* eye. You must do this to avoid bumping noses during the procedure. Place your free hand on the person's shoulder or forehead (Fig. 12–21*A*). This helps orient you in space, because once you have the ophthalmoscope in position, you only have a very narrow range of vision. Also, your thumb can anchor the upper lid and help prevent blinking.

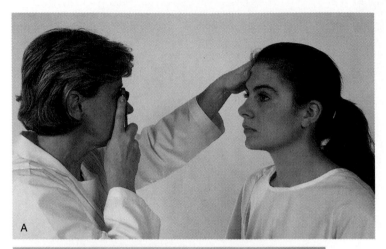

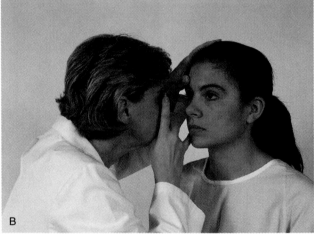

12–21

Begin about 25 cm (10 inches) away from the person at an angle about 15 degrees lateral to the person's line of vision. Note the red glow filling the person's pupil. This is the **red reflex,** caused by the reflection of your ophthalmoscope light off the inner retina. Keep sight of the red reflex, and steadily move closer to the eye. If you lose the red reflex, the light has wandered off the pupil and onto the iris or sclera. Adjust your angle to find it again.

As you advance, adjust the lens to +6 and note any opacities in the media. These appear as dark shadows or black dots interrupting the red reflex. Normally, none are present.

Progress toward the person until your foreheads almost touch (Fig. 12–21*B*). Adjust the diopter setting to bring the ocular fundus into sharp focus. If you and the person have normal vision, this should be at 0. Moving the diopters compensates for nearsightedness or farsightedness. Use the red lenses for nearsighted eyes and the black for farsighted eyes (Fig. 12–22).

Cataracts appear as opaque black areas against the red reflex (see Table 12–8).

NORMAL EYE

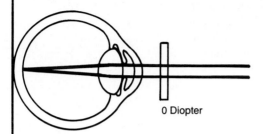

0 Diopter

The person's eye and your eye are normal. The 0 diopter (clear glass) will focus sharply on the retina

MYOPIA (nearsighted)

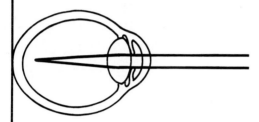

In myopia, the globe is longer than normal and light rays focus in *front* of the retina

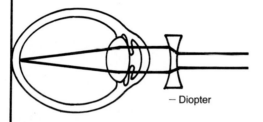

− Diopter

Compensate for myopia in yourself or the other person by using a negative diopter (red or concave lens). This corrects the focal point onto the retina

HYPEROPIA (farsighted)

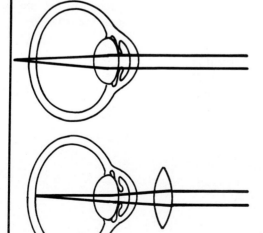

In hyperopia, the globe is shorter than normal. Light rays would focus behind the retina (if they could pass through)

+ Diopter

Compensate for hyperopia by using a positive diopter (black or convex lens). This bends the light rays so the focal point is on the retina

12–22

| ► Normal Range of Findings | Abnormal Findings |

Moving in on the 15-degree lateral line should bring your view just to the optic disc. If the disc is not in sight, track a blood vessel as it grows larger and it will lead you to the disc. Systematically inspect the structures in the ocular fundus: (1) optic disc, (2) retinal vessels, (3) general background, and (4) macula (Fig. 12–23). (Note the illustration here shows a large area of the fundus. Your actual view through the ophthalmoscope is much smaller, slightly larger than 1 disc diameter.)

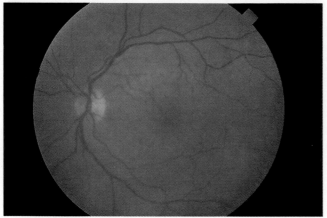

12–23

Normal ocular fundus

Optic Disc

The most prominent landmark is the optic disc, located on the nasal side of the retina. Explore these characteristics:

1. Color	Creamy yellow-orange to pink.	Pallor. Hyperemia.
2. Shape	Round or oval.	Irregular.
3. Margins	Distinct and sharply demarcated, although the nasal edge may be slightly fuzzy.	Blurred margins.
4. Cup-disc ratio	Distinctness varies. When visible, physiologic cup is a brighter yellow-white than rest of the disc. Its width is not more than one-half the disc diameter.	Cup extending to the disc border (see Table 12–9).

Two normal variations may occur around the disc margins. A **scleral crescent** is a gray-white new moon shape (Fig. 12–24). It occurs when pigment is absent in the choroid layer and you are looking directly at the sclera. A **pigment crescent** is black, and is due to accumulation of pigment in the choroid.

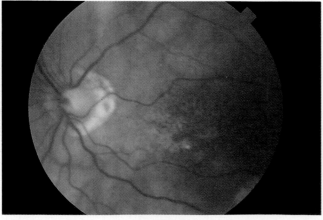

12–24

Scleral crescent and drusen

Chapter 12 / EYES   **321**

| ▶ Normal Range of Findings | Abnormal Findings |

The diameter of the disc, or DD, is a standard of measure for other fundus structures (Fig. 12–25). To describe a finding, note its clock-face position as well as its relationship to the disc in size and distance, e.g., ". . . at 5:00, 3 DD from the disc."

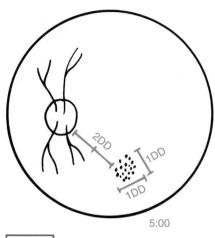

5:00

12–25

Retinal Vessels

This is the only place in the body where you can view blood vessels directly. Many systemic diseases that affect the vascular system show signs in the retinal vessels. Follow a paired artery and vein out to the periphery in the four quadrants (see Fig. 12–23), noting these points:

1. Number	A paired artery and vein pass to each quadrant. Vessels look straighter at the nasal side.	Absence of major vessels.
2. Color	Arteries are brighter red than veins. Also, they have the arterial light reflex, with a thin stripe of light down the middle.	
3. A:V ratio	The ratio comparing the artery-to-vein width is 2:3 or 4:5.	Arteries too constricted. Veins dilated.
4. Caliber	Arteries and veins show a regular decrease in caliber as they extend to periphery.	Focal constriction. Neovascularization.
5. A-V (arteriovenous) crossing	An artery and vein may cross paths. This is not significant if within 2 DD of disc and if no sign of interruption in blood flow is seen. There should be no indenting or displacing of vessel.	Crossings more than 2 DD away. Nicking or pinching of underlying vessel. Vessel engorged peripheral to crossing (see Table 12–10).
6. Tortuosity	Mild vessel twisting when present in both eyes is usually congenital and not significant.	Extreme tortuosity or marked asymmetry in two eyes.
7. Pulsations	Present in veins near disc as their drainage meets the intermittent pressure of arterial systole. (Often hard to see.)	Absent pulsations.

General Background of the Fundus

The color normally varies from light red to dark brown-red, generally corresponding with the person's skin color. Your view of the fundus should be clear; no lesions should obstruct the retinal structures.

Abnormal lesions: hemorrhages, exudates, microaneurysms (see Table 12–11).

Macula

The macula is 1 DD in size and located 2 DD temporal to the disc. Inspect this area last in the funduscopic examination. A bright light on this area of central vision causes some watering and discomfort and pupillary constriction. Note that the normal color of the area is somewhat darker than the rest of the fundus but is even and homogeneous. Clumped pigment may occur with aging.

Clumped pigment occurs with trauma or retinal detachment.

Within the macula, you may note the foveal light reflex. This is a tiny white glistening dot reflecting your ophthalmoscope light.

Hemorrhage or exudate in the macula occurs with senile macular degeneration.

 ## DEVELOPMENTAL CONSIDERATIONS

Infants and Children

The eye examination is often deferred at birth because of transient edema of the lids from birth trauma or from the instillation of silver nitrate for prophylaxis. The eyes should be examined within a few days and at every well child visit thereafter.

Visual Acuity

The child's age determines the screening measures used. With a newborn, test visual reflexes and attending behaviors. Test **light perception** using the blink reflex; the neonate blinks in response to bright light (Fig. 12–26). Also the pupillary light reflex shows that the pupils constrict in response to light. These reflexes indicate that the lower portion of the visual apparatus is intact. But you cannot infer that the infant can *see:* that requires later observation to show that the brain has received images and can interpret them.

Absent blinking.

Absent pupillary light reflex, especially after 3 weeks, indicates blindness.

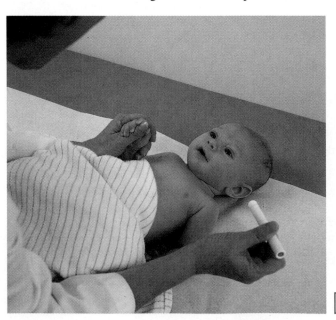

12–26

Normal Range of Findings	Abnormal Findings

As you introduce an object to the infant's line of vision, note these attending behaviors:

Birth to 2 weeks—Refusal to reopen eyes after exposure to bright light; increasing alertness to object; infant may fixate on an object.
By 2 to 4 weeks—Infant can fixate on an object.
By 1 month—Infant can fixate and follow a light or bright toy.
By 3 to 4 months—Infant can fixate, follow, and reach for the toy.
By 6 to 10 months—Infant can fixate and follow the toy in all directions.

The Allen test (picture cards) screens children from 2½ years to 2 years and 11 months of age and even is reliable with cooperative toddlers as young as 2 years of age. The test contains seven cards of familiar objects (birthday cake, teddy bear, tree, house, car, telephone, and horse and rider). First, show the pictures up close to the child to make sure the child can identify them. Then, present each picture at a distance of 15 ft. Results are normal if the child can name three out of seven cards within three to five trials.

Use a picture chart or the Snellen E chart for the preschooler from 3 to 6 years of age. The E chart shows the capital letter E in varying sizes pointing in different directions. The child points his or her fingers in the direction the "table legs" are pointing. By age 7 to 8 years of age when the child is familiar with reading letters, begin to use the standard Snellen alphabet chart. Normally, a child achieves 20/20 acuity by 6 to 7 years of age (Fig. 12–27).

The National Society for Prevention of Blindness states these criteria for referral:

1. Age 3—vision 20/50 or less in either eye.
2. Age 4 and over—20/40 or less in either eye.
3. Difference between two eyes is one line or more.
4. Child shows other signs of vision impairment, regardless of acuity.

Screen two separate times before referral.

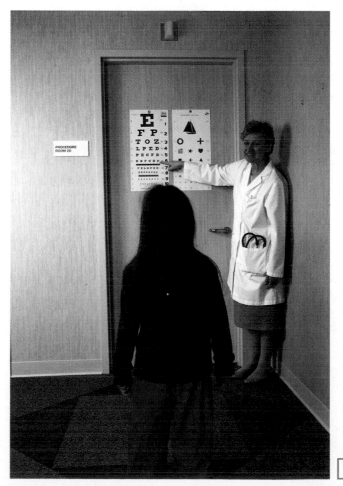

12–27

|

Visual Fields

Assess peripheral vision with the confrontation test in children older than 3 years when the preschooler is able to stay in position. As with the adult, the child should see the moving target at the same time your normal eyes do. Often a young child forgets to say "now" or "stop" as the moving object is seen. Rather, note the instant the child's eyes deviate or head shifts position to gaze at the moving object. Match this nearly automatic response with your own sighting.

Color Vision

Color blindness is an inherited recessive X-linked trait affecting about 8 percent of white males and 4 percent of black males. It is rare in females (0.4 percent). "Color deficient" is a more accurate term, because the condition is relative and not disabling. Often, it is just a social inconvenience, although it may affect the person's ability to discern traffic lights, or it may affect school performance in which color is a learning tool.

Test only boys for color vision, once between the ages of 4 and 8. Use Ishihara's test, a series of polychromatic cards. Each card has a pattern of dots printed against a background of many colored dots. Ask the child to identify each pattern. A boy with normal color vision can see each pattern. A color blind person cannot see the letter against the field color.

Extraocular Muscle Function

Testing for **strabismus** (squint, crossed eye) is an important screening measure to perform during early childhood. Strabismus causes disconjugate vision because one eye deviates off the fixation point. To avoid diplopia or unclear images, the brain begins to suppress data from the weak eye (a suppression scotoma). Then, visual acuity in this otherwise normal eye begins to deteriorate from disuse. Early recognition and treatment are essential to restore binocular vision. Diagnosis after age 6 years has a poor prognosis. Test malalignment by the corneal light reflex and the cover test.

Check the **corneal light reflex** by shining a light toward the child's eyes. The light should be reflected at exactly the same spot in the two corneas (see Fig. 12–33 on p. 328). Some asymmetry (where one light falls off center) under age 6 months is normal.

Perform the **cover test** on all children as described on p. 310. Some examiners omit the opaque card and place their hand on the child's head. The examiner's thumb extends down and blocks vision over the eye without actually touching the eye. One can use a familiar character puppet to attract the child's attention. The normal results are the same as those listed in the adult section.

Function of the extraocular muscles during movement can be assessed during the early weeks by the child's following a brightly colored toy as a target. An older infant can sit on the parent's lap as you move the toy in all directions. After age 2 years, direct the child's gaze through the six cardinal positions of gaze. You may stabilize the child's chin with your hand to prevent him or her from moving the entire head.

External Eye Structures

Inspect the ocular structures as described in the earlier section. A neonate usually holds the eyes tightly shut. Do not attempt to pry them open; that just increases contraction of the orbicularis oculi muscle. Hold the newborn supine

Untreated strabismus can lead to permanent visual damage. The resulting loss of vision due to disuse is **amblyopia ex anopsia.**

Asymmetry in the corneal light reflex after 6 months is abnormal and must be referred.

► **Normal Range of Findings**   **Abnormal Findings**

and gently lower the head; the eyes will open. Also the eyes will open when you hold the infant at arm's length and slowly turn the infant in one direction (Fig. 12–28). In addition to inspecting the ocular structures, this also tests the vestibular function reflex. That is, the baby's eyes will look in the same direction as the body is being turned. When the turning stops, the eyes will shift to the opposite direction after a few quick beats of nystagmus. Also termed "doll's eyes," this reflex disappears by 2 months of age.

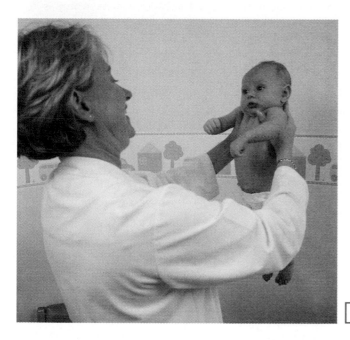

12–28

Eyelids and Lashes. Normally, the upper lids overlie the superior part of the iris. In newborns, the *setting-sun sign* is common. The eyes appear to deviate down, and you see a white rim of sclera over the iris. It may show as you rapidly change the neonate from a sitting to a supine position.

Many infants have an *epicanthal fold,* an excess skinfold extending over the inner corner of the eye, partly or totally overlapping the inner canthus. It occurs frequently in Asian children and in 20 percent of whites. In non-Asians it disappears as the child grows, usually by age 10 years. While they are present, epicanthal folds give a false appearance of malalignment, termed **pseudostrabismus** (Fig. 12–29). Yet the corneal light reflex is normal.

The setting-sun sign also occurs with hydrocephalus as the globes protrude.

Blank sunken eyes accompany malnutrition, dehydration, and a severe illness.

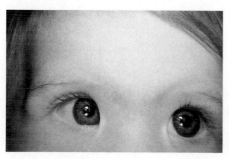

12–29

Pseudostrabismus

Normal Range of Findings

Abnormal Findings

Asian infants normally have an upward slant of the palpebral fissures. Entropion, a turning inward of the eyelid, is found normally in some Asian children. If the lashes do not abrade the corneas, it is not significant.

Conjunctiva and Sclera. A newborn may have a transient chemical conjunctivitis due to the instillation of silver nitrate. This appears within 1 hour and lasts not more than 24 hours after birth. The sclera should be white and clear, although it may have a blue tint due to thinness at birth. The lacrimal glands are not functional at birth.

Iris and Pupils. The iris normally is blue or slate gray in light-skinned newborns and brown in dark-skinned infants. By 6 to 9 months, the permanent color is differentiated. Brushfield's spots, or white specks around the edge of the iris, occasionally may be normal.

A searching nystagmus is common just after birth. The pupils are small but constrict to light.

The Ocular Fundus

The amount of data gathered during the funduscopic examination depends on the child's ability to hold the eyes still and on your ability to glean as much data as possible in a brief period of time.

A complete funduscopic examination is difficult to perform on an infant, but at least check the red reflex when the infant fixates at the bright light for a few seconds. Note any interruption.

Perform a funduscopic examination on an infant between 2 and 6 months of age. Position the infant (up to 18 months) lying on the table.

The fundus appears pale, and the vessels are not fully developed. There is no foveal light reflection because the macula area will not be mature until 1 year.

Inspect the fundus of the young child and school-age child as described in the adult section. Allow the child to handle the equipment. Explain why you are darkening the room and that you will leave a small light on. Assure the child that the procedure will not hurt. Direct the young child to look at an appealing picture, perhaps Mickey Mouse or an animal, during the examination.

The Aging Adult

Visual Acuity

Perform the same examination as described in the adult section. Central acuity may decrease, particularly after age 70. Peripheral vision may be diminished.

Mongolian slant—An upward lateral slope together with epicanthal folds and hypertelorism (large spacing between the eyes) occurs with Down syndrome.

Ophthalmia neonatorum (conjunctivitis of the newborn) is a purulent discharge due to a chemical irritant or a bacterial or viral agent acquired from the birth canal.

Absence of iris color occurs with albinism.

The occurrence of Brushfield's spots usually suggests Down syndrome.

Constant nystagmus, prolonged setting-sun sign, marked strabismus, and slow lateral movements suggest vision loss.

An interruption in the red reflex indicates an opacity in the cornea or lens. An absent red reflex occurs with congenital cataracts or retinal disorders.

Papilledema is rare in the infant because the fontanels and open sutures will absorb any increased intracranial pressure if it occurs.

▶ | Normal Range of Findings | | Abnormal Findings

Ocular Structures

The eyebrows may show a loss of the outer one-third to one-half of hair due to a decrease in hair follicles. The remaining brow hair is coarse (Fig. 12–30). Owing to atrophy of elastic tissues, the skin around the eyes may show wrinkles or crow's feet. The upper lid may be so elongated as to rest on the lashes, resulting in a pseudoptosis.

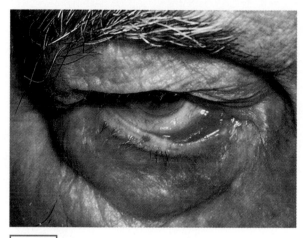

12–30

The eyes may appear sunken owing to atrophy of the orbital fat. Also, the orbital fat may herniate, causing bulging at the lower lids and inner third of the upper lids.

Atrophy of elastic and fibrous tissues may cause the lower lid to drop away from the globe, or **ectropion.** This compromises the globe structures because the tears cannot drain into the out-turned puncta. Alternately, **entropion,** or a turning inward of the lower lid, may irritate the eye from friction of lashes.

The lacrimal apparatus may decrease tear production, causing the eyes to look dry and lusterless and the person to report a burning sensation. **Pingueculae** commonly show on the sclera (Fig. 12–31). These yellowish elevated nodules are due to a thickening of the bulbar conjunctiva from prolonged exposure to sun, wind, and dust. Pingueculae appear at the 3 and 9 o'clock positions, first on the nasal side, then on the temporal side.

See ectropion and entropion (Table 12–3).

Distinguish from the abnormal **pterygium,** also an opacity on the bulbar conjunctiva, but one that grows over the cornea (see Table 12–6).

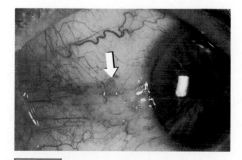

12–31

Pinguecula

The cornea may look cloudy with age. An **arcus senilis** commonly is seen around the cornea (Fig. 12–32). This is a gray-white arc or circle around the limbus and is due to deposition of lipid material. As more lipid accumulates, the cornea may look thickened and raised, but the arcus has no effect on vision.

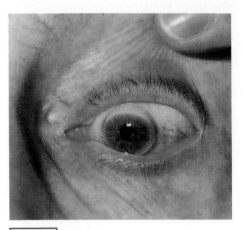

12–32

Arcus senilis

Xanthelasma are soft, raised yellow plaques occurring on the lids at the inner canthus (Fig. 12–33). They commonly occur around the fifth decade of life and more frequently in women. They occur with both high and normal blood levels of cholesterol and have no pathologic significance.

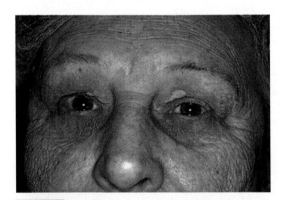

12–33

Xanthelasma

Pupils are small in old age, and the pupillary light reflex may be slowed. The lens loses transparency and looks opaque.

The Ocular Fundus

Retinal structures generally have less shine. The blood vessels look paler, narrower, and attenuated. Arterioles appear paler and straighter, with a narrower light reflex. More arteriovenous crossing defects occur.

Normal Range of Findings

Abnormal Findings

A normal development on the retinal surface is **drusen,** or benign degenerative hyaline deposits (Fig. 12–34). They are small, round, yellow dots that are scattered haphazardly on the retina. Although they do not occur in a pattern, they are usually symmetrically placed in the two eyes. They have no effect on vision.

Drusen are easily confused with the abnormal finding, *hard exudates* (see Table 12–11).

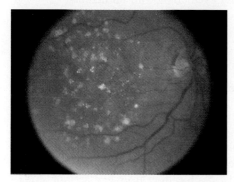

12–34

Drusen

 SUMMARY CHECKLIST: Eye Exam

1: Test visual acuity
Snellen eye chart
Near vision (those older than 40 years or those having difficulty reading)

2: Test visual fields— confrontation test

3: Inspect extraocular muscle function
Corneal light reflex (Hirschberg test)
Cover test
Diagnostic positions test

4: Inspect external eye structures
General
Eyebrows
Eyelids and lashes
Eyeball alignment
Conjunctiva and sclera
Lacrimal apparatus

5: Inspect anterior eyeball structures
Cornea and lens
Iris and pupil
    Size, shape, and equality
    Pupillary light reflex
    Accommodation

6: Inspect the ocular fundus
Optic disc (color, shape, margins, cup-disc ratio)
Retinal vessels (number, color, artery-vein [A:V] ratio, caliber, arteriovenous crossings, tortuosity, pulsations)
General background (color, integrity)
Macula

APPLICATION AND CRITICAL THINKING

SAMPLE CHARTING

Subjective

Vision reported good with no recent change. No eye pain, no inflammation, no discharge, no lesions. Wears no corrective lenses, vision last tested 1 year PTA, test for glaucoma at that time was normal.

Continued

Objective

Snellen chart—O.D. 20/20, O.S. 20/20 −1. Fields normal by confrontation. Corneal light reflex symmetric bilaterally. Diagnostic positions test shows EOMs intact. Brows and lashes present. No ptosis. Conjunctiva clear. Sclera white. No lesions. PERRLA.

Fundi: Red reflex present bilaterally. Discs flat with sharp margins. Vessels present in all quadrants without crossing defects. Retinal background has even color with no hemorrhages or exudates. Macula has even color.

CLINICAL CASE STUDY 1

Emma K. is a 34-year-old married, white, female homemaker, brought to the Emergency Department by police following a reported domestic quarrel.

Subjective

States husband struck her about the face and eyes with his fists about 1 hour PTA. "I ruined the dinner again. I can't do anything right." Pain in left cheek and both eyes felt immediately and continues. Alarmed at "bright red blood on eyeball." No bleeding from eye area or cheek. Vision intact just after trauma. Now reports difficulty opening lids.

Objective

Sitting quietly and hunched over, hands over eyes. Voice tired and flat. L cheek swollen and discolored, no laceration. Lids edematous and discolored both eyes. No skin laceration. L lid swollen almost shut. L eye—round 1-mm bright red patch over lateral aspect of globe. No active bleeding out of eye, iris intact, anterior chamber clear. R eye—conjunctiva clear, sclera white, cornea and iris intact, anterior chamber clear. PERRLA, Pupils R $\frac{4}{1}$ = $\frac{4}{1}$ L. Vision $\frac{14}{14}$ both eyes by Jaeger card.

ASSESSMENT

Ecchymoses L cheek and both eyes
Subconjunctival hemorrhage L eye
Pain R/T inflammation
Self-esteem disturbance R/T effects of domestic violence

CLINICAL CASE STUDY 2

Sam T. is a 63-year-old married, white, male postal carrier admitted to the Medical Center for surgery for suspected brain tumor. Following postanesthesia recovery, Sam T. is admitted to the Neuro ICU, awake, lethargic with slowed but correct verbal responses, oriented × 3, moving all four extremities, vital signs stable. Pupils R $\frac{4}{2}$ = $\frac{4}{2}$ L with sluggish response. Assessments are made q 15 minutes.

Subjective

No response now to verbal stimuli.

Objective

Semi-comatose—no response to verbal stimuli, does withdraw R arm and leg purposefully to painful stimuli. No movement L arm or leg. Pupils R $\frac{5}{5}$ ≠ L $\frac{4}{2}$. Vitals remain stable as noted on graphic sheet.

ASSESSMENT

Unilateral dilated and fixed R pupil
Clouding of consciousness
Focal motor deficit—no movement L side
Altered tissue perfusion: cerebral R/T interruption of flow

CLINICAL CASE STUDY 3

Trung Q. is a 4-year-old male born in Southeast Asia, who arrived in this country 1 month PTA. Lives with parents, 2 siblings. Speaks only native language, here with uncle to act as interpreter.

▶ Subjective

Seeks care because RN in church sponsoring family noted "crossed eyes." Uncle states vision seemed normal to parents. Plays with toys and manipulates small objects without difficulty. Identifies objects in picture books, does not read.

▶ Objective

With uncle interpreting directions for test to Trung, vision by Snellen E chart—O.D. 20/30, O.S. 20/50 −1. Fields seem intact by confrontation—jerks head to gaze at object entering field.

EOMs—asymmetric corneal light reflex with outward deviation L eye. Cover test—as R eye covered, L eye jerks to fixate, R eye steady when uncovered. As L eye covered, R eye holds steady gaze, L eye jerks to fixate as uncovered. Diagnostic positions—able to gaze in six positions, although L eye obviously malaligned at extreme medial gaze.

Eye structures—brows and lashes present and normal bilaterally. Upward palpebral slant, epicanthal folds bilaterally—consistent with racial heritage. Conjunctiva clear, sclera white, iris intact, PERRLA.

Fundi—discs flat with sharp margins. Observed vessels normal. Unable to see in all four quadrants, unable to see macular area.

▶ ASSESSMENT

L exotropia
Abnormal vision in L eye
Sensory/perceptual alteration: visual R/T effects of neurologic impairment

CLINICAL CASE STUDY 4

Vera K. is an 87-year-old widowed, black, female homemaker, living independently, who is admitted to hospital for observation and adjustment of digitalis medication. Cardiac status has been stable during hospital stay.

▶ Subjective

Reports desire to monitor own medication at home but fears problems owing to blurred vision. First noted distant vision blurred 5 years ago but near vision seemed to improve at that time, "I started to read better without my glasses!" Since then, blurring at distant vision has increased, near vision now blurred also.

Able to navigate home environment without difficulty. Fixes simple meals with cold foods. Receives hot meal from "Meals on Wheels" at lunch. Enjoys television, though it looks somewhat blurred. Unable to write letters, sew, or read paper, which she regrets.

▶ Objective

Vision by Jaeger card O.D. 20/200. O.S. 20/400−1, with glasses on. Fields intact by confrontation. EOMs intact. Brow hair absent lateral third. Upper lids have folds of redundant skin but lids do not droop. Lower lids and lashes intact. Xanthelasma present both inner canthi. Conjunctiva clear, sclera white, iris intact, L pupil looks cloudy, PERRLA, pupils R ½ = ½ L.

Fundi: Red reflex has central dark spot both eyes. Discs flat, with sharp margins. Observed vessels normal. Unable to see in all four quadrants or macular area owing to small pupils.

Continued

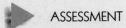

ASSESSMENT

Central opacity, both eyes
Central visual acuity deficit, both eyes
Diversional activity deficit R/T poor vision

NURSING DIAGNOSES COMMONLY ASSOCIATED WITH THE EYES AND VISUAL DISORDERS

Diagnosis	Related Factors (Etiology)	Defining Characteristics (Symptoms and Signs)

Sensory/perceptual alterations: visual	Restriction of head/neck motion
	Effects of
	   Aging
	   Stress
	   Neurologic impairment
	Failure to use protective eye devices
	Improper use of contact lens
	Difficulty in adjusting to corrective lens
	Persistent visual stimulation
		Headache
		Blurring
		Spots
		Double vision
		Excessive tearing
		Inflammation
		Lack of blink or corneal reflex
		Squinting
		Holding objects too close or at a distance for viewing
		Colliding with objects
		Abnormal results of vision testing

Diversional activity deficit	Effects of chronic illness Physical limitations Poor vision Social isolation Decreased economic resources Confined to bedrest Preoccupation with job	Restlessness Napping during day Apathy or hostility Complaints of boredom Verbalizes desire for activity Inability to participate in usual activities or hobbies because of physical limitations Depression Preoccupation with self Weight loss or gain
Impaired home maintenance management	Impaired mental status Effects of chronic debilitating disease (loss of vision) Inadequate support system Substance abuse Depression Lack of knowledge Lack of motivation Decreased financial resources	Offensive odors Presence of rodents or vermin Accumulation of dirt, food, dirty laundry, or hygienic wastes Reports by patient or family of difficulty maintaining home in comfortable fashion Inappropriate room temperature Lack of necessary equipment

Other Related Nursing Diagnoses

ACTUAL	RISK/WELLNESS
Anxiety Pain Self-care deficit Social isolation	**Risk** Risk for injury **Wellness** Progressive adjustment to vision changes Participating in satisfying activities

 ## ASSESSMENT VIDEO CRITICAL THINKING QUESTIONS

The Saunders *Physical Examination and Health Assessment* video series Head, Eyes, and Ears—will direct you to consider the following:

1. In addition to the screening vision test using the Snellen eye chart, what other vision tests could you use and why would you use them?

2. Describe the following abnormal findings, which may be found during inspection of the eyelids: exophthalmos, ptosis, ectropion, hordeolum, chalazion, and carcinoma.

▼ **Table 12–1 VISUAL FIELD LOSS**

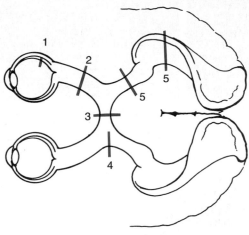

1. **Retinal damage**
   - Macula—central blind area, e.g., diabetes:

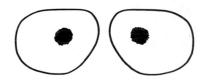

   - Localized damage—blind spot (scotoma) corresponding to particular area:

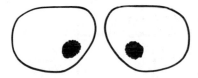

   - Increasing intraocular pressure—decrease in peripheral vision, e.g., glaucoma. Starts with paracentral scotoma in early stage:

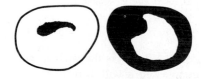

   - Retinal detachment. Person has shadow or diminished vision in one quadrant or one-half visual field:

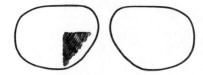

2. **Lesion in globe or optic nerve.**
   Injury here yields one blind eye, or unilateral blindness:

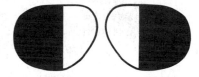

3. **Lesion at optic chiasm** (e.g., pituitary tumor)—Injury to crossing fibers only yields a loss of nasal part of each retina and a loss of both temporal visual fields. Bitemporal (heteronymous) hemianopsia:

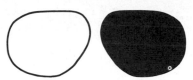

4. **Lesion of outer uncrossed fibers at optic chiasm,** e.g., aneurysm of left internal carotid artery exerts pressure on uncrossed fibers. Injury yields left nasal hemianopsia:

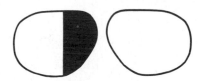

5. **Lesion R optic tract or R optic radiation.**
   Visual field loss in R nasal and L temporal fields. Loss of same half visual field in both eyes is homonymous hemianopsia:

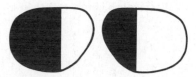

▼ Table 12–2   EXTRAOCULAR MUSCLE DYSFUNCTION

CORNEAL LIGHT REFLEX

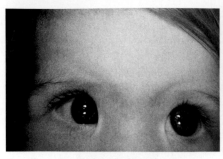

A   Pseudostrabismus

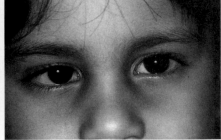

B   R Esotropia

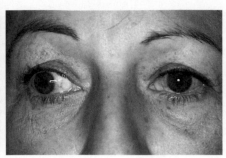

C   R Exotropia

Symmetric Corneal Light Reflex

A. **Pseudostrabismus** has the appearance of strabismus due to epicanthic fold but is normal for a young child.

Asymmetric Corneal Light Reflex

Strabismus is true disparity of the eye axes. This constant malalignment is also termed tropia and is likely to cause amblyopia.

B. Esotropia—inward turn of the eye.

C. Exotropia—outward turn of the eye.

COVER TEST

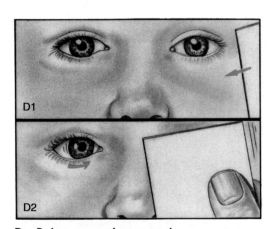

D   Right, uncovered eye is weaker

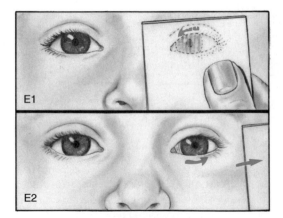

E   Left, covered eye is weaker

D. Uncovered eye—If it jumps to fixate on designated point, it was out of alignment before (i.e., when you cover the stronger eye, the weaker eye now tries to fixate).

Phoria—mild weakness, apparent only with the cover test and less likely to cause amblyopia than a tropia but still possible.

E. Covered eye—If this is the weaker eye, once macular image is suppressed it will drift to relaxed position.

As eye is uncovered—If it jumps to re-establish fixation, weakness exists.

Esophoria—nasal (inward) drift.

Exophoria—temporal (outward) drift.

Table 12-2 EXTRAOCULAR MUSCLE DYSFUNCTION *Continued*

DIAGNOSTIC POSITIONS TEST

(Paralysis apparent during movement through six cardinal positions of gaze.)

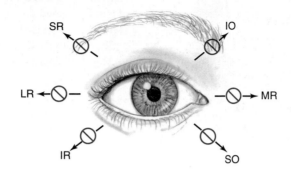

If eye will not turn:	Indicates paralysis in:	or cranial nerve
Straight nasal	Medial rectus	III
Up and nasal	Inferior oblique	III
Up and temporal	Superior rectus	III
Straight temporal	Lateral rectus	VI
Down and temporal	Inferior rectus	III
Down and nasal	Superior oblique	IV

 Table 12-3 ABNORMALITIES IN THE EYELIDS

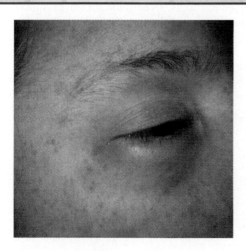

◀ **Periorbital Edema**

Lids are swollen and puffy. Lid tissues are loosely connected so excess fluid is easily apparent. This occurs with local infections, crying, and systemic conditions such as congestive heart failure, renal failure, allergy, hypothyroidism (myxedema).

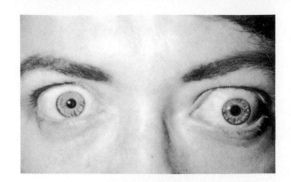

Exophthalmos (Protruding Eyes)

Exophthalmos is a forward displacement of the eyeballs and widened palpebral fissures. Note "lid lag," the upper lid rests well above the limbus and white sclera is visible. Acquired bilateral exophthalmos is associated with thyrotoxicosis.

Enophthalmos (Sunken Eyes) (not illustrated)

A look of narrowed palpebral fissures shows with enophthalmos, in which the eyeballs are recessed. Bilateral enophthalmos is caused by loss of fat in the orbits and occurs with dehydration and chronic wasting illnesses. For illustration, see Cachexia in Table 11–5.

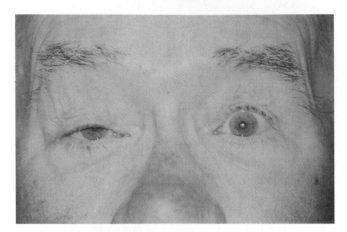

Ptosis (Drooping Upper Lid)

Ptosis occurs from neuromuscular weakness (e.g., myasthenia gravis with bilateral fatigue as the day progresses), oculomotor cranial nerve III damage, or sympathetic nerve damage (e.g., Horner's syndrome). It is a positional defect that gives the person a sleepy appearance and impairs vision.

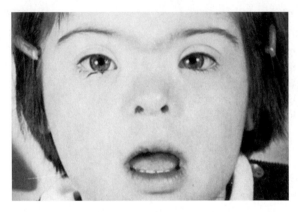

Upward Palpebral Slant

Although normal in many children, when combined with epicanthal folds, hypertelorism (large spacing between the eyes), and Brushfield spots (light-colored areas in outer iris) indicates Down syndrome.

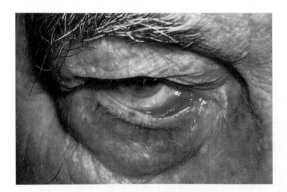

Ectropion

The lower lid is loose and rolling out, does not approximate to eyeball. Puncta cannot siphon tears effectively so excess tearing results. The eyes feel dry and itchy because the tears do not drain correctly over the corner and toward the medial canthus. Exposed palpebral conjunctiva increases risk for inflammation. Occurs most often in aging adults but may result from trauma.

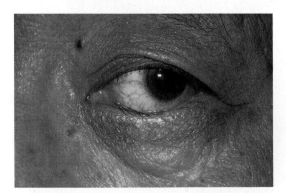

Entropion

The lower lid rolls in due to spasm of lids or scar tissue contracting. Constant rubbing of lashes may irritate cornea. The person feels a "foreign body" sensation.

Table 12-4   LESIONS ON THE EYELIDS

ABNORMAL FINDINGS

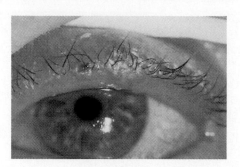

Blepharitis (Inflammation of the Eyelids)

Red, scaly, greasy flakes and thickened, crusted lid margins occur with staphylococcal infection or seborrheic dermatitis of the lid edge. Symptoms include burning, itching, tearing, foreign body sensation, and some pain.

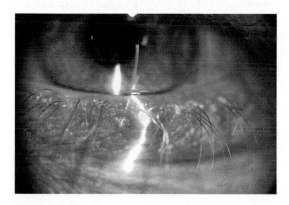

Hordeolum (Stye)

Hordeolum is a localized staphylococcal infection of the hair follicles at the lid margin. It is painful, red, and swollen—a pustule at the lid margin. Rubbing the eyes can cause cross-contamination and development of another stye.

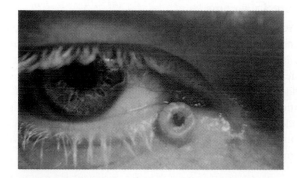

Basal Cell Carcinoma

Carcinoma is rare, but it occurs most often on the lower lid and medial canthus. It looks like a papule with an ulcerated center. Note the rolled-out pearly edges. Metastasis is rare but should be referred for removal.

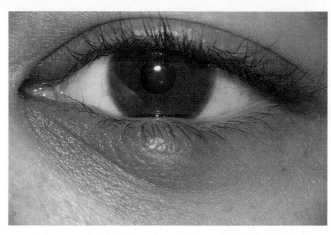

Chalazion

A beady nodule protruding on the lid, chalazion is an infection or retention cyst of a meibomian gland. It is a nontender, firm, discrete swelling with freely movable skin overlying the nodule. If it becomes inflamed, it points inside and not on lid margin (in contrast with stye).

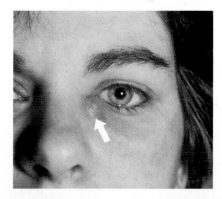

Dacryocystitis (Inflammation of the Lacrimal Sac)

Dacryocystitis is infection and blockage of sac and duct. Pain, warmth, redness, and swelling occur below the inner canthus toward nose. Tearing is present. Pressure on sac yields purulent discharge from puncta.

Dacryoadenitis (Inflammation of the Lacrimal Gland) (not illustrated)

Dacryoadenitis is an infection of the lacrimal gland. Pain, swelling, and redness occur in the outer third of upper lid. It occurs with mumps, measles, and infectious mononucleosis, or from trauma.

337

▼ Table 12-5 VASCULAR DISORDERS OF THE EXTERNAL EYE

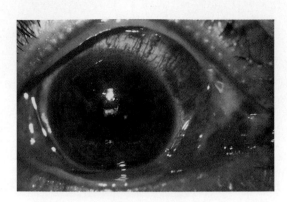

Conjunctivitis

Infection of the conjunctiva, "pink eye," has red beefy-looking vessels at periphery but usually looks clearer around iris (although here it is severe). This is a common disorder due to bacterial or viral infection, allergy, or chemical irritation. Purulent discharge accompanies bacterial infection. Preauricular lymph node is often swollen and painful. Often, the person has a history of an upper respiratory infection. Symptoms include itching, burning, foreign body sensation, and eyelids stuck together on awakening in the morning.

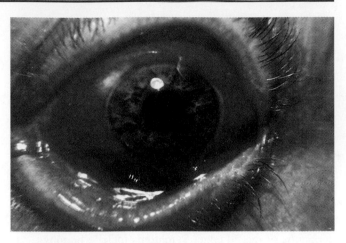

Subconjunctival Hemorrhage

A red patch on the sclera, subconjunctival hemorrhage looks alarming but is usually not serious. The red patch has sharp edges like a spot of paint, although here it is extensive. It occurs from increased intraocular pressure from coughing, sneezing, weight lifting, labor during childbirth, straining at stool, or trauma.

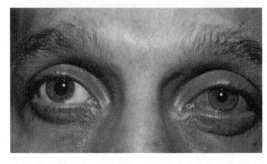

Iritis (Circumcorneal Redness)

Deep dull red halo around the iris and cornea. Note red is around iris, in contrast with conjunctivitis, in which redness is more prominent at the periphery. Pupil shape may be irregular from swelling of iris. Person also has marked photophobia, constricted pupil, blurred vision, and throbbing pain. Warrants immediate referral.

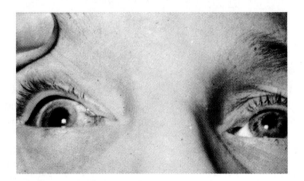

Acute Glaucoma

Acute, narrow-angle glaucoma shows a circumcorneal redness with a dilated pupil. The redness radiates around the iris. Pupil is oval, dilated, and cornea looks "steamy." Anterior chamber is shallow. Acute glaucoma occurs with sudden increase in intraocular pressure due to blocked outflow from anterior chamber. The person experiences a sudden clouding of vision, sudden eye pain, and halos around lights. This requires emergency treatment to avoid permanent vision loss.

▼ Table 12–6 ABNORMALITIES ON THE CORNEA AND IRIS

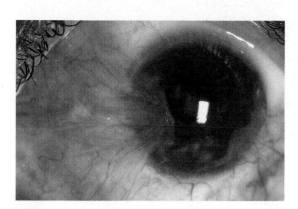

Pterygium

A triangular opaque wing of bulbar conjunctiva grows toward the center of the cornea. It usually invades from nasal side, and it may obstruct vision as it covers pupil. Occurs usually from chronic exposure to hot, dry, sandy climate, which stimulates the growth of a pinguecula into a pterygium.

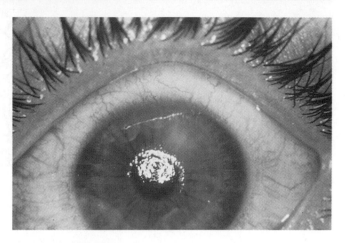

Corneal Abrasion

Irregular ridges are usually visible only when fluorescein stain reveals yellow-green branching. Top layer of corneal epithelium removed. A common disorder from scratches or poorly fitting or overworn contact lenses. Because the area is rich in nerve endings, the person feels intense pain, a foreign body sensation, and lacrimation, redness, and photophobia.

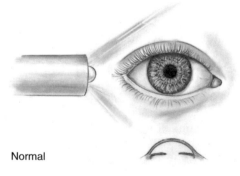

Normal

Normal Anterior Chamber (for Contrast)

A light directed across the eye from the temporal side illuminates the entire iris evenly because the normal iris is flat and creates no shadow.

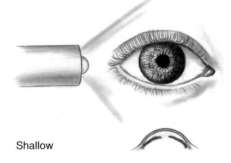

Shallow

Shallow Anterior Chamber

The iris is pushed anteriorly because of increased intraocular pressure. Because direct light is received from the temporal side, only the temporal part of iris is illuminated; the nasal side is shadowed, the "shadow sign." This may be a sign of acute angle-closure glaucoma.

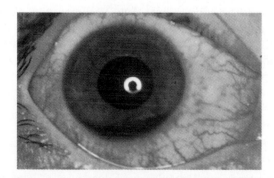

Hyphema

Blood in anterior chamber is a serious result of trauma or spontaneous hemorrhage. Suspect scleral rupture or major intraocular trauma. Note that gravity settles blood.

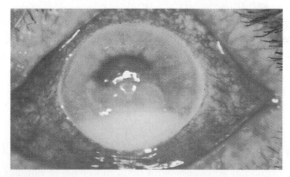

Hypopyon

Purulent matter in anterior chamber occurs with iritis, and inflammation in the anterior chamber.

Table 12-7 ABNORMALITIES IN THE PUPIL

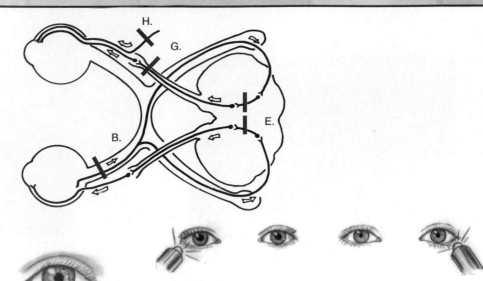

A. Unequal Pupil Size—Anisocoria

Although this exists normally in 5 percent of the population, consider central nervous system disease.

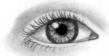
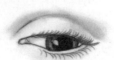

B. Monocular Blindness

When light is directed to the blind eye, no response occurs in either eye. When light is directed to normal eye, both pupils constrict (direct and consensual response to light) as long as the oculomotor nerve is intact.

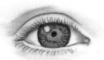

C. Constricted and Fixed Pupils—Miosis

Miosis occurs with the use of pilocarpine drops for glaucoma treatment, the use of narcotics, with iritis, and with brain damage of pons.

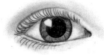

D. Dilated and Fixed Pupils—Mydriasis

Enlarged pupils occur with stimulation of the sympathetic nervous system, reaction to sympathomimetic drugs, use of dilating drops, acute glaucoma, past or recent trauma. Also, they herald central nervous system injury, circulatory arrest, or deep anesthesia.

E. Argyll Robertson Pupil

No reaction to light, pupil does constrict with accommodation. Small and irregular bilaterally. Argyll Robertson pupil occurs with central nervous system syphilis, brain tumor, meningitis, and chronic alcoholism.

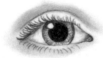

F. Tonic Pupil (Adie's Pupil)

Sluggish reaction to light and accommodation. Tonic pupil is usually unilateral, a large regular pupil that does react, but sluggishly after long latent time. No pathologic significance.

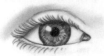

G. Cranial Nerve III Damage

Unilateral dilated pupil with no reaction to light or accommodation, occurs with oculomotor nerve damage. May also have ptosis with eye deviating down and laterally.

H. Horner's Syndrome

Unilateral, small, regular pupil does react to light and accommodation. Occurs with Horner's syndrome, a lesion of the sympathetic nerve. Also, note ptosis and absence of sweat (anhidrosis) on same side.

340

▼ Table 12-8 OPACITIES IN THE LENS

Senile Cataracts

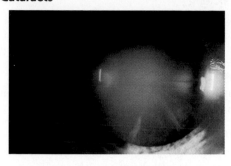

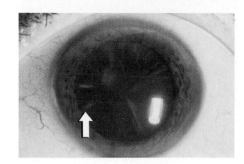

Central Gray Opacity—Nuclear Cataract

Nuclear cataract shows as an opaque gray surrounded by black background as it forms in the center of lens nucleus. Through the ophthalmoscope, it looks like a black center against the red reflex. It begins after age 40 and develops slowly, gradually obstructing vision.

Star-Shaped Opacity—Cortical Cataract

Cortical cataract shows as asymmetrical, radial, white spokes with black center. Through ophthalmoscope, black spokes are evident against the red reflex. This forms in outer cortex of lens, progressing faster than nuclear cataract.

▼ Table 12-9 ABNORMALITIES IN THE OPTIC DISC

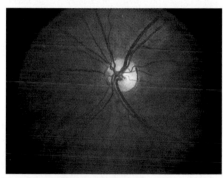

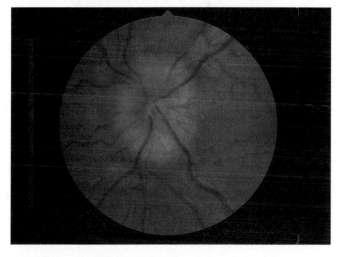

Optic Atrophy (Disc Pallor)

Optic atrophy is a white or gray color of the disc due to partial or complete death of the optic nerve. This results in decreased visual acuity, decreased color vision, and decreased contrast sensitivity.

Papilledema (Choked Disc)

Increased intracranial pressure causes venous stasis in the globe, showing redness, congestion, and elevation of the disc, blurred margins, hemorrhages, and absent venous pulsations. This is a serious sign of intracranial pressure, usually caused by a space-occupying mass, e.g., a brain tumor or hematoma. Visual acuity is not affected.

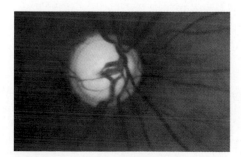 ◀ #### Excessive Cup-Disc Ratio

With primary, open-angle glaucoma, the increased intraocular pressure decreases blood supply to retinal structures. The physiologic cup enlarges to more than ½ of the disc diameter, vessels appear to plunge over edge of cup, and the vessels are displaced nasally. This is asymptomatic, although the person may experience decreased vision or visual field defects in the late stages of glaucoma.

Table 12–10   ABNORMALITIES IN THE RETINAL VESSELS

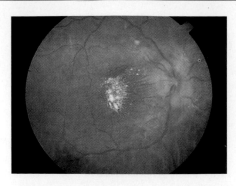

Arteriovenous Crossing

Arteriovenous crossing with interruption of blood flow. When vein is occluded, it dilates distal to crossing. This person also has disc edema and hard exudates in a macular star pattern that occur with malignant hypertension.

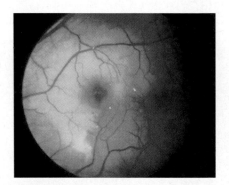

Narrowed Arteries

This is a generalized decrease in diameter. The light reflex also narrows. It occurs with severe hypertension, occlusion of central retinal artery, and retinitis pigmentosa.

Vessel Nicking

Nicking is a localized narrowing in vein caused by arteriole crossing. It is seen with hypertension and arteriosclerosis.

Silverwire Arteries

With hypertension, the arteriole wall thickens and becomes opaque so that no blood is seen inside it.

Copperwire Arteries

The light reflex widens, showing a metallic copper color. This is seen with hypertension.

Table 12–11   ABNORMALITIES IN THE GENERAL BACKGROUND

Diabetic Retinopathy

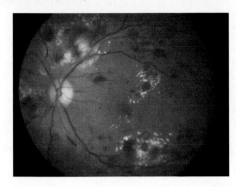

Microaneurysms

Microaneurysms are round punctate red dots that are localized dilatations of a small vessel. Their edges are smooth and discrete. The vessel itself is too small to view with the ophthalmoscope; only the isolated red dots are seen. This occurs with diabetes.

Dot-Shaped Hemorrhages

Deep intraretinal hemorrhages look splattered on. These occur with diabetes. They may be distinguished from microaneurysms by the blurred irregular edges.

Flame-Shaped Hemorrhages

Flame-shaped hemorrhages are superficial retinal hemorrhages that look linear and spindle shaped. They occur with hypertension.

Soft Exudates

"Cotton wool" areas look like fluffy gray-white cumulus clouds. They are arteriolar microinfarctions that envelop and obscure the vessels. They occur with diabetes, hypertension, subacute bacterial endocarditis, lupus, and papilledema of any cause.

Hard Exudates

These are numerous small yellow-white spots, having distinct edges and a smooth, solid-looking surface (illustrated in figure with microaneurysms on this page). They often form a circular pattern, clustered around a venous microinfarction. They also may form a linear or star pattern. (This is in contrast with the normal drusen, which have a scattered haphazard location [see Fig. 12–34].)

Bibliography

Bartunek CK, Brodell LP, Brodell RT: The skin and the eye: A multidisciplinary approach. Derm Nurs 8(4):263–284, Aug 1996.

Bedrossian E: Treatment of hordeolums: Styes and chalazia. Hosp Med 33(3):59–64, Mar 1997.

Boyd-Monk H: Improving the outlook for diagnosing visual disorders: Genes on the move. J Ophthalmol Nurs Tech 16(5):225–226, Sep–Oct 1997.

Carr L: Case history: Cornerstone in the neuro-ophthalmic examination. Optom Clin 5(3/4):17–32, 1996.

Coody D, Banks JM, Yetman RJ, Musgrove K: Eye trauma in children: Epidemiology, management, and prevention. J Pediatr Health Care 11(4):182–188, July–Aug 1997.

Easterbrook M, Johnston RH, Howcroft MJ: Assessment and management of ocular foreign bodies. Physician Sports Med 25(2):76–94, Feb 1997.

Friedman NJ, Pineda R, Kaiser PK: The Massachusetts Eye and Ear Infirmary Illustrated Manual of Ophthalmology. Philadelphia, W.B. Saunders Company, 1998.

Gaasterland DE, Ederer F, Sullivan K, et al: The advanced glaucoma intervention study (AGIS): 4. Comparison of treatment outcomes within race. Ophthalmology 105(7):1146–1164, July 1998.

Galant JJ: Differential diagnosis of decreased vision: A case study. J Am Acad Nurs Pract 9(9):421–425, Sep 1997.

Ghafouri A, Burgess SK, Hrdlicka AK, Zagelbaum BM: Air-bag related ocular trauma. Am J Emerg Med 15(4):389–392, July 1997.

Goldberg M: The diagnostic challenge. Emerg Med 29(9):34–39, Sep 1997.

Hartnett ME: Ocular complications of diabetes mellitus: Diagnosis, current management, and laboratory evaluation. Clin Lab Science 9(2):96–100, Mar–Apr 1996.

Heffner D: Allergic conjunctivitis. Lippincott's Primary Care Pract 1(2):217–219, May–June 1997.

Kane RT, Ouslander JG, Abrass IB: Essentials of Clinical Geriatrics, 3rd ed. New York, McGraw-Hill, 1994.

Kearney KM: Retinal detachment. Am J Nurs 97(8):50, Aug 1997.

Kingston L, Reynolds D, Phillips LP: Comprehensive assessment of the head and neck. J Nurse Midwifery 40(2):187–201, Mar–Apr 1995.

Lish AJ: Differentiating the causes of acute conjunctivitis in adults. Hosp Med 32(1):28–31, Jan 1996.

McGrory A: Eye injuries: A review of the literature with nursing implications. Int J Nurs Stud 34(2):87–92, Apr 1997.

Modica PA: Afferent pupillary defects and the swinging flashlight test: What you thought you already knew. Optometry Clin 5(3/4):1–15, 1996.

Pepper J: Eye injuries. Emergency 29(1):42–47, Jan 1997.

Ruppert SD: Differential diagnosis of pediatric conjunctivitis (red eye). Nurse Pract 21(7):12–16, July 1996.

Sapira JD, Ologinboba KA, Schneiderman H: The funduscopic examination: The more you know what to look for, the more you see. Consultant 35(10):1443–1446, Oct 1995.

Schmidt ER, Kramer J: Consumer product-related eye injuries. J Ophthalmol Nurs Tech 16(5):251–255, Sep–Oct 1997.

Servodidio CA, Abramson DH: Self-assessment quiz. J Ophthalmol Nurs Tech 14(1):36,39, Jan–Feb 1995.

Sher NA, Trobe JD, Weingeist TA: New options for vision loss. Patient Care 29(14):55–70, Sep 15 1995.

Small RG: Ophthalmology in primary care: Office workup for red eye. Consultant 35(3):321–327, Mar 1995.

Stromland K, Hellstrom A: Fetal alcohol syndrome: An ophthalmological and socioeducational prospective study. Pediatrics 96(6, Part 1):845–850, June 1996.

Tomask RL: An approach to acquired visual loss in adults. J Ophthalmol Nurs Tech 16(5):229–257, Sep–Oct 1997.

Vrabec TR: Ocular manifestations of AIDS. J Ophthalmol Nurs Tech 15(5):205–211, Sep–Oct 1996.

Weber CM, Eichenbaum JW: Acute red eye: Differentiating viral conjunctivitis from other, less common causes. Postgrad Med 101(5):189–196, May 1997.

Wehenmeyer J, Gallman E: Neuroscience Curriculum, 25th ed. Urbana–Champaign, University of Illinois, 1997.

West G: Care of the older person: Detecting and treating eye problems in later life. Community Nurse 3(5):24–27, June 1997.

Woods AD, Caputo MK: Neuro-ophthalmic manifestations of AIDS. Optometry Clin 5(3/4):113–152, 1996.

Yetman RJ, Coody DK: Conjunctivitis: A practice guideline. J Pediatr Health Care 11(5):238–241, Sep–Oct 1997.

CHAPTER THIRTEEN

Ears

The ear is the sensory organ for hearing and maintaining equilibrium. The ear has three parts: the external, middle, and inner ear. The external ear is called the **auricle** or **pinna** and consists of movable cartilage and skin (Fig. 13–1). Note the landmarks of the auricle and use these terms to describe your findings. The mastoid process, the bony prominence behind the lobule, is not part of the ear but is an important landmark.

EXTERNAL EAR

The external ear has a characteristic shape and serves to funnel sound waves into its opening, the **external auditory canal** (Fig. 13–2). The canal is a cul-de-sac 2.5 to 3 cm long in the adult and terminates at the eardrum, or tympanic membrane. The canal is lined with glands that secrete cerumen, a yellow waxy material that lubricates and protects the ear. The wax forms a sticky barrier that helps keep foreign bodies from entering. Cerumen migrates out to the meatus by the movements of chewing and talking. Two types of earwax exist among races: one looks wet, sticky, and honey colored and is seen in whites and blacks, and the other looks dry and flaky and is seen in Asians and Native Americans (see Transcultural Considerations).

The outer one-third of the canal is cartilage; the inner two-thirds consists of bone covered by thin sensitive skin. The canal has a slight S-curve in the adult. The outer one-third curves up and toward the back of the head, whereas the inner two-thirds angles down and forward toward the nose.

The **tympanic membrane,** or **eardrum,** separates the external and middle ear and is tilted obliquely to the ear canal, facing downward and somewhat forward. It is a translucent membrane with a pearly gray color and a prominent cone of light in the anteroinferior quadrant, which is the reflection of the otoscope light (Fig. 13–3). The drum is oval and slightly concave, pulled in at its center by one of the middle ear ossicles, the **malleus.** The parts of the malleus show through the translucent drum; these are the **umbo,** the **manubrium** (handle), and the **short process.** The small, slack, superior section of the tympanic membrane is called the **pars flaccida.** The remainder of the drum, which is thicker and more taut, is the **pars tensa.** The **annulus** is the outer fibrous rim of the drum.

Lymphatic drainage of the external ear flows to the parotid, mastoid, and superficial cervical nodes.

MIDDLE EAR

The middle ear is a tiny air-filled cavity inside the temporal bone (see Fig. 13–2). It contains tiny ear bones, or auditory ossicles: the **malleus, incus,** and **stapes.** Several openings into the middle ear are present. Its opening to the outer ear is covered by the tympanic membrane. The openings to the inner ear are the oval window at the end of the stapes and the round window. Another opening is the **eustachian tube,** which connects the middle ear with the nasopharynx and allows passage of air. The tube is normally closed, but it opens with swallowing or yawning.

The middle ear has three functions: (1) It conducts sound vibrations from the outer ear to the central hearing apparatus in the inner ear; (2) it protects the inner ear by reducing the amplitude of loud sounds; and (3) its eustachian tube allows equalization of air pressure on each side of the tympanic membrane so that the membrane does not rupture, e.g., during altitude changes in an airplane.

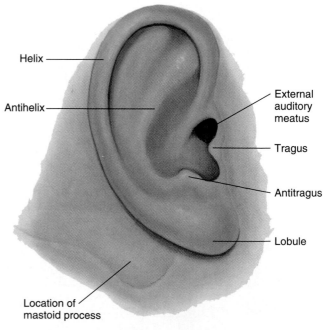

Helix

Antihelix

External auditory meatus

Tragus

Antitragus

Lobule

Location of mastoid process

AURICLE, OR PINNA

13–1

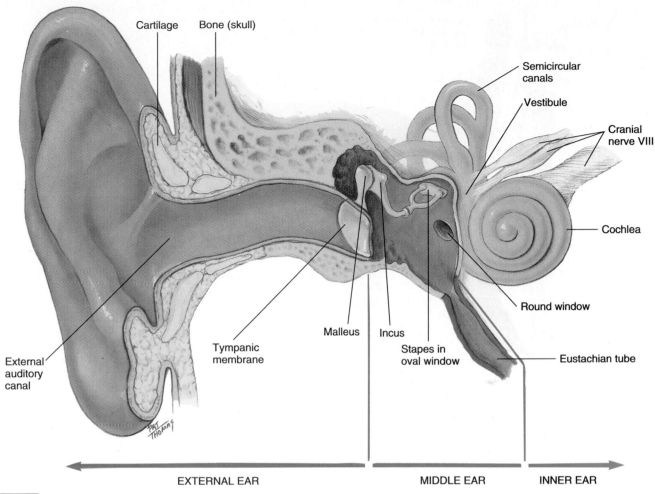

Cartilage   Bone (skull)

Semicircular canals

Vestibule

Cranial nerve VIII

Cochlea

Round window

Eustachian tube

Stapes in oval window

Incus

Malleus

Tympanic membrane

External auditory canal

EXTERNAL EAR   MIDDLE EAR   INNER EAR

13-2

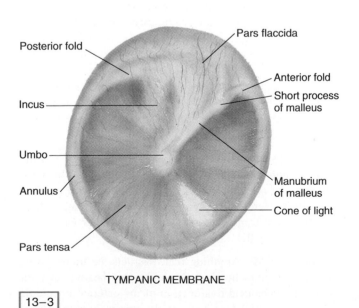

Pars flaccida

Posterior fold

Anterior fold

Short process of malleus

Incus

Umbo

Annulus

Manubrium of malleus

Cone of light

Pars tensa

TYMPANIC MEMBRANE

13-3

INNER EAR

The inner ear contains the **bony labyrinth,** which holds the sensory organs for equilibrium and hearing. Within the bony labyrinth, the **vestibule** and the **semicircular canals** compose the vestibular apparatus, and the **cochlea** (Latin for snail shell) contains the central hearing apparatus. Although the inner ear is not accessible to direct examination, its functions can be assessed.

HEARING

Concerning the function of hearing, the auditory system can be divided into three levels: peripheral, brain stem, and cerebral cortex. At the peripheral level, the ear transmits sound and converts its vibrations into electrical impulses, which can be analyzed by the brain. For example,

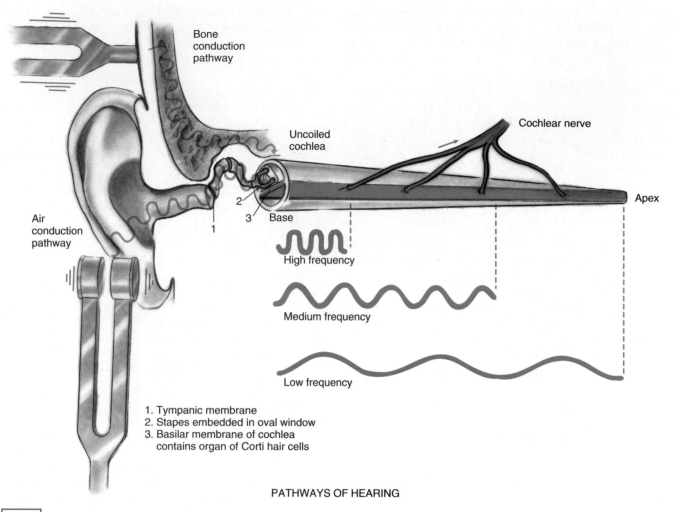

1. Tympanic membrane
2. Stapes embedded in oval window
3. Basilar membrane of cochlea contains organ of Corti hair cells

PATHWAYS OF HEARING

13–4

you hear an alarm bell ringing in the hall. Its sound waves travel instantly to your ears (Fig. 13–4). The *amplitude* is how loud the alarm is; its *frequency* is the pitch (in this case, high) or the number of cycles per second. The sound waves produce vibrations on your tympanic membrane. These vibrations are carried by the middle ear ossicles to your oval window. Then the sound waves travel through your cochlea, which is coiled like a snail's shell, and are dissipated against the round window. Along the way, the **basilar membrane** vibrates at a point specific to the frequency of the sound. In this case, the alarm's high frequency stimulates the basilar membrane at its base near the stapes. The numerous fibers along the basilar membrane are the receptor hair cells of the **organ of Corti,** the sensory organ of hearing. As the hair cells bend, they mediate the vibrations into electric impulses. The electric impulses are conducted by the auditory portion of cranial nerve VIII to the brain stem.

The function at the brain stem level is *binaural interaction,* which permits locating the direction of a sound in space as well as identifying the sound. How does this work? Each ear is actually one-half of the total sensory organ. The ears are located on each side of a movable head. The cranial nerve VIII from each ear sends signals to both sides of the brain stem. Areas in the brain stem are sensitive to differences in intensity and timing of the messages from the two ears, depending on the way the head is turned.

Finally, the function of the cortex is to interpret the meaning of the sound and begin the appropriate response. All this happens in the split second it takes you to react to the alarm.

Pathways of Hearing. The normal pathway of hearing is air conduction (AC) described above; it is the most efficient. An alternate route of hearing is by bone conduction (BC). Here, the bones of the skull vibrate. These vibrations are transmitted directly to the inner ear and to cranial nerve VIII.

Hearing Loss. Anything that obstructs the transmission of sound impairs hearing. A **conductive** hearing loss involves a mechanical dysfunction of the external or middle ear. It is a partial loss because the person is able to hear if the sound amplitude is increased enough to reach normal nerve elements in the inner ear. Conductive hearing loss may be caused by impacted cerumen, foreign bodies, a perforated tympanic membrane, pus or serum in the middle ear, and otosclerosis (a decrease in mobility of the ossicles).

Sensorineural (or perceptive) loss signifies pathology of the inner ear, cranial nerve VIII, or the auditory areas of the cerebral cortex. A simple increase in amplitude may not enable the person to understand words. Sensorineural hearing loss may be caused by *presbycusis,* a gradual nerve degeneration that occurs with aging, and by ototoxic drugs, which affect the hair cells in the cochlea.

A **mixed** loss is a combination of conductive and sensorineural types in the same ear.

Equilibrium. The labyrinth in the inner ear constantly feeds information to your brain about your body's position in space. It works like a plumb line to determine verticality or depth. The ear's plumb lines register the angle of your head in relation to gravity. If the labyrinth ever becomes inflamed, it feeds the wrong information to the brain, creating a staggering gait and a strong, spinning, whirling sensation called *vertigo.*

 DEVELOPMENTAL CONSIDERATIONS

Infants and Children

The inner ear starts to develop early in the 4th week of gestation. If maternal rubella infection occurs during the first trimester, it can damage the organ of Corti and impair hearing. The infant's eustachian tube is relatively shorter and wider, and its position is more horizontal than the adult's, so it is easier for pathogens from the nasopharynx to migrate through to the middle ear (Fig. 13–

5). The lumen is surrounded by lymphoid tissue, which increases during childhood; thus, the lumen is easily occluded. These factors place the infant at greater risk for middle ear infections than the adult.

The infant's and the young child's external auditory canal is shorter and has a slope opposite to that of the adult's (see Fig. 13–17).

The Adult

Otosclerosis is a common cause of conductive hearing loss in young adults between the ages of 20 and 40. It is a gradual hardening that causes the foot plate of the stapes to become fixed in the oval window, impeding the transmission of sound and causing progressive deafness.

The Aging Adult

In the aging person, cilia lining the ear canal become coarse and stiff. This condition may cause decreased hearing, since it impedes sound waves traveling toward the tympanic membrane. It also causes cerumen to accumulate and oxidize, which greatly reduces hearing. The cerumen itself is drier because of atrophy of the apocrine glands. Also, an older person with a life history of frequent ear infections may have noticeable scarring on the drum.

Impacted cerumen is a common but reversible cause of hearing loss in older people. Data from 226 hospitalized patients 65 years of age or older showed that 35% had impacted cerumen. Following removal of cerumen, 75% of these people had significantly improved hearing ability. This study suggests that nurses could improve the hearing health of older people by routinely performing otoscopic examinations and by performing ear canal irrigations when they find impacted cerumen (Lewis-Cullinan and Janken, 1990).

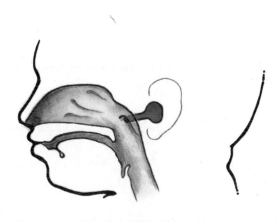

INFANT—HORIZONTAL
EUSTACHIAN TUBE

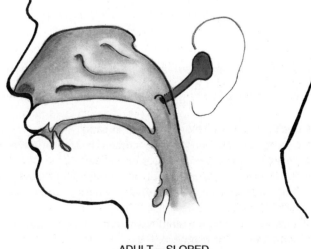

ADULT—SLOPED
EUSTACHIAN TUBE

13–5

A person living in a noise-polluted area (e.g., near an airport or a busy highway) has a greater risk of hearing loss. But **presbycusis** is a type of hearing loss that occurs with aging, even in people living in a quiet environment. It is a gradual sensorineural loss caused by nerve degeneration in the inner ear or auditory nerve. Its onset usually occurs in the fifth decade, and then it slowly progresses. The person first notices a high-frequency tone loss; it is harder to hear consonants (high-pitched components of speech) than vowels. This makes words sound garbled. The ability to localize sound is impaired also. This communication dysfunction is accentuated when background noise is present (e.g., with music, with dishes clattering, or at a large noisy party).

Lastly, the "auditory reaction time" increases after age 70 (Kane, Ouslander, and Abrass, 1994). That is, it takes longer for the older adult to process sensory input and to respond to it.

TRANSCULTURAL CONSIDERATIONS

Otitis media (middle ear infection) occurs because of obstruction of the eustachian tube and/or passage of nasopharyngeal secretions into the middle ear. Otitis media is one of the most common illnesses in children. The incidence and severity are increased in Native Americans, Alaskan and Canadian Inuits, and Hispanics (Terris, Magit, and Davidson, 1995).

The incidence of otitis media also is increased in premature infants, in those with Down syndrome, and in babies fed by bottle in a supine position. In the supine position, the effects of gravity and sucking tend to draw the nasopharyngeal contents directly into the middle ear. Urge the parent to hold the baby partly upright against the arm while feeding. Do not prop the bottle or let the baby take a bottle to bed. Encouraging breast-feeding helps prevent this problem.

The most important side effect of acute otitis media is the persistence of fluid in the middle ear after treatment. This middle ear effusion can impair hearing, placing the child at risk for delayed cognitive development.

Cerumen is genetically determined and comes in two major types: (1) dry cerumen, which is gray, flaky, and frequently forms a thin mass in the ear canal, and (2) wet cerumen, which is honey brown to dark brown and moist. Asians and Native Americans have an 84 percent frequency of dry cerumen, whereas blacks have a 99 percent and whites have a 97 percent frequency of wet cerumen (Overfield, 1995). The clinical significance of this occurs when examining or irrigating the ears. The presence and composition of cerumen are not related to poor hygiene. Take caution to avoid mistaking the flaky, dry cerumen for eczematous lesions.

SUBJECTIVE DATA

1. Earaches
2. Infections
3. Discharge
4. Hearing loss
5. Environmental noise
6. Tinnitus
7. Vertigo
8. Self-care behaviors

Examiner Asks	Rationale
1 Earache. Any **earache** or other pain in ears? • Location—feel close to the surface or deep in the head? • Does it hurt when you push on the ear? • Character—dull, aching or sharp, stabbing? Constant or come and go? Is it affected by changing position of head? Ever had this kind of pain before? • Any accompanying cold symptoms or sore throat? Any problems with sinuses or teeth? • Ever been hit on the ear or on the side of the head, or had any sport injury? Ever had any trauma from a foreign body? • What have you tried to relieve pain?	Otalgia may be directly due to ear disease or may be referred pain from a problem in teeth or oropharynx. Virus/bacteria from upper respiratory infection may migrate up eustachian tube to involve middle ear. Trauma may rupture the tympanic membrane. Assess effect of coping strategies.

Examiner Asks	Rationale

2 **Infections.** Any ear **infections?** As an adult, or in childhood?
  ● How frequent were they? How were they treated?

A history of chronic ear problems alerts you to possibility of sequelae.

3 **Discharge.** Any **discharge** from your ears?

Discharge (otorrhea) suggests infection; it may come from canal or may indicate a perforated eardrum. For example:

  ● Does it look like pus, or bloody?

External otitis—purulent, sanguineous, or watery discharge.
Acute otitis media with perforation—purulent discharge.

  ● Any odor to the discharge?

Cholesteatoma—dirty yellow/gray discharge, foul odor.

  ● Any relation between the discharge and the ear pain?

Typically with perforation—ear pain occurs first, stops with a popping sensation, then drainage occurs.

4 **Hearing loss.** Ever had any trouble hearing?
  ● Onset—Did the loss come on slowly or all at once?

Presbycusis has a gradual onset over years, whereas a hearing loss due to trauma is often sudden. Any sudden loss in one or both ears *not* associated with upper respiratory infection warrants referral.

  ● Character—Has all your hearing decreased, or just on hearing certain sounds?
  ● In what situations do you notice the loss: conversations, using the telephone, listening to TV, at a party?

Loss may be apparent when competition from background noise is present, e.g., at a party.

  ● Do people seem to shout at you?

Recruitment—a marked loss occurs when sound is at low intensity, but sound actually may become painful when repeated in a loud voice.

  ● Do ordinary sounds seem hollow, as if you are hearing in a barrel or under water?
  ● Recently traveled by airplane?
  ● Any family history of hearing loss?
  ● Effort to treat—any hearing aid or other device? Anything to help hearing?

Character of hearing loss when cerumen expands and becomes impacted, as in after swimming or showering.

  ● Coping strategies—how does the loss affect your daily life? Any job problem? Feel embarrassed? Frustrated? How do your family, friends react?

Hearing loss can cause social isolation and can lessen pleasure of leisure activities.

Note to examiner—during history, note these clues from normal conversation, which indicate possible hearing loss

1. Person lip reading or watching your face and lips closely rather than your eyes
2. Frowning or straining forward to hear
3. Posturing of head to catch sounds with better ear
4. Misunderstands your questions, or frequently asks you to repeat
5. Acts irritable or shows startle reflex when you raise your voice (recruitment)
6. Person's speech sounds garbled, possibly vowel sounds distorted
7. Inappropriately loud voice
8. Flat, monotonous tone of voice

Examiner Asks	Rationale

5 Environmental noise. Any loud noises at home or on the job? For example, do you live in a noise-polluted area, near an airport or busy traffic area? Now or in the past?

Old trauma to hearing initially goes unnoticed but results in further decibel loss in later years.

- Are you near other noises such as heavy machinery, loud persistent music, gunshots while hunting?
- Coping strategies—any steps to protect your ears, such as headphones or ear plugs?

6 Tinnitus. Ever felt ringing, crackling, or buzzing in your ears? When did this occur?

The sound of tinnitus originates within the person. Tinnitus accompanies some hearing loss or ear disorders.

- Seem louder at night?

Tinnitus seems louder when no competition from environmental noise exists.

- Are you taking any medications?

Consider medications with possible ototoxic sequelae: aspirin, aminoglycosides (streptomycin, gentamicin, kanamycin, neomycin), ethacrynic acid, furosemide, indomethacin, naproxen, quinine, vancomycin.

7 Vertigo. Ever felt **vertigo,** that is, the room spinning around or yourself spinning? (Vertigo is a true twirling motion.)

True rotational spinning occurs with dysfunction of labyrinth. Objective vertigo—feels like room spins. Subjective vertigo—person feels like she or he spins.

- Ever felt dizzy, like you are not quite steady, like falling or losing your balance? Giddy, lightheaded?

Distinguish true vertigo from dizziness or lightheadedness.

8 Self-care behaviors. How do you clean your ears?

Assess potential trauma from invasive instruments. Cleaning with cotton-tipped applicators can impact cerumen, causing hearing loss.

- Last time you had your hearing checked?
- If a hearing loss was noted, did you obtain a hearing aid? How long have you had it? Do you wear it? How does it work? Any trouble with upkeep, cleaning, changing batteries?

Prescribe frequency of hearing assessment according to person's age and/or risk factors.

ADDITIONAL HISTORY FOR INFANTS AND CHILDREN

1 Ear infections. At what age was the child's first episode? How many ear infections in the last 6 months? How many total? How were these treated?
- Has the child had any surgery, such as insertion of ear tubes or removal of tonsils?
- Are the infections increasing in frequency, in severity, or staying the same?
- Does anyone in the home smoke cigarettes?

If three or more episodes occur in the first 18 months of age, the child is "otitis-prone" and will have twice as many subsequent episodes as the child with one episode or no episodes during the first year (Prellner et al., 1994; Stenstrom and Ingvarsson, 1995).
Passive or secondhand smoke is a risk factor for ear infections.

Examiner Asks	Rationale

- Does your child receive child care outside your home? In a day care center or someone else's home? How many children in the group care?

Attendance at group day care, and bottle feeding compared with breastfeeding, are also risk factors for otitis media (Otitis Media Guideline Panel, 1994).

2 Does the child seem to be hearing well?
- Have you noticed that the infant startles with loud noise? Did the infant babble around 6 months? Does he or she talk; at what age did talking start? Was the speech intelligible?
- Ever had the child's hearing tested? If there was a hearing loss, did it follow any diseases in the child, or in the mother during pregnancy?

(Note: It is important to catch any problem early, because a child with hearing loss is at risk for delayed speech and social development and learning deficit.)

Children at risk for hearing deficit include those exposed to maternal rubella, syphilis, cytomegalovirus, or toxoplasmosis, or to maternal ototoxic drugs in utero; premature infants; low-birth-weight infants; trauma or hypoxia at birth; and infants with congenital liver or kidney disease.

In children, the incidence of meningitis, measles, mumps, otitis media, and any illness with persistent high fever may increase risk of hearing deficit.

3 Does the child tend to put objects in the ears? Is the older child or adolescent active in contact sports?

These children are at increased risk for trauma.

OBJECTIVE DATA

Preparation

Position the adult sitting up straight with his or her head at your eye level. Occasionally the ear canal is partially filled with cerumen, which obstructs your view of the tympanic membrane. If the eardrum is intact and no current infection is present, a preferred method of cleaning the adult canal is to soften the cerumen with a warmed solution of mineral oil and hydrogen peroxide. Then the canal is irrigated with warm water (body temperature) using a bulb syringe or a low-pulsatile dental irrigator (Water-Pik). Direct fluid to the posterior wall. Leave space around the irrigator tip for water to escape. Do not irrigate if the history or the examination suggests perforation or infection.

Equipment Needed

Otoscope with bright light (fresh batteries give off white—not yellow—light)

Pneumatic bulb attachment, sometimes used with infant or young child

Tuning forks in 512, 1024 Hz

Normal Range of Findings	Abnormal Findings

THE EXTERNAL EAR

Inspect and palpate the external ear
Size and Shape

The ears are of equal size bilaterally with no swelling or thickening. Ears of unusual size and shape may be a normal familial trait with no clinical significance.

Microtia—ears smaller than 4 cm vertically.
Macrotia—ears larger than 10 cm vertically.
Edema.

Normal Range of Findings

Abnormal Findings

Skin Condition

The skin color is consistent with the person's facial skin color. The skin is intact, with no lumps or lesions. On some people you may note **Darwin's tubercle,** a small painless nodule at the helix. This is a congenital variation and is not significant (see Table 13–2).

Reddened, excessively warm skin indicates inflammation (see Table 13–1).

Crusts and scaling occur with otitis externa and with eczema, contact dermatitis, and seborrhea.

Enlarged tender lymph nodes in the region indicate inflammation of the pinna for mastoid process.

Red-blue discoloration indicates frostbite.

Tophi, sebaceous cyst, chondrodermatitis, keloid, carcinoma (see Table 13–2).

Tenderness

Move the pinna and push on the tragus. They should feel firm, and movement should produce no pain. Palpating the mastoid process should also produce no pain.

Pain with movement occurs with otitis externa and furuncle.

Pain at the mastoid process may indicate mastoiditis or lymphadenitis of the posterior auricular node.

The External Auditory Meatus

Note the size of the opening to direct your choice of speculum for the otoscope. No swelling, redness, or discharge should be present.

Atresia—absence or closure of the ear canal.

A sticky yellow discharge accompanies otitis externa, or it may indicate otitis media if the drum has ruptured.

Some cerumen is usually present. The color varies from gray-yellow to light brown and black, and the texture varies from moist and waxy to dry and desiccated. A large amount of cerumen obscures visualization of the canal and drum.

Impacted cerumen is a common cause of conductive hearing loss.

THE OTOSCOPIC EXAMINATION

Inspect using the otoscope

As you inspect the external ear, note the size of the auditory meatus. Then choose the largest speculum that will fit comfortably in the ear canal, and attach it to the otoscope. Tilt the person's head slightly away from you toward the opposite shoulder. This method brings the obliquely sloping eardrum into better view.

Pull the pinna up and back on an adult or older child; this helps straighten the S-shape of the canal (Fig. 13–6). (Pull the pinna down on an infant and a child under 3 years of age [see Fig. 13–17].) Hold the pinna gently but firmly. Do not release traction on the ear until you have finished the examination and the otoscope is removed.

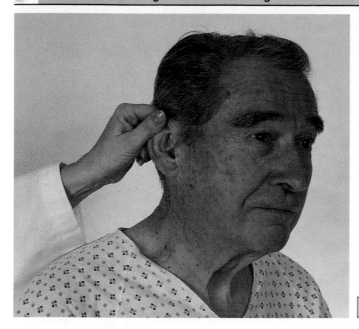

13–6

Hold the otoscope "upside down" along your fingers and have the dorsa (back) of your hand along the person's cheek braced to steady the otoscope (Fig. 13–7). This position feels awkward to you only at first. It soon will feel natural and you will find it useful to prevent forceful insertion. Also your stabilizing hand acts as a protecting lever if the person suddenly moves the head.

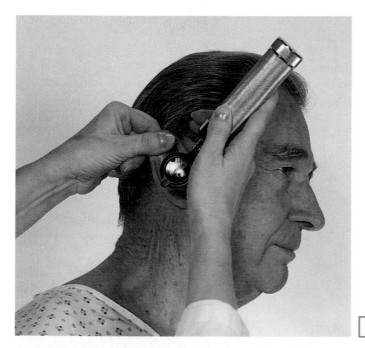

13–7

Insert the speculum slowly and carefully along the axis of the canal. Watch the insertion; then put your eye up to the otoscope. Avoid touching the inner "bony" section of the canal wall, which is covered by a thin epithelial layer and is sensitive to pain. Sometimes you cannot see anything but canal wall. If so, try to reposition the person's head, apply more traction on the pinna, and re-angle the otoscope to look forward toward the person's nose.

Once it is in place, you may need to rotate the otoscope slightly to visualize all of the drum; do this gently. Lastly, perform the otoscopic examination before you test hearing; ear canals with impacted cerumen give the erroneous impression of pathologic hearing loss.

The External Canal

Note any redness and swelling, lesions, foreign bodies, or discharge. If any discharge is present, note the color and odor. (Also, clean any discharge from the speculum before examining the other ear to avoid contamination with possibly infectious material.) For a person with a hearing aid, note any irritation on the canal wall from poorly fitting earmolds.

Redness and swelling occur with otitis externa; canal may be completely closed with swelling.

Purulent otorrhea suggests otitis externa, or may indicate otitis media if the drum has ruptured.

Frank blood or clear, watery drainage (cerebrospinal fluid leak) following trauma suggests basal skull fracture and warrants immediate referral. Cerebrospinal fluid feels oily and produces a positive glucose finding on TesTape.

Foreign body, exostosis, polyp, furuncle (see Table 13-3, Abnormalities in the Ear Canal).

The Tympanic Membrane

Color and Characteristics. Systematically explore its landmarks (Fig. 13-8). The normal eardrum is shiny and translucent, with a pearl-gray color. The cone-shaped light reflex is prominent in the anteroinferior quadrant (at 5 o'clock in the right drum and 7 o'clock in the left drum). This is the reflection of your otoscope light. Sections of the malleus are visible through the translucent drum: the umbo, manubrium, and short process. (Infrequently, you also may see the incus behind the drum; it shows as a whitish haze in the upper posterior area.) At the periphery, the annulus looks whiter and denser.

Yellow-amber color of the drum occurs with serous otitis media.

Red color occurs with acute otitis media.

Absent or distorted landmarks.

Air/fluid level or air bubbles behind drum indicate serous otitis media (see Tables 13-4 and 13-5).

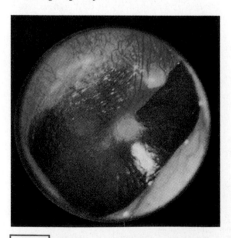

13-8 **Normal tympanic membrane, right**

Normal Range of Findings	Abnormal Findings

Position. The eardrum is flat, slightly pulled in at the center, and flutters when the person performs the Valsalva maneuver or holds the nose and swallows (insufflation). You may elicit these maneuvers to assess drum mobility. Avoid them with an aging person because they may disrupt equilibrium. Also avoid middle ear insufflation in a person with upper respiratory infection because it could propel infectious matter into the middle ear.

Retracted drum due to vacuum in middle ear with obstructed eustachian tube.

Bulging drum from increased pressure in otitis media.

Drum hypomobility is an early sign of otitis media (see Table 13–5).

Integrity of Membrane. Inspect the eardrum and the entire circumference of the annulus for perforations. The normal tympanic membrane is intact. Some adults may show scarring, which is a dense white patch on the drum. This is a sequela of repeated ear infections.

Perforation shows as a dark oval area or as a larger opening on the drum.

Vesicles on drum (see Table 13–5).

HEARING ACUITY

Test Hearing Acuity

Your screening for a hearing deficit begins during the history; how well does the person hear conversational speech? An audiometer gives a precise quantitative measure of hearing by assessing the person's ability to hear sounds of varying frequency. Since this equipment usually is not available in the clinical setting, you may use alternate screening measures. These are "crude" tests. They are nonquantitative; they are useful to document the *presence* of hearing loss but do not measure the degree of loss. Refer any abnormal findings for more accurate measures with pure tone audiometry.

Voice Test

Test one ear at a time while masking hearing in the other ear to prevent sound transmission around the head. This is done by placing one finger on the tragus and rapidly pushing it in and out of the auditory meatus. Shield your lips so the person cannot compensate for a hearing loss (consciously or unconsciously) by lip reading or using the "good" ear. With your head 30 to 60 cm (1 to 2 ft) from the person's ear, exhale and whisper slowly some two-syllable words, such as Tuesday, armchair, baseball, and fourteen. Normally, the person repeats each word correctly after you say it.

The person is unable to hear whispered words. A whisper is a high-frequency sound and is used to detect high-tone loss.

Tuning Fork Tests

Tuning fork tests measure hearing by air conduction (AC) or by bone conduction (BC), in which the sound vibrates through the cranial bones to the inner ear. The AC route through the ear canal and middle ear is usually the more sensitive route. To activate the tuning fork, hold it by the stem and strike the tines softly on the back of your hand (Fig. 13–9). A hard strike makes the tone too loud, and it takes a long time to fade out.

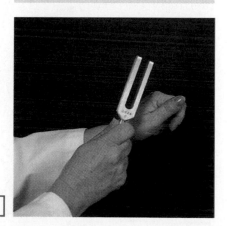

13–9

▶

The **Weber test** is valuable when a person reports hearing better with one ear than the other. Place a vibrating tuning fork in the midline of the person's skull and ask if the tone sounds the same in both ears or better in one (Fig. 13–10). The person should hear the tone by bone conduction through the skull, and it should sound equally loud in both ears.

Sound lateralizes to one ear (see Table 13–6).

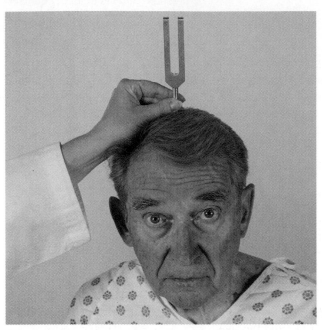

13–10
Weber test

The **Rinne test** compares air conduction and bone conduction sound (Fig.13–11). Place the stem of the vibrating tuning fork on the person's mastoid process and ask him or her to signal when the sound goes away. Quickly invert the fork so the vibrating end is near the ear canal; the person should still hear a sound (Fig. 13–12). Normally, the sound is heard twice as long by air conduction (next to ear canal) as by bone conduction (through the mastoid process). A normal response is a positive Rinne test, or "AC > BC." Repeat with the other ear.

Ratio of AC to BC is altered with hearing loss (see Table 13–6).

Sound is heard longer by bone conduction.

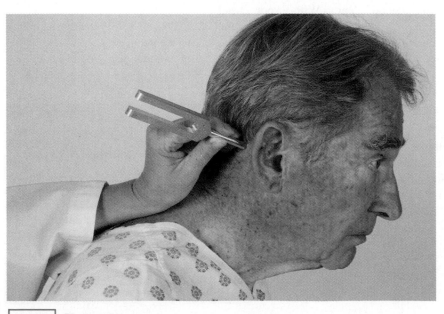

13–11 **Rinne test**

| Normal Range of Findings | Abnormal Findings |

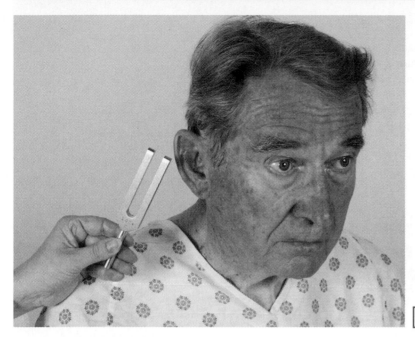

13–12

THE VESTIBULAR APPARATUS

The **Romberg test** assesses the ability of the vestibular apparatus in the inner ear to help maintain standing balance. Because the Romberg test also assesses intactness of the cerebellum and proprioception, it is discussed in Chapter 21, Neurologic System (see Fig. 21–17).

 ### DEVELOPMENTAL CONSIDERATIONS

Infants and Young Children

Examination of the external ear is similar to that described for the adult, with the addition of examination of position and alignment on head. Note the ear position. The top of the pinna should match an imaginary line extending from the corner of the eye to the occiput. Also, the ear should be positioned within 10 degrees of vertical (Fig. 13–13).

Low-set ears or deviation in alignment may indicate mental retardation or a genitourinary malformation.

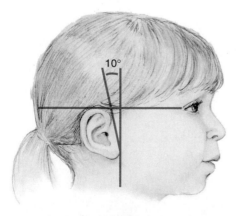

13–13   Normal alignment

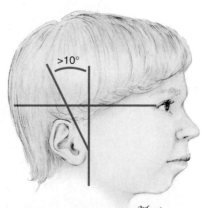

Low set ears and deviation in alignment

Otoscopic Examination

In addition to its place in the complete examination, eardrum assessment is mandatory for any infant or child requiring care for illness or fever. For the infant or young child, the timing of the otoscopic examination is best toward the end of the complete examination. Many young children protest vigorously during this procedure no matter how well you prepare, and it is difficult to reestablish cooperation afterward. Save the otoscopic examination until last. Then the parent can hold and comfort the child.

To help prepare the child, let the child hold your funny-looking "flashlight." You may wish to have the child look in the parent's ear as you hold the otoscope (Fig. 13–14).

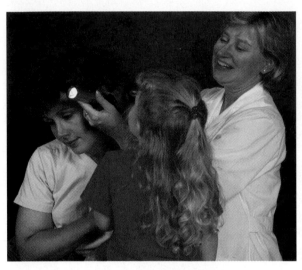

13–14

Positioning of the child is important. You need a clear view of the canal, and you must protect the eardrum from injury in case of sudden head movement. Enlist the aid of a cooperative parent. Prop an infant upright against the parent's chest or shoulder, with the parent's arm around the upper part of the head (Fig. 13–15). A toddler can be held in the parent's lap or may lie on the examining table with his or her arms secured (Fig. 13–16). In each case, the child's head is stabilized to avoid movement against the otoscope.

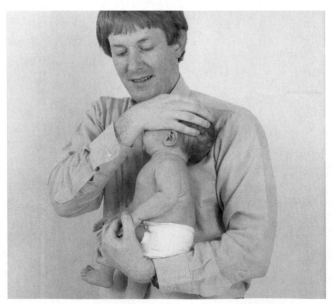

13–15

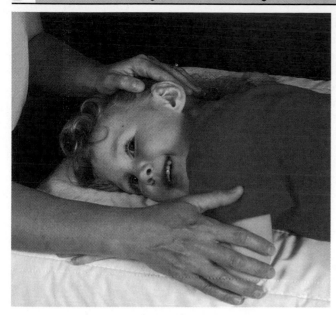

13–16

Remember to pull the pinna straight down on an infant or a child under 3 years old. This method will match the slope of the ear canal (Fig. 13–17).

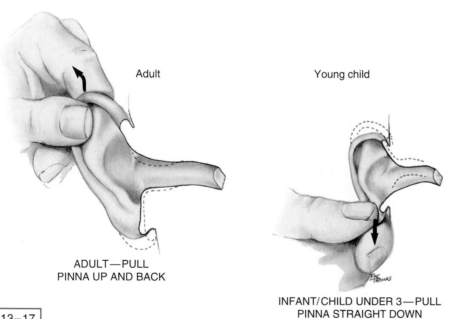

Adult

Young child

ADULT—PULL
PINNA UP AND BACK

INFANT/CHILD UNDER 3—PULL
PINNA STRAIGHT DOWN

13–17

At birth, the patency of the ear canal is determined, but the otoscopic examination is not performed because the canal is filled with amniotic fluid and vernix caseosa. After a few days, the tympanic membrane is examined. During the first few days, the tympanic membrane often looks thickened and opaque. It may look "injected" and have a mild redness due to increased vascularity. The drum also looks injected in infants after crying. The position of the eardrum is more horizontal in the neonate, making it more difficult to see completely and harder to differentiate from the canal wall. By 1 month of age, the drum is in the oblique (more vertical) position as in the older child, and examination is a bit easier.

When examining an infant or young child, a pneumatic bulb attachment enables you to direct a light puff of air toward the drum to assess vibratility (Fig. 13–18). Choose the largest speculum that will fit in the ear canal without causing pain, for a secure seal. A rubber tip on the end of the speculum gives a better seal. Give a small pump to the bulb (positive pressure), then release the bulb (negative pressure). Normally the tympanic membrane moves inward with a slight puff and outward with a slight release.

An abnormal response is no movement. Drum hypomobility indicates effusion or a high vacuum in the middle ear. For the newborn's first 6 weeks, drum immobility is the best indicator of middle ear infection.

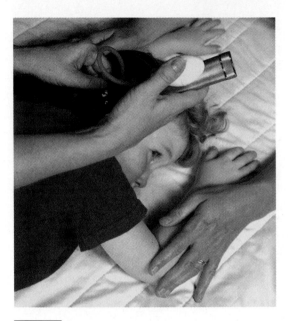

13–18

Normally, the tympanic membrane is intact. In a child being treated for chronic otitis media, you may note the presence of a tympanostomy tube in the central part of the drum. This is inserted surgically to equalize pressure and drain secretions. Finally, although the condition is not normal, it is not uncommon to note a foreign body in a child's canal, such as a small stone or a bead.

Tympanostomy tubes (see Table 13–5).

Foreign body (see Table 13–3).

Test Hearing Acuity

Use the developmental milestones mentioned in this section to assess hearing in an infant. Also, attend to the parents' concern over the infant's inability to hear; their assessment is usually well founded.

The room should be silent and the baby contented. Make a loud sudden noise (hand clap or squeeze toy) out of the baby's peripheral range of vision of about 30 cm (12 in). You may need to repeat a few times, but you should note these responses:

Newborn—startle (Moro) reflex, acoustic blink reflex
3 to 4 months—acoustic blink reflex, infant stops movement and appears to "listen," halts sucking, quiets if crying, cries if quiet

6 to 8 months—infant turns head to localize sound, responds to own name

Preschool and school-age child—child must be screened with audiometry

Absence of alerting behavior may indicate congenital deafness.

Failure to localize sound.

No intelligible speech by 2 years of age.

► Normal Range of Findings	Abnormal Findings

Note that a young child may be unaware of a hearing loss because the child does not know how one "ought" to hear. Note these behavioral manifestations of hearing loss:

1. The child is inattentive in casual conversation.
2. The child reacts more to movement and facial expression than to sound.
3. The child's facial expression is strained or puzzled.
4. The child frequently asks to have statements repeated.
5. The child confuses words that sound alike.
6. The child has an accompanying speech problem: Speech is monotonous or garbled; the child mispronounces or omits sounds.
7. The child appears shy and withdrawn and "lives in a world of his or her own."
8. The child frequently complains of earaches.
9. The child hears better at times when the environment is more conducive to hearing.

The Aging Adult

An aging person may have pendulous earlobes with linear wrinkling because of loss of elasticity of the pinna. Coarse, wiry hairs may be present at the opening of the ear canal. During otoscopy, the drum normally may be whiter in color and more opaque, duller than in the younger adult. It also may look thickened.

A high tone frequency hearing loss is apparent for those affected with presbycusis, the hearing loss that occurs with aging. This condition is revealed in difficulty hearing whispered words in the voice test and in difficulty hearing consonants during conversational speech.

►SUMMARY CHECKLIST: Ear Exam

1. Inspect external ear:
Size and shape of auricle
Position and alignment on head
Note skin condition—color, lumps, lesions
Check movement of auricle and tragus for tenderness
Evaluate external auditory meatus—note size, swelling, redness, discharge, cerumen, lesions, foreign bodies

2. Otoscopic examination:
External canal
Cerumen, discharge, foreign bodies, lesions
Redness or swelling of canal wall

3. Inspect tympanic membrane:
Color and characteristics
Note position (flat, bulging, retracted)
Integrity of membrane

4. Test hearing acuity:
Note behavioral response to conversational speech
Voice test
Tuning fork tests—Weber and Rinne

SAMPLE CHARTING

 Subjective

States hearing is good, no earaches, infections, discharge, hearing loss, tinnitus, or vertigo.

Objective

Pinna—skin intact with no masses, lesions, tenderness, or discharge.

Otoscope—external canals are clear with no redness, swelling, lesions, foreign body, or discharge. Both tympanic membranes are pearly gray in color, with light reflex and landmarks intact, no perforations.

Hearing—whispered words heard bilaterally. Weber test—tone heard midline without lateralization. Rinne test—AC > BC and = bilaterally.

CLINICAL CASE STUDY 1

Jamal K. is a 9-month-old black infant who is brought to the clinic by his mother because he "feels hot and was up crying all night."

Past History. Jamal is the third child of Mr. and Mrs. K. Mrs. K. received regular prenatal care. Jamal was born at 37 weeks gestation; labor and delivery were uncomplicated. Jamal weighed 3200 g at birth, and was discharged 2 days after delivery. Jamal has been bottle fed, with solids introduced at 5 months. Well baby care has been regular, immunizations are up-to-date. Jamal has had two prior episodes of otitis media, no other illnesses.

Social History. Jamal lives with his family in a two-bedroom apartment over their grocery store and shares a bedroom with a 4-year-old brother and a 2-year-old brother. Mr. K. works full time in their grocery store; Mrs. K. provides child care in her own home for her children and for her sister's two young children. Both parents smoke cigarettes, 1–2 packs per day.

 Subjective

1 day PTA—Mrs. K. put Jamal down for nap with a bottle of juice, as is usual for her. Jamal woke up in the middle of the nap crying furiously. Quieted somewhat when held upright but still fussy. Took juice from bottle, refused solid baby food. Temperature 38° C rectally. Crying and fussy all night. Mrs. K. has given no medications to Jamal.

 Objective

Vital signs—temp 38.4° C (tympanic), pulse 152, resp 36, Wt. 9.2 kg (50th percentile), Ht. 29 in. (75th percentile).

General—alert, active, crying, and fussy. Developmentally appropriate for age.

Skin—warm and dry, no rashes or lesions.

Head—anterior fontanel flat, 1 × 1.5 cm, posterior fontanel closed.

Eyes—no exudate, conjunctivae clear, sclerae white, red reflex present bilaterally.

Ears—both tympanic membranes dull red and bulging, no light reflex, no mobility on pneumatic otoscopy.

Mouth/throat—oral mucosa pink, no lesions or exudate, tonsils 1+.

Neck—supple, no lymphadenopathy.

Heart—regular rate and rhythm, no murmurs.

Lungs—breath sounds clear and equal bilaterally, unlabored.

Abdomen—bowel sounds present, abdomen soft, nontender.

 ASSESSMENT

Acute otitis media, both ears

Pain R/T inflammation in TMs

Risk for ear infection injury R/T supine bottle feeding, group child care, secondhand smoke
Knowledge deficit (parents) R/T lack of exposure to risk factors for otitis media

CLINICAL CASE STUDY 2

Todd R. is a 15-year-old high school student who comes to the Health Center to seek care for "cough off and on all winter and earache since last night."

Subjective

6 weeks PTA—nonproductive cough throughout day, no fever, no nasal congestion, no chest soreness. Todd's father gave him an over-the-counter decongestant, which helped, but cough continued off/on since. Does not smoke.
1 day PTA—intermittent cough continues, nasal congestion c̄ thick white mucus. Also earache R ear, treated self with heating pad, pain unrelieved. Pain is moderate, not deep and throbbing. Says R ear feels full, "hollow headed," voices sound muffled and far away, switches telephone to L ear to talk. No sore throat, no fever, no chest congestion or soreness.

Objective

Vital signs—T 37° C oral, P 76, B/P 106/72.
Ears—L ear, canal, TM normal. R ear and canal normal, R TM retracted, with multiple air bubbles, drum color is yellow/amber. No sinus tenderness.
Nose—turbinates bright red and swollen, mucopurulent discharge.
Throat—not reddened, tonsils 1+.
Neck—1 R anterior cervical node enlarged, firm, movable, tender. All others not palpable.
Lungs—Breath sounds clear to auscultation, resonant to percussion throughout.
Hearing—Weber lateralizes to R.

ASSESSMENT

Serous otitis media, R ear, with mild URI
Transient conductive hearing loss
Sensory/perceptual alteration (auditory) R/T excessive fluid in middle ear
Pain R/T middle ear pressure

CLINICAL CASE STUDY 3

Emma S., 78 years old, has a medical diagnosis of angina pectoris, which has responded to nitroglycerin prn and periods of rest between activity. She has been independent in her own home, is coping well with activity restrictions through help from neighbors and family. Now hospitalized for evaluation of acute chest pain episode; MI has been ruled out, pain diagnosed as anginal, to be released to own home with a beta-blocking medication and nitroglycerin prn.

Just before this hospitalization Mrs. S. received a hearing aid following evaluation by audiologist at senior center. Mrs. S. was born in Germany, immigrated to U.S. at age 5, considers English her primary language.

Complete Problem List

Problem No.	Title	Date Entered
1	Angina pectoris	5/20/
2	Hearing loss	6/3/

Progress Notes

Subjective

Since this hospitalization, feels "irritable and nervous." Relates this to worry about heart and also, "I get so mixed up in here, this room is so strange, and I just can't hear the nurses. They talk like cavemen, 'oo-i-ee-uou.'" Tried using her new hearing aid but no relief, "It just kept screeching in my ear, and it made the monitor beep so loud it drove me crazy." States no tinnitus, no vertigo.

Continued

Objective

Ears—pinna with elongated lobes, but no tenderness to palpation, no discharge, no masses or lesions. Both canals clear of cerumen. Both TM appear gray-white, slightly opaque and dull, although all landmarks visible. No perforation.

Hearing—unable to hear whispered voice bilaterally. Weber test—tone heard midline, although unable to hear 1024 Hz fork, used 512 Hz. Rinne test positive, AC > BC, but time reduced overall.

 ASSESSMENT

Knowledge deficit R/T lack of teaching on hearing aid
Sensory/perceptual alteration (auditory) R/T effects of aging
Anxiety R/T change in cardiovascular health status and inability to communicate effectively

NURSING DIAGNOSES COMMONLY ASSOCIATED WITH THE EARS AND HEARING DISORDERS

Diagnosis	Related Factors (Etiology)	Defining Characteristics (Symptoms and Signs)
Sensory/perceptual alteration; auditory	Effects of aging Neurologic impairment Effects of certain antibiotics Excessive earwax, fluid, or foreign body in ear Social isolation Stress Failure to use protective ear devices Continuous exposure to excessive noise Psychoses	Tinnitus Abnormal hearing test Lack of startle reflex Failure to respond to verbal stimuli Cupping of ears Inattentiveness Withdrawal Daydreaming Auditory hallucinations Inappropriate responses Delayed speech or language development

Impaired social interaction	Knowledge/skills deficit about ways to enhance mutuality
	Communication barriers
	Self-concept disturbances
	Limited physical mobility
	Therapeutic isolation
	Sociocultural dissonance
	Environmental barriers
		Verbalized or observed discomfort
		   In social situations
		   In receiving or communicating
		Observed use of unsuccessful socialization behaviors
		Dysfunctional interaction with peers, family, and/or others

Other Related Nursing Diagnoses

ACTUAL	RISK/WELLNESS
Impaired verbal communication Pain	**Risk** Risk for infection Risk for trauma related to balance difficulties **Wellness** Health-seeking behavior R/T ways to decrease ear infections in child

 ASSESSMENT VIDEO CRITICAL THINKING QUESTIONS

The Saunders *Physical Examination and Health Assessment* video series—Head, Eyes, and Ears—will direct you to consider the following:

1. Describe the following lumps or lesions that may occur on the external ear: sebaceous cyst, keloid, carcinoma, and otitis externa.

2. Contrast the way you would move the pinna to straighten the ear canal of an adult and of a very young child.

Table 13–1   ABNORMALITIES OF THE EXTERNAL EAR

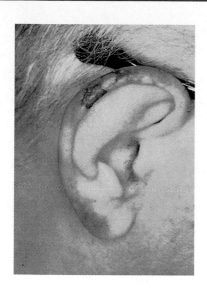

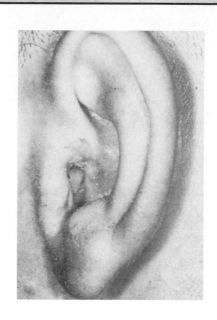

Frostbite

Reddish blue discoloration and swelling of auricle following exposure to extreme cold. Vesicles or bullae may develop, the person feels pain and tenderness, and ear necrosis may ensue.

Otitis Externa (Swimmer's Ear)

An infection of the outer ear, with severe painful movement of the pinna and tragus, redness and swelling of pinna and canal, scanty purulent discharge, scaling, itching, fever, and enlarged tender regional lymph nodes. Hearing is normal or slightly diminished. More common in hot humid weather. Swimming causes canal to become waterlogged and swell; skinfolds are set up for infection. Prevent by using rubbing alcohol or 2% acetic acid eardrops after every swim.

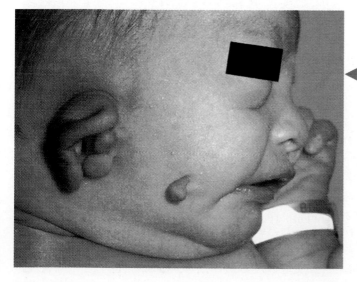

◀ Branchial Remnant and Ear Deformity

A facial remnant or leftover of the embryologic branchial arch usually appears as a skin tag, in this case one containing cartilage. They occur most often in the preauricular area, in front of the tragus. When bilateral, there is increased risk of renal anomalies.

Cerebrospinal Fluid Otorrhea (not illustrated)

Skull fracture of temporal bone causes cerebrospinal fluid to leak from ear canal and pool in concha when the person is supine. Cerebrospinal fluid feels oily and gives a positive glucose reaction on TesTape.

ABNORMAL FINDINGS

Table 13-2   LUMPS AND LESIONS ON THE EXTERNAL EAR

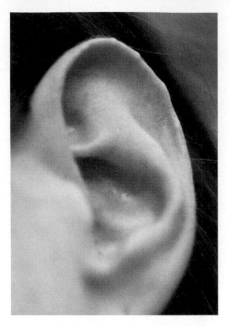

Darwin's Tubercle

Small painless nodule at the helix. It is a congenital variation and is not significant. Do not mistake it for a tophus.

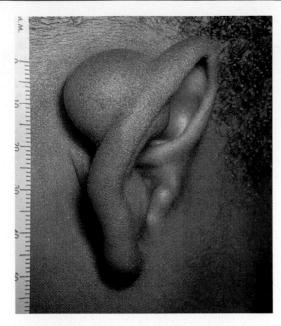

Sebaceous Cyst

Location is commonly behind lobule, in the postauricular fold. A nodule with central black punctum indicates blocked sebaceous gland. It is filled with waxy sebaceous material and is painful if it becomes infected. Often are multiple.

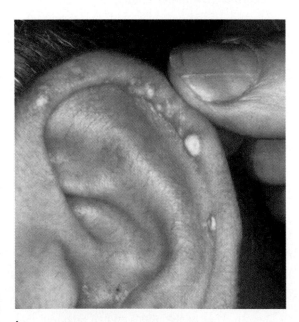

Tophi

Small, whitish-yellow, hard, nontender nodules in or near helix or antihelix. Contain greasy, chalky material of uric acid crystals and are a sign of gout.

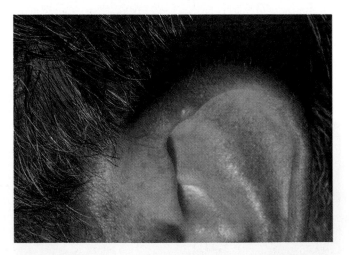

Chondrodermatitis Nodularis Helicus

Painful nodules develop on the rim of the helix (where there is no cushioning subcutaneous tissue) as a result of repetitive mechanical pressure or environmental trauma (sunlight). They are small, indurated, and very painful.

Table 13-2   LUMPS AND LESIONS ON THE EXTERNAL EAR *Continued*

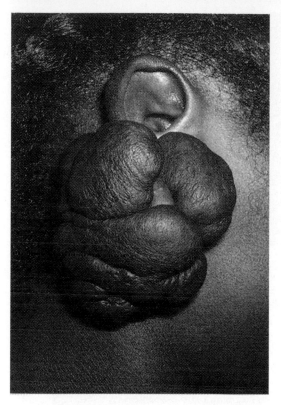

Carcinoma

Ulcerated crusted nodule with indurated base that fails to heal. Bleeds intermittently. Must refer for biopsy. Usually occurs on the superior rim of the pinna, which has the most sun exposure. May occur also in ear canal and show chronic discharge that is either serosanguineous or bloody.

Keloid

Overgrowth of scar tissue, which invades original site of trauma. It is more common in dark-skinned people, although it also occurs in whites. In the ear, it is most common at lobule at the site of a pierced ear. Overgrowth shown here is unusually large.

Table 13-3   ABNORMALITIES IN THE EAR CANAL

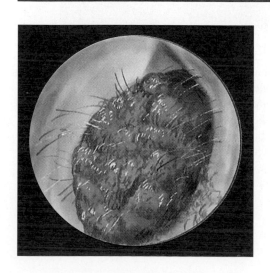

◀ Excessive Cerumen

Excessive cerumen is produced or is impacted owing to narrow tortuous canal or to poor cleaning method. May show as round ball partially obscuring drum or totally occluding canal. Even when canal is 90%–95% blocked, hearing stays normal. But when last 5%–10% is totally occluded (when cerumen expands after swimming or showering), person experiences ear fullness and sudden hearing loss.

Table continued on following page

Table 13-3   ABNORMALITIES IN THE EAR CANAL *Continued*

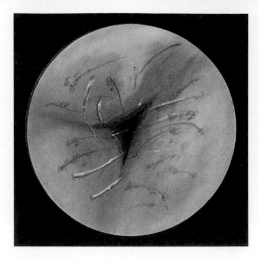

Otitis Externa

Severe swelling of canal, inflammation, tenderness. Here canal lumen is narrowed to one-quarter normal size. (See complete description in Table 13–1.)

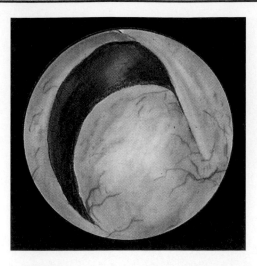

Osteoma

Single, stony hard, rounded nodule that obscures the drum; nontender; overlying skin appears normal. Attached to inner third, the bony part, of canal. Benign, but refer for removal.

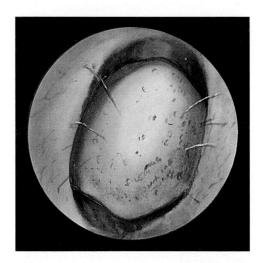

Foreign Body

Usually it is children who place a foreign body in the ear (here, a stone completely occludes the canal), which is later noted on routine examination. Common objects are beans, corn, jewelry beads, small stones, sponge rubber. Cotton is most common in adults and becomes impacted from cotton-tipped applicators. A trapped live insect is uncommon, but makes the person especially frantic.

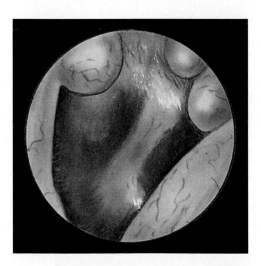

Exostosis

More common than osteoma. Small, bony hard, rounded nodules of hypertrophic bone, covered with normal epithelium. They arise near the drum but usually do not obstruct the view of the drum. They are usually multiple and bilateral. They may occur more frequently in cold-water swimmers. The condition needs no treatment, although it may cause accumulation of cerumen, which blocks the canal.

Table 13-3 ABNORMALITIES IN THE EAR CANAL *Continued*

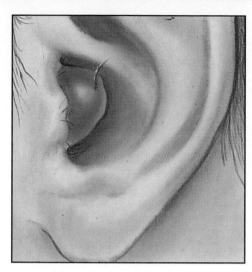

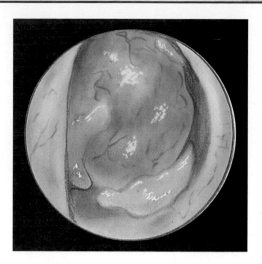

Furuncle

Exquisitely painful, reddened, infected hair follicle. Here, it occurs on the tragus but also may be on cartilaginous part of ear canal. Regional lymphadenopathy often accompanies a furuncle.

Polyp

Arises in canal from granulomatous or mucosal tissue; redder than surrounding skin and bleeds easily; bathed in foul purulent discharge; indicates chronic ear disease. Benign, but refer for excision.

Table 13-4 ABNORMAL FINDINGS SEEN ON OTOSCOPY

Appearance of Eardrum	Indicates	Suggested Condition
Yellow-amber color	Serum or pus	Serous otitis media or chronic otitis media
Prominent landmarks	Retraction of drum	Negative pressure in middle ear from an obstructed eustachian tube
Air/fluid level or air bubbles	Serous fluid	Serous otitis media
Absent or distorted light reflex	Bulging of eardrum	Acute otitis media
Bright red color	Infection in middle ear	Acute purulent otitis media
Blue or dark red color	Blood behind drum	Trauma, skull fracture
Dark oval areas	Perforation	Drum rupture
White dense areas	Scarring	Sequelae of infections
Diminished or absent landmarks	Thickened drum	Chronic otitis media
Black or white dots on drum or canal	Colony of growth	Fungal infection

Table 13–5 ABNORMALITIES OF THE TYMPANIC MEMBRANE

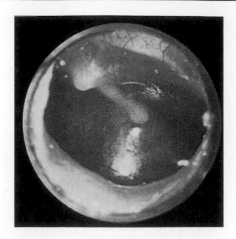

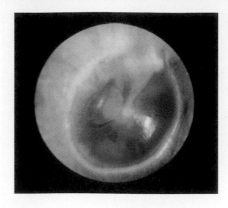

Retracted Drum

Landmarks look more prominent and well defined. Malleus handle looks shorter and more horizontal than normal. Short process is very prominent. Light reflex is absent or distorted. The drum is dull and lusterless and does not move. These signs indicate negative pressure and middle ear vacuum due to obstructed eustachian tube and serous otitis media.

Serous Otitis Media

An amber-yellow drum suggests serum in middle ear that transudates to relieve negative pressure from the blocked eustachian tube. You may note an air/fluid level with fine black dividing line, or air bubbles visible behind drum. Symptoms are feeling of fullness, transient hearing loss, popping sound with swallowing. Also called: secretory otitis media, middle ear effusion, glue ear.

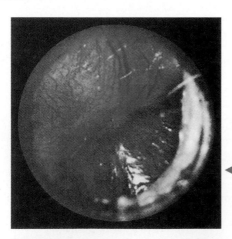

Early stage

◀ Acute Purulent Otitis Media

This results when the middle ear fluid is infected. An absent light reflex due to increasing middle ear pressure is an early sign. Redness and bulging are first noted in superior part of drum (pars flaccida), along with earache and fever. Then fiery red bulging of entire drum occurs; deep throbbing pain; fever; transient hearing loss. Pneumatic otoscopy reveals drum hypomobility.

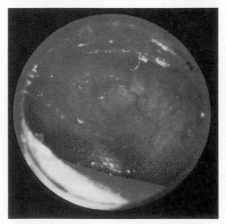

Later stage

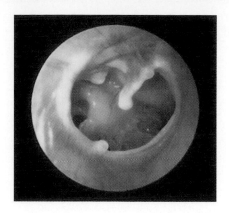

Perforation

If the acute otitis media is not treated, the drum may rupture from increased pressure. Perforations also occur from trauma (e.g., a slap on the ear). Usually, the perforation appears as a round or oval darkened area on the drum, but in this photo the perforation is very large. *Central* perforations occur in the pars tensa. *Marginal* perforations occur at the annulus. Marginal perforations are called attic perforations when they occur in superior part of the drum, the pars flaccida.

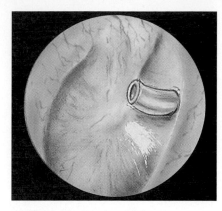

Insertion of Tympanostomy Tubes

Polyethylene tubes are inserted surgically into the eardrum to relieve middle ear pressure and promote drainage of chronic or recurrent middle ear infections. Number of acute infections tends to decrease because of improved aeration. Tubes extrude spontaneously in 12 to 18 months.

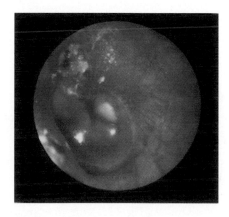

Cholesteatoma

A malignant overgrowth of epidermal tissue may result over the years following a marginal perforation. It has a pearly white, cheesy appearance. Growth of cholesteatoma can erode bone and produce hearing loss.

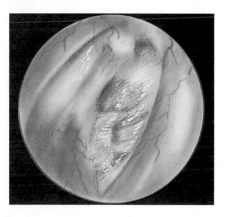

Scarred Drum

Dense white patches on the eardrum are sequelae of repeated ear infections. They do not necessarily affect hearing.

Table continued on following page

Table 13–5   ABNORMALITIES OF THE TYMPANIC MEMBRANE *Continued*

ABNORMAL FINDINGS

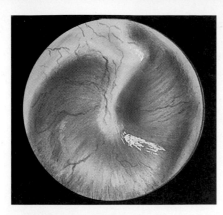

Blue Drum (Hemotympanum)

This indicates blood in the middle ear, as in trauma resulting in skull fracture.

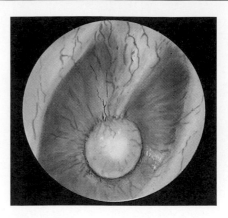

Bullous Myringitis

Small vesicles on the drum; accompany mycoplasma pneumonia and virus infections.

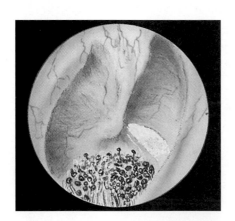

◀ ### Fungal Infection (Otomycosis)

Colony of black or white dots on drum or canal wall suggests a yeast or fungal infection.

▼ Table 13–6 TUNING FORK TESTS

Weber Test

Normal

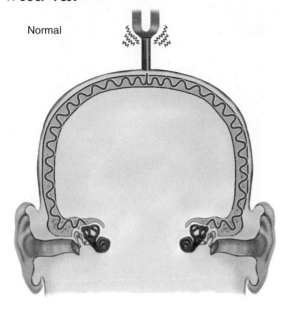

Normal—Sound is equally loud in both ears; sound does not lateralize.

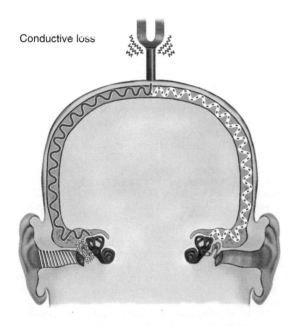

Conductive loss

Conductive loss—Sound lateralizes to "poorer" ear owing to background room noise, which masks hearing in normal ear. "Poorer" ear (the one with conductive loss) is not distracted by background noise, thus has a better chance to hear bone-conducted sound. Examples: transient conductive loss with serous or purulent otitis media.

Rinne Test

Normal

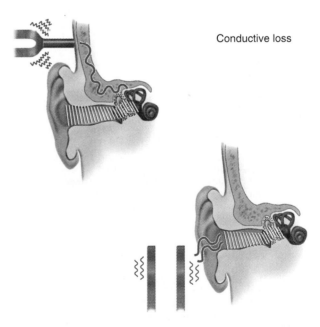

Normal—Sound is heard twice as long by air conduction (AC) as by bone conduction (BC); a "positive" Rinne, or AC > BC.

Conductive loss

Conductive loss—Person hears as long by bone conduction (AC = BC) or even longer (AC < BC), a "negative" finding on the Rinne test.

Table continued on following page

Table 13–6 TUNING FORK TESTS *Continued*

Weber Test

Sensorineural loss

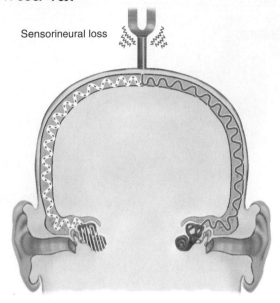

Sensorineural loss—Sound lateralizes to "better" ear or unaffected ear. Poor ear (the one with nerve loss) is unable to perceive the sound.

Rinne Test

Sensorineural loss

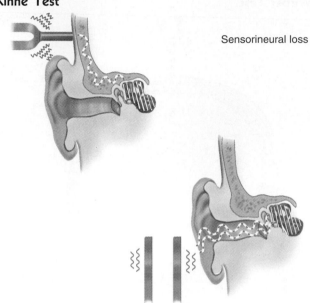

Sensorineural loss—Normal ratio of AC > BC is intact but is reduced overall. That is, person hears poorly both ways.

Bibliography

Abyad A: In-office screening for age-related hearing and vision loss. Geriatrics 52(6):51–57, June 1997.

Adams GL, Boies LR, Hilger PA: Boies Fundamentals of Otolaryngology, 6th ed. Philadelphia, W.B. Saunders Company, 1989.

Berman S: Otitis media in children. N Engl J Med 332(23): 1560–1565, June 8, 1995.

Bluestone CD: Otitis media: To treat or not to treat? Consultant 38(6): 1421–1427, June 1998.

Bluestone CD, Klein JO: Otitis Media in Infants and Children, 2nd ed. Philadelphia, W.B. Saunders Company, 1995.

Freeman RB: Impacted cerumen: How to safely remove earwax in an office visit. Geriatrics 50(6):52–53, June 1995.

Hanson MS: Acute otitis media in children. Nurse Pract 21(5):72–80, May 1996.

Hanson MS: Otitis media with effusion. Lippincott's Primary Care Practice 1(2):168–171, May–June 1997.

Hawke M, Martin RL: A photographic study of the normal and diseased ear. Hearing J 48(6):29–36, June 1995.

Kane RL, Ouslander JG, Abrass IB: Essentials of Clinical Geriatrics, 3rd ed. New York: McGraw-Hill, 1994.

Kingston L, Reynolds D, Phillips LP: Comprehensive assessment of the head and neck. J Nurse Midwifery 40(2):187–201, Mar–Apr 1995.

Levine N: Painful papules on the ear: Chondrodermatitis. Geriatrics 51(9):22, Sep 1996.

Lewis-Cullinan C, Janken JK: Effect of cerumen removal on the hearing ability of geriatric patients. J Adv Nurs 15(5):594–600, 1990.

Mallinson AI, Longridge NS, Peacock C: Dizziness, imbalance, whiplash. J Musculoskel Pain 4(4):105–112, 1996.

Naeem Z, Newton V: Prevalence of sensorineural hearing loss in Asian children. Br J Audiol 30(5):332–339, Oct 1996.

Ostrowski VB, Wiet RJ: Pathologic conditions of the external ear and auditory canal. Postgrad Med 100(3):223–229, 1996.

Otitis Media Guideline Panel: Otitis media with effusion in young children: Clinical practice guideline number 12 (AHCPR Publication No. 94-0622). Rockville, MD, Agency for Health Care Policy and Research, Public Health Services, U.S. Department of Health and Human Services, 1994.

Overfield T: Biologic Variation in Health and Illness: Race, Age, and Sex Differences, 2nd ed. New York, CRC Press, 1995.

Prellner K, Fogle-Hansson M, Jorgensen F, et al: Prevention of recurrent otitis media in otitis-prone children by intermittent prophylaxis with penicillin. Acta Otolaryngol 114(2):182–187, Mar 1994.

Quick G: Warm weather woes: Stemming the tide of swimmer's ear. Consultant 35(5):629–630, May 1995.

Shaw L: Protocol for detection and follow-up of hearing loss. Clin Nurs Spec 11(6):240–247, Nov 1997.

Smeltzer CD: Primary care screening and evaluation of hearing loss. Nurs Pract 18(8):50–55, 1993.

Stenstrom C, Ingvarsson L: Late effects on ear disease in otitis-prone children: A long-term follow-up study. Acta Otolaryngol 115(5): 658–663, Sep 1995.

Terris MH, Magit AE, Davidson TE: Otitis media with effusion in infants and children. Postgrad Med 97:137–151, 1995.

Waitzman, AA, Hawke M: Otoscopic examination: What to look for in the middle ear. Consultant 36(6):1299–1305, June 1996.

Wooldridge WE: Musculoskeletal photo diagnosis: A recurrently tender ear. J Musculoskel Med 14(2):78, 80, Feb 1997.

Zivic R, King S: Cerumen-impaction management for clients of all ages. Nurs Pract 18(3):29–38, Mar 1993.

CHAPTER FOURTEEN

Nose, Mouth, and Throat

NOSE

The **nose** is the first segment of the respiratory system. It warms, moistens, and filters the inhaled air, and it is the sensory organ for smell. The external nose is shaped like a triangle with one side attached to the face (Fig. 14–1). On its leading edge, the superior part is the *bridge* and the free corner is the *tip*. The oval openings at the base of the triangle are the *nares;* just inside, each naris widens into the *vestibule*. The *columella* divides the two nares and is continuous inside with the nasal septum. The *ala* is the lateral outside wing of the nose on either side. The upper third of the external nose is made up of bone; the rest is cartilage.

Inside, the **nasal cavity** is much larger than the external nose would indicate (Fig. 14–2). It extends back over the roof of the mouth. The anterior edge of the cavity is lined with numerous coarse nasal hairs, or vibrissae. The rest of the cavity is lined with a blanket of ciliated mucous membrane. The nasal hairs filter the coarsest matter from inhaled air, whereas the mucous blanket filters out dust and bacteria. Nasal mucosa appears redder than oral mucosa because of the rich blood supply present to warm the inhaled air.

The nasal cavity is divided medially by the **septum** into two slitlike air passages. The anterior part of the septum holds a rich vascular network, *Kiesselbach's plexus,* the most common site of nosebleeds. In many people, the nasal septum is not absolutely straight and may deviate toward one passage.

The lateral walls of each nasal cavity contain three parallel bony projections—the superior, middle, and inferior **turbinates.** They increase the surface area so that more blood vessels and mucous membranes are available to warm, humidify, and filter the inhaled air. Underlying each turbinate is a cleft, the **meatus**, which is named for the turbinate above. The sinuses drain into the middle meatus, and tears from the nasolacrimal duct drain into the inferior meatus.

The olfactory receptors (hair cells) lie at the roof of the nasal cavity and in the upper one-third of the septum. These receptors for smell merge into the olfactory nerve, cranial nerve I, which transmits to the temporal lobe of the brain. Although it is not necessary for human survival, the sense of smell adds to nutrition by enhancing the pleasure and taste of food.

The **paranasal sinuses** are air-filled pockets within the cranium (Fig. 14–3). They communicate with the nasal cavity and are lined with the same type of ciliated mucous membrane. They lighten the weight of the skull bones, serve as resonators for sound production, and provide mucus, which drains into the nasal cavity. The sinus openings are narrow and easily occluded, which may cause inflammation or sinusitis.

Two pairs of sinuses are accessible to examination: the **frontal** sinuses in the frontal bone above and medial to the orbits, and the **maxillary** sinuses in the maxilla

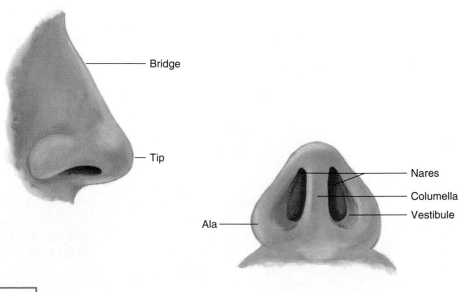

Bridge

Tip

Nares

Columella

Vestibule

Ala

14–1

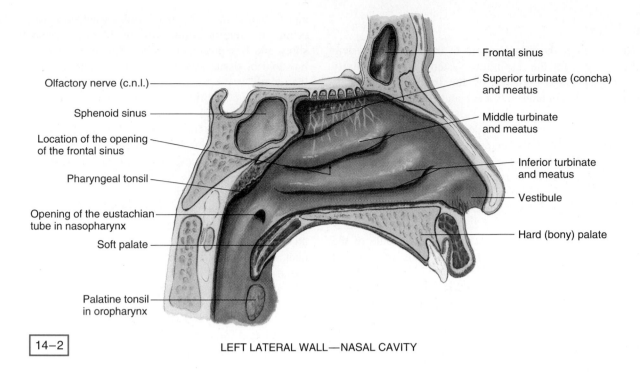

Frontal sinus

Superior turbinate (concha) and meatus

Middle turbinate and meatus

Inferior turbinate and meatus

Vestibule

Hard (bony) palate

Olfactory nerve (c.n.I.)

Sphenoid sinus

Location of the opening of the frontal sinus

Pharyngeal tonsil

Opening of the eustachian tube in nasopharynx

Soft palate

Palatine tonsil in oropharynx

14–2   LEFT LATERAL WALL—NASAL CAVITY

(cheekbone) along the side walls of the nasal cavity. The other two sets are smaller and deeper: the **ethmoid** sinuses between the orbits, and the **sphenoid** sinuses deep within the skull in the sphenoid bone.

Only the maxillary and ethmoid sinuses are present at birth. The maxillary sinuses reach full size after all permanent teeth have erupted. The ethmoid sinuses grow rapidly between 6 and 8 years of age and after puberty. The frontal sinuses are absent at birth, are fairly well developed between 7 and 8 years of age, and reach full size after puberty. The sphenoid sinuses are minute at birth and develop after puberty.

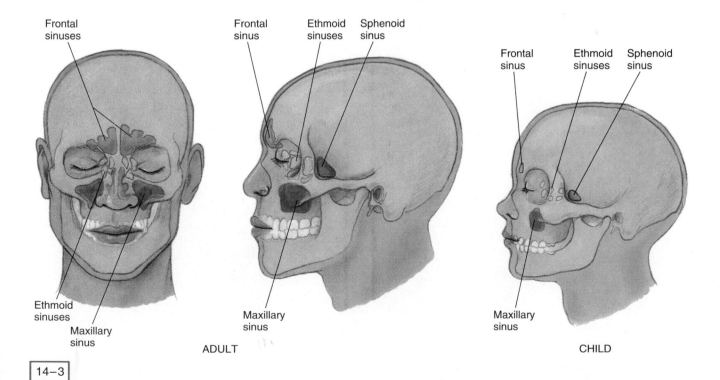

Frontal sinuses

Ethmoid sinuses

Maxillary sinus

ADULT

Frontal sinus   Ethmoid sinuses   Sphenoid sinus

Maxillary sinus

Frontal sinus   Ethmoid sinuses   Sphenoid sinus

Maxillary sinus

CHILD

14–3

MOUTH

The mouth is the first segment of the digestive system and an airway for the respiratory system. The **oral cavity** is a short passage bordered by the lips, palate, cheeks, and tongue. It contains the teeth and gums, tongue, and salivary glands (Fig. 14–4).

The lips are the anterior border of the oral cavity—the transition zone from the outer skin to the inner mucous membrane lining the oral cavity. The arching roof of the mouth is the palate; it is divided into two parts. The anterior **hard palate** is made up of bone and is a whitish color. Posterior to this is the **soft palate,** an arch of muscle that is pinker in color and mobile. The **uvula** is the free projection hanging down from the middle of the soft palate. The cheeks are the side walls of the oral cavity.

The floor of the mouth consists of the horseshoe-shaped mandible bone, the tongue, and underlying muscles. The **tongue** is a mass of striated muscle arranged in a crosswise pattern so that it can change shape and position. The papillae are the rough, bumpy elevations on its dorsal surface. Note the larger vallate papillae in an inverted V shape across the posterior base of the tongue,

and do not confuse them with abnormal growths. Underneath, the ventral surface of the tongue is smooth and shiny and has prominent veins. The **frenulum** is a midline fold of tissue that connects the tongue to the floor of the mouth.

The tongue's ability to change shape and position enhances its functions in mastication, swallowing, cleansing the teeth, and the formation of speech. The tongue also functions in taste sensation. Microscopic taste buds are in the papillae at the back and along the sides of the tongue and on the soft palate.

The mouth contains three pairs of salivary glands (Fig. 14–5). The largest, the **parotid** gland, lies within the cheeks in front of the ear extending from the zygomatic arch down to the angle of the jaw. Its duct, Stensen's duct, runs forward to open on the buccal mucosa opposite the second molar. The **submandibular** gland is the size of a walnut. It lies beneath the mandible at the angle of the jaw. Wharton's duct runs up and forward to the floor of the mouth and opens at either side of the frenulum. The smallest, the almond-shaped **sublingual** gland, lies within the floor of the mouth under the tongue. It has many small openings along the sublingual fold under the tongue.

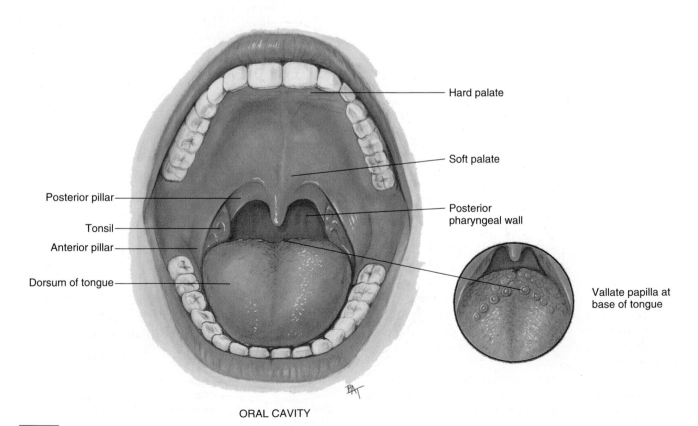

Hard palate

Soft palate

Posterior pillar

Tonsil

Anterior pillar

Dorsum of tongue

Posterior pharyngeal wall

Vallate papilla at base of tongue

ORAL CAVITY

14–4

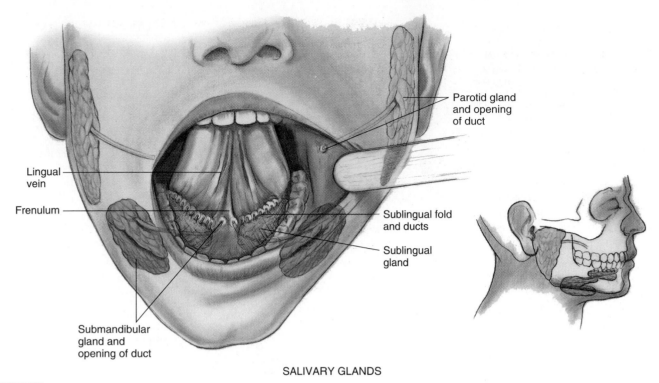

Parotid gland
and opening
of duct

Lingual
vein

Frenulum

Sublingual fold
and ducts

Sublingual
gland

Submandibular
gland and
opening of duct

SALIVARY GLANDS

14–5

The glands secrete saliva, the clear fluid that moistens and lubricates the food bolus, starts digestion, and cleans and protects the mucosa.

Adults have 32 **permanent** teeth, 16 in each arch. Each tooth has three parts: the crown, the neck, and the root. The gums (gingivae) collar the teeth. They are thick fibrous tissues covered with mucous membrane. The gums are different from the rest of the oral mucosa because of their pale pink color and stippled surface.

THROAT

The throat, or pharynx, is the area behind the mouth and nose. The **oropharynx** is separated from the mouth by a fold of tissue on each side, the anterior tonsillar pillar. Behind the folds are the **tonsils,** each a mass of lymphoid tissue. The tonsils are the same color as the surrounding mucous membrane, although they look more granular, and their surface shows deep crypts. Tonsillar tissue enlarges during childhood until puberty, then involutes. The posterior pharyngeal wall is seen behind these structures. Some small blood vessels may show on it.

The **nasopharynx** is continuous with the oropharynx, although it is above the oropharynx and behind the nasal cavity. The pharyngeal tonsils (adenoids) and the eustachian tube openings are located here (see Fig. 14–2).

The oral cavity and throat have a rich lymphatic network. Review the lymph nodes and their drainage patterns in Chapter 11, and keep this in mind when evaluating the mouth.

DEVELOPMENTAL CONSIDERATIONS

Infants and Children

In the infant, salivation starts at 3 months. The baby will drool periodically for a few months before learning to swallow the saliva. This drooling does not herald the eruption of the first tooth, although many parents think it does.

The teeth, both sets, begin development in utero. Children have 20 **deciduous,** or temporary, teeth. These erupt between 6 months and 24 months of age. All 20 teeth should appear by 2 ½ years of age. The deciduous teeth are lost beginning at age 6 years through age 12. They are replaced by the permanent teeth, starting with the central incisors (Fig. 14–6). The permanent teeth appear earlier in girls than in boys, and they erupt earlier in black children than in white children.

The nose develops during adolescence, along with other secondary sex characteristics. This growth starts at age 12 or 13, reaching full growth at age 16 in females and age 18 in males.

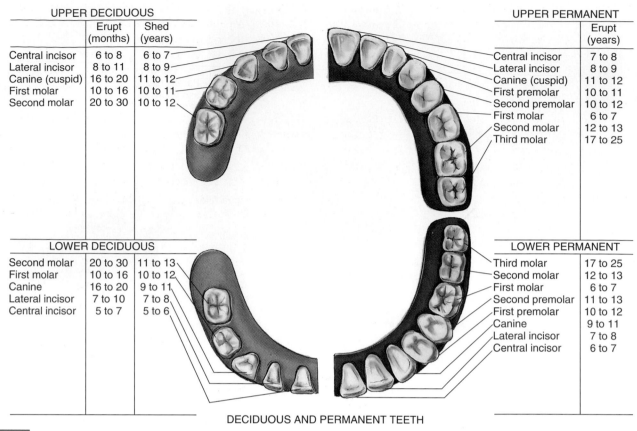

UPPER DECIDUOUS	Erupt (months)	Shed (years)
Central incisor	6 to 8	6 to 7
Lateral incisor	8 to 11	8 to 9
Canine (cuspid)	16 to 20	11 to 12
First molar	10 to 16	10 to 11
Second molar	20 to 30	10 to 12

UPPER PERMANENT	Erupt (years)
Central incisor	7 to 8
Lateral incisor	8 to 9
Canine (cuspid)	11 to 12
First premolar	10 to 11
Second premolar	10 to 12
First molar	6 to 7
Second molar	12 to 13
Third molar	17 to 25

LOWER DECIDUOUS	Erupt (months)	Shed (years)
Second molar	20 to 30	11 to 13
First molar	10 to 16	10 to 12
Canine	16 to 20	9 to 11
Lateral incisor	7 to 10	7 to 8
Central incisor	5 to 7	5 to 6

LOWER PERMANENT	Erupt (years)
Third molar	17 to 25
Second molar	12 to 13
First molar	6 to 7
Second premolar	11 to 13
First premolar	10 to 12
Canine	9 to 11
Lateral incisor	7 to 8
Central incisor	6 to 7

DECIDUOUS AND PERMANENT TEETH

14–6

The Pregnant Female

Nasal stuffiness and epistaxis may occur during pregnancy owing to increased vascularity in the upper respiratory tract. Also, the gums may be hyperemic and softened and may bleed with normal toothbrushing. Contrary to superstitious folklore, no evidence exists that pregnancy causes tooth decay or loss.

The Aging Adult

A gradual loss of subcutaneous fat starts during later middle adult years, making the nose appear more prominent in some people. The nasal hairs grow coarser and stiffer and may not filter the air as well. The hairs protrude and may cause itching and sneezing. Many older people clip these hairs, thinking them unsightly, but this practice can cause infection. The sense of smell may diminish because of a decrease in the number of olfactory nerve fibers. The decrease in the sensation of smell begins after age 60, and it continues progressively with age (Edelstein, 1996).

In the oral cavity, the soft tissues atrophy and the epithelium thins, especially in the cheek and tongue. This results in loss of taste buds, with about an 80 percent reduction in taste functioning. Further impairments to taste include a decrease in salivary secretion that is needed to dissolve flavoring agents, and the presence of upper dentures that cover secondary taste sites (Kane, Ouslander, and Abrass, 1994).

Atrophic tissues ulcerate easily, which places the older person at risk for infections such as oral moniliasis. An increased risk of malignant oral lesions is also present.

Many dental changes occur with aging. The tooth surface is abraded. The gums begin to recede and the teeth begin to erode at the gum line. A smooth V-shaped cavity forms around the neck of the tooth, exposing the nerve and making the tooth hypersensitive. Some tooth loss may occur owing to bone resorption (osteoporosis), which decreases the inner tooth structure and its outer support. Natural tooth loss is exacerbated by years of inadequate dental care, decay, poor oral hygiene, and tobacco use.

If tooth loss occurs, the remaining teeth drift, causing **malocclusion.** The stress of chewing with maloccluding teeth causes further problems: (1) Excessive bone resorption with further tooth loss occurs; (2) muscle imbalance results from a mandible and maxilla now out of alignment, which produces muscle spasms, tenderness of muscles of mastication, and chronic headaches; and (3) the temporomandibular joint is stressed, leading to osteoarthritis, pain, and inability to fully open the mouth.

A diminished sense of taste and smell decreases the aging person's interest in food and may contribute to malnutrition. Saliva production decreases; saliva acts as a solvent for food flavors and helps move food around the mouth. Decreased saliva also reduces the mouth's self-cleaning property. The major cause of decreased saliva flow is not the aging process itself but the use of medications that have anticholinergic effects (Lee, 1996). Over 250 medications have a side effect of dry mouth.

The absence of some teeth and trouble with mastication encourage the older person to eat soft foods (usually high in carbohydrates) and to decrease meat and fresh vegetable intake. This produces a risk of nutritional deficit for protein, vitamins, and minerals.

TRANSCULTURAL CONSIDERATIONS

Bifid uvula, a condition in which the uvula is split either completely or partially, occurs in 18 percent of some Native American groups and in 10 percent of Asians. The occurrence in whites and blacks is rare. **Cleft lip** and **cleft palate** are most common in Asians and Native Americans and least common in blacks (Overfield, 1995). **Torus palatinus,** a bony ridge running in the middle of the hard palate, is more common in Native Americans (55 percent) and in Inuits and Asians (up to 77 percent; Jarvis and Gorlin, 1972).

Leukoedema, a grayish white benign lesion occurring on the buccal mucosa, is present in 68 to 90 percent of blacks but in only 43 percent of whites (Martin and Crump, 1972). Oral hyperpigmentation also varies according to race. Usually absent at birth, hyperpigmentation increases with age. By age 50 years, 10 percent of whites and 50 to 90 percent of blacks will show oral hyperpig-mentation, a condition that is believed to be caused by a lifetime of accumulation of postinflammatory oral changes (Overfield, 1995).

Although it is rare for a white baby to be born with teeth (1 in 3000), the incidence rises to 1 in 11 among Tlingit Indians and to 1 or 2 in 100 among Canadian Inuit infants (Jarvis and Gorlin, 1972).

The size of teeth varies widely, with the teeth of whites being the smallest, followed by blacks, then Asians and Native Americans. The largest teeth are found among Inuits and Australian Aborigines (Overfield, 1995). Larger teeth cause some groups to have prognathic, or protruding, jaws, a condition that is seen more frequently in blacks and Asians. The condition is normal and does not reflect an orthodontic problem.

Agenesis (absence) of teeth varies by race, with absence of the third molar occurring in 18 to 35 percent of Asians, 9 to 25 percent of whites, and 1 to 11 percent of blacks (Overfield, 1995). Throughout life, whites have more tooth decay than blacks. The differences in tooth decay between blacks and whites occurs because blacks have harder and denser tooth enamel that makes their teeth less susceptible to the organisms that cause caries.

The incidence of tooth loss and edentulism has decreased substantially in the United States over the past several decades due to fluoridation, improved dental treatment, and better personal care. While the overall prevalence of edentulism has dropped to 10.5 percent of the population, there remain significant variations among subgroups in the population; that is, Mexican Americans had the lowest rate of tooth loss, while blacks had the highest rate of tooth loss (Marcus, Drury, Brown, and Zion, 1996).

SUBJECTIVE DATA

Nose

1. Discharge
2. Frequent colds (upper respiratory infections)
3. Sinus pain
4. Trauma
5. Epistaxis (nosebleeds)
6. Allergies
7. Altered smell

Mouth and Throat

1. Sores or lesions
2. Sore throat
3. Bleeding gums
4. Toothache
5. Hoarseness
6. Dysphagia
7. Altered taste
8. Smoking, alcohol consumption
9. Self-care behaviors
    Dental care pattern
    Dentures or appliances

Examiner Asks	Rationale

NOSE

❶ Discharge. Any **nasal discharge** or runny nose? Continuous?
- Is the discharge watery, purulent, mucoid, bloody?

Rhinorrhea occurs with colds, allergies, sinus infection, trauma.

❷ Frequent colds. Any unusually **frequent** or **severe colds (upper respiratory infections)?** How often do these occur?

Most people have occasional colds; thus, asking this more precise question yields more meaningful data.

❸ Sinus pain. Any **sinus pain** or sinusitis? How is this treated?
- Do you have chronic postnasal drip?

❹ Trauma. Ever had any **trauma** or a blow to the nose?
- Can you breathe through your nose? Are both sides obstructed or one?

Trauma may cause deviated septum, which may cause nares to be obstructed.

❺ Epistaxis (nosebleeds). Any nosebleeds? How often?
- How much bleeding—a teaspoonful or does it pour out?
- Color of the blood—red or brown? Clots?
- From one nostril or both?
- Aggravated by nose-picking or scratching?
- How do you treat the nosebleeds? Are they difficult to stop?

Epistaxis occurs with trauma, vigorous nose blowing, foreign body.

Person should sit up with head tilted forward, pinch nose between thumb and forefinger for 5 to 15 minutes.

❻ Allergies. Any **allergies** or hay fever? To what are you allergic, e.g., pollen, dust, pets?
- How was this determined?
- What type of environment makes it worse? Can you avoid exposure?
- Use inhalers, nasal spray, nose drops? How often? Which type?
- How long have you used this?

"Seasonal" rhinitis if due to pollen; "perennial" if allergen is dust.

Misuse of over-the-counter nasal medications irritates the mucosa and causes rebound swelling, a common problem.

❼ Altered smell. Experienced any **change in sense of smell?**

Sense of smell diminished with cigarette smoking or chronic allergies.

MOUTH AND THROAT

❶ Sores or lesions. Noticed any **sores** or **lesions** in the mouth, tongue, or gums?
- How long have you had it? Ever had this lesion before?
- Is it single or multiple?
- Does it seem to be associated with stress, season change, food?
- How have you treated the sore? Applied any local medication?

History helps to determine if oral lesions have infectious, traumatic, immunologic, or malignant etiology.

Examiner Asks	Rationale

2 **Sore throat.** How about **sore throats?** How frequently do you get them? Have a sore throat now? When did it start?
- Is it associated with cough, fever, fatigue, decreased appetite, head-ache, postnasal drip, or hoarseness?
- Is it worse when arising? What is the humidity level in the room where you sleep? Any dust or smoke inhaled at work?
- Usually get a throat culture for the sore throats? Were any documented as streptococcal?
- How have you treated this sore throat: medication, gargling? How effective are these? Have your tonsils or adenoids been taken out?

Untreated strep throat may lead to the complication of rheumatic fever.

3 **Bleeding gums.** Any **bleeding gums?** How long have you had this?

4 **Toothache.** Any **toothache?** Do your teeth seem sensitive to hot, cold? Have you lost any teeth?

5 **Hoarseness.** Any **hoarseness,** voice change? For how long?
- Feel like having to clear your throat? Or, like a "lump in your throat?"
- Use your voice a lot at work, recreation?
- Does the hoarseness seem associated with a cold, sore throat?

A disorder of the larynx due to many causes, e.g., overuse of the voice, upper respiratory infection, chronic inflammation, lesions, or a neoplasm.

6 **Dysphagia.** Any difficulty swallowing? How long have you had it?
- Feel like food gets stopped at a certain point?
- Any pain with this?

Dysphagia occurs with many conditions, including gastroesophageal reflux disease, pharyngitis, stroke and other neurologic diseases, and esophageal cancer.

7 **Altered taste.** Any **change in sense of taste?**

8 **Smoking, alcohol consumption.** Do you smoke? Pipe or cigarettes? Smokeless tobacco? How many packs per day? For how many years?

Chronic tobacco use is associated with tooth loss, coronal and root caries, and periodontal disease in older adults (Jette, Feldman, and Tennstedt, 1993).

- When was your last alcohol drink? How much alcohol did you drink that time? How much alcohol do you usually drink?

Chronic use of tobacco in any form and heavy alcohol consumption highly increase risk of oral and pharyngeal cancers (Shugars and Patton, 1997).

9 **Self-care behaviors.** Tell me about your daily dental care. How often do you use a toothbrush and floss?
- Last dental examination? Do dental problems affect which foods you eat?
- Do you have a dental appliance: braces, bridge, headgear?
- Wear dentures? All the time? How long have you had this set? How do they fit?
- Any sores or irritation on the palate or gums?
- Any problems with talking—Do the dentures whistle or drop? Can you chew all foods with them? How do you clean them?

Assess self-care behaviors for oral hygiene.
Periodic dental screening is necessary to note caries.

Lesions may arise from ill-fitting dentures, or the presence of dentures may mask the eruption of new lesion.

Examiner Asks	Rationale

ADDITIONAL HISTORY FOR INFANTS AND CHILDREN

1 Does the child have any mouth infections or sores, such as thrush or canker sores? How frequently do these occur?

2 Does the child have frequent sore throat, or tonsillitis? How often? How are these treated? Have they ever been documented as streptococcal infections?

3 Did the child's teeth erupt about on time?

Many delayed teeth may impair nutrition. Eruption is delayed with Down syndrome, cretinism, rickets.

- Do the teeth seem straight to you?

Malocclusion.

- Is the child using a bottle? How often during the day? Does the child go to sleep with a bottle at night?

Prolonged use of a bottle during day or when going to sleep places infant at risk for tooth decay and middle ear infections.

- Have you noticed any thumb-sucking after the child's secondary teeth came in?

Prolonged thumb-sucking (after age 6 to 7) may affect occlusion.

- Have you noticed the child grinding his or her teeth? Does this happen at night?

Bruxism—occurs in sleep, usually from nervous tension.

4 **Self-care behaviors.** How are the child's dental habits? Use a toothbrush regularly? How often does the child see a dentist?
- Do you use fluoridated water or fluoride supplement?

Evaluate child's self-care. Early self-care has best compliance.

ADDITIONAL HISTORY FOR THE AGING ADULT

1 Any dryness in the mouth? Are you taking any medications? (Note prescribed and over-the-counter medications.)

Xerostomia (dry mouth) is a side effect of many drugs used by older people: antidepressants, anticholinergics, antispasmodics, antihypertensives, antipsychotics, bronchodilators.

2 Have you had any loss of teeth? Can you chew all types of food?

Note a decrease in eating meat, fresh vegetables, and cleansing foods such as apples.

3 Are you able to care for your own teeth or dentures?

Ability to perform self-care may be decreased by physical disability (arthritis), vision loss, confusion, or depression.

4 Noticed a change in your sense of taste or smell?

Some people add condiments to enhance food when taste begins to wane. Note salt and sugar additives especially.

Also, diminished smell may decrease the person's ability to detect food spoilage, natural gas leaks, or smoke from a fire.

Preparation

Position the person sitting up straight with his or her head at your eye level. If the person wears dentures, offer a paper towel and ask the person to remove them.

 Equipment Needed

Otoscope with short, wide-tipped nasal speculum attachment or nasal speculum and penlight

Tongue blade

Cotton gauze pad (4 × 4 inches)

Gloves

Occasionally: long-stem light attachment for otoscope

Normal Range of Findings	Abnormal Findings

THE NOSE

Inspect and palpate the nose
External Nose

Normally, the nose is symmetric, in the midline, and in proportion to other facial features (Fig. 14–7). Inspect for any deformity, asymmetry, inflammation, or skin lesions. If an injury is reported or suspected, palpate gently for any pain or break in contour.

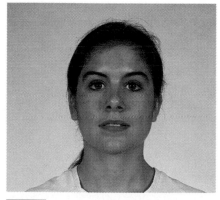

14–7

Test the patency of the nostrils by pushing each nasal wing shut with your finger while asking the person to sniff inward through the other naris. This reveals any obstruction, which later is explored using the nasal speculum. The sense of smell, mediated by cranial nerve I, is usually not tested in a routine examination. The procedure for assessing smell is presented with cranial nerve testing in Chapter 21.

Absence of sniff indicates obstruction, e.g., nasal polyps, rhinitis.

Nasal Cavity

Two possible techniques to explore the nasal cavity exist. You may use a nasal speculum to open the vestibule and a penlight to illuminate the cavity (Fig. 14–8). Hold the speculum in your left palm with its blades pointing away from you. Insert the closed blades 1 cm into the vestibule. Keep the blades vertical to avoid any pressure on the sensitive nasal septum. Keep your index finger on the nasal wing to stabilize the instrument. (Examiners with small hands may find this difficult to do.) Use your free hand to hold the penlight and to change position of the person's head.

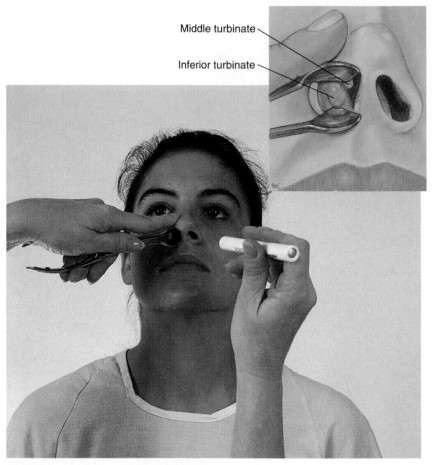

Middle turbinate

Inferior turbinate

14–8

An alternate technique is to attach the short wide-tipped speculum to the otoscope head and insert this combined apparatus into the nasal vestibule, again avoiding pressure on the nasal septum (Fig. 14–9). Gently lift up the tip of the nose with your finger before inserting.

▶ Normal Range of Findings

Abnormal Findings

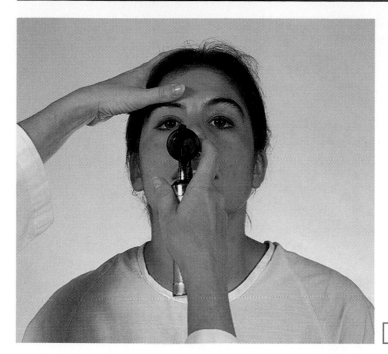

14-9

View each nasal cavity with the person's head erect, then with the head tilted back. Inspect the nasal mucosa, noting its normal red color and smooth moist surface (see Fig. 14-8). Note any swelling, discharge, bleeding, or foreign body.

Rhinitis—Nasal mucosa is swollen and bright red with an upper respiratory infection.

Discharge is common with rhinitis and sinusitis, varying from watery and copious to thick, purulent, and green-yellow.

With chronic allergy, mucosa looks swollen, boggy, pale, and gray.

Observe the nasal septum for deviation (Fig. 14-10). A deviated septum is common and is not significant unless airflow is obstructed. (If present in a hospitalized patient, document the deviated septum in the event that the person needs nasal suctioning or a nasogastric tube.) Also note any perforation or bleeding in the septum.

A deviated septum looks like a hump or shelf in one nasal cavity.

Perforation is seen as a spot of light from penlight shining in other naris.

Epistaxis commonly comes from anterior septum (see Table 14-1 on p. 405).

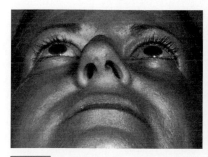 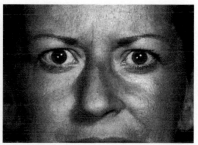

14-10

Normal Range of Findings	Abnormal Findings

Inspect the turbinates, the bony ridges curving down from the lateral walls. The superior turbinate will not be in your view, but the middle and inferior turbinates appear the same light red color as the nasal mucosa. Note any swelling but do not try to push the speculum past it. Turbinates are quite vascular and tender if touched.

Note any polyps, which are benign growths that accompany chronic allergy, and distinguish them from the normal turbinates.

Polyps are smooth, pale gray in color, avascular, mobile, and nontender (see Table 14–1).

THE SINUS AREAS

Palpate the sinus areas

Using your thumbs, press over the frontal sinuses below the eyebrows (Fig. 14–11A) and over the maxillary sinuses below the cheekbones (Fig. 14–11B). Take care not to press directly on the eyeballs. The person should feel firm pressure but no pain.

Sinus areas are tender to palpation in persons with chronic allergies and acute infection (sinusitis).

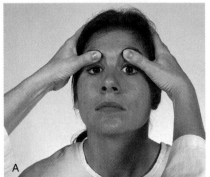
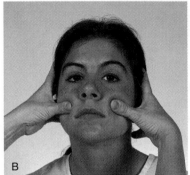

14–11

Transillumination

You may use this technique when you suspect sinus inflammation, although it is of limited usefulness. Darken the examining room. Affix a strong narrow light to the end of the otoscope, and hold it under the superior orbital ridge against the location of the frontal sinus area (Fig. 14–12). Cover with your hand. A diffuse red glow is a normal response. It comes from the light shining through the air in the healthy sinus. An inflamed sinus filled with fluid does not transilluminate.

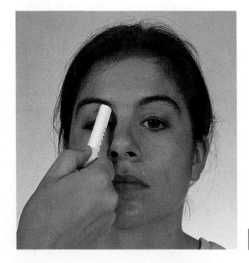

14–12

▶ Normal Range of Findings	Abnormal Findings

You may use the same technique with the maxillary sinuses, providing the person has no upper denture that would impede the light (Fig. 14–13). Ask the person to tilt the head back and open the mouth. Shine the light on each cheek just under the inner corner of the eye. Note a dull glow inside the mouth on the hard palate as the light transmits through the sinuses. Healthy sinuses contain air and may light up symmetrically. But be aware that asymmetry is not a reliable sign of sinus inflammation because many healthy sinuses normally will not transilluminate.

A significant finding is one sinus illuminated and the other clouded. If one has fluid, it looks darker than the healthy one.

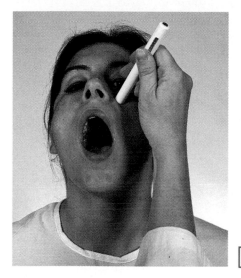

14–13

THE MOUTH

Inspect the mouth

Begin with anterior structures and move posteriorly. Use a tongue blade to retract structures and a bright light for optimal visualization.

Lips

Inspect the lips for color, moisture, cracking, or lesions. Retract the lips and note their inner surface as well (Fig. 14–14). Black persons normally may have bluish lips.

In light-skinned people: circumoral pallor occurs with shock and anemia; cyanosis with hypoxemia and chilling; cherry red lips with carbon monoxide poisoning, acidosis from aspirin poisoning, or ketoacidosis.

Cheilitis (perlèche)—cracking at the corners.

Herpes simplex, other lesions (see Table 14–2).

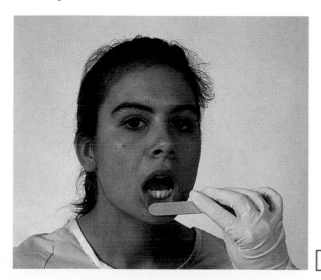

14–14

▶ | **Normal Range of Findings** | **Abnormal Findings**

Teeth and Gums

The condition of the teeth is an index of the person's general health. Your examination should not replace the regular dental examination, but you should note any diseased, absent, loose, or abnormally positioned teeth. The teeth normally look white, straight, and evenly spaced, and clean and free of debris or decay.

Compare the number of teeth with the number expected for the person's age. Ask the person to bite as if chewing something and note alignment of upper and lower jaw. Normal occlusion in the back is the upper teeth resting directly on the lowers; in the front, the upper incisors slightly override the lower incisors.

Discolored teeth appear brown with excessive fluoride use; yellow with tobacco use.

Grinding down of tooth surface.

Plaque—soft debris.

Caries—decay.

Malocclusion (poor biting relationship), e.g., protrusion of upper or lower incisors (see Table 14–3).

Normally, the gums look pink or coral with a stippled (dotted) surface. The gum margins at the teeth are tight and well defined. Check for swelling; retraction of gingival margins; and spongy, bleeding, or discolored gums. Black people normally may have a dark melanotic line along the gingival margin.

Gingival hypertrophy (see Table 14–3), crevices between teeth and gums, pockets of debris.

Gums bleed with slight pressure, indicating gingivitis.

Dark line on gingival margins occurs with lead and bismuth poisoning.

Tongue

Check the tongue for color, surface characteristics, and moisture. The color is pink and even. The dorsal surface is normally roughened from the papillae. A thin white coating may be present. Ask the person to touch the tongue to the roof of the mouth. Its ventral surface looks smooth, glistening, and shows veins. Saliva is present.

Beefy red swollen tongue. Smooth glossy areas (see Table 14–5).

Enlarged tongue occurs with mental retardation, hypothyroidism, acromegaly.

A small tongue accompanies malnutrition.

Dry mouth occurs with dehydration, fever; tongue has deep vertical fissures.

Saliva is decreased while the person is taking anticholinergic and other medication.

Excess saliva and drooling occur with gingivostomatitis and neurologic dysfunction.

Don a glove,* hold the tongue using a cotton gauze pad for traction, and swing the tongue out and to each side (Fig. 14–15). Inspect for any white patches or lesions—Normally none are present. If any occur, palpate these lesions for induration.

---

*Always wear gloves to examine mucous membranes. This follows Universal Precautions to prevent the spread of possible communicable disease.

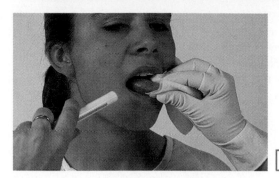

14–15

Inspect carefully the entire U-shaped area under the tongue. Oral malignancies are most likely to develop here. Note any white patches, nodules, or ulcerations. If lesions are present, or with any person over 50 or with a positive history of smoking or alcohol use, use your gloved hand to palpate the area. Place your other hand under the jaw to stabilize the tissue and to "capture" any abnormality (Fig. 14–16). Note any induration.

Any lesion or ulcer persisting for more than 2 weeks must be investigated.

An indurated area may be a mass or lymphadenopathy, and it must be investigated.

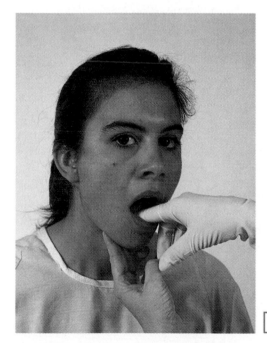

14–16

Buccal Mucosa

Hold the cheek open with a wooden tongue blade, and check the buccal mucosa for color, nodules, or lesions. It looks pink, smooth, and moist, although patchy hyperpigmentation is common and normal in dark-skinned people.

An expected finding is **Stensen's duct,** the opening of the parotid salivary gland. It looks like a small dimple opposite the upper second molar. You also may see a raised occlusion line on the buccal mucosa parallel with the level the teeth meet due to the teeth closing against the cheek.

Dappled brown patches present with Addison's disease (chronic adrenal insufficiency).

Orifice of Stensen's duct looks red with mumps.

Koplik's spots—a prodromal sign of measles.

Normal Range of Findings	Abnormal Findings

A larger patch also may be present along the buccal mucosa. This is **leukoedema,** a benign grayish opaque area, more common in blacks and East Indians. When it is mild, the patch disappears as you stretch the cheeks. The severity of the condition increases with age, looking grayish white and thickened. The cause of the condition is unknown. Do not mistake leukoedema for oral infections such as candidiasis (thrush).

Fordyce's granules are small, isolated white or yellow papules on the mucosa of cheek, tongue, and lips (Fig. 14–17). These little sebaceous cysts are painless and not significant.

The chalky white raised patch of **leukoplakia** is abnormal (see Table 14–4).

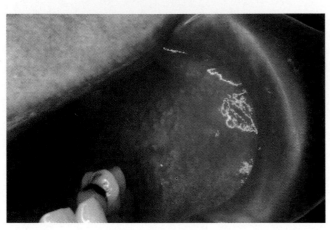

14–17

Fordyce's granules

Palate

Shine your light up to the roof of the mouth. The more anterior hard palate is white with irregular transverse rugae. The posterior soft palate is pinker, smooth, and upwardly movable. A normal variation is a nodular bony ridge down the middle of the hard palate, a **torus palatinus** (Fig. 14–18). This benign growth arises after puberty and is present in 25 percent of females and in 15 percent of males (Adams, Boies, and Hilger, 1989). It is a more common finding in Native Americans, Inuits, and Asians. Figure 14–18 uses a mirror to reflect the image of the torus palatinus, which actually lies in the roof of the mouth.

The hard palate appears yellow with jaundice. In blacks with jaundice, it may look yellow, muddy yellow, or green-brown.

Oral Kaposi's sarcoma is the most common early lesion in people with AIDS (see Table 14–6).

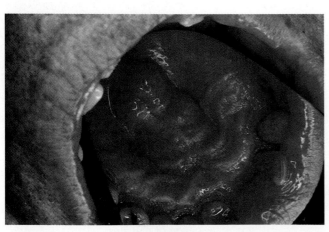

14–18

Torus palatinus

|

Observe the uvula; it normally looks like a fleshy pendant hanging in the midline (Fig. 14–19). Ask the person to say "ahhh" and note the soft palate and uvula rise in the midline. This tests one function of cranial nerve X, the vagus nerve.

A *bifid* uvula looks like it is split in two; more common in Native Americans (see Table 14–6).

Any deviation to the side or absent movement indicates nerve damage, which also occurs with poliomyelitis and diphtheria.

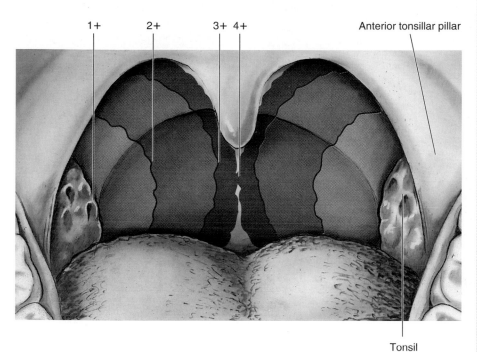

1+   2+   3+ 4+   Anterior tonsillar pillar

Tonsil

14–19

THE THROAT

Inspect the throat

Using your light, observe the oval, rough-surfaced **tonsils** behind the anterior tonsillar pillar (see Fig. 14–19). Their color is the same pink as the oral mucosa, and their surface is peppered with indentations, or crypts. In some people, the crypts collect small plugs of whitish cellular debris. This does not indicate infection. However, there should be no exudate on the tonsils. Tonsils are graded in size as:

With an acute infection tonsils are bright red, swollen, and may have exudate or large white spots.

A white membrane covering the tonsils may accompany infectious mononucleosis, leukemia, and diphtheria.

      1 + —visible
      2 + —halfway between tonsillar pillars and uvula
      3 + —touching the uvula
      4 + —touching each other

You may normally see 1+ or 2+ tonsils in healthy people, especially in children, because lymphoid tissue is proportionately enlarged until puberty.

Tonsils are enlarged to 2+, 3+, or 4+ with an acute infection.

▶

Enlarge your view of the posterior pharyngeal wall by depressing the tongue with a tongue blade (Fig. 14–20). Push down halfway back on the tongue; if you push on its tip, the tongue will hump up in back. Press slightly off center to avoid eliciting the gag reflex. You can help the person whose gag reflex is easily triggered by offering a tongue blade to depress his or her own tongue. (Some people can depress their own tongue so the tongue blade is not needed.) Scan the posterior wall for color, exudate, or lesions. When finished, discard the tongue blade.

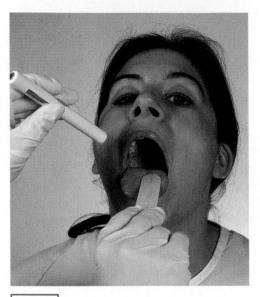

14–20

Although usually it is not done in the screening examination, touching the posterior wall with the tongue blade elicits the gag reflex. This tests cranial nerves IX and X, the glossopharyngeal and vagus.

Test cranial nerve XII, the hypoglossal nerve, by asking the person to stick out the tongue. It should protrude in the midline. Children enjoy this request! Note any tremor, loss of movement, or deviation to the side.

With damage to cranial nerve XII, the tongue deviates *toward* the paralyzed side.

A fine tremor of the tongue occurs with hyperthyroidism; a coarse tremor with cerebral palsy and alcoholism.

During the examination, notice any breath odor, *halitosis*. This is common and usually is due to a local cause, such as poor oral hygiene, consumption of odoriferous foods, alcohol consumption, heavy smoking, or dental infection. Occasionally, it may indicate a systemic disease.

Diabetic ketoacidosis has a sweet, fruity breath odor; this acetone smell also occurs in children with malnutrition or dehydration. Others are: an ammonia breath odor with uremia; a musty odor with liver disease; a foul, fetid odor with dental or respiratory infections; alcohol odor with alcohol ingestion or chemicals; a mouselike smell of the breath with diphtheria.

DEVELOPMENTAL CONSIDERATIONS

Infants and Children

Since the oral examination is intrusive for the infant or young child, the timing is best toward the end of the complete examination, along with the ear examination. But if any crying episodes occur earlier, seize the opportunity to examine the open mouth and oropharynx.

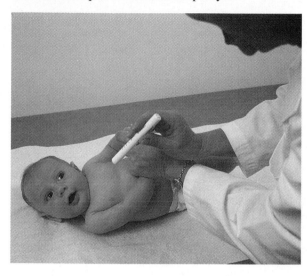

14–21

As with the ear examination, let the parent help position the child. Place the infant supine on the examining table, with the arms restrained (Fig. 14–21). The older infant and toddler may be held on the parent's lap with one of the parent's hands holding the arms down and the other hand restraining the child's head against the parent's chest. Although not often needed, the parent's leg can reach over and capture the child's legs between the parent's own (Fig. 14–22).

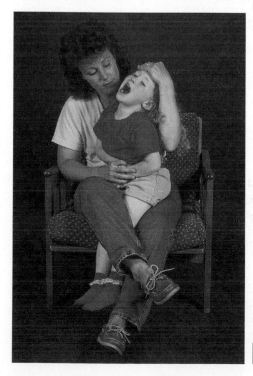

14–22

Use a game to help prepare the young child. Encourage the preschool child to use a tongue blade to look into a puppet's mouth. Or place a mirror so that the child can look into the mouth while you do. The school-age child is usually cooperative and loves to show off missing or new teeth (Fig. 14–23).

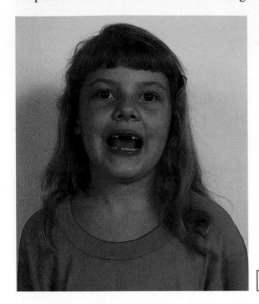

14–23

Be discriminating in your use of the tongue blade. It may be necessary for a full view of oral structures, but it produces a strong gag reflex in the infant. You may avoid the tongue blade completely with a cooperative preschooler and school-age child. Try asking the young child to open the mouth "as big as a lion" and to move the tongue in different directions. To enlarge your view of the oropharynx, ask the child to stick out the tongue and "pant like a dog."

At some point, you will encounter an uncooperative young child who clenches the teeth and refuses to open the mouth. If all your other efforts have failed, slide the tongue blade along the buccal mucosa and turn it between the back teeth. Push down to depress the tongue. This stimulates the gag reflex, and the child opens the mouth wide for a few seconds. You will have a *brief* look at the throat. Make the most of it.

Nose

The newborn may have milia across the nose. The nasal bridge may be flat in black and Asian children. There should be no nasal flaring or narrowing with breathing.

It is essential to determine the patency of the nares in the immediate newborn period because most newborns are obligate nose-breathers. Nares blocked with amniotic fluid are suctioned gently with a bulb syringe. If obstruction is suspected, a small lumen (5 to 10 Fr) catheter is passed down each naris to confirm patency.

Nasal flaring in the infant indicates respiratory distress.

A transverse ridge across the nose occurs in a child with chronic allergy from wiping the nose upward with palm (see Table 14–4). Nasal narrowing on inhalation is seen with chronic nasal obstruction and mouth-breathing.

Inability to pass catheter through nasal cavity indicates choanal atresia, which needs immediate intervention (see Table 14–1).

▶ Normal Range of Findings

Avoid the nasal speculum when examining the infant and young child. Instead, gently push up the tip of the nose with your thumb while using your other hand to shine the light into the naris. With a toddler, be alert for the possible foreign body lodged in the nasal cavity (see Table 14–1).

Only in children older than 8 years do you need to palpate the child's sinus areas. In younger children, sinus areas are too small for palpation.

Mouth and Throat

A normal finding in infants is the **sucking tubercle,** a small pad in the middle of the upper lip from friction of breast- or bottle-feeding. Note the number of teeth, and whether or not it is appropriate for the child's age. Also note pattern of eruption, position, condition, and hygiene. Use this guide for children under 2 years; the child's age in months minus the number 6 should equal the expected number of deciduous teeth. Normally, all 20 deciduous teeth are in by 2 ½ years. Saliva is present after 3 months of age and shows in excess with teething children.

Mobility should allow the tongue to extend at least as far as the alveolar ridge.

Note any bruising or laceration on the buccal mucosa or gums of the infant or young child.

On the palate, **Epstein's pearls** are a normal finding in newborns and infants (Fig. 14–24). They are small, yellow-white, glistening, pearly papules along the median raphe of the hard palate and on the gums where they look like teeth. They are small retention cysts and disappear in the first few weeks.

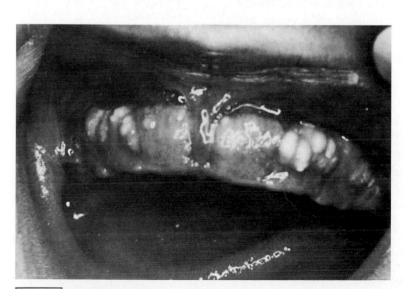

14–24 | **Epstein's pearls**

Abnormal Findings

No teeth by age 1 year.

Discolored teeth appear yellow or yellow-brown with infants taking tetracycline or whose mothers took the drug during the last trimester; appear green or black with excessive iron ingestion, although this reverses when the iron is stopped.

Malocclusion: upper or lower dental arches are out of alignment.

Ankyloglossia, a short lingual frenulum, can limit protrusion and impair speech development (see Table 14–5).

Trauma may indicate child abuse due to forced feeding of bottle or spoon.

A high-arched palate is usually normal in the newborn, but a very narrow or high arch also occurs with Tumer's syndrome, Ehlers-Danlos syndrome, Marfan's syndrome, and Treacher Collins syndrome, or develops in the mouth-breather in chronic allergies.

|

Bednar aphthae are traumatic areas or ulcers on the posterior hard palate on either side of the midline. They result from abrasions while sucking.

The tonsils are not visible in the newborn. They gradually enlarge during childhood, remaining proportionately larger until puberty. Tonsils appear still larger if the infant is crying or gagging. Normally, the newborn can produce a strong, lusty cry.

Insert your gloved finger into the baby's mouth and palpate the hard and soft palate as the baby sucks. The sucking reflex can be elicited in infants up to 12 months.

The Pregnant Female

Gum hypertrophy (surface looks smooth and stippling disappears) may occur normally at puberty or during pregnancy (pregnancy gingivitis).

The Aging Adult

The nose may appear more prominent on the face due to a loss of subcutaneous fat. In the edentulous person, the mouth and lips fold in, giving a "purse-string" appearance. The teeth may look slightly yellowed although the color is uniform. Yellowing results from the dentin visible through worn enamel. The surface of the incisors may show vertical cracks from a lifetime of exposure to extreme temperatures. The teeth may look longer as the gum margins recede.

The surfaces look worn down or abraded. Old dental work deteriorates, especially at the gum margins. The teeth loosen with bone resorption and may move with palpation.

The tongue looks smoother owing to papillary atrophy. The aging adult's buccal mucosa is thinned and may look shinier, as though it was "varnished."

SUMMARY CHECKLIST: NOSE, MOUTH, AND THROAT EXAM

NOSE

1: Inspect external nose for symmetry, any deformity, or lesions

2: Palpation—Test patency of each nostril

3: Inspect using nasal speculum:
Color and integrity of nasal mucosa
Septum—Note any deviation, perforation, or bleeding
Turbinates—Note color, any exudate, swelling, or polyps

4: Palpate the sinus areas— Note any tenderness

MOUTH AND THROAT

1: Inspect using penlight:
Lips, teeth and gums, tongue, buccal mucosa—Note color; if structures are intact, any lesions
Palate and uvula—Note integrity and mobility as person phonates
Grade tonsils
Pharyngeal wall—Note color, any exudate, or lesions

2: Palpation:
When indicated in adults, bimanual palpation of mouth
With the neonate, palpate for integrity of palate and to assess sucking reflex

SAMPLE CHARTING

▶ **Subjective**

Nose. No history of discharge, sinus problems, obstruction, epistaxis, or allergy. Colds 1–2 /yr, mild. Fractured nose during high school sports, treated by M.D.

Mouth and Throat. No pain, lesions, bleeding gums, toothache, dysphagia, or hoarseness. Occasional sore throat with colds. Tonsillectomy, age 8. Smokes cigarettes 1 PPD × 9 years. Alcohol—1–2 drinks socially, about 2 × /month. Visits dentist annually, dental hygienist 2 × /year, flosses daily. No dental appliance.

▶ **Objective**

Nose. Symmetric, no deformity or skin lesions. Nares patent. Mucosa pink, no discharge, lesions, or polyps; no septal deviation or perforation. Sinuses—no tenderness to palpation.

Mouth. Can clench teeth. Mucosa and gingivae pink, no masses or lesions. Teeth are all present, straight, and in good repair. Tongue smooth, pink, no lesions, protrudes in midline, no tremor.

Throat. Mucosa pink, no lesions or exudate. Uvula rises in midline on phonation. Tonsils out. Gag reflex present.

CLINICAL CASE STUDY 1

Brad D., a 34-year-old electrician, seeks care for "sore throat for 2 days."

▶ **Subjective**

2 days PTA experienced sudden onset of sore throat, swollen glands, fever 101° F, occasional shaking chills, extreme fatigue.

Today—symptoms remain. Cough productive of yellow sputum. Treated self with aspirin for minimal relief. Unable to eat last 2 days because "throat on fire." Taking adequate fluids, on bedrest. Not aware of exposure to other sick persons. Does not smoke.

▶ **Objective.**

Ears. Tympanic membranes pearl gray with landmarks intact.

Nose. No discharge. Mucosa pink, no swelling.

Mouth. Mucosa and gingivae pink, no lesions.

Throat. Tonsils 3+. Pharyngeal wall bright red with yellow-white exudate, exudate also on tonsils.

Neck. Enlarged anterior cervical nodes bilaterally, painful to palpation. No other lymph adenopathy.

Chest. Resonant to percussion throughout. Breath sounds clear anterior and posterior. No adventitious sounds.

▶ ASSESSMENT

Pharyngitis
Pain R/T inflammation
Altered nutrition: less than body requirements R/T dysphagia

Continued

CLINICAL CASE STUDY 2

Calvin W., a 53-year-old white businessman, is in the hospital awaiting coronary bypass surgery for coronary artery disease. As part of a preoperative teaching plan for coughing and deep breathing, a respiratory assessment is performed.

Problem List

No.	Title	Date Entered
1	Coronary artery disease	7/4/
2	Chronic allergy to dust or animal hair	7/4/

Progress Notes

▶ **Subjective**

States understanding of reason for admission to hospital and extent of coronary artery disease. Unaware of details of surgical procedure and postoperative care. Interested, "I do better when I know what I'm dealing with." History of exertional angina after walking one short block or climbing one flight of stairs, treats self with nitroglycerin. Does not smoke. Chronic watery nasal discharge, "comes and goes, but present most of time."

▶ **Objective**

Nose. Only R naris patent. Mucosa gray and boggy bilaterally. L naris has mobile, gray, nontender mass, obstructing view of turbinates and rest of nasal cavity.

Mouth and Throat. Mucosa pink, no lesions. Uvula midline, rises on phonation. Tonsils absent. No lumps or lesions on palpation.

Chest. Thorax symmetric, AP < transverse diameter, respirations 18/min, effortless. Resonant to percussion. Breath sounds are clear. No adventitious sounds.

▶ ASSESSMENT

L nasal mass, possibly polyp
Knowledge deficit for surgery and expected postop course R/T lack of exposure

CLINICAL CASE STUDY 3

Esther V. is a 61-year-old professor who has been admitted to the hospital for chemotherapy for carcinoma of the breast. This is her 5th day in the hospital. An oral assessment is performed when she complains of "soreness and a white coating" in the mouth.

▶ **Subjective**

Felt soreness on tongue and cheeks during night. Now pain persists, and E.V. can see a "white coating" on tongue and cheeks. "I'm worried. Is this more cancer?"

▶ **Objective**

E.V. generally appears restless and overly aware.

Oral mucosa pink. Large white, cheesy patches covering most of dorsal surface of tongue and buccal mucosa. Will scrape off with tongue blade, revealing red eroded area beneath.

Bleeds with slight contact. Posterior pharyngeal wall pink, no lesions. Patches are soft to palpation. No palpable lymph nodes.

▶ ASSESSMENT

Oral lesion, appears as candidiasis
Altered oral mucous membrane R/T effects of chemotherapy
Pain R/T infectious process
Anxiety R/T threat to health status

NURSING DIAGNOSES COMMONLY ASSOCIATED WITH NOSE, MOUTH, THROAT DISORDERS

Diagnosis	Related Factors (Etiology)	Defining Characteristics (Symptoms and Signs)

Altered oral mucous membrane	Dehydration
	Effects of
	    Chemotherapy
	    Medication
	    Radiation to head/neck
	    Diabetes mellitus
	    Oral cancer
	Immunosuppression
	Inadequate oral hygiene
	Infection
	Lack of knowledge
	Mouth-breathing
	Malnutrition/vitamin deficiency
	NPO for > 24 h
	Chemical trauma
	    Acidic foods
	    Alcohol
	    Drugs
	    Noxious agents
	    Tobacco
	Mechanical trauma
	    Braces
	    Broken teeth
	    Endotracheal tube
	    Fractured mandible
	    Ill-fitting dentures
	    Nasogastric tube
	Vomiting
		Atrophy of gums
		Coated tongue
		Dry mouth (xerostomia)
		Edema of mucosa
		Halitosis
		Hemorrhagic gingivitis
		Hyperemia
		Lack of or decreased salivation
		Leukoplakia
		Oral
		    Lesions
		    Pain or discomfort
		    Plaque
		Redness
		    Ulcers
		    Vesicles
		Purulent drainage
		Stomatitis

Impaired swallowing	Effects of
	    Cleft lip/palate
	    Cerebrovascular accident
	    Cranial nerve damage (V, VII, IX, X)
	Neuromuscular disorder (e.g., cerebral palsy, muscular dystrophy, Guillain-Barré syndrome, myasthenia gravis, poliomyelitis), oral/pharyngeal cancer
	Excessive/inadequate salivation
	Fatigue
	Limited awareness
	Mechanical obstruction
	    Edema
	    Tracheostomy tube
	    Tumor
	Neuromuscular impairment
	    Decreased/absent gag reflex
	    Decreased strength of muscles of mastication
	    Perceptual impairment
	    Facial paralysis
	Reddened, irritated oropharynx
		Coughing/choking
		Dehydration
		Evidence of aspiration
		Regurgitation of fluids/solids through mouth or nose
		Reported pain on swallowing
		Stasis of food in oral cavity
		Weight loss

Continued

Pain	Effects of surgery or trauma	Reports of pain
	Experiences during diagnostic tests	Anxiety
	Infectious process	Clutching of painful area
	Inflammation	Crying or moaning
	Muscle spasm	Distraction behavior
	Immobility	Focused on self
	Obstructive processes	Immobilization
	Overactivity	Painful response to palpation
	Pressure points	Facial mask of pain
		Changes in posture or gait
		Withdrawal reflex
		Changes in muscle tone—listless to rigid
		Autonomic responses
		Increased blood pressure, pulse, respirations
		Diaphoresis
		Dilated pupils
		Social withdrawal
		Impaired thought process
		Altered time perception
		Feelings of guilt, despair, or helplessness
Sensory/perceptual alterations: Olfactory	Effects of aging	Decreased sensitivity to smells
	Foreign body in nares	Decreased appetite
	Inflammation of nasal mucosa	
	Neurologic impairment	
	Obstruction in nares	
Gustatory	Effects of aging	Decreased sensitivity to tastes
	Effects of trauma to tongue	Decreased appetite
	Inflammation of nasal mucosa	Increased seasoning of foods
	Neurologic impairment	
	Side effects of specific medications	

Other Related Nursing Diagnoses

ACTUAL	RISK/WELLNESS
Impaired verbal communication	**Risk**
Ineffective airway clearance	Risk for aspiration
	Wellness
	Actively seeking knowledge about smoking cessation

ASSESSMENT VIDEO CRITICAL THINKING QUESTIONS

The Saunders Physical Examination and Health Assessment Video Series—Nose, Mouth, and Throat—will direct you to consider the following:

1. How may oral self-care affect mouth examination findings?

2. Describe abnormal findings that may be found during inspection of the internal nose.

3. How do mouth examination findings vary among darkly pigmented people?

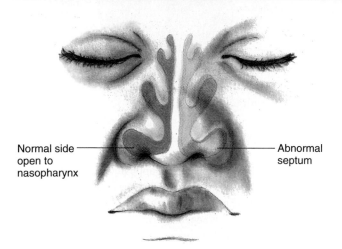

Normal side open to nasopharynx — Abnormal septum

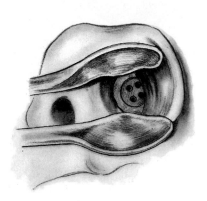

Choanal Atresia

A bony or membranous septum between the nasal cavity and the pharynx of the newborn. When the condition is bilateral, it requires the immediate insertion of an oral airway to prevent asphyxia because most newborns are obligate nose-breathers. When the condition is unilateral, the infant may be asymptomatic until the onset of his or her first respiratory infection.

Foreign Body

Children particularly are apt to put an object up the nose, producing unilateral purulent drainage and foul odor. Because some risk for aspiration exists, removal should be prompt.

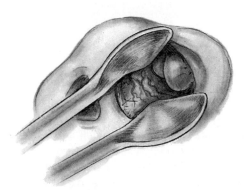

Epistaxis

The most common site of a nosebleed is Kiesselbach's plexus in the anterior septum. It may be spontaneous from a local cause or a sign of underlying illness. Causes include nose-picking, forceful coughing or sneezing, fracture, foreign body, rhinitis, following heavy exertion, or with a coagulation disorder. Bleeding from the anterior septum is easily controlled and rarely severe. A posterior hemorrhage is less common (< 10 percent) but is more profuse, harder to manage, and more serious.

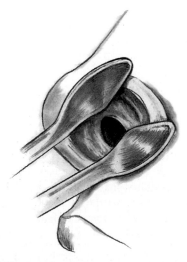

Perforated Septum

A hole in the septum, usually in the cartilaginous part, may be caused by chronic infection, trauma from continual picking of crusts, sniffing cocaine, or nasal surgery. It is seen as a spot of light when the penlight is directed into the other naris.

Table continued on following page

Table 14-1   ABNORMALITIES OF THE NOSE *Continued*

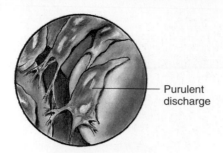
Purulent discharge

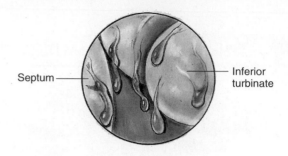
Septum — Inferior turbinate

Acute Rhinitis

The first sign is a watery discharge, rhinorrhea, which becomes purulent. This is accompanied by sneezing and swollen mucosa, which causes nasal obstruction. Turbinates are dark red and swollen.

Allergic Rhinitis

Rhinorrhea, itching of nose and eyes, lacrimation, nasal congestion, and sneezing are present. Note serous edema and swelling of turbinates to fill the air space. Turbinates are usually pale (although may appear violet), and their surface looks smooth and glistening. May be seasonal or perennial, depending on allergen. Individual has a strong family history of seasonal allergies.

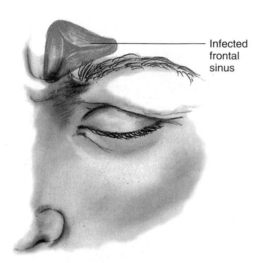
Infected frontal sinus

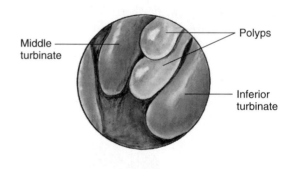
Middle turbinate — Polyps — Inferior turbinate

Sinusitis

Facial pain, following upper respiratory infection; signs include red swollen nasal mucosa, swollen turbinates, and purulent discharge. Person also experiences fever, chills, malaise. With maxillary sinusitis, dull throbbing pain occurs in cheeks and teeth on the same side, and pain with palpation is present. With frontal sinusitis, pain is above the supraorbital ridge.

Polyps

Smooth, pale gray nodules, which are overgrowths of mucosa, most commonly caused by chronic allergic rhinitis. May be stalked. A common site is protrusion from the middle meatus. Often multiple, they are mobile and nontender in contrast to turbinates. They may obstruct air passageways as they get larger. Symptoms include the absence of a sense of smell and a "valve that moves" in the nose as the person breathes.

ABNORMAL FINDINGS

Table 14–1 ABNORMALITIES OF THE NOSE *Continued*

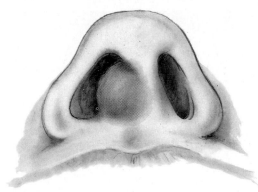

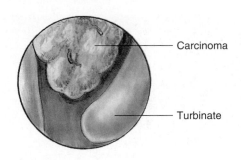

— Carcinoma

— Turbinate

Furuncle

A small boil located in the skin or mucous membrane; appears red and swollen and is quite painful. Avoid any manipulation or trauma that may spread the infection.

Carcinoma

This appears gray-white and nontender. It may produce slow bloody unilateral discharge, in contrast to the profuse bleeding that accompanies epistaxis. It is not a common lesion.

 Table 14–2 ABNORMALITIES OF THE LIPS

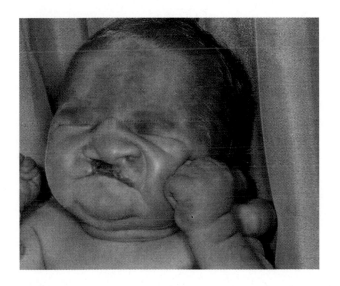

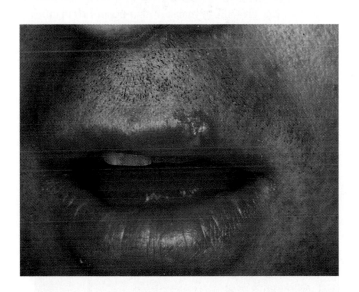

Cleft Lip

Maxillofacial clefts are the most common congenital deformities of the head and neck. The incidence varies among racial groups, being highest in Native North Americans and in the Japanese (1 in 300 to 400), and lowest in blacks (1 in 1300 to 1800). Although reliable birth registry is not present in all countries, birth records do show a relatively high incidence in Scandinavia and middle European countries, e.g., 1 in 550 in Denmark and Finland, 1 in 575 in Poland and the former Czechoslovakia (Bluestone, Stool, and Kenna, 1996). Early treatment preserves the functions of speech and language formation and deglutition (swallowing).

Herpes Simplex I

The cold sores are groups of clear vesicles with a surrounding indurated erythematous base. These evolve into pustules, which rupture, weep, and crust, and heal in 4 to 10 days. The most likely site is the lip-skin junction; infection often recurs in same site. Caused by the herpes simplex virus (HSV-1), the lesion is highly contagious and is spread by direct contact. Recurrent herpes infections may be precipitated by sunlight, fever, colds, allergy. It is a very common lesion, affecting 50 percent of adults.

Table continued on following page

Table 14–2   ABNORMALITIES OF THE LIPS *Continued*

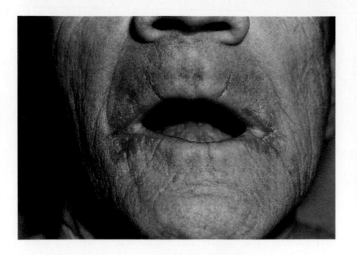

Angular Cheilitis (Stomatitis, Perlèche)

Erythema, scaling, shallow and painful fissures at the corners of the mouth occur with excess salivation and *Candida* infection. It is often seen in edentulous persons and in those with poorly fitting dentures causing folding in of corners of mouth, creating a warm, moist environment favoring growth of yeast. It also occurs from riboflavin deficiency (rare).

Carcinoma

The initial lesion is round and indurated, then it becomes crusted and ulcerated with an elevated border. The vast majority occur between the outer and middle thirds of lip. Any lesion that is still unhealed after 2 weeks should be referred.

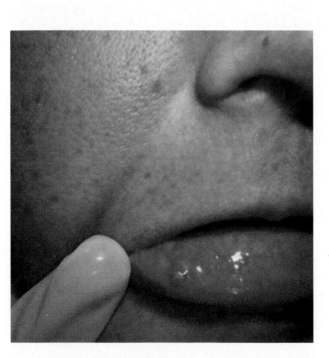

◀ Retention "Cyst" (Mucocele)

A round, well-defined nodule that may be very small or up to 1 or 2 cm. It is a pocket of mucus that forms when a duct of a minor salivary gland ruptures. The benign lesion also may occur on the buccal mucosa, on the floor of the mouth, or under the tip of the tongue.

Table 14–3 ABNORMALITIES OF THE TEETH AND GUMS

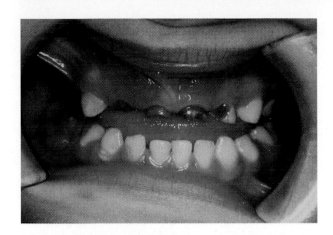

Baby Bottle Tooth Decay

Destruction of numerous deciduous teeth may occur in older infants and toddlers who take a bottle of milk, juice, or sweetened drink to bed and prolong bottle feeding past the age of 1 year. Liquid pools around the upper front teeth. Mouth bacteria act on carbohydrates in the liquid, especially sucrose, forming metabolic acids. Acids break down tooth enamel and destroy its protein.

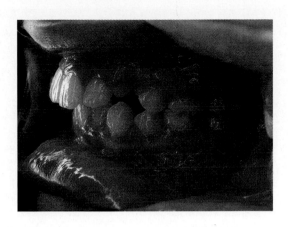

Malocclusion

Upper or lower dental arches are out of alignment and incisors protrude owing to developmental problem of mandible or maxilla, or incompatibility between jaw size and tooth size. The condition increases risk of facial deformity, negative body image, chewing problems, or speech dysfluency.

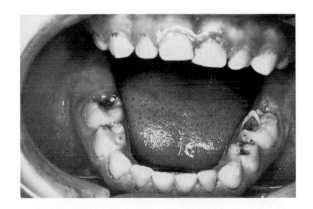

Dental Caries

Progressive destruction of tooth. Decay initially looks chalky white. Later, it turns brown or black and forms a cavity. Early decay is apparent only on x-ray study. Susceptible sites are tooth surfaces where food debris, bacterial plaque, and saliva collect.

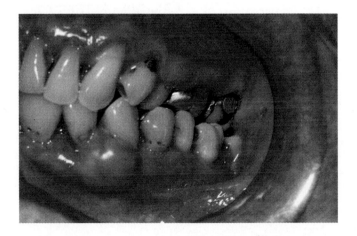

Epulis

A nontender, fibrous nodule of the gum, seen emerging between the teeth; an inflammatory response to injury or hemorrhage.

Table continued on following page

409

Table 14—3   ABNORMALITIES OF THE TEETH AND GUMS *Continued*

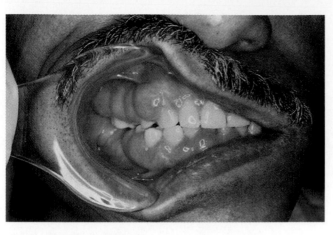

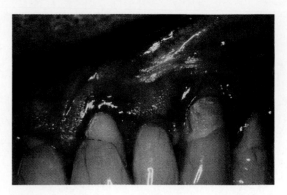

Gingival Hyperplasia

Painless enlargement of the gums, sometimes over-reaching the teeth. This occurs with puberty, pregnancy, leukemia, and with long therapeutic use of phenytoin (Dilantin).

Gingivitis

Gum margins are red, swollen, and bleed easily. This case is severe; gingival tissue has desquamated, exposing roots or teeth. Inflammation is usually due to poor dental hygiene or vitamin C deficiency. The condition may occur in pregnancy and puberty because of changing hormonal balance.

Table 14—4   ABNORMALITIES OF THE BUCCAL MUCOSA

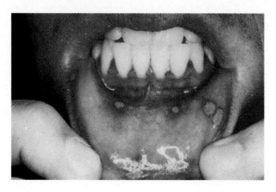

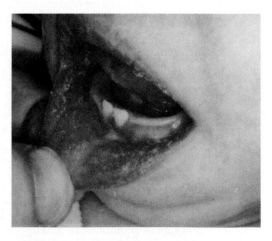

Aphthous Ulcers

A "canker sore" is a vesicle at first, then a small, round, "punched-out" ulcer with white base surrounded by a red halo. It is quite painful and lasts for 1 to 2 weeks. The cause is unknown, although it is associated with stress, fatigue, and food allergy. It is common, affecting 20 to 60 percent of the population.

Koplik's Spots

Small blue-white spots with irregular red halo scattered over mucosa opposite the molars. An early sign, and pathognomonic, of measles.

Table 14-4   ABNORMALITIES OF THE BUCCAL MUCOSA *Continued*

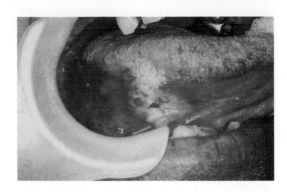

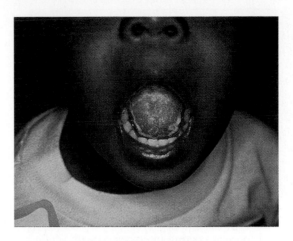

Leukoplakia

Chalky white, thick, raised patch with well-defined borders. The lesion is firmly attached and does not scrape off. It may occur on the lateral edges of tongue. It is due to chronic irritation, and occurs more frequently with heavy smoking and heavy alcohol use. Lesions are precancerous, and the person should be referred. (Here, the lesion is associated with squamous carcinoma.)

Candidiasis or Monilial Infection

A white, cheesy, curdlike patch on the buccal mucosa and tongue. It scrapes off, leaving raw, red surface that bleeds easily. Termed "thrush" in the newborn. It also occurs after the use of antibiotics, corticosteroids, and in immunosuppressed persons.

Table 14-5   ABNORMALITIES OF THE TONGUE

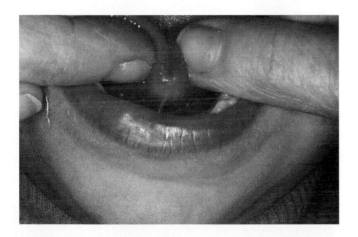

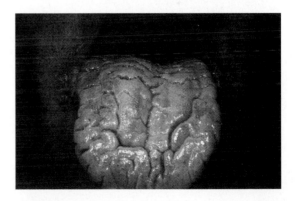

Ankyloglossia

(Tongue-tie.) A short lingual frenulum, here fixing the tongue tip to the floor of the mouth and gums. This limits mobility and will affect speech (pronunciation of a, d, n) if the tongue tip cannot be elevated to the alveolar ridge. A congenital defect.

Fissured or Scrotal Tongue

Deep furrows divide the papillae into small irregular rows. The condition is congenital and is not significant. The incidence increases with age. (Vertical, or longitudinal, fissures also occur with dehydration because of reduced volume of the tongue.)

Table continued on following page

Table 14–5 ABNORMALITIES OF THE TONGUE *Continued*

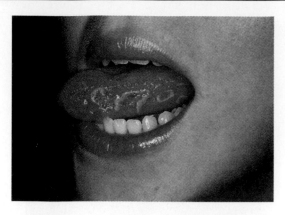

Geographic Tongue (Migratory Glossitis)

Pattern of normal coating interspersed with bright red, shiny, circular bald areas, having raised pearly borders. Pattern resembles a map, and changes in a few days. Not significant, and its cause is not known.

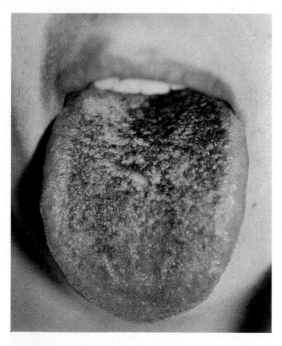

Black Hairy Tongue

This is not really hair but the elongation of filiform papillae and painless overgrowth of mycelial threads of fungus infection on the tongue. It occurs following use of antibiotics, which inhibit normal bacteria and allow proliferation of fungus.

Carcinoma

An ulcer with rolled edges; indurated. Occurs particularly at sides, base, and under the tongue. When it is in the floor of mouth, it may cause painful movement or limited movement of tongue. Risk of early metastasis is present due to rich lymphatic drainage. Heavy smoking and heavy alcohol use place persons at greater risk.

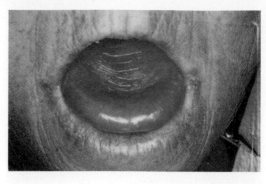

Smooth, Glossy Tongue (Atrophic Glossitis)

The surface is slick and shiny; the mucosa thins and looks red from decreased papillae. Accompanied by dryness of tongue and burning. Occurs with vitamin B_{12} deficiency (pernicious anemia), folic acid deficiency, and iron deficiency anemia. Here, also note angular cheilitis.

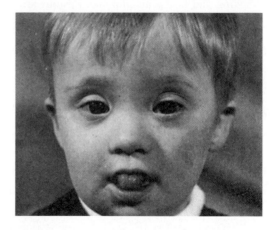

Enlarged Tongue (Macroglossia)

The tongue is enlarged and may protrude from mouth. The condition is not painful but may impair speech development. Here, it occurs with Down syndrome; it also occurs with cretinism, myxedema, acromegaly. Also a transient swelling occurs with local infections.

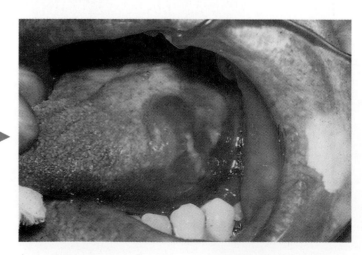

Table 14-6 ABNORMALITIES OF THE OROPHARYNX

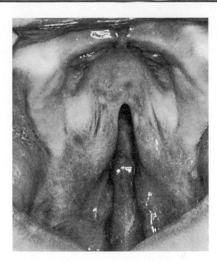

Cleft Palate

A congenital defect, the failure of fusion of the maxillary processes. Wide variation occurs in the extent of cleft formation, from upper lip only, palate only, uvula only, to cleft of the nostril and the hard and soft palates.

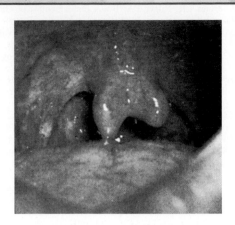

Bifid Uvula

The uvula looks partly severed. May indicate a submucous cleft palate, which feels like a notch at the junction of the hard and soft palates. The submucous cleft palate may affect speech development because it prevents necessary air trapping. The incidence of bifid uvula varies among racial groups: It is common in Native Americans, uncommon in whites, and rare in blacks.

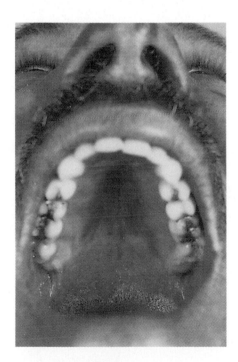

Oral Kaposi's Sarcoma

Bruiselike, dark red or violet, confluent macule, usually on the hard palate, may be on soft palate or gingival margin. Oral lesions may be among the earliest lesions to develop with AIDS.

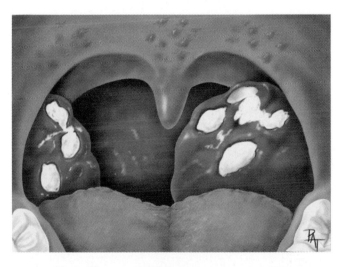

Acute Tonsillitis and Pharyngitis

Bright red throat, swollen tonsils, white or yellow exudate on tonsils and pharynx, swollen uvula, and enlarged, tender anterior cervical and tonsillar nodes. Accompanied by severe sore throat, painful swallowing, fever > 101° F of sudden onset.

Caution: One cannot discriminate bacterial from viral infection on clinical data alone; all sore throats need a throat culture. Bacterial pharyngitis caused by group A beta-hemolytic streptococcus, if untreated, may lead to the complication of rheumatic fever. This is a serious complex illness characterized by fever, malaise, swollen joints, rash, and scarring on the heart valves.

Bibliography

Adams GL, Boies LR, Hilger PA: Boies Fundamentals of Otolaryngology, 6th ed. Philadelphia, W.B. Saunders Company, 1989.

Berrey MM, Corey L: Diagnosing oral manifestations of sexually transmitted diseases. Consultant 37(5):1243–1244, May 1997.

Bluestone CD, Stool SE, Kenna MA: Pediatric Otolaryngology, 3rd ed. Philadelphia, W.B. Saunders Company, 1996.

Brothwell DR, Carbonell VM, Goose DH: Congenital absence of teeth in human populations. *In* Brothwell DR (Ed): Dental Anthropology. New York, Pergamon Press, 1963, pp 179–189.

Davidson TM, Davidson D: Immediate management of epistaxis: Bloody nuisance or ominous sign? Phys Sports Med 24(8):74–95, Aug 1996.

Edelstein DR: Aging of the normal nose in adults. Laryngoscope 106(9, Part 2, Suppl 81):1–25, Sep 1996.

Evans WB, White GL, Wood SD, et al: Managing dysphagia: Fundamentals of primary care. Clin Rev 8(8):47–71, Aug 1998.

Finney LS, Gonzalez-Campoy JM: What the mouth has to say about diabetes: Careful examinations can avert serious complications. Postgrad Med 102(6): 117–126, Dec 1997.

Gauwitz DF: How to protect the dysphagic stroke patient. AM J Nurs 95(8):34–38, Aug 1995.

Hollingsworth HM: Allergic rhinoconjunctivitis: Current therapy. Hosp Pract 31(6):61–72, June 15, 1996.

Jarvis A, Gorlin R: Minor orofacial abnormalities in an Eskimo population. Oral Surg 33:417–426, 1972.

Jette AM, Feldman HA, Tennstedt SL: Tobacco use: A modifiable risk factor for dental disease among the elderly. Am J Public Health 83(9): 1271–1276, Sep 1993.

Kadish HA, Corneli HM: Removal of nasal foreign bodies in the pediatric population. Am J Emerg Med 15(1):54–56, Jan 1997.

Kane RL, Ouslander JG, Abrass IB: Essentials of Clinical Geriatrics, 3rd ed. New York: McGraw-Hill, 1994.

Killen JM: Understanding dysphagia: Interventions for care. Medsurg Nurs 5(2):99–105, Apr 1996.

Kingston L, Reynolds D, Phillips LP: Primary care for women: Comprehensive assessment of the head and neck. J Nurse Midwifery 40(2):187–201, Mar–Apr 1995.

Lee M: Drugs and the elderly: Do you know the risks? Am J Nurs 96(7):25–32, July 1996.

Logemann JA: Dysphagia: Evaluation and treatment. Folia Phoniatr Logop 47(3): 140–164, 1995.

Mackin LA, Antonini CH: Acute sinusitis. Prim Care Pract 3(1):65–69, Jan–Feb 1999.

Marcus SE, Drury TF, Brown LJ, Zion GR: Tooth retention and tooth loss in the permanent dentition of adults, United States, 1988–1991. J Dent Res 75 (Spec No):684–695, Feb 1996.

Martin J, Crump E: Leukoedema of the buccal mucosa in Negro children and youth. Oral Surg 34:49–58, 1972.

Newland JA: Epistaxis. Am J Nurs 98(3): 16HHH, Mar 1998.

Overfield T: Biologic Variation in Health and Illness: Race, Age, and Sex Differences, 2nd ed. New York, CRC Press, 1995.

Petersen MJ, Baughman RA: Recurrent aphthous stomatitis: Primary care management. Nurs Pract 21(5):36–47, May 1996.

Phillips LP, Campbell LR, Barger MK: Primary care for women: Management of common problems of the head and neck. J Nurse Midwifery 41(2):101–116, Mar–Apr 1996.

Shay K, Ship JA: The importance of oral health in the older patient. J Am Geriatr Soc 42(12):1414–1422, Dec 1995.

Shugars DC, Patton LL: Detecting, diagnosing, and preventing oral cancer. Nurs Pract 22(6):105–132, June 1997.

Templer J: Removing foreign bodies from the nose. Hosp Med 31(5): 37–40, May 1995.

Templer J: Removing foreign bodies from the throat. Hosp Med 31(3): 51–53, Mar 1995.

Touger-Decker R, Sirois DA: Physical assessment of the oral cavity. Support Line 18(5):1–6, Oct 1996.

Walpole J: Oral candidiasis. Am J Nurs Pract 2(1):37–43, 1998.

CHAPTER FIFTEEN

Breasts and
Regional Lymphatics

The breasts, or mammary glands, are present in both females and males, although in the male they are rudimentary throughout life. The female breasts are accessory reproductive organs whose function is to produce milk for nourishing the newborn.

SURFACE ANATOMY

The **breasts** lie anterior to the pectoralis major and serratus anterior muscles (Fig. 15–1). The breasts are located between the second and sixth ribs, extending from the side of the sternum to the midaxillary line. The superior lateral corner of breast tissue, called the axillary **tail of Spence,** projects up and laterally into the axilla.

The **nipple** is just below the center of the breast. It is rough, round, and usually protuberant; its surface looks wrinkled and indented with tiny milk duct openings. The **areola** surrounds the nipple for a 1- to 2-cm radius. In the areola are small elevated sebaceous glands, called Montgomery's glands. These secrete a protective lipid material during lactation. The areola also has smooth muscle fibers that cause nipple erection when stimulated. Both the nipple and areola are more darkly pigmented than the rest of the breast surface; the color varies from pink to brown depending on the person's skin color and parity.

INTERNAL ANATOMY

The breast is composed of (1) glandular tissue, (2) fibrous tissue including the suspensory ligaments, and (3) adipose tissue (Fig. 15–2). First, the **glandular tissue** contains 15 to 20 lobes radiating from the nipple, and these are composed of lobules. Within each lobule are

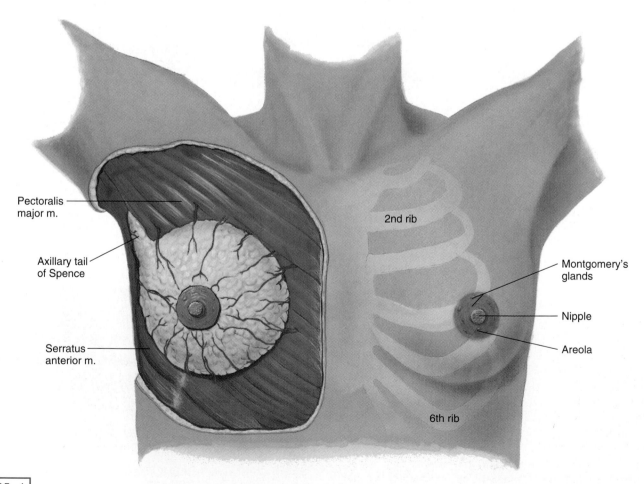

Pectoralis major m.

Axillary tail of Spence

Serratus anterior m.

2nd rib

Montgomery's glands

Nipple

Areola

6th rib

15–1

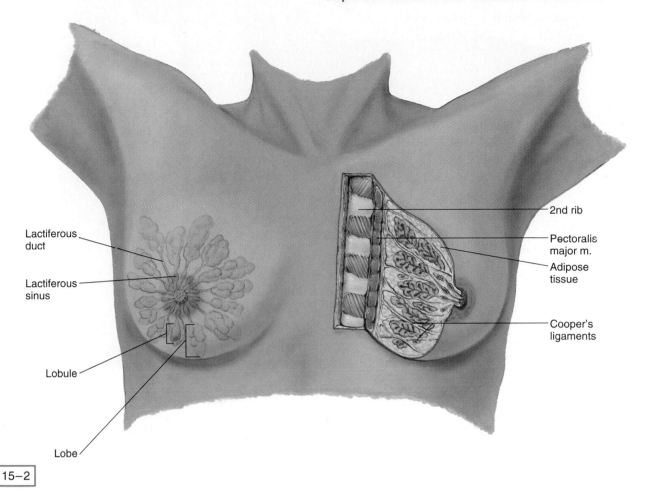

Lactiferous duct

Lactiferous sinus

Lobule

Lobe

2nd rib

Pectoralis major m.

Adipose tissue

Cooper's ligaments

15–2

clusters of alveoli that produce milk. Each lobe empties into a lactiferous duct. The 15 to 20 lactiferous ducts form a collecting duct system converging toward the nipple. There, the ducts form ampullae, or lactiferous sinuses, behind the nipple, which are reservoirs for storing milk.

Second, the suspensory ligaments, or **Cooper's ligaments,** are fibrous bands extending vertically from the surface to attach on chest wall muscles. These support the breast tissue. They become contracted in cancer of the breast, producing pits or dimples in the overlying skin.

Finally, the lobes are embedded in **adipose tissue.** These layers of subcutaneous and retromammary fat actually provide most of the bulk of the breast. The relative proportion of glandular, fibrous, and fatty tissue varies depending on age, cycle, pregnancy, lactation, and general nutritional state.

The breast may be divided into four quadrants by imaginary horizontal and vertical lines intersecting at the nipple (Fig. 15–3). This makes a convenient map to describe clinical findings. In the upper outer quadrant, note the axillary **tail of Spence,** the cone-shaped breast tissue that projects up into the axilla, close to the pectoral group of axillary lymph nodes. The upper outer quadrant is the site of most breast tumors.

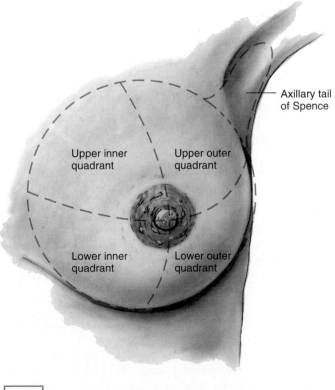

Axillary tail of Spence

Upper inner quadrant

Upper outer quadrant

Lower inner quadrant

Lower outer quadrant

15–3

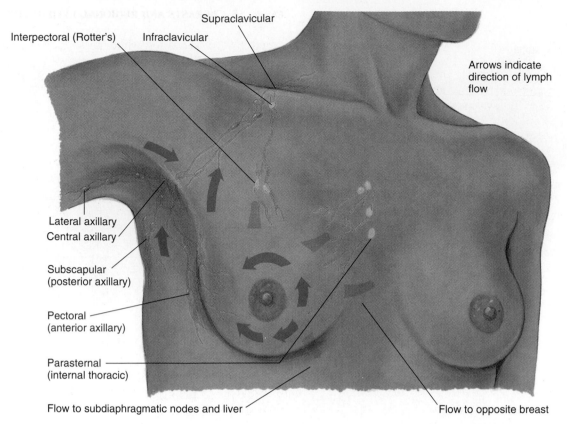

Supraclavicular

Interpectoral (Rotter's) Infraclavicular

Arrows indicate direction of lymph flow

Lateral axillary
Central axillary

Subscapular
(posterior axillary)

Pectoral
(anterior axillary)

Parasternal
(internal thoracic)

15–4

Flow to subdiaphragmatic nodes and liver

Flow to opposite breast

LYMPHATICS

The breast has extensive lymphatic drainage. Most of the lymph, more than 75 percent, drains into the ipsilateral axillary nodes. Four groups of axillary nodes are present (Fig. 15–4):

1. **Central axillary nodes**—high up in the middle of the axilla, over the ribs and serratus anterior muscle. These receive lymph from the other three groups of nodes:
2. **Pectoral** (anterior)—along the lateral edge of the pectoralis major muscle, just inside the anterior axillary fold
3. **Subscapular** (posterior)—along the lateral edge of the scapula, deep in the posterior axillary fold
4. **Lateral**—along the humerus, inside the upper arm

From the central axillary nodes, drainage flows up to the infraclavicular and supraclavicular nodes.

A smaller amount of lymphatic drainage does not take these channels but flows directly up to the infraclavicular group, deep into the chest, or into the abdomen, or directly across to the opposite breast.

 DEVELOPMENTAL CONSIDERATIONS

During embryonic life, ventral epidermal ridges, or "milk lines," are present; these curve down from the axilla to the groin bilaterally (Fig. 15–5). The breast develops along the ridge over the thorax, and the rest of the ridge usually atrophies. Occasionally a *supernumerary nipple* (i.e., an extra nipple) persists and is visible somewhere along the track of the mammary ridge (see Fig. 15–8).

At birth, the only breast structures present are the lactiferous ducts within the nipple. No alveoli have developed. Little change occurs until puberty.

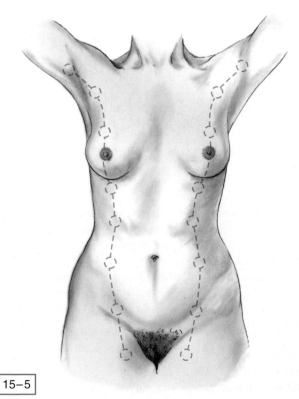

15–5

The Adolescent

At puberty, the estrogen hormones stimulate breast changes. The breasts enlarge, mostly due to extensive fat deposition. The duct system also grows and branches, and masses of small, solid cells develop at the duct endings. These are potential alveoli.

A 1997 study of 17,077 girls in the United States aged 3 through 12 indicates that puberty is occurring earlier than classically used norms (Herman-Giddens et al., 1997). The onset of breast development occurred at an average (mean) age between 8 and 9 years for black girls and by 10 years for white girls. Earlier studies cited breast development beginning at an average age of 10 to 11 years (Harlan, Harlan, and Grillo, 1980; Marshall and Tanner, 1969).

Occasionally, one breast may grow faster than the other, producing a temporary asymmetry. This may cause some distress; reassurance is necessary. Tenderness is common also. Although the age of onset varies widely, the five stages of breast development follow this classic description of Marshall and Tanner's (1969) sexual maturity rating, or Tanner staging (Table 15–1).

Table 15–1 • Sexual Maturity Rating in Girls

Stage

1 Preadolescent
  Only a small elevated nipple

2 Breast bud stage
  A small mound of breast and nipple develops; the areola widens

3 The breast and areola enlarge
  The nipple is flush with the breast surface

4 The areola and nipple form a secondary mound over the breast

5 Mature breast
  Only the nipple protrudes, the areola is flush with the breast contour (the areola may continue as a secondary mound in some normal women)

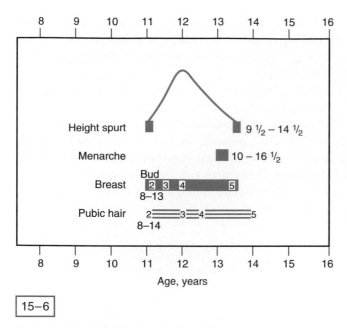

15–6

Pattern of pubertal changes in girls

Full development from stage 2 to stage 5 takes an average of 3 years, although the range is 1.5 to 6 years. During this time, pubic hair develops, and axillary hair appears 2 years after the onset of pubic hair. The beginning of breast development precedes menarche by about 2 years. Menarche occurs in breast development stage 3 or 4, usually just after the peak of the adolescent growth spurt, which occurs around age 12. Note the relationship of these events (Fig. 15–6). This knowledge aids in assessing the development of adolescent girls and increasing their knowledge about their own development.

Breasts of the nonpregnant woman change with the ebb and flow of hormones during the monthly menstrual cycle. Nodularity increases from midcycle up to menstruation. During the 3 to 4 days before menstruation, the breasts feel full, tight, heavy, and occasionally sore. The breast volume is smallest on days 4 to 7 of the menstrual cycle.

The Pregnant Female

During pregnancy, breast changes start during the 2nd month and are an early sign of pregnancy for most women. Pregnancy stimulates the expansion of the ductal system and supporting fatty tissue as well as development of the true secretory alveoli. Thus the breasts enlarge and feel more nodular. The nipples are larger, darker, and more erectile. The areolae become larger and grow a darker brown as pregnancy progresses, and the tubercles become more prominent. (The brown color fades after lactation, but the areolae never return to the original color.) A venous pattern is prominent over the skin surface.

After the 4th month, **colostrum** may be expressed. This thick yellow fluid is the precursor of milk, containing the same amount of protein and lactose but practically no fat. The breasts produce colostrum for the first few days after delivery. It is rich with antibodies that protect the newborn against infection, so breastfeeding is important. Milk production (lactation) begins 1 to 3 days postpartum. The whitish color is from emulsified fat and calcium caseinate.

The Aging Female

After menopause, ovarian secretion of estrogen and progesterone decreases, which causes the breast glandular tissue to atrophy. This is replaced with fibrous connective tissue. The fat envelope atrophies also, beginning in the middle years and becoming marked in the eighth and ninth decades. These changes decrease breast size and elasticity so the breasts droop and sag, looking flattened and flabby. Drooping is accentuated by the kyphosis in some older women.

The decreased breast size makes inner structures more prominent. A breast lump may have been present for years but is suddenly palpable. Around the nipple the lactiferous ducts are more palpable and feel firm and stringy because of fibrosis and calcification. The axillary hair decreases.

THE MALE BREAST

The male breast is a rudimentary structure consisting of a thin disc of undeveloped tissue underlying the nipple. The areola is well developed, although the nipple is relatively very small. During adolescence, it is common for the breast tissue to temporarily enlarge, producing **gynecomastia.** This condition is usually unilateral and temporary. Reassurance is necessary for the adolescent male, whose attention is riveted on his body image. Gynecomastia may reappear in the aging male and may be due to testosterone deficiency.

TRANSCULTURAL **CONSIDERATIONS**

Marshall and Tanner's data on sexual maturity are derived from studies of white British females and do not generalize to other racial groups. The 1997 study of secondary sexual characteristics in 17,077 young American girls shows that black girls begin puberty about 1 to 1.5 years earlier than white girls and start menstruating about 8.5 months earlier (Herman-Giddens et al., 1997). The onset of breast development occurred at an average (mean) age of 8.87 years for black girls and 9.96 years for white girls (Hispanic ethnicity occurs in both groups). At age 7, 27.2 percent of black girls and 6.7 percent of white girls had begun breast and/or pubic hair develop-ment, and at age 8 this increased to 48.3 percent of black girls and 14.7 percent of white girls. Menses began at an average age of 12.16 years for black girls and at 12.88 years for white girls.

Breast Cancer. The incidence of breast cancer var-ies with different cultural groups. In the search for an environmental influence to account for this difference, researchers suspect that a diet rich in certain fats has a strong promoting effect on breast cancer (Weisburger, 1997). The high incidence of breast cancer rates in the United States, Canada, Britain, and the Netherlands corre-lates with a high amount of fat in the diet of those nations. In Japan, China, Singapore, and Romania, where people eat a lean diet, the incidence of breast cancer is one-sixth to one-half that in the United States (American Cancer Society [ACS], 1998). However, migratory studies show that when Japanese move to the United States, their previously low incidence rises as they adapt to a western diet (Secretary's Task Force on Black & Minority Health, 1986).

Although breast cancer is the second leading cause of cancer death in women in the United States, it is the leading cause of cancer death among black women (Phil-lips, 1996). This racial difference in mortality may relate to insufficient use of early-detection procedures, including breast self-examination and mammograms. Barriers to breast cancer screening among black women include cost, accessibility, availability, lack of knowledge, and lack of community involvement (Brown and Williams, 1994).

SUBJECTIVE DATA

Breast

1. Pain
2. Lump
3. Discharge
4. Rash
5. Swelling
6. Trauma
7. History of breast disease

8. Surgery
9. Self-care behaviors
   Perform breast self-examination
   Last mammogram

Axilla

1. Tenderness, lump, or swelling
2. Rash

In Western culture, the female breasts signify more than their primary purpose of lactation. Women are surrounded by messages that feminine norms of beauty and desir-ability are enhanced by and dependent on the size of the breasts and their appearance. More recently, women leaders have tried to refocus this attitude, stressing women's self-worth as individual human beings, not as stereotyped sexual objects. The intense cultural emphasis is gradually changing, yet the breasts still are crucial to a woman's self-concept and her perception of her femininity. Matters pertaining to the breast affect a woman's body image and generate deep emotional responses.

This emotionality may take strong forms that you observe as you discuss the woman's history. One woman may be acutely embarrassed talking about the breasts, as evidenced by lack of eye contact, minimal response, nervous gestures, or inappropriate humor. Another woman may talk wryly and disparagingly about the size or development of her breasts. A young adolescent is acutely aware of her own development in relation to her peers. Or, a woman who has found a breast lump may come to you with fear, high anxiety, and even panic. Although a high percentage of breast lumps are benign, many women initially assume the worst possible outcome—cancer, disfigurement, and death. While you are collecting the subjective data, tune in to cues for these behaviors that call for a straightforward and reasoned attitude.

Examiner Asks	Rationale

BREAST

1 **Pain.** Any **pain** or tenderness in the breasts? When did you first notice it?
- Where is the pain? Localized or all over?
- Is the painful spot sore to touch? Do you feel a burning or pulling sensation?
- Is the pain cyclic? Any relation to your menstrual period?

- Is the pain brought on by strenuous activity, especially involving one arm; a change in activity; manipulation during sex; part of underwire bra; exercise?

Mastalgia occurs with trauma, inflammation, infection, and benign breast disease.

Cyclic pain is common with normal breasts, use of oral contraceptives, and benign breast (fibrocystic) disease.

Is pain related to specific cause?

2 **Lump.** Ever noticed a **lump or thickening** in the breast? Where?
- When did you first notice it? Changed at all since then?
- Does the lump have any relation to your menstrual period?
- Noticed any change in the overlying skin: redness, warmth, dimpling, swelling?

The presence of any lump must be carefully explored. A lump that has been present for many years and is exhibiting no change may not be serious but still should be explored. Approach any recent change or new lump with suspicion.

3 **Discharge.** Any **discharge** from the nipple?
- When did you first notice this?
- What color is the discharge?
- Consistency—thick or runny?
- Odor?

Galactorrhea. Note use of medications that may cause clear nipple discharge, such as oral contraceptives, phenothiazines, diuretics, digitalis, and steroids. Also, reserpine, methyldopa, calcium channel blockers.

Bloody or blood-tinged discharge always is significant. Any discharge in the presence of a lump is significant.

4 **Rash.** Any **rash** on the breast?
- When did you first notice this?
- Where did it start? On the nipple, areola, or surrounding skin?

Paget's disease starts with a small crust on the nipple apex, then spreads to areola.

Eczema or other dermatitis rarely starts at nipple unless it is due to breastfeeding. It usually starts on the areola or surrounding skin and then spreads to the nipple.

5 **Swelling.** Any **swelling** in the breasts? In one spot or all over?
- Seem to be related to your menstrual period, pregnancy, or breastfeeding?
- Any change in bra size?

6 **Trauma.** Any **trauma** or injury to the breasts?
- Did it result in any swelling, lump, or break in skin?

A lump from an injury is due to local hematoma or edema and should resolve shortly. Or, trauma may cause a woman to feel the breast and find a lump that really was there before.

Examiner Asks	Rationale
7 **History of breast disease.** Any **history of breast disease** yourself? ● What type? How was this diagnosed? ● When did this occur? ● How is it being treated? ● Any breast cancer in your family? Who? Sister, mother, maternal grandmother, maternal aunts, daughter? ● At what age did this relative have breast cancer?	A history of breast cancer increases the risk of recurrent cancer (see Risk Factors for Breast Cancer, p. 425). The presence of fibrocystic disease makes it more difficult to examine the breasts; the general lumpiness of the breast conceals a new lump. The finding of breast cancer occurring before menopause in certain family members increases risk for this woman (see Risk Factors for Breast Cancer, p. 425).
8 **Surgery.** Ever had **surgery** on the breasts? Was this a biopsy? What were the biopsy results? ● Mastectomy? Mammoplasty—augmentation or reduction?	
9 **Self-care behaviors.** ● Have you ever been taught **breast self-examination?** ● **(If so.)** How often do you perform it? What helps you remember? That is an excellent way to be in charge of your own health. I would like you to show me your technique after we do your examination. ● **(If not.)** This will be an excellent way that you can take charge of your own health. You can make breast self-examination a very routine health habit, just like brushing your teeth. I will teach you the technique after we do your examination. ● Ever had **mammography,** a screening x-ray examination of the breasts? When was the last x-ray?	The monthly practice of breast self examination (BSE), and routine clinical breast examination and mammograms are complementary screening measures. Good BSE practice is associated with a smaller size of tumor at diagnosis, which may reduce breast cancer mortality (Champion, 1995). Mammography can reveal cancers too small to be detected by the woman or by the most experienced examiner. However, mammography does not detect *all* palpable lumps, and interval lumps may become palpable between mammograms (Cole, 1998). The American Cancer Society recommends a baseline mammogram for all women between the ages of 35 and 39. Women ages 20 to 39 should perform monthly BSE and have a clinical breast exam (CBE) every 3 years; women 40 and older should perform monthly BSE, with an annual mammogram and an annual CBE conducted close to the same time (ACS, 1998).

AXILLA

1 **Tenderness, lump, or swelling.** Any **tenderness** or **lump** in the underarm area? ● Where? When did you first notice this? **2** **Rash.** Any axillary **rash?** Please describe it. ● Seem to be a reaction to deodorant?	Breast tissue extends up into the axilla. Also, the axilla contains numerous lymph nodes.

Examiner Asks	Rationale

ADDITIONAL HISTORY FOR THE PREADOLESCENT

1 Have you noticed your breasts changing?
  - How long has this been happening?

2 Many girls notice other changes in their bodies too that come with growing up. What have you noticed?
  - What do you think about all this?

Developing breasts are the most obvious sign of puberty. This is the focus of attention for most girls, especially in comparison to their peers. Assess each adolescent's perception of her own development and provide teaching and reassurance as indicated.

ADDITIONAL HISTORY FOR THE PREGNANT FEMALE

1 Have you noticed any enlargement or fullness in the breasts?
  - Is there any tenderness or tingling?

  - Do you have a history of inverted nipples?

2 Are you planning to breastfeed your baby?

Breast changes are expected and normal during pregnancy. Assess the woman's knowledge and provide reassurance.
Inverted nipples may need special care in preparation for breastfeeding.

In addition to providing the perfect food and antibodies for the baby, promoting bonding, and providing relaxation, lactation is also associated with a slight reduction in the risk of breast cancer among premenopausal women (Newcomb et al., 1994).

ADDITIONAL HISTORY FOR THE MENOPAUSAL WOMAN

1 Have you noticed any change in the breast contour, size, or firmness? (Note: Change may not be as apparent to the obese woman or to the woman whose earlier pregnancies already have produced breast changes.)

Decreased estrogen level causes decreased firmness. Rapid decrease in estrogen level causes actual shrinkage.

RISK FACTOR PROFILE FOR BREAST CANCER

Breast cancer is the second major cause of death from cancer in women. One of nine women will acquire breast cancer at some point in her lifetime; however, early detection and improved treatment have increased survival rates. The 5-year survival rate for localized breast cancer has increased from 78 percent in the 1940s to 97 percent today. If the cancer

Examiner Asks	Rationale

has spread regionally, the survival rate is 76 percent; if the cancer has distant metastases, the survival rate is 21 percent (ACS, 1998).

Table 15–2 • Breast Cancer Factors

Most Significant Risk Factors	Other Risk Factors
Female gender, age >50	Nulliparity or first child after 30 years of age
Personal history of breast cancer	Menstruation before age 12
Atypical hyperplasia on biopsy	Menopause after age 55
First-degree relative with breast cancer (mother, sister, daughter)	Second-degree relative with breast cancer (aunt, grandmother)
	Exposure to high doses of ionizing radiation
	Alcohol intake of 1–2 drinks a day or more*
	Tobacco smoking, particularly as an adolescent* when breast tissue is most susceptible to carcinogens
	Exposure to environmental hazards*
	High-fat diet and obesity
	Decreased exercise*
	Oral contraceptive or estrogen replacement therapy*

*Suspected (conflicting data).
Original data from Colditz et al., 1995; Love & Lindsey, 1995; Marchant, 1994; Thune et al., 1997; White et al., 1996.
Modified from Ziegfeld CR: Differential diagnosis of a breast mass. Prim Care Pract 2 (2):121–128, March–Apr 1998.

The best way to detect a person's risk for breast cancer is by asking the right history questions. Table 15–2 highlights risk factors for breast cancer, and from these you can fashion your questions. Be aware, however, that about 70 percent of breast cancers occur in women with no identifiable risk factors except gender and age (Love and Lindsey, 1995; Sherman and Seremetis, 1997). Just because a woman does not report the cited risk factors does not mean that you or she should fail to consider breast cancer seriously.

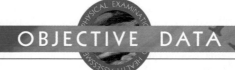

OBJECTIVE DATA

Preparation

The woman is sitting up, disrobed to the waist, facing the examiner. An alternative draping method is to use a short gown, open at the back, and lift it up to the woman's shoulders during inspection. During palpation when the woman is supine, cover one breast with the gown while examining the other. Be aware that many women are embarrassed to have their breasts examined; use a sensitive but matter-of-fact approach.

Following your examination, be prepared to teach the woman breast self-examination.

 ## Equipment Needed

Small pillow
Ruler marked in centimeters
Pamphlet or teaching aid for BSE

THE BREASTS

Inspect the breasts
General Appearance

Note symmetry of size and shape (Fig. 15–7). It is common to have a slight asymmetry in size; often the left breast is slightly larger than the right.

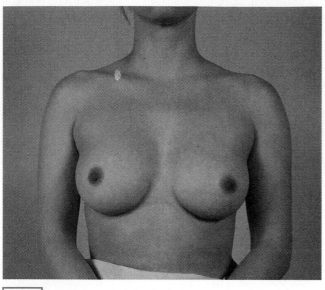

15–7

A sudden increase in the size of one breast signifies inflammation or new growth.

Skin

The skin normally is smooth and of even color. Note any localized areas of redness, bulging, or dimpling. Also, note any skin lesions or focal vascular pattern. A fine blue vascular network is visible normally during pregnancy. Pale linear striae, or stretch marks, often follow pregnancy.

Normally no edema is present. Edema exaggerates the hair follicles, giving a "pig-skin" or "orange-peel" look (also called *peau d'orange*).

Hyperpigmentation.

Redness and heat with inflammation.

Unilateral dilated superficial veins in a nonpregnant woman. Edema, see Table 15–3 p. 440.

Lymphatic Drainage Areas

Observe the axillary and supraclavicular regions. Note any bulging, discoloration, or edema.

Nipple

The nipples should be symmetrically placed on the same plane on the two breasts. Nipples usually protrude, although some are flat and some are inverted. They tend to stay in their original condition. Distinguish a recently retracted nipple from one that has been inverted for many years or since puberty. Normal nipple inversion may be unilateral or bilateral and usually can be pulled out (i.e., it is not fixed).

Deviation in pointing (see Table 15–3).

Recent nipple retraction signifies acquired disease (see Table 15–3).

▶ Normal Range of Findings	Abnormal Findings

Note any dry scaling, any fissure or ulceration, and bleeding or other discharge.

A normal variation in about 1 percent of men and women is a **supernumerary nipple** (Fig. 15–8). An extra nipple along the embryonic "milk line" on the thorax or abdomen is a congenital finding. Usually, it is 5 to 6 cm below the breast near the midline and has no associated glandular tissue. It looks like a mole, although a close look reveals a tiny nipple and areola. It is not significant; merely distinguish it from a mole.

Any discharge must be explored, especially in the presence of a breast mass.

Rarely, glandular tissue, a supernumerary breast, or polymastia is present.

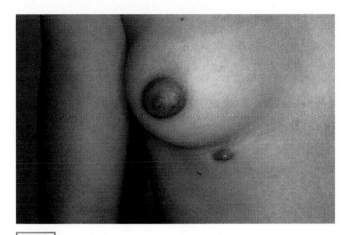

15–8

Supernumerary nipple and areolar complex

Maneuvers to Screen for Retraction

Direct the woman to change position while you check the breasts for skin retraction signs. First ask her to lift the arms slowly over the head. Both breasts should move up symmetrically (Fig. 15–9).

Retraction signs are due to fibrosis in the breast tissue, usually caused by growing neoplasms. The fibrosis shortens with time, causing contrasting signs with the normally loose breast tissue.

Note a lag in movement of one breast.

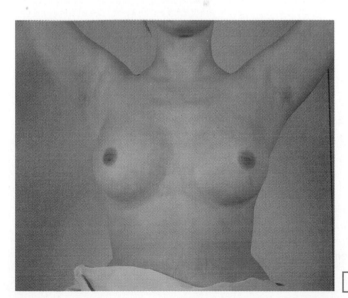

15–9

▶ Normal Range of Findings	Abnormal Findings

Next ask her to push her hands onto her hips (Fig. 15–10) and to push her two palms together (Fig. 15–11). These maneuvers contract the pectoralis major muscle. A slight lifting of both breasts will occur.

Note a dimpling or a pucker, which indicates skin retraction (see Table 15–3).

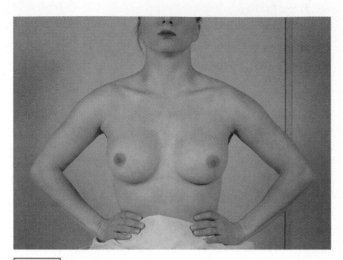

15–10

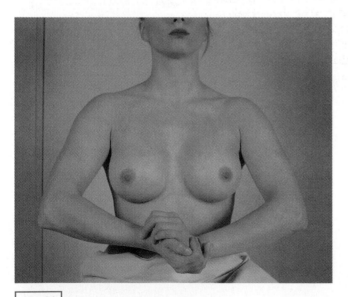

15–11

Ask the woman with large pendulous breasts to lean forward while you support her forearms. Note the symmetric free-forward movement of both breasts (Fig. 15–12).

Note fixation to chest wall or skin retraction (see Table 15–3).

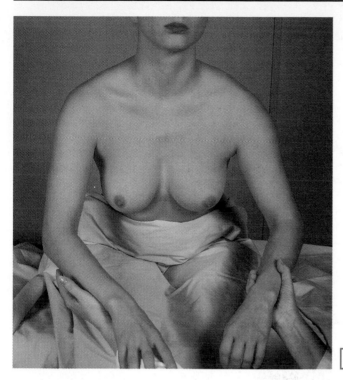

15-12

THE AXILLAE

Inspect and palpate the axillae

Examine the axillae while the woman is sitting. Inspect the skin, noting any rash or infection. Lift the woman's arm and support it yourself, so that her muscles are loose and relaxed. Use your right hand to palpate the left axilla (Fig. 15–13). Reach your fingers high into the axilla. Move them firmly down in four directions: down the chest wall in a line from the middle of the axilla, along the anterior border of the axilla, along the posterior border, and along the inner aspect of the upper arm. Move the woman's arm through range-of-motion to increase the surface area you can reach.

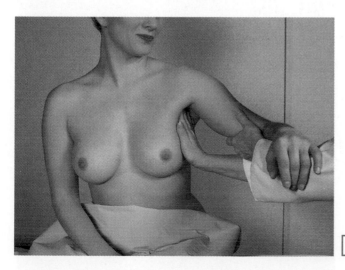

15-13

Normal Range of Findings	Abnormal Findings

Usually nodes are not palpable, although you may feel a small, soft, non-tender node in the central group. Expect some tenderness when palpating high in the axilla. Note any enlarged and tender lymph nodes.

BREAST PALPATION

Palpate the breasts

Help the woman to a supine position. Tuck a small pad under the side to be palpated and raise her arm over her head. These maneuvers will flatten the breast tissue and displace it medially. Any significant lumps will then feel more distinct (Fig. 15–14).

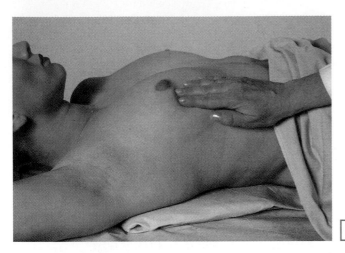

15–14

Use the pads of your first three fingers and make a gentle rotary motion on the breast. Choose one of two patterns for palpation: (1) You may start at the nipple and palpate out to the periphery as if following spokes on a wheel (Fig. 15–15); or (2) start at the nipple and palpate in concentric circles, increasing out

Abnormal Findings (right column):

Nodes enlarge with any local infection of the breast, arm, or hand, and with breast cancer metastases.

Heat, redness, and swelling in nonlactating and nonpostpartum breasts indicate inflammation.

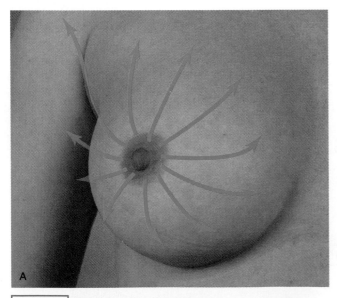

15–15A **Spokes-on-a-wheel pattern of palpation**

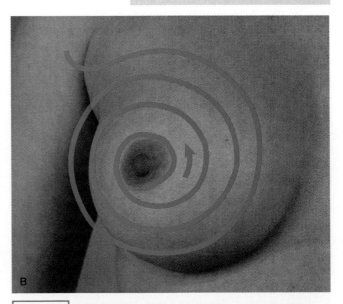

15–15B **Concentric circles of pattern of palpation**

to the periphery. With either pattern, move in a clockwise direction, taking care to examine every square inch of the breast. Also, take care to palpate the tail of Spence extending from the upper outer quadrant into the axilla. It does not matter which method of palpation you use, but be consistent and thorough.

In nulliparous women, normal breast tissue feels firm, smooth, and elastic. After pregnancy, the tissue feels softer and looser. Premenstrual engorgement is normal owing to increasing progesterone. This consists of a slight enlargement, a tenderness to palpation, and a generalized nodularity; the lobes feel prominent and their margins more distinct.

Also, normally you may feel a firm transverse ridge of compressed tissue in the lower quadrants. This is the **inframammary ridge,** and it is especially noticeable in large breasts. Do not confuse it with an abnormal lump.

After palpating over the four breast quadrants, palpate the nipple (Fig. 15–16). Note any induration or subareolar mass. Use your thumb and forefinger to apply gentle pressure or a stripping action to the nipple. Starting at the outside of the areola, "milk" your fingers toward the nipple—repeat, from a few different directions. If any discharge appears, note its color and consistency.

Except in pregnancy and lactation, discharge is abnormal (see Table 15–6). Note the number of discharge droplets and the quadrant(s) producing them. Blot the discharge on a white tissue to ascertain its color. Test any abnormal discharge for the presence of blood.

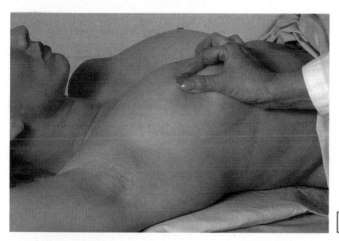

15–16

For the woman with large pendulous breasts, you may palpate using a bimanual technique (Fig. 15–17). The woman is in a sitting position, leaning forward. Support the inferior part of the breast with one hand. Use your other hand to palpate the breast tissue against your supporting hand.

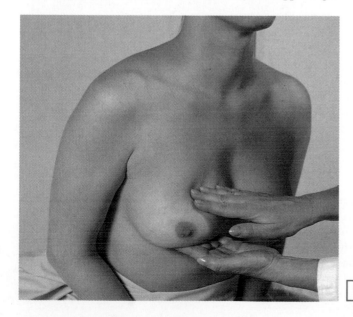

15–17

If the woman mentions a breast lump that she has discovered herself, examine the unaffected breast first to learn a baseline of normal consistency for this individual. If you do feel a lump or mass, note these characteristics (Fig. 15–18):

1. Location—Using the breast as a clock face, describe the distance in centimeters from the nipple, e.g., "7:00, 2 cm from the nipple." Or, diagram the breast in the woman's record and mark in the location of the lump.
2. Size—Judge in centimeters in three dimensions: width × length × thickness.
3. Shape—State if the lump is oval, round, lobulated, or indistinct.
4. Consistency—State if the lump is soft, firm, or hard.
5. Movable—Is the lump freely movable, or is it fixed when you try to slide it over the chest wall?
6. Distinctness—Is the lump solitary or multiple?
7. Nipple—Is it displaced or retracted?
8. Note the skin over the lump—Is it erythematous, dimpled, or retracted?
9. Tenderness—Is the lump tender to palpation?
10. Lymphadenopathy—Are any regional lymph nodes palpable?

See Tables 15–4 and 15–5 for description of common breast lumps using these characteristics.

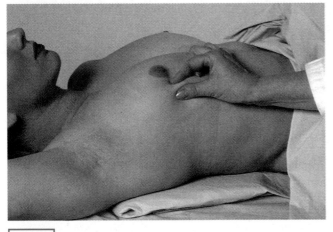

15–18

A procedure called the *friction-free examination* incorporates hot, soapy lather applied to the breasts before palpation. The soap acts as a lubricant and greatly enhances the breast features. Talcum powder also can be used. Some high-risk breast clinics advocate this technique as a valuable tool for detection of lumps because the details are so clearly defined. The heat also enhances detection of any nipple secretions. Following the examination, the breasts are cleaned with a hot wet towel.

TEACH THE BREAST SELF-EXAMINATION

Finish your own assessment first, then teach the self-examination. You need to focus your skill and concentration on the examination, and you may be diverted by teaching at the same time. The same is true for the woman. She waits to hear that your examination of her affirms that she is healthy. Once reassured, she can relax about the findings and concentrate on your teaching.

Help each woman establish a regular schedule of self-care. The best time to conduct BSE is right after the menstrual period, or the 4th through 7th day of the menstrual cycle, when the breasts are the smallest and least congested. Advise the pregnant or menopausal woman who is not having menstrual periods to select a familiar date to examine her breasts each month, for example, her birthdate or the day the rent is due.

Stress that a regular monthly self-examination will familiarize the woman with her own breasts and their normal variation. This is a positive step that will reassure her of her healthy state. Emphasize the absence of lumps (not the presence of them). However, do encourage her to report any unusual finding promptly.

While teaching, focus on the positive aspects of BSE. Avoid citing frightening mortality statistics about breast cancer. This may generate excessive fear and denial that actually obstructs a woman's self-care action. Rather, be selective in your choice of factual material:

The majority of women will never get breast cancer.
The great majority of breast lumps are benign.
Early detection of breast cancer is important; if the cancer is not invasive, the
    survival rate is close to 100 percent.

Emphasize self-care through knowledge of risk factors, regular performance of BSE to increase confidence in detecting abnormalities, and early referral for any suspicious findings.

Keep your teaching simple! The simpler the plan, the more likely the person is to comply. Describe the correct technique and rationale and the expected findings to note as the woman inspects her own breasts (Fig. 15–19). Teach the woman to do this in front of a mirror while she is disrobed to the waist. At home, she can start palpation in the shower where soap and water assist palpation. Then, palpation should be performed while lying supine. Encourage the woman to palpate her own breasts while you are there to monitor her technique. Use the return demonstration to assess her technique and understanding of the procedure.

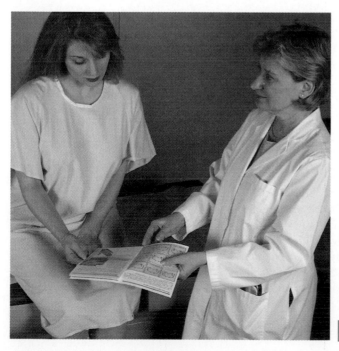

15–19

Many examiners use a simulated breast model so that the woman can palpate a "lump." Pamphlets also are helpful reinforcers; just be sure they conform to the method you teach, e.g., circular approach versus radiating line approach to palpation. Give the woman two pamphlets to take home and encourage her to give one to a relative or friend. This may promote discussion, which is reinforcing.

THE MALE BREAST

Your examination of the male breast can be much more abbreviated, but do not omit it. Inspect the chest wall noting the skin surface and any lumps or swelling. Palpate the nipple area for any lump or tissue enlargement (Fig. 15–20). It should feel even, with no nodules.

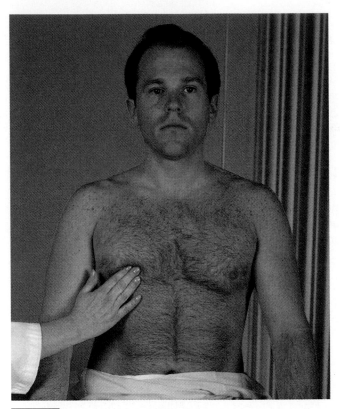

15–20

The normal male breast has a flat disc of undeveloped breast tissue beneath the nipple. **Gynecomastia** is an enlargement of this breast tissue, making it clinically distinguishable from the other tissues in the chest wall (Fig. 15–21). It feels like a smooth, firm, movable disc. This occurs normally during puberty. It usually affects only one breast and is temporary. The adolescent male is acutely aware of his body image. Reassure him that this change is normal, common, and temporary.

An obese male has an increase of fatty, not glandular, tissue.

Gynecomastia also occurs with use of anabolic steroids, some medications, and some disease states. See Table 15–8.

▶ 　　　　　

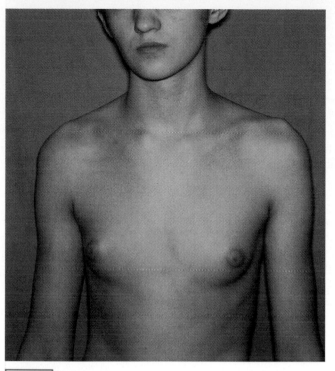

15–21

Adolescent gynecomastia

 DEVELOPMENTAL CONSIDERATIONS

Infants and Children

In the neonate of either sex, the breasts may be enlarged and visible owing to maternal estrogen crossing the placenta. They may secrete a clear or white fluid, called "witch's milk." These signs are not significant and are resolved within a few days to a few weeks.

Note the position of the nipples on the prepubertal child. They should be symmetric, just lateral to the midclavicular line, between the fourth and fifth ribs. The nipple is flat, and the areola is darker pigmented.

Premature thelarche is early breast development with no other hormone-dependent signs (pubic hair, menses).

The Adolescent

Adolescent breast development usually begins on an average between 8 and 10 years of age. Expect some asymmetry during growth. (Distinguish breast development from extra adipose tissue present in obese children.) Record the stage of development using Tanner's staging described on p. 419. Use the chart to teach the adolescent normal developmental stages and to assure her of her own normal progress.

Note precocious development, occurring before age 8. It is usually normal but also occurs with thyroid dysfunction, stilbestrol ingestion, or ovarian or adrenal tumor.

▶ Normal Range of Findings	Abnormal Findings
	Note delayed development, occurring with hormonal failure or anorexia nervosa beginning before puberty, or with severe malnutrition.
With maturing adolescents, palpate the breasts as you would with the adult. The breasts normally feel firm and uniform. Note any mass.	At this age, a mass is almost always a benign fibroadenoma or a cyst (see Table 15–4).
Teach BSE now, so that the technique will become a natural, comfortable habit by the time the girl becomes an adult and will be at higher risk.	

The Pregnant Female

A delicate blue vascular pattern is visible over the breasts. The breasts increase in size as do the nipples. Jagged linear stretch marks, or striae, may develop if the breasts have a large increase. The nipples also become darker and more erectile. The areolae widen, grow darker, and contain the small, scattered, elevated Montgomery's glands. On palpation, the breasts feel more nodular, and thick yellow colostrum can be expressed after the first trimester.

The Lactating Female

Colostrum changes to milk production around the 3rd postpartum day. At this time, the breasts may become engorged, appearing enlarged, reddened, and shiny and feeling warm and hard. Frequent nursings help drain the ducts and sinuses and stimulate milk production. Nipple soreness is normal, appearing around the twentieth nursing, lasting 24 to 48 hours, then disappearing rapidly. The nipples may look red and irritated. They may even crack but will heal rapidly if kept dry and exposed to air. Again, frequent nursings are the best treatment for nipple soreness.

One section of the breast surface appearing red and tender indicates a plugged duct (see Table 15–7).

The Aging Female

On inspection, the breasts look pendulous, flattened, and sagging. Nipples may be retracted but can be pulled outward. On palpation, the breasts feel more granular, and the terminal ducts around the nipple feel more prominent and stringy. Thickening of the inframammary ridge at the lower breast is normal, and it feels more prominent with age.

Reinforce the value of the breast self-examination. Women over 50 years have an increased risk of breast cancer. Older women may have problems with arthritis, limited range of motion, or decreased vision that may inhibit self-care. Suggest aids to the self-examination, e.g., talcum powder helps fingers glide over skin.

Since atrophy causes shrinkage of normal glandular tissue, cancer detection is somewhat easier. Any palpable lump that cannot be positively identified as a normal structure should be referred.

SUMMARY CHECKLIST: Breasts and Regional Lymphatics

1. **Inspect breasts as the woman sits, raises arms overhead, pushes hands on hips, leans forward**

2. **Inspect the supraclavicular and infraclavicular areas**

3. **Palpate the axillae and regional lymph nodes**

4. **With woman supine, palpate the breast tissue, including tail of Spence, the nipples, and areolae**

5. **Teach BSE**

SAMPLE CHARTING

FEMALE

▶ **Subjective**

States no breast pain, lump, discharge, rash, swelling, or trauma. No history of breast disease herself, does have mother with fibrocystic disease. No history of breast surgery. Never been pregnant. Performs BSE monthly.

▶ **Objective**

Inspection. Breasts symmetric. Skin smooth with even color and no rash or lesions. Arm movement shows no dimpling or retractions. No nipple discharge, no lesions.

Palpation. Breast contour and consistency firm and homogeneous. No masses or tenderness. No lymphadenopathy.

MALE

▶ **Subjective**

No pain, lump, rash, or swelling.

▶ **Objective**

No masses or tenderness. No lymphadenopathy.

CLINICAL CASE STUDY 1

J.G. is a 32-year-old white female high school teacher, married, with no children. She reports good health until finding "lump in right breast 2 weeks ago."

▶ **Subjective**

2 weeks PTA—noticed lump in R breast on self-examination. Lump firm, nonmovable area "the size of a quarter," in upper outer quadrant of breast, tender on touch only. No skin changes, no nipple discharge, on no medications. Last breast exam by M.D. 3 months before was reported normal. Did not notice lump on previous self-exam 1 month before. No history of breast disease in self or family.

2 days PTA—saw M.D., who confirmed presence of lump and recommended biopsy as outpatient. Last menstrual period 1/25/ (2 1/2 weeks PTA). States the last 2 days has been so nervous has been unable to sleep well or to concentrate at work. "I just know it's cancer."

▶ **Objective**

Voice trembling and breathless during history. Sitting posture stiff and rigid. B/P 148/78. 37°-92-16.

Inspection. Breasts symmetric, nipples everted. No skin lesions, no dimpling, no retraction, no fixation.

Palpation. Left breast firm, no mass, no tenderness, no discharge. Right breast firm, with 2 cm × 2 cm × 1 cm mass at 10:00 position, 5 cm from the nipple. Lump is firm, oval, with smooth discrete borders, nonmovable, tender to palpation. No other mass. No discharge. No lymphadenopathy.

▶ ASSESSMENT

Lump in R breast
Anxiety R/T threat to health status

Continued

CLINICAL CASE STUDY 2

D.B. is a 62-year-old black female bank comptroller, married, with no children. History of hypertension, managed by diuretic medication and diet. No other health problems until yearly company physical exam 3 days PTA, when M.D. "found a lump in my right breast."

 Subjective

3 days PTA—M.D. noted lump in R breast during yearly physical exam. M.D. did not describe lump but told D.B. it was "serious" and needed immediate biopsy. D.B. has not felt it herself. States has noted no skin changes, no nipple discharge. No previous history of breast disease. Mother died age 54 of breast cancer, no other relative with breast disease. D.B. has had no full-term pregnancies; two spontaneous abortions, ages 28, 31. Menopause completed at age 52.

Aware of BSE but has never performed it. "I feel so bad. If only I had been doing it. I should have found this myself." Married 43 years. States husband supportive, but "I just can't talk to him about this. I can't even go near him now."

 Objective

Inspection. Breasts symmetric when sitting, arms down. Nipples flat. No lesions, no discharge. As lifts arms, left breast elevates, right breast stays fixed. Dimple in right breast, 9:00 position, apparent at rest and with muscle contraction. Leaning forward reveals left breast falls free, right breast flattens.

Palpation. Left breast feels soft and granular throughout, no mass. Right breast soft and granular, with large, stony hard mass in outer quadrant. Lump is 5 cm × 4 cm × 2 cm, at 9:00 position, 3 cm from nipple. Borders irregular, mass fixed to tissues, no pain with palpation.

One firm, palpable lymph node in center of right axilla. No palpable nodes on the left.

 ASSESSMENT

Lump in R breast
Ineffective individual coping R/T effects of breast lump

NURSING DIAGNOSES COMMONLY ASSOCIATED WITH BREAST DISORDERS

Diagnosis	Related Factors (Etiology)	Defining Characteristics (Symptoms and Signs)
Ineffective breastfeeding	Prematurity Infant receiving supplemental feedings with artificial nipple Poor infant sucking reflex Nonsupportive partner/family Knowledge deficit Interruption of breastfeeding Maternal anxiety or ambivalence	Unsatisfactory breastfeeding process Actual or perceived inadequate milk supply Infant inability to attach onto maternal breast correctly Nonsustained suckling at the breast Persistence of sore nipples beyond 1st week of breastfeeding Observable signs of inadequate infant intake Insufficient emptying of each breast per feeding Insufficient opportunity for suckling at the breast Infant arching and crying at the breast, resisting latching on

Ineffective individual coping	Effects of acute or chronic illness	Change in communication pattern
	Loss of control over body part or body system	Inability to meet or be responsible for basic needs
	Lack of support systems	Fear of pain, death
	Low self-esteem	Frequent headaches
	Major change in lifestyle	Emotional tension
	Unrealistic perceptions	Insomnia
	Situational or maturational crisis	Verbalizes inability to cope or inability to ask for help
	Knowledge deficit about	Inability to perform expected roles
	Disease process	Physical inactivity
	Therapeutic regimen	Stress-related disorders
	Prognosis	Ulcers
	Separation from or loss of significant other	Hypertension
	Sensory overload	Irritable bowel
		Substance abuse
		Inappropriate use of defense mechanisms
		Withdrawal
		Depression
		Overeating
		Blaming
		Scapegoating
		Manipulative behavior
		Self-pity
		Chronic anxiety
		Indecisiveness
Knowledge deficit: breast self-examination	Lack of exposure or recall	Expresses inaccurate perception of potential problem
	Information misinterpretation	Repeatedly requests information
	Unfamiliarity with information resources	Inadequate performance of examination
	Lack of interest in learning	Verbalizes the problem
	Denial	Inaccurate use of health-related vocabulary
	Effects of aging	Inability to explain therapeutic regimen or describe personal health status
	Sensory deficits	
	Language barrier	
	Cognitive limitations	
	Inadequate economic resources	

Other Related Nursing Diagnosis

ACTUAL	RISK/WELLNESS
Anxiety	**Risk**
Body image disturbance (see example in Chapter 11)	Risk for loneliness
Interrupted breastfeeding	**Wellness**
	Actively seeking knowledge about BSE
	Effective breastfeeding
	Increasing compliance with prescribed regimen

 ## ASSESSMENT VIDEO CRITICAL THINKING QUESTIONS

Saunders *Physical Examination and Health Assessment* Video Series—BREASTS AND REGIONAL LYMPHATICS—will direct you to consider the following:

1. How do breast assessment findings differ between older women and younger adult women?

2. How should you modify breast palpation in a woman with large, pendulous breasts?

3. Which conditions may be associated with a breast lump? Nipple rash? Enlarged axillary lymph nodes?

4. How does breast examination in men differ from that in women?

▼ **Table 15–3** SIGNS OF RETRACTION AND INFLAMMATION IN THE BREAST

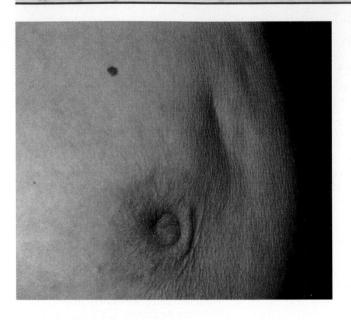

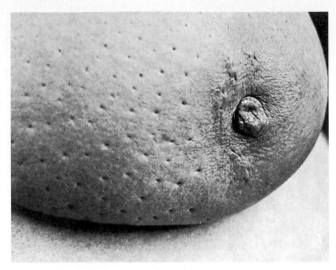

Dimpling

The shallow dimple (also called a skin tether) shown here is a sign of skin retraction. Cancer causes fibrosis, which contracts the suspensory ligaments. The dimple may be apparent at rest, with compression, or with lifting of the arms. Also, note the distortion of the areola here as the fibrosis pulls the nipple toward it.

Nipple Retraction

The retracted nipple looks flatter and broader, like an underlying crater. A recent retraction suggests cancer, which causes fibrosis of the whole duct system and pulls in the nipple. It also may occur with benign lesions such as ectasia of the ducts. Do not confuse retraction with the normal long-standing type of nipple inversion, which has no broadening and is not fixed.

Edema (Peau d'Orange)

Lymphatic obstruction produces edema. This thickens the skin and exaggerates the hair follicles, giving a pig-skin or orange-peel look. This condition suggests cancer. Edema usually begins in the skin around and beneath the areola, the most dependent area of the breast. Also note nipple retraction and dimpling here.

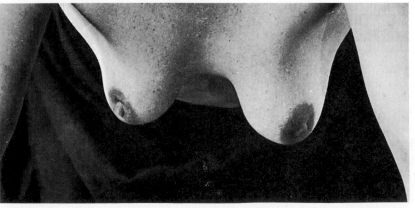

◄ **Fixation**

Asymmetry, distortion, or decreased mobility with the forward-bending maneuver. As cancer becomes invasive, the fibrosis fixes the breast to the underlying pectoral muscles. Here, note the right breast is held against the chest wall, with lateral deviation of the nipple and areola.

Table 15–3 SIGNS OF RETRACTION AND INFLAMMATION IN THE BREAST
Continued

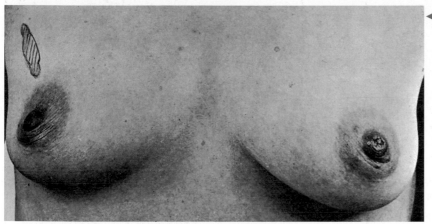

◀ Deviation in Nipple Pointing

An underlying cancer causes fibrosis in the mammary ducts, which pulls the nipple angle toward it. Here, note that the horizontal level of the right nipple is elevated and the nipple tilts upward and laterally.

Prominent Venous Pattern (not illustrated)

An obvious venous pattern that is unilateral occurs with some types of breast tumors.

 Table 15–4 BREAST LUMP

Benign Breast Disease (Formerly Fibrocystic Breast Disease)

Multiple tender masses. "Fibrocystic disease" is a meaningless term because it covers too many entities. Actually, six diagnostic categories exist, based on symptoms and physical findings (Love and Lindsey, 1995):

- Swelling and tenderness (cyclic discomfort)
- Mastalgia (severe pain, both cyclic and noncyclic)
- Nodularity (significant lumpiness, both cyclic and noncyclic)
- Dominant lumps (including cysts and fibroadenomas)
- Nipple discharge (including intraductal papilloma and duct ectasia)
- Infections and inflammations (including subareolar abscess, lactational mastitis, breast abscess, and Mondor's disease)

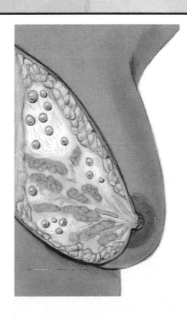

About 50 percent of all women have some form of benign breast disease. Nodularity occurs bilaterally; regular, firm nodules that are mobile, well demarcated, and feel rubbery, like small water balloons. Pain may be dull, heavy, and cyclic or just before menses as nodules enlarge. Some women have nodularity but no pain, and vice versa. Cysts are discrete, fluid-filled sacs. Dominant lumps and nipple discharge must be investigated carefully and may need biopsy to rule out cancer. Nodularity itself is not premalignant, but may produce difficulty in detecting other cancerous lumps.

Table continued on following page

Table 15–4 • BREAST LUMP *Continued*

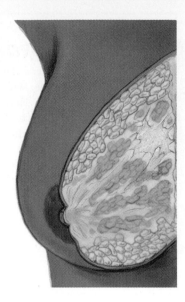 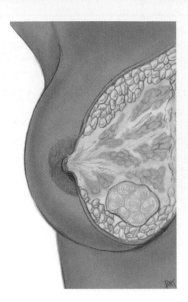

Cancer

Solitary unilateral nontender mass. Single focus in one area, although it may be interspersed with other nodules. Solid, hard, dense, and fixed to underlying tissues or skin as cancer becomes invasive. Borders are irregular and poorly delineated. Grows constantly. Often painless, although the person may have pain. Most common in upper outer quadrant. Usually found in women 30 to 80 years of age; increased risk in ages 40 to 44 and in women older than 50 years. As cancer advances, signs include firm or hard irregular axillary nodes; skin dimpling; nipple retraction, elevation, and discharge.

Fibroadenoma

Solitary nontender mass. A category of benign breast disease that deserves mention due to its frequency and characteristic appearance. Solid, firm, rubbery, and elastic. Round, oval, or lobulated; 1 to 5 cm. Freely movable, slippery; fingers slide it easily through tissue. Most common between 15 and 30 years of age, but can occur up to age 55 years. Grows quickly and constantly. Benign, although it must be diagnosed by biopsy.

Table 15–5 • DIFFERENTIATING BREAST LUMPS

	Fibroadenoma	Benign Breast Disease	Cancer
Likely age	15–30, can occur up to 55	30–55, decreases after menopause	30–80, risk increases after 50
Shape	Round, lobular	Round, lobular	Irregular, star-shaped
Consistency	Usually firm, rubbery	Firm to soft, rubbery	Firm to stony hard
Demarcation	Well demarcated, clear margins	Well demarcated	Poorly defined
Number	Usually single	Usually multiple, may be single	Single
Mobility	Very mobile, slippery	Mobile	Fixed
Tenderness	Usually none	Tender, usually increases before menses, may be noncyclic	Usually none, can be tender
Skin retraction	None	None	Usually
Pattern of growth	Grows quickly and constantly	Size may increase or decrease rapidly	Grows constantly
Risk to health	None; they are benign—must diagnose by biopsy	Benign, although general lumpiness may mask other cancerous lump	Serious, needs early treatment

Table 15-6 ABNORMAL NIPPLE DISCHARGE

Mammary Duct Ectasia (not illustrated)

Pastelike matter in subareolar ducts produces sticky, purulent discharge that may be white, gray, brown, green, or bloody, usually bilateral and from multiple ducts. It is thought to be caused by stagnation of cellular debris and secretions in the ducts, leading to obstruction, inflammation, and infection. Occurs in women who have lactated in the past; usually occurs in perimenopausal age.

Itching, burning, or drawing pain occurs around nipple. May have subareolar redness and swelling, possibly nipple retraction and dimpling. Ducts are palpable as rubbery, twisted tubules under areola. May have palpable mass, soft or firm, poorly delineated. Not malignant, but needs biopsy.

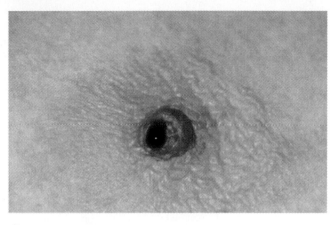

Carcinoma

Bloody nipple discharge that is unilateral and from a single duct requires further investigation. Although there was no palpable lump associated with the discharge shown here, mammography revealed a 1-cm, centrally located, ill-defined mass.

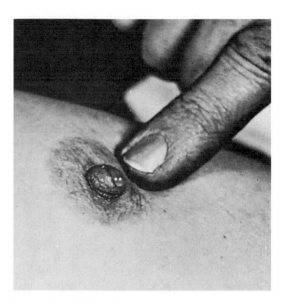

Intraductal Papilloma

Serous or serosanguineous discharge, which is spontaneous, unilateral, and from a single duct. Lesion consists of tiny tumors, 2 to 3 mm, which are too small to palpate. If you can palpate a mass, it is soft, poorly delineated. Moderate pain.

Papillomas affect women 40 to 60 years of age. Some papillomas are associated with concurrent or subsequent cancer, although most are benign. Refer any bloody discharge for careful evaluation, including biopsy, to rule out cancer.

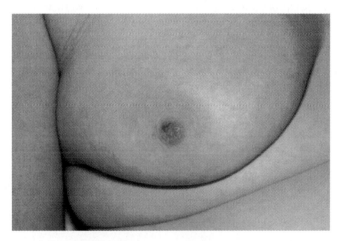

Paget's Disease (Intraductal Carcinoma)

Early lesion has clear yellow discharge and dry, scaling crusts, friable at nipple apex. Spreads to areola with erythematous halo on areola and crusted, eczematous, retracted nipple. Later lesion shows nipple reddened, excoriated, ulcerated, with bloody discharge when surface is eroded, and an erythematous plaque surrounding the nipple. Symptoms include tingling, burning, itching.

Except for the redness and occasional cracking due to initial breastfeeding, any dermatitis of the nipple area must be carefully explored and referred immediately.

Table 15–7   DISORDERS OCCURRING DURING LACTATION

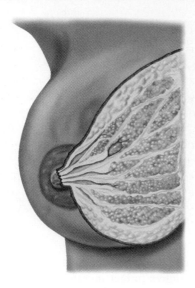

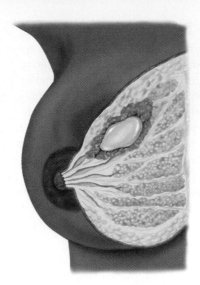

Plugged Duct

A fairly common and not serious condition. One milk duct is clogged. One section of the breast is tender; may be reddened. No infection. It is important to keep breast as empty as possible and milk flowing. The woman should nurse her baby frequently, on affected side first to ensure complete emptying, and manually express any remaining milk. A plugged duct usually resolves in less than 1 day.

Breast Abscess

A rare complication of generalized infection, e.g., mastitis if untreated. A pocket of pus accumulates in one local area. Must temporarily discontinue nursing on affected breast; manually express milk and discard. Continue to nurse on unaffected side. Treat with antibiotics, surgical incision, and drainage.

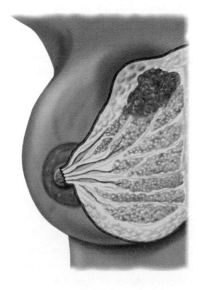

◀ Mastitis

This is uncommon; an inflammatory mass. Usually occurs in single quadrant. Area is red, swollen, tender, very hot, and hard. Also the woman has a headache, malaise, fever, chills and sweating, increased pulse, flulike symptoms. May occur during first 4 months of lactation from infection or from stasis due to plugged duct. Treat with rest, local heat to area, antibiotics, and frequent nursing to keep breast as empty as possible. Must not wean now or the breast will become engorged and the pain will increase. Mother's antibiotic not harmful to infant. Usually resolves in 2 to 3 days.

▼ Table 15-8   ABNORMALITIES IN THE MALE BREAST

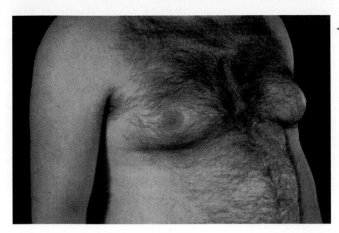

◄ Gynecomastia

Noninflammatory enlargement of male breast tissue. This is physiologic at puberty, unilateral, usually mild and transient. Gynecomastia occurs commonly in aging males owing to changing hormone levels. It is bilateral and may be tender.

It also occurs bilaterally from hormone stimulation, e.g., on estrogen for cancer of prostate; Cushing's syndrome; cirrhosis of liver as unable to metabolize estrogen completely; leukemia occasionally; and sometimes with medication—digitalis, isoniazid, spironolactone, phenothiazines, digitalis, and marijuana; testicular tumor, lung cancer; adrenal disease; and thyrotoxicosis.

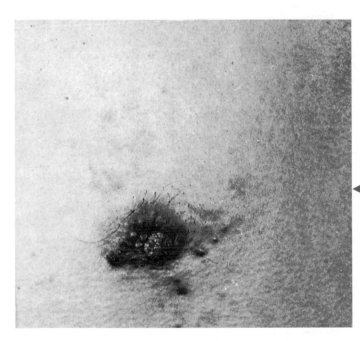

◄ Carcinoma

Less than 1 percent of all breast cancer occurs in men. The lesion is a hard, irregular, nontender mass, most often directly under the areola, fixed to the area, and may have nipple retraction. Mass is noticeable early owing to minimal breast tissue. There is also early spread to axillary lymph nodes owing to minimal breast tissue. The ulcerating mass shown here had been present for 3½ years and is advanced carcinoma.

Bibliography

Adderley-Kelly B, Green PM: Breast cancer education, self-efficacy, and screening in older African American women. J Natl Black Nurs Assoc 9(1):45–57, 1997.

American Cancer Society: Cancer Facts and Figures—1998 Atlanta, GA, American Cancer Society, 1998.

Appling SE: Mastitis. Prim Care Pract 2(2):184–188, Mar–Apr 1998.

Appling SE: One in nine: Risks and prevention strategies for breast cancer. Medsurg Nurs 5(1):62–64, Feb 1996.

Appling SE: Prevention, early detection, and treatment of breast cancer: A collaborative approach. Prim Care Pract 2(2):111–120, Mar–Apr 1998.

Arnold GJ, Neiheisel MB: A comprehensive approach to evaluating nipple discharge. Nurse Pract 22(7):96–111, July 1997.

Brown LW, Williams RD: Culturally sensitive breast cancer screening programs for older black women. Nurs Pract 19(3):21–33, Mar 1994.

Champion VL: Results of a nurse-delivered intervention on proficiency and nodule detection with breast self-examination. Oncol Nurs Forum 22(5):819–824, 1995.

Champion VL, Scott CR: Reliability and validity of breast cancer screening belief scales in African American women. Nurs Res 46(6):331–337, Nov 1997.

Colditz G, Hankinson S, Hunter D, et al: The use of estrogens and progestins and the risk of breast cancer in postmenopausal women. N Engl J Med 332(24): 1589–1593, June 15, 1995.

Colditz GA, Willett WC, Hunter DJ, et al: Family history, age, and risk of breast cancer—Prospective data from the Nurses' Health Study. JAMA 270(3):338–343, July 21, 1993.

Cole CF: Issues in breast imaging. Prim Care Pract 2(2):141–148, Mar–Apr 1998.

Costanza ME, Greene HL, McManus D, et al: Can practicing physicians improve their counseling and physical examination skills in breast cancer screening? J Cancer Educ 10(1):14–21, Spring 1995.

Damsky DD: Common questions about ductal carcinoma in situ. Am J Nurs 97(5):61–66, May 1997.

Dienger MJ, Llewellyn J: Increasing compliance with breast self-examination. Medsurg Nurs 4(5):359–366, Oct 1995.

Gross RE: Women at high risk for breast cancer. Am J Nurs 98(4):55–56, Apr, 1998.

Harlan WR, Harlan EA, Grillo GP: Secondary sex characteristics of girls 12 to 17 years of age: The U.S. Health Examination Survey. J Pediatr 96(6): 1074–1078, 1980.

Herman-Giddens ME, Slora EJ, Wasserman RC, et al: Secondary sexual characteristics and menses in young girls seen in office practice: A study from the pediatric research in office settings network. Pediatrics 99(4):505–512, Apr 1997.

Hoskins KF, Stopfer JE, Calzone KA, et al: Assessment and counseling for women with a family history of breast cancer. JAMA 273(7): 577–585, Feb 15, 1995.

Leslie NS: Role of the nurse practitioner in breast and cervical cancer prevention. Cancer Nurs 18(4):251–257, 1995.

Leslie NS, Roche BG: The effectiveness of the breast self-examination facilitation shield. Oncol Nurs Forum 24(10): 1759–1765, Nov–Dec 1997.

Lester J, Fulton JS: Breast cancer: Advances in diagnosis and surgical treatment. Am J Nurs 98(Suppl):8–11, Apr 1998.

Love S, Lindsey K: Dr. Susan Love's Breast Book, 2nd ed. New York, Addison-Wesley, 1995.

Lu ZJ: Variables associated with breast self-examination among Chinese women. Cancer Nurs 18(1):29–34, 1995.

Mahon SM: Comparison of methods for the early detection of breast cancer. Image 29(3):292, 1997.

Marchant DJ: Breast Disease. Philadelphia, W.B. Saunders Company, 1997.

Marchant DJ: Risk factors. Obstet Gynecol Clin North Am 21(4):561–586, Dec 1994.

Marshall WA, Tanner JM: Variations in pattern of pubertal changes in girls. Arch Dis Child 44:291–303, June 1969.

Maurer F: A peer education model for teaching breast self-examination to undergraduate college women. Cancer Nurs 20(1):49–61, Feb 1997.

McCance KL, Jorde LB: Evaluating the genetic risk of breast cancer. Nurs Pract 23(8):14–29, Aug 1998.

Miller AM, Champion VL: Mammography in older women: One time and three year adherence to guidelines. Nurs Res 45(4):239–244, July–Aug 1996.

Morrison C: Determining crucial correlates of breast self-examination in older women with low incomes. Oncol Nurs Forum 23(1):83–93, Jan–Feb 1996.

Morrison C: The significance of nipple discharge: Diagnosis and treatment regimes. Prim Care Pract 2(2):129–140, Mar–Apr 1998.

Newcomb PA, et al: Lactation and a reduced risk of premenopausal breast cancer. N Engl J Med 330(2):81–87 1994.

Phillips JM: Breast cancer and African-American women. In Dow KH (Ed): Contemporary Issues in Breast Cancer. Sudbury, MA, Jones and Bartlett, 1996, pp 219–228.

Ryan AS: The resurgence of breastfeeding in the United States. Pediatrics 99(4):12, 1997.

Secretary's Task Force on Black & Minority Health: Report. Volume III: Cancer. Washington, DC, U.S. Department of Health and Human Services, 1986.

Sensiba ME, Stewart DS: Relationship of perceived barriers to breast self-examination in women of varying ages and levels of education. Oncol Nurs Forum 22(8):1265–1268, 1995.

Shapiro TJ, Clark PM: Breast cancer: What the primary care provider needs to know. Nurse Pract 20(3):36–53, 1995.

Sherman F, Seremetis S: Breast health at midlife: Guidelines for screening and patient evaluation. Geriatrics 52(6):58–60, June 1997.

Sherman JJ, Abel E, Tavakoli A: Demographic predictors of clinical breast examination, mammography, and Pap test screening among older women. J Am Acad Nurs Pract 8(5):231–236, May 1996.

Sloand E: Pediatric and adolescent breast health. Prim Care Pract 2(2): 170–175, Mar–Apr 1998.

Tanner JM: Growth at Adolescence, 2nd ed. Oxford, England, Blackwell Scientific, 1962.

Thune I, Brenn T, Lund E, Gaard M: Physical activity and the risk of breast cancer. N Engl J Med 336(18): 1269–1275, May 1997.

Weber ES: Questions & answers about breast cancer diagnosis. Am J Nurs 97(10):34–38, Oct 1997.

Weisburger JH: Dietary fat and risk of chronic disease: Mechanistic insights from experimental studies. J Am Diet Assoc 97(7, Suppl): S16–23, July 1997.

Ziegfeld CR: Differential diagnosis of a breast mass. Prim Care Pract 2(2): 121–128, Mar–Apr 1998.

CHAPTER SIXTEEN

Thorax and Lungs

POSITION AND SURFACE LANDMARKS

The **thoracic cage** is a bony structure with a conical shape, which is narrower at the top (Fig. 16–1). It is defined by the **sternum,** 12 pairs of **ribs** and 12 thoracic **vertebrae.** Its "floor" is the **diaphragm,** a musculotendinous septum that separates the thoracic cavity from the abdomen. The first seven ribs attach directly to the sternum via their costal cartilages; ribs 8, 9, and 10 attach to the costal cartilage above, and ribs 11 and 12 are "floating," with free palpable tips. The **costochondral junctions** are the points at which the ribs join their cartilages. They are not palpable.

Anterior Thoracic Landmarks

Surface landmarks on the thorax are signposts for underlying respiratory structures. Knowledge of landmarks will help you localize a finding and will facilitate communication of your findings to others.

Suprasternal Notch. Feel this hollow U-shaped depression just above the sternum, in between the clavicles.

Sternum. The "breastbone" has three parts—the manubrium, the body, and the xiphoid process. Walk your fingers down the manubrium a few centimeters until you feel a distinct bony ridge, the manubriosternal angle.

Manubriosternal Angle. Often called the sternal angle or the "angle of Louis," this is the articulation of the manubrium and body of the sternum, and it is continuous with the second rib. The angle of Louis is a useful place to start counting ribs, which helps localize a respiratory finding horizontally. Identify the angle of Louis, palpate lightly to the second rib, and slide down to the second intercostal space. Each intercostal space is numbered by the rib above it. Continue counting down the ribs in the middle of the hemithorax, not close to the sternum where the costal cartilages lie too close together to count. You can palpate easily down to the 10th rib.

The angle of Louis also marks the site of tracheal bifurcation into the right and left main bronchi; it corresponds with the upper border of the atria of the heart, and it lies above the fourth thoracic vertebra on the back.

Costal Angle. The right and left costal margins form an angle where they meet at the xiphoid process. Usually 90 degrees or less, this angle increases when the rib cage is chronically overinflated, as in emphysema.

Posterior Thoracic Landmarks

Counting ribs and intercostal spaces on the back is a bit harder due to the muscles and soft tissue surrounding the ribs and spinal column (Fig. 16–2).

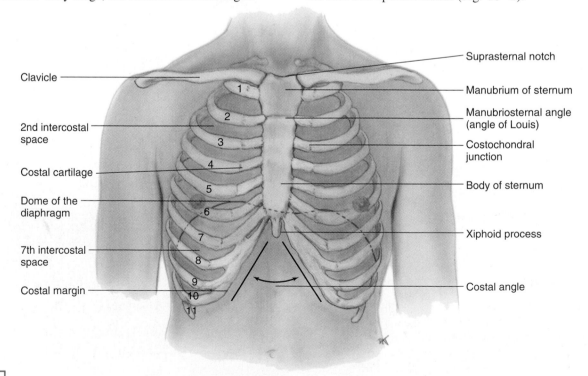

Clavicle

2nd intercostal space

Costal cartilage

Dome of the diaphragm

7th intercostal space

Costal margin

Suprasternal notch

Manubrium of sternum

Manubriosternal angle (angle of Louis)

Costochondral junction

Body of sternum

Xiphoid process

Costal angle

ANTERIOR THORACIC CAGE

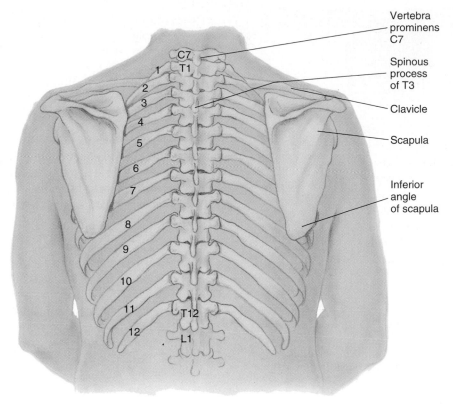

POSTERIOR THORACIC CAGE

16–2

Vertebra Prominens. Start here. Flex your head and feel for the most prominent bony spur protruding at the base of the neck. This is the spinous process of C7. If two bumps seem equally prominent, the upper one is C7 and the lower one is T1.

Spinous Processes. Count down these knobs on the vertebrae, which stack together to form the spinal column. Note that the spinous processes align with their same numbered ribs only down to T4. After T4, the spinous processes angle downward from their vertebral body and overlie the vertebral body and rib below.

Inferior Border of the Scapula. The scapulae are located symmetrically in each hemithorax. The lower tip is usually at the seventh or eighth rib.

Twelfth Rib. Palpate midway between the spine and the person's side to identify its free tip.

Reference Lines

Use the reference lines to pinpoint a finding vertically on the chest. On the anterior chest, note the **midsternal** line and the **midclavicular** line. The midclavicular line bisects the center of each clavicle at a point halfway between the palpated sternoclavicular and acromioclavicular joints (Fig. 16–3).

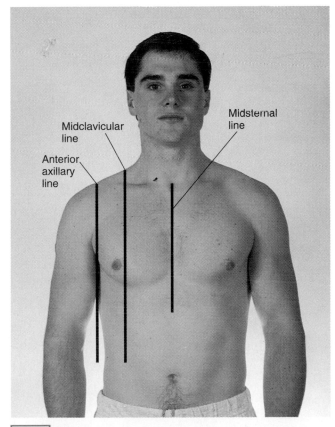

16–3

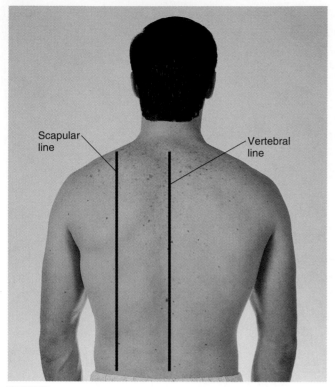

16–4

The posterior chest wall has the **vertebral** (or mid-spinal) line and the **scapular** line, which extends through the inferior angle of the scapula when the arms are at the sides of the body (Fig. 16–4).

Lift up the person's arm 90 degrees, and divide the lateral chest by three lines: The **anterior axillary** line

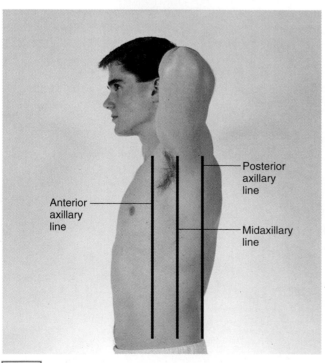

16–5

extends down from the anterior axillary fold where the pectoralis major muscle inserts; the **posterior axillary** line continues down from the posterior axillary fold where the latissimus dorsi muscle inserts; and the **mid-axillary** line runs down from the apex of the axilla and lies between and parallel to the other two (Fig. 16–5).

THE THORACIC CAVITY

The **mediastinum** is the middle section of the thoracic cavity containing the esophagus, trachea, heart, and great vessels. The right and left **pleural cavities,** on either side of the mediastinum, contain the lungs.

Lung Borders. In the anterior chest, the **apex,** or highest point, of lung tissue is 3 or 4 cm above the inner third of the clavicles. The **base,** or lower border, rests on the diaphragm at about the sixth rib in the midclavicular line. Laterally, lung tissue extends from the apex of the axilla down to the seventh or eighth rib. Posteriorly, the location of C7 marks the apex of lung tissue, and T10 usually corresponds to the base. Deep inspiration expands the lungs, and their lower border drops to the level of T12.

Lobes of the Lungs

The lungs are paired but not precisely symmetric structures (Fig. 16–6). The right lung is shorter than the left lung because of the underlying liver. The left lung is narrower than the right lung because the heart bulges to the left. The right lung has three lobes, and the left lung has two lobes. These lobes are not arranged in horizontal bands like dessert layers in a parfait glass. Rather, they stack in diagonal sloping segments and are separated by **fissures** that run obliquely through the chest.

Anterior. On the anterior chest, the **oblique** (the major, or diagonal) fissure crosses the fifth rib in the midaxillary line and terminates at the sixth rib in the midclavicular line. The right lung also contains the **horizontal** (minor) fissure, which divides the right upper and middle lobes. This fissure extends from the fifth rib in the right midaxillary line to the third intercostal space or fourth rib at the right sternal border.

Posterior. The most remarkable point about the posterior chest is that it is almost all lower lobe (Fig. 16–7). The upper lobes occupy a smaller band of tissue from their apices at T1 down to T3 or T4. At this level, the lower lobes begin, and their inferior border reaches down to the level of T10 on expiration and to TI2 on inspiration. Note that the right middle lobe does not project onto the posterior chest at all. If the person abducts the arms and places the hands on the back of the head, the division between upper and lower lobes corresponds to the medial border of the scapulae.

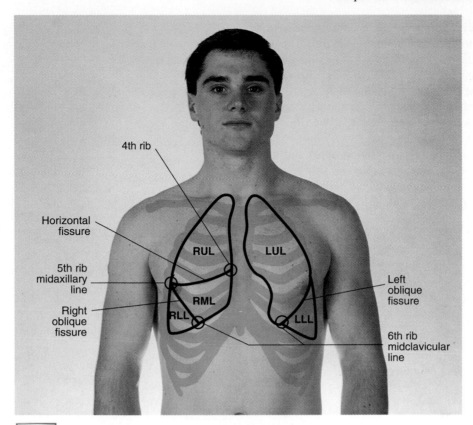

4th rib

Horizontal
fissure

5th rib
midaxillary
line

Right
oblique
fissure

RUL

LUL

RML

RLL   LLL

Left
oblique
fissure

6th rib
midclavicular
line

16–6

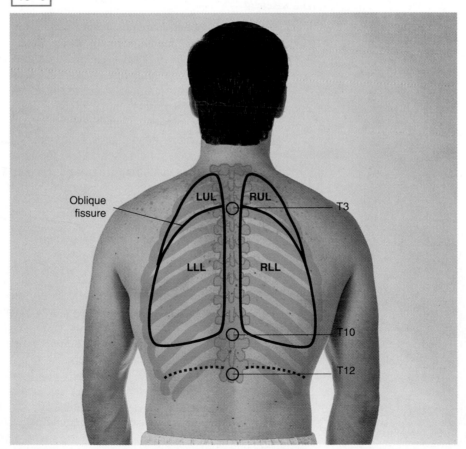

Oblique
fissure

LUL   RUL   T3

LLL   RLL

T10

T12

16–7

Lateral. Laterally, lung tissue extends from the apex of the axilla down to the seventh or eighth rib. The right upper lobe extends from the apex of the axilla down to the horizontal fissure at the fifth rib (Fig. 16–8). The right middle lobe extends from the horizontal fissure down and forward to the sixth rib at the midclavicular line. The right lower lobe continues from the fifth rib to the eighth rib in the midaxillary line.

The left lung contains only two lobes, upper and lower (Fig. 16–9). These are seen laterally as two triangular areas separated by the oblique fissure. The left upper lobe extends from the apex of the axilla down to the fifth rib at the midaxillary line. The left lower lobe continues down to the eighth rib in the midaxillary line.

Using these landmarks, take a grease pencil and try tracing the outline of each lobe on a willing partner. Take special note of the three points that commonly confuse beginning examiners:

1. The left lung has no middle lobe.
2. The anterior chest contains mostly upper and middle lobe with very little lower lobe.
3. The posterior chest contains almost all lower lobe.

Pleurae

The thin, slippery **pleurae** form an envelope between the lungs and the chest wall (Fig. 16–10). The **visceral** pleura lines the outside of the lungs, dipping down into the fissures. It is continuous with the **parietal** pleura lining the inside of the chest wall and diaphragm.

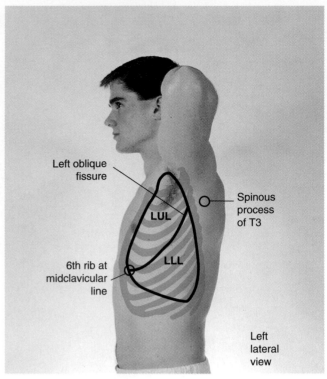

16–9

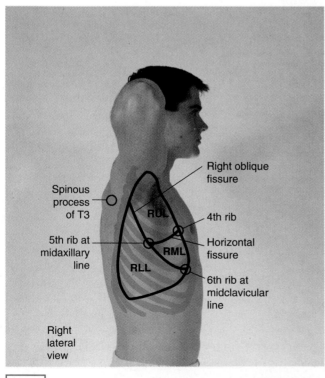

16–8

The inside of the envelope, the pleural cavity, is a potential space filled only with a few milliliters of lubricating fluid. It normally has a vacuum, or negative pressure, which holds the lungs tightly against the chest wall. The lungs slide smoothly and noiselessly up and down during respiration, lubricated by a few milliliters of fluid. Think of this as similar to two glass slides with a drop of water between them; although it is difficult to separate the slides, they slide smoothly back and forth. The pleurae extend about 3 cm below the level of the lungs, forming the **costodiaphragmatic recess.** This is a potential space; when it abnormally fills with air or fluid, it compromises lung expansion.

Trachea and Bronchial Tree

The **trachea** lies anterior to the esophagus and is 10 to 11 cm long in the adult. It begins at the level of the cricoid cartilage in the neck and bifurcates just below the sternal angle into the right and left main bronchi. Posteriorly, tracheal bifurcation is at the level of T4 or T5. The right main bronchus is shorter, wider, and more vertical than the left main bronchus.

The **trachea** and **bronchi** transport gases between the environment and the lung parenchyma. They constitute the *dead space,* or space that is filled with air but is not available for gaseous exchange. This is about 150 ml in the adult. The bronchial tree also protects alveoli from small particulate matter in the inhaled air. The bronchi are lined with goblet cells, which secrete mucus that en-

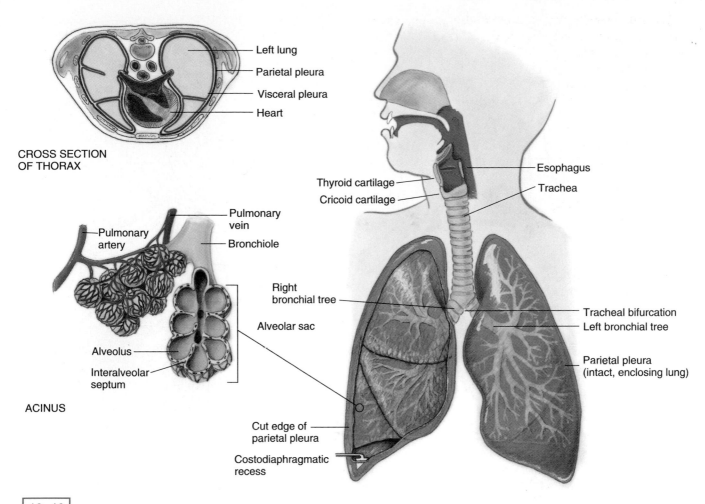

CROSS SECTION
OF THORAX

- Left lung
- Parietal pleura
- Visceral pleura
- Heart

Pulmonary
artery
Pulmonary
vein
Bronchiole
Alveolus
Interalveolar
septum

ACINUS

Right
bronchial tree
Alveolar sac
Cut edge of
parietal pleura
Costodiaphragmatic
recess

Thyroid cartilage
Cricoid cartilage
Esophagus
Trachea
Tracheal bifurcation
Left bronchial tree
Parietal pleura
(intact, enclosing lung)

16–10

traps the particles. The bronchi also are lined with cilia, which sweep particles upward where they can be swallowed or expelled.

An **acinus** is a functional respiratory unit and consists of the bronchioles, alveolar ducts, alveolar sacs, and the alveoli. Gaseous exchange occurs across the respiratory membrane in the alveolar duct and in the millions of alveoli. Note how the alveoli are clustered like grapes around each alveolar duct. This creates millions of interalveolar septa (walls) that increase tremendously the working space available for gas exchange. This bunched arrangement creates a surface area for gas exchange that is as large as a tennis court.

MECHANICS OF RESPIRATION

There are four major functions of the respiratory system: 1) Supply oxygen to the body for energy production; 2) remove carbon dioxide as a waste product of energy reactions; 3) maintain homeostasis (acid-base balance) of arterial blood; and 4) maintain heat exchange (less important in humans).

By supplying oxygen to the blood and eliminating excess carbon dioxide, respiration maintains the pH or the acid-base balance of the blood. The body tissues are bathed by blood that normally has a narrow acceptable range of pH. Although a number of compensatory mechanisms regulate the pH, the lungs help maintain the balance by adjusting the level of carbon dioxide through respiration. That is, hypoventilation (slow, shallow breathing) causes carbon dioxide to build up in the blood, and hyperventilation (rapid, deep breathing) causes carbon dioxide to be blown off.

Changing Chest Size

Respiration is the physical act of breathing; air rushes into the lungs as the chest size increases (inspiration) and is expelled from the lungs as the chest recoils (expiration). The mechanical expansion and contraction of the chest cavity alters the size of the thoracic container in two dimensions: (1) The vertical diameter lengthens or shortens, which is accomplished by downward or upward movement of the diaphragm; and (2) the anteroposterior diameter increases or decreases, which is accomplished by elevation or depression of the ribs (Fig. 16–11).

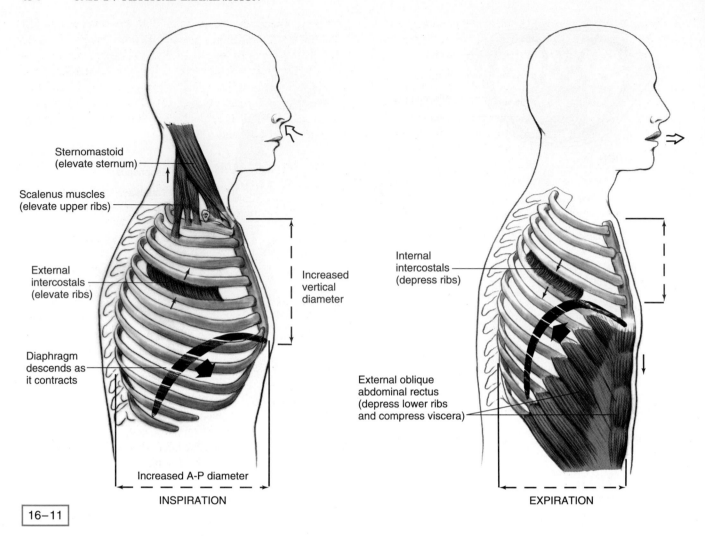

Sternomastoid (elevate sternum)

Scalenus muscles (elevate upper ribs)

External intercostals (elevate ribs)

Diaphragm descends as it contracts

Increased vertical diameter

Increased A-P diameter

INSPIRATION

Internal intercostals (depress ribs)

External oblique abdominal rectus (depress lower ribs and compress viscera)

EXPIRATION

16–11

In inspiration, increasing the size of the thoracic container creates a slightly negative pressure in relation to the atmosphere, so air rushes in to fill the partial vacuum. The major muscle responsible for this increase is the diaphragm. During inspiration, contraction of the bell-shaped diaphragm causes it to descend and flatten. This lengthens the vertical diameter. Intercostal muscles lift the sternum and elevate the ribs, making them more horizontal. This increases the anteroposterior diameter.

Expiration is primarily passive. As the diaphragm relaxes, elastic forces within the lung, chest cage, and abdomen cause it to dome up. All this squeezing creates a relatively positive pressure within the alveoli, and the air flows out.

Forced inspiration, such as that following heavy exercise or occurring pathologically with respiratory distress, commands the use of the accessory neck muscles to heave up the sternum and rib cage. These neck muscles are the sternomastoids, the scaleni, and the trapezii. In forced expiration, the abdominal muscles contract powerfully to push the abdominal viscera forcefully in and up against the diaphragm, making it dome upward, and making it squeeze against the lungs.

Control of Respirations

Normally, our breathing pattern changes without our awareness in response to cellular demands. This involuntary control of respirations is mediated by the respiratory center in the brain stem (pons and medulla). The major feedback loop is humoral regulation, or the change in carbon dioxide and oxygen levels in the blood, and, less importantly, the hydrogen ion level. The *normal stimulus to breathe* for most of us is an increase of carbon dioxide in the blood, or **hypercapnia.** A decrease of oxygen in the blood (**hypoxemia**) also increases respirations but is less effective than hypercapnia.

 DEVELOPMENTAL CONSIDERATIONS

Infants and Children

During the first 5 weeks of fetal life, the primitive lung bud emerges; by 16 weeks, the conducting airways reach the same number as in the adult; at 32 weeks, **surfactant,** the complex lipid substance needed for sustained inflation of the air sacs, is present in adequate amounts; and by birth the lungs have 70 million primitive alveoli ready to start the job of respiration.

Breath is life. When the newborn inhales the first breath, the lusty cry that follows reassures straining parents that their baby is all right (Fig. 16–12). The baby's body systems all develop in utero, but the respiratory system alone does not function until birth. Birth demands its instant performance.

When the cord is cut, blood is cut off from the placenta, and it gushes into the pulmonary circulation. Relatively less resistance exists in the pulmonary arteries than in the aorta, so the foramen ovale in the heart closes just after birth. (See the discussion of fetal circulation in Chapter 17.) The ductus arteriosus (linking the pulmonary artery and the aorta) contracts and closes some hours later, and pulmonary and systemic circulation are functional.

Respiratory development continues throughout childhood, with increases in diameter and length of airways, and increases in size and number of alveoli, reaching the adult range of 300 million by adolescence.

The relatively smaller size and immaturity of children's pulmonary systems, as well as the presence of older caregivers who smoke, result in enormously increased risks to child health. "Each year, among American children, tobacco is associated with an estimated 284 to 360 deaths from lower respiratory tract illnesses and fires initiated by

smoking materials, more than 300 fire-related injuries, 354,000 to 2.2 million episodes of otitis media, 5200 to 165,000 tympanostomies, 14,000 to 21,000 tonsillectomies and/or tympanostomies, 529,000 physician visits for asthma, 1.3 to 2 million visits for coughs, and in children younger than 5 years of age, 260,000 to 436,000 episodes of bronchitis and 115,000 to 190,000 episodes of pneumonia" (DiFranza and Lew, 1996).

The Pregnant Female

The enlarging uterus elevates the diaphragm 4 cm during pregnancy. This decreases the vertical diameter of the thoracic cage, but this decrease is compensated for by an increase in the horizontal diameter. The increase in estrogen level relaxes the chest cage ligaments. This allows an increase in the transverse diameter of the chest cage by 2 cm, and the costal angle widens. The total circumference of the chest cage increases by 6 cm. Although the diaphragm is elevated, it is not fixed. It moves with breathing even more during pregnancy, which results in an increase in tidal volume (Cunningham et al., 1997).

The growing fetus increases the oxygen demand on the mother's body. This is met easily by the increasing tidal volume (deeper breathing). Little change occurs in the respiratory rate. An increased awareness of the need to breathe develops, even early in pregnancy, and some pregnant women may interpret this as dyspnea even though structurally nothing is wrong.

The Aging Adult

The costal cartilages become calcified, which produces a less mobile thorax. Respiratory muscle strength declines after age 50 and continues to decrease into the 70s (Berry, Vitalo, Larson et al., 1996). A more significant change is the decrease in elastic properties within the lungs, making them less distensible and lessening their tendency to collapse and recoil. In all, the aging lung is a more rigid structure that is harder to inflate.

These changes result in an increase in small airway closure, and that yields a *decreased vital capacity* (the maximum amount of air that a person can expel from the lungs after first filling the lungs to maximum) and an *increased residual volume* (the amount of air remaining in the lungs even after the most forceful expiration).

With aging histologic changes, i.e., a gradual loss of intraalveolar septa and a decreased number of alveoli, also occur so less surface area is available for gas exchange. Also the lung bases become less ventilated due to closing off of a number of airways. This increases the older person's risk of dyspnea with exertion beyond his or her usual workload.

The histologic changes also increase the older person's risk of postoperative pulmonary complications. That is, the older person has a greater risk of postoperative atelectasis and infection due to a decreased ability to cough, a

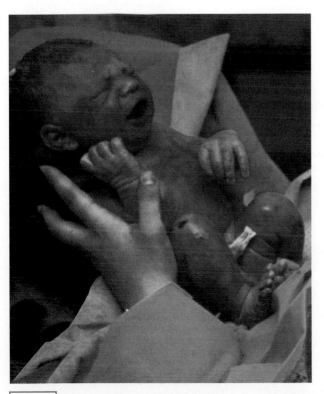

16–12

loss of protective airway reflexes, and increased secretions (Bezanson, 1997; Fraser, 1997).

TRANSCULTURAL CONSIDERATIONS

The incidence of **tuberculosis** (TB) is higher in Asian Americans, and this occurs primarily in those who have recently immigrated to the United States from countries with a high endemic rate of TB (Makinodan and Harada, 1996). Their TB incidence peaked in the first 2 months of entry to the United States. Relative to the risk for the U.S. general population, the risk is increased by 112 times for newly arrived Vietnamese, 60 times for newly arrived Filipinos, 37 times for those from mainland China, and 28 times for those from Korea.

Biocultural differences in the **size of the thoracic cavity** significantly influence pulmonary functioning as determined by vital capacity and forced expiratory volume. In descending order, the largest chest volumes are found in whites, blacks, Asians, and Native Americans. Even when the shorter height of Asians is considered, their chest volume remains significantly lower than whites and blacks.

Some biocultural differences are present even before birth. The **lecithin/sphingomyelin ratio** is a laboratory measurement of the amniotic fluid that indicates fetal pulmonary maturation. The ratio is used to calculate the risk of respiratory distress syndrome in premature infants. This ratio differs between blacks and whites, as does the pulmonary maturity it predicts (Olowe and Akinkugbe, 1978). Blacks have higher ratios than whites from 23 to 42 weeks of gestation. Lung maturity, measured by a lecithin/sphingomyelin ratio of 2.0, is reached 1 week earlier in blacks than in whites, i.e., at 34 versus 35 weeks. The risk of respiratory distress syndrome is 40 to 50 percent for a ratio score between 1.5 and 1.9 for premature white infants but not for premature blacks. Premature black infants have a much lower risk of respiratory distress syndrome at the same low ratio scores. When the lecithin/sphingomyelin ratio is determined before induction of labor or elective cesarean section, the racial difference should be considered in making the decision (Overfield, 1995).

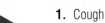

SUBJECTIVE DATA

1. Cough
2. Shortness of breath
3. Chest pain with breathing
4. Past history of respiratory infections
5. Smoking history
6. Environmental exposure
7. Self-care behaviors

Examiner Asks	Rationale

Cough. Do you have a **cough?** When did it start? Gradual or sudden?
• How long have you had it?
• How often do you cough? At any special time of day or just on arising? Cough wake you up at night?
	Some conditions have a characteristic timing of a cough:
	    Continuous throughout day—associated with acute illness, e.g., respiratory infection.
	    Afternoon/evening—may reflect exposure to irritants at work
	    Night—postnasal drip, sinusitis
	    Early morning—chronic bronchial inflammation of smokers

• Do you cough up any phlegm or sputum? How much? What color is it?	Chronic bronchitis is characterized by a history of productive cough for 3 months of the year for 2 years in a row.
• Cough up any blood? Does this look like streaks or frank blood? Does the sputum have a foul odor?	Hemoptysis.

Examiner Asks	Rationale

Although sputum is not diagnostic alone, some conditions have characteristic sputum production: white or clear mucoid—colds, bronchitis, viral infections; yellow or green—bacterial infections; rust colored—tuberculosis, pneumococcal pneumonia; pink, frothy—pulmonary edema, some sympathomimetic medications have a side effect of pink-tinged mucus.

- How would you describe your cough: hacking, dry, barking, hoarse, congested, bubbling?

Although not mutually exclusive, some conditions have a characteristic cough: mycoplasma pneumonia—hacking; early congestive heart failure—dry; croup—barking; colds, bronchitis, pneumonia—congested.

- Cough seem to come with anything: activity, position (lying), fever, congestion, talking, anxiety?
- Activity make it better or worse?
- What treatment have you tried? Prescription or over-the-counter medications, vaporizer, rest, position change?

Assess effectiveness of coping strategies.

- Does the cough bring on anything: chest pain, ear pain? Is it tiring? Are you concerned about it?

Note severity.

2 **Shortness of breath.** Ever had any **shortness of breath** or hard breathing spells? What brings it on? How severe is it? How long does it last?

Determine exactly how much activity precipitates the shortness of breath—state specific number of blocks walked, number of stairs.

- Is it affected by position, like lying down?

Orthopnea is difficulty breathing when supine. State number of pillows the person sleeps with to achieve comfort, e.g., "two-pillow orthopnea."

- Occur at any specific time of day or night?

Paroxysmal nocturnal dyspnea is awakening from sleep with shortness of breath and needing to be upright to achieve comfort.

- Shortness of breath episodes associated with night sweats?
- Or cough, chest pain, or bluish color around lips or nails? Wheezing sound?

Diaphoresis.

Cyanosis.

- Episodes seem to be related to food, pollen, dust, animals, season, or emotion?

Asthma attacks are associated with a specific allergen.

- What do you do in a hard-breathing attack? Take a special position, or use pursed-lip breathing? Use any oxygen, inhalers, or medications?

Assess effect of coping strategies and the need for more teaching.

- How does the shortness of breath affect your work or home activities? Getting better or worse or staying about the same?

Assess effect on activities of daily living.

3 **Chest pain with breathing.** Any **chest pain with breathing?** Please point to the exact location.
- When did it start? Constant or does it come and go?
- Describe the pain: burning, stabbing?
- Brought on by respiratory infection, coughing, or trauma? Is it associated with fever, deep breathing, unequal chest inflation?
- What have you done to treat it? Medication or heat application?

Examiner Asks	Rationale
4 **Past history of respiratory infections.** Any **past history** of breathing trouble or lung diseases like bronchitis, emphysema, asthma, pneumonia?	Consider sequelae following these conditions.
• Any unusually frequent or unusually severe colds?	Since most people have had some colds, it is more meaningful to ask about excess number or severity.
• Any family history of allergies, tuberculosis, or asthma?	Assess possible risk factors.
5 **Smoking history.** Do you **smoke** cigarettes or cigars? At what age did you start? How many packs per day do you smoke now? For how long?	State number of packs per day and the number of years.
• Have you ever tried to quit? What helped? Why do you think it did not work? What activities do you associate with smoking? • Live with someone who smokes?	Most people already know they should quit smoking. Instead of admonishing, assess smoking behavior and ways to modify daily smoking activities.
6 **Environmental exposure.** Are there any **environmental conditions** that may affect your breathing? Where do you work? At a factory, chemical plant, coal mine, farming, outdoors in a heavy traffic area?	Pollution exposure. Farmers may be at risk for grain inhalation, pesticide inhalation. People in the rural midwest have a risk of histoplasmosis exposure; those in the southwest and Mexico have a risk of coccidioidomycosis. Coal miners have a risk of pneumoconiosis. Stone cutters, miners, potters—silicosis. Other irritants: asbestos, beryllium.
• Do anything to protect your lungs, such as wear a mask or have the ventilatory system checked at work? Do anything to monitor your exposure? Have periodic examinations, pulmonary function tests, x-ray examination?	Assess **self-care** measures.
• Do you know what specific symptoms to note that may signal breathing problems?	General symptoms: cough, shortness of breath. Exposure to some gases produces specific symptoms: carbon monoxide—dizziness, headache, fatigue; sulfur dioxide—cough, congestion.
7 **Self-care behaviors.** Last tuberculosis skin test, chest x-ray study, pneumonia or influenza immunization?	Self-care measures.

ADDITIONAL HISTORY FOR INFANTS AND CHILDREN

1 Has the child had any frequent or very severe colds?	Limit of four to six uncomplicated upper respiratory infections per year is expected in early childhood.
2 Is there any history of allergy in the family? • (For child under 2 years of age): At what age were new foods introduced? Was the child breast fed or bottle fed?	Consider new foods as possible allergens. Consider formula as allergen.
3 Does the child have a cough? Seem congested? Have noisy breathing or wheezing? (Further questions similar to those listed in the section on adults.)	Screen for onset and follow course of childhood chronic respiratory problems: asthma, bronchitis.

Examiner Asks	Rationale

4 What measures have you taken to child-proof your home? Yard? Is there any possibility of the child inhaling or swallowing toxic substances?
  ● Has anyone taught you emergency care measures in case of accidental choking or a hard-breathing spell?

Self-care behaviors. Young child is at risk for accidental aspiration, poisoning, and injury.
Assess knowledge level of parent and caregivers.

5 Any smokers in the home or in the car with child?

Second-hand smoke enormously increases the risk of upper and lower respiratory infections in children (DiFranza and Lew, 1996).

ADDITIONAL HISTORY FOR THE AGING ADULT

1 Have you noticed any shortness of breath or fatigue with your daily activities?

Some older adults have a less efficient respiratory system (decreased vital capacity, less surface area for gas exchange), so they experience less tolerance for activity.

2 Tell me about your usual amount of physical activity.

Assess self-care behaviors.
  May have reduced capacity to perform exercise because of pulmonary function deficits of aging.
  Sedentary or bedridden people are at risk for respiratory dysfunction.

3 (For those with a history of chronic obstructive pulmonary disease, lung cancer, or tuberculosis): How are you getting along each day? Any weight change in the last 3 months? How much?
  ● How about energy level? Do you tire more easily? How does your illness affect you at home? At work?

Assess coping strategies.

Activities may decrease because of increasing shortness of breath or because of pain.

4 Do you have any chest pain with breathing?

  ● Any chest pain after a bout of coughing? After a fall?

Some older adults feel pleuritic pain less intensely than younger adults.
Precisely localized sharp pain (when person points to it with one finger)—consider fractured rib or muscle injury.

OBJECTIVE DATA

Preparation

Ask the person to sit upright and the male to disrobe to the waist. For the female, leave the gown on and open at the back. When examining the anterior chest, lift up the gown and drape it on her shoulders rather than removing it completely. This promotes comfort by giving her the feeling of

▶ Equipment Needed

Stethoscope
Small ruler, marked in centimeters
Marking pen
Alcohol swab

being somewhat clothed. These provisions will ensure further comfort: a warm room, a warm diaphragm endpiece, and a private examination time with no interruptions.

For smooth choreography in a complete examination, begin the respiratory examination just after palpating the thyroid gland when you are standing behind the person. Perform the inspection, palpation, percussion, and auscultation on the posterior and lateral thorax. Then move to face the person and repeat the four maneuvers on the anterior chest. This avoids repetitiously moving front-to-back around the person.

Finally, clean your stethoscope endpiece with an alcohol swab. Since your stethoscope touches many people, it could be a possible vector for both aerobic and anaerobic bacteria (Assadian et al., 1998). Cleaning with an alcohol swab is very effective.

▶ Normal Range of Findings	Abnormal Findings

THE POSTERIOR CHEST

Inspect the posterior chest
Thoracic Cage

Note the **shape and configuration** of the chest wall. The spinous processes should appear in a straight line. The thorax is symmetric, in an elliptical shape, with downward sloping ribs, about 45 degrees relative to the spine. The scapulae are placed symmetrically in each hemithorax.

Skeletal deformities may limit thoracic cage excursion: scoliosis, kyphosis (see Table 16–4 on p. 484).

The anteroposterior diameter should be less than the transverse diameter. The ratio of anteroposterior:transverse diameter is from 1:2 to 5:7.

Anteroposterior = transverse diameter, or "barrel chest." Ribs are horizontal, chest appears as if held in continuous inspiration. This occurs in chronic emphysema due to hyperinflation of the lungs (see Table 16–4).

The neck muscles and trapezius muscles should be developed normally for age and occupation.

Neck muscles are hypertrophied in chronic obstructive pulmonary disease from aiding in forced respirations.

Note the **position** the person takes to breathe. This includes a relaxed posture and the ability to support one's own weight with arms comfortably at the sides or in the lap.

People with chronic obstructive pulmonary disease often sit in a tripod position, leaning forward with arms braced against their knees, chair, or bed. This gives them leverage so that their rectus abdominis, intercostal, and accessory neck muscles all can aid in expiration.

Assess the **skin color and condition.** Color should be consistent with person's genetic background, with allowance for sun-exposed areas on the chest and the back. No cyanosis or pallor should be present. Note any lesions. Inquire as to any change in a nevus on the back, for example, where the person may have difficulty monitoring (see Chapter 10, Skin, Hair, and Nails).

Normal Range of Findings	Abnormal Findings

Palpate the posterior chest
Symmetric Expansion

Confirm **symmetric chest expansion** by placing your warmed hands on the posterolateral chest wall with thumbs at the level of T9 or T10. Slide your hands medially to pinch up a small fold of skin between your thumbs (Fig. 16–13).

Ask the person to take a deep breath. Your hands serve as mechanical amplifiers; as the person inhales deeply, your thumbs should move apart symmetrically. Note any lag in expansion.

Unequal chest expansion occurs with marked atelectasis or pneumonia; with thoracic trauma, such as fractured ribs; or with pneumothorax.

Pain accompanies deep breathing when the pleurae are inflamed.

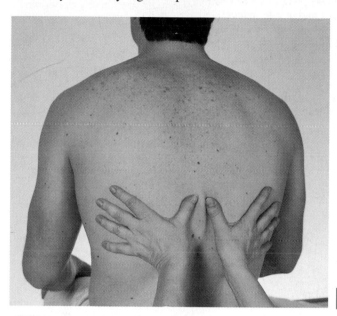

16–13

Tactile Fremitus

Assess **tactile (or vocal) fremitus.** Fremitus is a palpable vibration. Sounds generated from the larynx are transmitted through patent bronchi and through the lung parenchyma to the chest wall where you feel them as vibrations.

Use either the palmar base (the ball) of the fingers or the ulnar edge of one hand, and touch the person's chest while he or she repeats the words "ninety-nine" or "blue moon." These are resonant phrases that generate strong vibrations. Start over the lung apices and palpate from one side to another (Fig. 16–14).

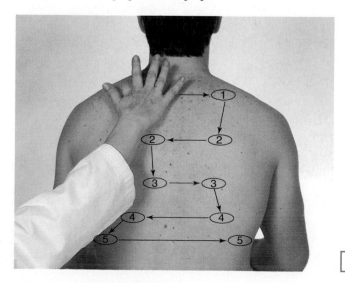

16–14

Fremitus varies among persons but symmetry is most important; the vibrations should feel the same in the corresponding area on each side. However, just between the scapulae, fremitus may feel stronger on the right side than on the left side because the right side is closer to the bronchial bifurcation. Avoid palpating over the scapulae because bone damps out sound transmission.

The following factors affect the normal intensity of tactile fremitus:

- Relative location of bronchi to the chest wall
  Normally, fremitus is most prominent between the scapulae and around the sternum, sites where the major bronchi are closest to the chest wall. Fremitus normally decreases as you progress down because more and more tissue impedes sound transmission.
- Thickness of the chest wall
  Fremitus feels greater over a thin chest wall than over an obese or heavily muscular one where thick tissue damps the vibration.
- Pitch and intensity
  A loud, low-pitched voice generates more fremitus than a soft, high-pitched one.

Note any areas of abnormal fremitus. Sound is conducted better through a uniformly dense structure than through a porous one, which changes in shape and solidity (as does the lung tissue during normal respiration). Thus, conditions that increase the density of lung tissue make a better conducting medium for sound vibrations and increase tactile fremitus.

Decreased fremitus occurs when anything obstructs transmission of vibrations, e.g., obstructed bronchus, pleural effusion or thickening, pneumothorax, or emphysema. Any barrier that comes between the sound and your palpating hand will decrease fremitus.

Increased fremitus occurs with compression or consolidation of lung tissue, e.g., lobar pneumonia. This is present only when the bronchus is patent and when the consolidation extends to the lung surface. Note that only gross changes increase fremitus. Small areas of early pneumonia do not significantly affect fremitus.

Rhonchal fremitus is palpable with thick bronchial secretions.

Pleural friction fremitus is palpable with inflammation of the pleura (see Table 16–6).

Crepitus is a coarse crackling sensation palpable over the skin surface. It occurs in subcutaneous emphysema when air escapes from the lung and enters the subcutaneous tissue, as following open thoracic injury or surgery.

Using the fingers, gently **palpate the entire chest wall.** This enables you to note any areas of tenderness, to note skin temperature and moisture, to detect any superficial lumps or masses, and to explore any skin lesions noted on inspection.

Percuss the posterior chest
Lung Fields

Determine the **predominant note over the lung fields.** Start at the apices and percuss the band of normally resonant tissue across the tops of both shoulders (Fig. 16–15). Then, percussing in the interspaces, make a side-to-side comparison all the way down the lung region. Percuss at 5-cm intervals. Avoid the damping effect of the scapulae and ribs.

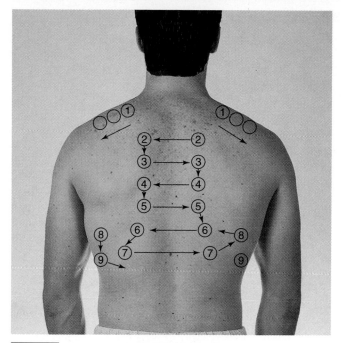

16–15   **Sequence for percussion**

Resonance predominates in healthy lung tissue in the adult (Fig. 16–16). However, resonance is a relative term and has no constant standard. The resonant note may be modified somewhat in the athlete with a heavily muscular chest wall and in the heavily obese adult in whom subcutaneous fat produces scattered dullness.

Hyperresonance is found when too much air is present, as in emphysema or pneumothorax.

A **dull** note signals abnormal density in the lungs, as with pneumonia, pleural effusion, atelectasis, or tumor.

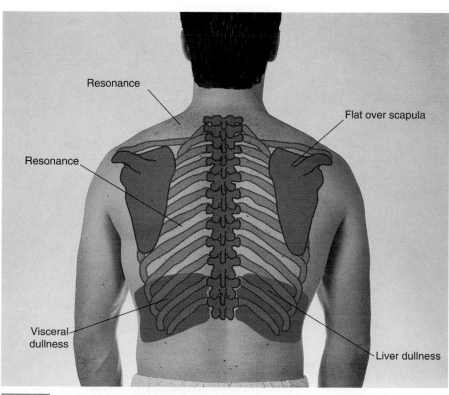

16–16   **Expected percussion notes**

The depth of penetration of percussion has limits. Percussion sets into motion only the outer 5 to 7 cm of tissue. It will not penetrate to reveal any change in density deeper than that. Also, an abnormal finding must be 2 to 3 cm wide to yield an abnormal percussion note. Lesions smaller than that are not detectable by percussion.

Diaphragmatic Excursion

Determine **diaphragmatic excursion** (Fig. 16–17). Percuss to map out the lower lung border, both in expiration and in inspiration. First, ask the person to "exhale and hold it" briefly while you percuss down the scapular line until the sound changes from resonant to dull on each side. This estimates the level of the diaphragm separating the lungs from the abdominal viscera. It may be somewhat higher on the right side (about 1 to 2 cm) due to the presence of the liver. Mark the spot.

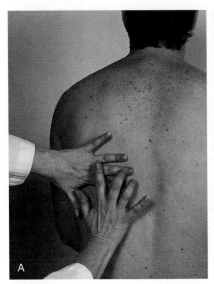 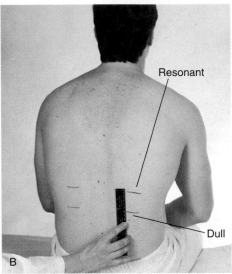

16–17

Now ask the person to "take a deep breath and hold it." Continue percussing down from your first mark and mark the level where the sound changes to dull on this deep inspiration. Measure the difference. This diaphragmatic excursion should be equal bilaterally and measure about 3 to 5 cm in adults, although it may be up to 7 to 8 cm in well-conditioned people.

Often, the beginning examiner becomes so involved in the subtle differences of percussion notes that she or he extends the patient's limits of breathholding. Always hold your own breath when you ask your patient to. When you run out of air, the other person surely has too, especially if that person has a respiratory problem.

Auscultate the posterior chest

The passage of air through the tracheobronchial tree creates a characteristic set of noises that are audible through the chest wall. These noises also may be modified by obstruction within the respiratory passageways or by changes in the lung parenchyma, the pleura, or the chest wall.

An abnormally high level of dullness, as well as absence of excursion, occurs with pleural effusion or atelectasis of the lower lobes.

► Normal Range of Findings	Abnormal Findings

Breath Sounds

Evaluate the presence and quality of **normal breath sounds.** The person is sitting, leaning forward slightly, with arms resting comfortably across the lap. Instruct the person to breathe through the mouth, a little bit deeper than usual, but to stop if he or she begins to feel dizzy. Be careful to monitor the breathing throughout the examination, and offer times for the person to rest and breathe normally. The person is usually willing to comply with your instructions in an effort to please you and to be a "good patient." Watch that he or she does not hyperventilate to the point of fainting.

Use the flat diaphragm endpiece of the stethoscope and hold it firmly on the person's chest wall. Listen to at least one full respiration in each location. Side-to-side comparison is most important.

Do not confuse background noise with lung sounds. Become familiar with these extraneous noises that may be confused with lung pathology if not recognized:

1. Examiner's breathing on stethoscope tubing
2. Stethoscope tubing bumping together
3. Patient shivering
4. Patient's hairy chest; movement of hairs under stethoscope sounds like crackles (rales) (see p. 487)—minimize this by pressing harder or by wetting the hair with a damp cloth
5. Rustling of paper gown or paper drapes

While standing behind the person, listen to the following lung areas—posterior from the apices at C7 to the bases (around T10), and laterally from the axilla down to the seventh or eighth rib. Use the sequence illustrated in Figure 16–18.

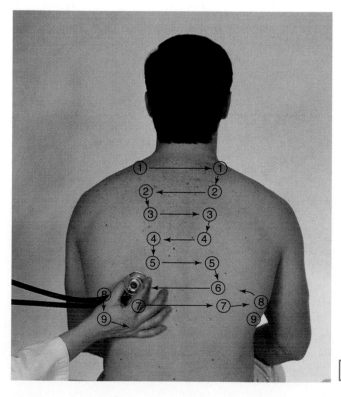

16–18

▶ Normal Range of Findings   Abnormal Findings

Continue to visualize approximate locations of the lobes of each lung so that you correlate your findings to anatomic areas. As you listen, think (1) What am I hearing over this spot, and (2) What should I EXPECT to be hearing? You should expect to hear three types of normal breath sounds in the adult and older child: bronchial (sometimes called tracheal or tubular), bronchovesicular, and vesicular. Study the description of the characteristics of these normal breath sounds in Table 16–1.

Table 16–1 · Characteristics of Normal Breath Sounds

	Pitch	Amplitude	Duration	Quality	Normal Location
Bronchial (Tracheal) 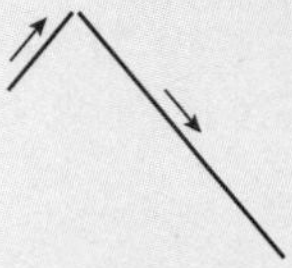	High	Loud	Inspiration < expiration	Harsh, hollow tubular	Trachea and larynx
Bronchovesicular 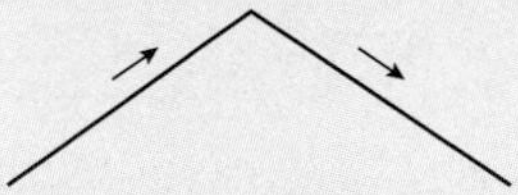	Moderate	Moderate	Inspiration = expiration	Mixed	Over major bronchi where fewer alveoli are located: posterior, between scapulae especially on right; anterior, around upper sternum in first and second intercostal spaces
Vesicular 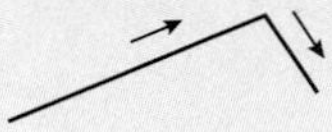	Low	Soft	Inspiration > expiration	Rustling, like the sound of the wind in the trees	Over peripheral lung fields where air flows through smaller bronchioles and alveoli

Note the normal location of the three types of breath sounds on the chest wall of the adult and older child (Figs. 16–19 and 16–20).

Decreased or **absent breath sounds** occur

1. When the bronchial tree is obstructed at some point by secretions, mucous plug, or a foreign body
2. In emphysema due to loss of elasticity in the lung fibers and decreased force of inspired air; also the lungs are already hyperinflated so the inhaled air does not make as much noise
3. When anything obstructs transmission of sound between the lung and your stethoscope, such as pleurisy or pleural thickening, or air (pneumothorax) or fluid (pleural effusion) in the pleural space

▶ Normal Range of Findings

Abnormal Findings

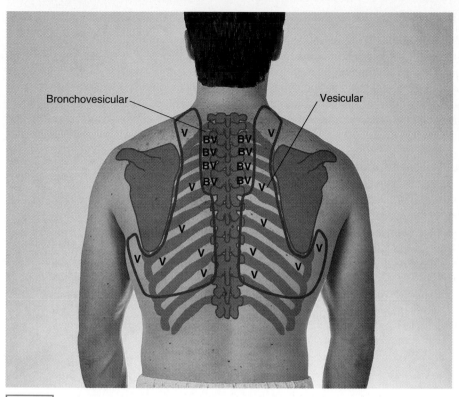

Bronchovesicular

Vesicular

16–19

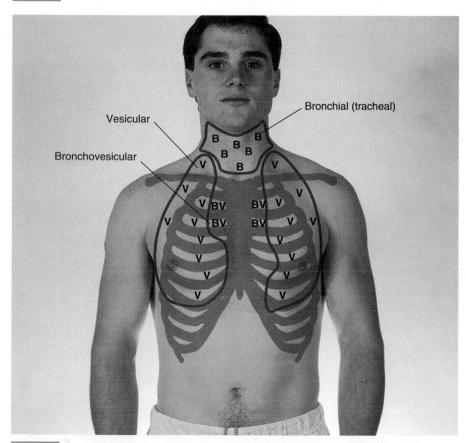

Bronchial (tracheal)

Vesicular

Bronchovesicular

16–20

A silent chest means no air is moving in or out, which is an ominous sign.

Increased breath sounds mean that sounds are louder than they should be, e.g., bronchial sounds are abnormal when they are heard over an abnormal location, the peripheral lung fields. They have a high-pitched tubular quality, with a prolonged expiratory phase and a distinct pause between inspiration and expiration. They sound very close to your stethoscope, as if they were right *in* the tubing close to your ear. They occur when consolidation (e.g., pneumonia) or compression (e.g., fluid in the intrapleural space) yields a dense lung area that enhances the transmission of sound from the bronchi. When the inspired air reaches the alveoli, it hits solid lung tissue that conducts sound more efficiently to the surface.

▶ **Normal Range of Findings**   **Abnormal Findings**

Adventitious Sounds

Note the presence of any **adventitious sounds.** These are added sounds that are *not* normally heard in the lungs. If present, they are heard as being superimposed on the breath sounds. They are caused by moving air colliding with secretions in the tracheobronchial passageways, or by the popping open of previously deflated airways. Sources differ as to the classification and nomenclature of these sounds (see Table 16–7), but **crackles** (or rales) and **wheeze** (or rhonchi) are terms commonly used by most examiners.

One type of adventitious sound, **atelectatic crackles,** is not pathologic. They are short, popping, crackling sounds that sound like fine crackles but do not last beyond a few breaths. When sections of alveoli are not fully aerated (as in people who are asleep, or in the elderly), they deflate slightly and accumulate secretions. Crackles are heard when these sections are reexpanded by a few deep breaths. Atelectatic crackles are heard only in the periphery, usually in dependent portions of the lungs, and disappear after the first few breaths or after a cough.

In the past, persons were asked to "take a deep breath and blow it out hard" to screen for the presence of wheezing. However, this maneuver is futile because it is known that wheezing may occur on maximal forced exhalation in normal people (King et al., 1989).

Voice Sounds

Determine the quality of **voice sounds** or **vocal resonance.** The spoken voice can be auscultated over the chest wall just as it can be felt in tactile fremitus described earlier. Ask the person to repeat a phrase while you listen over the chest wall. Normal voice transmission is soft, muffled, and indistinct; you can hear sound through the stethoscope but cannot distinguish exactly what is being said. Pathology that increases lung density enhances transmission of voice sounds.

Eliciting the voice sounds is usually not done in the routine examination. Rather, these are supplemental maneuvers that are performed if you suspect lung pathology based on earlier data. When they are performed, you are testing for possible presence of **bronchophony, egophony,** and **whispered pectoriloquy** (Table 16–2).

Study Table 16–7 on p. 487 for a complete description of these abnormal adventitious breath sounds.

During normal tidal flow, wheezing indicates asthma.

Consolidation or compression of lung tissue will enhance the voice sounds.

▶ | Normal Range of Findings | Abnormal Findings |

Table 16–2 • Voice Sounds

Technique	Normal Finding	Abnormal Finding
Bronchophony Ask the person to repeat "ninety-nine" while you listen with the stethoscope over the chest wall; listen especially if you suspect pathology	Normal voice transmission is soft, muffled, and indistinct; you can hear sound through the stethoscope but cannot distinguish exactly what is being said	Pathology that increases lung density will enhance transmission of voice sounds. You auscultate a clear "ninety-nine" The words are more distinct than normal and sound close to your ear

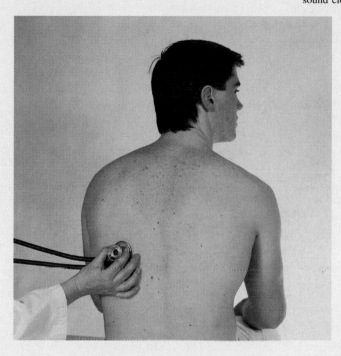

Egophony (Greek: the voice of a goat) Auscultate the chest while the person phonates a long "ee-ee-ee-ee" sound	Normally, you should hear "eeeeee" through your stethoscope	Over areas of consolidation or compression, the spoken "eeee" sound changes to a bleating long "aaaaa" sound If this is present, record, "E → A changes"
Whispered pectoriloquy Ask the person to whisper a phrase like "one-two-three" as you auscultate	The normal response is faint, muffled, and almost inaudible	With only small amounts of consolidation, the whispered voice is transmitted very clearly and distinctly, although still somewhat faint; it sounds as if the person is whispering right into your stethoscope, "one-two-three"

THE ANTERIOR CHEST

Inspect the anterior chest

Note the **shape and configuration** of the chest wall. The ribs are sloping downward with symmetric interspaces. The costal angle is within 90 degrees. Development of abdominal muscles is as expected for the person's age, weight, and athletic condition.

Barrel chest has horizontal ribs and costal angle >90 degrees.

▶ N o r m a l   R a n g e   o f   F i n d i n g s   A b n o r m a l   F i n d i n g s

Note the person's **facial expression.** The facial expression should be relaxed and benign, indicating an unconscious effort of breathing.

Assess the **level of consciousness.** The level of consciousness should be alert and cooperative.

Note skin **color and condition.** The lips and nail beds are free of cyanosis or unusual pallor. The nails are of normal configuration. Explore any skin lesions.

Assess the quality of **respirations.** Normal relaxed breathing is automatic and effortless, regular and even, and produces no noise. The chest expands symmetrically with each inspiration. Note any localized lag on inspiration.

No retraction or bulging of the interspaces should occur on inspiration.

Normally, accessory muscles are not used to augment respiratory effort. However, with very heavy exercise, the accessory neck muscles (scalene, sternomastoid, trapezius) are used momentarily to enhance inspiration.

Hypertrophy of abdominal muscles occurs in chronic emphysema.

Tense, strained, tired facies accompany chronic obstructive pulmonary disease (COPD).

The person with COPD may purse the lips in a whistling position. By exhaling slowly and against a narrow opening, the pressure in the bronchial tree remains positive, and fewer airways collapse.

Cerebral hypoxia may be reflected by excessive drowsiness or by anxiety, restlessness, and irritability.

Clubbing of distal phalanx occurs with chronic respiratory disease.

Cutaneous angiomas (spider nevi) associated with liver disease or portal hypertension may be evident on the chest.

Noisy breathing occurs with severe asthma or chronic bronchitis.

Unequal chest expansion occurs when part of the lung is obstructed or collapsed, as with pneumonia, or when guarding to avoid postoperative incisional pain or the pleurisy pain.

Retraction suggests obstruction of respiratory tract or increased inspiratory effort is needed as with atelectasis. Bulging indicates trapped air as in the forced expiration associated with emphysema or asthma.

Accessory muscles must be used in acute airway obstruction and massive atelectasis.

Rectus abdominis and internal intercostal muscles are used to force expiration in COPD.

▶ Normal Range of Findings	Abnormal Findings

The respiratory rate is within normal limits for the person's age (see Table 9–3) and the pattern of breathing is regular. Occasional sighs normally punctuate breathing.

Tachypnea and hyperventilation, bradypnea and hypoventilation, periodic breathing (see Table 16–5).

Palpate the anterior chest

Palpate **symmetric chest expansion.** Place your hands on the anterolateral wall with the thumbs along the costal margins and pointing toward the xiphoid process (Fig. 16–21).

An abnormally wide costal angle with little inspiratory variation occurs with emphysema.

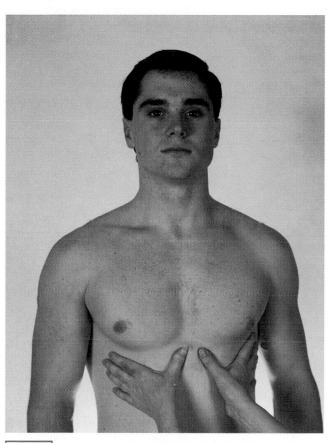

16–21

Ask the person to take a deep breath. Watch your thumbs move apart symmetrically, and note smooth chest expansion with your fingers. Any limitation in thoracic expansion is easier to detect on the anterior chest because greater range of motion exists with breathing here.

A lag in expansion occurs with atelectasis, pneumonia, and postoperative guarding.

A palpable grating sensation with breathing indicates pleural friction fremitus (see Table 16–6).

Assess **tactile (vocal) fremitus.** Begin palpating over the lung apices in the supraclavicular areas (Fig. 16–22). Compare vibrations from one side to the other as the person repeats "ninety-nine." Avoid palpating over female breast tissue because breast tissue normally damps the sound.

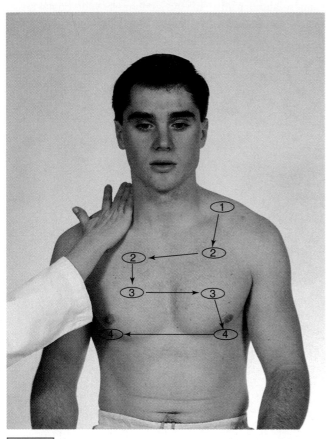

16–22

Palpate the anterior chest wall to note any tenderness (normally none is present) and to detect any superficial lumps or masses (again, normally none are present). Note skin mobility and turgor, and note skin temperature and moisture.

Percuss the anterior chest

Begin percussing the apices in the supraclavicular areas. Then, percussing the interspaces and comparing one side to the other, move down the anterior chest.

Interspaces are easier to palpate on the anterior chest than on the back. Do not percuss directly over female breast tissue because this would produce a dull note. Shift the breast tissue over slightly using the edge of your stationary hand. In females with large breasts, percussion may yield little useful data. With all people, use the sequence illustrated in Figure 16–23.

Normal Range of Findings	Abnormal Findings

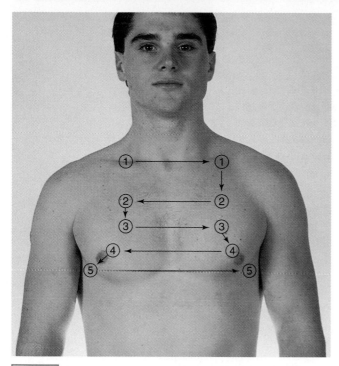

16-23 | **Sequence for percussion and auscultation**

Note the borders of cardiac dullness normally found on the anterior chest and do not confuse these with suspected lung pathology (Fig. 16-24). In the right hemithorax, the upper border of liver dullness is located in the fifth intercostal space in the right midclavicular line. On the left, tympany is evident over the gastric space.

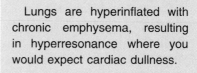

Lungs are hyperinflated with chronic emphysema, resulting in hyperresonance where you would expect cardiac dullness.

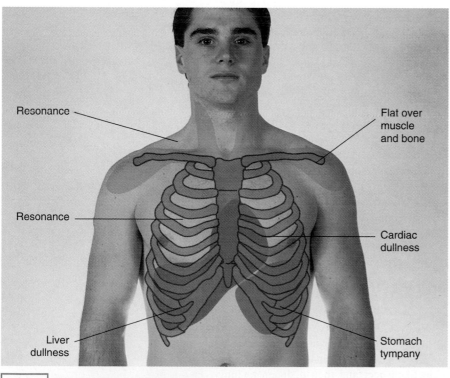

Resonance

Resonance

Liver dullness

Flat over muscle and bone

Cardiac dullness

Stomach tympany

16-24 | **Expected percussion notes**

Auscultate the anterior chest

Breath Sounds

Auscultate the lung fields over the anterior chest from the apices in the supraclavicular areas down to the sixth rib. Progress from side to side as you move downward, and listen to one full respiration in each location. Use the sequence indicated for percussion. Do not place your stethoscope directly over the female breast. Displace the breast and listen directly over the chest wall.

Evaluate normal breath sounds, noting any abnormal breath sounds and any adventitious sounds. If the situation warrants, assess the voice sounds on the anterior chest.

Study Table 16–8 for a complete description of abnormal respiratory conditions.

Measurement of Pulmonary Function Status

The **forced expiratory time** is the number of seconds it takes for the person to exhale from total lung capacity to residual volume. It is a screening measure of airflow obstruction. Although the test usually is not performed in the respiratory assessment, it is useful when you wish to screen for pulmonary function.

Ask the person to inhale the deepest breath possible and then to blow it all out hard, as quickly as possible, with the mouth open. Listen with your stethoscope over the sternum. The normal time for full expiration is 4 seconds or less.

A forced expiration of 6 seconds or more occurs with obstructive lung disease. Refer this person for more precise pulmonary function studies.

The **pulse oximeter** is a noninvasive method to assess arterial oxygen saturation (SpO_2). A sensor attached to the person's finger or ear has a diode that emits light and a detector that measures the relative amount of light absorbed by oxyhemoglobin (HbO_2) and unoxygenated (reduced) hemoglobin (Hb). The pulse oximeter compares the ratio of light emitted to light absorbed and converts this ratio into the percentage of oxygen saturation. Since it only measures light absorption of pulsatile flow, the result is arterial oxygen saturation. A healthy person with no lung disease and no anemia normally has an SpO_2 of 97 to 98 percent. However, every SpO_2 result must be evaluated in the context of the person's hemoglobin level, acid-base balance, and ventilatory status.

The **12-minute distance (12MD) walk** is a simple, inexpensive, clinical measure of functional status in people with COPD (Larson et al., 1996). The 12MD is used as an outcome measure for people in pulmonary rehabilitation because it mirrors conditions that are used in everyday life. Locate a flat-surfaced corridor that has little foot traffic, is wide enough to permit comfortable turns, and has a controlled environment. Ensure that the person is wearing comfortable shoes, and equip him or her with a pulse oximeter to monitor oxygen saturation. Ask the person to set his or her own pace to cover as much ground as possible in 12 minutes, and assure the person it is all right to slow down or to stop to rest at any time. Use a stopwatch to time the walk.

Ask the person to stop the walk if you notice an SpO_2 below 85% to 88% or if extreme breathlessness occurs.

 DEVELOPMENTAL CONSIDERATIONS

Infants and Children

To prepare, let the parent hold an infant supported against the chest or shoulder. Do not let the usual sequence of the physical examination restrain you; seize the opportunity with a sleeping infant to inspect and then to listen to lung

Normal Range of Findings	Abnormal Findings

sounds next. This way you can concentrate on the breath sounds before the baby wakes up and possibly cries. Infant crying does not have to be a problem for you though, because it actually enhances palpation of tactile fremitus and auscultation of breath sounds.

A child may sit upright on the parent's lap. Offer the stethoscope and let the child handle it. This reduces any fear of the equipment. Promote the child's participation; school-age children usually are delighted to hear their own breath sounds when you place the stethoscope properly. While listening to breath sounds, ask the young child to take a deep breath and "blow out" your penlight while you hold the stethoscope with your other hand. Time your letting go of the penlight button so the light goes off after the child blows. Or, ask the child to "pant like a dog" while you auscultate.

Inspection. The infant has a rounded thorax with an equal anteroposterior-to-transverse chest diameter (Fig. 16–25). By age 6, the thorax reaches the adult ratio of 1:2 (anteroposterior-to-transverse diameter). The newborn's chest circumference is 30 to 36 cm and is 2 cm smaller than the head circumference until 2 years of age. The chest wall is thin with little musculature. The ribs and the xiphoid are prominent; you can see as well as feel the sharp tip of the xiphoid process. The thoracic cage is soft and flexible.

Note a barrel shape persisting after age 6, which may develop with chronic asthma or cystic fibrosis.

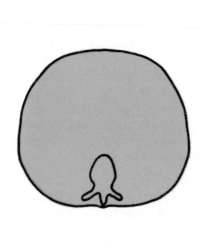
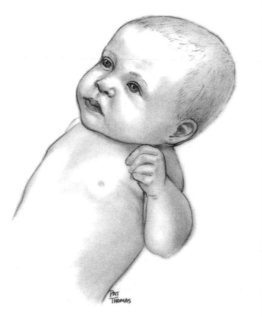

16–25

Round thorax in an infant

In newborn males and females the breasts may look enlarged by the 2nd or 3rd day due to maternal estrogen. Occasionally, a white fluid, called by the slang expression "witch's milk," can be expressed. This resolves within a week.

In some children, "Harrison's groove" occurs normally. This is a horizontal groove in the rib cage at the level of the diaphragm, extending from the sternum to the midaxillary line.

Harrison's groove also occurs with rickets.

Table 16–3 • Apgar Scoring System

	2	1	0	
Heart rate	Over 100	Slow (below 100)	Absent	_____
Respiratory effort	Good, sustained cry; regular respirations	Slow, irregular, shallow	Absent	_____
Muscle tone	Active motion, spontaneous flexion	Some flexion of extremities; some resistance to extension	Limp, flaccid	_____
Reflex irritability (response to catheter nares)	Sneeze, cough, cry	Grimace, frown	No response	_____
Color	Completely pink	Body pink, extremities pale	Cyanotic, pale	_____
			Total score	_____

The newborn's first respiratory assessment is part of the **Apgar scoring system** to measure the successful transition to extrauterine life (Table 16–3). The five standard parameters are scored at 1 minute and at 5 minutes after birth. A 1-minute Apgar with a total score of 7 to 10 indicates a newborn in good condition, needing only suctioning of the nose and mouth and otherwise routine care.

The infant breathes through the nose rather than the mouth, and is an obligate nose-breather until 3 months. Slight flaring of the lower costal margins may occur with respirations, but normally no flaring of the nostrils and no sternal retractions or intercostal retractions occur. The diaphragm is the newborn's major respiratory muscle. Intercostal muscles are not well developed. Thus, you observe the abdomen bulge with each inspiration but see little thoracic expansion.

Count the respiratory rate for 1 full minute. Normal rates for the newborn are 30 to 40 breaths per minute but may spike up to 60 per minute. Obtain the most accurate respiratory rate by counting when the infant is asleep, because infants reach rapid rates with very little excitation when awake. The respiratory pattern may be irregular when extremes in room temperature occur or with feeding or sleeping. Brief periods of apnea less than 10 or 15 seconds are common. This periodic breathing is more common in premature infants.

Palpation. Palpate symmetric chest expansion by encircling the infant's thorax with both hands. Further palpation should yield no lumps, masses, or crepitus, although you may feel the costochondral junctions in some normal infants.

In the immediate newborn period, depressed respirations are due to maternal drugs, interruption of the uterine blood supply, or obstruction of the tracheo-bronchial tree with mucus or fluid.

A 1-minute Apgar with a total score of 3 to 6 indicates a moderately depressed newborn needing more resuscitation and subsequent close observation. A score of 0 to 2 indicates a severely depressed newborn needing full resuscitation, ventilatory assistance, and subsequent intensive care.

Marked retractions of sternum and intercostal muscles indicate increased inspiratory effort, as in atelectasis, pneumonia, asthma, and acute airway obstruction.

Rapid respiratory rates accompany pneumonia, fever, pain, heart disease, and anemia.

In an infant, tachypnea of 50 to 100 per minute during sleep may be an early sign of congestive heart failure.

Asymmetric expansion occurs with diaphragmatic hernia or pneumothorax.

▶ Normal Range of Findings

Abnormal Findings

Percussion. Percussion is of limited usefulness in the newborn and especially in the premature newborn because the adult's fingers are too large in relation to the tiny chest. The percussion note of hyperresonance occurs normally in the infant and young child owing to the relatively thin chest wall. Anything less than hyperresonance would have the same clinical significance as would dullness in the adult. If measured, diaphragmatic excursion measures about one to two rib interspaces in children.

Auscultation. Auscultation normally yields bronchovesicular breath sounds in the peripheral lung fields of the infant and young child up to age 5 to 6. Their relatively thin chest walls with underdeveloped musculature do not damp off the sound as do the thicker walls of adults, so breath sounds are louder and harsher.

Fine crackles are the adventitious sounds commonly heard in the immediate newborn period due to opening of the airways and clearing of fluid. Since the newborn's chest wall is so thin, transmission of sounds is enhanced and is heard easily all over the chest, making localization of breath sounds a problem. Even bowel sounds are easily heard in the chest. Try using the smaller pediatric diaphragm endpiece, or place the bell over the infant's interspaces and not over the ribs. Use the pediatric diaphragm on an older infant or toddler (Fig. 16–26).

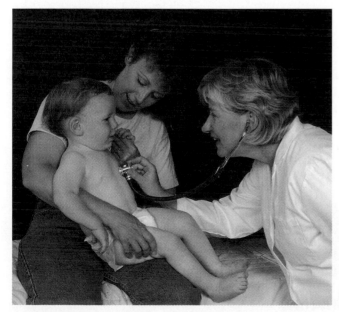

16–26

The Pregnant Female

The thoracic cage may appear wider, and the costal angle may feel wider than in the nonpregnant state. Respirations may be deeper, although this can be quantified only with pulmonary function tests.

Crepitus is palpable around a fractured clavicle, which may occur with difficult forceps delivery.

Rachitic rosary—prominent round knobs at costochondral junctions—is seen in infants with rickets or scurvy.

Diminished breath sounds occur with pneumonia, atelectasis, pleural effusion, or pneumothorax.

Persistent fine crackles that are scattered over the chest occur with pneumonia, bronchiolitis, or atelectasis.

Crackles only in upper lung fields occur with cystic fibrosis; crackles only in lower lung fields occur with heart failure.

Expiratory wheezing occurs with lower airway obstruction, e.g., asthma or bronchiolitis. When unilateral, it may be foreign body aspiration.

Persistent peristaltic sounds with diminished breath sounds on the same side may indicate diaphragmatic hernia.

Stridor is a high-pitched inspiratory crowing sound heard without the stethoscope, occurring with upper airway obstruction, e.g., croup, foreign body aspiration, or acute epiglottitis.

Normal Range of Findings	Abnormal Findings

The Aging Adult

The chest cage commonly shows an increased anteroposterior diameter, giving a round barrel shape, and **kyphosis** or an outward curvature of the thoracic spine (see Table 16–4). The person compensates by holding the head extended and tilted back. You may palpate marked bony prominences because of decreased subcutaneous fat. Chest expansion may be somewhat decreased with the older person, although it still should be symmetric. The costal cartilages become calcified with aging, resulting in a less mobile thorax.

The older person may fatigue easily, especially during auscultation when deep mouth breathing is required. Take care that this person does not hyperventilate and become dizzy. Allow brief rest periods or quiet breathing. If the person does feel faint, holding the breath for a few seconds will restore equilibrium.

The Acutely Ill Person

Ask a second examiner to hold the person's arms and to support him or her in the upright position. If no one else is available, you need to roll the person from side to side, examining the uppermost half of the thorax. This obviously prevents you from comparing findings from one side to another. Also, side flexion of the trunk alters percussion findings because the ribs of the upward side may flex closer together.

SUMMARY CHECKLIST: Thorax and Lung Exam

1: Inspection
Thoracic cage
Respirations
Skin color and condition
Person's position
Facial expression
Level of consciousness

2: Palpation
Confirm symmetric expansion
Tactile fremitus
Detect any lumps, masses, tenderness

3: Percussion
Percuss over lung fields
Estimate diaphragmatic excursion

4: Auscultation
Assess normal breath sounds
Note any abnormal breath sounds
If so, perform bronchophony, whispered pectoriloquy, egophony
Note any adventitious sounds

APPLICATION AND CRITICAL THINKING

SAMPLE CHARTING

Subjective

No cough, shortness of breath, or chest pain with breathing. No past history of respiratory diseases. Has "one or no" colds per year. Has never smoked. Works in well-ventilated office—smoking coworkers are restricted to smoke in lounge. Last TB skin test 4 years PTA, negative. Never had chest x-ray.

▶ **Objective**

Inspection. AP < transverse diameter. Respirations 16/min, relaxed and even.

Palpation. Chest expansion symmetric. Tactile fremitus equal bilaterally. No tenderness to palpation. No lumps or lesions.

Percussion. Resonant to percussion over lung fields. Diaphragmatic excursion 5 cm and = bilaterally.

Auscultation. Vesicular breath sounds clear over lung fields. No adventitious sounds.

CLINICAL CASE STUDY

Thomas G. is a 58-year-old, thin, white, male traffic patrolman who appears older than stated age. Face is anxious and tense, although in no acute distress at this time. Seeks care for "increasing SOB and fatigue in last couple months."

▶ **Subjective**

1 year PTA—noticed more "winded" than usual when walking > 3–4 blocks. Early morning cough present daily × 10 years, but now increased sputum production to 2 T per morning, frothy white.

6 mo. PTA—had a "cold" with severe harsh coughing, productive of ½ cup thick white sputum/day. Noted midsternal chest pain (mild) with cough. Lasted 2 weeks. Treated self with humidifier and OTC cough syrup—minimal relief.

3 mo. PTA—noticed increasing SOB with less activity. Fatigue and SOB when working outside during traffic rush hours. Unable to take evening walks (usually 2–3 blocks) due to SOB and fatigue. Has two-pillow orthopnea. Wakes 3–4 times during night.

Now—feels he is "worse and needs some help." Continues with 2-pillow orthopnea. Unable to walk > two blocks or climb > one flight stairs without resting. Unable to blow out birthday candles on cake last week. Morning cough productive of ¼ cup thin white sputum, cough continues sporadically during day.

No chest pain, hemoptysis, night sweats, or paroxysmal nocturnal dyspnea. No history of allergies, hospitalizations, or injuries to chest. No family history of TB, allergies, asthma, or cancer. Smokes cigarettes 2 packs per day × 30 years. Alcohol < one 6-pack beer/week summer months only.

▶ **Objective**

Inspection. Sitting on side of bed with arms propped on bedside table. Resp. resting 24/min, regular, shallow with prolonged expiration; resp. 34/min ambulating. Increased use of accessory muscles, AP = transverse diameter with widening of costal angle, slightly flushed face, tense expression.

Palpation. Minimal but symmetric chest expansion. Tactile fremitus = bilaterally. No lumps, masses, or tenderness to palpation.

Percussion. Diaphragmatic excursion is 1 cm and = bilaterally. Hyperresonance over lung fields.

Auscultation. Breath sounds diminished. Expiratory wheeze throughout posterior chest, R > L. No crackles.

▶ ASSESSMENT

Chronic and increasing SOB
Ineffective airway clearance R/T bronchial secretions and obstruction
Activity intolerance R/T imbalance between oxygen supply and demand
Sleep pattern disturbance R/T dyspnea and decreased mobility
Anxiety R/T change in health status

Continued

NURSING DIAGNOSES COMMONLY ASSOCIATED WITH THE THORAX AND LUNGS/RESPIRATORY DISORDERS

Diagnosis	Related Factors (Etiology)	Defining Characteristics (Symptoms and Signs)
Activity intolerance	Imbalance between oxygen supply and demand Deconditioned status Pain Fatigue Bedrest Sedentary lifestyle Electrolyte imbalance Hypovolemia Malnourishment Interrupted sleep Impaired sensory or motor function Effects of aging Generalized weakness Side effects of sedatives, tranquilizers, or narcotics Immobility Depression Lack of motivation	Increased or decreased heart rate, blood pressure, respirations Exertional discomfort or dyspnea Redness, cyanosis, or pallor of skin during activity Dizziness during activity Requiring frequent rest periods Worried or uneasy facial expression Verbal report of fatigue or weakness Impaired ability to change position or stand or walk without support Weakness Confusion

Ineffective breathing pattern	Decreased energy, lung expansion
	Effect of
	  Anesthesia
	  Medication (narcotics, sedatives, tranquilizers)
	  Obesity
	Fatigue
	Immobility, inactivity
	Impairment
	  Cognitive
	  Musculoskeletal
	  Neuromuscular
	  Perceptual
	Inflammatory processes
	Pain
	Tracheobronchial obstruction
	Anxiety
		Abnormal blood gases
		Altered chest excursion
		Assumption of three-point position
		Cough
		Cyanosis
		Dyspnea
		Fremitus
		Nasal flaring
		Pursed-lip breathing and prolonged expiratory phase
		Respiratory rate, depth changes
		Shortness of breath
		Tachypnea
		Use of accessory muscles

Ineffective airway clearance	Decreased energy, fatigue
	Effects of
	  Anesthesia
	  Infection
	  Medication (narcotics, sedatives, tranquilizers)
	Inability to cough effectively
	Perceptual or cognitive impairment
	Presence of artificial airway
	Tracheobronchial secretions or obstruction
	Aspiration of foreign matter
	Environmental pollutants
	Inhalation of toxic fumes or substances
	Trauma
		Absent or adventitious sounds
		Air hunger
		Change in respiratory rate or depth
		Cough, effective or ineffective, with or without spasm
		Cyanosis
		Diaphoresis
		Dyspnea
		Fever
		Nasal flaring
		Restlessness
		Stridor
		Substernal, intercostal retraction
		Tachycardia
		  Tachypnea
		Anxiety

Impaired gas exchange	Altered
	  Blood flow
	  Oxygen-carrying capacity of blood
	  Oxygen supply
		Clubbing of fingers
		Confusion
		Cyanosis
		Fatigue and lethargy

	Alveolar-capillary membrane changes
	Aspiration of foreign matter
	Decreased surfactant production
	Effects of
	  Anesthesia
	  Medications (narcotics, sedatives, tranquilizers)
	Hypoventilation or hyperventilation
	Inhalation of toxic fumes or substances
		Hypercapnia
		Hypoxia
		Inability to move secretions
		Irritability
		Restlessness
		Somnolence
		Tachycardia
		Use of accessory muscles

Fluid volume excess	Compromised regulatory mechanisms
	  Aldosterone
	  Antidiuretic hormone
	  Renin-angiotensin
	Effects of
	  Age extremes
	  Medications
	  Pregnancy
	Excessive fluid or sodium intake
		Abnormal breath sounds, rales
		Changes in
		  Respiratory pattern
		  Blood pressure
		  Central venous pressure
		  Mental status
		  Pulmonary artery pressure
		  Specific gravity
		  Edema
		Pulmonary congestion on x-ray study
		Shortness of breath, orthopnea
		Restlessness and anxiety
		Altered electrolytes
		Anasarca
		Azotemia
		Intake greater than output
		Jugular vein distention
		Nausea and/or vomiting
		Oliguria
		Positive finding of hepatojugular reflex
		S_3 heart sound
		Weight gain

Anxiety	Threat to or change in health status, relationships, role functioning, self-concept, socioeconomic status Threat of death Lack of knowledge Loss of control Actual or perceived loss of significant others Situational or maturational crises Unmet needs Unconscious conflict about essential values and goals of life Feelings of failure Disruptive family life Interpersonal transmission and contagion	Trembling Increased blood pressure Rapid respiration and pulse Feelings of helplessness, apprehensiveness, inadequacy, dread, worry Focus on self Irritability Restlessness Inability to concentrate Crying Change in appetite Diaphoresis Lack of eye contact Extraneous movements, foot shuffling, hand or arm movements Nausea Headache Increased wariness Lack of awareness of surroundings Regret Uncertainty Change in sleeping patterns Agitated Worried Feeling of dread Difficulty expressing self Change in voice quality Fear of unspecific consequences Expressed concern regarding changes in life events

Table continued on following page

Fatigue	Decreased/increased metabolic energy production
	Increased energy requirements to perform activities of daily living
	Overwhelming psychological or emotional demands
	Excessive social and/or role demands
	States of discomfort
	Altered body chemistry
	  Medications
	  Drug withdrawal
	  Chemotherapy
		Verbalization of an unremitting and over-whelming lack of energy
		Inability to maintain usual routines
		Increase in physical complaints
		Inability to concentrate
		Decreased performance
		Accident prone
		Lethargy or listlessness
		Disinterest in surroundings/introspection
		Decreased libido

Other Related Nursing Diagnoses

ACTUAL	RISK/WELLNESS
Impaired home maintenance management (see Chapter 12) Pain (see Chapter 14) Sleep pattern disturbance Altered role performance Altered tissue perfusion Dysfunctional ventilatory weaning response Inability to sustain spontaneous ventilation Impaired home maintenance management Pain Self-care deficit Sleep pattern disturbance	**Risk** Risk for infection **Wellness** Health-seeking behavior about smoking cessation strategies

ASSESSMENT VIDEO CRITICAL THINKING QUESTIONS

Saunders *Physical Examination and Health Assessment* Video Series—THORAX AND LUNGS—will direct you to consider the following:

1. Which conditions are associated with a productive cough?

2. Describe the characteristics of the following adventitious sounds: fine crackles, coarse crackles, wheezes, and rhonchi.

3. What assessment findings are normal variations in a pregnant woman?

4. Which nursing diagnoses are most appropriate for a person with wheezes, dyspnea, and tachypnea?

Table 16–4   CONFIGURATIONS OF THE THORAX

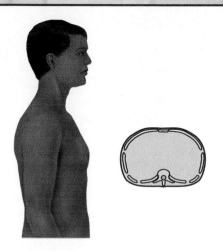

Normal Adult (for Comparison)

The thorax has an elliptical shape with an anteroposterior : transverse diameter of 1 : 2 or 5 : 7.

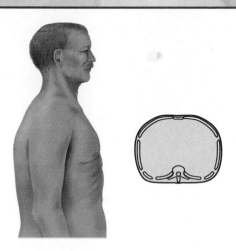

Barrel Chest

Note anteroposterior 5 transverse diameter and that ribs are horizontal instead of the normal downward slope. This is associated with normal aging and also with chronic emphysema and asthma due to hyperinflation of lungs.

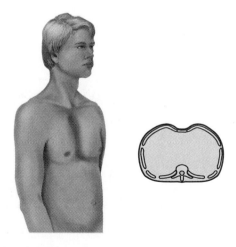

Pectus Excavatum

A markedly sunken sternum and adjacent cartilages (also called funnel breast). Depression begins at second intercostal space, becoming depressed most at junction of xiphoid with body of sternum. More noticeable on inspiration. Congenital, usually not symptomatic. When severe, sternal depression may cause embarrassment and a negative self-concept. Surgery may be indicated for cosmetic purposes.

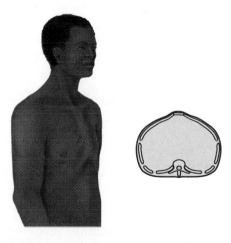

Pectus Carinatum

A forward protusion of the sternum, with ribs sloping back at either side and vertical depressions along costochondral junctions (pigeon breast). Less common than pectus excavatum, this minor deformity requires no treatment. If severe, surgery may be indicated for cosmetic purposes.

Table continued on following page

Table 16-4   CONFIGURATIONS OF THE THORAX *Continued*

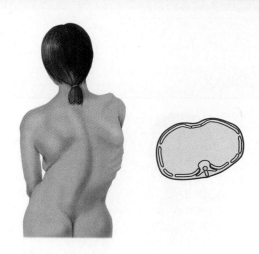

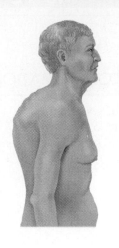

Scoliosis

A lateral S-shaped curvature of the thoracic and lumbar spine, usually with involved vertebrae rotation. Note unequal shoulder and scapular height and unequal hip levels, rib interspaces flared on convex side. More prevalent in adolescent age groups, especially girls. Mild deformities are asymptomatic. If severe (>45 degrees) deviation is present, scoliosis may reduce lung volume, then person is at risk for impaired cardiopulmonary function. Primary impairment is cosmetic deformity, negatively affecting self-image. Refer early for treatment, often surgery.

Kyphosis

An exaggerated posterior curvature of the thoracic spine (humpback) that causes significant back pain and limited mobility. Severe deformities impair cardiopulmonary function. Compensation may occur by hyperextension of head to maintain level of vision.

Kyphosis has been associated with aging, especially the familiar "dowager's hump" of postmenopausal osteoporotic women. However, it is common well before menopause. It is related to physical fitness; women with adequate exercise habits have less kyphosis (Cutler et al., 1993).

Table 16-5   RESPIRATION PATTERNS*

Inspiration   Expiration

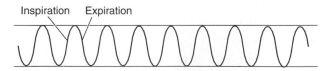

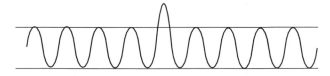

Normal Adult (for Comparison)

Rate—10 to 20 breaths per minute.
Depth—500 ml to 800 ml.
Pattern—even.

The ratio of pulse to respirations is fairly constant, about 4:1. Both values increase as a normal response to exercise, fear, or fever.
Depth—air moving in and out with each respiration.

Sigh

Occasional sighs punctuate the normal breathing pattern and are purposeful to expand alveoli. Frequent sighs may indicate emotional dysfunction. Frequent sighs also may lead to hyperventilation and dizziness.

*Assess the (1) rate, (2) depth (tidal volume), and (3) pattern.

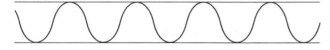

Tachypnea

Rapid shallow breathing. Increased rate >24 per minute. This is a normal response to fever, fear, or exercise. Rate also increases with respiratory insufficiency, pneumonia, alkalosis, pleurisy, and lesions in the pons.

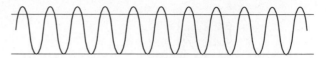

Hyperventilation

Increase in both rate and depth. Normally occurs with extreme exertion, fear, or anxiety. Also occurs with diabetic ketoacidosis (Kussmaul's respirations), hepatic coma, salicylate overdose (producing a respiratory alkalosis to compensate for the metabolic acidosis), lesions of the midbrain, and alteration in blood gas concentration (either an increase in carbon dioxide or decrease in oxygen). Hyperventilation blows off carbon dioxide, causing a decreased level in the blood (alkalosis).

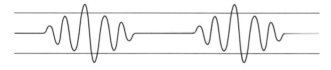

Bradypnea

Slow breathing. A decreased but regular rate (less than 10 per minute), as in drug-induced depression of the respiratory center in the medulla, increased intracranial pressure, and diabetic coma.

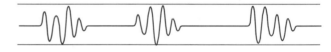

Hypoventilation

An irregular shallow pattern caused by an overdose of narcotics or anesthetics. May also occur with prolonged bedrest or conscious splinting of the chest to avoid respiratory pain.

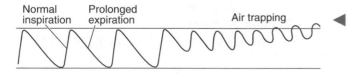

Cheyne-Stokes Respiration

A cycle in which respirations gradually wax and wane in a regular pattern, increasing in rate and depth and then decreasing. The breathing periods last 30 to 45 seconds, with periods of apnea (20 seconds) alternating the cycle. The most common cause is severe congestive heart failure; other causes are renal failure, meningitis, drug overdose, and increased intracranial pressure. Occurs normally in infants and aging persons during sleep.

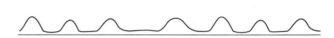

Biot's Respiration

Similar to Cheyne-Stokes respiration, except that the pattern is irregular. A series of normal respirations (3 to 4) is followed by a period of apnea. The cycle length is variable, lasting anywhere from 10 seconds to 1 minute. Seen with head trauma, brain abscess, heat stroke, spinal meningitis, and encephalitis.

Normal inspiration   Prolonged expiration   Air trapping ◄

Chronic Obstructive Breathing

Normal inspiration and prolonged expiration to overcome increased airway resistance. In a person with chronic obstructive lung disease, any situation calling for increased heart rate (exercise) may lead to dyspneic episode (air trapping), because then the person does not have enough time for full expiration.

▼ Table 16–6 ABNORMAL TACTILE FREMITUS

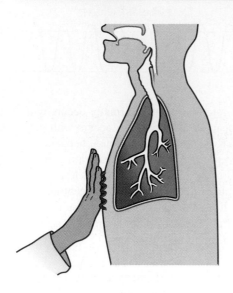

Increased Tactile Fremitus

Occurs with conditions that increase the density of lung tissue, thereby making a better conducting medium for vibrations, e.g., compression or consolidation (pneumonia). There must be a patent bronchus, and consolidation must extend to lung surface for increased fremitus to be apparent.

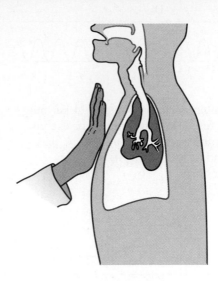

Decreased Tactile Fremitus

Occurs when anything obstructs transmission of vibrations, e.g., an obstructed bronchus, pleural effusion or thickening, pneumothorax, and emphysema. Any barrier that gets in the way of the sound and your palpating hand decreases fremitus.

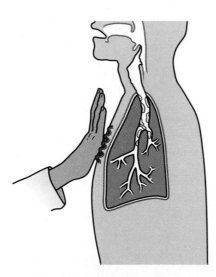

Rhonchal Fremitus

Vibration felt when inhaled air passes through thick secretions in the larger bronchi. This may decrease somewhat by coughing.

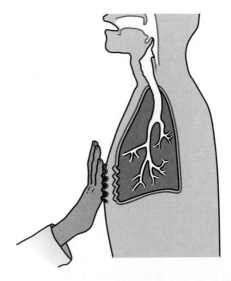

Pleural Friction Fremitus

Produced when inflammation of the parietal or visceral pleura causes a decrease in the normal lubricating fluid. Then the opposing surfaces make a coarse grating sound when rubbed together during breathing. Although this sound is best detected by auscultation, it may sometimes be palpable and feels like two pieces of leather grating together. It is synchronous with respiratory excursion. Also called a palpable friction rub.

Table 16-7 ADVENTITIOUS LUNG SOUNDS

Sound	Description	Mechanism	Clinical Example

(1) Discontinuous Sounds
These are discrete, crackling sounds.

Crackles—fine (formerly called rales)

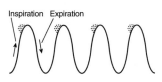

Inspiration Expiration

Discontinuous, high-pitched, short crackling, popping sounds heard during inspiration that are not cleared by coughing; you can simulate this sound by rolling a strand of hair between your fingers near your ear, or by moistening your thumb and index finger and separating them near your ear

Inhaled air collides with previously deflated airways; airways suddenly pop open, creating crackling sound as gas pressures between the two compartments equalize (Forgacs, 1978a)

Late inspiratory crackles occur with restrictive disease: pneumonia, heart failure, and interstitial fibrosis
Early inspiratory crackles occur with obstructive disease: chronic bronchitis, asthma, and emphysema
Posturally induced crackles (PICs) are fine crackles that appear with a change from sitting to the supine position, or with a change from supine to supine with legs elevated. PIC that appear after acute myocardial infarction have been associated with increased mortality (Deguchi et al., 1993).

Crackles—coarse (coarse rales)

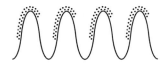

Loud, low-pitched, bubbling and gurgling sounds that start in early inspiration and may be present in expiration; may decrease somewhat by suctioning or coughing but will reappear shortly—sounds like opening a Velcro fastener

Inhaled air collides with secretions in the trachea and large bronchi

Pulmonary edema, pneumonia, pulmonary fibrosis, and the terminally ill who have a depressed cough reflex

Atelectatic crackles (atelectatic rales)

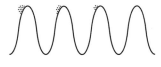

Sounds like fine crackles, but do not last and are not pathologic; disappear after the first few breaths; heard in axillae and bases (usually dependent) of lungs

When sections of alveoli are not fully aerated, they deflate and accumulate secretions. Crackles are heard when these sections reexpand with a few deep breaths

In aging adults, bed-ridden persons, or in persons just aroused from sleep

Pleural friction rub

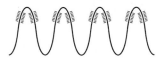

A very superficial sound that is coarse and low pitched; it has a grating quality as if two pieces of leather are being rubbed together; sounds just like crackles, but *close* to the ear; sounds louder if you push the stethoscope harder onto the chest wall; sound is inspiratory and expiratory

Caused when pleurae become inflamed and lose their normal lubricating fluid; their opposing roughened pleural surfaces rub together during respiration; heard best in anterolateral wall where greatest lung mobility exists

Pleuritis, accompanied by pain with breathing (rub disappears after a few days if pleural fluid accumulates and separates pleurae)

Table continued on following page

Sound	Description	Mechanism	Clinical Example
(2) Continuous Sounds These are connected, musical sounds.			
Wheeze—high-pitched (sibilant) 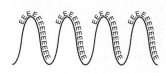	High-pitched, musical squeaking sounds that sound polyphonic (multiple notes as in a musical chord); predominate in expiration but may occur in both expiration and inspiration	Air squeezed or compressed through passageways narrowed almost to closure by collapsing, swelling, secretions, or tumors; the passageway walls oscillate in apposition between the closed and barely open positions; the resulting sound is similar to a vibrating reed (Forgacs, 1978a)	Diffuse airway obstruction from acute asthma or chronic emphysema
Wheeze—low-pitched (sonorous rhonchi) 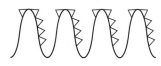	Low-pitched; monophonic single note, musical snoring, moaning sounds; they are heard throughout the cycle, although they are more prominent on expiration; may clear somewhat by coughing	Airflow obstruction as described by the vibrating reed mechanism above; the pitch of the wheeze cannot be correlated to the size of the passageway that generates it	Bronchitis, single bronchus obstruction from airway tumor
Stridor 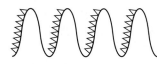	High-pitched, monophonic, inspiratory, crowing sound, louder in neck than over chest wall	Originating in larynx or trachea, upper airway obstruction from swollen, inflamed tissues or lodged foreign body	Croup and acute epiglottitis in children, and foreign inhalation, obstructed airway may be life threatening

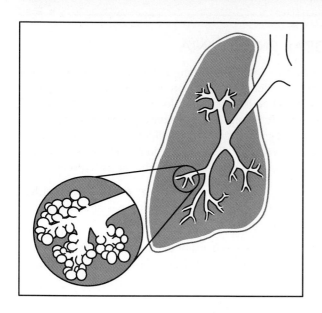

◄ NORMAL LUNG

Inspection   Anteroposterior < transverse diameter, relaxed posture, normal musculature; rate 10 to 18 breaths per minute, regular, no cyanosis or pallor

Palpation   Symmetric chest expansion. Tactile fremitus present and equal bilaterally, diminishing toward periphery. No lumps, masses, or tenderness

Percussion   Resonant. Diaphragmatic excursion 3 to 5 cm and equal bilaterally

Auscultation   Vesicular over peripheral fields. Bronchovesicular parasternally (anterior) and between scapulae (posterior). Infant and young child—bronchovesicular throughout

Adventitious Sounds   None

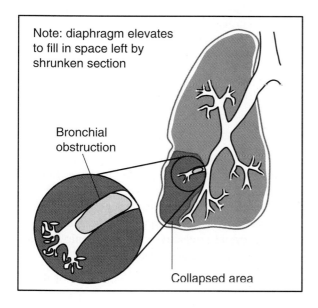

Note: diaphragm elevates to fill in space left by shrunken section

Bronchial obstruction

Collapsed area

◄ ATELECTASIS (IMPAIRED EXPANSION)

Condition   Collapsed shrunken section of alveoli, or an entire lung, due to (1) airway obstruction (e.g., the bronchus is completely blocked by thick exudate, aspirated foreign body, or tumor), the alveolar air beyond it is gradually absorbed by the pulmonary capillaries, and the alveolar walls cave in; (2) compression on the lung; and (3) lack of surfactant (hyaline membrane disease)

Inspection   Cough. Lag on expansion on affected side. Increased respiratory rate. Increased pulse. Possible cyanosis

Palpation   Chest expansion decreased on affected side. Tactile fremitus decreased or absent over area. With large collapse, tracheal shift toward affected side

Percussion   Dull over area (remainder of thorax sometimes may have hyperresonant note)

Auscultation   Breath sounds decreased vesicular or absent over area. Voice sounds variable, usually decreased or absent over affected area

Adventitious Sounds   None if bronchus is obstructed. Occasional fine crackles if bronchus is patent

Table continued on following page

Table 16–8   ASSESSMENT OF COMMON RESPIRATORY CONDITIONS
Continued

ABNORMAL FINDINGS

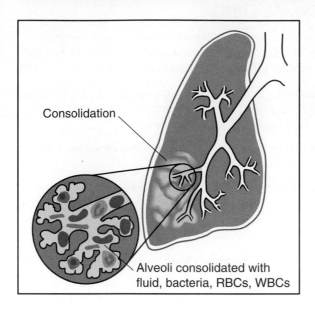

Consolidation

Alveoli consolidated with
fluid, bacteria, RBCs, WBCs

LOBAR PNEUMONIA

Condition   Infection in lung parenchyma leaves alveolar membrane edematous and porous, so red blood cells and white blood cells pass from blood to alveoli. Alveoli progressively fill up (become consolidated) with bacteria, solid cellular debris, fluid, and blood cells, all of which replace alveolar air. This results in decreased surface area of the respiratory membrane, which causes hypoxemia.

Inspection   Increased respiratory rate. Guarding and lag on expansion on affected side. Children—sternal retraction, nasal flaring

Palpation   Chest expansion decreased on affected side. Tactile fremitus increased if bronchus patent, decreased if bronchus obstructed

Percussion   Dull over lobar pneumonia

Auscultation   Breath sounds louder with patent bronchus, as if coming directly from larynx. Voice sounds have increased clarity, bronchophony, egophony, whispered pectoriloquy present. Children—diminished breath sounds may occur early in pneumonia

Adventitious Sounds   Crackles, fine to medium

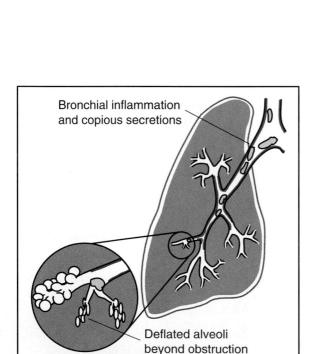

Bronchial inflammation
and copious secretions

Deflated alveoli
beyond obstruction

BRONCHITIS

Condition   Proliferation of mucous glands in the passageways, resulting in excessive mucus secretion. Inflammation of bronchi with partial obstruction of bronchi by secretions or constrictions. Sections of lung distal to obstruction may be deflated. Bronchitis may be acute or chronic with recurrent productive cough. Chronic bronchitis is usually caused by cigarette smoking.

Inspection   Hacking, rasping cough productive of thick mucoid sputum. Chronic—dyspnea, fatigue, cyanosis, possible clubbing of fingers

Palpation   Tactile fremitus normal

Percussion   Resonant

Auscultation   Normal vesicular. Voice sounds normal. Chronic—prolonged expiration

Adventitious Sounds   Crackles over deflated areas. May have wheeze

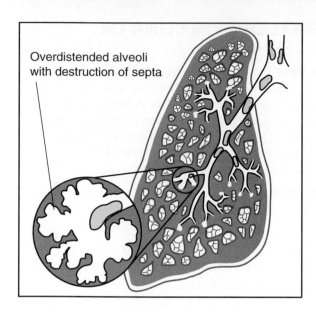

Overdistended alveoli with destruction of septa

◀ EMPHYSEMA

Condition   Emphysema is caused by destruction of pulmonary connective tissue (elastin, collagen) and is characterized by permanent enlargement of air sacs distal to terminal bronchioles and rupture of interalveolar walls. This increases airway resistance, especially on expiration—producing a hyperinflated lung and an increase in lung volume. Cigarette smoking accounts for 80%–90% of cases of emphysema.

Inspection   Increased anteroposterior diameter. Barrel chest. Use of accessory muscles to aid respiration. Tripod position. Shortness of breath, especially on exertion. Respiratory distress. Tachypnea

Palpation   Tactile fremitus decreased. Chest expansion decreased

Percussion   Hyperresonant. Decreased diaphragmatic excursion

Auscultation   Decreased breath sounds. May have prolonged expiration. Muffled heart sounds secondary to overdistention of lungs.

Adventitious Sounds   Usually none. Occasionally you may hear wheeze

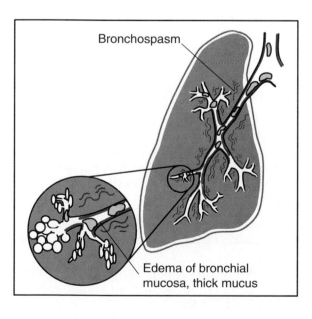

Bronchospasm

Edema of bronchial mucosa, thick mucus

◀ ASTHMA

Condition   An allergic hypersensitivity to certain inhaled allergens (pollen), irritants (tobacco, ozone), microorganisms, stress, or exercise that produces an early-phase response characterized by bronchospasm. This induces a late-phase response several hours later, characterized by inflammation, edema in walls of bronchioles, and secretion of highly viscous mucus into airways. All these factors greatly increase airway resistance, especially during expiration, and produce the symptoms in both phases of wheezing, dyspnea, and chest tightness.

Inspection   During severe attack. Increased respiratory rate, shortness of breath with audible wheeze. Use of accessory neck muscles. Cyanosis. Apprehension. Retraction of intercostal spaces. Expiration labored, prolonged. When chronic may have barrel chest

Palpation   Tactile fremitus decreased, tachycardia

Percussion   Resonant. May be hyperresonant if chronic

Auscultation   Diminished air movement. Breath sounds decreased, with prolonged expiration. Voice sounds decreased

Adventitious Sounds   Bilateral wheezing on expiration, sometimes inspiratory and expiratory wheezing.

Table continued on following page

Table 16–8 ASSESSMENT OF COMMON RESPIRATORY CONDITIONS
Continued

ABNORMAL FINDINGS

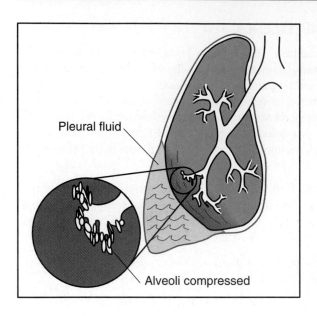

Pleural fluid

Alveoli compressed

◄ PLEURAL EFFUSION (FLUID) OR THICKENING

Condition Collection of excess fluid in the intrapleural space, with compression of overlying lung tissue. Effusion may contain watery capillary fluid (transudative), protein (exudative), purulent matter (empyemic), blood (hemothorax), or milky lymphatic fluid (chylothorax). Gravity settles fluid in dependent areas of thorax. Presence of fluid subdues all lung sounds

Inspection Increased respiratory rate, dyspnea, may have dry cough, tachycardia, cyanosis, abdominal distention

Palpation Tactile fremitus decreased or absent. Tracheal shift away from affected side. Chest expansion decreased on affected side

Percussion Dull to flat. No diaphragmatic excursion on affected side

Auscultation Breath sounds decreased or absent. Voice sounds decreased or absent. When remainder of lung is compressed near the effusion, may have bronchial breath sounds over the compression along with bronchophony, egophony, whispered pectoriloquy

Adventitious Sounds None

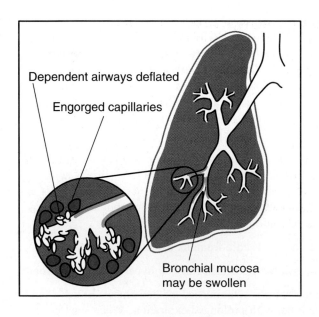

Dependent airways deflated

Engorged capillaries

Bronchial mucosa may be swollen

◄ CONGESTIVE HEART FAILURE

Condition Pump failure with increasing pressure of cardiac overload causes pulmonary congestion or an increased amount of blood present in pulmonary capillaries. Dependent air sacs are deflated. Pulmonary capillaries engorged. Bronchial mucosa may be swollen

Inspection Increased respiratory rate, shortness of breath on exertion, orthopnea, paroxysmal nocturnal dyspnea, nocturia, ankle edema, pallor in light-skinned people

Palpation Skin moist, clammy. Tactile fremitus normal

Percussion Resonant

Auscultation Normal vesicular. Heart sounds include S_3 gallop

Adventitious Sounds Crackles at lung bases

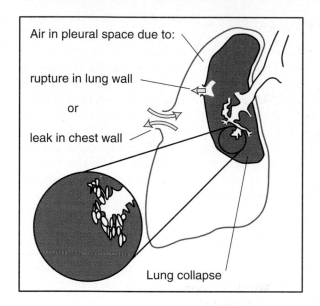

Air in pleural space due to:

rupture in lung wall

or

leak in chest wall

Lung collapse

◀ **PNEUMOTHORAX**

Condition Free air in pleural space causes partial or complete lung collapse. Air in pleural space neutralizes the usual negative pressure present, thus lung collapses. Usually unilateral

Pneumothorax can be (1) spontaneous (air enters pleural space through rupture in lung wall; (2) traumatic (air enters through opening or injury in chest wall); or (3) tension (trapped air in pleural space increases, compressing lung and shifting mediastinum to the unaffected side)

Inspection Unequal chest expansion. If large, increased respiratory rate, cyanosis, apprehension, bulging in interspaces

Palpation Tactile fremitus decreased or absent. Tracheal shift to opposite side (unaffected side). Chest expansion decreased on affected side. Tachycardia, decreased BP

Percussion Hyperresonant. Decreased diaphragmatic excursion

Auscultation Breath sounds decreased or absent. Voice sounds decreased or absent

Adventitious Sounds None

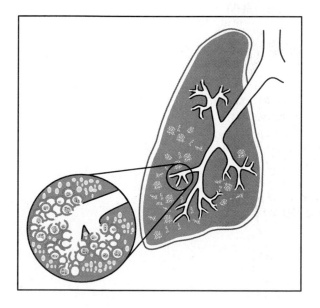

◀ *PNEUMOCYSTIS CARINII* PNEUMONIA

Condition This virulent form of pneumonia is a protozoal infection associated with AIDS. The parasite *P. carinii* is common in the United States and harmless to most people, except to the immunocompromised in whom a diffuse interstitial pneumonitis ensues. Cysts containing the organism and macrophages form in alveolar spaces, alveolar walls thicken, and the disease spreads to bilateral interstitial infiltrates of foamy, protein-rich fluid

Inspection Anxiety, shortness of breath, dyspnea on exertion, malaise are common; also tachypnea; fever; a dry, nonproductive cough; intercostal retractions in children; cyanosis

Palpation Decreased chest expansion

Percussion Dull over areas of diffuse infiltrate

Auscultation Breath sounds may be diminished

Adventitious Sounds Crackles may be present, but often are absent

Table continued on following page

493

▼ Table 16–8   ASSESSMENT OF COMMON RESPIRATORY CONDITIONS
Continued

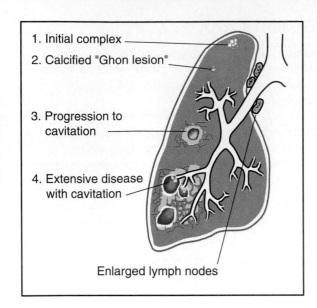

1. Initial complex
2. Calcified "Ghon lesion"
3. Progression to cavitation
4. Extensive disease with cavitation

Enlarged lymph nodes

◀ **TUBERCULOSIS**

Condition   Inhalation of tubercle bacilli into the alveolar wall starts the process. (1) Initial complex is acute inflammatory response—macrophages engulf bacilli but do not kill them. Tubercle forms around bacilli. (2) Scar tissue forms, lesion calcifies and shows on x-ray. (3) Reactivation of previously healed lesion. Dormant bacilli now multiply, producing necrosis, cavitation, and caseous lung tissue (cheeselike). (4) Extensive destruction as lesion erodes into bronchus, forming air-filled cavity. Apex usually has the most damage

Subjective   Primary tuberculosis usually is asymptomatic, showing as positive skin test or on x-ray. Progressive tuberculosis involves weight loss, anorexia, easy fatigability, low-grade afternoon fevers, night sweats. May have pleurisy with or without effusion, recurrent lower respiratory infections

Inspection   Cough initially nonproductive, later productive of purulent, yellow-green sputum, may be blood-tinged. Dyspnea, orthopnea, fatigue, weakness

Palpation   Skin moist at night from night sweats

Percussion   Resonant initially. Dull over effusion (if present)

Auscultation   Normal or decreased vesicular breath sounds

Adventitious Sounds   Crackles over upper lobes common, persist following full expiration and cough

Bibliography

Apgar V: A proposal for a new method of evaluating the newborn infant. Curr Res Anesth Analg Jul–Aug:260, 1953.

Ares C, Fein AM: Pneumothorax. Emerg Med 27(12):62–70, Dec 1995.

Assadian O, Assadian A, Aspock C, Killer W: The stethoscope as a potential source of transmission of bacteria. Infec Control Hosp Epidemiol 19(5):298–299, May 1998.

Autio L, Rosenow D: Effectively managing asthma in young and middle adulthood. Nurs Pract 24(1):100–113, Jan 1999.

Avila PC: Differential diagnosis of wheezing in children. Prim Care Pract 2(6):559–577, Nov–Dec 1998.

Barrow S, Higgins B: Asthma-related arrest. Am J Nurs 98(1):50, Jan 1998.

Basfield-Holland ES: Assessing pulmonary status: It's more than listening to breath sounds. Nursing97 27(8):32hh1–32hh9, Aug 1997.

Bechler-Karsch A: Assessment and management of status asthmaticus. Pediatr Nurs 20(3):217–223, May–June 1994.

Berry JK, Vitalo CA, Larson JL, et al: Respiratory muscle strength in older adults. Nurs Res 45(3):154–159, May–June 1996.

Bezanson J: Respiratory care of older adults after cardiac surgery. J Cardiovasc Nurs 12(1):71–83, Oct 1997.

Borkgren MW, Gronkiewicz CA: Update your asthma care from hospital to home. Am J Nurs 95(1):26–35, Jan 1995.

Brooks-Brunn J: Postoperative atelectasis and pneumonia. Heart Lung 24(2):94–115, Mar–Apr 1995.

Carlson-Catalano J: Clinical validation of ineffective breathing pattern, ineffective airway clearance, and impaired gas exchange. Image 30(3):243–248, 1998.

Carroll P: Using pulse oximetry in the home. Home Healthcare Nurse 15(2):88–97, Feb 1997.

Chiramannil A: Lung cancer. Am J Nurs 98(4):46–47, Apr 1998.

Christie F: Pulmonary embolism. Am J Nurs 98(11):36–37, Nov 1998.

Coakley-Maller C, Shea M: Respiratory infections in children. Adv Nurs Pract 5(9):21–27, Sep 1997.

Collins PM: Pleural effusion. Am J Nurs 96(7):38–39, July 1996.

Corcoran CA, Pierce JD: Evaluating diaphragm activity in trauma patients. J Trauma Nurs 2(2):36–42, Apr–Jun 1995.

Cunningham FG, MacDonald PC, Gant NF: Williams Obstetrics, 20th ed. Norwalk, CT, Appleton-Lange, 1997.

Cutler WB, Friedmann E, Genovese-Stone E: Prevalence of kyphosis in a healthy sample of pre- and postmenopausal women. Am J Phys Med Rehabil 72(4):219–225, 1993.

Deguchi F, Hirakawa S, Gotoh K, et al: Prognostic significance of posturally induced crackles: Long term follow-up of patients after recovery from acute myocardial infarction. Chest 103:1457–1462, 1993.

DeLorenzo RA: Sneezes, wheezes, and breezes: Listening to the chest. J Emerg Med Serv 20(10):58–71, Oct 1995.

DiFranza JR, Lew RA: Morbidity and mortality in children associated with the use of tobacco products by other people. Pediatrics 97(4):560–568, Apr 1996.

Ferrin MS, Tino G: Acute dyspnea. AACN Clin Issues 8(3):398–410, Aug 1997.

Forgacs P: The functional basis of pulmonary sounds. Chest 73:399–405, 1978a.

Forgacs P: Lung Sounds. London, Ballière Tindall, 1978b.

Fraser D: Assessing the elderly for infections. J Gerontol Nurs 23(4):5–10, Nov 1997.

Gravil JH, Al-Rawas OA, Cotton MM, et al: Home treatment of exacerbations of chronic obstructive pulmonary disease by an acute respiratory assessment service. Lancet 351(9119):1853–1855, June 20, 1998.

Hayden C: Spontaneous pneumothorax. Am J Nurs 98(4):16BB–16EE, Apr 1998.

Hendell M: Mycobacterial infections in patients with HIV: A review of disease and care. Nurse Pract 23(10):75–83, Oct 1998.

Johannsen JM: Chronic obstructive pulmonary disease: Current comprehensive care for emphysema and bronchitis. Nurse Pract 19(1):59–67, 1994.

Keep NB: Identifying pulmonary embolism. Am J Nurs 95(4):52, Apr 1995.

Kelly M: Acute respiratory failure. Am J Nurs 96(12):46, Dec 1996.

King RP, Thompson BT, Johnson DC: Wheezing on maximal forced exhalation in the diagnosis of atypical asthma. Ann Intern Med 110(6):451–455, 1989.

Kwiatkowski M, Jain M: Current trends and treatments in chronic obstructive pulmonary disease. Prim Care Pract 2(6):545–558, Nov–Dec 1998.

Lapp NL: Lung volumes and flow rates in black and white subjects. Thorax 29:185–188, 1974.

Larson JL, Covey MK, Vitalo CA, et al: Reliability and validity of the 12-minute distance walk in patients with chronic obstructive pulmonary disease. Nurs Res 45(4):203–210, Jul–Aug 1996.

Laskowski-Jones L: Meeting the challenge of chest trauma. Am J Nurs 95(9):23–30, Sep 1995.

Lehrer S: Understanding Lung Sounds, 2nd ed. Philadelphia, W.B. Saunders Company, 1993.

Leidy NK: Functional performance in people with chronic obstructive pulmonary disease. Image 27(1):23–34, Spring 1995.

Leiner S, Mays M: Diagnosing latent and active pulmonary tuberculosis: A review for clinicians. Nurs Pract 21(2):86–111, Feb 1996.

Lisanti P, Zwolski K: Understanding the devastation of AIDS. Am J Nurs 97(7):26–35, July 1997.

Loudon RG: The lung exam. Clin Chest Med 8:265–272, 1987.

Mackin LA: Screening for tuberculosis in the primary care setting. Prim Care Pract 2(6):599–610, Nov–Dec 1998.

Makinodan T, Harada N: Medical health outcome studies in the Asian and Pacific Islander American population. Asian Am Pacific Islander J Health 4(1–3):97–104, 1996.

Manganelli D, Palla A, Donnamaria V, Giuntini C: Clinical features of pulmonary embolism. Chest 107(1):255–325, Jan 1995.

Marchese TW, Diamond FB: Comprehensive assessment of the respiratory system. J Nurse Midwifery 40(2):150–162, Mar–Apr 1995.

Mays M, Leiner S: Asthma—A comprehensive review. J Nurse Midwifery 40(3):256–268, May–June 1995.

Mays M, Leiner S: Management of common respiratory problems. J Nurse Midwifery 41(2):139–154, Mar–Apr 1996.

McDermott TD, Chestnut T, Schumann L: A comparison of conventional percussion and auscultation percussion in the detection of pleural effusions of hospitalized patients. J Am Acad Nurs Pract 9(10):483–486, Oct 1997.

McKinney G: Under new management: Asthma and the elderly. J Gerontol Nurs 21(1):39–45, Nov 1995.

Moccia JM: Pulmonary embolism. Nursing96 26(4):26–31, Apr 1996.

Naylor CD, McCormack DG, Sullivan SN: The midclavicular line: A wandering landmark. Can Med Assoc J 136:48–50, 1987.

Nelson RS, Rickman LS, Mathews WC, et al: Rapid clinical diagnosis of pulmonary abnormalities in HIV-seropositive patients by auscultatory percussion. Chest 105(2):402–407, Feb 1994.

O'Hanlon-Nichols T: The adult pulmonary system. Am J Nurs 98(2):39–45, Feb 1998.

O'Hanlon-Nichols T: Adult respiratory distress syndrome. Am J Nurs 95(8):42–43, Aug 1995.

Olowe SA, Akinkugbe A: Amniotic fluid lecithin/sphingomyelin ratio: Comparison between an African and a North American community. Pediatrics 62(1):38–41, 1978.

Oscherwitz R: Differences in pulmonary functions in various racial groups. Am J Epidemiol 96(5):319–327, 1972.

Overfield T: Biologic Variation in Health and Illness: Race, Age, and Sex Differences, 2nd ed. New York, CRC Press, 1995.

Owen A: Respiratory assessment revisited. Nursing98 28(4):48–49, Apr 1998.

Repasky TM: Epiglottitis. Am J Nurs 95(9):52, Sep 1995.

Schwartz R: Respiratory syncytial virus in infants and children. Nurs Pract 20(9):24–29, Sep 1995.

Skelskey C, Leshem OA: Tuberculosis surveillance in long-term care. Am J Nurs 97(10):16BBBB–16DDDD, Oct 1997.

Stein P, Henry JW, Gopalakrishman D, Relyea B: Asymmetry of the calves in the assessment of patients with suspected acute pulmonary embolism. Chest 107(4):936–939, Apr 1995.

Tallon RW: Oximetry: State of the art. Nurs Manage 27(11):43–44, Nov 1996.

Wagner C, Lung CL: Asthma management in the primary care setting. Am J Nurs 97(Suppl):8–16, Nov 1997.

Walsek C, Boler AM, Zwerski S: Lower respiratory tract infections in the pediatric patient. Prim Care Pract 3(1):93–107, Jan–Feb 1999.

Wintermeyer SF: Occupational asthma. Prim Care Pract 2(6):614–624, Nov–Dec 1998.

Zitkus BS: Sarcoidosis. Am J Nurs 97(10):40–41, Oct 1997.

CHAPTER SEVENTEEN

Heart and Neck Vessels

The cardiovascular system consists of the **heart,** a muscular pump, and the **blood vessels.** The blood vessels are arranged in two continuous loops, the *pulmonary circulation* and the *systemic circulation* (Fig. 17–1). When the heart contracts, it pumps blood simultaneously into both loops.

POSITION AND SURFACE LANDMARKS

The **precordium** is the area on the anterior chest overlying the heart and great vessels (Fig. 17–2). The great vessels are the major arteries and veins connected to the heart. The heart and the great vessels are located between the lungs in the middle third of the thoracic cage, called the **mediastinum.** The heart extends from the second to the fifth intercostal space and from the right border of the sternum to the left midclavicular line.

Think of the heart as an upside-down triangle in the chest. The "top" of the heart is the broader *base,* and the "bottom" is the *apex,* which points down and to the left.

During contraction, the apex beats against the chest wall, producing an apical impulse. This is palpable in most people, normally at the fifth intercostal space, 7 to 9 cm from the midsternal line.

Inside the body, the heart is rotated so that its right side is anterior and its left side is mostly posterior. Of the heart's four chambers, the right ventricle forms the greatest area of anterior cardiac surface (Fig. 17–3). The left ventricle lies behind the right ventricle and forms the apex and slender area of left border. The right atrium lies to the right and above the right ventricle and forms the right border. The left atrium is located posteriorly, with only a small portion, the left atrial appendage, showing anteriorly.

The **great vessels** lie bunched above the base of the heart. The **superior** and **inferior vena cava** return unoxygenated venous blood to the right side of the heart. The **pulmonary artery** leaves the right ventricle, bifurcates, and carries the venous blood to the lungs. The **pulmonary veins** return the freshly oxygenated blood to the left side of the heart, and the **aorta** carries it out to the body. The aorta ascends from the left ventricle, arches back at the level of the sternal angle, and descends behind the heart.

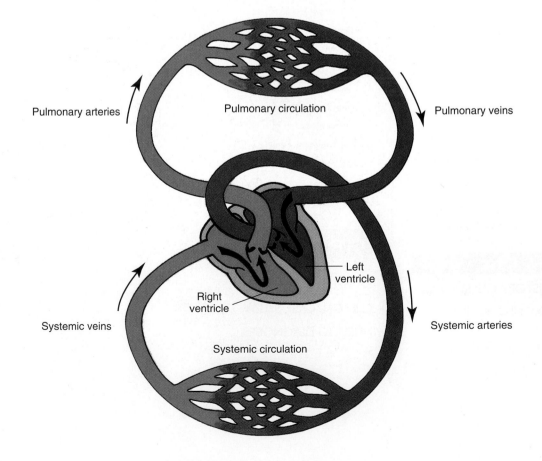

Pulmonary arteries   Pulmonary circulation   Pulmonary veins

Left ventricle

Right ventricle

Systemic veins   Systemic arteries

Systemic circulation

17–1

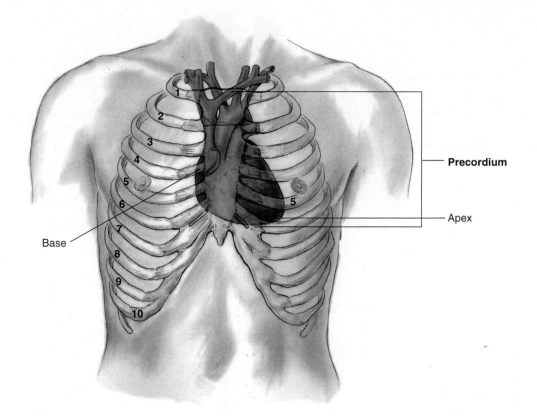

1
2
3
4
5
6
7
8
9
10

Precordium

Apex

Base

5

17–2

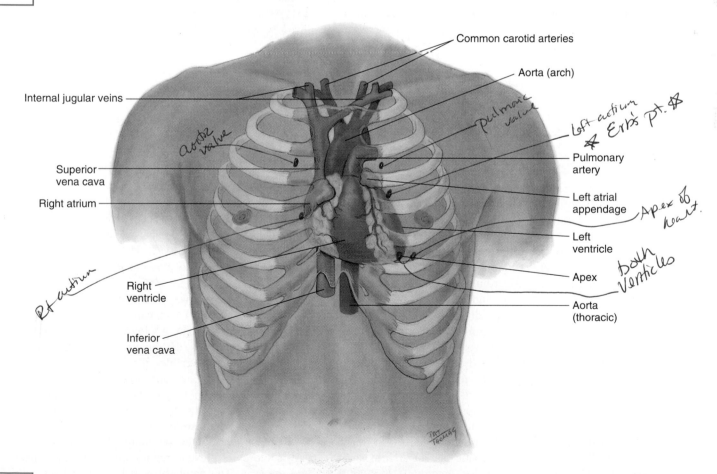

Common carotid arteries

Aorta (arch)

Internal jugular veins

Superior
vena cava

Right atrium

Right
ventricle

Inferior
vena cava

Pulmonary
artery

Left atrial
appendage

Left
ventricle

Apex

Aorta
(thoracic)

Aortic valve

Pulmonic valve

Left atrium & Erb's pt.

Apex of heart.

Both Ventricles

Rt atrium

17–3

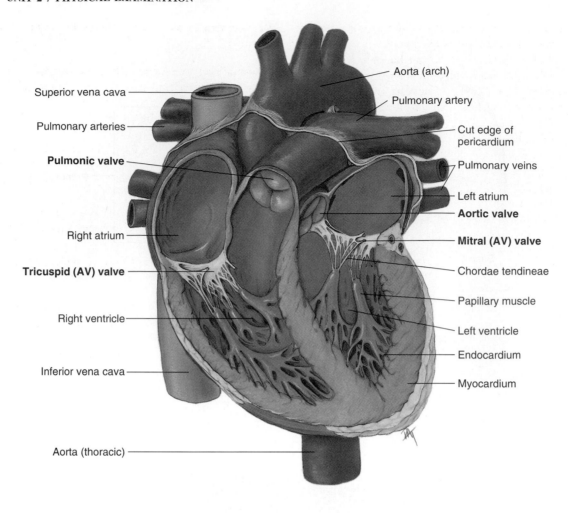

Aorta (arch)

Pulmonary artery

Cut edge of pericardium

Pulmonary veins

Left atrium

Aortic valve

Mitral (AV) valve

Chordae tendineae

Papillary muscle

Left ventricle

Endocardium

Myocardium

Superior vena cava

Pulmonary arteries

Pulmonic valve

Right atrium

Tricuspid (AV) valve

Right ventricle

Inferior vena cava

Aorta (thoracic)

17–4

HEART WALL, CHAMBERS, AND VALVES

The **heart wall** has numerous layers. The **pericardium** is a tough, fibrous, double-walled sac that surrounds and protects the heart (see its cut edge in Fig. 17–4). It has two layers that contain a few milliliters of serous *pericardial fluid.* This ensures smooth, friction-free movement of the heart muscle. The pericardium is adherent to the great vessels, esophagus, sternum, and pleurae and is anchored to the diaphragm. The **myocardium** is the muscular wall of the heart; it does the pumping. The **endocardium** is the thin layer of endothelial tissue that lines the inner surface of the heart chambers and valves.

The common metaphor is to think of the heart as a pump. But consider that the heart actually is *two* pumps; the right side of the heart pumps blood into the lungs, and the left side of the heart simultaneously pumps blood into the body. The two pumps are separated by an impermeable wall, the septum. Each side has an **atrium** and a **ventricle.** The atrium (Latin for anteroom) is a thin-

walled reservoir for holding blood, and the thick-walled ventricle is the muscular pumping chamber. (It is common to use the following abbreviations to refer to the chambers: RA, right atrium; RV, right ventricle; LA, left atrium; and LV, left ventricle.)

The four **chambers** are separated by swinging doorlike structures, called *valves,* whose main purpose is to prevent backflow of blood. The valves are unidirectional; they can only open one way. The valves open and close *passively* in response to pressure gradients in the moving blood.

There are four **valves** in the heart (Fig. 17–4). The two **atrioventricular** (AV) valves separate the atria and the ventricles. The right AV valve is the **tricuspid,** and the left AV valve is the bicuspid or **mitral** valve (so named because it resembles a bishop's mitred cap). The valves' thin leaflets are anchored by collagenous fibers (**chordae tendineae**) to papillary muscles embedded in the ventricle floor. The AV valves open during the heart's filling phase, or **diastole,** to allow the ventricles to fill with blood. During the pumping phase, or **systole,** AV valves close to prevent regurgitation of blood back up into the atria. The papillary muscles contract at this time, so that the valve leaflets meet and unite to form a perfect seal without turning themselves inside out.

The **semilunar** (SL) valves are set between the ventricles and the arteries. Each valve has three cusps that look like half-moons. The SL valves are the **pulmonic** valve in the right side of the heart and the **aortic** valve in the left side of the heart. They open during pumping, or **systole,** to allow blood to be ejected from the heart.

Note that no valves are present between the vena cava and the right atrium, nor between the pulmonary veins and the left atrium. For this reason, abnormally high pressure in the left side of the heart gives a person symptoms of pulmonary congestion, and abnormally high pressure in the right side of the heart shows in the neck veins and abdomen.

DIRECTION OF BLOOD FLOW

Think of an unoxygenated red blood cell being drained downstream into the vena cava. It is swept along with the flow of venous blood and follows the route illustrated in Figure 17–5.

1. From liver to RA via inferior vena cava
   Superior vena cava drains venous blood from head and upper extremities
   From RA, venous blood travels through tricuspid valve to RV
2. From RV, venous blood flows through pulmonic valve to pulmonary artery
   Pulmonary artery delivers unoxygenated blood to lungs
3. Lungs oxygenate blood
   Pulmonary veins return fresh blood to LA
4. From LA, arterial blood travels through mitral valve to LV
   LV ejects blood through aortic valve into aorta
5. Aorta delivers oxygenated blood to body

Remember that the circulation is a continuous loop. The blood is kept moving along by continually shifting pressure gradients. The blood flows from an area of higher pressure to one of lower pressure.

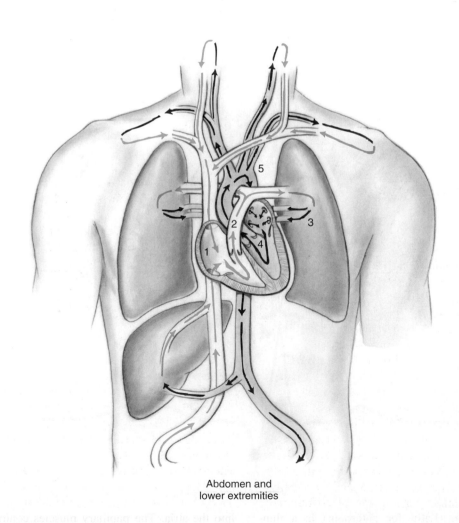

Abdomen and
lower extremities

17–5

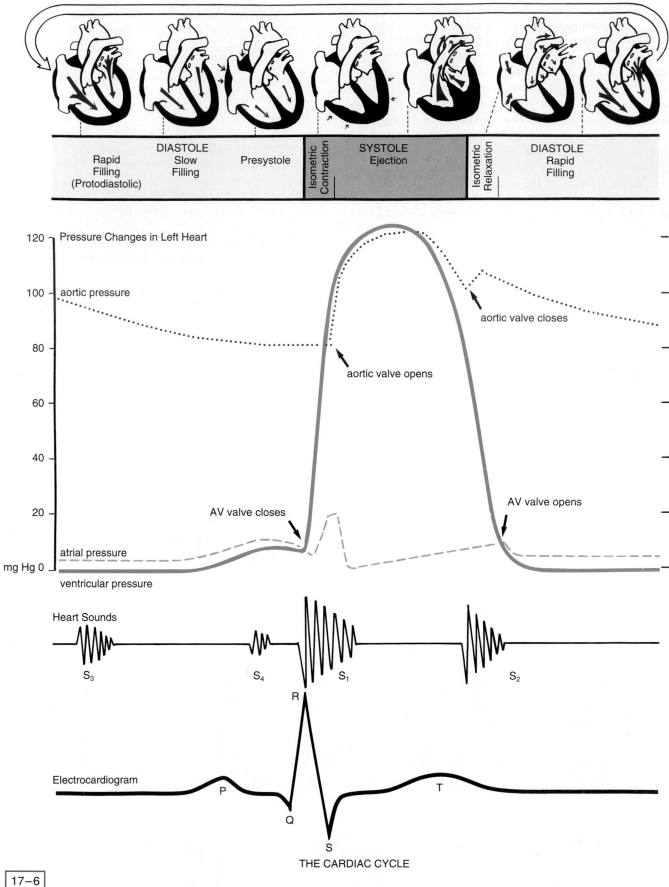

THE CARDIAC CYCLE

17-6

CARDIAC CYCLE

The rhythmic movement of blood through the heart is the **cardiac cycle.** It has two phases, **diastole** and **systole.** In **diastole,** the ventricles relax and fill with blood. This takes up two-thirds of the cardiac cycle. The heart's contraction is **systole.** During systole, blood is pumped from the ventricles and fills the pulmonary and systemic arteries. This is one-third of the cardiac cycle.

Diastole. In diastole, the ventricles are relaxed, and the AV valves, i.e., the tricuspid and mitral, are open (Fig. 17–6). (Opening of the normal valve is acoustically silent.) The pressure in the atria is higher than that in the ventricles, so blood pours rapidly into the ventricles. This first passive filling phase is called *early* or *protodiastolic filling.*

Toward the end of diastole, the atria contract and push the last amount of blood (about 25 percent of stroke volume) into the ventricles. This active filling phase is called *presystole,* or *atrial systole,* or sometimes the "atrial kick." It causes a small rise in left ventricular pressure. (Note that atrial systole occurs during ventricular diastole, a confusing but important point.)

Systole. Now so much blood has been pumped into the ventricles that ventricular pressure is finally higher than that in the atria, so the mitral and tricuspid valves swing shut. The closure of the AV valves contributes to the first heart sound (S_1) and signals the beginning of systole. The AV valves close to prevent any regurgitation of blood back up into the atria during contraction.

For a very brief moment, all four valves are closed. The ventricular walls contract. This contraction against a closed system works to build pressure inside the ventricles to a high level *(isometric contraction).* Consider first the left side of the heart. When the pressure in the ventri-

cle finally exceeds pressure in the aorta, the aortic valve opens and blood is ejected rapidly.

After the ventricle's contents are ejected, its pressure falls. When pressure falls below pressure in the aorta, some blood flows backward toward the ventricle, causing the aortic valve to swing shut. This closure of the semilunar valves causes the second heart sound (S_2) and signals the end of systole.

Diastole Again. Now all four valves are closed and the ventricles relax (called *isometric* or *isovolumic relaxation*). Meanwhile, the atria have been filling with blood delivered from the lungs. Atrial pressure is now higher than the relaxed ventricular pressure. The mitral valve drifts open and diastolic filling begins again.

Events in the Right and Left Sides. The same events are happening in the right side of the heart, but pressures in the right side of the heart are much lower than those of the left side because less energy is needed to pump blood to its destination, the pulmonary circulation. Also, events occur just slightly later in the right side of the heart due to the route of myocardial depolarization. As a result, two distinct components to each of the heart sounds exist, and sometimes you can hear them separately. In the first heart sound, the mitral component (M_1) closes just before the tricuspid component (T_1). And with S_2, aortic closure (A_2) occurs slightly before pulmonic closure (P_2).

HEART SOUNDS

Events in the cardiac cycle generate sounds that can be heard through a stethoscope over the chest wall. These include normal heart sounds and, occasionally, extra heart sounds and murmurs (Fig. 17–7).

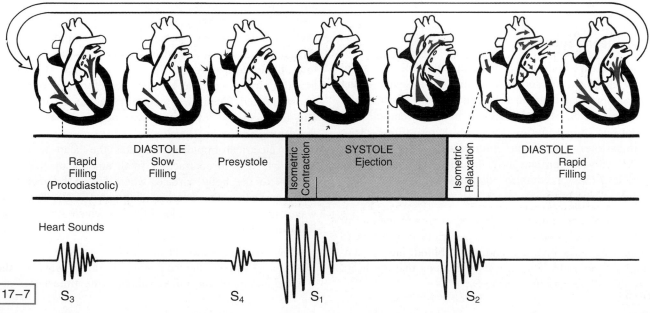

DIASTOLE			Isometric Contraction	SYSTOLE	Isometric Relaxation	DIASTOLE
Rapid Filling (Protodiastolic)	Slow Filling	Presystole		Ejection		Rapid Filling

Heart Sounds

S_3 S_4 S_1 S_2

17–7

Normal Heart Sounds

The **first heart sound** (S_1) occurs with closure of the AV valves and thus signals the beginning of systole. The mitral component of the first sound (M_1) slightly precedes the tricuspid component (T_1), but you usually hear these two components fused as one sound. You can hear S_1 over all the precordium, but usually it is loudest at the apex.

The **second heart sound** (S_2) occurs with closure of the semilunar valves and signals the end of systole. The aortic component of the second sound (A_2) slightly precedes the pulmonic component (P_2). Although it is heard over all the precordium, S_2 is loudest at the base.

Effect of Respiration. The volume of right and left ventricular systole is just about equal, but this can be affected by respiration. To learn this, consider the phrase:

MoRe to the Right heart,
Less to the Left

That means that during inspiration, intrathoracic pressure is decreased. This pushes more blood into the vena cava, increasing venous return to the right side of the heart, which increases right ventricular stroke volume. The increased volume prolongs right ventricular systole and delays pulmonic valve closure.

Meanwhile on the left side, a greater amount of blood is sequestered in the lungs during inspiration. This momentarily decreases the amount returned to the left side of the heart, decreasing left ventricular stroke volume. The decreased volume shortens left ventricular systole and allows the aortic valve to close a bit earlier. When the aortic valve closes significantly earlier than the pulmonic valve, you can hear the two components separately. This is a *split* S_2.

Extra Heart Sounds

Third Heart Sound (S_3). Normally diastole is a silent event. However, in some conditions, ventricular filling creates vibrations that can be heard over the chest. These vibrations are S_3. The S_3 occurs when the ventricles are resistant to filling during the early rapid filling phase (protodiastole). This occurs immediately after S_2, when the AV valves open and atrial blood first pours into the ventricles. (See a complete discussion of S_3 in Table 17–6.)

Fourth Heart Sound (S_4). The S_4 occurs at the end of diastole, at presystole, when the ventricle is resistant to filling. The atria contract and push blood into a noncompliant ventricle. This creates vibrations that are heard as S_4. The S_4 occurs just before S_1.

Murmurs

Blood circulating through normal cardiac chambers and valves usually makes no noise. However, some conditions create turbulent blood flow and collision currents. These result in a murmur, much like a pile of stones or a sharp turn in a stream creates a noisy water flow. A murmur is a gentle, blowing, swooshing sound that can be heard on the chest wall. Conditions resulting in a murmur are as follows:

1. Velocity of blood increases (flow murmur), e.g., in exercise, thyrotoxicosis
2. Viscosity of blood decreases, e.g., in anemia
3. Structural defects in the valves or unusual openings occur in the chambers

Characteristics of Sound

All heart sounds are described by:

1. Frequency (pitch)—heart sounds are described as high pitched or low pitched, although these terms are relative because all are low-frequency sounds, and you need a good stethoscope to hear them
2. Intensity (loudness)—loud or soft
3. Duration—very short for heart sounds; silent periods are longer
4. Timing—systole or diastole

CONDUCTION

Of all organs, the heart has a unique ability—automaticity. The heart can contract by itself, independent of any signals or stimulation from the body. The heart contracts in response to an electrical current conveyed by a conduction system (Fig. 17–8). Specialized cells in the sinoatrial (SA) node near the superior vena cava initiate an electrical impulse. (Because the SA node has an intrinsic rhythm, it is the "pacemaker.") The current flows in an orderly sequence, first across the atria to the AV node low in the atrial septum. There, it is delayed slightly so that the atria have time to contract before the ventricles are stimulated. Then, the impulse travels to the bundle of His, the right and left bundle branches, and then through the ventricles.

The electrical impulse stimulates the heart to do its work, which is to contract. A small amount of electricity spreads to the body surface, where it can be measured and recorded on the electrocardiograph (ECG). The ECG waves are arbitrarily labeled PQRST, which stand for the following elements:

P wave—depolarization of the atria
PR interval—from the beginning of the P wave to the beginning of the QRS complex (the time necessary

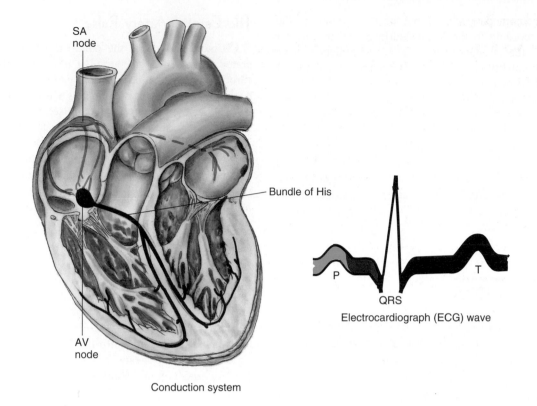

SA node

Bundle of His

AV node

QRS

P

T

Electrocardiograph (ECG) wave

17–8

Conduction system

for atrial depolarization plus time for the impulse to travel through the AV node to the ventricles)

QRS complex—depolarization of the ventricles

T wave—repolarization of the ventricles

Electrical events slightly *precede* the mechanical events in the heart. The ECG juxtaposed on the cardiac cycle is illustrated in Figure 17–6.

PUMPING ABILITY

In the resting adult, the heart normally pumps between 4 and 6 L of blood per minute throughout the body. This **cardiac output** equals the volume of blood in each sys-

tole (called the stroke volume) times the number of beats per minute (rate). This is described as:

$$CO = SV \times R$$

The heart can alter its cardiac output to adapt to the metabolic needs of the body. Preload and afterload affect the heart's ability to increase cardiac output.

Preload is the venous return that builds during diastole. It is the length to which the ventricular muscle is stretched at the end of diastole (Fig. 17–9).

When the volume of blood returned to the ventricles is increased (as when exercise stimulates skeletal muscles to contract and force more blood back to the heart), the muscle bundles are stretched beyond their normal resting

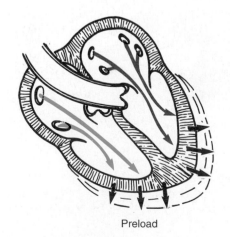

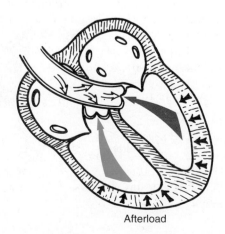

17–9

Preload

Afterload

state to accommodate. The force of this stretch is the preload. According to the Frank-Starling law, the greater the stretch, the stronger is the heart's contraction. This increased contractility results in an increased volume of blood ejected (increased stroke volume).

Afterload is the opposing pressure the ventricle must generate to open the aortic valve against the higher aortic pressure. It is the resistance against which the ventricle must pump its blood. Once the ventricle is filled with blood, the ventricular end diastolic pressure is 5 to 10 mm Hg, whereas that in the aorta is 70 to 80 mm Hg. To overcome this difference, the ventricular muscle *tenses* (isovolumic contraction). After the aortic valve opens, rapid ejection occurs.

THE NECK VESSELS

Cardiovascular assessment includes the survey of vascular structures in the neck—the carotid artery and the jugular veins (Fig. 17–10). These vessels reflect the efficiency of cardiac function.

The Carotid Artery Pulse

Chapter 9 describes the pulse as a pressure wave generated by each systole pumping blood into the aorta. The carotid artery is a central artery, i.e., it is close to the heart. Its timing closely coincides with ventricular systole. (Assessment of the peripheral pulses is found in Chapter 18, and blood pressure assessment is found in Chapter 9.)

The **carotid artery** is located in the groove between the trachea and the sternomastoid muscle, medial to and alongside that muscle. Note the characteristics of its waveform (Fig. 17–11): a smooth rapid upstroke, a summit that is rounded and smooth, and a downstroke that is more gradual and that has a dicrotic notch caused by closure of the aortic valve (marked D in the figure).

Jugular Venous Pulse and Pressure

The **jugular veins** empty unoxygenated blood directly into the superior vena cava. Since no cardiac valve exists to separate the superior vena cava from the right atrium, the jugular veins give information about activity on the right side of the heart. Specifically, they reflect filling pressure and volume changes. Since volume and pressure

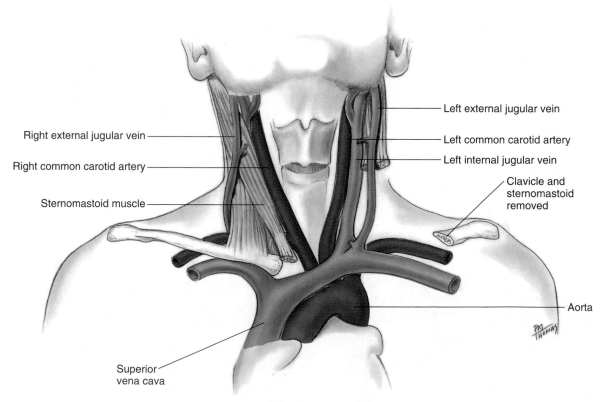

Right external jugular vein

Right common carotid artery

Sternomastoid muscle

Left external jugular vein

Left common carotid artery

Left internal jugular vein

Clavicle and sternomastoid removed

Aorta

Superior vena cava

NECK VESSELS

17–10

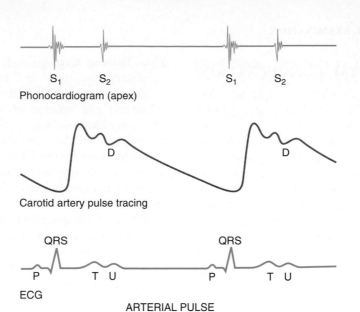

Phonocardiogram (apex)

Carotid artery pulse tracing

ECG

17–11

ARTERIAL PULSE

increase when the right side of the heart fails to pump efficiently, the jugular veins expose this.

Two jugular veins are present in each side of the neck (see Fig. 17–10). The larger **internal jugular** lies deep and medial to the sternomastoid muscle. It is usually not visible, although its diffuse pulsations may be seen in the sternal notch when the person is supine. The **external jugular** vein is more superficial; it lies lateral to the sternomastoid muscle, above the clavicle.

Although an arterial pulse is caused by a forward propulsion of blood, the jugular pulse is different. The jugular pulse results from a backwash, a waveform moving backward caused by events upstream. The jugular pulse has five components (Fig. 17–12):

Jugular Pulse	Reflects	Results from
A wave	Atrial contraction	Some blood flows backward to the vena cava during right atrial contraction
C wave	Ventricular contraction	Backflow from bulging upward of tricuspid valve when it closes at beginning of ventricular systole (not from neighboring carotid artery pulsation)
X descent	Atrial relaxation	Right ventricle contracts (systole) and pulls bottom of atria downward
V wave	Passive atrial filling	Increasing volume of atrial filling and increased pressure
Y descent	Passive ventricular filling	Tricuspid valve opens and blood flows from RA to RV

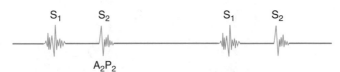

Phonocardiogram

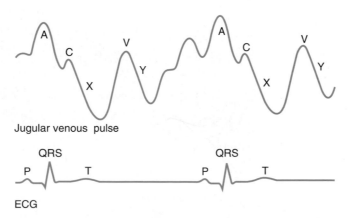

Jugular venous pulse

ECG

17–12

VENOUS PULSE

DEVELOPMENTAL CONSIDERATIONS

Infants and Children

The fetal heart functions early; it begins to beat at the end of 3 weeks gestation. The lungs are nonfunctional, but the fetal circulation compensates for this (Fig. 17–13). Oxygenation takes place at the placenta, and the arterial blood is returned to the right side of the heart. There is no point in pumping all this freshly oxygenated blood through the lungs, so it is rerouted in two ways. First, about two-thirds of it is shunted through an opening in the atrial septum, the **foramen ovale**, into the left side of the heart, where it is pumped out through the aorta. Second, the rest of the oxygenated blood is pumped by the right side of the heart out via the pulmonary artery, but it is detoured through the **ductus arteriosus** to the aorta. Because they are both pumping into the systemic circulation, the right and left ventricles are equal in weight and muscle wall thickness.

Inflation and aeration of the lungs at birth produces circulatory changes. Now the blood is oxygenated through the lungs rather than through the placenta. The foramen ovale closes within the 1st hour because of the new lower pressure in the right side of the heart than in the left side. The ductus arteriosus closes later, usually within 10 to 15 hours of birth. Now, the left ventricle has the greater workload of pumping into the systemic circulation, so that when the baby has reached 1 year of age, the left ventricle's mass increases to reach the adult ratio of 2:1, left ventricle to right ventricle.

The heart's position in the chest is more horizontal in the infant than in the adult; thus the apex is higher, located at the fourth left intercostal space (Fig. 17–14). It reaches the adult position when the child reaches age 7.

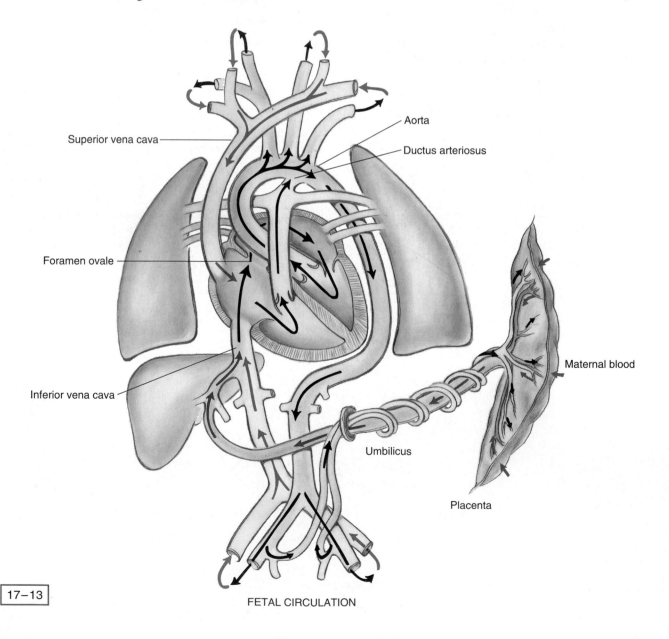

17–13

FETAL CIRCULATION

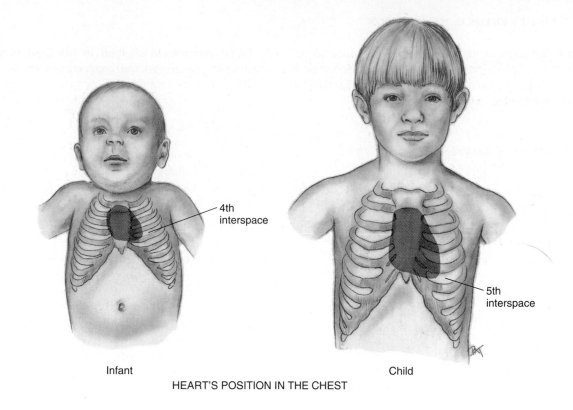

4th
interspace

5th
interspace

Infant   Child

17–14   HEART'S POSITION IN THE CHEST

The Pregnant Female

Blood volume increases by 30 to 40 percent during pregnancy, with the most rapid expansion occurring during the second trimester. This creates an increase in stroke volume and cardiac output and an increased pulse rate of 10 to 15 beats per minute. Despite the increased cardiac output, arterial blood pressure decreases in pregnancy due to peripheral vasodilatation. The blood pressure drops to its lowest point during the second trimester, then rises after that. The blood pressure varies with the person's position, as described on p. 531.

The Aging Adult

It is difficult to isolate the "aging process" of the cardiovascular system *per se* because it is so closely interrelated with lifestyle, habits, and diseases. We now know that lifestyle is a modifying factor in the development of cardiovascular disease; smoking, diet, alcohol use, exercise patterns, and stress have an influence on coronary artery disease. Lifestyle also affects the aging process; cardiac changes once thought to be due to aging are partially due to the sedentary lifestyle accompanying aging (Fig. 17–15).

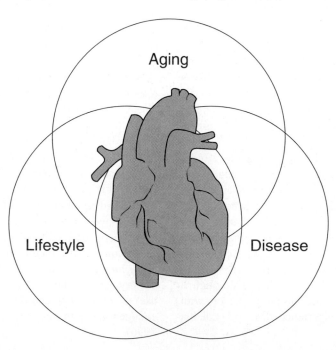

Aging

Lifestyle   Disease

17–15

What is left to be attributed to the aging process alone? When studies exclude people with clinical or occult heart disease (Lakatta, Gerstenblith, Weisfeldt, 1997), the following hemodynamic "aging process" emerges.

Hemodynamic Changes with Aging

- From age 20 to 60, systolic blood pressure tends to increase by about 20 mm Hg, and by another 20 mm Hg between ages 60 and 80, (Wei, 1992). This is due to stiffening of the large arteries, which, in turn, is due to calcification of vessel walls (arteriosclerosis). This stiffening creates an increase in pulse wave velocity because the less compliant arteries cannot store the volume ejected.
- The overall size of the heart does not increase with age, but left ventricular wall thickness increases somewhat. This is an adaptive mechanism to accommodate the vascular stiffening mentioned earlier that creates an increased workload on the heart.
- No significant change in diastolic pressure occurs with age. A rising systolic pressure with a relatively constant diastolic results in an increase in pulse pressure (the difference between the two).
- No change in resting heart rate occurs with aging.
- Cardiac output at rest is not changed with aging.
- There is a decreased ability of the heart to augment cardiac output with exercise. This is shown by a decreased maximum heart rate with exercise and diminished sympathetic response. Noncardiac factors also cause a decrease in maximum work performance with aging: decrease in skeletal muscle performance, increase in muscle fatigue, increased sense of dyspnea. Chronic exercise conditioning will modify many of the aging changes in cardiovascular function (Lakatta, et al., 1997).

Arrhythmias. The presence of supraventricular and ventricular arrhythmias increases with age. Ectopic beats are common in aging people; while these are usually asymptomatic in healthy older people, they may compromise cardiac output and blood pressure when disease is present (Lakatta, et al., 1997).

Tachyarrhythmias may not be tolerated as well in older people. The myocardium is thicker and less compliant, and early diastolic filling is impaired at rest (Wei, 1992). Thus, it may not tolerate a tachycardia as well because of shortened diastole. Another consequence is that tachyarrhythmias may further compromise a vital organ whose function already has been affected by aging or disease. For example, a ventricular tachycardia produces a 40 to 70 percent decrease in cerebral blood flow. Although a younger person may tolerate this, an older person with cerebrovascular disease may experience syncope (Lakatta et al., 1997).

ECG. Age-related changes in the ECG occur due to histologic changes in the conduction system. These include:

- Prolonged P-R interval (first-degree AV block) and prolonged Q-T interval, but the QRS interval is unchanged
- Left axis deviation due to age-related mild LV hypertrophy and fibrosis in left bundle branch
- Increased incidence of bundle branch block (Lakatta et al., 1997).

Although the hemodynamic changes associated with aging alone do not seem severe or portentous, the fact remains that the incidence of cardiovascular disease increases with age. The incidence of coronary artery disease increases sharply with advancing age and accounts for about half of the deaths of older people. Hypertension (systolic > 160 mm Hg and diastolic > 95 mm Hg) and heart failure also increase with age (Wei, 1992). Certainly, lifestyle habits (smoking, lack of exercise, diet) play a significant role in the acquisition of heart disease. Also, increasing the physical activity of older adults, even at a moderate level, is associated with a reduced risk of death from cardiovascular diseases and respiratory illnesses (Kushi et al., 1997). Both points underscore the need for health teaching as an important treatment parameter.

TRANSCULTURAL CONSIDERATIONS

Heart disease and stroke account for more than one-third of all deaths among individuals from culturally diverse backgrounds. Under age 35, heart disease mortality for Native Americans is approximately twice as high as that for all other Americans. Black men are nearly twice as likely to die from stroke as white men, and their death rate from stroke is more than double that of other ethnic groups (Office of Minority Health, 1990).

The National Health and Nutrition Examination Survey (NHANES I) showed that the incidence of coronary heart disease (CHD) differed between blacks and whites (Gillum, Mussolino, Madans, 1997). Middle-aged black women (25 to 54 years) were at a significantly higher risk for CHD than white women, while older black women (65 to 74 years) were at a significantly lower risk for CHD than white women. For men in both age groups, blacks had a lower risk of CHD than their white counterparts. However, death from CHD did not differ significantly between racial groups.

The major risk factors for heart disease and stroke are high blood pressure, smoking, high cholesterol levels, obesity, and diabetes. In addition, for some women, the use of oral contraceptives and lack of postmenopausal endogenous estrogen are risk factors (Arnstein et al., 1996).

Hypertension. Blacks, Puerto Ricans, Cubans, and Mexicans have a higher incidence of hypertension than whites. The prevalence of hypertension in blacks is 1.4 times greater than in whites despite a decline in mean blood pressure in blacks between 1960 and 1980. Reduction of blood pressure can reduce the incidence of CHD among both whites and blacks. Although data pertaining to Asian Americans are scarce, Filipinos of all gender and age categories have higher blood pressure than whites. Data available on Japanese Americans and Native Americans indicate that a lower prevalence of hypertension exists among members of these groups (Office of Minority Health, 1990).

Smoking. More black and Hispanic men smoke than white men, although whites tend to be heavier smokers. The prevalence of smoking in other ethnic groups tends to be lower than in whites (Office of Minority Health, 1990).

Serum Cholesterol. Serum cholesterol levels among blacks and whites are approximately the same at birth, but during childhood, blacks have higher serum cholesterol levels than whites (5 mg/100 ml). These differences reverse during adulthood when blacks have lower serum cholesterol levels than whites. Black men tend to have higher rates of high-density lipoprotein (HDL), which reduces cardiovascular risks. Certain Hispanic subgroups, such as Mexican Americans and Puerto Ricans, exhibit higher cholesterol levels than whites. Both Native Americans and Japanese Americans show lower cholesterol levels than whites (Office of Minority Health, 1990).

Obesity. Obesity is defined as an excess of 20 percent of standard weight for age and height. This risk factor for cardiovascular disease is more common among black women than other groups, but obesity is also problematic among many Hispanic women.

Diabetes. Diabetes is a contributing factor to 300,000 deaths per year. It has been ranked seventh among leading causes of death in the United States. In many Native American tribes, more than 20 percent of members have diabetes, ten times the incidence found among the general population. A dramatic increase in obesity among Native Americans has accompanied the increase in diabetes that has been documented during the past 50 years. In one tribe, the Pima Indians, nearly 50 percent of those over 35 years of age are affected. The complications of diabetes, especially kidney disease, blindness, and amputation, are known to have increased severity in Native Americans (Office of Minority Health, 1990).

Diabetes is 33 percent more common among blacks than among whites, with black women having an incidence of 50 percent more cases of diabetes than white women. Obesity among diabetic black women is also higher than the incidence found among nonblack women. The complications of diabetes, such as blindness and kidney disease, are more frequent in blacks than in whites. Unfortunately, the infants of pregnant diabetic black women also are at greater risk, with the death rate being three times higher for infants born to black diabetic mothers than to white diabetic mothers (Office of Minority Health, 1990).

Hispanics in the United States have three times the risk of developing diabetes as do non-Hispanic whites. Research-based data on Hispanics are scarce because early studies included Hispanics as part of the white population.

Among Japanese men in the United States 40 years of age or older, researchers find the diabetes rate to be as high as 10 to 14 percent, and Japanese living in the United States have, as a group, more than twice the incidence of diabetes as Japanese living in Japan. Japanese, Chinese, and Filipino Americans who are born in the United States have higher death rates from diabetes than their native-born counterparts. The blame for what these statistics reveal is being placed on the high-fat content of a typical American diet. Japanese diets in the United States, for example, are much higher in both animal and total fat content than those in Japan.

SUBJECTIVE DATA

1. Chest pain
2. Dyspnea
3. Orthopnea
4. Cough
5. Fatigue
6. Cyanosis or pallor

7. Edema
8. Nocturia
9. Past cardiac history
10. Family cardiac history
11. Personal habits (cardiac risk factors)

Examiner Asks	Rationale

1 **Chest pain.** Any **chest pain** or tightness?

- Onset: When did it start? How long have you had it *this* time? Had this type of pain before? How often?
- Location: where did the pain start? Does the pain radiate to any other spot?
- Character: How would you describe it? Crushing, stabbing, burning, viselike? (Allow the person to offer adjectives before you suggest them.) (Note if uses clenched fist to describe pain.)

- Pain brought on by: activity—what type; rest; emotional upset; after eating; during sexual intercourse; with cold weather?
- Any associated symptoms: sweating, ashen gray or pale skin, heart skips beat, shortness of breath, nausea or vomiting, racing of heart?

- Pain made worse by moving the arms or neck, breathing, lying flat?

- Pain relieved by rest or nitroglycerin? How many tablets?

Angina, an important cardiac symptom, occurs when heart's vascular supply cannot keep up with metabolic demand. Chest pain also may have pulmonary, musculoskeletal, or gastrointestinal origin; it is important to differentiate.

"Clenched fist" sign is characteristic of angina.

Diaphoresis, pallor.
Palpitations, dyspnea, nausea, tachycardia.
Try to differentiate pain of cardiac versus noncardiac origin.

2 **Dyspnea.** Any shortness of breath?

- What type of activity and how much brings on shortness of breath? How much activity brought it on 6 months ago?
- Onset: Does the shortness of breath come on unexpectedly?
- Duration: constant or does it come and go?
- Seem to be affected by position: lying down?
- Awaken you from sleep at night?

- Does the shortness of breath interfere with activities of daily living?

Dyspnea. Dyspnea on exertion (DOE)—Quantify exactly, e.g., DOE after walking two level blocks.
Paroxysmal.
Constant or intermittent.
Recumbent.
Paroxysmal nocturnal dyspnea (PND) occurs with heart failure. Lying down increases volume of intrathoracic blood, and the weakened heart cannot accommodate the increased load. Classically, the person awakens after 2 hours of sleep, arises, and flings open a window with the perception of needing fresh air.

3 **Orthopnea.** How many pillows do you use when sleeping or lying down?

Orthopnea is the need to assume a more upright position to breathe. Note the exact number of pillows used.

4 **Cough.** Do you have a **cough?**

- Duration: How long have you had it?
- Frequency: Is it related to time of day?
- Type: dry, hacking, barky, hoarse, or congested?
- Do you cough up mucus? Color? Any odor? Blood tinged?

Sputum production, mucoid or purulent. Hemoptysis is often of a pulmonary disorder but also occurs with mitral stenosis.

- Associated with: activity, position (lying down), anxiety, talking?
- Does activity make it better or worse (sit, walk, exercise)?
- Relieved by rest or medication?

5 **Fatigue.** Do you seem to tire easily? Able to keep up with your family and coworkers?

- Onset: When did fatigue start? Sudden or gradual? Has any *recent* change occurred in energy level?

Examiner Asks	Rationale
• Fatigue related to time of day: all day, morning, evening?	Fatigue due to decreased cardiac output is worse in the evening, whereas fatigue from anxiety or depression occurs all day or is worse in the morning.
6 **Cyanosis or pallor.** Ever noted your facial skin turn blue or ashen?	**Cyanosis** or **pallor** occurs with myocardial infarction or low cardiac output states due to decreased tissue perfusion.
7 **Edema.** Any swelling of your feet and legs? • Onset: When did you first notice this? • Any recent change? • What time of day does the swelling occur? Do your shoes feel tight at the end of day? • How much swelling would you say there is? Are both legs equally swollen? • Does the swelling go away with: rest, elevation, after a night's sleep? • Any associated symptoms, such as shortness of breath? If so, does the shortness of breath occur before leg swelling or after?	**Edema** is dependent when due to congestive heart failure. Cardiac edema is worse at evening and better in morning after elevating legs all night.
8 **Nocturia.** Do you awaken at night with an urgent need to urinate? How long has this been occurring? Any recent change?	**Nocturia**—Recumbency at night promotes fluid reabsorption and excretion; this occurs with heart failure in the person who is ambulatory during the day.
9 **Past cardiac history.** Any **past history** of: hypertension, elevated blood cholesterol or triglycerides, heart murmur, congenital heart disease, rheumatic fever or unexplained joint pains as child or youth, recurrent tonsillitis, anemia? • Ever had heart disease? When was this? Treated by medication or heart surgery? • Last ECG, stress ECG, serum cholesterol measurement, other heart tests?	
10 **Family cardiac history.** Any **family history** of: hypertension, obesity, diabetes, coronary artery disease (CAD), sudden death at younger age?	
11 **Personal habits (cardiac risk factors).** • Nutrition: Please describe your usual daily diet. (Note if this diet is representative of the basic food groups, the amount of calories, cholesterol, and any additives such as salt.) What is your usual weight? Has there been any recent change? • Smoking: Do you smoke cigarettes or other tobacco? At what age did you start? How many packs per day? For how many years have you smoked this amount? Have you ever tried to quit? If so, how did this go? • Alcohol: How much alcohol do you usually drink each week, or each day? When was your last drink? What was the number of drinks that episode? Have you ever been told you had a drinking problem? • Exercise: What is your usual amount of exercise each day or week? What type of exercise (state type or sport)? If a sport, what is your usual amount (light, moderate, heavy)? • Drugs: Do you take any antihypertensives, beta-blockers, calcium channel blockers, digoxin, diuretics, aspirin/anticoagulants, over-the-counter, or street drugs?	**Risk factors for coronary artery disease**—Collect data regarding elevated serum cholesterol, elevated blood pressure, blood sugar levels above 130 or known diabetes mellitus, obesity, cigarette smoking, low activity level. Also, postmenopausal women have an increased risk of CAD due to loss of the protective effect of estrogen on the lipid profile.

Examiner Asks	Rationale

ADDITIONAL HISTORY FOR INFANTS

1 How was the mother's health during pregnancy: any unexplained fever, rubella first trimester, other infection, hypertension, drugs taken?

2 Have you noted any cyanosis while nursing, crying? Is the baby able to eat, nurse, or finish bottle without tiring?

To screen for heart disease in infant, focus on feeding. Note fatigue during feeding. Infant with congestive heart failure takes fewer ounces each feeding; becomes dyspneic with sucking; may be diaphoretic, then falls into exhausted sleep; awakens after a short time hungry again.

3 **Growth:** Has this baby grown as expected by growth charts and about the same as siblings or peers?

Poor weight gain.

4 **Activity:** Were this baby's motor milestones achieved as expected? Is the baby able to play without tiring? How many naps does the baby take each day? How long does a nap last?

ADDITIONAL HISTORY FOR CHILDREN

1 **Growth:** Has this child grown as expected by growth charts?

Poor weight gain.

2 **Activity:** Is this child able to keep up with siblings or age-mates? Is the child willing or reluctant to go out to play? Is the child able to climb stairs, ride a bike, walk a few blocks? Does the child squat to rest during play or to watch television, or assume a knee-chest position while sleeping?
Have you noted "blue spells" during exercise?

Fatigue. Record specific limitations.

Cyanosis.

3 Has the child had any unexplained joint pains or unexplained fever?

4 Does the child have frequent headaches, nosebleeds?

5 Does the child have frequent respiratory infections? How many per year? How are they treated? Have any of these proved to be streptococcal infections?

6 **Family history:** Does the child have a sibling with heart defect?

7 **Past history:** Is anyone in the child's family known to have chromosomal abnormalities, e.g., Down syndrome?

ADDITIONAL HISTORY FOR THE PREGNANT FEMALE

1 Have you had any high blood pressure during this or earlier pregnancies?
   ● What was your usual blood pressure level before pregnancy? How has your blood pressure been monitored during the pregnancy?
   ● If high blood pressure, what treatment has been started?

Examiner Asks	Rationale

- Any associated symptoms: weight gain, protein in urine, swelling in feet, legs, or face?

2 Have you experienced any faintness or dizziness with this pregnancy?

ADDITIONAL HISTORY FOR THE AGING ADULT

1 Do you have any known heart or lung disease: hypertension, CAD, chronic emphysema, or bronchitis?
- What efforts to treat this have been started?
- Usual symptoms changed recently? Does your illness interfere with activities of daily living?

2 Do you take any medications for your illness such as digitalis? Aware of side effects? Have you recently stopped taking your medication? Why?

Noncompliance may be related to side effects or lack of finances.

3 **Environment:** Does your home have any stairs? How often do you need to climb them? Does this have any effect on activities of daily living?

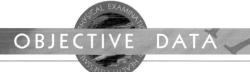

OBJECTIVE DATA

Preparation

To evaluate the carotid arteries, the person can be sitting up. To assess the jugular veins and the precordium, the person should be supine with the head and chest slightly elevated.

Stand on the person's right side; this will facilitate your hand placement and auscultation of the precordium.

The room must be warm—chilling makes the person uncomfortable, and shivering interferes with heart sounds. Take scrupulous care to ensure *quiet;* heart sounds are very soft, and any ambient room noise masks them.

Ensure the female's privacy by keeping her breasts draped. The female's left breast overrides part of the area you will need to examine. Gently displace the breast upward, or ask the woman to hold it out of the way.

When performing a regional cardiovascular assessment, use this order:

1. Pulse and blood pressure (see Chapter 9)
2. Extremities (see Peripheral Vascular Assessment, Chapter 18)
3. Neck vessels
4. Precordium

The logic of this order is that you will begin observations peripherally and move in toward the heart. For choreography of these steps in the complete physical examination, see Chapter 26.

Equipment Needed

Marking pen
Small centimeter ruler
Stethoscope with diaphragm and bell endpieces
Alcohol swab (to clean endpiece)

THE NECK VESSELS

The Carotid Arteries

Palpate the carotid artery

Located central to the heart, the carotid artery yields important information on cardiac function.

Palpate each carotid artery medial to the sternomastoid muscle in the neck (Fig. 17–16). Avoid excessive pressure on the carotid sinus area higher in the neck; excessive vagal stimulation here could slow down the heart rate, especially in older adults. Take care to palpate gently. Palpate only one carotid artery at a time to avoid compromising arterial blood to the brain.

Carotid sinus hypersensitivity is the condition in which pressure over the carotid sinus leads to a decreased heart rate, decreased BP, and cerebral ischemia with syncope. This may occur in older adults with hypertension or occlusion of the carotid artery.

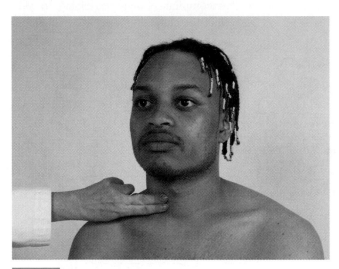

17–16

Feel the contour and amplitude of the pulse. Normally the contour is smooth with a rapid upstroke and slower downstroke, and the normal strength is 2+ or moderate (see Chapter 18). Your findings should be the same bilaterally.

Diminished pulse feels small and weak; occurs with decreased stroke volume.

Increased pulse feels full and strong; occurs with hyperkinetic states (see Table 18–1).

Auscultate the carotid artery

For persons middle-aged or older, or who show symptoms or signs of cardiovascular disease, auscultate each carotid artery for the presence of a **bruit** (Fig. 17–17). This is a blowing, swishing sound indicating blood flow turbulence; normally none is present.

A bruit indicates turbulence due to a local vascular cause, e.g., atherosclerotic narrowing.

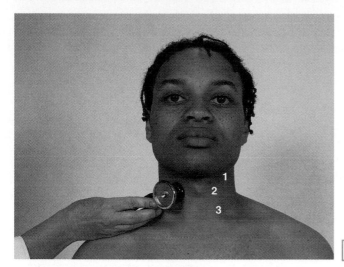

17–17

Keep the neck in a neutral position. Lightly apply the bell of the stethoscope over the carotid artery at three levels: 1) the angle of the jaw, 2) the midcervical area, and 3) the base of the neck (see Fig. 17–17). Avoid compressing the artery because this could create an artificial bruit, and it could compromise circulation if the carotid artery is already narrowed by atherosclerosis. Ask the person to hold his or her breath briefly while you listen so that tracheal breath sounds do not mask or mimic a carotid artery bruit. Sometimes you can hear normal heart sounds transmitted to the neck; do not confuse these with a bruit.

A carotid bruit is audible when the lumen is occluded by one-half to two-thirds. Bruit loudness increases as the atherosclerosis worsens until the lumen is occluded by two-thirds. After that, bruit loudness decreases. When the lumen is completely occluded, the bruit disappears. Thus, absence of a bruit does not ensure absence of a carotid lesion.

A murmur sounds much the same but is caused by a cardiac disorder. Some aortic valve murmurs radiate to the neck and must be distinguished from a local bruit.

The Jugular Veins

Inspect the jugular venous pulse

From the jugular veins you can assess the **central venous pressure (CVP)** and thus the heart's efficiency as a pump. Although the external jugular vein is easier to see, the internal (especially the right) is attached more directly to the superior vena cava and thus is more reliable for assessment. You cannot see the internal jugular vein itself, but you can see its pulsation.

Position the person supine anywhere from a 30- to a 45-degree angle, wherever you can best see the pulsations. In general, the higher the venous pressure, the higher the position you need. Remove the pillow to avoid flexing the neck; the head should be in the same plane as the trunk. Turn the person's head slightly away from the examined side, and direct a strong light tangentially onto the neck to highlight pulsations and shadows.

Normal Range of Findings

Abnormal Findings

Note the external jugular veins overlying the sternomastoid muscle. In some persons, the veins are not visible at all; whereas in others, they are full in the supine position. As the person is raised to a sitting position, these external jugulars flatten and disappear, usually at 45 degrees.

Now look for pulsations of the internal jugular veins in the area of the suprasternal notch or around the origin of the sternomastoid muscle around the clavicle. You must be able to distinguish internal jugular vein pulsation from that of the carotid artery. It is easy to confuse them because they lie close together. Use the guidelines shown in Table 17–1.

Table 17–1 · Characteristics of Jugular Versus Carotid Pulsations

	Internal Jugular Pulse	Carotid Pulse
1. **Location**	Lower, more lateral, under or behind the sternomastoid muscle	Higher and medial to this muscle
2. **Quality**	Undulant and diffuse, two visible waves per cycle	Brisk and localized, one wave per cycle
3. **Respiration**	Varies with respiration; its level descends during inspiration when intrathoracic pressure is decreased	Does not vary
4. **Palpable**	No	Yes
5. **Pressure**	Light pressure at the base of the neck easily obliterates	No change
6. **Position of person**	Level of pulse drops and disappears as the person is brought to a sitting position	Unaffected

Estimate the jugular venous pressure

Think of the jugular veins as a CVP manometer attached directly to the right atrium. You can "read" the CVP at the highest level of pulsations (Fig. 17–18). Use the angle of Louis (sternal angle) as an arbitrary reference point, and compare it with the highest level of venous pulsation. Hold a vertical ruler on the sternal angle. Align a straight edge on the ruler like a T-square, and adjust the level of the horizontal straight edge to the level of pulsation. Read the level of intersection on the vertical ruler; normal jugular venous pulsation is 2 cm or less above the sternal angle. Also state the person's position, e.g., "internal jugular vein pulsations 3 cm above sternal angle when elevated 30 degrees."

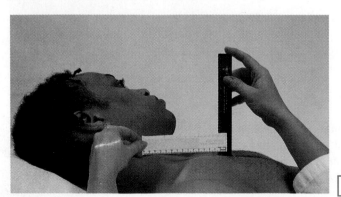

17–18

Unilateral distention of external jugular veins is due to local cause, e.g., kinking or aneurysm.

Full distended external jugular veins above 45 degrees signify increased CVP.

Elevated pressure is a level of pulsation that is more than 3 cm above the sternal angle while at 45 degrees. This occurs with heart failure.

▶ Normal Range of Findings	Abnormal Findings

If you cannot find the internal jugular veins, use the external jugular veins and note the point where they look collapsed. Be aware that the technique of estimating venous pressure is difficult and is not always a reliable predictor of CVP. Consistency in grading among examiners is difficult to achieve.

If venous pressure is elevated, or if you suspect congestive heart failure, perform **hepatojugular reflux** (Fig. 17–19). Position the person comfortably supine and instruct him or her to breathe quietly through an open mouth. Hold your right hand on the right upper quadrant of the person's abdomen just below the rib cage. Watch the level of jugular pulsation as you push in with your hand. Exert firm sustained pressure for 30 seconds. This empties venous blood out of the liver sinusoids and adds its volume to the venous system. If the heart is able to pump this additional volume (i.e., if no elevated CVP is present), the jugular veins will rise for a few seconds, then recede back to previous level.

If heart failure is present, the jugular veins will elevate and stay elevated as long as you push.

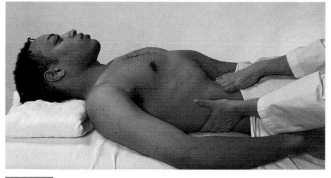

17–19

Hepatojugular Reflux

THE PRECORDIUM

Inspection

Inspect the anterior chest

Arrange tangential lighting to accentuate any flicker of movement.

Pulsations. You may or may not see the **apical impulse,** the pulsation created as the left ventricle rotates against the chest wall during systole. When visible, it occupies the fourth or fifth intercostal space, at or inside the midclavicular line. It is easier to see in children and in those with thinner chest walls.

A **heave** or **lift** is a sustained forceful thrusting of the ventricle during systole. It occurs with ventricular hypertrophy due to increased workload. A right ventricular heave is seen at the sternal border; a left ventricular heave is seen at the apex (see Table 17–7.)

Palpation

Palpate the apical impulse

(This used to be called the point of maximal impulse, or PMI. Since some abnormal conditions may cause a maximal impulse to be felt elsewhere on the chest, use the term **apical impulse** specifically for the apex beat.)

Localize the apical impulse precisely using one finger pad (Fig. 17–20). Asking the person to "exhale and then hold it" aids the examiner in locating the pulsation. You may need to roll the person midway to the left to find it; note that this also displaces the apical impulse farther to the left.

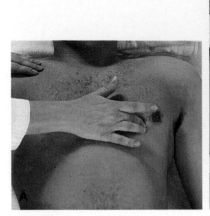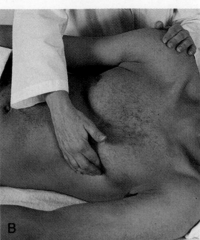

17–20

The Apical Impulse

Note

- Location—The apical impulse should occupy only one interspace, the fourth or fifth, and be at or medial to the midclavicular line
- Size—normally 1 cm × 2 cm
- Amplitude—normally a short, gentle tap
- Duration—short, normally occupies only first half of systole

Cardiac enlargement:

- Left ventricular dilatation (volume overload) displaces impulse down and to left, and increases size more than one space.
- Increased force and duration but no change in location occurs with left ventricular hypertrophy and no dilatation (pressure overload) (see Table 17–7).

Not palpable with pulmonary emphysema due to overriding lungs.

The apical impulse is palpable in about half of adults. It is not palpable in obese persons or in persons with thick chest walls. With high cardiac output states (anxiety, fever, hyperthyroidism, anemia), the apical impulse increases in amplitude and duration.

Palpate across the precordium

Using the palmar aspects of your four fingers, gently palpate the apex, the left sternal border, and the base, searching for any other pulsations (Fig. 17–21). Normally none occur. If any are present, note the timing. Use the carotid artery pulsation as a guide, or auscultate as you palpate.

A **thrill** is a palpable vibration. It feels like the throat of a purring cat. The thrill signifies turbulent blood flow and accompanies loud murmurs. Absence of a thrill, however, does not necessarily rule out the presence of a murmur.

Normal Range of Findings	Abnormal Findings

Accentuated first and second heart sounds and extra heart sounds also may cause abnormal pulsations.

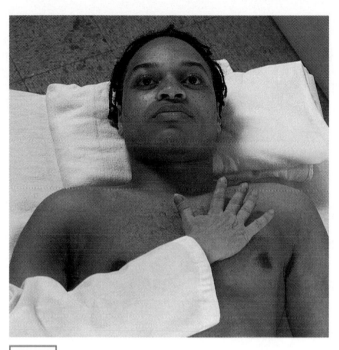

17–21

Percussion

Percussion is used to outline the heart's borders, but it often has been displaced by the chest x-ray study. The x-ray study is much more accurate in detecting heart enlargement. When the right ventricle enlarges, it does so in the anteroposterior diameter, which is better seen on x-ray film. Also, percussion is of limited usefulness with the female breast tissue or in an obese person or a person with a muscular chest wall.

However, there are times when your percussing hands are the only tools you have with you, such as in an outpatient setting, extended care facility, or the person's home. When you need to search for cardiac enlargement, place your stationary finger in the person's fifth intercostal space over on the left side of the chest near the anterior axillary line. Slide your stationary hand toward yourself, percussing as you go, and note the change of sound from resonance over the lung to dull (over the heart). Normally, the left border of cardiac dullness is at the midclavicular line in the fifth interspace and slopes in toward the sternum as you progress upward so that by the second interspace the border of dullness coincides with the left sternal border. The right border of dullness normally matches the sternal border.

Cardiac enlargement is due to increased ventricular volume or wall thickness, and occurs with hypertension, CAD, heart failure, and cardiomyopathy.

Auscultation

Identify the auscultatory areas where you will listen. These include the four traditional valve "areas" (Fig. 17–22). The valve areas are not over the actual anatomic locations of the valves but are the sites on the chest wall where sounds produced by the valves are best heard. The sound radiates with the direction of blood flow.

- Second right interspace—aortic valve area
- Second left interspace—pulmonic valve area
- Left lower sternal border—tricuspid valve area
- Fifth interspace at around left midclavicular line—mitral valve area

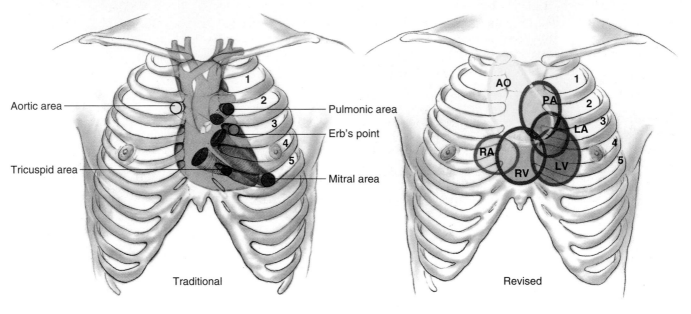

AUSCULTATORY AREAS

17–22

Do not limit your auscultation to only four locations. Sounds produced by the valves may be heard all over the precordium. (For this reason, many experts even discourage the naming of the valve areas.) Thus, learn to inch your stethoscope in a **Z** pattern, from the base of the heart across and down, then over to the apex. Or start at the apex and work your way up. Include the sites shown in Figure 17–22.

Recall the characteristics of a good stethoscope (see Chapter 8). Clean the endpieces with an alcohol swab; you will use both endpieces. Although all heart sounds are low frequency, the diaphragm is for relatively higher pitched sounds, and the bell is for relatively lower pitched ones.

Before you begin, alert the person, "I always listen to the heart in a number of places on the chest. Just because I am listening a long time, it does not necessarily mean that something is wrong."

Concentrate, and listen selectively to *one sound at a time.* Consider that at least two, and perhaps three or four, sounds may be happening in less than 1 second. You cannot process everything at once. Begin with the diaphragm endpiece and use the following routine: (1) Note the rate and rhythm; (2) identify S_1

▶ | N o r m a l   R a n g e   o f   F i n d i n g s | A b n o r m a l   F i n d i n g s

and S_2; (3) assess S_1 and S_2 separately; (4) listen for extra heart sounds; and (5) listen for murmurs.

Note the rate and rhythm

The rate ranges normally from 60 to 100 beats per minute. (Review the full discussion of the pulse in Chapter 9 and the normal rates across age groups.) The rhythm should be regular, although **sinus arrhythmia** occurs normally in young adults and children. With sinus arrhythmia, the rhythm varies with the person's breathing, increasing at the peak of inspiration and slowing with expiration. Note any other irregular rhythm. If one occurs, check if it has any pattern, or if it is totally irregular.

When you notice any irregularity, check for a **pulse deficit** by auscultating the apical beat while simultaneously palpating the radial pulse. Count a serial measurement (one after the other) of apical beat and radial pulse. Normally, every beat you hear at the apex should perfuse to the periphery and be palpable. The two counts should be identical. When different, subtract the radial rate from the apical and record the remainder as the pulse deficit.

Identify S_1 and S_2

This is important because S_1 is the start of systole and thus serves as the reference point for the timing of all other cardiac sounds. Usually, you can identify S_1 instantly because you hear a pair of sounds close together (lub-dup), and S_1 is the first of the pair. This guideline works, except in the cases of the tachyarrhythmias (rates > 100 per minute). Then the diastolic filling time is shortened, and the beats are too close together to distinguish. Other guidelines to distinguish S_1 from S_2 are

- S_1 is louder than S_2 at the apex; S_2 is louder than S_1 at the base.
- S_1 coincides with the carotid artery pulse. Feel the carotid gently as you auscultate at the apex; the sound you hear as you feel each pulse is S_1 (Fig. 17–23).
- S_1 coincides with the R wave (the upstroke of the QRS complex) if the person is on an ECG monitor.

Premature beat—an isolated beat is early, or a pattern occurs in which every third or fourth beat sounds early.

Irregularly irregular—no pattern to the sounds; beats come rapidly and at random intervals.

A **pulse deficit** signals a weak contraction of the ventricles, and occurs with atrial fibrillation, premature beats, and heart failure.

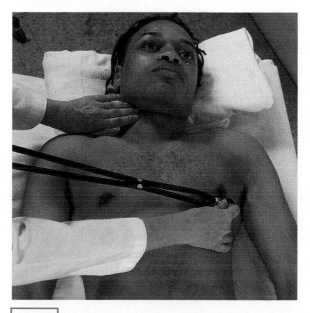

17–23

▶ |

Listen to S_1 and S_2 separately

Note whether each heart sound is normal, accentuated, diminished, or split. Inch your diaphragm across the chest as you do this.

First Heart Sound (S_1). Caused by closure of the AV valves, S_1 signals the beginning of systole. You can hear it over the entire precordium, although it is loudest at the apex (Fig. 17–24). (Sometimes the two sounds are equally loud at the apex, because S_1 is lower pitched than S_2.)

Causes of accentuated or diminished S_1 (see Table 17–2).
Both heart sounds are diminished with conditions that place an increased amount of tissue between the heart and your stethoscope: emphysema (hyperinflated lungs), obesity, pericardial fluid.

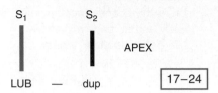

You can hear S_1 with the diaphragm with the person in any position and equally well in inspiration and expiration. A split S_1 is normal, but it occurs rarely. A split S_1 means you are hearing the mitral and tricuspid components separately. It is audible in the tricuspid valve area, the left lower sternal border. The split is very rapid, with the two components only 0.03 second apart.

Second Heart Sound (S_2). The S_2 is associated with closure of the semilunar valves. You can hear it with the diaphragm, over the entire precordium, although S_2 is loudest at the base (Fig. 17–25).

Accentuated or diminished S_2 (see Table 17–3).

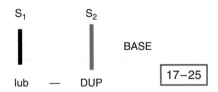

Splitting of S_2. A split S_2 is a normal phenomenon that occurs toward the end of inspiration in some people. Recall that closure of the aortic and pulmonic valves is nearly synchronous. Because of the effects of respiration on the heart described earlier, inspiration separates the timing of the two valves' closure, and the aortic valve closes 0.06 second before the pulmonic valve. Instead of one DUP, you hear a split sound—T-DUP (Fig. 17–26). During expiration, synchrony returns, and the aortic and pulmonic components fuse together. A split S_2 is heard only in the pulmonic valve area, the second left interspace.

SPLITTING OF THE SECOND HEART SOUND

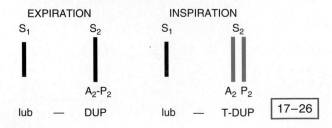

▶ Normal Range of Findings

Abnormal Findings

When you first hear the split S_2, do *not* be tempted to ask the person to hold his or her breath so that you can concentrate on the sounds. Breath-holding will only equalize ejection times in the right and left sides of the heart and cause the split to go away. Instead, concentrate on the split as you watch the person's chest rise up and down with breathing. The split S_2 occurs about every fourth heartbeat, fading in with inhalation and fading out with exhalation.

A **fixed split** is unaffected by respiration; the split is always there.

A **paradoxical split** is the opposite of what you would expect; the sounds fuse on inspiration and split on expiration (see Table 17–4).

Focus on systole, then on diastole, and listen for any extra heart sounds

Listen with the diaphragm, then switch to the bell, covering all auscultatory areas (Fig. 17–27). Usually, these are silent periods. When you do detect an extra heart sound, listen carefully to note its timing and characteristics. During systole, the **midsystolic click** (which is associated with mitral valve prolapse) is the most common extra sound (see Table 17–5). The third and fourth heart sounds occur in diastole; either may be normal or abnormal (see Table 17–6).

A pathologic S_3 (ventricular gallop) occurs with heart failure and volume overload; a pathologic S_4 (atrial gallop) occurs with CAD (see Table 17–6 for a full description).

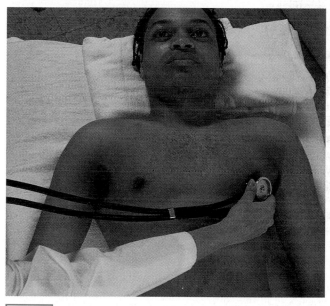

17–27

Listen for murmurs

A murmur is a blowing, swooshing sound that occurs with turbulent blood flow in the heart or great vessels. Except for the innocent murmurs described on the following page, murmurs are abnormal. If you hear a murmur, describe it by indicating these following characteristics:

Timing. It is crucial to define the murmur by its occurrence in systole or diastole. You must be able to identify S_1 and S_2 accurately to do this. Try to further describe the murmur as being in early, mid-, or late systole or diastole; throughout the cardiac event (termed pansystolic or holosystolic/pandiastolic or holodiastolic); and whether it obscures or muffles the heart sounds.

Study Tables 17–8 and 17–9 for a complete description of murmurs due to congenital defects and acquired valvular defects.

A systolic murmur may occur with a normal heart or with heart disease; a diastolic murmur always indicates heart disease.

|

Loudness. Describe the intensity in terms of six "grades." For example, record a grade ii murmur as "ii/vi."

Grade i—barely audible, heard only in a quiet room and then with difficulty
Grade ii—clearly audible, but faint
Grade iii—moderately loud, easy to hear
Grade iv—loud, associated with a thrill palpable on the chest wall
Grade v—very loud, heard with one corner of the stethoscope lifted off the chest wall
Grade vi—loudest, still heard with entire stethoscope lifted just off the chest wall

Pitch. Describe the pitch as high, medium, or low. The pitch depends on the pressure and the rate of blood flow producing the murmur.

Pattern. The intensity may follow a pattern during the cardiac phase, growing louder (crescendo), tapering off (decrescendo), or increasing to a peak and then decreasing (crescendo-decrescendo, or diamond shaped). Since the whole murmur is just milliseconds long, it takes practice to diagnose any pattern.

Quality. Describe the quality as musical, blowing, harsh, or rumbling.

> The murmur of mitral stenosis is rumbling, whereas that of aortic stenosis is harsh (see Table 17–9).

Location. Describe the area of maximum intensity of the murmur (where it is best heard) by noting the valve area or intercostal spaces.

Radiation. The murmur may be transmitted downstream in the direction of blood flow and may be heard in another place on the precordium, the neck, the back, or the axilla.

Posture. Some murmurs disappear or are enhanced by a change in position.
Some murmurs are common in healthy children or adolescents and are termed *innocent* or *functional*. **Innocent** indicates having no valvular or other pathologic cause; **functional** is due to increased blood flow in the heart, e.g., in anemia, fever, pregnancy, hyperthyroidism. The contractile force of the heart is greater in children. This increases blood flow velocity. The increased velocity plus a smaller chest measurement makes an audible murmur.

The innocent murmur is generally soft (grade ii), midsystolic, short, crescendo-decrescendo, and with a vibratory or musical quality ("vooot" sound like fiddle strings). Also, the innocent murmur is heard at the second or third left intercostal space and disappears with sitting, and the young person has no associated signs of cardiac dysfunction.

Although it is important to distinguish innocent murmurs from pathologic ones, it is best to suspect all murmurs as pathologic until they are proved otherwise. Diagnostic tests such as ECG, phonocardiogram, and echocardiogram are needed to establish an accurate diagnosis.

Change position

After auscultating in the supine position, roll the person toward his or her left side. Listen with the bell at the apex for the presence of any diastolic filling sounds i.e., the S_3 or S_4 (Fig. 17–28).

> S_3 and S_4, and the murmur of mitral stenosis sometimes may be heard only when on the left side.

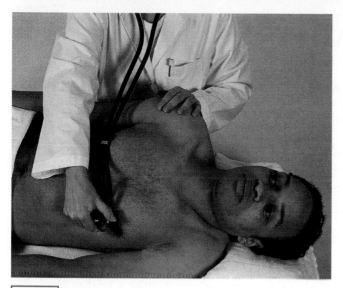

17–28

Ask the person to sit up, lean forward slightly, and exhale. Listen with the diaphragm firmly pressed at the base, right, and left sides. Check for the soft, high-pitched, early diastolic murmur of aortic or pulmonic regurgitation (Fig. 17–29).

Murmur of aortic regurgitation sometimes may be heard only when the person is leaning forward in the sitting position.

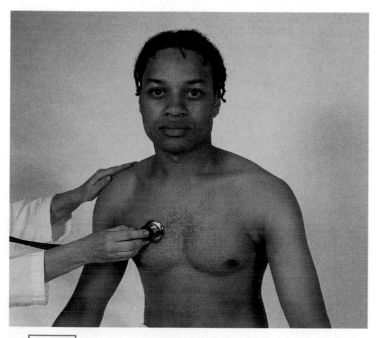

17–29

Normal Range of Findings	Abnormal Findings

 DEVELOPMENTAL CONSIDERATIONS

Infants

The transition from fetal to pulmonic circulation occurs in the immediate newborn period. Fetal shunts normally close within 10 to 15 hours but may take up to 48 hours. Thus, you should assess the cardiovascular system during the first 24 hours and again in 2 to 3 days.

Note any extracardiac signs that may reflect heart status (particularly in the skin), liver size, and respiratory status. The skin color should be pink to pinkish brown, depending on the infant's genetic heritage. If cyanosis occurs, determine its first appearance—at or shortly after birth versus after the neonatal period. Normally, the liver is not enlarged, and the respirations are not labored. Also, note the expected parameters of weight gain throughout infancy.

Palpate the apical impulse to determine the size and position of the heart. Since the infant's heart has a more horizontal placement, expect to palpate the apical impulse at the fourth intercostal space just lateral to the midclavicular line. It may or may not be visible.

The heart rate is best auscultated because radial pulses are hard to count accurately. Use the small (pediatric size) diaphragm and bell (Fig. 17–30). The heart rate may range from 100 to 180 per minute immediately after birth, then stabilize to an average of 120 to 140 per minute. Infants normally have wide fluctuations with activity, from 170 per minute or more with crying or being active to 70 to 90 per minute with sleeping. Variations are greatest at birth and are even more so with premature babies (see Table 9–3).

Failure of shunts to close, e.g., patent ductus arteriosus (PDA), atrial septal defect (ASD; see Table 17–8).

Cyanosis signals oxygen desaturation of congenital heart disease. Cyanosis at or just after birth suggests Fallot tetralogy, transposition of great vessels, severe septal defect, severe pulmonic stenosis, or tricuspid atresia.

The most important signs of heart failure in an infant are persistent tachycardia, tachypnea, and liver enlargement. Engorged veins, gallop rhythm, and pulsus alternans also are signs. Respiratory crackles (rales) is an important sign in adults but not in infants.

Failure to thrive occurs with cardiac disease.

The apex is displaced with:

- Cardiac enlargement, shifts to the left
- Pneumothorax, shifts away from affected side
- Diaphragmatic hernia, shifts usually to right because this hernia occurs more often on the left
- Dextrocardia, a rare anomaly in which the heart is located on right side of chest

Persistent tachycardia is >200 per minute in newborns, or >150 per minute in infants.

Bradycardia is <90 per minute in newborns or <60 in older infants or children. This causes a serious drop in cardiac output because the small muscle mass of their hearts cannot increase stroke volume significantly.

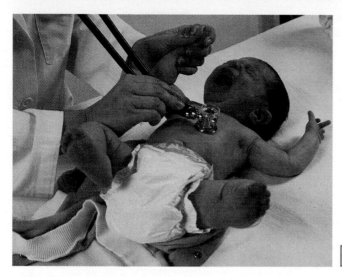

17–30

Expect the heart rhythm to have sinus arrhythmia, the phasic speeding up or slowing down with the respiratory cycle.

Rapid rates make it more challenging to evaluate heart sounds. Expect heart sounds to be louder in infants than in adults because of the infant's thinner chest wall. Also, S_2 has a higher pitch and is sharper than S_1. Splitting of S_2 just after the height of inspiration is common, not at birth, but beginning a few hours after birth.

Murmurs in the immediate newborn period do not necessarily indicate congenital heart disease. Murmurs are relatively common in the first 2 to 3 days because of fetal shunt closure. These murmurs are usually grade i or ii, systolic, accompany no other signs of cardiac disease, and disappear in 2 to 3 days. The murmur of PDA is a continuous machinery murmur, which disappears by 2 to 3 days. On the other hand, absence of a murmur in the immediate newborn period does not ensure a perfect heart; congenital defects can be present that are not signaled by an early murmur. It is best to listen frequently and to note and describe any murmur according to the characteristics listed on p. 526.

Children

Note any extracardiac or cardiac signs that may indicate heart disease: poor weight gain, developmental delay, persistent tachycardia, tachypnea, dyspnea on exertion, cyanosis, and clubbing. Note that clubbing of fingers and toes usually does not appear until late in the 1st year, even with severe cyanotic defects.

The apical impulse is sometimes visible in children with thin chest walls. Note any obvious bulge or any heave—These are not normal.

Investigate any irregularity except sinus arrhythmia.

Fixed split S_2 indicates ASD (see Table 17–8).

Persistent murmur after 2 to 3 days, holosystolic murmurs or those that last into diastole, and those that are loud all warrant further evaluation.

A precordial bulge to the left of the sternum with a hyperdynamic precordium signals cardiac enlargement. The bulge occurs because the cartilaginous rib cage is more compliant.

A substernal heave occurs with right ventricular enlargement, and an apical heave occurs with left ventricular hypertrophy.

▶ Normal Range of Findings

Abnormal Findings

Palpate the apical impulse: in the fourth intercostal space to the left of the midclavicular line until age 4; at the fourth interspace at the midclavicular line from age 4 to 6; and in the fifth interspace to the right of the midclavicular line at age 7 (Fig. 17–31).

The apical impulse moves laterally with cardiac enlargement.

Thrill (palpable vibration).

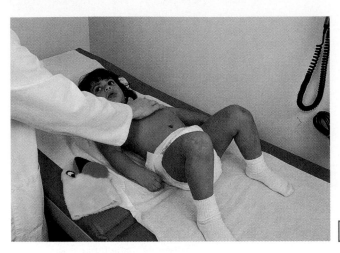

17–31

The average heart rate slows as the child grows older, although it is still variable with rest or activity (see Table 9–2).

The heart rhythm remains characterized by sinus arrhythmia. Physiologic S_3 is common in children (see Table 17–6). It occurs in early diastole, just after S_2, and is a dull soft sound that is best heard at the apex.

A **venous hum,** due to turbulence of blood flow in the jugular venous system, is common in normal children and has no pathologic significance. It is a continuous, low-pitched, soft hum, heard throughout the cycle, although it is loudest in diastole. Listen with the bell over the supraclavicular fossa at the medial third of the clavicle, especially on the right, or over the upper anterior chest. The venous hum is usually not affected by respiration, may sound louder when the child stands, and is easily obliterated by occluding the jugular veins in the neck with your fingers. The latter maneuver helps differentiate the insignificant venous hum from other organic cardiac murmurs, e.g., PDA.

Heart murmurs that are innocent (or functional) in origin are very common through childhood. Some authors say they have a 30 percent occurrence, and some authors say nearly all children may demonstrate a murmur at some time. Most innocent murmurs have these characteristics: soft, relatively short systolic ejection murmur; medium pitch; vibratory; best heard at the left lower sternal or midsternal border, with no radiation to the apex, base, or back.

It is important to distinguish innocent murmurs from pathologic ones. This may involve referral to another examiner or the performance of diagnostic tests such as the ECG or echocardiogram.

For the child whose murmur has been shown to be innocent, it is very important that the parents understand this completely. They need to believe that this murmur is just a "noise" and has no pathologic significance. Otherwise, the parents may become overprotective and limit activity for the child, which may result in the child developing a negative self-concept.

The Pregnant Female

The vital signs usually yield an increase in resting pulse rate of 10 to 15 beats per minute and a drop in blood pressure from the normal prepregnancy

▶ Normal Range of Findings	Abnormal Findings

level. The blood pressure decreases to its lowest point during the second trimester and then slowly rises during the third trimester. The blood pressure varies with position. It is usually lowest in left lateral recumbent position, a bit higher when supine (except for some who experience hypotension when supine), and highest when sitting (Cunningham et al., 1997).

Inspection of the skin often shows a mild hyperemia in light-skinned women because the increased cutaneous blood flow tries to eliminate the excess heat generated by the increased metabolism. Palpation of the apical impulse is higher and lateral compared with the normal position, as the enlarging uterus elevates the diaphragm and displaces the heart up and to the left and rotates it on its long axis.

Auscultation of the heart sounds shows changes due to the increased blood volume and workload:

- Heart sounds
  Exaggerated splitting of S_1 and increased loudness of S_1
  A loud, easily heard S_3
- Heart murmurs
  A systolic murmur in 90 percent, which disappears soon after delivery
  A soft, diastolic murmur heard transiently in 19 percent
  A continuous murmur arising from breast vasculature in 10 percent (Cunningham et al., 1997).

The last-mentioned murmur is termed a **mammary souffle** (pronounced SOOF′ f′l), which occurs near term or when the mother is lactating; it is due to increased blood flow through the internal mammary artery. The murmur is heard in the second, third, or fourth intercostal space, and it is continuous, although it is accented in systole. You can obliterate it by pressure with the stethoscope or one finger lateral to the murmur. This distinguishes it from the murmur of aortic stenosis, aortic insufficiency, or PDA.

The ECG has no changes except for a slight left axis deviation due to the change in the heart's position.

The Aging Adult

A gradual rise in systolic blood pressure is common with aging; the diastolic blood pressure stays fairly constant with a resulting widening of pulse pressure. Some older adults experience **orthostatic hypotension,** a sudden drop in blood pressure when rising to sit or stand.

Use caution in palpating and auscultating the carotid artery. Avoid pressure in the carotid sinus area, which could cause a reflex slowing of the heart rate. Also, pressure on the carotid artery could compromise circulation if the artery is already narrowed by atherosclerosis.

When measuring jugular venous pressure, view the right internal jugular vein. The aorta stiffens, dilates, and elongates with aging, which may compress the left neck veins and obscure pulsations on the left side (Fleg, 1990).

The chest often increases in anteroposterior diameter with aging. This makes it more difficult to palpate the apical impulse and to hear the splitting of S_2. The S_4 often occurs in older people with no known cardiac disease. Systolic murmurs are common, occuring in over 50% of aging people (Fleg, 1990).

Occasional premature ectopic beats are common and do not necessarily indicate underlying heart disease. When in doubt, obtain an ECG. However, consider that the ECG only records for one isolated minute in time and may need to be supplemented by a test of 24-hour ambulatory heart monitoring.

Abnormal Findings column:

Suspect pregnancy-induced hypertension with a sustained rise of 30 mm Hg systolic or 15 mm diastolic under basal conditions.

The S_3 is associated with heart failure and is always abnormal over age 35 (see Table 17–10).

SUMMARY CHECKLIST: Heart and Neck Vessels Exam

1: Neck

Carotid pulse—Observe and palpate

Observe jugular venous pulse

Estimate jugular venous pressure

2: Precordium

Inspection and palpation

   (1) Describe location of apical impulse

   (2) Note any heave (lift) or thrill

Auscultation

   (1) Identify anatomic areas where you listen

   (2) Note rate and rhythm of heartbeat

   (3) Identify S_1 and S_2 and note any variation

   (4) Listen in systole and diastole for any extra heart sounds

   (5) Listen in systole and diastole for any murmurs

   (6) Repeat sequence with bell

   (7) Listen at the apex with person in left lateral position

   (8) Listen at the base with person in sitting position

APPLICATION AND CRITICAL THINKING

SAMPLE CHARTING

 Subjective

No chest pain, dyspnea, orthopnea, cough, fatigue, or edema. No past history of hypertension, abnormal blood tests, heart murmur, or rheumatic fever in self. Last ECG 2 yrs. PTA, result normal. No stress ECG or other heart tests.

Family history: father with obesity, smoking, and hypertension, treated c̄ diuretic medication. No other family history significant for cardiovascular disease.

Personal habits: diet balanced in 4 food groups, 2 to 3 c. regular coffee/day; no smoking; alcohol, 1 to 2 beers occasionally on weekend; exercise, runs 2 miles, 3 to 4 ×/week; no prescription or OTC medications or street drugs.

 Objective

Neck. Carotids 2 + and = bilaterally. Internal jugular vein pulsations present when supine, and disappear when elevated to a 45° position.

Precordium. Inspection. No visible pulsations, no heave or lift.

Palpation. Apical impulse in 5th ics at left midclavicular line, no thrill.

Auscultation. Rate 68 beats per minute, rhythm regular, S_1–S_2 are normal, not diminished or accentuated, no S_3, no S_4 or other extra sounds, no murmurs.

CLINICAL CASE STUDY

Mr. N.V. is a 53-year-old white male woodcutter admitted to the CCU at University Medical Center (UMC) with chest pain.

▶ Subjective

1 year PTA—N.V. admitted to UMC with crushing substernal chest pain, radiating to L shoulder, accompanied by nausea, vomiting, diaphoresis.

Diagnosed as MI, hospitalized 7 days, discharged with nitroglycerin prn for anginal pain.

Did not return to work. Activity included walking 1 mile/day, hunting. Had occasional episodes of chest pain with exercise, relieved by rest.

1 day PTA—had increasing frequency of chest pain, about every 2 hours, lasting few minutes, saw pain as warning to go to MD.

Day of admission—severe substernal chest pain ("like someone sitting on my chest") unrelieved by rest. Saw personal MD, while in office had episode of chest pain as last year's, accompanied by diaphoresis, no N & V or SOB, relieved by 1 nitroglycerin. Transferred to UMC by paramedics. No further pain since admission 2 hours ago.

Family hx.—mother died of MI at age 57.

Personal habits—smokes 1½ pack cigarettes daily × 34 years, no alcohol, diet—trying to limit fat and fried food, still high in added salt.

▶ Objective

Extremities. Skin pink, no cyanosis. Upper extrem.—capillary refill sluggish, no clubbing. Lower extrem.—no edema, no hair growth 10 cm below knee bilaterally.

Pulses—

carotid	brachial	radial	femoral	popliteal	P.T.	D.P.	
2+	2+	2+	2+	0	0	1+	all = bilaterally

B/P R arm 104/66

Neck. External jugulars flat. Internal jugular pulsations present when supine and absent when elevated to 45°.

Precordium. Inspection. Apical impulse visible 5th ics, 7 cm left of midsternal line, no heave.

Palpation. Apical impulse palpable in 5th and 6th ics. No thrill.

Auscultation. Apical rate 92 regular, S_1-S_2 are normal, not diminished or accentuated, no S_3 or S_4, grade iii/vi systolic murmur present at left lower sternal border.

▶ ASSESSMENT

Substernal chest pain
Systolic murmur
Alteration in tissue perfusion R/T interruption in flow
Decreased cardiac output R/T reduction in stroke volume

NURSING DIAGNOSES COMMONLY ASSOCIATED WITH CARDIOVASCULAR DISORDERS

Diagnosis	Related Factors (Etiology)	Defining Characteristics (Symptoms and Signs)

Decreased cardiac output	Reduction in stroke volume as a result of
	  Electrical malfunction (alteration in conduction, rate, or rhythm)
	  Mechanical malfunction (alteration in afterload, inotropic changes in heart, or preload)
	  Structural problems secondary to congenital abnormalities, trauma
		Abnormal heart sounds
		Altered blood gases
		Changes in mental status
		Cool, clammy skin
		Cough
		Crackles (rales)
		Cyanosis or pallor
		Decreased peripheral pulses
		Dyspnea
		Dysrhythmias, electrocardiographic changes
		Edema, dependent
		Fatigue
		Frothy sputum
		Jugular vein distention
		Orthopnea
		Restlessness
		Syncope
		Tachycardia
		Urine output decreased
		Variations in hemodynamic readings
		Weight gain, sudden

Altered tissue perfusion	Exchange problems
	Hypervolemia
	Hypovolemia
	Interruption of flow
		Cardiopulmonary
		  Chest pain (relieved by rest)
		  Increased heart rate
		  Increased respiratory rate
		  Shortness of breath
		Cerebral
		  Alteration in thought processes
		  Blurred vision
		  Changes in level of consciousness
		  Confusion
		  Restlessness
		  Syncope/vertigo

Dysfunctional grieving	Effects of loss of function or body part Absence of anticipatory grieving Actual or perceived loss of health or social status, significant other, or valued object Multiple losses or crises Changes in lifestyle Decreased support system Thwarted grieving in response to a loss Lack of resolution of previous grieving response Ambivalent feelings toward loss	Changes in sleep patterns Feelings of anger, guilt, worthlessness, denial, sorrow Decreased interest in personal appearance Interference with life functioning Difficulty in expressing loss Fear of future Absence of emotion Suicidal thoughts Social withdrawal Weight loss Amenorrhea Decreased level of activity Reliving of past experiences Alteration in concentration Developmental regression Hyperactivity

Other Related Nursing Diagnoses

ACTUAL	RISK/WELLNESS
Activity intolerance (see Chapter 16)	**Risk**
Altered role performance	Risk for Injury
Altered sexuality patterns	
Anxiety (see Chapter 16)	**Wellness**
Fatigue	Health-seeking behavior R/T learning a low-fat diet
Fear	
Fluid volume deficit	
Fluid volume excess	
Impaired home maintenance management (see Chapter 12)	
Impaired physical mobility	
Ineffective breathing pattern	
Ineffective individual coping	
Noncompliance	
Pain (see Chapter 14)	
Powerlessness	
Self-care deficit	

ASSESSMENT VIDEO CRITICAL THINKING QUESTIONS

Saunders *Physical Examination and Health Assessment* Video Series—CARDIOVASCU-
LAR SYSTEM: HEART AND NECK VESSELS—will direct you to consider the following:

1. What cardiac risk factors are important to explore during the health history? How do they
affect cardiovascular function?

2. How would you modify your technique when assessing an older adult's neck vessels?

3. How do you describe sinus arrhythmia and what does it signify?

4. What heart sounds should you expect to hear in a person with aortic stenosis?

Table 17–2 VARIATIONS IN S₁

The intensity of S_1 depends on three factors: (1) position of AV valve at the start of systole, (2) structure of the valve leaflets, and (3) how quickly pressure rises in the ventricle.

	FACTOR	EXAMPLES
Loud (Accentuated) S_1 S_1 S_2	1. Position of AV valve at start of systole—wide open and no time to drift together 2. Change in valve structure—calcification of valve, needs increasing ventricular pressure to close the valve against increased atrial pressure	Hyperkinetic states where blood velocity is increased: exercise, fever, anemia, hyperthyroidism Mitral stenosis with leaflets still mobile
Faint (Diminished) S_1 S_1 S_2	1. Position of AV valve—delayed conduction from atria to ventricles. Mitral valve drifts shut before ventricular contraction closes it 2. Change in valve structure—extreme calcification, which limits mobility 3. More forceful atrial contraction into noncompliant ventricle; delays or diminishes ventricular contraction	First-degree heart block (prolonged PR interval) Mitral insufficiency Severe hypertension—systemic or pulmonary
Varying Intensity of S_1 S_1 S_2 S_1 S_2	1. Position of AV valve varies before closing from beat to beat 2. Atria and ventricles beat independently	Atrial fibrillation—irregularly-irregular rhythm Complete heart block with changing PR interval
Split S_1 S_1 S_2 T M	Mitral and tricuspid components are heard separately	Normal but uncommon

Table 17-3   VARIATIONS IN S₂

	CONDITION	EXAMPLE
Accentuated S₂ 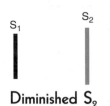	1. Higher closing pressure	Systemic hypertension, ringing or booming S_2
	2. Exercise and excitement increase pressure in aorta	
	3. Pulmonary hypertension	Mitral stenosis, heart failure
	4. Semilunar valves calcified but still mobile	Aortic or pulmonic stenosis
Diminished S₂	1. A fall in systemic blood pressure causes a decrease in valve strength	Shock
	2. Semilunar valves thickened and calcified, with decreased mobility	Aortic or pulmonic stenosis

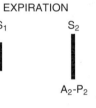 **Table 17-4   VARIATIONS IN SPLIT S₂**

Normal Splitting

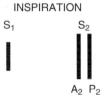

EXPIRATION S_1 S_2 A_2-P_2

INSPIRATION S_1 S_2 A_2 P_2

	CONDITION	EXAMPLE
Fixed Split 	A fixed split is unaffected by respiration; the split is always there	Atrial septal defect Right ventricular failure
Paradoxical Split 	Conditions that delay aortic valve closure cause the opposite of a normal split. In inspiration, P_2 is normally delayed so with a paradoxical split, the sounds fuse. In expiration you hear the split, in the order of P_2A_2.	Aortic stenosis Left bundle branch block Patent ductus arteriosus
Wide Split 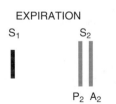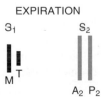	When the right ventricle has delayed electrical activation, the split is very wide on inspiration and is still there on expiration	Right bundle branch block (which delays P_2)

Table 17–5   SYSTOLIC EXTRA SOUNDS

Early systolic	Mid-/late systolic
Ejection click	Midsystolic (mitral) click
Aortic prosthetic valve sounds	

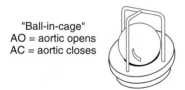

Aortic ejection click (apex and base)

Pulmonic ejection click (base only)

Expiration / Inspiration — S₁, S₂, Eⱼ

Ejection Click

The ejection click occurs early in systole at the start of ejection, because it results from opening of the semilunar valves. Normally, the SL valves open silently, but in the presence of stenosis (e.g., aortic stenosis, pulmonic stenosis) their opening makes a sound. It is short and high pitched, with a click quality, and is heard better with the diaphragm.

The aortic ejection click is heard at the second right interspace and apex, and may be loudest at the apex. Its intensity does not change with respiration. The pulmonic ejection click is best heard in the second left interspace and often grows softer with inspiration.

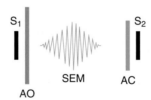

"Ball-in-cage"
AO = aortic opens
AC = aortic closes

S₁   AO   SEM   AC   S₂

Aortic Prosthetic Valve Sounds

As a sequela of modern technologic intervention for heart problems, some people now have *iatrogenically* induced heart sounds. The opening of an aortic ball-in-cage prosthesis (e.g., Starr-Edwards prosthesis) produces an early systolic sound. This sound is less intense with a tilting disc prosthesis (e.g., Bjork-Shiley prosthesis) and is absent with a tissue prosthesis (e.g., porcine).

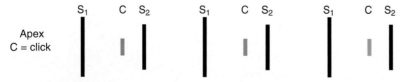

Apex
C = click

S₁   C   S₂   S₁   C   S₂   S₁   C   S₂

Midsystolic Click

Although it is systolic, this is not an ejection click. It is associated with **mitral valve prolapse,** in which the mitral valve leaflets not only close with contraction but balloon back up into the left atrium. During ballooning, the sudden tensing of the valve leaflets and the chordae tendineae creates the click.

The sound occurs mid- to late systole and is short and high pitched, with a click quality. It is best heard with the diaphragm, at the apex, but also may be heard at the left lower sternal border. The click usually is followed by a systolic murmur. The click and murmur move with postural change; when the person assumes a squatting position, the click may move closer to **S₂,** and the murmur may sound louder and delayed. The Valsalva maneuver also moves the click closer to **S₂.**

Table 17–6   DIASTOLIC EXTRA SOUNDS

Early diastole	Mid-diastole	Late diastole
Opening snap	Third heart sound	Fourth heart sound
Mitral prosthetic valve sound	Summation sound ($S_3 + S_4$)	Pacemaker-induced sound

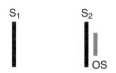

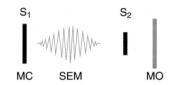 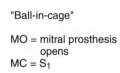

Opening Snap

Normally, the opening of the AV valves is silent. In the presence of stenosis, increasingly higher atrial pressure is required to open the valve. The deformed valve opens with a noise, the opening snap. It is sharp and high pitched, with a snapping quality. It sounds after S_2 and is best heard with the diaphragm at the third or fourth left interspace at the sternal border, less well at the apex.

The opening snap usually is not an isolated sound. As a sign of mitral stenosis, the opening snap usually ushers in the low-pitched diastolic rumbling murmur of that condition.

Mitral Prosthetic Valve Sound

An iatrogenic sound, the opening of a ball-in-cage mitral prosthesis gives an early diastolic sound, an opening click just after S_2. It is loud, is heard over the whole precordium, and is loudest at the apex and left lower sternal border.

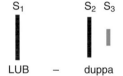 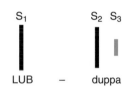

Third Heart Sound

The S_3 is a ventricular filling sound. It occurs in early diastole during the rapid filling phase. Your hearing quickly accommodates to the S_3, so it is best heard when you listen initially. It sounds after S_2 but later than an opening snap would be. It is a dull, soft sound, and it is low pitched, like "distant thunder." It is heard best in a quiet room, at the apex, with the bell held lightly (just enough to form a seal), and with the person in the left lateral position.

The S_3 can be confused with a split S_2. Use these guidelines to distinguish the S_3:

- Location—the S_3 is heard at the apex or left lower sternal border; the split S_2 at the base.
- Respiratory variation—the S_3 does not vary in timing with respirations; the split S_2 does.
- Pitch—the S_3 is lower pitched; the pitch of the split S_2 stays the same.

The S_3 may be normal (physiologic) or abnormal (pathologic). The **physiologic S_3 is heard frequently in children and young adults**; it occasionally may persist after age 40, especially in women. The normal S_3 usually disappears when the person sits up.

In adults, the S_3 is usually abnormal. The **pathologic S_3** is also called a **ventricular gallop** or an **S_3 gallop** and it persists when sitting up. The S_3 indicates decreased compliance of the ventricles, as in congestive heart failure. The S_3 may be the earliest sign of heart failure. The S_3 may originate from either the left or the right ventricle; a left-sided S_3 is heard at the apex in the left lateral position, and a right-sided S_3 is heard at the left lower sternal border with the person supine and is louder in inspiration.

The S_3 occurs also with conditions of volume overload, e.g., mitral regurgitation, aortic or tricuspid regurgitation. The S_3 is also found in high cardiac output states in the absence of heart disease, such as hyperthyroidism, anemia, and pregnancy. When the primary condition is corrected, the gallop disappears.

Table continued on following page

539

Table 17–6   DIASTOLIC EXTRA SOUNDS *Continued*

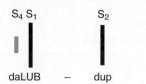

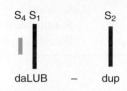

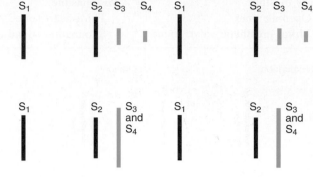

Fourth Heart Sound

The S_4 is a ventricular filling sound. It occurs when the atria contract late in diastole. It is heard immediately before S_1. This is a very soft sound, of very low pitch. You need a good bell, and you must listen for it. It is heard best at the apex, with the person in left lateral position.

A **physiologic** S_4 may occur in adults older than 40 or 50 with no evidence of cardiovascular disease, especially after exercise.

A **pathologic** S_4 is termed an **atrial gallop** or an S_4 **gallop.** It occurs with decreased compliance of the ventricle, e.g., coronary artery disease, cardiomyopathy, and with systolic overload (afterload), including outflow obstruction to the ventricle (aortic stenosis) and systemic hypertension. A left-sided S_4 occurs with these conditions. It is heard best at the apex, in the left lateral position.

A right-sided S_4 is less common. It is heard at the left lower sternal border and may increase with inspiration. It occurs with pulmonary stenosis or pulmonary hypertension.

Summation Sound

When both the pathologic S_3 and S_4 are present, a quadruple rhythm is heard. Often, in cases of cardiac stress, one response is tachycardia. During rapid rates, the diastolic filling time shortens and the S_3 and S_4 move closer together. They sound superimposed in mid-diastole, and you hear one loud, prolonged, summated sound, often louder than either S_1 or S_2.

EXTRACARDIAC SOUNDS

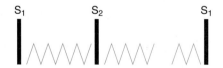

◀ Pericardial Friction Rub

Inflammation of the precordium gives rise to a friction rub. The sound is high pitched and scratchy, like sandpaper being rubbed. It is best heard with the diaphragm, with the person sitting up and leaning forward, and with the breath held in expiration.

A friction rub can be heard any place on the precordium but usually is best heard at the apex and left lower sternal border, places where the pericardium comes in close contact with the chest wall. Timing may be systolic and diastolic. The friction rub of pericarditis is common during the 1st week following a myocardial infarction and may last only a few hours.

▼ Table 17–7   ABNORMAL PULSATIONS ON THE PRECORDIUM

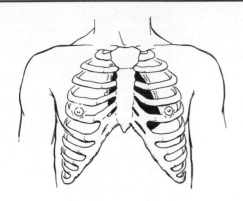

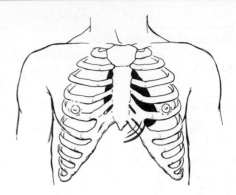

Base

A **thrill** in the second and third right interspaces occurs with severe aortic stenosis and systemic hypertension.

A **thrill** in the second and third left interspaces occurs with pulmonic stenosis and pulmonic hypertension.

Left Sternal Border

A **lift (heave)** occurs with right ventricular hypertrophy, as found in pulmonic valve disease, pulmonic hypertension, and chronic lung disease. You feel a diffuse lifting impulse during systole at the left lower sternal border. It may be associated with retraction at the apex, because the left ventricle is rotated posteriorly by the enlarged right ventricle.

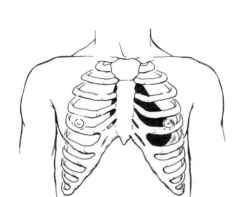

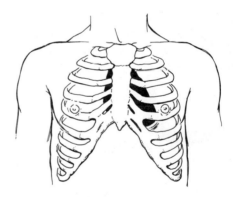

Apex

Cardiac enlargement displaces the apical impulse laterally and over a wider area when left ventricular hypertrophy and dilatation are present. This is **volume overload,** as in mitral regurgitation, aortic regurgitation, and left-to-right shunts.

Apex

The apical impulse is increased in force and duration but is not necessarily displaced to the left when left ventricular hypertrophy occurs alone without dilatation. This is **pressure overload,** as found in aortic stenosis or systemic hypertension.

Table 17–8 CONGENITAL HEART DEFECTS

	Description	Clinical Data

Patent Ductus Arteriosus (PDA)

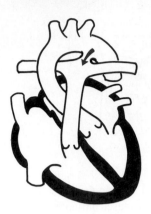

Persistence of the channel joining left pulmonary artery to aorta. This is normal in the fetus, and usually closes spontaneously within hours of birth.

S: Usually no symptoms in early childhood; growth and development are normal.

O: Blood pressure has wide pulse pressure and bounding peripheral pulses owing to rapid runoff of blood into low-resistance pulmonary bed during diastole. Thrill often palpable at left upper sternal border. The continuous murmur heard in systole and diastole is called a machinery murmur.

Atrial Septal Defect (ASD)

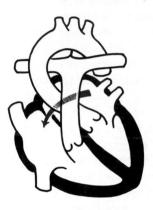

Abnormal opening in the atrial septum resulting usually in left-to-right shunt, and causing large increase in pulmonary blood flow.

S: Defect is remarkably well tolerated. Symptoms in infant are rare; growth and development normal. Children and young adults have mild fatigue and DOE.

O: Sternal lift often present. S_2 has fixed split, with P_2 often louder than A_2. Murmur is systolic, ejection, medium pitch, best heard at base in second left interspace. Murmur caused not by shunt itself but by increased blood flow through pulmonic valve.

Ventricular Septal Defect (VSD)

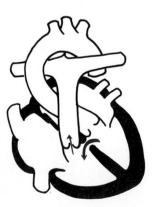

Abnormal opening in septum between the ventricles, usually subaortic area. The size and exact position vary considerably.

S: Small defects are asymptomatic. Infants with large defects have poor growth, slow weight gain, later look pale, thin, delicate. May have feeding problems, DOE, frequent respiratory infections, and, when the condition is severe, heart failure.

O: Loud, harsh holosystolic murmur, best heard at left lower sternal border, may be accompanied by thrill. Large defects also have soft diastolic murmur at apex (mitral flow murmur) owing to increased blood flow through mitral valve.

S = subjective data; O = objective data.

Table 17–8 CONGENITAL HEART DEFECTS *Continued*

	Description	Clinical Data
Tetralogy of Fallot 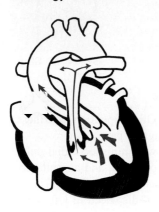	Four components: (1) right ventricular outflow stenosis, (2) VSD, (3) right ventricular hypertrophy, and (4) over-riding aorta. Result: shunts a lot of venous blood directly into aorta away from pulmonary system, so blood never gets oxygenated.	S: Severe cyanosis, not in first months of life but develops as infant grows and RV outflow (i.e., pulmonic) stenosis gets worse. Cyanosis with crying and exertion at first, then at rest. Uses squatting posture after starts walking. DOE common. Development is slowed. O: Thrill palpable at left lower sternal border. S_1 normal, S_2 has A_2 loud and P_2 diminished or absent. Murmur is systolic, loud, crescendo-decrescendo.
Coarctation of the Aorta 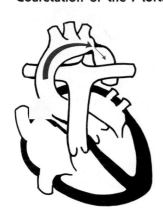	Severe narrowing of descending aorta, usually at the junction of the ductus arteriosus and the aortic arch, just distal to the origin of the left subclavian artery. Results in increased work load on left ventricle. Associated with defects of aortic valve in most cases, as well as associated patent ductus arteriosus; and associated ventricular septal defect (Braunwald, 1997).	S: In infants with associated lesions or symptoms, diagnosis occurs in first few months as symptoms of heart failure develop. For asymptomatic children and adolescents, growth and development are normal. Diagnosis usually accidental due to blood pressure findings. Adolescents may complain of vague lower extremity cramping that is worse with exercise. O: Upper extremity hypertension over 20 mm Hg higher than lower extremity measures is a hallmark of coarctation. Another important sign is absent or greatly diminished femoral pulses. A systolic murmur is heard best at the left sternal border, radiating to the back.

S = subjective data; O = objective data.

Table 17–9   MURMURS DUE TO VALVULAR DEFECTS

Midsystolic Ejection Murmurs

Due to forward flow through semilunar valves

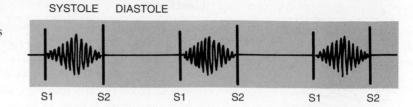

	Description	Clinical Data
Aortic Stenosis 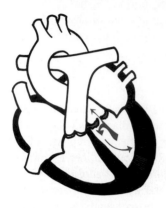	Calcification of aortic valve cusps restricts forward flow of blood during systole; LV hypertrophy develops.	S: Fatigue, DOE, palpitation, dizziness, fainting, anginal pain. O: Pallor, slow diminished radial pulse, low blood pressure, and auscultatory gap are common. Apical impulse sustained and displaced to left. Thrill in systole over second and third right interspaces and right side of neck. S_1 normal, often ejection click present, often paradoxical split S_2, S_4 present with LV hypertrophy. Murmur: Loud, harsh, midsystolic, crescendo-decrescendo, loudest at second right interspace, radiates widely to side of neck, down left sternal border, or apex.
Pulmonic Stenosis 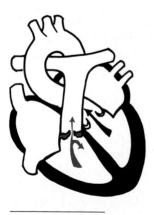	Calcification of pulmonic valve restricts forward flow of blood.	O: Thrill in systole at second and third left interspace, ejection click often present after S_1, diminished S_2 and usually with wide split, S_4 common with RV hypertrophy. Murmur: Systolic, medium pitch, coarse, crescendo-descrescendo (diamond shape), best heard at second left interspace, radiates to left and neck.

S = subjective data; O = objective data.

Pansystolic Regurgitant Murmurs

Due to backward flow of blood from area of higher pressure to one of lower pressure

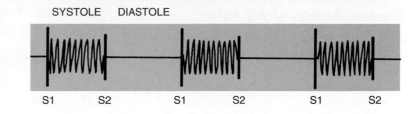

	Description	Clinical Data
Mitral Regurgitation 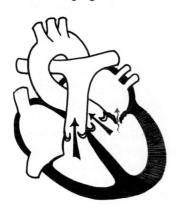	Stream of blood regurgitates back into LA during systole through incompetent mitral valve. In diastole, blood passes back into LV again along with new flow; results in LV dilatation and hypertrophy.	S: Fatigue, palpitation, orthopnea, PND O: Thrill in systole at apex. Lift at apex. Apical impulse displaced down and to left. S_1 diminished, S_2 accentuated, S_3 at apex often present. Murmur: Pansystolic, often loud, blowing, best heard at apex, radiates well to left axilla.
Tricuspid Regurgitation 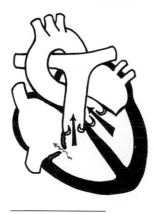	Backflow of blood through incompetent tricuspid valve into RA.	O: Engorged pulsating neck veins, liver enlarged. Lift at sternum if RV hypertrophy present, often thrill at left lower sternal border. Murmur: Soft, blowing, pansystolic, best heard at left lower sternal border, increases with inspiration.

S = subjective data; O = objective data.

Table continued on following page

Table 17-9   MURMURS DUE TO VALVULAR DEFECTS *Continued*

Diastolic Rumbles of AV Valves

Filling murmurs at low pressures, best heard with bell lightly touching skin

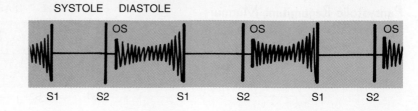

	Description	Clinical Data
Mitral Stenosis 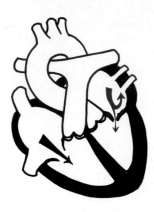	Calcified mitral valve will not open properly, impedes forward flow of blood into LV during diastole. Results in LA enlarged and LA pressure increased.	S: Fatigue, palpitations, DOE, orthopnea, occasional PND or pulmonary edema. O: Diminished, often irregular arterial pulse. Lift at apex, diastolic thrill common at apex. S_1 accentuated, opening snap after S_2 heard over wide area of precordium, followed by murmur. Murmur: Low-pitched diastolic rumble, best heard at apex, with person in left lateral position; does not radiate.
Tricuspid Stenosis 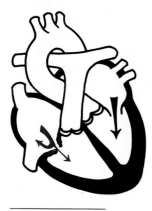	Calcification of tricuspid valve impedes forward flow into RV during diastole.	O: Diminished arterial pulse, jugular venous pulse prominent. Murmur: Diastolic rumble; best heard at left lower sternal border; louder in inspiration.

S = subjective data; O = objective data.

Table 17-9   MURMURS DUE TO VALVULAR DEFECTS *Continued*

Early Diastolic Murmurs

Due to SL valve incompetence

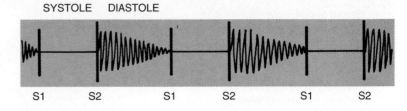

SYSTOLE   DIASTOLE

S1   S2   S1   S2   S1   S2

	Description	Clinical Data
Aortic Regurgitation 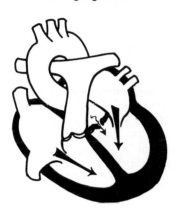	Stream of blood regurgitates back through incompetent aortic valve into LV during diastole. LV dilatation and hypertrophy due to increased LV stroke volume. Rapid ejection of large stroke volume into poorly filled aorta, then rapid runoff in diastole as part of blood pushed back into LV.	S: Only minor symptoms for many years, then rapid deterioration: DOE, PND, angina, dizziness. O: Bounding "water-hammer" pulse in carotid, brachial, and femoral arteries. Blood pressure has wide pulse pressure. Pulsations in cervical and suprasternal area, apical impulse displaced to left and down, apical impulse feels brief. Murmur starts almost simultaneously with S_2: soft high pitched, blowing diastolic, decrescendo, best heard at third left interspace at base, as person sits up and leans forward, radiates down.
Pulmonic Regurgitation 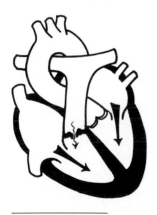	Backflow of blood through incompetent pulmonic valve, from pulmonary artery to RV.	Murmur has same timing and characteristics as that of aortic regurgitation, and is hard to distinguish on physical examination.

S = subjective data; O = objective data.

▼ Table 17–10   CLINICAL PORTRAIT OF CONGESTIVE HEART FAILURE

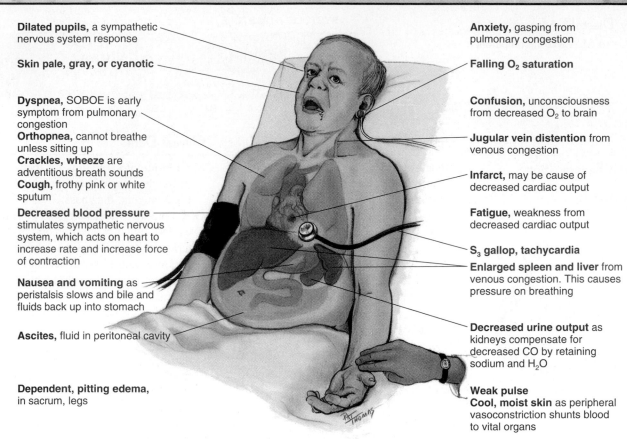

Dilated pupils, a sympathetic nervous system response

Skin pale, gray, or cyanotic

Dyspnea, SOBOE is early symptom from pulmonary congestion
Orthopnea, cannot breathe unless sitting up
Crackles, wheeze are adventitious breath sounds
Cough, frothy pink or white sputum

Decreased blood pressure stimulates sympathetic nervous system, which acts on heart to increase rate and increase force of contraction

Nausea and vomiting as peristalsis slows and bile and fluids back up into stomach

Ascites, fluid in peritoneal cavity

Dependent, pitting edema, in sacrum, legs

Anxiety, gasping from pulmonary congestion

Falling O$_2$ saturation

Confusion, unconsciousness from decreased O$_2$ to brain

Jugular vein distention from venous congestion

Infarct, may be cause of decreased cardiac output

Fatigue, weakness from decreased cardiac output

S$_3$ gallop, tachycardia

Enlarged spleen and liver from venous congestion. This causes pressure on breathing

Decreased urine output as kidneys compensate for decreased CO by retaining sodium and H$_2$O

Weak pulse
Cool, moist skin as peripheral vasoconstriction shunts blood to vital organs

   Decreased cardiac output occurs when the heart fails as a pump, and the circulation becomes backed up and congested.

   Signs and symptoms of congestive heart failure come from two basic mechanisms: (1) the heart's inability to pump enough blood to meet the metabolic demands of the body, and (2) the kidney's compensatory mechanisms of abnormal retention of sodium and water to compensate for the decreased cardiac output. This increases blood volume and venous return, which causes further congestion.

   Onset of heart failure may be: (1) acute, e.g., following a myocardial infarction when direct damage to the heart's contracting ability has occurred, or (2) chronic, e.g., with hypertension, when the ventricles must pump against chronically increased pressure.

Bibliography

Allen HD, Golinko RJ, Williams RG: Heart murmurs in children: When is a workup needed? Patient Care 28(7):123–150, Apr 15, 1994.

Arnstein PM, Buselli EF, Rankin SH: Women and heart attacks: Prevention, diagnosis, and care. Nurse Pract 21(5):57–69, May 1996.

Asprey DP: Evaluation of children with heart murmurs. Primary Care Pract 2(5):505–513, Sep–Oct 1998.

Behrman RE (Ed): Nelson Textbook of Pediatrics, 15th ed. Philadelphia, W.B. Saunders Company, 1996.

Braunwald E: Heart Disease: A Textbook of Cardiovascular Medicine, 5th ed. Philadelphia, W.B. Saunders Company, 1997.

Burnette MM, Meilahn E, Wing RR, Kuller LH: Smoking cessation, weight gain, and changes in cardiovascular risk factors during menopause: The healthy women study. Am J Public Health 88(1): 93–96, Jan 1998.

Campbell C: Comprehensive cardiovascular assessment. J Nurse Midwifery 40(2):137–149, Mar–Apr 1995.

Cunningham FG, MacDonald PC, Gant NF: Williams Obstetrics, 20th ed. Norwalk, CT, Appleton-Century-Crofts, 1997.

Daly TM, Dempster JS: Mitral valve prolapse. J Am Acad Nurse Pract 8(9):437–443, Sep 1996.

Davis L, Stecy P: Pharmacologic management of cardiovascular problems in women. J Nurse Midwifery 42(3):176–185, May–June 1997.

DeJong MJ: Cardiogenic shock. Am J Nurs 97(6):40–41, June 1997.

Evanoski CM: Myocardial infarction: The number one killer of women. Crit Care Nurs Clin North Am 9(4):489–496, Dec 1997.

Fleg JL: Diagnostic evaluations. *In* Abrams WB, Berkow R (Eds): The Merck Manual of Geriatrics. Rahway, NJ, Merck, Sharp and Dohme Research Laboratories, 1990.

Garrett AP: Assessing cardiovascular status in the older adult with cognitive impairments. J Cardiovasc Nurs 11(4):1–11, Jul 1997.

Gillum RF, Mussolino ME, Madans JH: Coronary heart disease incidence and survival in African-American women and men: The NHANES I epidemiologic follow-up study. Ann Intern Med 127(2):111–118, July 1997.

Gomel MK, Oldenburg B, Simpson JM, et al: Composite cardiovascular risk outcomes of a work-site intervention trial. Am J Public Health 87(4):673–676, Apr 1997.

Grenier M, Gagnon K, Genest J, Durand J, Durand L: Clinical comparison of acoustic and electronic stethoscopes and design of a new electronic stethoscope. Am J Cardiol 81(5):653–656, Mar 1, 1998.

Hanson MJ: Modifiable risk factors for coronary heart disease in women. Am J Critical Care 3(3): 177–186, 1994.

Hart ND, McLeod MF, Fruh S: Cardiovascular disease in women with diabetes. Adv Nurs Pract 5(8):32–35, Aug 1997.

Heckerling PS, Wiener SL, Wolfkiel CJ, et al: Precordial percussion for cardiomegaly. JAMA 270:1943, 1993.

Howes DG: Cardiovascular disease and women. Primary Care Pract 2(5):514–524, Sep–Oct 1998.

Hu FB, Stampfer MJ, Manson JE, et al: Dietary fat intake and the risk of coronary heart disease in women. N Engl J Med 337(21):1491–1499, Nov 1997.

Ishii K: Physical capacity assessment of the acute cardiovascular patient. J Cardiovasc Nurs 9(4):53–63, July 1995.

Karz JR, Kraft P, Fox K: Assessing a murmur, saving a life: Current trends in the management of hypertrophic cardiomyopathy. Nurse Pract 21(11):62–74, Nov 1996.

Kushi LH, Fee RM, Folsom AR, et al: Physical activity and mortality in postmenopausal women. JAMA 277(16):1287–1292, Apr 23/30, 1997.

Lakatta EG, Gerstenblith G, Weisfeldt ML: The aging heart: Structure, function, and disease. *In* Braunwald E (Ed): Heart Disease: A Textbook of Cardiovascular Medicine, 5th ed. Philadelphia, W.B. Saunders Company, 1997.

Mangione S, Nieman LZ: Cardiac auscultatory skills of internal medicine and family practice trainees. JAMA 278(9):717–722, Sep 3, 1997.

McGrath D: Coronary artery disease in women. Am J Nurse Pract 2(6): 7–23, 1998.

McGrath D: Mitral valve prolapse. Am J Nurs 97(5):40–41, May 1997.

Minarik PA: Cognitive assessment of the cardiovascular patient in the acute care setting. J Cardiovasc Nurs 9(4):36–52, July 1995.

Moody LY: Pediatric cardiovascular assessment and referral in the primary care setting. Nurse Pract 22(1):120–134, Jan 1997.

Nowazek V, Neeley M: Health assessment of the older patient. Crit Care Nurs Q 19(2):1–6, 1996.

Ober K, Carlson L, Anderson P: Cardiovascular risk factors in homeless adults. J Cardiovasc Nurs 11(4):50–59, Jul 1997.

Office of Minority Health: Heart Disease, Stroke, and Minorities. Closing the Gap. Public Health Service, Department of Health and Human Services. Washington, DC, Government Printing Office, 1990, pp 1–5.

O'Brien L: Angina pectoris. Am J Nurs 98(1):48–49, Jan 1998.

O'Hanlon-Nichols T: The adult cardiovascular system. Am J Nurs 97(12):34–40, Dec 1997.

O'Neal PV: How to spot early signs of cardiogenic shock. Am J Nurs 94(5):36–41, May 1994.

Perloff JK: Physical Examination of the Heart and Circulation, 2nd ed. Philadelphia, W.B. Saunders Company, 1990.

Reisz WG, Robinson, DJ: Evaluating nontraumatic chest pain. Primary Care Pract 2(5):455–471, Sep–Oct 1998.

Roberts C, Banning M: Risk factors for hypertension and cardiovascular disease. Nurs Standard 12(22):39–42, Feb 1998.

Talbot L, Curtis L: Cardiovascular assessment of the patient with renal problems. Am Nephrol Nurs Assoc J 23(5):445–456, Oct 1996.

Thompson PD: Cardiovascular screening: Tailoring the preparticipation exam. Phys Sports Med 24(6):47–50, June 1996.

Thurau R: Perceived gender bias in the treatment of cardiovascular disease. J Vasc Nurs 15(4):124–127, Dec 1997.

Tilkian AG, Conover MB: Understanding Heart Sounds and Murmurs, 3rd ed. Philadelphia, W.B. Saunders Company, 1993.

Trichopoulou A, Lagiou P: Worldwide patterns of dietary lipids intake and health implications. Am J Clin Nutr 66(45, Suppl):961S–964S, Oct 1997.

Verklan MT: Diagnostic techniques in cardiac disorders: Part I. Neonat Network 16(4):9–15, June 1997.

Verklan MT: Diagnostic techniques in cardiac disorders: Part II. Neonat Network 16(5):7–13, Aug 1997.

Wei JY: Age and the cardiovascular system. N Engl J Med 327(14): 1735–1739, Dec 10, 1992.

CHAPTER EIGHTEEN

Peripheral Vascular System and Lymphatic System

The vascular system consists of the vessels of the body. Vessels are tubes for transporting fluid, such as the blood or lymph. Any disease in the vascular system creates problems with delivery of oxygen and nutrients to the tissues and/or elimination of waste products from cellular metabolism.

ARTERIES

The heart pumps freshly oxygenated blood through the arteries to all body tissues. The pumping heart makes this a high-pressure system. The artery walls are strong, tough, and tense to withstand pressure demands. Arteries contain elastic fibers, which allow their walls to stretch with systole and recoil with diastole. Arteries also contain muscle fibers (vascular smooth muscle, or VSM), which control the amount of blood delivered to the tissues. The VSM contracts or dilates, which changes the diameter of the arteries to control the rate of blood flow.

Each heartbeat creates a pressure wave, which makes the arteries expand and then recoil. It is the recoil that propels blood through like a wave. All arteries have this pressure wave, or **pulse,** throughout their length, but you can feel it only at body sites where the artery lies close to the skin and over a bone. The following arteries are accessible to examination.

Temporal Artery. The temporal artery is palpated in front of the ear, as discussed in Chapter 11 with the head and neck.

Carotid Artery. The carotid artery is palpated in the groove between the sternomastoid muscle, and the trachea and is covered in Chapter 17 with the great vessels.

Arteries in the Arm. The major artery supplying the arm is the **brachial** artery, which runs in the biceps-triceps furrow of the upper arm and surfaces at the antecubital fossa in the elbow medial to the biceps tendon (Fig. 18–1). Immediately below the elbow, the brachial artery bifurcates into the **ulnar** and **radial** arteries. These run distally and form two arches supplying the hand, called the *superficial* and *deep palmar arches.* The radial pulse lies just medial to the radius at the wrist; the ulnar artery is in the same relation to the ulna, but it is deeper and often difficult to feel.

Arteries in the Leg. The major artery to the leg is the **femoral** artery, passing under the inguinal ligament (Fig. 18–2). The femoral artery travels down the thigh. At the lower thigh, it courses posteriorly; then it is termed the **popliteal** artery. Below the knee, the popliteal artery divides. The anterior tibial artery travels down the front of the leg on to the dorsum of the foot, where it becomes the **dorsalis pedis.** In back of the leg, the **posterior tibial** artery travels down behind the medial malleolus and in the foot forms the plantar arteries.

The function of the arteries is to supply oxygen and essential nutrients to the tissues. *Ischemia* is a deficient supply of oxygenated arterial blood to a tissue caused by obstruction of a blood vessel. A complete blockage leads to death of the distal tissue. A partial blockage creates an insufficient supply, and the ischemia may be apparent only at exercise when oxygen needs increase.

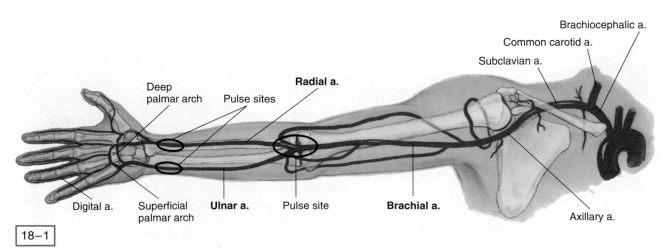

18–1

VEINS

The course of veins parallels that of arteries, but the body has more veins, and they lie closer to the skin surface. The following veins are accessible to examination.

Jugular Veins. Assessment of the jugular veins is presented in Chapter 17.

Veins in the Arm. Each arm has two sets of veins: superficial and deep. The superficial veins are in the subcutaneous tissue and are responsible for most of the venous return.

Veins in the Leg. The legs have three types of veins (Fig. 18–3).

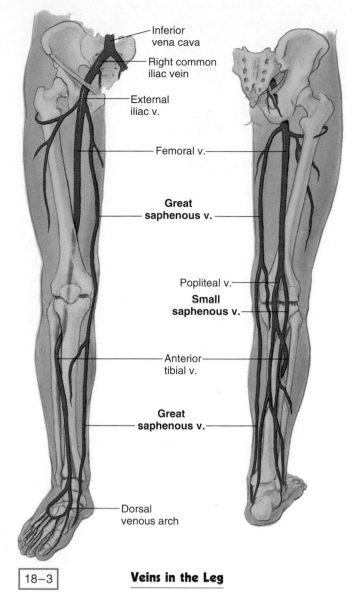

18–3   **Veins in the Leg**

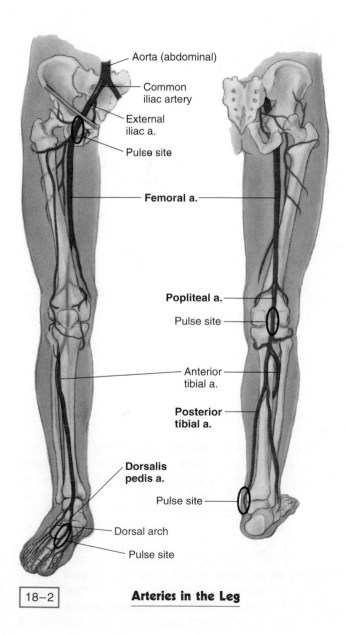

18–2   **Arteries in the Leg**

(1) The **deep veins** run alongside the deep arteries and conduct most of the venous return from the legs. These are the **femoral** and **popliteal** veins. As long as these veins remain intact, the superficial veins can be excised without harming the circulation.

(2) The **superficial veins** are the **great** and **small saphenous** veins. The great saphenous vein, inside the leg, starts at the medial side of the dorsum of the foot. You can see it ascend in front of the medial malleolus, then it crosses the tibia obliquely and ascends along the medial side of the thigh. The small saphenous vein, outside the leg, starts on the lateral side of the dorsum of the foot, ascends behind the lateral malleolus, up the back of the leg, where it joins the popliteal vein.

(3) **Perforators** (not illustrated) are connecting veins

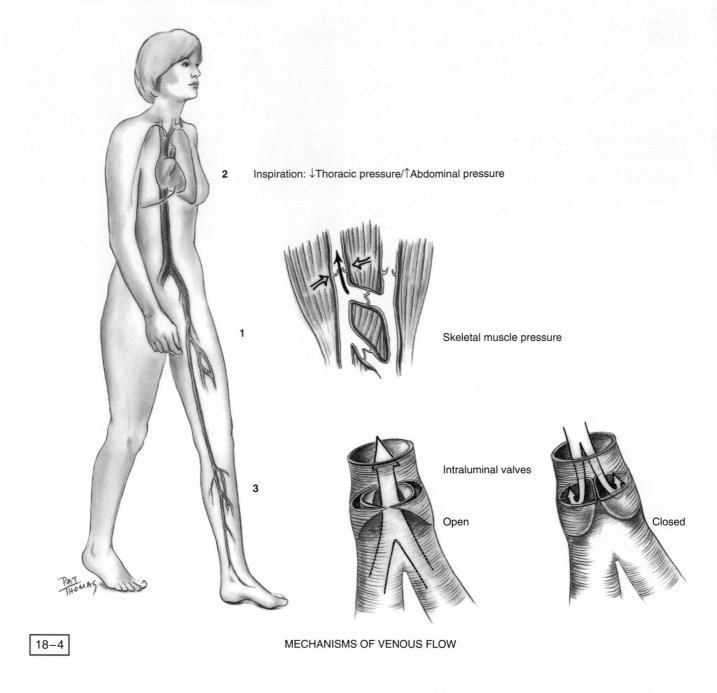

2 Inspiration: ↓Thoracic pressure/↑Abdominal pressure

Skeletal muscle pressure

Intraluminal valves

Open

Closed

18–4   MECHANISMS OF VENOUS FLOW

that join the two sets. They also have one-way valves that route blood from the superficial into the deep veins.

Veins drain the deoxygenated blood and its waste products from the tissues and return it to the heart. Unlike the arteries, veins are a low-pressure system. Because veins do not have a pump to generate their blood flow, the veins need a mechanism to keep blood moving (Fig. 18–4). This is accomplished by (1) the contracting skeletal muscles that milk the blood proximally, back toward the heart; (2) the pressure gradient caused by breathing, in which inspiration makes the thoracic pressure decrease and the abdominal pressure increase; and (3) the intraluminal valves, which ensure unidirectional flow. Each valve is a paired semilunar pocket that opens toward the

heart and closes tightly when filled to prevent backflow of blood.

In the legs, this mechanism is called the "calf pump," or "peripheral heart." While walking, the calf muscles alternately contract (systole) and relax (diastole). In the contraction phase, the gastrocnemius and soleus muscles squeeze the veins and direct the blood flow proximally. Because of the valves, venous blood flows just one way, toward the heart.

Besides the presence of intraluminal valves, venous structure differs from arterial structure. Because venous pressure is lower, walls of the veins are thinner than those of the arteries. Veins have a larger diameter and are more distensible; they can expand and hold more blood when blood volume increases. This is a compensatory mechanism to reduce stress on the heart. Because of this ability to stretch, veins are called **capacitance vessels.**

Efficient venous return is dependent on contracting skeletal muscles, competent valves in the veins, and patent lumen. Problems with any of these three elements lead to venous stasis. At risk for venous disease are people who undergo prolonged standing, sitting, or bedrest because they do not benefit from the milking action that walking accomplishes. Hypercoagulable states and vein wall trauma are other factors that place the person at risk for venous disease. Also, dilated and tortuous (varicose) veins create *incompetent valves*—The lumen is so wide the valve cusps cannot approximate. This condition increases venous pressure, which further dilates the vein. Some people have a genetic predisposition to varicose veins, but obesity and pregnancy are increased risk factors.

LYMPHATICS

The lymphatics form a completely separate vessel system, which retrieves excess fluid from the tissue spaces and returns it to the blood stream (Fig. 18–5). During circulation of the blood, somewhat more fluid leaves the capillaries than the veins can absorb. Without lymphatic drainage, fluid would build up in the interstitial spaces and produce edema.

The vessels drain into two main trunks, which empty into the venous system at the subclavian veins (see Fig. 18–5): (1) The **right lymphatic duct** empties into the right subclavian vein. It drains the right side of the head and neck, right arm, right side of thorax, right lung and pleura, right side of the heart, and right upper section of the liver. (2) The **thoracic duct** drains the rest of the body. It empties into the left subclavian vein.

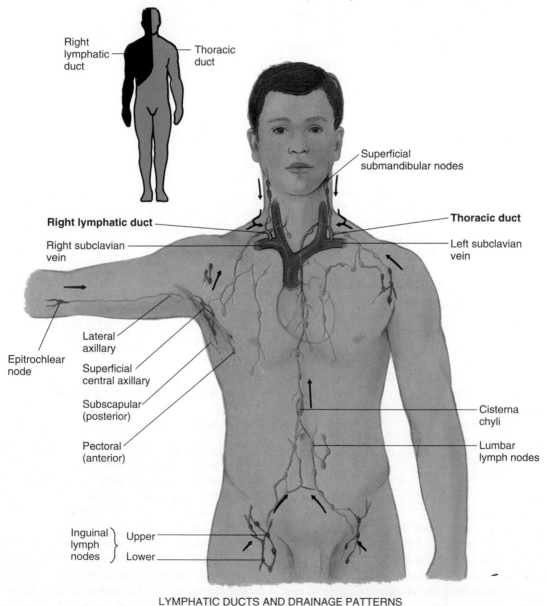

18–5   LYMPHATIC DUCTS AND DRAINAGE PATTERNS

The functions of the lymphatic system are (1) to conserve fluid and plasma proteins that leak out of the capillaries, (2) to form a major part of the immune system that defends the body against disease, and (3) to absorb lipids from the intestinal tract.

The processes of the immune system are complicated and not fully understood. The immune system detects and eliminates foreign pathogens, both those that come in from the environment and those arising from inside (abnormal or mutant cells). It accomplishes this by phagocytosis (digestion) of the substances by neutrophils and monocytes/macrophages, and by production of specific antibodies or specific immune responses by the lymphocytes.

The lymphatic vessels have a unique structure. Lymphatic capillaries start as microscopic open-ended tubes, which siphon interstitial fluid. The capillaries converge to form vessels. The vessels, like veins, drain into larger ones. The vessels have valves, so flow is one way from the tissue spaces into the blood stream. The many valves make the vessels look beaded. The flow of lymph is slow compared with that of the blood. Lymph flow is propelled by contracting skeletal muscles, by pressure changes secondary to breathing, and by contraction of the vessel walls themselves.

Lymph nodes are small oval clumps of lymphatic tissue located at intervals along the vessels. Most nodes are arranged in groups, both deep and superficial in the body. Nodes filter the fluid before it is returned to the blood stream and filter out microorganisms that could be harmful to the body. The pathogens are exposed to lymphocytes in the lymph nodes. The lymphocytes mount an antigen-specific response to eliminate the pathogens. With local inflammation, the nodes in that area become swollen and tender.

The superficial groups of nodes are accessible to inspection and palpation and give clues to the status of the lymphatic system:

- Cervical nodes drain the head and neck and are described in Chapter 11.
- Axillary nodes drain the breast and upper arm. They are described in Chapter 15.
- The epitrochlear node is in the antecubital fossa and drains the hand and lower arm.
- The inguinal nodes in the groin drain most of the lymph of the lower extremity, the external genitalia, and the anterior abdominal wall.

Related Organs

The spleen, tonsils, and thymus aid the lymphatic system (Fig. 18–6). The **spleen** is located in the left upper quadrant of the abdomen. It has four functions: (1) to destroy old red blood cells, (2) to produce antibodies, (3) to store red blood cells, and (4) to filter microorganisms from the blood.

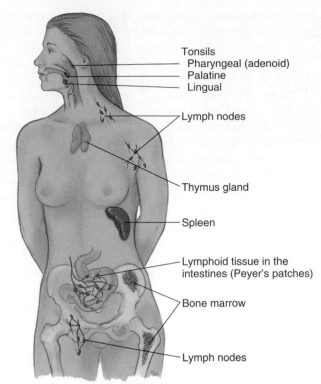

RELATED ORGANS IN IMMUNE SYSTEM

18–6

The **tonsils** (palatine, adenoid, and lingual) are located at the entrance to the respiratory and gastrointestinal tracts and respond to local inflammation.

The **thymus** is the flat, pink-gray gland located in the superior mediastinum behind the sternum and in front of the aorta. It is relatively large in the fetus and young child and atrophies after puberty. It is important in developing the T-lymphocytes of the immune system in children, but it serves no function in adults. The T-lymphocytes and B-lymphocytes originate in the bone marrow and mature in the lymphoid tissue.

 ## DEVELOPMENTAL CONSIDERATIONS

Infants and Children

The lymphatic system has the same function in children as in adults. Lymphoid tissue has a unique growth pattern when compared with other body systems (Fig. 18–7). It is well developed at birth and grows rapidly until age 10 or 11. By age 6, the lymphoid tissue reaches adult size, it surpasses adult size by puberty, and then it slowly atrophies. It is possible that the excessive antigen stimulation in children causes the early rapid growth.

Lymph nodes are relatively large in children, and the superficial ones often are palpable even when the child is healthy. With infection, excessive swelling and hyperpla-

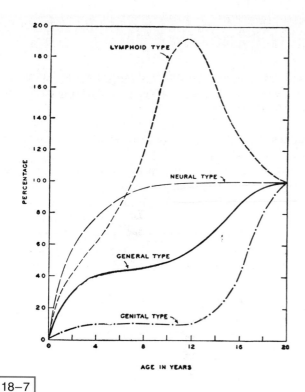

18-7

Comparison of Growth Rates of Three Types of Tissues and the Body as a Whole

sia occur. Enlarged tonsils are familiar signs in respiratory infections. The excessive lymphoid response also may account for the common childhood symptom of abdominal pain with seemingly unrelated problems such as upper respiratory infections (Johnson et al., 1978). Possibly the inflammation of mesenteric lymph nodes produces the abdominal pain.

The Pregnant Female

Hormonal changes cause vasodilatation and the resulting drop in blood pressure described in Chapter 17. The growing uterus obstructs drainage of the iliac veins and the inferior vena cava. This condition causes low blood flow and increases venous pressure. This, in turn, causes dependent edema, varicosities in the legs and vulva, and hemorrhoids.

The Aging Adult

Peripheral blood vessels grow more rigid with age, resulting in a condition called *arteriosclerosis*. This condition produces the rise in systolic blood pressure discussed in Chapter 9. Do not confuse this process with another one, *atherosclerosis*, or the deposition of fatty plaques on the intima of the arteries.

Aging produces a progressive enlargement of the intramuscular calf veins. Prolonged bedrest, prolonged sitting, and heart failure increase the risk of deep venous thrombosis and subsequent pulmonary embolism. These conditions are common in aging, and also occur following myocardial infarction (MI). However, care for MI now includes early mobilization and low-dose anticoagulant medication, which reduce the risk of pulmonary embolism (Braunwald, 1997).

Loss of lymphatic tissue leads to fewer numbers of lymph nodes in older people and to a decrease in the size of remaining nodes.

SUBJECTIVE DATA

1. Leg pain or cramps
2. Skin changes on arms or legs
3. Swelling
4. Lymph node enlargement
5. Medications

Examiner Asks	Rationale
1 **Leg pain or cramps.** Any leg pain (cramps)? Where? • Describe the type of pain, e.g., burning, aching, cramping, stabbing? Did this come on gradually or suddenly? • Is it aggravated by activity, walking?	Peripheral vascular disease (PVD)—see Table 18–3, History Profiles, p. 576.

Examiner Asks	Rationale
• How many blocks (stairs) does it take to produce this pain?	*Claudication distance* is the number of blocks walked or stairs climbed to produce pain.
• Has this amount changed recently? • Is the pain worse with elevation? Worse with cool temperatures?	Note sudden decrease in claudication distance, or pain suddenly not relieved by rest.
• Does the pain wake you up at night?	Night leg pain is common in aging adults. It may indicate the ischemic rest pain of peripheral vascular disease, severe night muscle cramping (usually the calf), or the restless leg syndrome.
• Any recent change in exercise, a new exercise, increasing exercise?	Pain of musculoskeletal origin rather than vascular.
• What relieves this pain: dangling, walking, rubbing? Is the leg pain associated with any skin changes? • Is it associated with any change in sexual function (males)?	Aortoiliac occlusion is associated with impotence (Leriche's syndrome).
• Any past history of: vascular problems, heart problems, diabetes, obesity, pregnancy, smoking, trauma, prolonged standing, or bedrest?	
❷ Skin changes on arms or legs. Any **skin changes** in arms or legs? What color: redness, pallor, blueness, brown discolorations? • Any change in temperature—excess warmth or coolness?	Coolness is associated with arterial disease.
• Do your leg veins look bulging and crooked? How have you treated these? Do you use support hose?	Varicose veins.
• Any leg sores or ulcers? Where on the leg? Any pain with the leg ulcer?	Leg ulcers occur with chronic arterial and chronic venous disease.
❸ Swelling in the arms or legs. Swelling in one or both legs? When did this swelling start? • What time of day is the swelling at its worst: morning, or after up most of day? • Does the swelling come and go, or is it constant? • What seems to bring it on: trauma, standing all day, sitting? • What relieves swelling: elevation, support hose? • Is swelling associated with pain, heat, redness, ulceration, hardened skin?	**Edema** is bilateral when caused by a systemic problem such as heart failure, or unilateral when due to a local obstruction or inflammation.
❹ Lymph node enlargement. Any "swollen glands" (lumps, kernels)? Where in body? How long have you had them? • Any recent change? • How do they feel to you: hard, soft? • Are the swollen glands associated with: pain, local infection?	**Enlarged lymph nodes** occur with infectious diseases, immunologic diseases, and malignant diseases.
❺ Medications. What medications are you taking, e.g., oral contraceptives?	

Preparation

During a complete physical examination, examine the arms at the very beginning when you are checking the vital signs—the person is sitting. Examine the legs directly after the abdominal examination while the person is still supine. Then stand the person up to evaluate the leg veins.

Examination of the arms and legs includes peripheral vascular characteristics (following here), the skin (see Chapter 10), musculoskeletal findings (Chapter 20), and neurologic findings (Chapter 21). A method of integrating these steps is discussed in Chapter 26.

Room temperature should be about 22° C (72° F) and draftless to prevent vasodilatation or vasoconstriction.

Use inspection and palpation. Compare your findings with the opposite extremity.

► Equipment Needed

Occasionally need: paper tape measure
Tourniquet or blood pressure cuff
Stethoscope
Doppler ultrasonic stethoscope

Normal Range of Findings	Abnormal Findings

THE ARMS

Inspect and palpate the arms

Lift both the person's hands in your hands. Inspect, then turn the person's hands over, noting color of skin and nailbeds; temperature, texture, and turgor of skin; and the presence of any lesions, edema, or clubbing. Use the *profile sign* (viewing the finger from the side) to detect early clubbing. The normal nail bed angle is 160 degrees. (See Chapter 10, Skin, Hair, and Nails, for a full discussion of skin color, lesions, and clubbing.)

Flattening of angle and clubbing (diffuse enlargement of terminal phalanges) occur with congenital cyanotic heart disease, cor pulmonale, and subacute bacterial endocarditis.

With the person's hands near the level of his or her heart, check **capillary refill.** This is an index of peripheral perfusion and cardiac output. Depress and blanch the nail beds; release and note the time for color return. Usually, the vessels refill within a fraction of a second. Consider it normal if the color returns in less than 1 or 2 seconds. Note these conditions that can skew your findings: a cool room, decreased body temperature, cigarette smoking, peripheral edema, and anemia.

The two arms should be symmetric in size.

Refill lasting more than 1 or 2 seconds signifies vasoconstriction or decreased cardiac output (hypovolemia, heart failure, shock). The hands are cold, clammy, and pale.

Edema of upper extremities occurs when lymphatic drainage is obstructed, which may occur following breast surgery (see Table 18-2).

Note the presence of any scars on hands and arms. Many occur normally with usual childhood abrasions or with occupations involving hand tools.

Needle tracks in antecubital fossae occur with intravenous drug use; linear scars in wrists may signify past self-inflicted injury.

▶ Normal Range of Findings | Abnormal Findings

Palpate both radial pulses, noting rate, rhythm, elasticity of vessel wall, and equal force (Fig. 18–8). Grade the force (amplitude) on a four-point scale:

4 +, bounding
3 +, increased
2 +, **normal**
1 +, weak
0, absent

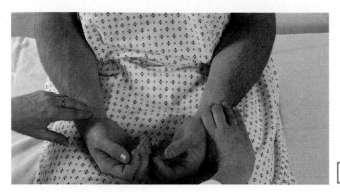

18–8

It usually is not necessary to palpate the ulnar pulses. If indicated, palpate along the medial side of the inner forearm (Fig. 18–9), although the ulnar pulses often are not palpable in the normal person.

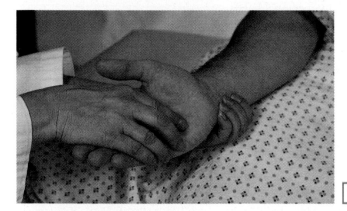

18–9

Palpate the brachial pulses—Their force should be equal bilaterally (Fig. 18–10).

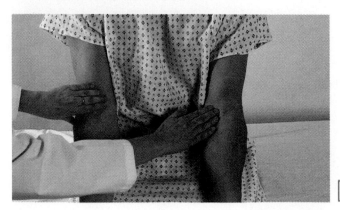

18–10

Full, bounding pulse (3+ or 4+) occurs with hyperkinetic states (exercise, anxiety, fever), anemia, and hyperthyroidism. Weak, "thready" pulse occurs with shock and peripheral arterial disease. See Table 18–1 on p. 574 for illustrations of these and irregular pulse rhythms.

▶ Normal Range of Findings	Abnormal Findings

Check the epitrochlear lymph node in the depression above and behind the medial condyle of the humerus. Do this by "shaking hands" with the person and reaching your other hand under the person's elbow to the groove between the biceps and triceps muscles, above the medial epicondyle (Fig. 18–11). This node is not palpable normally.

An enlarged epitrochlear node occurs with infection of the hand or forearm.

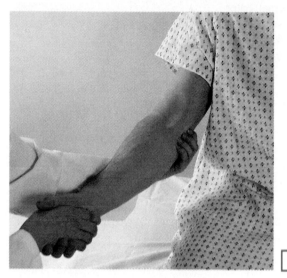

18–11

The Allen Test. Determine the patency of the radial and ulnar arteries by performing the Allen test (Fig. 18–12). Ask the person to rest the hands on the knees, palms up. (A) Compress both radial arteries with your thumbs, and ask the person to open and close the fists several times. (B) Continue to compress the arteries and have the person open the hands (without hyperextending them). Look at the palms; they should turn pink promptly as long as the ulnar artery is patent. Repeat the test while occluding the ulnar arteries.

(C) Pallor persists if ulnar artery or its arch is occluded.

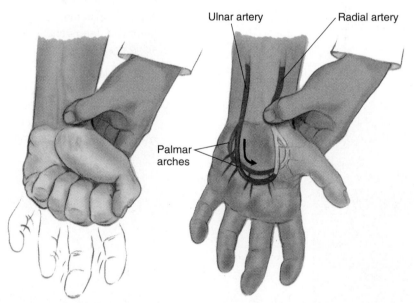
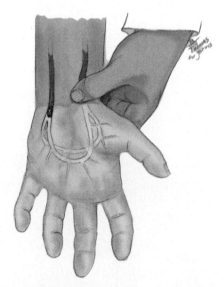

Ulnar artery   Radial artery

Palmar arches

A Depress radial artery—person opens and closes fist

B Normal—blood returns via ulnar artery

C Occluded ulnar artery— no blood return

18–12

▶ Normal Range of Findings	Abnormal Findings

Modified Allen Test. The modified Allen test is used to evaluate the adequacy of collateral circulation prior to cannulating the radial artery. Firmly occlude both the ulnar and radial arteries of one hand while the person makes a fist. This causes the hand to blanch. Ask the person to open the hand; then release pressure on the ulnar artery while maintaining pressure on the radial artery. Adequate circulation is suggested by a return to the hand's normal color in approximately 3 to 5 seconds. Although this test is simple and useful, it is relatively crude and subject to error, i.e., you must occlude both arteries uniformly with 11 pounds of pressure for the test to be accurate (Fuhrman et al, 1992; Gelberman and Blasingame, 1981).

A sluggish or an absent return to color suggests occlusion of the collateral circulation.

THE LEGS

Inspect and palpate the legs

Uncover the legs while keeping the genitalia draped. Inspect both legs together, noting skin color, hair distribution, venous pattern, size (swelling or atrophy), and any skin lesions or ulcers.

Pallor with vasoconstriction; erythema with vasodilatation; cyanosis.

Normally hair covers the legs. Even if leg hair is shaved, you will still note hair on the dorsa of the toes.

Malnutrition: thin, shiny atrophic skin, thick-ridged nails, loss of hair, ulcers, gangrene. Malnutrition, pallor, and coolness occur with arterial insufficiency.

The venous pattern normally is flat and barely visible. Note obvious varicosities, although these are best assessed while standing.

Both legs should be symmetric in size without any swelling or atrophy. If the lower legs look asymmetric or if deep venous thrombosis is suspected, measure the calf circumference with a nonstretchable tape measure (Fig. 18–13). Measure at the widest point, taking care to measure the other leg in exactly the same place, the same number of centimeters down from the patella or other landmark. If lymphedema is suspected, measure also at the ankle, distal calf, knee, and thigh. Record your findings in centimeters.

Diffuse bilateral edema occurs with systemic illnesses.

Unilateral swelling indicates a local acute problem. Asymmetry of calves of 1 cm or more is abnormal; refer the person to determine if deep venous thrombosis is present.

Asymmetry of 1 to 3 cm occurs with mild lymphedema; 3 to 5 cm with moderate lymphedema; and more than 5 cm with severe lymphedema (see Table 18–2).

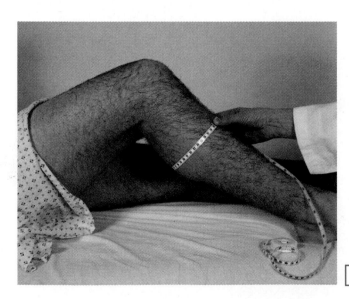

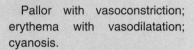
18–13

▶ Normal Range of Findings	Abnormal Findings

In the presence of skin discoloration, skin ulcers, or gangrene, note the size and the exact location.

Brown discoloration occurs with chronic venous stasis due to hemosiderin deposits (a by-product of red blood cell degradation).

Venous ulcers occur usually at medial malleolus because of bacterial invasion of poorly drained tissues (see Table 18–4).

With arterial deficit, ulcers occur on tips of toes, metatarsal heads, and lateral malleoli.

Palpate for temperature along the legs down to the feet, comparing symmetric spots (Fig. 18–14). The skin should be warm and equal bilaterally. Bilateral cool feet may be due to environmental factors such as cool room temperature, apprehension, and cigarette smoking. If any increase in temperature is present up the leg, note if it is gradual or abrupt.

A unilateral cool foot or leg or a sudden temperature drop as you move down the leg occurs with arterial deficit.

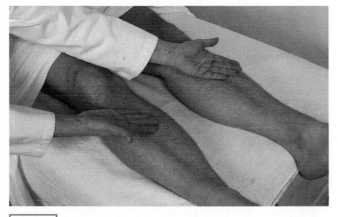

18–14

Flex the person's knee, then gently compress the gastrocnemius (calf) muscle anteriorly against the tibia; no tenderness should be present. Or you may sharply dorsiflex the foot toward the tibia. Flexing the knee first exerts pressure on the posterior tibial vein. Normally this does not cause pain.

Calf pain with these maneuvers is a positive **Homans' sign,** which occurs in about 35 percent of cases of deep vein thrombosis. It is not specific for this condition because it occurs also with superficial phlebitis, Achilles tendinitis, gastrocnemius and plantar muscle injury, and lumbosacral disorders.

Palpate the inguinal lymph nodes. It is not unusual to find palpable nodes that are small (1 cm or less), movable, and nontender.

Enlarged nodes, tender, or fixed in area.

▶

Palpate these peripheral arteries in both legs: femoral, popliteal, dorsalis pedis, and posterior tibial. Grade the force on the four-point scale. Locate the **femoral arteries** just below the inguinal ligament halfway between the pubis and anterior superior iliac spines (Fig. 18–15). To help expose the femoral area, particularly in obese people, ask the person to bend his or her knees to the side in a froglike position. Press firmly and then slowly release, noting the pulse tap under your fingertips. Should this pulse be weak or diminished, auscultate the site for a bruit.

A bruit occurs with turbulent blood flow, indicating partial occlusion (see Table 18–5).

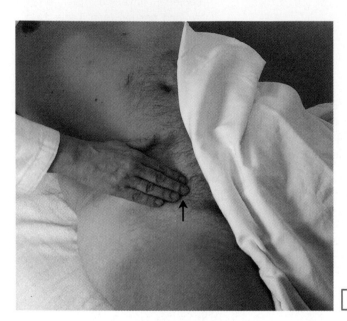

18–15

The **popliteal pulse** is a more diffuse pulse and can be difficult to localize. With the leg extended but relaxed, anchor your thumbs on the knee, and curl your fingers around into the popliteal fossa (Fig. 18–16). Press your fingers forward hard to compress the artery against the bone (the lower edge of the femur or the upper edge of the tibia). Often it is just lateral to the medial tendon.

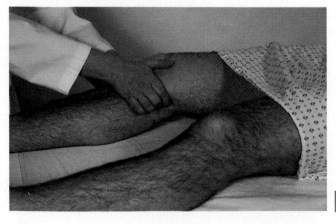

18–16

If you have difficulty, turn the person prone and lift up the lower leg (Fig. 18–17). Let the leg relax against your arm and press in deeply with your two thumbs. Often a normal popliteal pulse is impossible to palpate.

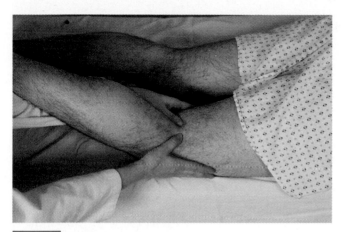

18–17

For the **posterior tibial** pulse, curve your fingers around the medial malleolus (Fig. 18–18). You will feel the tapping right behind it in the groove between the malleolus and the Achilles tendon. If you cannot, try passive dorsiflexion of the foot to make the pulse more accessible.

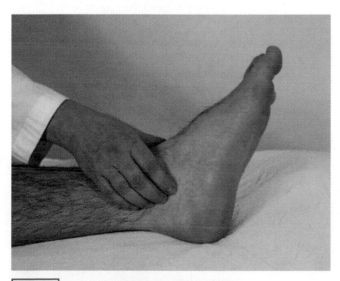

18–18   **Posterior Tibial Pulse**

▶ | Normal Range of Findings | Abnormal Findings

The **dorsalis pedis** pulse requires a very light touch. Normally it is just lateral to and parallel with the extensor tendon of the big toe (Fig. 18–19). Do not mistake the pulse in your own fingertips for that of the person.

In adults over 45 years, occasionally either the dorsalis pedis or the posterior tibial pulse may be hard to find, but not both on the same foot.

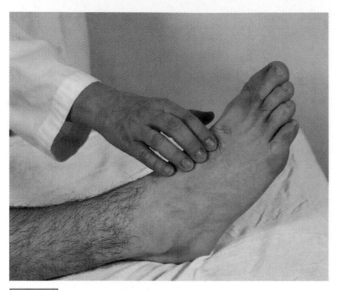

18–19   **Dorsalis Pedis Pulse**

Check for pretibial edema. Firmly depress the skin over the tibia or the medial malleolus for 5 seconds and release (Fig. 18–20A). Normally, your finger should leave no indentation, although a pit commonly is seen if the person has been standing all day or during pregnancy.

Bilateral, dependent, pitting edema occurs with heart failure and hepatic cirrhosis (see Fig. 18–20B).

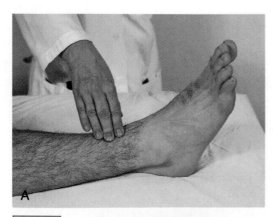

18–20A   **Check Pretibial Edema**

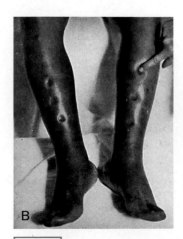

18–20B

▶ | Normal Range of Findings | Abnormal Findings

If pitting edema is present, grade it on this scale:

1+ Mild pitting, slight indentation, no perceptible swelling of the leg
2+ Moderate pitting, indentation subsides rapidly
3+ Deep pitting, indentation remains for a short time, leg looks swollen
4+ Very deep pitting, indentation lasts a long time, leg is very swollen

This scale is subjective and qualitative. The amount of pressure used is arbitrary, as is the judgment of the depth and rate of pitting. Clinicians need a standard quantified scale in order to ensure consistent clinical measurements and management. Many classify the edema by measuring the depth of the pitting in centimeters (1+ = 1 cm, 2+ = 2 cm, etc.) (Welsh, Arzouman, and Holm, 1996). Some measure with a millimeter scale, others by an increase in weight; still others try to quantify the rate of time the pitting remains after release of pressure. Check with your institution to determine a consistently used scale.

Ask the person to stand so that you can assess the venous system. Note any visible, dilated, and tortuous veins.

Manual Compression Test. While the person is still standing, test the length of the varicose vein to determine if its valves are competent (Fig. 18–21). Place one hand on the lower part of the varicose vein, and compress the vein with your other hand about 15 to 20 cm higher. Competent valves will prevent a wave transmission and your distal fingers will feel nothing.

Abnormal Findings

Unilateral edema occurs with occlusion of a deep vein. Unilateral or bilateral edema occurs with lymphatic obstruction. With these factors, it is "brawny" or nonpitting and feels hard to the touch.

Varicosities occur in the saphenous veins (see Table 18–4).

A palpable wave transmission occurs when the valves are incompetent.

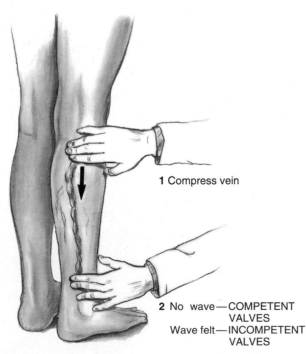

1 Compress vein

2 No wave—COMPETENT VALVES
Wave felt—INCOMPETENT VALVES

MANUAL COMPRESSION TEST

18–21

ADDITIONAL TECHNIQUES

The Trendelenburg Test. When varicosities are present in the legs, use the Trendelenburg test to determine valve competence (Fig. 18–22). Return the person to supine position, elevate the involved leg 90 degrees until the veins empty, and place a tourniquet high on the thigh. Help the person to stand up, and watch for venous filling. The saphenous veins should fill slowly from below in about 30 seconds.

Rapid filling of veins from above indicates incompetent valves.

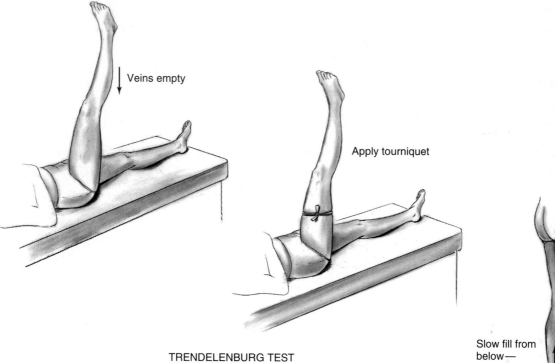

Veins empty

Apply tourniquet

TRENDELENBURG TEST

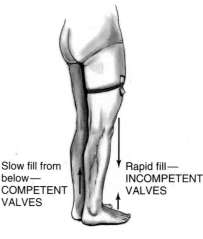

Slow fill from below—COMPETENT VALVES

Rapid fill—INCOMPETENT VALVES

18–22

After 30 seconds, take the tourniquet off. Now observe whether or not the varicose veins fill suddenly from above. Normally no sudden filling occurs.

Sudden filling after removing the tourniquet indicates retrograde flow past incompetent saphenous valves.

Color Changes. If you suspect an arterial deficit, raise the legs about 30 cm (12 inches) off the table and ask the person to wag the feet to drain off venous blood (Fig. 18–23). The skin color now reflects only the contribution of arterial blood. A light-skinned person's feet normally will look a little pale but still should be pink. A dark-skinned person's feet are more difficult to evaluate, but the soles should reveal extreme color change.

Elevational pallor (marked) indicates arterial insufficiency.

|

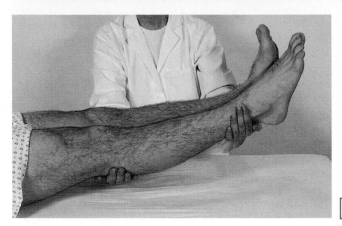

18–23

Now have the person sit up with the legs over the side of the table (Fig. 18–24). Compare the color of both feet. Note the time it takes for color to return to the feet. Normally, this is 10 seconds or less. Note also the time it takes for the superficial veins around the feet to fill—the normal time is about 15 seconds. This test is unreliable if the person has concomitant venous disease with incompetent valves.

Dependent rubor (deep blue-red color) occurs with severe arterial insufficiency. Chronic hypoxia produces a loss of vasomotor tone and a pooling of blood in the veins.

Delayed venous filling occurs with arterial insufficiency.

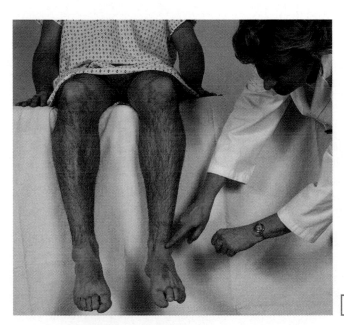

18–24

Test the lower legs for strength (see Chapter 20). Test the lower legs for sensation (see Chapter 21).

Motor loss occurs with severe arterial deficit.

Sensory loss occurs with arterial deficit, especially with diabetes.

The Doppler Ultrasonic Stethoscope. Use this device to detect a weak peripheral pulse, to monitor blood pressure in infants or children, or to measure a low blood pressure or blood pressure in a lower extremity (Fig. 18–25). The Doppler stethoscope magnifies pulsatile sounds from the heart and blood vessels. Position the person supine, with the legs externally rotated so you can reach the medial ankles easily. Place a drop of coupling gel on the end of the handheld transducer. Place the transducer over a pulse site, swiveled at a 45-degree angle. Apply very light pressure; locate the pulse site by the swishing, whooshing sound.

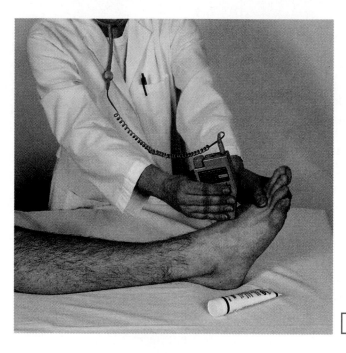

18–25

The Ankle-Brachial Index (ABI). Use of the Doppler stethoscope is a noninvasive way to determine the extent of peripheral vascular disease. Apply a regular arm blood pressure cuff above the ankle and determine the systolic pressure in either the posterior tibial or dorsalis pedis artery. Then divide that figure by the systolic pressure of the brachial artery. (Take brachial systolic pressures in both arms and use the higher measurement.) The normal ankle pressure is slightly greater than or equal to the brachial pressure; thus, a normal ABI is usually 1.0 to 1.2. For example,

$$\frac{132 \text{ ankle systolic pressure}}{124 \text{ arm systolic pressure}}$$

= 1.06 or 106%, indicating no flow reduction

In people with diabetes mellitus, the ABI may be less reliable because of calcification, which makes their arteries noncompressible, and may give a falsely high measurement (Cantwell-Gab, 1996).

An ABI of 90 percent or less indicates the presence of peripheral vascular disease:

- 0.90 to 0.70—mild claudication
- 0.70 to 0.40—moderate to severe claudication
- 0.40 to 0.30—severe claudication, usually with rest pain except in the presence of diabetic neuropathy
- <0.30—ischemia, with impending loss of tissue

Normal Range of Findings	Abnormal Findings

DEVELOPMENTAL CONSIDERATIONS

Infants and Children

Transient acrocyanosis and skin mottling at birth are discussed in Chapter 10. Pulse force should be normal and symmetric. Pulse force also should be the same in the upper and lower extremities.

Weak pulses occur with vaso-constriction or diminished cardiac output.

Full, bounding pulses occur with patent ductus arteriosus due to the large left-to-right shunt.

Diminished or absent femoral pulses while upper extremity pulses are normal suggest co-arctation of aorta.

Palpable lymph nodes occur often in normal infants and children. They are small, firm (shotty), mobile, and nontender. They may be the sequelae of past infection, e.g., inguinal nodes from a diaper rash or cervical nodes from a respiratory infection. Vaccinations also can produce local lymphadenopathy. Note characteristics of any palpable nodes and whether they are local or generalized.

Enlarged, warm, tender nodes indicate current infection. Look for source of infection.

The Pregnant Female

Expect diffuse bilateral pitting edema in the lower extremities, especially at the end of the day and into the third trimester. Varicose veins in the legs also are common in the third trimester.

The Aging Adult

The dorsalis pedis and posterior tibial pulses may become more difficult to find. Trophic changes associated with arterial insufficiency (thin, shiny skin, thick-ridged nails, loss of hair on lower legs) also occur normally with aging.

SUMMARY CHECKLIST: Peripheral Vascular Exam

1: Inspect arms for color, size, any lesions

2: Palpate pulses: radial, brachial

3: Check epitrochlear node

4: Inspect legs for color, size, any lesions, trophic skin changes

5: Palpate temperature of feet and legs

6: Palpate inguinal nodes

7: Palpate pulses: femoral, popliteal, posterior tibial, dorsalis pedis

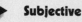
SAMPLE CHARTING

▶ **Subjective**

No leg pain, no skin changes, no swelling or lymph node enlargement. No past history of heart or vascular problems, diabetes, or obesity. Does not smoke. On no medications.

▶ **Objective**

Inspection. Extremities have pink-tan color without redness, cyanosis, or any skin lesions. Extremity size is symmetric without swelling or atrophy.

Palpation. Temperature is warm and = bilaterally. All pulses present, 2+ and = bilaterally. No lymphadenopathy.

CLINICAL CASE STUDY

James K. is a 43-year-old married white male city sanitation worker, admitted to University Medical Center today for "bypass surgery tomorrow to fix my aorta and these black toes."

▶ **Subjective**

6 yrs PTA: motorcycle accident with handle bars jammed into groin. Treated and released at local hospital. No apparent injury, although M.D. now thinks accident may have precipitated present stenosis of aorta.

1 yr PTA: radiating pain in right calf on walking 1 mile. Pain relieved by stopping walking.

3 months PTA: problems with sex, unable to maintain erection during intercourse.

1 month PTA: leg pain present after walking two blocks. Numbness and tingling in right foot and calf. Tips of three toes on right foot look black. Saw M.D. Diagnostic studies showed stenosis of aorta "below vessels that go to my kidneys."

Present: leg pain at rest, constant and severe, worse at night, partially relieved by dangling leg over side of bed.

Past history: No history of heart or vessel disease, hypertension, diabetes, obesity.

Personal habits: smokes cigarettes three packs/day × 23 years. Now cut down to 1 ppd.

Walking is part of occupation, although has been driving city truck last 3 months due to leg pain. On no medications.

▶ **Objective**

Inspection. Lower extremity size = bilaterally with no swelling or atrophy. No varicosities. Color L leg pink, R leg pink when supine, but marked pallor to R foot on elevation. Black gangrene at tips of R 2nd, 3rd, 4th toes. Leg hair present but absent on involved toes.

Palpation. R foot cool and temperature gradually warms as proceed palpating up R leg.

Pulses. Femorals, both 1+; popliteals, both 0; posterior tibial, both 0 but present with Doppler; dorsalis pedis 0, but left dorsalis pedis is present with Doppler, and right is not present with Doppler.

▶ ASSESSMENT

Ischemic rest pain R leg
Altered peripheral tissue perfusion R/T interruption of flow
Impaired tissue integrity R/T altered circulation
Activity intolerance R/T leg pain
Sexual dysfunction R/T effects of disease

NURSING DIAGNOSES COMMONLY ASSOCIATED WITH PERIPHERAL VASCULAR SYSTEM AND LYMPHATIC DISORDERS

Diagnosis	Related Factors (Etiology)	Defining Characteristics (Symptoms and Signs)
Altered tissue perfusion (peripheral)	Exchange problems Hypervolemia Hypovolemia Interruption of flow	Altered sensory or motor function Burning Changes in hair pattern Claudication Coolness of skin Diminished pulse quality Edema Erythema Extremity pain Inflammation Pallor Positive Homans' sign Tissue necrosis Trophic skin changes Ulcerated skin/poorly healing areas
Sensory/perceptual alteration (tactile)	Circulatory impairment Inflammation Effects of anesthesia Nutritional deficiencies Effects of aging Effects of burns Neurologic impairment Pain Persistent tactile stimulation	Paresthesias Hyperesthesias Anesthesias

Other Related Nursing Diagnoses

ACTUAL	RISK/WELLNESS
Activity intolerance (see Chapter 16) Body image disturbance Fatigue (see Chapter 16) Impaired bed mobility Impaired tissue integrity Impaired walking Pain (see Chapters 14 and 20) Risk for peripheral neurovascular dysfunction Sleep pattern disturbance Sexual dysfunction (see Chapter 24)	**Risk** Risk for infection Risk for peripheral neurovascular dysfunction **Wellness** Health-seeking behavior about beginning an exercise program

 ## ASSESSMENT VIDEO CRITICAL THINKING QUESTIONS

The Saunders *Physical Examination and Health Assessment* Video Series—CARDIOVAS-CULAR SYSTEM: PERIPHERAL VASCULAR SYSTEM AND LYMPHATICS—will direct you to consider the following:

1. Which assessment findings are you likely to see in a patient who seeks care because of leg pain or cramps?

2. How do ulcers caused by chronic arterial insufficiency compare to those of chronic venous insufficiency?

3. How may aging affect your findings when examining an older adult's peripheral vascular and lymphatic systems?

4. What nursing diagnoses commonly are related to abnormal findings in the peripheral vascular system?

ABNORMAL FINDINGS

▼ Table 18–1   VARIATIONS IN ARTERIAL PULSE

DESCRIPTION	ASSOCIATED WITH
Weak, "Thready" Pulse—1+ Hard to palpate, need to search for it, may fade in and out, easily obliterated by pressure	Decreased cardiac output; peripheral arterial disease; aortic valve stenosis
Full, Bounding Pulse—3+ or 4+ Easily palpable, pounds under your fingertips	Hyperkinetic states (exercise, anxiety, fever), anemia, hyperthyroidism
Water-Hammer (Corrigan's) Pulse—4+ Greater than normal force, then collapses suddenly	Aortic valve regurgitation; patent ductus arteriosus
Pulsus Bigeminus Rhythm is coupled, every other beat comes early, or normal beat followed by premature beat. Force of premature beat is decreased due to shortened cardiac filling time	Conduction disturbance, e.g., premature ventricular contraction, premature atrial contraction
Pulsus Alternans Rhythm is regular, but force varies with alternating beats of large and small amplitude	Heart failure

Table 18-1 VARIATIONS IN ARTERIAL PULSE *Continued*

DESCRIPTION	ASSOCIATED WITH

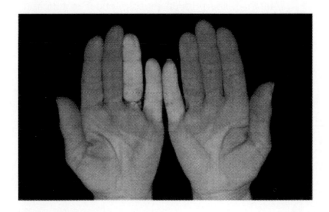

Pulsus Paradoxus

Beats have weaker amplitude with inspiration, stronger with expiration. Best determined during blood pressure measurement; reading decreases (> 10 mm Hg) during inspiration and increases with expiration

Any condition that blocks venous return to the right side of the heart, or blocks left ventricular filling, e.g., cardiac tamponade; constrictive pericarditis, pulmonary embolism

Pulsus Bisferiens

Each pulse has two strong systolic peaks, with a dip in between. Best assessed at the carotid artery

Aortic valve stenosis plus regurgitation

 ## Table 18-2 PERIPHERAL VASCULAR DISEASE IN THE ARMS

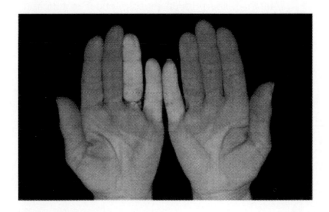

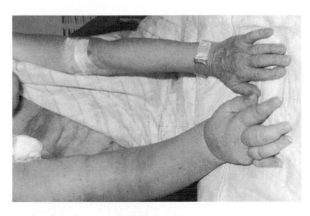

Raynaud's Syndrome

Episodes of abrupt progressive tricolor change of the fingers in response to cold, vibration, or stress: first white (pallor) from arteriospasm and resulting deficit in supply; then blue (cyanosis) due to slight relaxation of the spasm that allows a slow trickle of blood through the capillaries and increased oxygen extraction of hemoglobin; finally red (rubor) due to return of blood into the dilated capillary bed or reactive hyperemia.

May have cold, numbness, or pain along with pallor or cyanosis stage; then burning, throbbing pain, swelling along with rubor. Lasts minutes to hours; occurs bilaterally.

Lymphedema

Removal of lymph nodes with breast surgery, or damage to lymph nodes and channels with radiation therapy for breast cancer, can impede drainage of lymph. Protein-rich lymph builds up in the interstitial spaces, which further raises local colloid oncotic pressure and promotes more fluid leakage. Stagnant lymphatic fluid can lead to infection, delayed wound healing, chronic inflammation, and fibrosis of surrounding tissue. Chronic lymphedema is unilateral swelling, nonpitting brawny edema, with overlying skin indurated, and is psychologically demoralizing as a threat to body image and constant reminder of the cancer.

Table 18–3 HISTORY PROFILES OF PAIN OF PERIPHERAL VASCULAR DISEASE

SYMPTOM ANALYSIS	CHRONIC ARTERIAL SYMPTOMS	ACUTE ARTERIAL SYMPTOMS
Location	Deep muscle pain, usually in calf, but may be lower leg or dorsum of foot	Varies, distal to occlusion, may involve entire leg
Character	Intermittent claudication, feels like "cramp," "numbness and tingling," "feeling of cold"	Throbbing
Onset and duration	Chronic pain, onset gradual following exertion	Sudden onset (within 1 hr)
Aggravating factors	Activity (walking, stairs) "Claudication distance" is specific number of blocks, stairs it takes to produce pain. Elevation (Rest pain indicates severe involvement)	
Relieving factors	Rest (usually within 2 min; e.g., standing) Dangling (severe involvement)	
Associated symptoms	Cool pale skin *loss of hair, shiny skin. Thick nails*	Six Ps: pain, pallor, pulselessness, paresthesia, poikilothermia (coldness), paralysis (indicates severe)
Those at risk	Older adults, more males than females, inherited predisposition, history of hypertension, smoking, diabetes, hypercholesterolemia, obesity, vascular disease	History of vascular surgery, arterial invasive procedure, abdominal aneurysm (emboli), trauma, including injured arteries, chronic atrial fibrillation

ĉ Activity

	CHRONIC VENOUS SYMPTOMS	ACUTE VENOUS SYMPTOMS
Location	Calf, lower leg	Calf
Character	Aching, tiredness, feeling of fullness	Intense, sharp; deep muscle tender to touch
Onset and duration	Chronic pain, increases at end of day	Sudden onset (within 1 hr)
Aggravating factors	Prolonged standing, sitting	Pain may increase with sharp dorsiflexion of foot
Relieving factors	Elevation, lying, walking	
Associated symptoms	Edema, varicosities, weeping ulcers at ankles	Red, warm, swollen leg
Those at risk	Job with prolonged standing or sitting; obesity; pregnancy; prolonged bedrest; history of congestive heart failure, varicosities, or thrombophlebitis; veins crushed by trauma or surgery	

Skin—brown discoloration dry, cracked,

veins prompting

Deep Venous Thrombosis
Temp- warm
   Swollen
   Red
   painful ↑ ĉ dorsiflex
Homan Sign posthe

Table 18–4 PERIPHERAL VASCULAR DISEASE IN THE LEGS

CHRONIC ARTERIAL INSUFFICIENCY

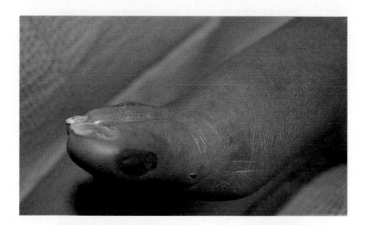

Arteriosclerosis — Ischemic Ulcer

Build-up of fatty plaques on intima (atherosclerosis) plus hardening and calcification of arterial wall (arteriosclerosis).

S: Deep muscle pain in calf or foot, claudication (pain with walking), pain at rest indicates worsening of condition.

O: Coolness, pallor, elevational pallor, and dependent rubor; diminished pulses; systolic bruits; trophic skin; signs of malnutrition (thin, shiny skin, thick-ridged nails, absence of hair, atrophy of muscles); xanthoma formation; distal gangrene.

Ulcers occur at toes, metatarsal heads, heels, lateral ankle, and are characterized by pale ischemic base, well-defined edges, and no bleeding.

Diabetes hastens changes described above, with generalized dysfunction in all arterial areas: peripheral, coronary, cerebral, retina, kidney. Peripheral involvement is associated with diabetic neuropathy and local infection.

CHRONIC VENOUS INSUFFICIENCY

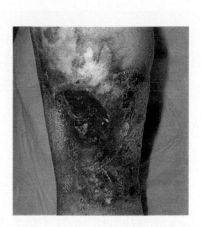

Venous (Stasis) Ulcer

Following acute deep vein thrombosis or following chronic incompetent valves in deep veins.

S: Aching pain in calf or lower leg, worse at end of the day, worse with prolonged standing or sitting.

O: Firm brawny edema; coarse, thickened skin; pulses normal; brown pigment discoloration; petechiae; dermatitis. Venous stasis causes increased venous pressure, which then causes red blood cells (RBCs) to leak out of veins and into the skin. As these RBCs break down, they leave hemosiderin (iron deposits) behind, which are the brown pigment deposits.

Ulcers occur at medial malleolus and are characterized by bleeding, uneven edges.

Table 18–4   PERIPHERAL VASCULAR DISEASE IN THE LEGS *Continued*

CHRONIC VENOUS DISEASE

ACUTE VENOUS DISEASE

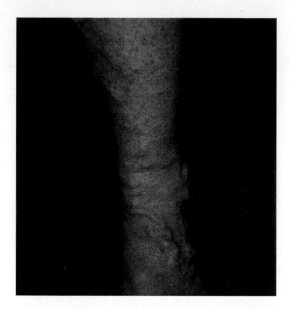

Superficial Varicose Veins

Incompetent valves permit reflux of blood, producing dilated, tortuous veins. Unremitting hydrostatic pressure causes distal valves to be incompetent and causes worsening of the varicosity.

Occurrence is three times more common in women than in men over age 45.

S: Aching, heaviness in calf, easy fatigability, night leg or foot cramps.
O: Dilated, tortuous veins.

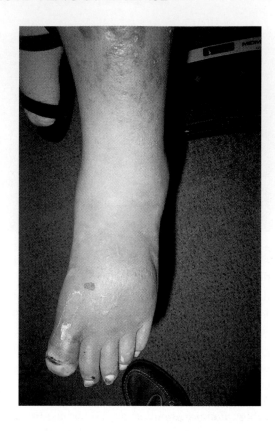

Deep Vein Thrombophlebitis

A deep vein is occluded by a thrombus, causing inflammation, blocked venous return, cyanosis, and edema. Cause may be prolonged bedrest, history of varicose veins, trauma, infection, cancer, and, in younger women, the use of oral estrogenic contraceptives (Dockery, 1997).

S: Sudden onset of intense, sharp, deep muscle pain, may increase with sharp dorsiflexion of foot.
O: Increased warmth; swelling (to compare swelling, observe the usual shoe size); redness; dependent cyanosis is mild or may be absent; tender to palpation; Homans' sign is present only in few cases.

Requires emergency referral due to risk of pulmonary embolism.

ABNORMAL FINDINGS

▼ **Table 18–5** PERIPHERAL ARTERY DISEASE

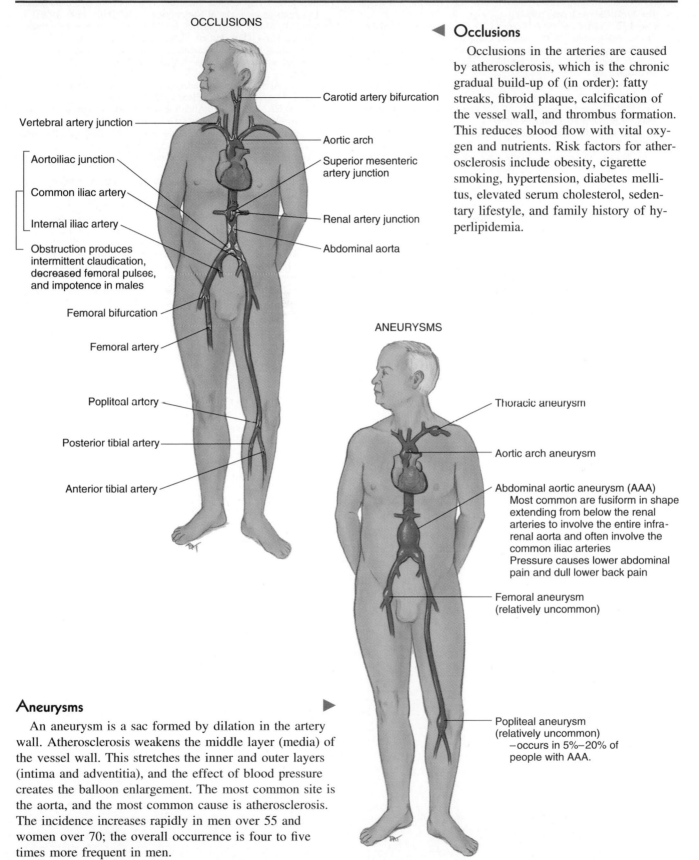

OCCLUSIONS

- Carotid artery bifurcation
- Vertebral artery junction
- Aortic arch
- Aortoiliac junction
- Superior mesenteric artery junction
- Common iliac artery
- Internal iliac artery
- Renal artery junction
- Obstruction produces intermittent claudication, decreased femoral pulses, and impotence in males
- Abdominal aorta
- Femoral bifurcation
- Femoral artery
- Popliteal artery
- Posterior tibial artery
- Anterior tibial artery

ANEURYSMS

- Thoracic aneurysm
- Aortic arch aneurysm
- Abdominal aortic aneurysm (AAA)
  Most common are fusiform in shape extending from below the renal arteries to involve the entire infra-renal aorta and often involve the common iliac arteries
  Pressure causes lower abdominal pain and dull lower back pain
- Femoral aneurysm (relatively uncommon)
- Popliteal aneurysm (relatively uncommon) —occurs in 5%–20% of people with AAA.

◀ Occlusions

Occlusions in the arteries are caused by atherosclerosis, which is the chronic gradual build-up of (in order): fatty streaks, fibroid plaque, calcification of the vessel wall, and thrombus formation. This reduces blood flow with vital oxygen and nutrients. Risk factors for atherosclerosis include obesity, cigarette smoking, hypertension, diabetes mellitus, elevated serum cholesterol, sedentary lifestyle, and family history of hyperlipidemia.

Aneurysms ▶

An aneurysm is a sac formed by dilation in the artery wall. Atherosclerosis weakens the middle layer (media) of the vessel wall. This stretches the inner and outer layers (intima and adventitia), and the effect of blood pressure creates the balloon enlargement. The most common site is the aorta, and the most common cause is atherosclerosis. The incidence increases rapidly in men over 55 and women over 70; the overall occurrence is four to five times more frequent in men.

ABNORMAL FINDINGS

579

Bibliography

Barbers RG: Inserting an arterial line: Protocol and precautions. J Respir Dis 15(5):429–432, May 1994.

Braunwald E: Heart Disease: A Textbook of Cardiovascular Medicine, 5th ed. Philadelphia, W.B. Saunders Company, 1997.

Bright LD: Deep vein thrombosis. Am J Nurs 95(6):48–49, June 1995.

Cameron J: Venous and arterial leg ulcers. Elderly Care 7(6):23–30, Dec–Jan 1995.

Cantwell-Gab K: Identifying chronic peripheral arterial disease. Am J Nurs 96(7):40–47, Jul 1996.

Dockery GL: Cutaneous Disorders of the Lower Extremity. Philadelphia, W.B. Saunders Company, 1997.

Dumas MS: Intermittent claudication. Am J Nurs 95(12):34–35, Dec 1995.

Erick L: Partners in prevention: Foot care for patients with diabetes. Advan Nurse Pract 5(9):29–33, Sep 1997.

Fahey VA: Vascular Nursing, 2nd ed. Philadelphia, W.B. Saunders Company, 1994.

Fuhrman TM, Pippin WD, Talmage LA, Reilley TE: Evaluation of collateral circulation of the hand. J Clin Monit 8(1):28–32, Jan 1992.

Gelberman RH, Blasingame JP: The timed Allen test. J Trauma 21(6):477–479, June 1981.

Harris AH, Brown-Etris M, Troyer-Caudle J: Managing vascular leg ulcers. Part 1: Assessment. Am J Nurs 96(1):38–44, Jan 1996.

Heitman B, Irizarry A: Infectious disease causes of lymphadenopathy: Localized versus diffuse. Primary Care Pract 3(1):19–38, Jan–Feb 1999.

Hodges H. Raynaud's disease: Pathophysiology, diagnosis, and treatment. J Am Acad Nurse Pract 7(4):159–164, Apr 1995.

Humble CA: Lymphedema: Incidence, pathophysiology, management, and nursing care. Oncol Nurs Forum 22(10):1503–1509, 1995.

Johnson TR, Moore WM, Jeffries JE: Children Are Different: Developmental Physiology, 2nd ed. Columbus, OH, Ross Labs, 1978.

Krenzer ME: Peripheral vascular assessment: Finding your way through arteries and veins. AACN Clin Issues 6(4):631–634, Nov 1995.

Longo DL, Arun B: Cervical adenopathy: A clinical approach to diagnosis. Consultant 36(11):2345–2352, Nov 1996.

McConnell EA: Performing Allen's test . . . whether ulnar and radial arteries are patent. Nursing97 27(11):26, Nov 1997.

Price J, Purtell JR: Prevention and treatment of lymphedema after breast cancer. Am J Nurs 97(9):34–37, Sep 1997.

Sandler RL: Abdominal aortic aneurysm. Am J Nurs 95(1):38–39, Jan 1995.

Stein PD, Henry JW, Gopalakrishnan D, Relyea B: Asymmetry of the calves in the assessment of patients with suspected acute pulmonary embolism. Chest 107(4):936–939, Apr 1995.

Welsh JR, Arzouman JM, Holm K: Nurses' assessment and documentation of peripheral edema. Clin Nurs Spec 10(1):7–10, Jan 1996.

Wheeler EC, Brenner ZR: Peripheral vascular anatomy, physiology, and pathophysiology. AACN Clin Issues 6(4):505–514, Nov 1995.

Whitaker L, Kelleher A: Raynaud's syndrome: Diagnosis and treatment. J Vasc Nurs XII(1):10–13, 1994.

Wills EM, Sloan HL: Assessing peripheral arterial disorders in the home: A multidisciplinary clinical guide. Home Healthcare Nurse 14(9):669–681, 1996.

CHAPTER NINETEEN

Abdomen

SURFACE LANDMARKS

The **abdomen** is a large oval cavity extending from the diaphragm down to the brim of the pelvis. It is bordered in back by the vertebral column and paravertebral muscles, and at the sides and front by the lower rib cage and abdominal muscles (Fig. 19–1). Four layers of large, flat muscles form the ventral abdominal wall. These are joined at the midline by a tendinous seam, the **linea alba.** One set, the **rectus abdominis,** forms a strip extending the length of the midline, and its edge is often palpable.

INTERNAL ANATOMY

Inside the abdominal cavity, all the internal organs are the **viscera.** It is important that you know the location of these organs so well that you could draw a roadmap on the skin (Fig. 19–2). You must be able to visualize each organ that you listen to or palpate through the abdominal wall.

The **solid viscera** are those that maintain a characteristic shape (liver, pancreas, spleen, adrenal glands, kidneys, ovaries, and uterus). The liver fills most of the right upper quadrant (RUQ) and extends over to the left midclavicular line. The lower edge of the liver and the right kidney may be palpable normally. The ovaries normally are palpable only on bimanual examination during the pelvic examination.

The shape of the **hollow viscera** (stomach, gallbladder, small intestine, colon, and bladder) depends on the contents. They usually are not palpable, although you may feel a colon distended with feces or a bladder distended with urine. The stomach is just below the diaphragm, between the liver and spleen. The gallbladder rests under the posterior surface of the liver, just lateral to the right midclavicular line. Note that the small intestine is located in all four quadrants. It extends from the stomach's pylo-

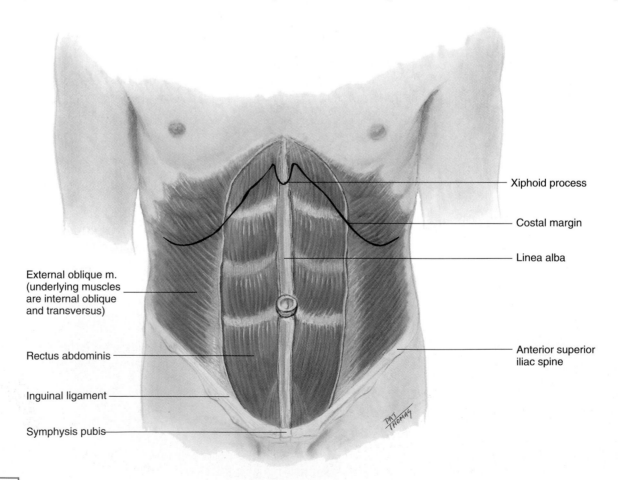

Xiphoid process

Costal margin

Linea alba

External oblique m. (underlying muscles are internal oblique and transversus)

Rectus abdominis

Inguinal ligament

Symphysis pubis

Anterior superior iliac spine

19–1

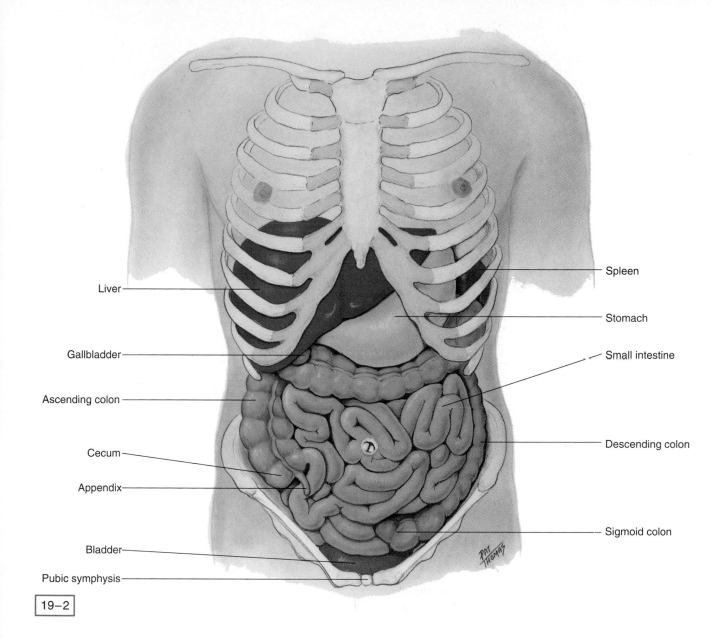

Liver

Gallbladder

Ascending colon

Cecum

Appendix

Bladder

Pubic symphysis

Spleen

Stomach

Small intestine

Descending colon

Sigmoid colon

PAT THOMAS

19–2

ric valve to the ileocecal valve in the right lower quadrant (RLQ) where it joins the colon.

The **spleen** is a soft mass of lymphatic tissue on the posterolateral wall of the abdominal cavity, immediately under the diaphragm (Fig. 19–3). It lies obliquely with its long axis behind and parallel to the 10th rib, lateral to the midaxillary line. Its width extends from the 9th to the 11th rib, about 7 cm. It is not palpable normally. If it becomes enlarged, its lower pole moves downward and toward the midline.

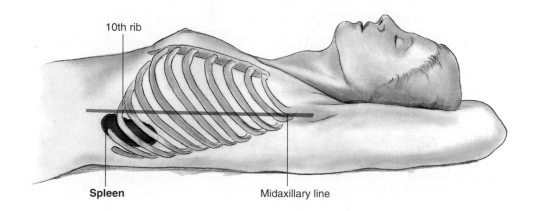

10th rib

Spleen

Midaxillary line

19–3

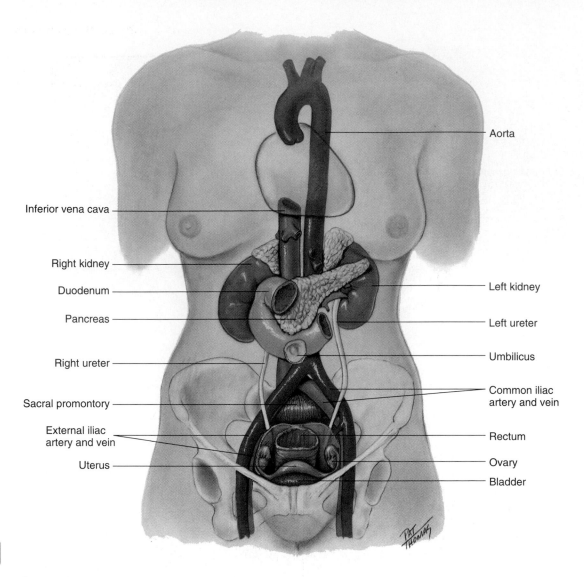

Aorta

Inferior vena cava

Right kidney

Duodenum

Pancreas

Right ureter

Sacral promontory

External iliac
artery and vein

Uterus

Left kidney

Left ureter

Umbilicus

Common iliac
artery and vein

Rectum

Ovary

Bladder

19–4

The **aorta** is just to the left of midline in the upper part of the abdomen (Fig. 19–4). It descends behind the peritoneum and at 2 cm below the umbilicus, it bifurcates into the right and left common iliac arteries opposite the fourth lumbar vertebra. You can palpate the aortic pulsations easily in the upper anterior abdominal wall. The right and left iliac arteries become the femoral arteries in the groin area. Their pulsations are easily palpated as well, at a point halfway between the anterior superior iliac spine and the symphysis pubis.

The **pancreas** is a soft, lobulated gland located behind the stomach. It stretches obliquely across the posterior abdominal wall to the left upper quadrant.

The bean-shaped **kidneys** are retroperitoneal, or posterior to the abdominal contents (Fig. 19–5). They are well protected by the posterior ribs and musculature. The 12th rib forms an angle with the vertebral column, the **costovertebral angle.** The left kidney lies here at the 11th and 12th ribs. Because of the placement of the liver, the right kidney rests 1 to 2 cm lower than the left kidney and sometimes may be palpable.

For convenience in description, the abdominal wall is divided into **four quadrants** by a vertical and a horizon-

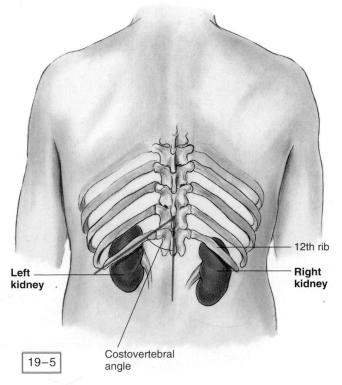

12th rib

**Left
kidney**

**Right
kidney**

Costovertebral
angle

19–5

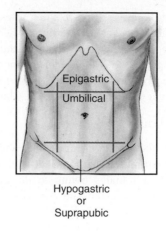

Epigastric
Umbilical

Hypogastric
or
Suprapubic

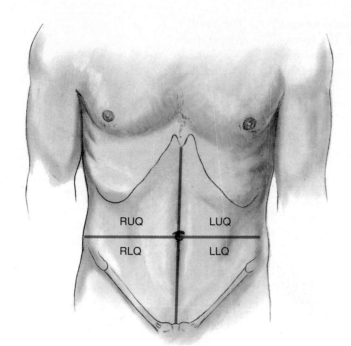

RUQ   LUQ
RLQ   LLQ

Four quadrants

19-6

tal line bisecting the umbilicus (Fig. 19–6). (An older, more complicated scheme divided the abdomen into nine regions. Although the old system generally is not used, some regional names persist, such as *epigastric* for the area between the costal margins, *umbilical* for the area around the umbilicus, and *hypogastric* or *suprapubic* for the area above the pubic bone.)

The anatomic location of the organ by quadrants is

Right Upper Quadrant (RUQ)	Left Upper Quadrant (LUQ)
Liver	Stomach
Gallbladder	Spleen
Duodenum	Left lobe of liver
Head of pancreas	Body of pancreas
Right kidney and adrenal	Left kidney and adrenal
Hepatic flexure of colon	Splenic flexure of colon
Part of ascending and transverse colon	Part of transverse and descending colon

Right Lower Quadrant (RLQ)	Left Lower Quadrant (LLQ)
Cecum	Part of descending colon
Appendix	Sigmoid colon
Right ovary and tube	Left ovary and tube
Right ureter	Left ureter
Right spermatic cord	Left spermatic cord

Midline
Aorta
Uterus (if enlarged)
Bladder (if distended)

DEVELOPMENTAL CONSIDERATIONS

Infants and Children

In the newborn, the umbilical cord shows prominently on the abdomen. It contains two arteries and one vein. The liver takes up proportionately more space in the abdomen at birth than in later life. In normal full-term neonates, the lower edge may be palpated 0.5 to 2.5 cm below the right costal margin. Age-related values of expected liver span are listed in the Objective Data section. The urinary bladder is located higher in the abdomen than in the adult. It lies between the symphysis and the umbilicus. Also during early childhood, the abdominal wall is less muscular, so the organs may be easier to palpate.

The Pregnant Female

Nausea and vomiting, or "morning sickness," is an early sign of pregnancy for 50 to 75 percent of pregnant women, starting between the first and second missed periods. The cause is unknown but may be due to hormone changes such as the production of human chorionic gonadotropin (hCG). Another symptom is "acid indigestion" or heartburn (pyrosis) caused by esophageal reflux. Gastrointestinal motility decreases, which prolongs gastric emptying time. The decreased motility also causes more water to be reabsorbed from the colon, which leads to constipation. The constipation, as well as increased venous pressure in the lower pelvis, may lead to hemorrhoids.

The enlarging uterus displaces the intestines upward and posteriorly. Bowel sounds are diminished. The appendix is displaced upward and to the right, which may complicate diagnosis of a possible appendicitis. Skin changes on the abdomen, such as striae and linea nigra, are discussed later in this chapter and in Chapter 10.

The Aging Adult

Aging alters the appearance of the abdominal wall. During and after middle age, some fat accumulates in the suprapubic area in females owing to decreased estrogen levels. Males also show some fat deposits in the abdominal area, resulting in the "spare tire," or "bay window." This is accentuated in adults with a more sedentary lifestyle.

With further aging, adipose tissue is redistributed away from the face and extremities and to the abdomen and hips. The abdominal musculature relaxes.

Changes of aging occur in the gastrointestinal system but do not significantly affect function as long as no disease is present.

- Salivation decreases, causing the aging person to have a dry mouth and a decreased sense of taste. Further changes involving the mouth and dentition are discussed in Chapter 14.
- Esophageal emptying is delayed. If an aging person is fed in the supine position, this may increase the risk of aspiration.
- Gastric acid secretion decreases with aging. This may cause pernicious anemia (because it interferes with vitamin B_{12} absorption), iron deficiency anemia, and malabsorption of calcium.
- The incidence of gallstones increases with age, occurring in 10 to 15 percent of men and in 20 to 40 percent of women after age 60 (Johnston and Kaplan, 1993).
- Liver size decreases with age, particularly after 80 years, although most liver function remains normal. Drug metabolism by the liver is impaired, in part because by age 60 to 80 years, blood flow through the liver is decreased by 55 to 60 percent (Katzung, 1995). Therefore, the liver metabolism that is responsible for the enzymatic oxidation, reduction, and hydrolysis of drugs is substantially decreased with age. Some of the drugs whose metabolism is decreased due to age-related changes include

Acetaminophen
Amitriptyline
Barbiturates
Chlordiazepoxide
Diazepam
Diphenhydramine
Flurazepam
Ibuprofen
Labetalol
Meperidine
Nortriptyline
Phenytoin
Propranolol
Quinidine
Theophylline
Tolbutamide

This is clinically significant because prolonged liver metabolism causes increased side effects. For example, the long-acting benzodiazepines such as flurazepam (Dalmane) have been shown to increase the risk of hip fracture in older people, whereas the short-acting benzodiazepines do not (Ray, 1992).

- Aging persons frequently report constipation. However, a greater number use laxatives regularly (up to 30 percent of healthy older people) than actually are constipated (<10 percent of healthy, ambulatory, aged people). Reasons for the disparity in rates of perceived and actual constipation include a mistaken opinion about how often a healthy person should defecate (true constipation is having a bowel movement less often than every 3rd day) and confusing the passage of hard or small stools, the feeling of incomplete evacuation, or the need to strain at stool for constipation (Stone, Wyman, and Salisbury, 1999).

Of those aging people who actually are constipated, two-thirds have been found to have slowed passage in the distal colon and delayed rectal emptying (Wald, 1990). Common causes of constipation include decreased physical activity, inadequate intake of water, a low-fiber diet, side effects of medications, irritable bowel syndrome, bowel obstruction, hypothyroidism, inadequate toilet facilities (i.e., difficulty ambulating to the toilet may cause the person to deliberately retain the stool until it becomes hard and difficult to pass), and colorectal dysmotility.

TRANSCULTURAL CONSIDERATIONS

Lactase is the digestive enzyme necessary for the absorption of the carbohydrate lactose (milk sugar). In some racial groups, lactase activity is high at birth but declines to low levels by adulthood. These people are *lactose intolerant* (or lactase deficient), and experience abdominal pain, bloating, and flatulence when milk products are consumed. The incidence of lactose intolerance is 70 to 90 percent in blacks, Native Americans, Asians, and Mediterranean groups. However, in Europeans and Americans of northern and western European descent, the level of lactase activity remains high through adulthood, and the incidence of milk intolerance is only about 15 percent (Ganong, 1995).

1. Appetite
2. Dysphagia
3. Food intolerance
4. Abdominal pain
5. Nausea/vomiting

6. Bowel habits
7. Past abdominal history
8. Medications
9. Nutritional assessment

Examiner Asks	Rationale

1 Appetite.
- Any change in **appetite?** Is this a loss of appetite?
- Any change in weight? How much weight gained or lost? Over what time period? Is the weight loss due to diet?

Anorexia is a loss of appetite for food that occurs with gastrointestinal disease or as a side effect to some medications, with pregnancy, or with psychological disorders.

2 Dysphagia.
- Any difficulty swallowing? When did you first notice this?

Dysphagia occurs with disorders of the throat or esophagus.

3 Food intolerance.
- Are there any foods you cannot eat? What happens if you do eat them: allergic reaction, heartburn, belching, bloating, indigestion?
- Do you use antacids? How often?

Food intolerance, e.g., lactase deficiency resulting in bloating or excessive gas after taking milk products.

Pyrosis (heartburn), a burning sensation in esophagus and stomach, owing to reflux of gastric acid.

Eructation (belching).

4 Abdominal pain.
- Any **abdominal pain?** Please point to it.
- Is the pain in one spot or does it move around?
- How did it start? How long have you had it?
- Constant or does it come and go? Occur before or after meals? Does it peak? When?
- How would you describe the character: cramping (colic type), burning in pit of stomach, dull, stabbing, aching?
- Is the pain relieved by food, or worse after eating?
- Is the pain associated with: menstrual period or irregularities, stress, dietary indiscretion, fatigue, nausea and vomiting, gas, fever, rectal bleeding, frequent urination, vaginal or penile discharge?
- What makes the pain worse: food, position, stress, medication, activity?
- What have you tried to relieve pain: rest, heating pad, change in position, medication?

Abdominal pain may be *visceral* from an internal organ (dull, general, poorly localized), *parietal* from inflammation of overlying peritoneum (sharp, precisely localized, aggravated by movement), or *referred* from a disorder in another site (see Table 19–2 on p. 616).

Aggravating factors.

Alleviating factors.

5 Nausea/vomiting.
- Any **nausea** or **vomiting?** How often? How much comes up? What is the color? Is there an odor?

Nausea/vomiting is a common side effect of many medications and occurs with gastrointestinal disease as well as early pregnancy.

Examiner Asks	Rationale
● Is it bloody?	Hematemesis occurs with ulcers of the stomach or duodenum and esophageal varices.
● Is the nausea and vomiting associated with colicky pain, diarrhea, fever, chills?	
● What foods did you eat in the last 24 hours? Where? At home, school, restaurant? Is there anyone else in the family with same symptoms in last 24 hours?	Consider food poisoning.
6 Bowel habits.	
● How often do you have a **bowel movement?**	Assess usual **bowel habits.**
● What is the color? Consistency?	Black stools may be tarry due to passage of occult blood (melena) from gastrointestinal bleeding or nontarry from injection of iron medications.
● Any diarrhea or constipation? How long?	
● Any recent change in bowel habits?	
● Use laxatives? Which ones? How often do you use them?	Red blood in stools occurs with gastrointestinal bleeding or localized bleeding around the anus.
7 Past abdominal history.	
● Any **past history** of gastrointestinal problems: ulcer, gallbladder disease, hepatitis/jaundice, appendicitis, colitis, hernia?	
● Ever had any operations in the abdomen? Please describe.	
● Any problems after surgery?	
● Any abdominal x-ray studies? How were the results?	
8 Medications.	
● What **medications** are you currently taking?	Consider gastrointestinal side effects of certain medications, e.g., aspirin.
● How about alcohol—How much would you say you drink each day? Each week? When was your last alcoholic drink?	
● How about cigarettes—Do you smoke? How many packs per day? For how long?	Cigarette smoking is a common cause of gastric ulcers.
9 Nutritional assessment.	
● Now I would like to ask you about your diet. Please tell me all the food you ate yesterday, starting with breakfast.	**Nutritional assessment,** via 24-hour recall (see Chapter 7 for a complete discussion).

ADDITIONAL HISTORY FOR INFANTS AND CHILDREN

1 Are you breast- or bottle-feeding the baby? If bottle-feeding, how does baby tolerate the formula?

2 What table foods have you introduced? How does the infant tolerate the food?

With allergies, consider a new food as a possible allergen. Adding only one new food at a time to the infant's diet helps identify any possible allergies.

3 How often does your toddler/child eat? Does he or she eat regular meals? How do you feel about your child's eating patterns?
   ● Please describe all that your child had to eat yesterday, starting with breakfast. What foods does the child eat for snacks?

Irregular eating patterns, although common at this age, can be a source of parental anxiety. As long as child shows normal growth and development and only nutritious foods are offered, parents may be reassured.

Examiner Asks	Rationale

- Does toddler/child ever eat nonfoods: grass, dirt, paint chips?

Pica—Although a toddler may attempt nonfoods at some time, he or she should recognize edibles by age 2.

4 Does your child have constipation: How long?
- What are the number of stools/day? Stools/week?
- How much water, juice is in the diet?
- Does the constipation seem to be associated with toilet training?
- What have you tried to treat the constipation?

5 Does the child have abdominal pain? Please describe what you have noticed and when it started.

This symptom is hard to assess with young children. Many conditions of unrelated organ systems are associated with vague abdominal pain (e.g., otitis media). Young children do not have the capacity to articulate specific symptoms and often focus on "the tummy." Abdominal pain accompanies inflammation of the bowel, as well as constipation, urinary tract infection, and anxiety.

6 For the overweight child: How long has weight been a problem?
- At what age did the child first seem overweight? Did any change in diet pattern occur then?
- Describe the diet pattern now.
- Do any others in family have similar problem?
- How does child feel about his or her own weight?

Alteration in nutrition: more than body overweight requirements.

Family history of obesity.
Assess body image.

ADDITIONAL HISTORY FOR ADOLESCENTS

1 What do you eat at regular meals? Do you eat breakfast? What do you eat for snacks?

Adolescent takes control of eating and may reject family values, e.g., skipping breakfast, consuming junk foods, soda pop. The only control parents have is to control what food is in the house.

- How many calories do you figure you consume?

You probably cannot change adolescent eating pattern, but you can supply nutritional facts.

2 What is your exercise pattern?

Boys need an average 4000 cal/day to maintain weight; more calories are needed if exercise is pursued. Girls need 20 percent fewer calories and the same nutrients as boys. Fast food is a problem because it is high in fat, calories, and salt and has no fiber.

3 If weight is less than body requirements: How much have you lost? By diet, exercise, or how?

Screen any extremely thin teenage girl for *anorexia nervosa,* a serious psychosocial disorder that includes loss of appetite, voluntary starvation, and grave weight loss. This person may augment weight loss by purging (self-induced vomiting) and use of laxatives.

Examiner Asks	Rationale
● How do you feel? Tired, hungry? How do you think your body looks?	Denial of these feelings is common. Though thin, this person insists she looks fat, "disgusting." Distorted body image.
● What is your activity pattern?	The anorectic may participate in normal activity and exercise but often is hyperactive.
● Is the weight loss associated with any other body change, such as menstrual irregularity?	Amenorrhea is common with anorexia nervosa.
● What do your parents say about your eating? Your friends?	This is a family problem involving control issues. Anyone at risk warrants immediate referral to a physician or psychologist.

ADDITIONAL HISTORY FOR THE AGING ADULT

1 How do you acquire your groceries and prepare your meals?	Assess if at risk for nutritional deficit due to limited access to grocery store, limited income, limited cooking facilities, physical disability (impaired vision, decreased mobility, decreased strength, neurologic deficit).
2 Do you eat alone or share meals with others?	Assess if at risk for nutritional deficit if living alone; may not bother to prepare all meals; social isolation; depression.
3 Please tell me all that you had to eat yesterday, starting with breakfast.	Note: 24-hour recall may not be sufficient because pattern may vary from day to day. Attempt week-long diary of intake. Food pattern may be different at the end of the month if monthly income, i.e., social security check, runs out.
● Do you have any trouble swallowing these foods?	
● What do you do right after eating: walk, take a nap?	
4 How often do your bowels move?	
● If the person reports constipation: What do you mean by constipation? How much liquid is in your diet? How much bulk or fiber?	
● Do you take anything for constipation, such as laxatives? Which ones? How often?	
● What medications do you take?	Consider gastrointestinal side effects; e.g., nausea, upset stomach, anorexia, dry mouth.

Preparation

The lighting should include a strong overhead light and a secondary stand light. Expose the abdomen so that it is fully visible. Drape the genitalia and female breasts.

The following measures will enhance abdominal wall relaxation:

- The person should have emptied the bladder, saving a urine specimen if needed.
- Keep the room warm to avoid chilling and tensing of muscles.
- Position the person supine, with the head on a pillow, the knees bent or on pillow, and the arms at the sides or across the chest. (Note: Discourage the person from placing his or her arms over the head because this tenses abdominal musculature.)
- To avoid abdominal tensing, the stethoscope endpiece must be warm, your hands must be warm, and your fingernails must be very short.
- Inquire about any painful areas. Examine such an area last to avoid any muscle guarding.
- Finally, learn to use distraction: Enhance muscle relaxation through breathing exercises; emotive imagery; your low, soothing voice; and the person relating his or her abdominal history while you palpate.

Equipment Needed

Stethoscope
Small centimeter ruler
Skin-marking pen
Alcohol swab (to clean endpiece)

Normal Range of Findings	Abnormal Findings

INSPECTION

Inspect the abdomen
Contour

Stand on the person's right side and look down on the abdomen. Then stoop or sit to gaze across the abdomen. Your head should be slightly higher than the abdomen. Determine the profile from the rib margin to the pubic bone. The contour describes the nutritional state and normally ranges from flat to rounded (Fig. 19–7).

Protuberant abdomen, abdominal distention (see Table 19–3).

Flat

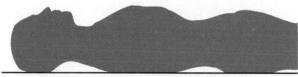
Scaphoid

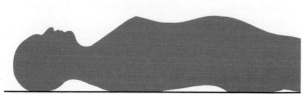
Rounded

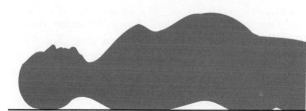
Protuberant

▶ | **N o r m a l   R a n g e   o f   F i n d i n g s** | **A b n o r m a l   F i n d i n g s**

Symmetry

Shine a light across the abdomen toward you, or shine it lengthwise across the person. The abdomen should be symmetric bilaterally (Fig. 19–8). Note any localized bulging, visible mass, or asymmetric shape. Even small bulges are highlighted by shadow. Step to the foot of the examination table to recheck symmetry.

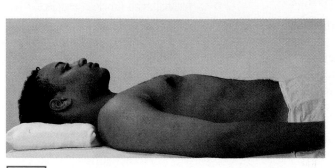

19–8

Ask the person to take a deep breath to further highlight any change. The abdomen should stay smooth and symmetric. Or ask the person to perform a sit-up without pushing up with his or her hands.

Umbilicus

Normally it is midline and inverted, with no sign of discoloration, inflammation, or hernia. It becomes everted and pushed upward with pregnancy.

Skin

The surface is smooth and even, with homogeneous color. This is a good area to judge pigment because it is often protected from sun.

One common pigment change is **striae** (lineae albicantes), silvery white, linear, jagged marks about 1 to 6 cm long (Fig. 19–9). They occur when elastic fibers in the reticular layer of the skin are broken following rapid or prolonged stretching, as in pregnancy or excessive weight gain. Recent striae are pink or blue, then they turn silvery white.

Abnormal Findings

Bulges, masses.

Hernia—protrusion of abdominal viscera through abnormal opening in muscle wall (see Table 19–4).

Note any localized bulging.

Hernia, enlarged liver or spleen may show.

Everted with acites, or underlying mass (see Table 19–3).

Deeply sunken with obesity.

Enlarged and everted with umbilical hernia.

Bluish periumbilical color occurs with intraabdominal bleeding (Cullen sign).

Redness with localized inflammation.

Jaundice (shows best in natural daylight).

Skin glistening and taut occurs with ascites.

Striae also occur with ascites.

Striae look purple-blue with Cushing's syndrome (excess adrenocortical hormone causes the skin to be fragile and easily broken from normal stretching).

▶ | **N o r m a l R a n g e o f F i n d i n g s** | **A b n o r m a l F i n d i n g s**

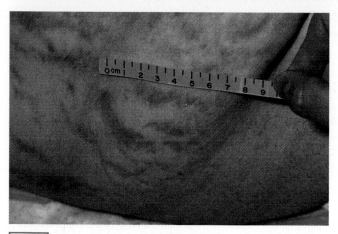

19–9

Striae

Moles, circumscribed brown macular or papular areas, are common on the abdomen.

Normally, no lesions are present, although you may note well-healed surgical scars. If a scar is present, draw its location in the person's record, indicating the length in centimeters (Fig. 19–10). (Not infrequently, a person forgets a past operation while providing the history. If you note a scar now, ask about it.) A surgical scar alerts you to the possible presence of underlying adhesions and excess fibrous tissue.

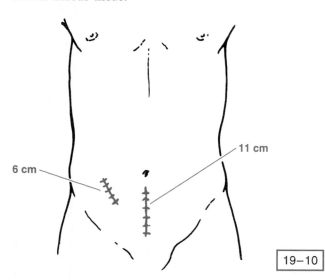

19–10

Veins usually are not seen, but a fine venous network may be visible in thin persons.

Unusual color or change in shape of mole (see Chapter 10).

Petechiae.

Cutaneous angiomas (spider nevi) occur with portal hypertension or liver disease.

Lesions, rashes (see Chapter 10).

Prominent, dilated veins occur with portal hypertension, cirrhosis, ascites, or vena caval obstruction. Veins are more visible with malnutrition due to thinned adipose tissue.

Normal Range of Findings

Abnormal Findings

Good skin turgor reflects healthy nutrition. Gently pinch up a fold of skin; then release to note the skin's immediate return to original position.

Poor turgor occurs with dehydration, which often accompanies gastrointestinal disease.

Pulsation or Movement

Normally, you may see the pulsations from the aorta beneath the skin in the epigastric area, particularly in thin persons with good muscle wall relaxation. Respiratory movement also shows in the abdomen, particularly in males. Finally, waves of peristalsis sometimes are visible in very thin persons. They ripple slowly and obliquely across the abdomen.

Marked pulsation of the aorta occurs with widened pulse pressure (e.g., hypertension, aortic insufficiency, thyrotoxicosis) and with aortic aneurysm.

Marked visible peristasis, together with a distended abdomen, indicates intestinal obstruction.

Hair Distribution

The pattern of pubic hair growth normally has a diamond shape in adult males and an inverted triangle shape in adult females (see Chapters 22 and 24).

Patterns alter with endocrine or hormone abnormalities and with chronic liver disease.

Demeanor

A comfortable person is relaxed quietly on the examining table and has a benign facial expression and slow, even respirations.

Restlessness and constant turning to find a comfortable position occur with the colicky pain of gastroenteritis or bowel obstruction.

Absolute stillness, resisting any movement, is demonstrated with the pain of peritonitis.

Knees flexed up, facial grimacing, and rapid, uneven respirations also indicate pain.

AUSCULTATION

Auscultate bowel sounds and vascular sounds

Depart from the usual examination sequence and auscultate the abdomen next. This is done because percussion and palpation can increase peristalsis, which would give a false interpretation of bowel sounds. Use the diaphragm endpiece because bowel sounds are relatively high pitched. Hold the stethoscope lightly against the skin; pushing too hard may stimulate more bowel sounds (Fig. 19–11). Begin in the RLQ at the ileocecal valve area, because bowel sounds are always present here normally.

Normal Range of Findings	Abnormal Findings

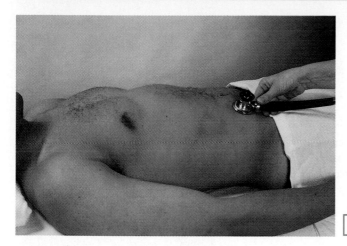

19–11

Bowel Sounds

Note the character and frequency of bowel sounds. Bowel sounds originate from the movement of air and fluid through the small intestine. Depending on the time elapsed since eating, a wide range of normal sounds can occur. Bowel sounds are high pitched, gurgling, cascading sounds, occurring irregularly anywhere from 5 to 30 times per minute. Do not bother to count them. Judge if they are normal, hypoactive, or hyperactive.

One type of hyperactive bowel sounds is fairly common. This is the hyperperistalsis when you feel your "stomach growling," termed *borborygmus*. A perfectly "silent abdomen" is uncommon; you must listen for 5 minutes by your watch before deciding bowel sounds are completely absent.

Two distinct patterns of abnormal bowel sounds may occur:

1. **Hyperactive sounds** are loud, high-pitched, rushing, tinkling sounds that signal increased motility.

2. **Hypoactive or absent sounds** follow abdominal surgery or with inflammation of the peritoneum (see Table 19–5).

Vascular Sounds

As you listen to the abdomen, note the presence of any vascular sounds or **bruits.** Using firmer pressure, check over the aorta, renal arteries, iliac and femoral arteries, especially in people with hypertension (Fig. 19–12). Usually, no such sound is present.

Note location, pitch, and timing of a vascular sound.

A systolic bruit is a pulsatile blowing sound and occurs with stenosis or occlusion of an artery.

Venous hum and peritoneal friction rub are rare (see Table 19–6).

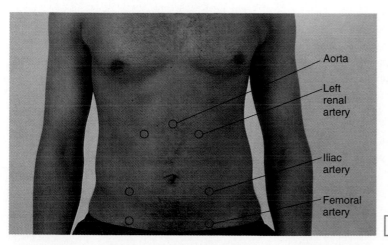

Aorta
Left renal artery
Iliac artery
Femoral artery

19–12

Normal Range of Findings	Abnormal Findings

PERCUSSION

Percuss general tympany, liver span, and splenic dullness

Percuss to assess the relative density of abdominal contents, to locate organs, and to screen for abnormal fluid or masses.

General Tympany

First, percuss lightly in all four quadrants to determine the prevailing amount of tympany and dullness (Fig. 19–13). Tympany should predominate because air in the intestines rises to the surface when the person is supine.

Dullness occurs over a distended bladder, adipose tissue, fluid, or a mass.

Hyperresonance is present with gaseous distention.

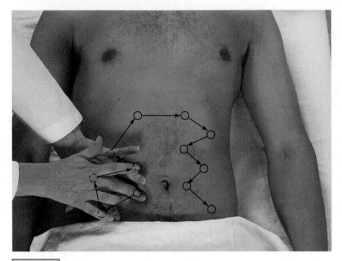

19–13

Liver Span

Next, percuss to map out the boundaries of certain organs. Measure the height of the liver in the right midclavicular line. (For a consistent placement of the midclavicular line landmark, remember to palpate the acromioclavicular and the sternoclavicular joints and judge the line at a point midway between the two.)

Begin in the area of lung resonance, and percuss down the interspaces until the sound changes to a dull quality (Fig. 19–14). Mark the spot, usually in the fifth intercostal space. Then find abdominal tympany and percuss up in the midclavicular line. Mark where the sound changes from tympany to a dull sound, normally at the right costal margin.

▶ Normal Range of Findings | Abnormal Findings

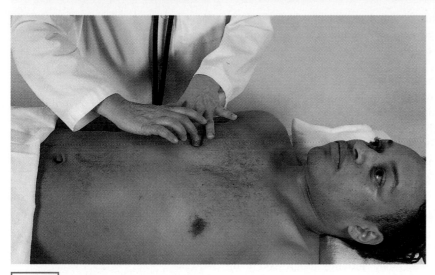

19-14

Measure the distance between the two marks; the normal liver span in the adult ranges from 6 to 12 cm (Fig. 19–15). The height of the liver span correlates with the height of the person; taller people have longer livers. Also males have a larger liver span than females of the same height. Overall, the mean liver span is 10.5 cm for males and 7 cm for females.

An enlarged liver span indicates liver enlargement or **hepatomegaly.**

Accurate detection of liver borders is confused by dullness above the fifth intercostal space, which occurs with lung disease, e.g., pleural effusion or consolidation. Accurate detection at the lower border is confused when dullness is pushed up with ascites or pregnancy or with gas distention in colon, which obscures lower border.

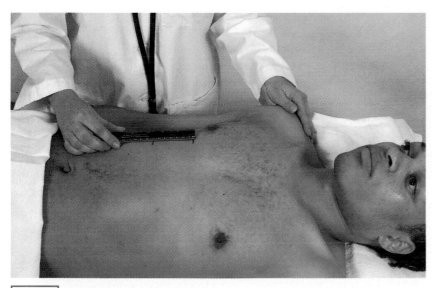

19-15

One variation occurs in people with chronic emphysema, in which the liver is displaced downward by the hyperinflated lungs. Although you hear a dull percussion note well below the right costal margin, the overall span is still within normal limits.

Clinical estimation of liver span is important to screen for hepatomegaly and to monitor changes in liver size. However, this measurement is a gross estimate; the liver span may be underestimated because of inaccurate detection of the upper border. *Direct* percussion, lightly tapping the body surface directly with the index finger, may be more sensitive to changes in pitch and vibration than the traditional method of indirect percussion (Skrainka et al., 1986). The bedside estimate of liver span by this direct percussion method was confirmed to be as accurate as ultrasound study.

Scratch Test. One final technique is the *scratch test,* which may help define the liver border when the abdomen is distended or the abdominal muscles are tense. Place your stethoscope over the liver. With one fingernail, scratch short strokes over the abdomen, starting in the RLQ and moving progressively up toward the liver (Fig. 19–16). When the scratching sound in your stethoscope becomes magnified, you will have crossed the border from over a hollow organ to a solid one.

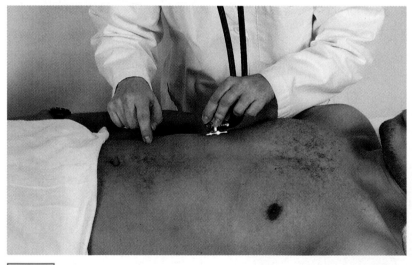

19–16

Splenic Dullness

Often the spleen is obscured by stomach contents, but you may locate it by percussing for a dull note from the 9th to 11th intercostal space just behind the left mid-axillary line (Fig. 19–17). The area of splenic dullness normally is not wider than 7 cm in the adult and should not encroach on the normal tympany over the gastric air bubble.

A dull note forward of the mid-axillary line indicates enlargement of the spleen, as occurs with mononucleosis, trauma, and infection.

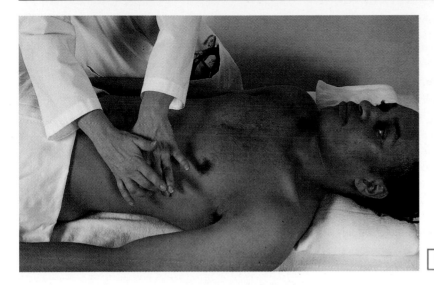

19–17

Now percuss in the lowest interspace in the left *anterior* axillary line. Tympany should result. Ask the person to take a deep breath. Normally, tympany remains through full inspiration.

In this site, the *anterior* axillary line, a change in percussion from tympany to a dull sound with full inspiration is a **positive spleen percussion sign,** indicating splenomegaly. This method will detect mild to moderate splenomegaly before the spleen becomes palpable, as in mononucleosis, malaria, or hepatic cirrhosis.

Costovertebral Angle Tenderness

Indirect fist percussion causes the tissues to vibrate instead of producing a sound. To assess the kidney, place one hand over the 12th rib at the costovertebral angle on the back (Fig. 19–18). Thump that hand with the ulnar edge of your other fist. The person normally feels a thud but no pain. (Although this step is explained here with percussion techniques, its usual sequence in a complete examination is with thoracic assessment, when the person is sitting up and you are standing behind.)

Sharp pain occurs with inflammation of the kidney or paranephric area.

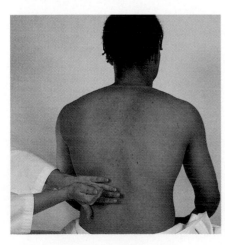

19–18

▶

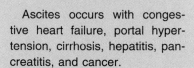

Special Procedures

At times, you may suspect that a person has ascites (free fluid in the peritoneal cavity) because of a distended abdomen, bulging flanks, and an umbilicus that is protruding and displaced downward. You can differentiate ascites from gaseous distention by performing two percussion tests.

Fluid Wave. First, test for a **fluid wave** by standing on the person's right side. Place the ulnar edge of another examiner's hand or the patient's own hand firmly on the abdomen in the midline (Fig. 19–19). (This will stop transmission across the skin of the upcoming tap.) Place your left hand on the person's right flank. With your right hand, reach across the abdomen and give the left flank a firm strike. If acites is present, the blow will generate a fluid wave through the abdomen and you will feel a distinct tap on your left hand. If the abdomen is distended from gas or adipose tissue, you will feel no change.

Ascites occurs with congestive heart failure, portal hypertension, cirrhosis, hepatitis, pancreatitis, and cancer.

A positive fluid wave test occurs with large amounts of ascitic fluid.

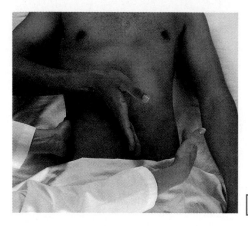

19–19

Shifting Dullness. The second test for ascites is percussing for **shifting dullness.** In a supine person, ascitic fluid settles by gravity into the flanks, displacing the air-filled bowel upward. You will hear a tympanitic note as you percuss over the top of the abdomen because gas-filled intestines float over the fluid (Fig. 19–20). Then percuss down the side of the abdomen. If fluid is present, the note will change from tympany to dull as you reach its level. Mark this spot.

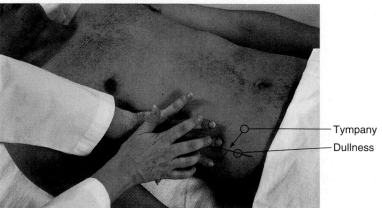

— Tympany
— Dullness

19–20

Now turn the person onto the right side (roll the person toward you) (Fig. 19–21). The fluid will gravitate to the dependent (in this case, right) side, displacing the lighter bowel upward. Begin percussing the upper side of the abdomen and move downward. The sound changes from tympany to a dull sound as you reach the fluid level, but this time the level of dullness is higher, upward toward the umbilicus. This *shifting level of dullness* indicates the presence of fluid.

Shifting dullness is positive with a large volume of ascitic fluid: It will not detect less than 500 ml of fluid.

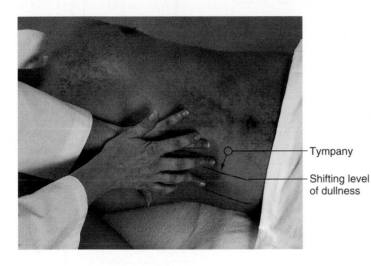

— Tympany

— Shifting level of dullness

19–21

Both tests, fluid wave and shifting dullness, are not reliable. Ultrasound study is the definitive tool.

PALPATION

Palpate surface and deep areas

Perform palpation to judge the size, location, and consistency of certain organs and to screen for an abnormal mass or tenderness. Review comfort measures on p. 591. Since most people are naturally inclined to protect the abdomen, you need to use additional measures to enhance complete muscle relaxation.

1. Bend the person's knees.
2. Keep your palpating hand low and parallel to the abdomen. Holding the hand high and pointing down would make anyone tense up.
3. Teach the person to breathe slowly (in through the nose, and out through the mouth).
4. Keep your own voice low and soothing. Conversation may relax the person.
5. Try "emotive imagery." For example, you might say, "Now I want you to imagine you are dozing on the beach, with the sun warming your muscles and the sound of the waves lulling you to sleep. Let yourself relax."
6. With a very ticklish person, keep the person's hand under your own with your fingers curled over his or her fingers. Move both hands around as you palpate; people are not ticklish to themselves.
7. Alternatively, perform palpation just after auscultation. Keep the stethoscope in place and curl your fingers around it, palpating as you pretend to auscultate. People·do not perceive a stethoscope as a ticklish object. You can slide the stethoscope out when the person is used to being touched.

▶ Normal Range of Findings

Abnormal Findings

Light and Deep Palpation

Begin with **light palpation.** With the first four fingers close together, depress the skin about 1 cm (Fig. 19–22). Make a gentle rotary motion, sliding the fingers and skin together. Then lift the fingers (do not drag them) and move clockwise to the next location around the abdomen. The objective here is not to search for organs but to form an overall impression of the skin surface and superficial musculature. Save the examination of any identified tender areas until last. This method avoids pain and the resulting muscle rigidity that would obscure deep palpation later in the examination.

Muscle guarding.

Rigidity.

Large masses.

Tenderness.

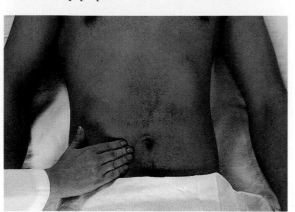

19–22

As you circle the abdomen, discriminate between voluntary muscle guarding and involuntary rigidity. **Voluntary guarding** occurs when the person is cold, tense, or ticklish. It is bilateral, and you will feel the muscles relax slightly during exhalation. Use the relaxation measures to try to eliminate this type of guarding, or it will interfere with deep palpation. If the rigidity persists, it is probably involuntary.

Involuntary rigidity is a constant boardlike hardness of the muscles. It is a protective mechanism accompanying acute inflammation of the peritoneum. It may be unilateral, and the same area usually becomes painful when the person increases intraabdominal pressure by attempting a sit-up.

Now perform **deep palpation** using the same technique described earlier, but push down about 5 to 8 cm (2 to 3 inches) (Fig. 19–23). Moving clockwise, explore the entire abdomen.

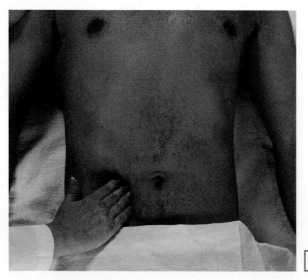

19–23

Normal Range of Findings	Abnormal Findings

To overcome the resistance of a very large or obese abdomen, use a bimanual technique. Place your two hands on top of each other (Fig. 19–24). The top hand does the pushing; the bottom hand is relaxed and can concentrate on the sense of palpation. With either technique, note the location, size, consistency, and mobility of any palpable organs and the presence of any abnormal enlargement, tenderness, or masses.

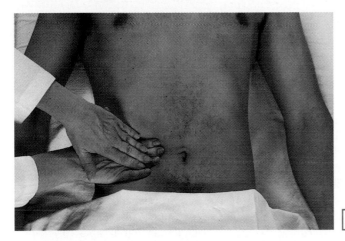

19–24

Making sense of what you are feeling is more difficult than it looks. Inexperienced examiners complain that the abdomen "all feels the same," as if they are pushing their hand into a soft sofa cushion. It helps to memorize the anatomy and visualize what is under each quadrant as you palpate. Also remember that some structures are normally palpable, as illustrated in Figure 19–25.

Mild tenderness normally is present when palpating the sigmoid colon. Any other tenderness should be investigated.

Tenderness occurs with local inflammation, with inflammation of the peritoneum or underlying organ, and with an enlarged organ whose capsule is stretched.

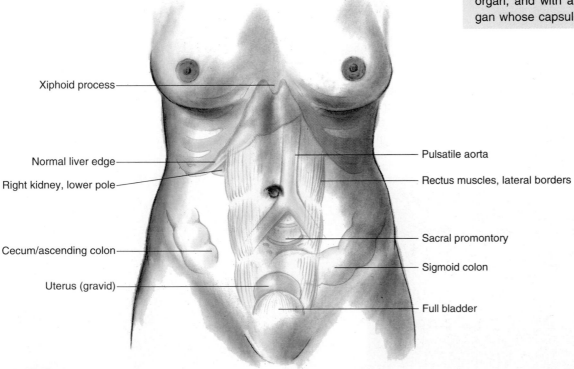

Xiphoid process

Normal liver edge

Right kidney, lower pole

Cecum/ascending colon

Uterus (gravid)

Pulsatile aorta

Rectus muscles, lateral borders

Sacral promontory

Sigmoid colon

Full bladder

19–25

NORMALLY PALPABLE STRUCTURES

If you identify a mass, first distinguish it from a normally palpable structure or an enlarged organ. Then note its

1. Location
2. Size
3. Shape
4. Consistency (soft, firm, hard)
5. Surface (smooth, nodular)
6. Mobility (including movement with respirations)
7. Pulsatility
8. Tenderness

Liver

Next, palpate for specific organs, beginning with the liver in the RUQ (Fig. 19–26). Place your left hand under the person's back parallel to the 11th and 12th ribs and lift up to support the abdominal contents. Place your right hand on the RUQ, with fingers parallel to the midline. Push deeply down and under the right costal margin. Ask the person to take a deep breath. It is normal to feel the edge of the liver bump your fingertips as the diaphragm pushes it down during inhalation. It feels like a firm regular ridge. Often, the liver is not palpable and you feel nothing firm.

Except with a depressed diaphragm, a liver palpated more than 1 to 2 cm below the right costal margin is enlarged. Record the number of centimeters it descends and note its consistency (hard, nodular) and tenderness (see Table 19–7.)

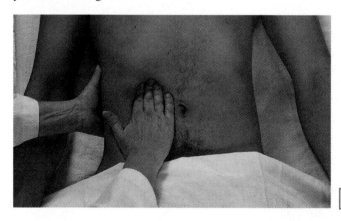

19–26

Hooking Technique. An alternative method of palpating the liver is to stand up at the person's shoulder and swivel your body to the right so that you face the person's feet (Fig. 19–27). Hook your fingers over the costal margin from above. Ask the person to take a deep breath. Try to feel the liver edge bump your fingertips.

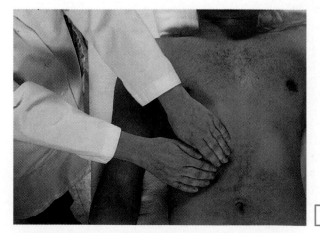

19–27

▶ Normal Range of Findings

Abnormal Findings

Spleen

Normally, the spleen is not palpable and must be enlarged three times its normal size to be felt. To search for it, reach your left hand over the abdomen and behind the left side at the 11th and 12th ribs (Fig. 19–28*A*). Lift up for support. Place your right hand obliquely on the LUQ with the fingers pointing toward the left axilla and just inferior to the rib margin. Push your hand deeply down and under the left costal margin and ask the person to take a deep breath. You should feel nothing firm.

The spleen enlarges with mononucleosis and trauma (see Table 19–7). If you feel an enlarged spleen, refer the person but do not continue to palpate it. An enlarged spleen is friable and can rupture easily with overpalpation.

Describe the number of centimeters it extends below the left costal margin.

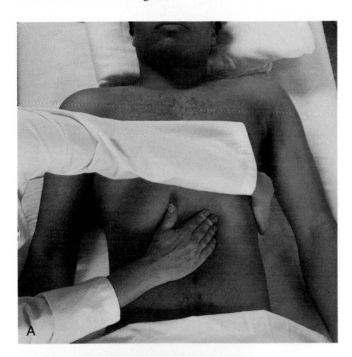

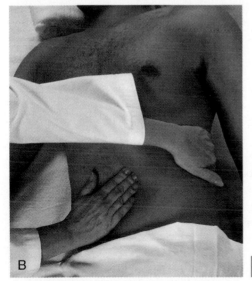

19–28

When enlarged, the spleen slides out and bumps your fingertips. It can grow so large that it extends into the lower quadrants. When this condition is suspected, start low so you will not miss it. An alternative position is to roll the person onto his or her right side to displace the spleen more forward and downward (Fig. 19–28*B*). Then palpate as described earlier.

Kidneys

Search for the right kidney by placing your hands together in a "duck-bill" position at the person's right flank (Fig. 19–29A). Press your two hands together firmly (you need deeper palpation than that used with the liver or spleen) and ask the person to take a deep breath. In most people, you will feel no change. Occasionally, you may feel the lower pole of the right kidney as a round, smooth mass slide between your fingers. Either condition is normal.

Enlarged kidney.

Kidney mass.

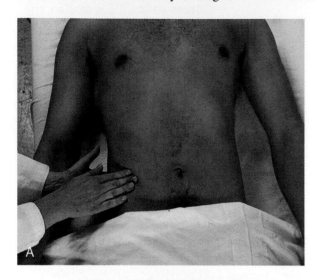

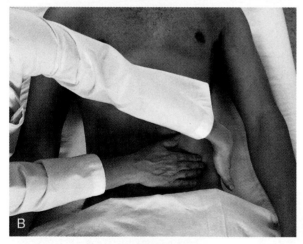

19–29

The left kidney sits 1 cm higher than the right kidney and is not palpable normally. Search for it by reaching your left hand across the abdomen and behind the left flank for support (Fig. 19–29B). Push your right hand deep into the abdomen and ask the person to breathe deeply. You should feel no change with the inhalation.

Aorta

Using your opposing thumb and fingers, palpate the aortic pulsation in the upper abdomen slightly to the left of midline (Fig. 19–30). Normally, it is 2.5 to 4 cm wide in the adult and pulsates in an anterior direction.

Widened with aneurysm (see Tables 19–6 and 19–7).

Prominent lateral pulsation with aortic aneurysm.

► Normal Range of Findings	Abnormal Findings

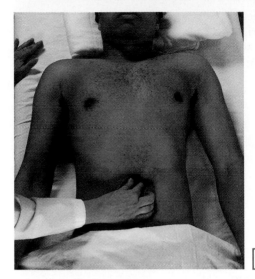

19–30

Special Procedures

Rebound Tenderness (Blumberg Sign). Assess rebound tenderness when the person reports abdominal pain or when you elicit tenderness during palpation. Choose a site away from the painful area. Hold your hand 90 degrees, or perpendicular, to the abdomen. Push down slowly and deeply; then lift up *quickly* (Fig. 19–31*A, B*). This makes structures that are indented by palpation rebound suddenly. A normal, or negative, response is no pain on release of pressure. Perform this test at the end of the examination, because it can cause severe pain and muscle rigidity.

Pain on release of pressure confirms rebound tenderness, which is a reliable sign of peritoneal inflammation. Peritoneal inflammation accompanies appendicitis.

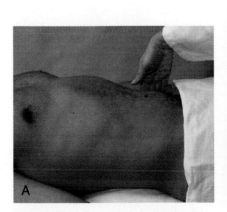
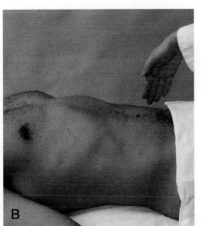

A   B

19–31

Inspiratory Arrest (Murphy's Sign). Normally, palpating the liver causes no pain. In a person with inflammation of the gallbladder, or cholecystitis, pain occurs. Hold your fingers under the liver border. Ask the person to take a deep breath. A normal response is to complete the deep breath without pain.

When the test is positive, as the descending liver pushes the inflamed gallbladder onto the examining hand, the person feels sharp pain and abruptly stops inspiration midway.

Normal Range of Findings	Abnormal Findings

Iliopsoas Muscle Test. Perform the iliopsoas muscle test when the acute abdominal pain of appendicitis is suspected. With the person supine, lift the right leg straight up, flexing at the hip (Fig. 19–32); then push down over the lower part of the right thigh as the person tries to hold the leg up. When the test is negative, the person feels no change.

When the iliopsoas muscle is inflamed (which occurs with an inflamed or perforated appendix), pain is felt in the right lower quadrant.

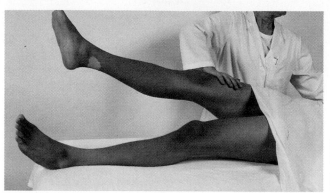

19–32

Iliopsoas Muscle Test

Obturator Test. The obturator test also is performed when appendicitis is suspected. With the person supine, lift the right leg, flexing at the hip and 90 degrees at the knee (Fig. 19–33). Hold the ankle and rotate the leg internally and externally. A negative or normal response is no pain.

A perforated appendix irritates the obturator muscle, producing pain.

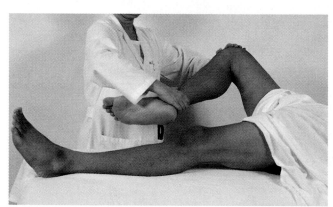

19–33

Obturator Test

 ## DEVELOPMENTAL CONSIDERATIONS

The Infant

Inspection. The contour of the abdomen is protuberant because of the immature abdominal musculature. The skin contains a fine, superficial venous pattern. This may be visible in lightly pigmented children up to the age of puberty.

Inspect the umbilical cord throughout the neonatal period. At birth, it is white and contains two umbilical arteries and one vein surrounded by mucoid connective tissue, called Wharton's jelly. The umbilical stump dries within a week, hardens, and falls off by 10 to 14 days. Skin covers the area by 3 to 4 weeks.

Scaphoid shape occurs with dehydration.

Dilated veins.

The presence of only one artery signals the risk of congenital defects.

Inflammation.

Drainage after cord falls off.

Normal Range of Findings	Abnormal Findings

The abdomen should be symmetric, although two bulges are common. You may note an **umbilical hernia.** It appears at 2 to 3 weeks and is especially prominent when the infant cries. The hernia reaches maximum size at 1 month (up to 2.5 cm or 1 inch), and usually disappears by 1 year. Another common variation is **diastasis recti,** a separation of the rectus muscles with a visible bulge along the midline. The condition is more common with black infants, and it usually disappears by early childhood.

Refer any umbilical hernia larger than 2.5 cm; continuing to grow after 1 month; or lasting for more than 2 years in a white child or for more than 7 years in a black child.

Refer diastasis recti lasting more than 6 years of age.

The abdomen shows respiratory movement. The only other abdominal movement you should note is occasional peristalsis, which may be visible because of the thin musculature.

Marked peristalsis with pyloric stenosis (see Table 19–4).

Auscultation. Auscultation yields only bowel sounds, the metallic tinkling of peristalsis. No vascular sounds should be heard.

Bruit.
Venous hum.

Percussion. Percussion finds tympany over the stomach (the infant swallows some air with feeding) and dullness over the liver. Percussing the spleen is not done. The abdomen sounds tympanitic, although it is normal to percuss dullness over the bladder. This dullness may extend up to the umbilicus.

Palpation. Aid palpation by flexing the baby's knees with one hand while palpating with the other (Fig. 19–34). Alternatively, you may hold the upper back and flex the neck slightly with one hand. Offer a pacifier to a crying baby.

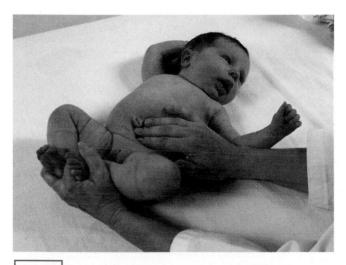

19–34

The liver fills the RUQ. It is normal to feel the liver edge at the right costal margin or 1 to 2 cm below. Normally, you may palpate the spleen tip and both kidneys as well as the bladder. Also easily palpated are the cecum in the RLQ, and the sigmoid colon, which feels like a sausage in the left inguinal area.

Make note of the newborn's first stool, a sticky, greenish-black meconium stool within 24 hours of birth. By the fourth day, stools of breast-fed babies are golden-yellow, pasty, and smell like sour milk, whereas those of formula-fed babies are brown-yellow, firmer, and more fecal smelling.

▶ Normal Range of Findings

Abnormal Findings

The Child

Under age 4 years, the abdomen looks protuberant when the child is both supine and standing. After age 4 years, the potbelly remains when standing because of lumbar lordosis, but the abdomen looks flat when supine. Normal movement on the abdomen includes respirations, which remain abdominal until 7 years of age.

To palpate the abdomen, position the young child on the parent's lap as you sit knee-to-knee with the parent (Fig. 19–35). Flex the knees up, and elevate the head slightly. The child can "pant like a dog" to further relax abdominal muscles. Hold your entire palm flat on the abdominal surface for a moment before starting palpation. This accustoms the child to being touched. If the child is very ticklish, hold his or her hand under your own as you palpate.

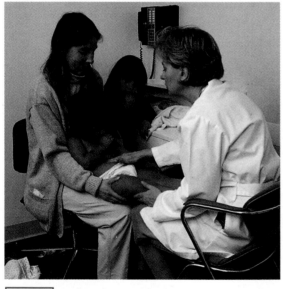

19–35

The liver remains easily palpable 1 to 2 cm below the right costal margin. The edge is soft and sharp and moves easily. On the left, the spleen also is easily palpable with a soft, sharp, movable edge. Usually you can feel 1 to 2 cm of the right kidney and the tip of the left kidney.

In assessing abdominal tenderness, remember that the young child often answers this question affirmatively no matter how the abdomen actually feels. Use objective signs to aid assessment, such as a cry changing in pitch as you palpate, facial grimacing, moving away from you, and guarding.

The school-age child has a slim abdominal shape as she or he loses the potbelly. This slimming trend continues into adolescence. See Table 19–1 for age-related values of liver span by percussion.

The adolescent easily is embarrassed with exposure of the abdomen, and adequate draping is necessary. The physical findings are the same as those listed for the adult.

A scaphoid abdomen is associated with dehydration or malnutrition.

Under 7 years of age, the absence of abdominal respirations occurs with inflammation of the peritoneum.

► Normal Range of Findings | Abnormal Findings

Table 19–1 • Expected Liver Span by Percussion Through Childhood and Adolescence		
	Mean Estimated Liver Span (cm)	
Age	*Males*	*Females*
6 mo	2.4	2.8
1 yr	2.8	3.1
2 yr	3.5	3.6
3 yr	4.0	4.0
4 yr	4.4	4.3
5 yr	4.8	4.5
6 yr	5.1	4.8
8 yr	5.6	5.1
10 yr	6.1	5.4
12 yr	6.5	5.6
14 yr	6.8	5.8
16 yr	7.1	6.0
18 yr	7.4	6.1
20 yr	7.7	6.3

Modified from Lawson EE, Grand RJ, Neff RK, Cohen LF: Clinical estimation of liver span in infants and children. Am J Dis Child 132:474–476, 1978. Copyright 1978, American Medical Association.

The Aging Adult

On inspection, you may note increased deposits of subcutaneous fat on the abdomen and hips, as it is redistributed away from the extremities. The abdominal musculature is thinner and has less tone than that of the younger adult, so in the absence of obesity you may note peristalsis.

Because of the thinner, softer abdominal wall, the organs may be easier to palpate (in the absence of obesity). The liver is easier to palpate. Normally, you will feel the liver edge at or just below the costal margin. With distended lungs and a depressed diaphragm, the liver is palpated lower, descending 1 to 2 cm below the costal margin with inhalation. The kidneys are easier to palpate.

Abdominal rigidity with acute abdominal conditions is less common in aging persons.

With an acute abdomen, the aging person often complains of less pain than a younger person would.

 SUMMARY CHECKLIST: Abdomen Exam

1: Inspection
Contour
Symmetry
Umbilicus
Skin
Pulsation or movement
Hair distribution
Demeanor

2: Auscultation
Bowel sounds
Note any vascular sounds

3: Percussion
Percuss all four quadrants
Percuss borders of liver, spleen

4: Palpation
Light palpation in all four quadrants
Deeper palpation in all four quadrants
Palpate for liver, spleen, kidneys

SAMPLE CHARTING

▶ **Subjective**

States appetite is good with no recent change, no dysphagia, no food intolerance, no pain, no nausea/vomiting. Has one formed BM/day. Takes vitamins, no other prescribed or over-the-counter medication. No history of abdominal disease, injury, or surgery. Diet recall of last 24 hours listed at end of history.

▶ **Objective**

Inspection. Abdomen flat, symmetric with no apparent masses. Skin smooth with no striae, scars, or lesions.

Auscultation. Bowel sounds present, no bruits.

Percussion. Tympany predominates in all four quadrants, liver span is 8 cm in right midclavicular line. Splenic dullness located at 10th intercostal space in left midaxillary line.

Palpation. Abdomen soft, no organomegaly, no masses, no tenderness.

CLINICAL CASE STUDY 1

George E. is a 58-year-old unemployed divorced white male with chronic alcoholism, who enters the chemical dependency treatment center.

▶ **Subjective**

States last 6 months has been drinking 1 pint whiskey/day. Last alcohol use 1 week PTA, with "5 or 6" drinks that episode. Estranged from family, lives alone. Makes a few meals on hot plate. States never has appetite. Has fatigue and weakness.

▶ **Objective**

Inspection. Appears older than stated age. Oriented, although verbal response time slowed. Weight loss of 12 lb in last 3 mo.

Abdomen protuberant, symmetric, no visible masses. Poor skin turgor. Dilated venous pattern over abdominal wall. Hair sparse in axillary, pubic area.

Auscultation. Bowel sounds present. No vascular sounds.

Percussion. Tympany predominates over abdomen. Liver span is 16 cm in right mid-clavicular line. No fluid wave. No shifting dullness.

Palpation. Soft. Liver palpable 10 cm below right costal margin, smooth and non-tender. No other organomegaly or masses.

▶ ASSESSMENT

Alcohol dependence, severe, with physiologic dependence
Altered nutrition: less than body requirements R/T impaired absorption
Ineffective individual coping R/T effects of chronic alcoholism
Social isolation

CLINICAL CASE STUDY 2

Edith J. is a 63-year-old retired homemaker with a history of lung cancer with metastases to the liver.

▶ **Subjective**

Feeling "puffy and bloated" for the past week. States unable to get comfortable. Also short of breath "all the time now." Difficulty sleeping. "I feel like crying all the time now."

▶ **Objective**

Inspection. Weight increase of 8 lb in 1 week. Abdomen is distended with everted umbilicus and bulging flanks. Girth at umbilicus is 85 cm. Prominent dilated venous pattern present over abdomen.

Auscultation. Bowel sounds present, no vascular sounds.

Percussion. When supine, tympany present at dome of abdomen, dullness over flanks. Shifting dullness present. Positive fluid wave present. Liver span is 12 cm in right midclavicular line.

Palpation. Abdominal wall firm, able to feel liver with deep palpation at 6 cm below right costal margin. Liver feels firm, nodular, nontender. 4 + pitting edema in both ankles.

▶ ASSESSMENT

Anticipatory grieving
Ascites
Ineffective breathing pattern R/T increased intraabdominal pressure
Pain R/T distended abdomen
Risk for impaired skin integrity: R/T ascites, edema, and faulty metabolism
Sleep pattern disturbance

CLINICAL CASE STUDY 3

Dan G. is a 17-year-old black male high school student who enters the emergency department with abdominal pain for 2 days.

▶ **Subjective**

Two days PTA Dan noted general abdominal pain in umbilical region. Now pain is sharp and severe, and Dan points to location in right lower quadrant. No BM for 2 days. Nausea and vomiting off and on 1 day.

▶ **Objective**

Inspection. BP 112/70 Temp 38° C, pulse 116, resp 18.
Lying on side with knees drawn up under chin. Resists any movement. Face tight and occasionally grimacing. Cries out with any sudden movement.

Auscultation. No bowel sounds present. No vascular sounds.

Percussion. Tympany. Percussion over RLQ leads to tenderness.

Palpation. Abdominal wall is rigid and boardlike. Extreme tenderness to palpation in RLQ.
Rebound tenderness is present in RLQ. Positive iliopsoas muscle test.

▶ ASSESSMENT

Acute abdominal pain in RLQ

Continued

NURSING DIAGNOSES COMMONLY ASSOCIATED WITH ABDOMINAL DISORDERS

Diagnosis	Related Factors (Etiology)	Defining Characteristics (Symptoms and Signs)

Constipation	Less than adequate dietary intake and bulk
	Neuromuscular or musculoskeletal impairment
	Pain/discomfort on defecation
	Effects of
	  Diagnostic procedures
	  Pregnancy
	  Aging
	  Medication
	  Stress or anxiety
	Weak abdominal musculature
	Immobility or less-than-adequate physical activity
	Chronic use of laxatives and enemas
	Gastrointestinal lesions
	Ignoring urge to defecate
	Fear of rectal or cardiac pain
		Frequency less than usual pattern
		Hard, formed stools
		Palpable mass
		Straining at stool
		Less than usual amount of stool
		Decreased bowel sounds
		Gas pain and flatulence
		Abdominal or back pain
		Reported feeling of abdominal or rectal fullness or pressure
		Impaired appetite
		Headache
		Nausea
		Irritability
		Palpable hard stool on rectal examination

Diarrhea	Effects of
	  Medications
	  Radiation
	  Surgical intervention
	Infectious process
	Inflammatory process
	Malabsorption syndrome
	Stress and anxiety
	Dietary alterations
	  Food intolerances
	  Increased caffeine consumption
	Excessive use of laxatives
	Allergies
	Nutritional disorders
	Ingestion of contaminated water or food
	Hyperosmolar tube feeding
		Abdominal pain
		Anorexia
		Change in color or odor of stool
		Chills
		Cramping
		Fatigue
		Increased frequency of bowel sounds
		Loose, liquid stools
		Increased frequency of stool
		Irritated anal area
		Fever
		Malaise
		Muscle weakness
		Thirst
		Urgency
		Weight loss

Urinary retention	Diminished or absent sensory and/or motor impulses
	Effects of some medications
	  Anesthetics
	  Opiates
	  Psychotropics
	Strong sphincter
	Urethral blockage associated with fecal impaction, postpartum edema, prostate hypertrophy, or surgical swelling
	Anxiety (fear of postoperative pain)
		Bladder distention
		Diminished force of urinary stream
		Dribbling
		Dysuria
		Hesitancy
		High residual urine
		Nocturia
		Sensation of bladder fullness
		Small, frequent voiding or absence of urine output

Altered tissue perfusion (renal, gastrointestinal)	Exchange problems
	Hypervolemia
	Hypovolemia
	Interruption of flow
		Renal
		  Diminished urine output
		  Edema
		Gastrointestinal
		  Constipation
		  Nausea and vomiting
		  Pain

Other Related Nursing Diagnoses

ACTUAL	RISK/WELLNESS
Altered nutrition: less than body requirements	**Risk**
Altered nutrition: more than body requirements	Risk for constipation
Altered nutrition: potential for more than body requirements	Risk for infection
Altered urinary elimination	**Wellness**
Bowel incontinence	Health-seeking behavior regarding weight-loss diet
Colonic constipation	
Functional incontinence	
Pain	
Perceived constipation	
Reflex incontinence	
Stress incontinence	
Total incontinence	
Urge incontinence	

 ASSESSMENT VIDEO CRITICAL THINKING QUESTIONS

The Saunders *Physical Examination and Health Assessment* Video Series—ABDOMEN—will direct you to consider the following:

1. Describe common sites of referred abdominal pain.

2. What bowel sounds would you expect to hear in a patient with diarrhea?

3. What abnormal findings can be detected by light palpation of the abdomen?

4. What should you suspect if your palpation detects an enlarged spleen? What should you do next?

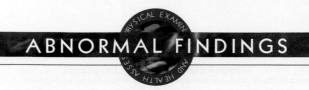

▼ Table 19–2   COMMON SITES OF REFERRED ABDOMINAL PAIN

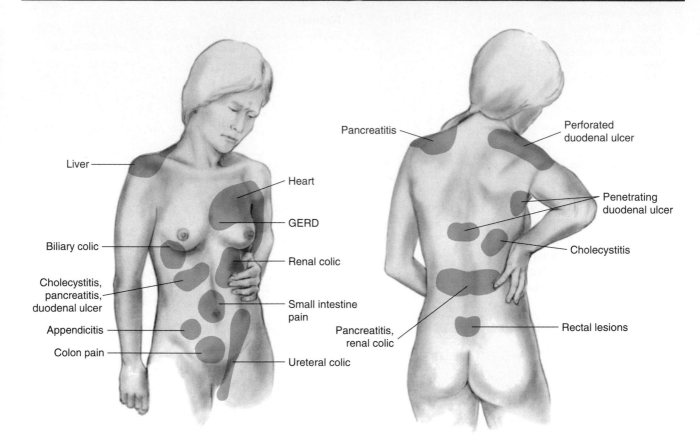

When a person gives a history of abdominal pain, the pain's location may not necessarily be directly over the involved organ. That is because the human brain has no felt image for internal organs. Rather, pain is referred to a site where the organ was located in fetal development. Although the organ migrates during fetal development, its nerves persist in referring sensations from the former location. The following are examples, not a complete list.

Liver. Hepatitis may have mild-to-moderate, dull pain in right upper quadrant or epigastrium, along with anorexia, nausea, malaise, low-grade fever.

Esophagus. Gastroesophageal reflux disease (GERD) is a complex of symptoms of esophagitis, including burning pain in midepigastrium or behind lower sternum that radiates upward, or "heartburn." Occurs 30 to 60 minutes after eating; aggravated by lying down or bending over.

Gallbladder. Cholecystitis is biliary colic, sudden pain in right upper quadrant that may radiate to right or left scapula, and which builds over time, lasting 2 to 4 hours, following ingestion of fatty foods, alcohol, or caffeine. Associated with nausea and vomiting, and positive Murphy's sign or sudden stop in inspiration with RUQ palpation.

Pancreas. Pancreatitis has acute, boring midepigastric pain radiating to the back and sometimes to the left scapula or flank, severe nausea, and vomiting.

Duodenum. Duodenal ulcer typically has dull, aching, gnawing pain, does not radiate, may be relieved by food, and may awaken the person from sleep.

Stomach. Gastric ulcer pain is dull, aching, gnawing epigastric pain, usually brought on by food, radiates to back or substernal area. Pain of perforated ulcer is burning epigastric pain of sudden onset that refers to one or both shoulders.

Appendix. Appendicitis typically starts as dull, diffuse pain in periumbilical region that later shifts to severe, sharp, persistent pain and tenderness localized in RLQ (McBurney's point). Pain is aggravated by movement, coughing, deep breathing; associated with anorexia, then nausea and vomiting, fever.

Kidney. Kidney stones prompt a sudden onset of severe, colicky flank or lower abdominal pain.

Small intestine. Gastroenteritis has diffuse, generalized abdominal pain, with nausea, diarrhea.

Colon. Large bowel obstruction has moderate, colicky pain of gradual onset in lower abdomen, bloating. Irritable bowel syndrome (IBS) has sharp or burning, cramping pain over a wide area; does not radiate. Brought on by meals, relieved by bowel movement.

 Table 19-3   ABDOMINAL DISTENTION*

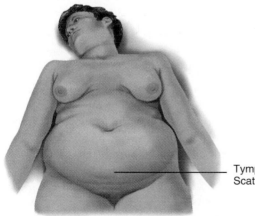

Tympany
Scattered dullness

Obesity

Inspection. Uniformly rounded. Umbilicus sunken (it adheres to peritoneum, and layers of fat are superficial to it).

Auscultation. Normal bowel sounds.

Percussion. Tympany. Scattered dullness over adipose tissue.

Palpation. Normal. May be hard to feel through thick abdominal wall.

---

* A mnemonic device to recall the common causes of abdominal distention is the seven Fs: fat, flatus, fluid, fetus, feces, fetal growth, and fibroid.

Table continued on following page

Table 19–3 ABDOMINAL DISTENTION *Continued*

ABNORMAL FINDINGS

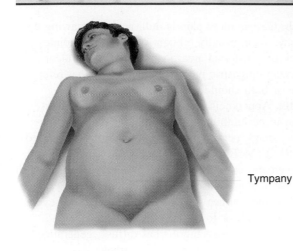

Air or Gas

Inspection. Single round curve.

Auscultation. Depends on cause of gas, e.g., decreased or absent bowel sounds with ileus; hyperactive with early intestinal obstruction.

Percussion. Tympany over large area.

Palpation. May have muscle spasm of abdominal wall.

Tympany

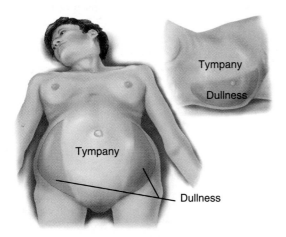

Tympany

Dullness

Tympany

Dullness

Ascites

Inspection. Single curve. Everted umbilicus. Bulging flanks when supine. Taut, glistening skin, recent weight gain, increase in abdominal girth.

Auscultation. Normal bowel sounds over intestines. Diminished over ascitic fluid.

Percussion. Tympany at top where intestines float. Dull over fluid. Produces fluid wave and shifting dullness.

Palpation. Taut skin and increased intraabdominal pressure limit palpation.

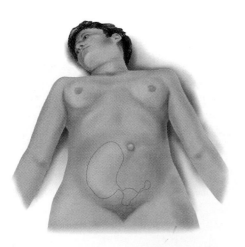

Ovarian Cyst (Large)

Inspection. Curve in lower half of abdomen, midline. Everted umbilicus.

Auscultation. Normal bowel sounds over upper abdomen where intestines pushed superiorly.

Percussion. Top dull over fluid. Intestines pushed superiorly. Large cyst produces fluid wave and shifting dullness.

Palpation. Transmits aortic pulsation while ascites does not.

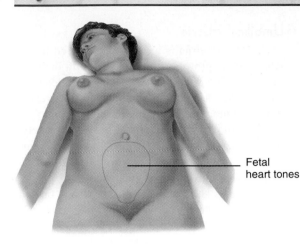

Fetal
heart tones

Pregnancy*

Inspection. Single curve. Umbilicus protruding. Breasts engorged.

Auscultation. Fetal heart tones. Bowel sounds diminished.

Percussion. Tympany over intestines. Dull over enlarging uterus.

Palpation. Fetal parts. Fetal movements.

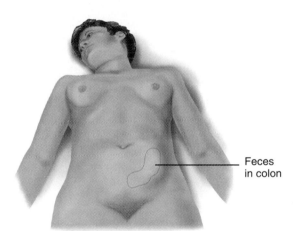

Feces
in colon

Feces

Inspection. Localized distention.

Auscultation. Normal bowel sounds.

Percussion. Tympany predominates. Scattered dullness over fecal mass.

Palpation. Plastic- or ropelike mass with feces in intestines.

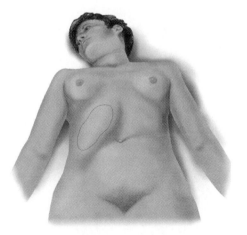

Tumor

Inspection. Localized distention.

Auscultation. Normal bowel sounds.

Percussion. Dull over mass if reaches up to skin surface.

Palpation. Define borders. Distinguish from enlarged organ or normally palpable structure.

---

* Obviously a normal finding, pregnancy is included for comparison of conditions causing abdominal distention.

Table 19–4   ABNORMALITIES ON INSPECTION

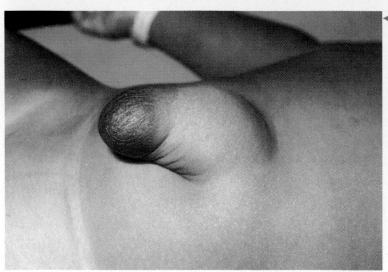

◄ Umbilical Hernia

Umbilical hernia is a soft, skin-covered mass, which is the protrusion of the omentum or intestine through a weakness or incomplete closure in the umbilical ring. It is accentuated by increased intraabdominal pressure as with crying, coughing, vomiting, or straining, but the bowel rarely incarcerates or strangulates. It is more common in black, Chinese, and premature infants. Most umbilical hernias resolve spontaneously by 1 year; parents should avoid affixing a belt or coin at the hernia because this will not help closure and may cause contact dermatitis.

In an adult, it occurs with pregnancy, chronic ascites, or from chronic intrathoracic pressure (e.g., asthma, chronic bronchitis).

Epigastric Hernia (not illustrated)

A small, fatty nodule at epigastrium in midline, through the linea alba. Usually one can feel it rather than observe it. May be palpable only when standing.

Incisional Hernia (not illustrated)

A bulge near an old operative scar that may not show when person is supine, but is apparent when the person increases intraabdominal pressure by a sit-up, stand, or Valsalva maneuver.

Diastasis Recti (not illustrated)

Diastasis recti, or a midline longitudinal ridge, is a separation of the abdominal rectus muscles. Ridge is revealed when intraabdominal pressure is increased by raising head while supine. Occurs congenitally and as a result of pregnancy or marked obesity in which prolonged distention or a decrease in muscle tone has occurred. It is not clinically significant.

▼ Table 19—5 ABNORMAL BOWEL SOUNDS

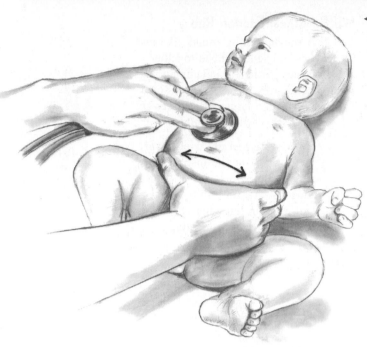

◄ Succussion Splash

Unrelated to peristalsis, this is a very loud splash auscultated over the upper abdomen when the infant is rocked side to side. It indicates increased air and fluid in the stomach, as seen with pyloric obstruction or large hiatus hernia.

Marked peristalsis, together with projectile vomiting in the newborn, suggests pyloric stenosis, an obstruction of the stomach's pyloric valve. Pyloric stenosis is a congenital defect and appears in the 2nd or 3rd week. After feeding, pronounced peristaltic waves cross from left to right, leading to projectile vomiting. Then one can palpate an olive-sized mass in the RUQ midway between the right costal margin and umbilicus. Refer promptly because of the risk of weight loss.

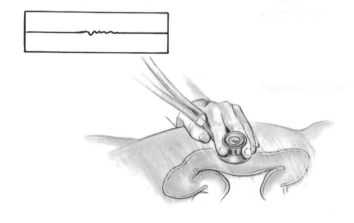

Hypoactive Bowel Sounds

Diminished or absent bowel sounds signal decreased motility due to inflammation as seen with peritonitis, from paralytic ileus as following abdominal surgery, or from late bowel obstruction. Occurs also with pneumonia.

Hyperactive Bowel Sounds

Loud, gurgling sounds, "borborygmi," signal increased motility. They occur with early mechanical bowel obstruction (high pitched), gastroenteritis, brisk diarrhea, laxative use, and subsiding paralytic ileus.

Table 19–6 ABDOMINAL FRICTION RUBS AND VASCULAR SOUNDS

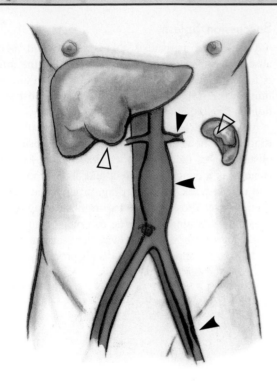

◁ Peritoneal Friction Rub

A rough, grating sound, like two pieces of leather rubbed together, indicates peritoneal inflammation. Occurs rarely. Usually occurs over organs with a large surface area in contact with the peritoneum.

Liver—friction rub over lower right rib cage, due to abscess or metastatic tumor.

Spleen—friction rub over lower left rib cage in left anterior axillary line, from abscess, infection, or tumor.

◀ Vascular Sounds

Arterial—a **bruit** indicates turbulent blood flow, as found in constricted, abnormally dilated, or tortuous vessels. Listen with the bell. Occurs with the following three conditions:

Aortic aneurysm—murmur is harsh, systolic, or continuous and accentuated with systole. Note in person with hypertension.

Renal artery stenosis—murmur is midline or toward flank, soft, low-to-medium pitch.

Partial occlusion of femoral arteries

Venous hum—occurs rarely. Heard in periumbilical region. Originates from inferior vena cava. Medium pitch, continuous sound, pressure on bell may obliterate it. May have palpable thrill. Occurs with portal hypertension and cirrhotic liver.

Table 19-7 ABNORMALITIES ON PALPATION OF ENLARGED ORGANS

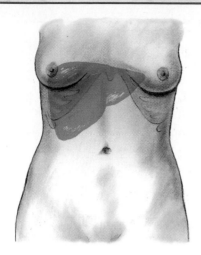

Enlarged Liver

An enlarged, smooth and nontender liver occurs with fatty infiltration, portal obstruction or cirrhosis, high obstruction of inferior vena cava, and lymphocytic leukemia.

The liver feels enlarged and smooth, but is tender to palpation with early congestive heart failure, acute hepatitis, or hepatic abscess.

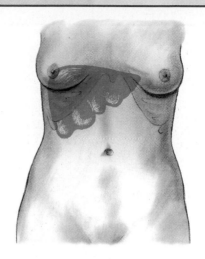

Enlarged Nodular Liver

An enlarged and nodular liver occurs with late portal cirrhosis, metastatic cancer, or tertiary syphilis.

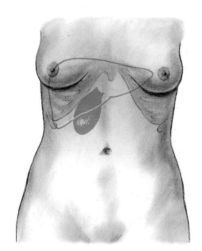

Enlarged Gallbladder

An enlarged, tender gallbladder suggests acute cholecystitis. Feel it behind the liver border as a smooth and firm mass like a sausage, although it may be difficult to palpate due to involuntary rigidity of abdominal muscles. The area is exquisitely painful to fist percussion, and inspiratory arrest (Murphy's sign) is present.

An enlarged, nontender gallbladder also feels like a smooth, sausagelike mass. It occurs when the gallbladder is filled with stones, as with common bile duct obstruction.

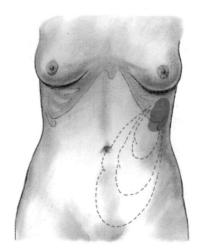

Enlarged Spleen

Since any enlargement superiorly is stopped by the diaphragm, the spleen enlarges down and to the midline. When extreme, it can extend down to the left pelvis. It retains the splenic notch on the medial edge. When splenomegaly occurs with acute infections (mononucleosis), it is moderately enlarged and soft, with rounded edges. When due to a chronic cause, the enlargement is firm or hard, with sharp edges. An enlarged spleen is usually not tender to palpation; it is tender only if the peritoneum is also inflamed.

Table continued on following page

Table 19–7 ABNORMALITIES ON PALPATION OF ENLARGED ORGANS
Continued

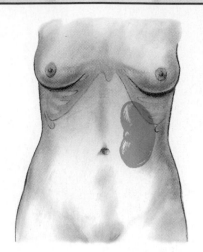

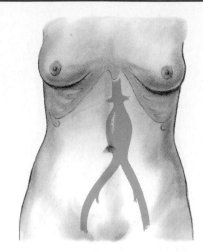

Enlarged Kidney

Enlarged with hydronephrosis, cyst, or neoplasm. May be difficult to distinguish an enlarged kidney from an enlarged spleen because they have a similar shape. Both extend forward and down. However, the spleen may have a sharp edge, whereas the kidney never does. The spleen retains the splenic notch, whereas the kidney has no palpable notch. Percussion over the spleen is dull, whereas over the kidney it is tympanitic due to the overriding bowel.

Aortic Aneurysm

Most aortic aneurysms (more than 95 percent) are located below the renal arteries and extend to the umbilicus. About 80 percent of these are palpable during routine physical examination and feel like a pulsating mass in the upper abdomen just to the left of midline. You will hear a bruit. Femoral pulses are present but decreased.

Additional information on abdominal aneurysm is illustrated in Table 18–5.

Bibliography

Alexander IM: Viral hepatitis: Primary care diagnosis and management. Nurse Pract 23(10):13–45, Oct 1998.

Allison OC, Porter ME, Briggs GC: Chronic constipation: Assessment and management in the elderly. J Am Acad Nurse Pract 6(7):311–317, 1994.

Bode C, Bode JC: Alcohol's role in gastrointestinal tract disorders. Alcohol Health Res World 21(1):76–96, 1997.

Brenner H, Rothenbacher D, Bode G, Adler G: Relation of smoking and alcohol and coffee consumption to active *Helicobacter pylori* infection: Cross sectional study. BMJ 315(7121):1489–1492, Dec 1997.

Caprio S, Hyman LD, McCarthy S, et al: Fat distribution and cardiovascular risk factors in obese adolescent girls: Importance of the intra-abdominal fat depot. Am J Clin Nutr 64:12–17, 1996.

Carlson E: Irritable bowel syndrome. Nurse Pract 23(1):82–93, Jan 1998.

Causey AL, Seago K, Wahl NG, Voelker CL: Pregnant adolescents in the emergency department: Diagnosed and not diagnosed. Am J Emerg Med 15(2):125–129, Mar 1997.

Driver DS: Renal assessment: Back to basics. ANNA J 23(4):361–368, Aug 1996.

Ganong WF: Review of Medical Physiology, 17th ed. Norwalk, CT, Appleton & Lange, 1995.

Goldberg EA: Physical assessment of children ages 1 to 10 years with renal disease. ANNA J 24(2):222–230, Apr 1997.

Goldsmith C: Gastroesophageal reflux disease. Am J Nurs 98(9):44–45, Sep 1998.

Johnston DE, Kaplan MM: Pathogenesis and treatment of gallstones. N Engl J Med 328:412–421, 1993.

Katzung BG: Basic & Clinical Pharmacology, 6th ed. Norwalk, CT, Appleton & Lange, 1995.

Langan JC: Abdominal assessment in the home: From A to Z. Home Healthcare Nurse 16(1):50–58, Jan 1998.

Lawson EE, Grand RJ, Neff RK, Cohen LF: Clinical estimation of liver span in infants and children. Am J Dis Child 132:474–476, 1978.

Martin FL: Ulcerative colitis. Am J Nurs 97(8):38–39, Aug 1997.

Middlemiss C: Gastroesophageal reflux disease: A common condition in the elderly. Nurse Pract 22(11):51–61, Nov 1997.

Muscari ME, Milks CJ: Assessing acute abdominal pain in adolescent females. Pediatr Nurs 21(3):215–220, May–June 1995.

Nicholson ML, Byrne RL, Steele GA, Callum KG: Predictive value of bruits and Doppler pressure measurements in detecting lower limb arterial stenosis. Eur J Vasc Surg 7(1):59–62, Jan 1993.

O'Hanlon-Nichols T: Basic assessment series: Gastrointestinal system. Am J Nurs 98(4):48–53, Apr 1998.

Ray WA: Psychotrophic drugs and injuries among the elderly: A review. J Clin Psychopharmacol 12:386, 1992.

Ray WA, Griffin MR, Downey W: Benzodiazepines of long and short elimination half-life and the risk of hip fracture. JAMA 262(23):3303, 1989.

Shaw B: Comprehensive assessment of gastrointestinal disorders. J Nurse Midwifery 40(2):216–230, Mar–Apr 1995.

Shaw B: Management and treatment of gastrointestinal disorders. J Nurse Midwifery 41(2): 155–172, Mar–Apr 1996.

Skrainka B, Stahlhut J, Fulbeck CL, et al: Measuring liver span: Bedside examination versus ultrasound and scintiscan. J Clin Gastroenterol 8(3):267–270, 1986.

Stone JK, Wyman JF, Salisbury SA: Clinical Gerontological Nursing—A Guide to Advanced Practice, 2nd ed. Philadelphia, W.B. Saunders Company. 1999.

Town J: Bringing acute abdomen into focus. Nursing97 27(5):52–58, May 1997.

Wald A: Constipation and fecal incontinence in the elderly. Gastroenterol Clin North Am 19:405, 1990.

Wright JA: Seven abdominal assessment signs every emergency nurse should know. J Emerg Nurs 23(5):446–450, Oct 1997.

CHAPTER TWENTY

Musculoskeletal System

Structure and Function

COMPONENTS OF THE MUSCULOSKELETAL SYSTEM

Nonsynovial or Synovial Joints

Muscles

Temporomandibular Joint

Spine

Shoulder

Elbow

Wrist and Carpals

Hip

Knee

Ankle and Foot

DEVELOPMENTAL CONSIDERATIONS

Infants and Children

The Pregnant Female

The Aging Adult

TRANSCULTURAL CONSIDERATIONS

Subjective Data

HEALTH HISTORY QUESTIONS

ADDITIONAL HISTORY FOR INFANTS AND CHILDREN

ADDITIONAL HISTORY FOR ADOLESCENTS

ADDITIONAL HISTORY FOR THE AGING ADULT

Objective Data

PREPARATION

ORDER OF THE EXAMINATION

Inspection

Palpation

Range of Motion (ROM)

Muscle Testing

TEMPOROMANDIBULAR JOINT

CERVICAL SPINE

UPPER EXTREMITY

Shoulders

Elbow

Wrist and Hand

LOWER EXTREMITY

Hip

Knee

Special Test for Meniscal Tears

Ankle and Foot

SPINE

DEVELOPMENTAL CONSIDERATIONS

Infants

Preschool- and School-Age Children

Adolescents

The Pregnant Female

The Aging Adult

Functional Assessment

SUMMARY CHECKLIST: MUSCULOSKELETAL EXAM

Application and Critical Thinking

SAMPLE CHARTING

CLINICAL CASE STUDY

NURSING DIAGNOSES

ASSESSMENT VIDEO CRITICAL THINKING QUESTIONS

Abnormal Findings

ABNORMALITIES AFFECTING MULTIPLE JOINTS

ABNORMALITIES OF THE SHOULDER

ABNORMALITIES OF THE ELBOW

ABNORMALITIES OF THE WRIST AND HAND

ABNORMALITIES OF THE KNEE

ABNORMALITIES OF THE ANKLE AND FOOT

ABNORMALITIES OF THE SPINE

COMMON CONGENITAL OR PEDIATRIC ABNORMALITIES

The musculoskeletal system consists of the body's **bones, joints,** and **muscles.** Humans need this system (1) for *support* to stand erect and (2) for *movement.* The musculoskeletal system also functions (3) to encase and *protect* the inner vital organs (e.g., brain, spinal cord, heart), (4) to *produce* the red blood cells in the bone marrow (hematopoiesis), and (5) as a *reservoir* for *storage* of essential minerals, such as calcium and phosphorus in the bones.

COMPONENTS OF THE MUSCULOSKELETAL SYSTEM

The skeleton is the bony framework of the body. It has 206 bones, which support the body like the posts and beams of a building. **Bone** and cartilage are specialized forms of connective tissue. Bone is hard, rigid, and very dense. Its cells are continually turning over and remodeling. The **joint** (or articulation) is the place of union of two or more bones. Joints are the functional units of the musculoskeletal system because they permit the mobility needed for activities of daily living.

Nonsynovial or Synovial Joints

In **nonsynovial** joints, the bones are united by fibrous tissue or cartilage and are immovable (e.g., the sutures in the skull) or only slightly movable (e.g., the vertebrae). **Synovial** joints are freely movable because they have bones that are separated from each other and are enclosed in a joint cavity (Fig. 20–1). This cavity is filled with a lubricant, or synovial fluid. Just like grease on gears, synovial fluid allows sliding of opposing surfaces, and this sliding permits movement.

In synovial joints, a layer of resilient **cartilage** covers the surface of opposing bones. Cartilage is avascular; it receives nourishment from synovial fluid that circulates during joint movement. It is a very stable connective tissue with a slow cell turnover. It has a tough, firm consistency, yet is flexible. This cartilage cushions the bones and gives a smooth surface to facilitate movement.

The joint is surrounded by a fibrous capsule and is supported by ligaments. **Ligaments** are fibrous bands running directly from one bone to another that strengthen the joint and help prevent movement in undesirable directions. A **bursa** is an enclosed sac filled with viscous synovial fluid, much like a joint. Bursae are located in areas of potential friction (e.g., subacromial bursa of the shoulder, prepatellar bursa of the knee) and help muscles and tendons glide smoothly over bone.

Muscles

Muscles account for 40 to 50 percent of the body's weight. When they contract, they produce movement.

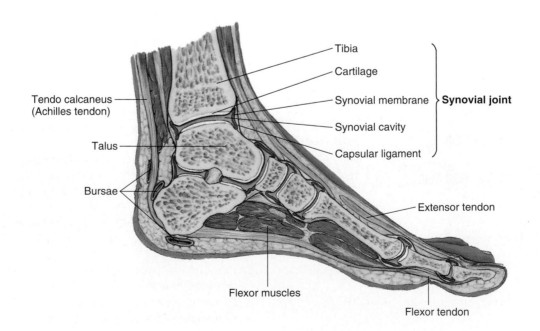

20–1

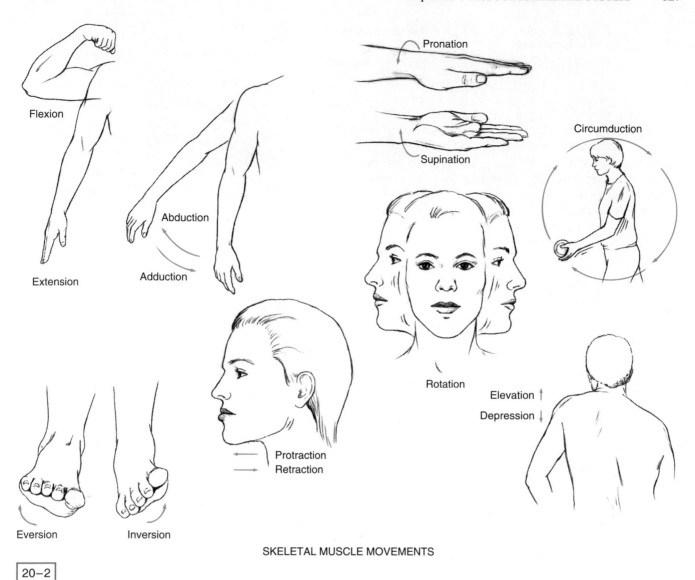

SKELETAL MUSCLE MOVEMENTS

20-2

Muscles are of three types: skeletal, smooth, and cardiac. This chapter is concerned with **skeletal,** or voluntary, muscles, those under conscious control.

Each **skeletal muscle** is composed of bundles of muscle fibers, or **fasciculi.** The skeletal muscle is attached to bone by a **tendon**—a strong fibrous cord. Skeletal muscles produce the following movements (Fig. 20–2):

1. Flexion—bending a limb at a joint
2. Extension—straightening a limb at a joint
3. Abduction—moving a limb away from the midline of the body
4. Adduction—moving a limb toward the midline of the body
5. Pronation—turning the forearm so that the palm is down
6. Supination—turning the forearm so that the palm is up
7. Circumduction—moving the arm in a circle around the shoulder
8. Inversion—moving the sole of the foot inward at the ankle
9. Eversion—moving the sole of the foot outward at the ankle
10. Rotation—moving the head around a central axis
11. Protraction—moving a body part forward and parallel to the ground
12. Retraction—moving a body part backward and parallel to the ground
13. Elevation—raising a body part
14. Depression—lowering a body part

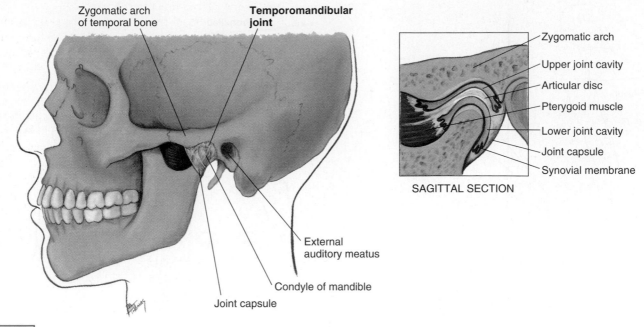

Zygomatic arch of temporal bone

Temporomandibular joint

Zygomatic arch

Upper joint cavity

Articular disc

Pterygoid muscle

Lower joint cavity

Joint capsule

Synovial membrane

SAGITTAL SECTION

External auditory meatus

Condyle of mandible

Joint capsule

20-3

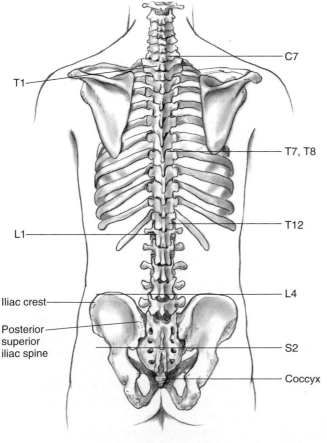

C7

T1

T7, T8

L1

T12

L4

Iliac crest

Posterior superior iliac spine

S2

Coccyx

LANDMARKS OF THE SPINE

20-4

Temporomandibular Joint

The temporomandibular joint (TMJ) is the articulation of the mandible and the temporal bone (Fig. 20–3). You can feel it in the depression anterior to the tragus of the ear. The TMJ permits jaw function for speaking and chewing. The joint allows three motions: (1) hinge action to open and close the jaws, (2) gliding action for protrusion and retraction, and (3) gliding for side-to-side movement of the lower jaw.

Spine

The **vertebrae** are 33 connecting bones stacked in a vertical column (Fig. 20–4). You can feel their spinous processes in a furrow down the midline of the back. The furrow has paravertebral muscles mounded on either side down to the sacrum, where it flattens. Humans have 7 cervical, 12 thoracic, 5 lumbar, 5 sacral, and 3 to 4 coccygeal vertebrae. The following surface landmarks will orient you to their levels:

- The spinous processes of C7 and T1 are prominent at the base of the neck.
- The inferior angle of the scapula normally is at the level of the interspace between T7 and T8.
- An imaginary line connecting the highest point on each iliac crest crosses L4.
- An imaginary line joining the two symmetric dimples that overlie the posterior superior iliac spines crosses S2.

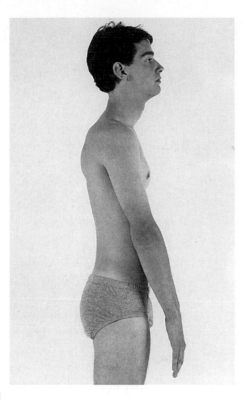

A lateral view shows that the vertebral column has four curves (a double S shape) (Fig. 20–5). The cervical and lumbar curves are concave (inward), and the thoracic and sacrococcygeal curves are convex. The balanced or compensatory nature of these curves, together with the resilient intervertebral discs, allows the spine to absorb a great deal of shock.

The **intervertebral discs** are elastic fibrocartilaginous plates that constitute one-quarter of the length of the column (Fig. 20–6). Each disc center has a **nucleus pulposus,** made of soft, semi-fluid, mucoid material that has the consistency of toothpaste in the young adult. The discs cushion the spine like a shock absorber and help it move. As the spine moves, the elasticity of the discs allows compression on one side, with compensatory expansion on the other. Sometimes compression can be too great. The disc then can rupture and the nucleus pulposus can herniate out of the vertebral column, compressing on the spinal nerves and causing pain.

The unique structure of the spine enables both upright posture and flexibility for motion. The motions of the vertebral column are flexion (bending forward), extension (bending back), abduction (to either side), and rotation.

20–5

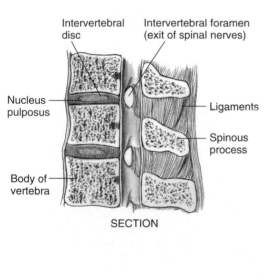

Intervertebral disc

Intervertebral foramen (exit of spinal nerves)

Nucleus pulposus

Ligaments

Spinous process

Body of vertebra

SECTION

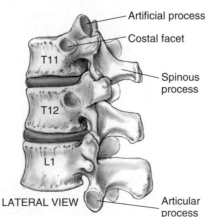

Artificial process

Costal facet

Spinous process

T11

T12

L1

LATERAL VIEW

Articular process

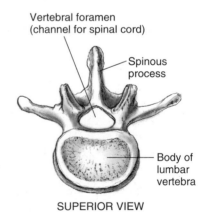

Vertebral foramen (channel for spinal cord)

Spinous process

Body of lumbar vertebra

SUPERIOR VIEW

20–6

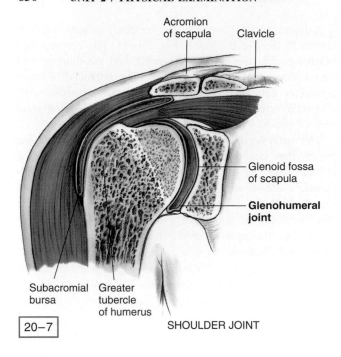

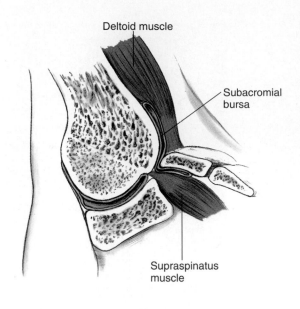

20-7   SHOULDER JOINT

SHOULDER WITH ARM ABDUCTED

Shoulder

The **glenohumeral joint** is the articulation of the humerus with the glenoid fossa of the scapula (Fig. 20–7). Its ball and socket action allows great mobility of the arm on many axes. The joint is enclosed by a group of four powerful muscles and tendons that support and stabilize it. Together these are called the **rotator cuff** of the shoulder. The large **subacromial bursa** helps during abduction of the arm, so that the greater tubercle of the humerus moves easily under the acromion process of the scapula.

The bones of the shoulder have palpable landmarks to guide your examination (Fig. 20–8). The scapula and the clavicle connect to form the shoulder girdle. You can feel the bump of the scapula's **acromion process** at the very

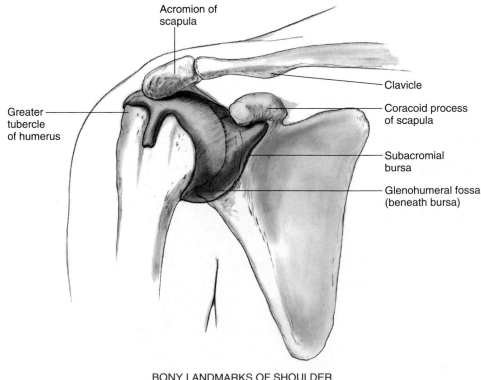

20-8   BONY LANDMARKS OF SHOULDER

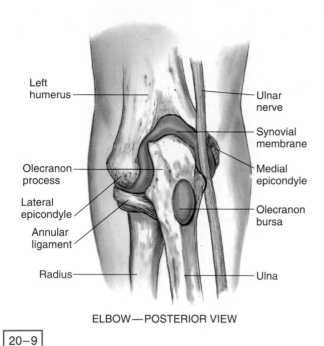

ELBOW—POSTERIOR VIEW

20–9

Elbow

The elbow joint contains the three bony articulations of the humerus, radius, and ulna of the forearm (Fig. 20–9). Its hinge action moves the forearm (radius and ulna) on one plane, allowing flexion and extension. The olecranon bursa lies between the olecranon process and the skin.

Palpable landmarks are the **medial** and **lateral epicondyles** of the humerus and the large **olecranon process** of the ulna in between them. The sensitive ulnar nerve runs between the olecranon process and the medial epicondyle.

The radius and ulna articulate with each other at two radioulnar joints, one at the elbow and one at the wrist. These move together to permit pronation and supination of the hand and forearm.

Wrist and Carpals

Of the body's 206 bones, over half are in the hands and feet. The wrist or **radiocarpal joint** is the articulation of the radius (on the thumb side) and a row of carpal bones (Fig. 20–10). Its condyloid action permits movement in two planes at right angles: flexion and extension, and side-to-side deviation. You can feel the groove of this joint on the dorsum of the wrist.

The **midcarpal** joint is the articulation between the two parallel rows of carpal bones. It allows flexion, extension, and some rotation. The **metacarpophalangeal** and the **interphalangeal** joints permit finger flexion and extension. The flexor tendons of the wrist and hand are enclosed in synovial sheaths.

top of the shoulder. Move your fingers in a small circle outward, down, and around. The next bump is the **greater tubercle** of the humerus a few centimeters down and laterally, and from that the **coracoid process** of the scapula is a few centimeters medially. These surround the deeply situated joint.

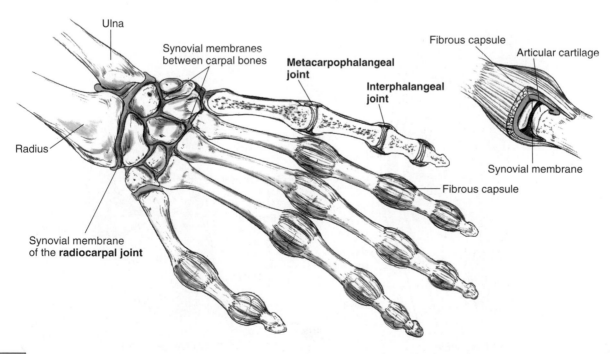

20–10

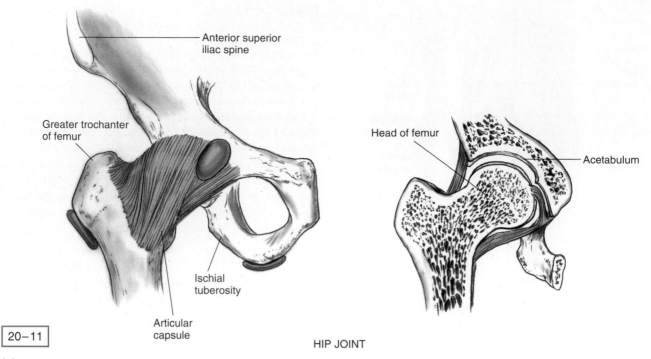

Anterior superior iliac spine

Greater trochanter of femur

Ischial tuberosity

Articular capsule

Head of femur

Acetabulum

20–11

HIP JOINT

Hip

The hip joint is the articulation between the acetabulum and the head of the femur (Fig. 20–11). Like the shoulder, its ball and socket action permits a wide range of motion on many axes. The hip has somewhat less range of motion (ROM) than the shoulder, but it has more stability as befits its weight-bearing function. Hip stability is due to powerful muscles that spread over the joint, a strong fibrous articular capsule, and the very deep inser-

tion of the head of the femur. Three bursae facilitate movement.

Palpation of these bony landmarks will guide your examination. You can feel the entire iliac crest, from the **anterior superior iliac spine** to the posterior. The **ischial tuberosity** lies under the gluteus maximus muscle and is palpable when the hip is flexed. The **greater trochanter** of the femur is normally the width of the person's palm below the iliac crest and halfway between the anterior

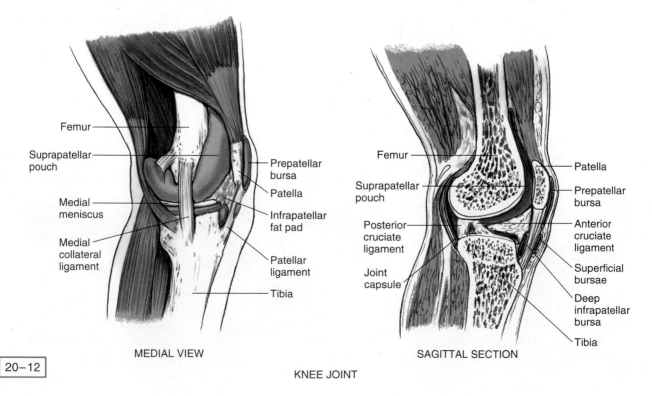

Femur

Suprapatellar pouch

Medial meniscus

Medial collateral ligament

Prepatellar bursa

Patella

Infrapatellar fat pad

Patellar ligament

Tibia

Femur

Suprapatellar pouch

Posterior cruciate ligament

Joint capsule

Patella

Prepatellar bursa

Anterior cruciate ligament

Superficial bursae

Deep infrapatellar bursa

Tibia

MEDIAL VIEW

SAGITTAL SECTION

20–12

KNEE JOINT

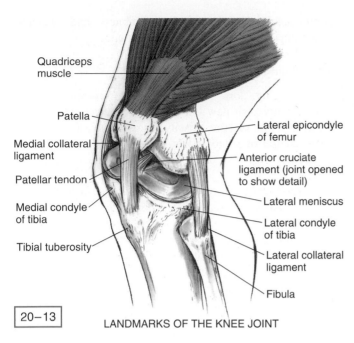

Quadriceps
muscle

Patella

Medial collateral
ligament

Patellar tendon

Medial condyle
of tibia

Tibial tuberosity

Lateral epicondyle
of femur

Anterior cruciate
ligament (joint opened
to show detail)

Lateral meniscus

Lateral condyle
of tibia

Lateral collateral
ligament

Fibula

20–13   LANDMARKS OF THE KNEE JOINT

cushion the tibia and femur. The joint is stabilized by two sets of ligaments. The **cruciate ligaments** (not shown) crisscross within the knee; they give anterior and posterior stability and help control rotation. The **collateral ligaments** connect the joint at both sides; they give medial and lateral stability and prevent dislocation. Numerous bursae prevent friction. One, the **prepatellar bursa,** lies between the patella and the skin. The **infrapatellar fat pad** is a small, triangular fat pad below the patella behind the patellar ligament.

Landmarks of the knee joint start with the large **quadriceps** muscle, which you can feel on your anterior and lateral thigh (Fig. 20–13). The muscle's four heads merge into a common tendon that continues down to enclose the round bony patella. Then the tendon inserts down on the **tibial tuberosity,** which you can feel as a bony prominence in the midline. Move to the sides and a bit superiorly and note the lateral and medial condyles of the tibia. Superior to these on either side of the patella are the medial and lateral epicondyles of the femur.

superior iliac spine and the ischial tuberosity. Feel it when the person is standing, in a flat depression on the upper lateral side of the thigh.

Knee

The knee joint is the articulation of three bones, the femur, the tibia, and the patella (kneecap), in one common articular cavity (Fig. 20–12). It is the largest joint in the body and is complex. It is a hinge joint, permitting flexion and extension of the lower leg on a single plane.

The knee's synovial membrane is the largest in the body. It forms a sac at the superior border of the patella, called the **suprapatellar pouch,** which extends up as much as 6 cm behind the quadriceps muscle. Two wedge-shaped cartilages, called the **medial** and **lateral menisci,**

Ankle and Foot

The ankle or **tibiotalar joint** is the articulation of the tibia, fibula, and talus (Fig. 20–14). It is a hinge joint, limited to flexion (dorsiflexion) and extension (plantar flexion) on one plane. Landmarks are two bony prominences on either side—the **medial malleolus** and the **lateral malleolus.** Strong, tight medial and lateral ligaments extend from each malleolus onto the foot. These help the lateral stability of the ankle joint, although they may be torn in eversion or inversion sprains of the ankle.

Joints distal to the ankle give additional mobility to the foot. The subtalar joint permits inversion and eversion of the foot. The foot has a longitudinal arch with weight-bearing distributed between the parts that touch the ground—the heads of the metatarsals and the calcaneus (heel).

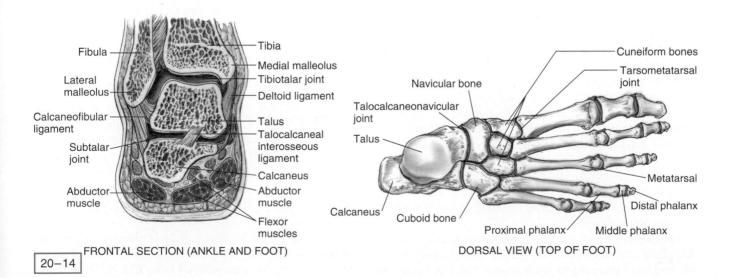

Fibula

Lateral
malleolus

Calcaneofibular
ligament

Subtalar
joint

Abductor
muscle

Tibia

Medial malleolus

Tibiotalar joint

Deltoid ligament

Talus

Talocalcaneal
interosseous
ligament

Calcaneus

Abductor
muscle

Flexor
muscles

20–14   FRONTAL SECTION (ANKLE AND FOOT)

Cuneiform bones

Tarsometatarsal
joint

Navicular bone

Talocalcaneonavicular
joint

Talus

Metatarsal

Distal phalanx

Calcaneus   Cuboid bone

Proximal phalanx   Middle phalanx

DORSAL VIEW (TOP OF FOOT)

DEVELOPMENTAL CONSIDERATIONS

Infants and Children

By 3 months gestation, the fetus has formed a "scale model" of the skeleton that is made up of cartilage. During succeeding months in utero, the cartilage ossifies into true bone and starts to grow. Bone growth continues after birth—rapidly during infancy and then steadily during childhood—until adolescence, when both boys and girls experience a rapid growth spurt.

Long bones grow in two dimensions. They increase in width or diameter by deposition of new bony tissue around the shafts. Lengthening occurs at the **epiphyses,** or growth plates. These specialized growth centers are transverse discs located at the ends of long bone. Any trauma or infection at this location puts the growing child at risk for bone deformity. This longitudinal growth continues until closure of the epiphyses; the last closure occurs at about age 20.

Skeletal contour changes are apparent at the vertebral column. At birth, the spine has a single C-shaped curve. At 3 to 4 months, raising the baby's head from prone position develops the anterior curve in the cervical neck region. From 1 year to 18 months, standing erect develops the anterior curve in the lumbar region.

Whereas the skeleton contributes to linear growth, muscles and fat are significant for weight increase. Individual muscle fibers grow through childhood, but growth is marked during the adolescent growth spurt. Then muscles respond to increased secretion of growth hormone, adrenal androgens, and in boys, to further stimulation by testosterone. Muscles vary in size and strength in different people. This is due to genetic programming, nutrition, and exercise. All through life, muscles increase with use and atrophy with disuse.

The Pregnant Female

Increased levels of circulating hormones (estrogen, relaxin from the corpus luteum, and corticosteroids) presumably cause increased mobility in the joints. Increased mobility in the sacroiliac, sacrococcygeal, and symphysis pubis joints in the pelvis may contribute to the noticeable changes in maternal posture. The most characteristic change in posture is progressive **lordosis.** Lordosis compensates for the enlarging fetus; otherwise, the center of balance would shift forward. Lordosis compensates by shifting the weight farther back on the lower extremities. This shift in balance in turn creates strain on the low back muscles, felt as low back pain during late pregnancy in some women.

Anterior flexion of the neck and slumping of the shoulder girdle are other postural changes that compensate for the lordosis. These upper back changes may put pressure on the ulnar and median nerves during the third trimester.

Nerve pressure creates aching, numbness, and weakness in the upper extremities in some women.

The Aging Adult

With aging, loss of bone matrix (resorption) occurs more rapidly than new bone growth (deposition). The net effect is a loss of bone density, or **osteoporosis.** Although some degree of osteoporosis is nearly universal, females experience it more than males, and whites more than blacks.

Postural changes are evident with aging, and decreased height is the most noticeable. Long bones do not shorten with age. Decreased height is due to shortening of the vertebral column. This is caused by loss of water content and thinning of the intervertebral discs, which occurs more in the middle years, and a decrease in height of individual vertebrae, which occurs in later years from osteoporosis. Both men and women can expect a progressive decrease in height beginning at age 40 in males and age 43 in females, although this is not significant until age 60 (Cline et al., 1989). A greater decrease occurs in the 70s and 80s owing to osteoporotic collapse of the vertebrae. The result is a shortening of the trunk and comparatively long extremities. Other postural changes are kyphosis, a backward head tilt to compensate for kyphosis, and a slight flexion of hips and knees.

The distribution of subcutaneous fat changes through life. Usually, men and women gain weight in their 40s and 50s. The contour is different, even if the weight is the same as when younger. They begin to lose fat in the face and deposit it in abdomen and hips. In the 80s and 90s, fat further decreases in the periphery, especially noticeable in the forearms, although it is still apparent over the abdomen and hips.

Loss of subcutaneous fat leaves bony prominences more marked (e.g., tips of vertebrae, ribs, iliac crests), and body hollows deeper (e.g., cheeks, axillae). An absolute loss in muscle mass occurs; some muscles decrease in size, and some atrophy, producing weakness. The contour of muscles becomes more prominent, and muscle bundles and tendons feel more distinct.

It has become more apparent that lifestyle affects musculoskeletal changes. A sedentary lifestyle hastens musculoskeletal changes of aging. However, physical exercise increases skeletal mass. This helps prevent or delay osteoporosis. Physical activity delays or prevents bone loss in postmenopausal and older women (Ebrahim et al., 1997; Gregg et al., 1998).

TRANSCULTURAL CONSIDERATIONS

The long bones of blacks are significantly longer, narrower, and denser than those of whites (Farrally and Moore, 1975). Measurement of bone density by race and sex reveals that black males have the densest bones, thus

Table 20-1 • Biocultural Variations in the Musculoskeletal System

Bone	Variations
Frontal	Thicker in black males than in white males.
Parietal occiput	Thicker in white males than in black males.
Palate	Tori (protuberances) along the suture line of the hard palate; problematic for denture wearers. Incidence: blacks—20 percent; whites—24 percent; Asians—up to 50 percent; Native Americans—up to 50 percent.
Mandible	Tori (protuberances) on the lingual surface of the mandible near the canine and premolar teeth; problematic for denture wearers; most common in Asians and Native Americans; incidence exceeds 50 percent in some Inuit groups.
Humerus	Torsion or rotation of proximal end with muscle pull; whites have a greater incidence than blacks; torsion in blacks is symmetric; torsion in whites greater on the right side than on the left side.
Radius	Length at the wrist variable.
Ulna	Ulna or radius may be longer. Equal length in Swedes—61 percent; in Chinese—16 percent. Ulna longer than radius in Swedes—16 percent; in Chinese—48 percent. Radius longer than ulna in Swedes—23 percent; in Chinese—10 percent.
Vertebrae	Twenty-four vertebrae (cervical, thoracic, lumbar) are found in 85 to 93 percent of all people. Racial and sex differences reveal 23 or 25 vertebrae in select groups; 11 percent of black females have 23, and 12 percent of Inuit and Native American males have 25. Increased number is related to lower back pain and lordosis.
Pelvis	Hip width is 1.6 cm (0.6 in) smaller in black women than in white women; Asian women have significantly smaller pelvises.
Femur	The femur has a convex anterior curve in Native Americans, is straight in blacks, and has an intermediate curve in whites.
Second tarsal	Second toe longer than the great toe—incidence: whites—8%–34%; blacks—8%–12%; Vietnamese—31%; Melanesians—21%–57%. Clinical significance for joggers and athletes, who reported increased foot problems.
Height	White males are 1.27 cm (0.5 in) taller than black males and 7.6 cm (2.9 in) taller than Asian males. White females have the same height as black females. Asian females are 4.14 cm (1.6 in) shorter than white or black females.
Composition of long bones	Longer, narrower, and denser in blacks than whites; bone density in whites is greater than in Chinese, Japanese, and Inuits. Osteoporosis incidence is lowest in black males; highest in white females.

Muscle	Variations
Peroneus tertius	Responsible for dorsiflexion of foot—muscle absent in 3%–10% of Asians, Native Americans, and whites; in 10%–15% of blacks; and in 24% of Berbers (Sahara desert). No clinical significance because the tibialis anterior also dorsiflexes the foot.
Palmaris longus	Responsible for wrist flexion—muscle absent in 12%–20% of whites; in 2%–12% of Native Americans; in 5% of blacks; and in 3% of Asians. No clinical significance because three other muscles are also responsible for flexion.

Data from Overfield T: Biologic Variation in Health and Illness: Race, Age, and Sex Differences, 2nd ed. New York, CRC Press, 1995; Andrews MM, Boyle JS (Eds): Transcultural Concepts in Nursing Care. Philadelphia, Lippincott-Raven, 1998.

accounting for the relatively low incidence of osteoporosis in this population. Bone density in the Chinese, Japanese, and Inuits is below that of white Americans (Garn, 1964).

Curvature of the long bones varies widely among culturally diverse groups. Native Americans have anteriorly convex femurs, blacks have markedly straight femurs, and in whites the femoral curvature is intermediate. This characteristic is related to both genetics and body weight. Thin blacks and whites have less curvature than average, whereas obese blacks and whites display increased curvatures. It is possible that the heavier density of the bones of blacks helps to protect them from increased curvature due to obesity.

Table 20-1 summarizes reported biocultural variations occurring in the musculoskeletal system.

SUBJECTIVE DATA

1. Joints
   Pain
   Stiffness
   Swelling, heat, redness
   Limitation of movement

2. Muscles
   Pain (cramps)
   Weakness

3. Bones
   Pain
   Deformity
   Trauma (fractures, sprains, dislocations)

4. Functional assessment (ADL)

5. Self-care behaviors

Examiner Asks	Rationale

1 Joints.

- Any problems with your joints? Any **pain?**

Joint pain and loss of function are the most common musculoskeletal concerns that prompt a person to seek care.

- Location—Which joints? On one side or both sides?

Rheumatoid arthritis (RA) involves symmetric joints; other musculoskeletal illnesses involve isolated or unilateral joints.

Exquisitely tender with acute inflammation.

- Quality—What does the pain feel like: aching, stiff, sharp or dull, shooting? Severity—How strong is the pain?
- Onset—When did this pain start?
- Timing—What time of day does the pain occur? How long does it last? How often does it occur?

RA pain is worse in morning when the person gets up; osteoarthritis is worse later on in the day; tendinitis is worse in morning, improves during the day.

- Is the pain aggravated by: movement, rest, position, weather? Is the pain relieved by: rest, medications, application of heat or ice?

Movement increases most joint pain except in RA, in which movement decreases pain.

- Is the pain associated with: chills, fever, recent sore throat, trauma, repetitive activity?

Joint pain occurring 10 to 14 days after a sore throat suggests rheumatic fever.

Joint injury occurs from trauma, repetitive motion.

- Any **stiffness** in your joints?

RA stiffness occurs in morning and after rest periods.

- Any **swelling, heat, redness** in the joints?
- Any **limitation of movement** in any joint? Which joint?
- Which activities give you problems? (See Functional assessment.)

Suggests acute inflammation.

Decreased ROM may be due to joint problems (injury to cartilage or capsule) or to muscle contracture.

2 Muscles.

- Any problems in the muscles, such as any **pain or cramping?** Which muscles?

Muscle pain usually is felt as cramping or aching.

- If in calf muscles: Is the pain with walking? Does it go away with rest?

Suggests intermittent claudication (see Chapter 18).

- Are your muscle aches associated with: fever, chills, the "flu"?

Viral illness often includes muscle aches (myalgia).

- Any **weakness** in muscles?
- Location—Where is the weakness? How long have you noticed weakness?

Weakness may involve musculoskeletal or neurologic systems (see also Chapter 21).

- Do the muscles look smaller there?

Atrophy.

3 Bones.

- Any **bone pain?** Is the pain affected by movement?

A fracture causes sharp pain that increases with movement. Other bone pain usually feels "dull" and "deep" and is unrelated to movement.

- Any **deformity** of any bone or joint? Is the deformity due to injury or trauma? Does the deformity affect ROM?
- Any **accidents or trauma** ever affected the bones or joints: fractures, joint strain, sprain, dislocation? Which ones?
- When did this occur? What treatment was given? Any problems or limitations now as a result?
- Any back pain? In which part of your back? Is pain felt anywhere else, e.g., shooting down leg?
- Any numbness and tingling? Any limping?

Examiner Asks	Rationale
4 **Functional assessment (ADL).** Do your joint (muscle, bone) problems create any limits on your usual activities of daily living (ADLs)? Which ones? (Note: Ask about each category; if the person answers "yes," ask specifically about each activity in category.)	**Functional assessment** is important to screen the safety of independent living, the need for home health care services, and quality of life. Assess any self-care deficit.
● Bathing—getting in and out of the tub, turning faucets?	
● Toileting—urinating, moving bowels, able to get self on/off toilet, wipe self?	
● Dressing—doing buttons, zipper, fasten opening behind neck, pulling dress or sweater over head, pulling up pants, tying shoes, getting shoes that fit?	
● Grooming—shaving, brushing teeth, brushing or fixing hair, applying make-up?	
● Eating—preparing meals, pouring liquids, cutting up foods, bringing food to mouth, drinking?	
● Mobility—walking, walking up or down stairs, getting in/out of bed, getting out of house?	Impaired physical mobility.
● Communicating—talking, using phone, writing?	Impaired verbal communication.
5 **Self-care behaviors.** Any occupational hazards that could affect the muscles and joints? Does your work involve heavy lifting? Or any repetitive motion or chronic stress to joints? Any efforts to alleviate these?	Assess risk for back pain or carpal tunnel syndrome.
● Tell me about your exercise program. Describe the type of exercise, frequency, the warm-up program.	**Self-care** behaviors.
● Any pain during exercise? How do you treat it?	
● Have you had any recent weight gain? Please describe your usual daily diet. (Note the person's usual caloric intake, all four food groups, daily amount of protein, calcium.)	
● Are you taking any medications for musculoskeletal system: aspirin, anti-inflammatory, muscle relaxant, pain reliever?	
● If person has chronic disability or crippling illness: How has your illness affected　Your interaction with family　Your interaction with friends　The way you view yourself	Assess for ● Self-esteem disturbance ● Loss of independence ● Body image disturbance ● Role performance disturbance ● Social isolation

ADDITIONAL HISTORY FOR INFANTS AND CHILDREN

1 Were you told about any trauma to infant during labor and delivery? Did the baby come head first? Was there a need for forceps?	Traumatic delivery increases risk for fractures, e.g., humerus, clavicle.
2 Did the baby need resuscitation?	Period of anoxia may result in hypotonia of muscles.
3 Were the baby's motor milestones achieved at about the same time as siblings or age-mates?	
4 Has your child ever broken any bones? Any dislocations? How were these treated?	
5 Have you ever noticed any bone deformity? Spinal curvature? Unusual shape of toes or feet? At what age? Have you ever sought treatment for any of these?	

Examiner Asks	Rationale

ADDITIONAL HISTORY FOR ADOLESCENTS

1 Involved in any sports at school or after school? How frequently (times per week)?

Assess safety of sport for child. Note if child's height and weight are adequate for the particular sport, e.g., football.

2 Do you use any special equipment? Does any training program exist for your sport?

Use of safety equipment and presence of adult supervision decreases risk of sports injuries.

3 What is the nature of your daily warm-up?

Lack of adequate warm-up increases risk of sports injury.

4 What do you do if you get hurt?

Some students will not report injury or pain for fear of limiting participation in sport.

5 How does your sport fit in with other school demands and other activities?

ADDITIONAL HISTORY FOR THE AGING ADULT

Use the functional assessment history (pp 86–88) questions to elicit any loss of function, self-care deficit, or safety risk that may occur as a process of aging or musculoskeletal illness. (If needed, review the section on functional assessment in Chapter 5 for further details.)

1 Any change in weakness over the past months or years?

2 Any increase in falls or stumbling over the past months or years?

3 Do you use any mobility aids to help you get around: cane, walker?

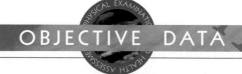

OBJECTIVE DATA

Preparation

The purpose of the musculoskeletal examination is to assess function for ADL, as well as to screen for any abnormalities. You already will have considerable data regarding ADL through the history. Note additional ADL data as the person goes through the motions necessary for an examination: gait, posture, how the person sits in a chair, raises from chair, takes off jacket, manipulates small object such as a pen, raises from supine.

A **screening** musculoskeletal examination suffices for most people:

- Inspection and palpation of joints integrated with each body region
- Observation of ROM as person proceeds through motions described earlier

 Equipment Needed

Tape measure
Goniometer, to measure joint angles
Skin marking pen

- Age-specific screening measures, e.g., Ortolani's sign for infants, or scoliosis screening for adolescents

A **complete** musculoskeletal examination, as described in this chapter, is appropriate for persons with articular disease, a history of musculoskeletal symptoms, or any problems with ADL.

Make the person comfortable before and throughout the examination. Drape for full visualization of the body part you are examining without needlessly exposing the person.

Take an orderly approach—head to toe, proximal to distal.

The joint to be examined should be supported at rest. Muscles must be soft and relaxed to assess the joints under them accurately. Take care when examining any inflamed area where rough manipulation could cause pain and muscle spasm. To avoid this, use firm support, gentle movement, and gentle return to a relaxed state.

Compare corresponding paired joints. Expect symmetry of structure and function, as well as normal parameters for that joint.

Normal Range of Findings	Abnormal Findings

ORDER OF THE EXAMINATION

Use the following order for each specific joint.

Inspection

Note the **size** and **contour** of the joint. Inspect the skin and tissues over the joints for **color, swelling,** and any **masses** or **deformity.** Presence of swelling is significant and signals joint irritation.

Swelling may be due to excess joint fluid (effusion), thickening of the synovial lining, inflammation of surrounding soft tissue (bursae, tendons) or bony enlargement.

Deformities include **dislocation** (one or more bones in a joint being out of position), **subluxation** (partial dislocation of a joint), **contracture** (shortening of a muscle leading to limited ROM of joint), or **ankylosis** (stiffness or fixation of a joint).

Palpation

Palpate each joint, including its skin for temperature, its muscles, bony articulations, and area of joint capsule. Notice any heat, tenderness, swelling, or masses. Joints normally are not tender to palpation. If any tenderness does occur, try to localize it to specific anatomic structures (e.g., skin, muscles, bursae, ligaments, tendons, fat pads, or joint capsule).

The synovial membrane normally is not palpable. When thickened, it feels "doughy" or "boggy." A small amount of fluid is present in the normal joint, but it is not palpable.

Palpable fluid is abnormal. Because fluid is contained in an enclosed sac, if you push on one side of the sac, the fluid will shift and cause a visible bulging on another side.

Range of Motion (ROM)

Ask for **active ROM** while stabilizing the body area proximal to that being moved. Familiarize yourself with the type of each joint and its normal ROM so that you can recognize limitations. If you see a limitation, gently attempt **passive motion.** Anchor the joint with one hand while your other hand slowly moves it to its limit. The normal ranges of active and passive motion should be the same.

If any limitation or any increase in ROM occurs, use a goniometer to measure the angles precisely (Fig. 20–15). First extend the joint to neutral or 0 degrees. Center the 0 point of the goniometer on the joint. Keep the fixed arm of the goniometer on the 0 line and use the movable arm to measure; then flex the joint and measure through the goniometer to determine the angle of greatest flexion.

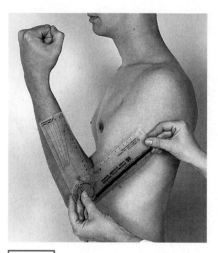

20–15

Joint motion normally causes no tenderness, pain, or crepitation. Do not confuse crepitation with the normal discrete "crack" heard as a tendon or ligament slips over bone during motion, such as when you do a knee bend.

Crepitation is an audible and palpable crunching or grating that accompanies movement. It occurs when the articular surfaces in the joints are roughened, as with rheumatoid arthritis (see Table 20–3).

Muscle Testing

Test the strength of the prime mover muscle groups for each joint. Repeat the motions you elicited for active ROM. Now ask the person to flex and hold as you apply opposing force. Muscle strength should be equal bilaterally and should fully resist your opposing force. (Note: Muscle status and joint status are interdependent and should be interpreted together. Chapter 21 discusses the examination of muscles for size and development, tone, and presence of tenderness.)

A wide variability of strength exists among people. You may wish to use a grading system from no voluntary movement to full strength, as shown in Table 20–2.

| ▶ Normal Range of Findings | Abnormal Findings |

Table 20–2 • Grading Muscle Strength

Grade	Description	Percent Normal	Assessment
5	Full ROM against gravity, full resistance	100	Normal
4	Full ROM against gravity, some resistance	75	Good
3	Full ROM with gravity	50	Fair
2	Full ROM with gravity eliminated (passive motion)	25	Poor
1	Slight contraction	10	Trace
0	No contraction	0	Zero

ROM = range of motion.

TEMPOROMANDIBULAR JOINT

With the person seated, **inspect** the area just anterior to the ear. Place the tips of your first two fingers in front of each ear and ask the person to open and close the mouth. Drop your fingers into the depressed area over the joint, and note smooth motion of the mandible. An audible and palpable snap or click occurs in many normal people as the mouth opens (Fig. 20–16).

Swelling looks like a round bulge over the joint, although it must be moderate or marked to be visible.

Crepitus and pain occur with temporomandibular joint dysfunction.

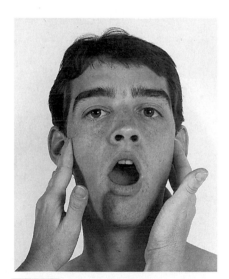

20–16

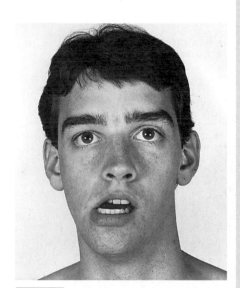

20–17

Ask the person to perform these motions (Fig. 20–17):

INSTRUCTIONS TO PERSON	MOTION AND EXPECTED RANGE
• Open mouth maximally.	Vertical motion. You can measure the space between the upper and lower incisors. Normal is 3 to 6 cm, or three fingers inserted sideways.
• Partially open mouth, protrude lower jaw, and move it side to side.	Lateral motion. Normal extent is 1 to 2 cm.
• Stick out lower jaw.	Protrude without deviation.

Lateral motion may be lost earlier and more significantly than vertical.

▶

Palpate the contracted temporalis and masseter muscles as the person clenches the teeth. Compare right and left sides for size, firmness, and strength. Ask the person to move the jaw forward and laterally against your resistance, open mouth against your resistance. This also tests the integrity of cranial nerve V (trigeminal).

CERVICAL SPINE

Inspect the alignment of head and neck. The spine should be straight and the head erect. **Palpate** the spinous processes and the sternomastoid, trapezius, and paravertebral muscles. They should feel firm, with no muscle spasm or tenderness.

Ask the person to follow these motions (Fig. 20–18):*

Head tilted to one side.

Asymmetry of muscles.

Tenderness and hard muscles with muscle spasm.

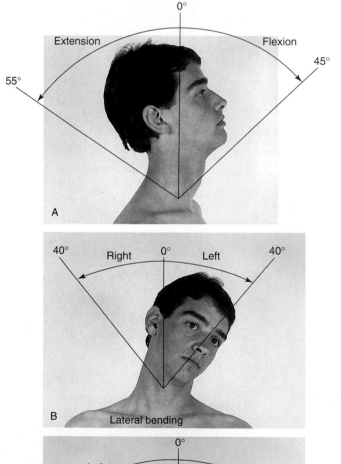

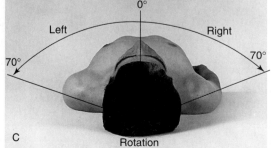

20–18

*DO NOT ATTEMPT IF YOU SUSPECT NECK TRAUMA.

|

INSTRUCTIONS TO PERSON   **MOTION AND EXPECTED RANGE**

- Touch chin to chest.
- Lift the chin toward the ceiling.
- Touch each ear toward the corresponding shoulder. Do not lift up the shoulder.
- Turn the chin toward each shoulder.

Flexion of 45 degrees (Fig. 20–18A).
Hyperextension of 55 degrees.
Lateral bending of 40 degrees (Fig. 20–18B).

Rotation of 70 degrees (Fig. 20–18C).

Repeat the motions while applying opposing force. The person normally can maintain flexion against your full resistance. This also tests integrity of cranial nerve XI (spinal).

UPPER EXTREMITY

Shoulders

Inspect and compare both shoulders posteriorly and anteriorly. Check the size and contour of the joint and compare shoulders for equality of bony landmarks. Normally, no redness, muscular atrophy, deformity, or swelling is present. Check the anterior aspect of the joint capsule and the subacromial bursa for abnormal swelling.

If the person reports any shoulder pain, ask that he or she point to the spot with the hand of the unaffected side. Be aware that shoulder pain may be from local causes or it may be referred pain due to a hiatal hernia or a cardiac or pleural condition, which could be potentially serious. Pain from a local cause is reproducible during the examination by palpation or motion.

While standing in front of the person, **palpate** both shoulders, noting any muscular spasm or atrophy, swelling, heat, or tenderness. Start at the clavicle and methodically explore the acromioclavicular joint, scapula, greater tubercle of the humerus, area of the subacromial bursa, the biceps groove, and the anterior aspect of the glenohumeral joint. Palpate the pyramid-shaped axilla; no adenopathy or masses should be present.

Limited ROM.

Pain with movement.

The person cannot hold flexion.

Redness.

Inequality of bony landmarks.

Atrophy, shows as lack of fullness.

Dislocated shoulder loses the normal rounded shape and looks flattened laterally.

Swelling from excess fluid is best seen anteriorly. Considerable fluid must be present to cause a visible distention because the capsule normally is so loose (see Table 20–4).

Swelling of subacromial bursa is localized under deltoid muscle and may be accentuated when the person tries to abduct the arm.

Swelling.

Hard muscles with muscle spasm.

Tenderness or pain.

Test ROM by asking the person to perform four motions (Fig. 20–19). Cup one hand over the shoulder during ROM to note any crepitation; normally none is present.

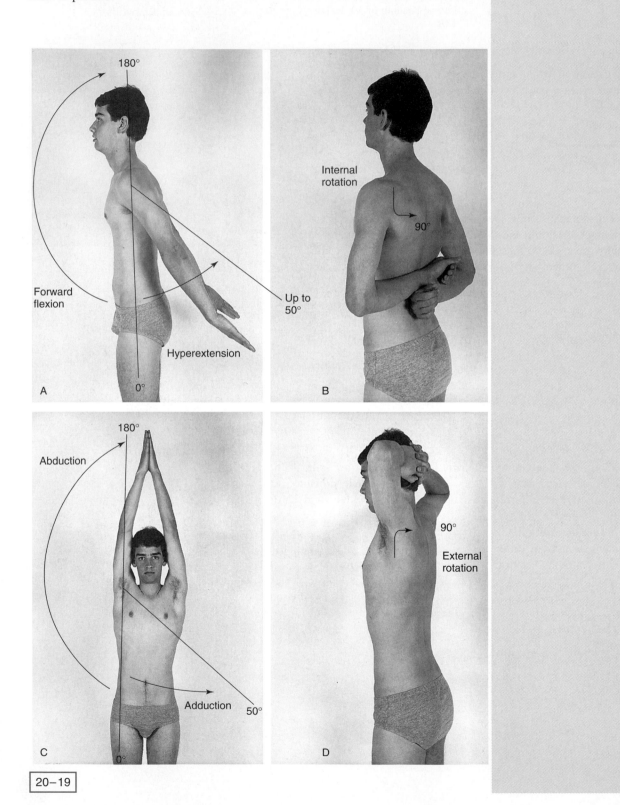

20–19

► Normal Range of Findings	Abnormal Findings

INSTRUCTIONS TO PERSON	**MOTION AND EXPECTED RANGE**	
• With arms at sides and elbows extended, move both arms forward and up in wide vertical arcs, then move them back.	Forward flexion of 180 degrees. Hyperextension up to 50 degrees (Fig. 20–19*A*).	Limited ROM.
		Asymmetry.
• Rotate arms internally behind back, place back of hands as high as possible toward the scapulae.	Internal rotation of 90 degrees (Fig. 20–19*B*).	Pain with motion.
		Crepitus with motion.
• With arms at sides and elbows extended, raise both arms in wide arcs in the coronal plane. Touch palms together above head.	Abduction of 180 degrees. Adduction of 50 degrees (Fig. 20–19*C*).	Rotator cuff lesions may cause limited ROM, pain, and muscle spasm during abduction, whereas forward flexion stays fairly normal.
• Touch both hands behind the head with elbows flexed and rotated posteriorly.	External rotation of 90 degrees (Fig. 20–19*D*).	

Test the strength of the shoulder muscles by asking the person to shrug the shoulders, flex forward and up, and abduct against your resistance. The shoulder shrug also tests the integrity of cranial nerve XI, the spinal accessory.

Elbow

Inspect the size and contour of the elbow in both flexed and extended positions. Look for any deformity, redness, or swelling. Check the olecranon bursa and the normally present hollows on either side of the olecranon process for abnormal swelling.

Subluxation of the elbow shows the forearm dislocated posteriorly.

Swelling and redness of olecranon bursa are localized and easy to observe because of the close proximity of the bursa to skin.

Effusion or synovial thickening shows first as a bulge or fullness in groove on either side of the olecranon process, and it occurs with gouty arthritis.

Epicondyles, head of radius, and tendons are common sites of inflammation and local tenderness, or "tennis elbow."

Palpate with the elbow flexed about 70 degrees and as relaxed as possible (Fig. 20–20). Use your left hand to support the person's left forearm and palpate the extensor surface of the elbow—the olecranon process and the medial and lateral epicondyles of humerus—with your right thumb and fingers.

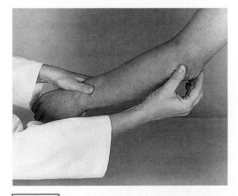

20–20

Normal Range of Findings	Abnormal Findings

With your thumb in the lateral groove and your index and middle fingers in the medial groove, palpate either side of the olecranon process using varying pressure. Normally present tissues and fat pads feel fairly solid. Check for any synovial thickening, swelling, nodules, or tenderness.

Palpate the area of the olecranon bursa for heat, swelling, tenderness, consistency, or nodules.

Test ROM by asking the person to do the following:

INSTRUCTIONS TO PERSON	MOTION AND EXPECTED RANGE
● Bend and straighten the elbow (Fig. 20–21).	Flexion of 150 to 160 degrees, extension at 0. Some normal people lack 5 to 10 degrees of full extension, and others have 5 to 10 degrees of hyperextension.
● Movement of 90 degrees in pronation and supination (Fig. 20–22).	Hold the hand midway, then touch front and back sides of hand to table.

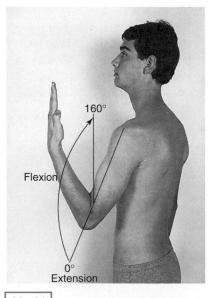

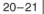

20–21

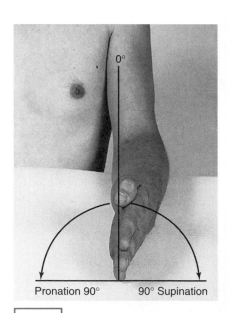

20–22

While testing **muscle strength,** stabilize the person's arm with one hand (Fig. 20–23). Have the person flex the elbow against your resistance applied just proximal to the wrist. Then ask the person to extend the elbow against your resistance.

Soft, boggy, or fluctuant swelling in both grooves occurs with synovial thickening or effusion.

Local heat or redness (signs of inflammation) can extend beyond synovial membrane.

Subcutaneous nodules are raised, firm, and nontender, and overlying skin moves freely. Common sites are in the olecranon bursa and along extensor surface of the ulna. These nodules occur with rheumatoid arthritis (see Table 20–5).

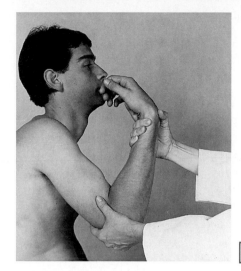

20–23

Wrist and Hand

Inspect the hands and wrists on the dorsal and palmar sides, noting position, contour, and shape. The normal functional position of the hand shows the wrist in slight extension. This way the fingers can flex efficiently, and the thumb can oppose them for grip and manipulation. The fingers lie straight in the same axis as the forearm. Normally, no swelling or redness, deformity, or nodules are present.

Subluxation of wrist.

Ulnar deviation; fingers list to ulnar side.

Ankylosis; wrist in extreme flexion.

Dupuytren's contracture; flexion contracture of finger(s).

The skin looks smooth with knuckle wrinkles present and no swelling or lesions. Muscles are full, with the palm showing a rounded mound proximal to the thumb (the **thenar eminence**) and a smaller rounded mound proximal to the little finger.

Swan-neck or boutonnière deformity in fingers.

Atrophy of the thenar eminence (see Table 20–6, Abnormalities of the Wrist and Hand).

Palpate each joint in the wrist and hands. Facing the person, support the hand with your fingers under it and palpate the wrist firmly with both your thumbs on its dorsum (Fig. 20–24). Make sure the person's wrist is relaxed and in straight alignment. Move your palpating thumbs side to side to identify the normal depressed areas that overlie the joint space. Use gentle but firm pressure. Normally, the joint surfaces feel smooth, with no swelling, bogginess, nodules, or tenderness.

Ganglion in wrist.

Synovial swelling on dorsum.

Generalized swelling.

Tenderness.

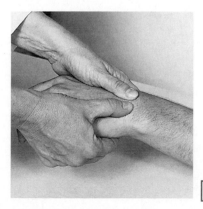

20–24

Palpate the metacarpophalangeal joints with your thumbs, just distal to and on either side of the knuckle (Fig. 20–25).

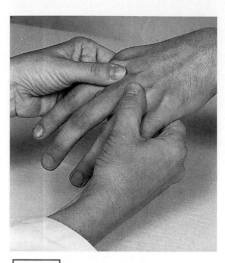

20–25

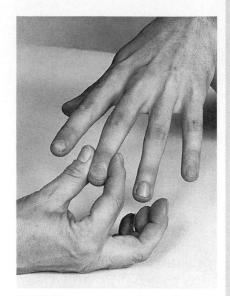

20–26

Use your thumb and index finger in a pinching motion to palpate the sides of the interphalangeal joints (Fig. 20–26). Normally, no synovial thickening, tenderness, warmth, or nodules are present.

Heberden's and Bouchard's nodules are hard and nontender and occur with osteoarthritis (see Table 20–6).

Test ROM (Fig. 20–27) by asking the person to do the following:

INSTRUCTIONS TO PERSON	MOTION AND EXPECTED RANGE
● Bend the hand up at the wrist.	Hyperextension of 70 degrees (Fig. 20–27A).
● Bend hand down at the wrist.	Palmar flexion of 90 degrees.
● Bend the fingers up and down at metacarpophalangeal joints.	Flexion of 90 degrees. Hyperextension of 30 degrees (Fig. 20–27B).
● With palms flat on table, turn them outward and in.	Ulnar deviation of 50–60 degrees, and radial deviation of 20 degrees (Fig. 20–27C).
● Spread fingers apart; make a fist.	Abduction of 20 degrees; fist tight. The responses should be equal bilaterally (Fig. 20–27D, E).
● Touch the thumb to each finger and to the base of little finger.	The person is able to perform, and the responses are equal bilaterally (Fig. 20–27F).

Loss of ROM here is the most common and the most significant type of functional loss of the wrist.

Limited motion.

Pain on movement.

▶ Normal Range of Findings   Abnormal Findings

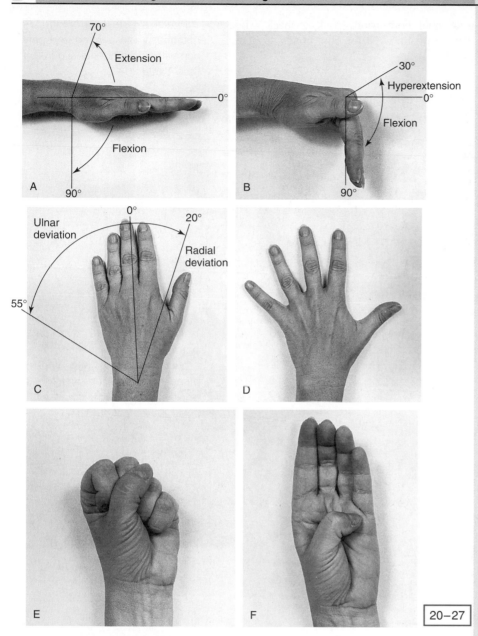

20–27

For **muscle testing,** position the person's forearm supinated (palm up) and resting on a table (Fig. 20–28). Stabilize by holding your hand at the person's mid-forearm. Ask the person to flex the wrist against your resistance at the palm.

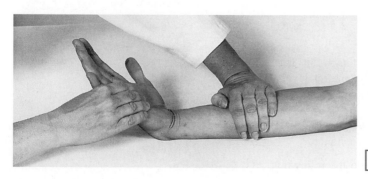

20–28

Phalen's Test. Ask the person to hold both hands back to back while flexing the wrists 90 degrees. Acute flexion of the wrist for 60 seconds produces no symptoms in the normal hand (Fig. 20–29).

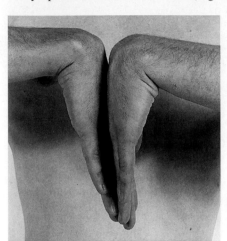

20–29

Phalen's Test

Phalen's test reproduces numbness and burning in a person with carpal tunnel syndrome (see Table 20–6).

Tinel's Sign. Direct percussion of the location of the median nerve at the wrist produces no symptoms in the normal hand (Fig. 20–30).

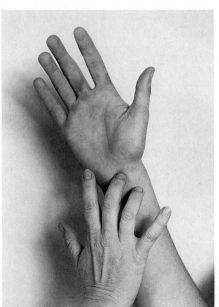

20–30

Tinel's Sign

In carpal tunnel syndrome, percussion of the median nerve produces burning and tingling along its distribution, which is a positive Tinel's sign.

LOWER EXTREMITY

Hip

Wait to **inspect** the hip joint together with the spine a bit later in the examination as the person stands. At that time, note symmetric levels of iliac crests, gluteal folds, and equally sized buttocks. A smooth, even gait reflects equal leg lengths and functional hip motion.

Help the person into a supine position and **palpate** the hip joints. The joints should feel stable and symmetric, with no tenderness or crepitance.

Assess ROM (Fig. 20–31) by asking the person to do the following:

Pain with palpation.

Crepitation.

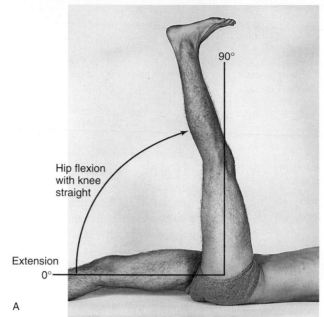

A

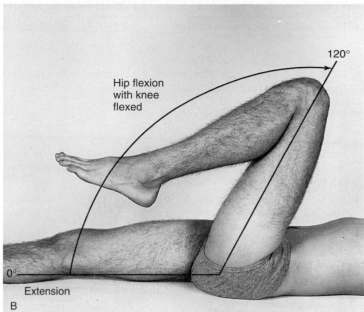

B

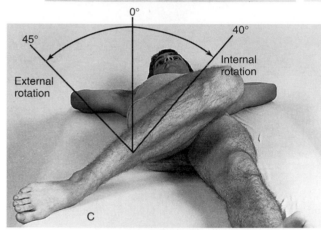

C

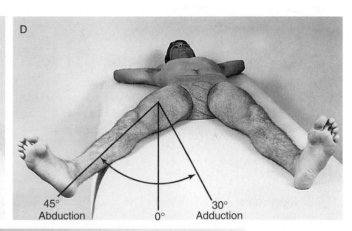

D

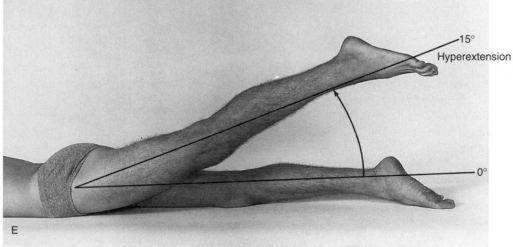

E

20–31

▶ | Normal Range of Findings | Abnormal Findings

INSTRUCTIONS TO PERSON	MOTION AND EXPECTED RANGE
• Raise each leg with knee extended.	Hip flexion of 90 degrees (Fig. 20–31A).
• Bend each knee up to the chest while keeping the other leg straight.	Hip flexion of 120 degrees. The opposite thigh should remain on the table (Fig. 20–31B).
• Flex knee and hip to 90 degrees. Stabilize by holding the thigh with one hand and the ankle with the other hand. Swing the foot outward. Swing the foot inward. (Foot and thigh move in opposite directions.)	Internal rotation of 40 degrees. External rotation of 45 degrees (Fig. 20–31C).
• Swing leg laterally, then medially, with knee straight. Stabilize pelvis by pushing down on the opposite anterior superior iliac spine.	Abduction of 40 to 45 degrees. Adduction of 20 to 30 degrees (Fig. 20–31D).
• When standing (later in examination), swing straight leg back behind body. Stabilize pelvis to eliminate exaggerated lumbar lordosis. The most efficient way is to ask person to bend over the table and to support the trunk on the table. Or the person can lie prone on the table.	Hyperextension of 15 degrees when stabilized (Fig. 20–31E).

Abnormal Findings

Limited motion.

Pain with motion.

Flexion flattens the lumbar spine; if this reveals a flexion deformity in the opposite hip, it represents a positive *Thomas test.*

Limited internal rotation of hip is an early and reliable sign of hip disease.

Limitation of abduction of the hip while supine is the most common motion dysfunction found in hip disease.

Knee

The person should remain supine with legs extended, although some examiners prefer the knees to be flexed and dangling for **inspection.** The skin normally looks smooth, with even coloring and no lesions.

Shiny and atrophic skin.

Swelling or inflammation (see Table 20–7).

Lesions, e.g., psoriasis.

Inspect lower leg alignment. The lower leg should extend in the same axis as the thigh.

Angulation deformity:

• Genu varum (bow-legs)
• Genu valgum (knock knees)
• Flexion contracture

Inspect the knee's shape and contour. Normally, distinct concavities, or hollows, are present on either side of the patella. Check them for any sign of fullness or swelling. Note other locations, such as the prepatellar bursa and the suprapatellar pouch, for any abnormal swelling.

Check the quadriceps muscle in the anterior thigh for any atrophy. Since it is the prime mover of knee extension, this muscle is important for joint stability during weight-bearing.

Hollows disappear, then they may bulge with synovial thickening or effusion.

Atrophy occurs with disuse or chronic disorders. First, it appears in the medial part of the muscle, although it is difficult to note because the vastus medialis is relatively small.

Normal Range of Findings	Abnormal Findings

Enhance **palpation** with the knee in the supine position with complete relaxation of the quadriceps muscle. Start high on the anterior thigh, about 10 cm above the patella. Palpate with your left thumb and fingers in a grasping fashion (Fig. 20–32). Proceed down toward the knee, exploring the region of the suprapatellar pouch. Note the consistency of the tissues. The muscles and soft tissues should feel solid, and the joint should feel smooth, with no warmth, tenderness, thickening, or nodularity.

Feels fluctuant or boggy with synovitis of suprapatellar pouch.

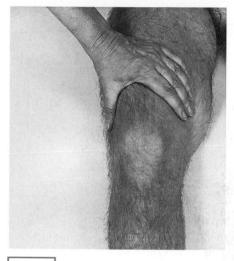

20–32

When swelling occurs, you need to distinguish whether it is due to soft tissue swelling or increased fluid in the joint. The tests for the bulge sign and ballottement of the patella aid this assessment.

Bulge Sign. For swelling in the suprapatellar pouch, the bulge sign confirms the presence of fluid. Firmly stroke up on the medial aspect of the knee two or three times to displace any fluid (Fig. 20–33A). Tap the lateral aspect (Fig. 20–33B). Watch the medial side in the hollow for a distinct bulge from a fluid wave. Normally, none is present.

The bulge sign occurs with very small amounts of effusion, 4 to 8 ml.

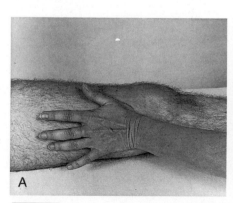
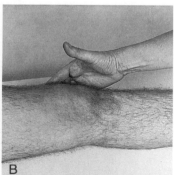

20–33

Bulge Sign

▶ |

Ballottement of the Patella. This test is reliable when larger amounts of fluid are present. Use your left hand to compress the suprapatellar pouch. With your right hand, push the patella sharply against the femur. If no fluid is present, the patella already is snug against the femur (Fig. 20–34).

If fluid has collected, your tap on the patella displaces the fluid, and you will hear a tap as the patella bumps up on the femur.

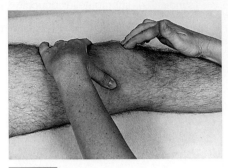

20–34

Ballottement

Continue palpation and explore the tibiofemoral joint (Fig. 20–35). Note smooth joint margins and absence of pain. Palpate the infrapatellar fat pad and the patella. Check for crepitus by holding your hand on the patella as the knee is flexed and extended. Some crepitus in an otherwise asymptomatic knee is not uncommon.

Irregular bony margins, occur with osteoarthritis.

Pain at joint line.

Pronounced crepitus is significant and it occurs with degenerative diseases of the knee.

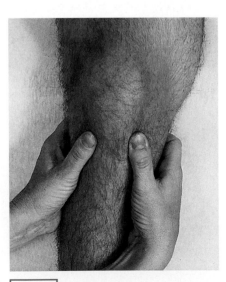

20–35

Check ROM (Fig. 20–36) by asking the person to do the following:

Normal Range of Findings	Abnormal Findings

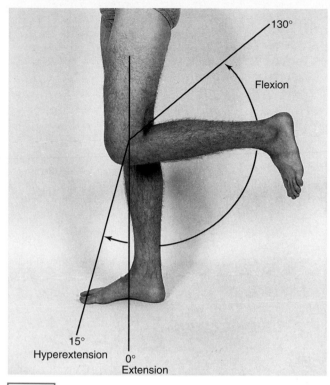

130°

Flexion

15°
Hyperextension   0°
Extension

20–36

INSTRUCTIONS TO PERSON	MOTION AND EXPECTED RANGE	
• Bend each knee.	Flexion of 130 to 150 degrees.	Limited ROM.
• Extend each knee.	A straight line of 0 degrees in some persons; a hyperextension of 15 degrees in others.	Contracture.
		Pain with motion.
• Check knee ROM during ambulation.		Limp.

Sudden locking—the person is unable to extend the knee fully. This usually occurs with a painful and audible "pop" or "click." Sudden buckling, or "giving way," occurs with ligament injury, which causes weakness and instability.

Check **muscle strength** by asking the person to maintain knee flexion while you oppose by trying to pull the leg forward. Muscle extension is demonstrated by the person's success in rising from a seated position in a low chair or by rising from a squat without using the hands for support.

▶ **Normal Range of Findings** | **Abnormal Findings**

Special Test for Meniscal Tears

McMurray's Test. Perform this test when the person has reported a history of trauma followed by locking, giving way, or local pain in the knee. Position the person supine, as you stand on the affected side. Hold the heel and flex the knee and hip. Place your other hand on the knee with fingers on the medial side. Rotate the leg in and out to loosen the joint. Externally rotate the leg and push a valgus (inward) stress on the knee. Then, slowly extend the knee. Normally, the leg extends smoothly with no pain (Fig. 20–37).

If you hear or feel a "click," the McMurray test is positive for a torn meniscus.

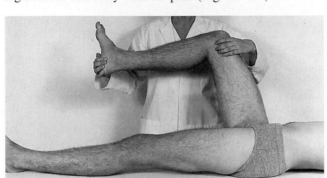

20–37

Ankle and Foot

Inspect while the person is in a sitting, non–weight-bearing position, as well as when standing and walking. Compare both feet, noting position of feet and toes, contour of joints, and skin characteristics. The foot should align with the long axis of the lower leg; an imaginary line would fall from mid-patella to between the first and second toes.

Weight-bearing should fall on the middle of the foot, from the heel, along the mid-foot, to between the second and third toes. Most feet have a longitudinal arch, although that can vary normally from "flat feet" to a high instep.

The toes point straight forward and lie flat. The ankles (malleoli) are smooth bony prominences. Normally, the skin is smooth with even coloring and no lesions. Note the locations of any calluses or bursal reactions because they reveal areas of abnormal friction. Examining well-worn shoes helps assess areas of wear and accommodation.

Support the ankle by grasping the heel with your fingers while palpating with your thumbs (Fig. 20–38). Explore the joint spaces. They should feel smooth and depressed, with no fullness, swelling, or tenderness.

Hallux valgus (see Table 20–8).

Hammer toes. Claw toes.

Swelling or inflammation.

Calluses. Ulcers.

Swelling or inflammation.

Tenderness.

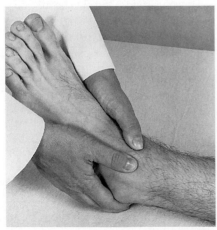

20–38

Normal Range of Findings	Abnormal Findings

Palpate the metatarsophalangeal joints between your thumb on the dorsum and your fingers on the plantar surface (Fig. 20–39).

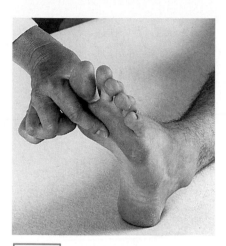

20–39

Using a pinching motion of your thumb and forefinger, palpate the interphalangeal joints on the medial and lateral sides of the toes.

Test ROM (Fig. 20–40) by asking the person to do the following:

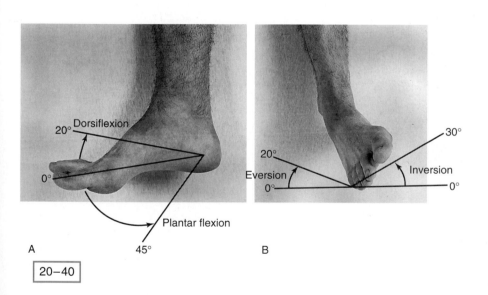

20–40

INSTRUCTIONS TO PERSON	MOTION AND EXPECTED RANGE
• Point toes toward the floor.	Plantar flexion of 45 degrees.
• Point toes toward your nose.	Dorsiflexion of 20 degrees (Fig. 20–40A).
• Turn soles of feet out, then in. (Stabilize the ankle with one hand, hold heel with the other to test the subtalar joint.)	Eversion of 20 degrees. Inversion of 30 degrees (Fig. 20–40B).
• Flex and straighten toes.	

Assess **muscle strength** by asking the person to maintain dorsiflexion and plantar flexion against your resistance.

Abnormal Findings (right column):

Swelling or inflammation; tenderness.

Limited ROM.

Pain with motion.

Unable to hold flexion.

▶

SPINE

The person should be standing, draped in a gown open at the back. Place yourself far enough back so that you can see the entire back. **Inspect** and note if the spine is straight by following an imaginary vertical line from the head through the spinous processes and down through the gluteal cleft, and by noting equal horizontal positions for the shoulders, scapulae, iliac crests, and gluteal folds, and equal spaces between arm and lateral thorax on the two sides (Fig. 20–41A). The person's knees and feet should be aligned with the trunk and should be pointing forward.

A difference in shoulder elevation and in level of scapulae and iliac crests occurs with scoliosis (see Table 20–9).

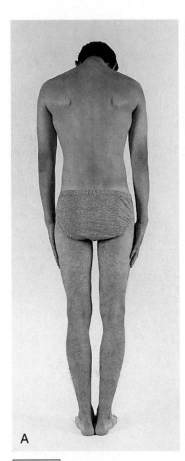
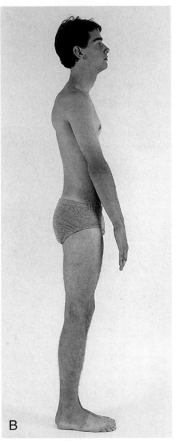

A   B

20–41

From the side, note the normal convex thoracic curve and concave lumbar curve (Fig. 20–41B). An enhanced thoracic curve, or kyphosis, is common in aging people. A pronounced lumbar curve, or lordosis, is common in obese people.

Lateral tilting and forward bending occur with a herniated nucleus pulposus (see Table 20–9).

Normal Range of Findings	Abnormal Findings

Palpate the spinous processes. Normally, they are straight and not tender. Palpate the paravertebral muscles; they should feel firm with no tenderness or spasm.

Check **ROM** of the spine by asking the person to bend forward and touch the toes (Fig. 20–42). Look for flexion of 75 to 90 degrees and smoothness and symmetry of movement. Note that the concave lumbar curve should disappear with this motion, and the back should have a single convex C-shaped curve.

Spinal curvature.

Tenderness. Spasm of para-vertebral muscles.

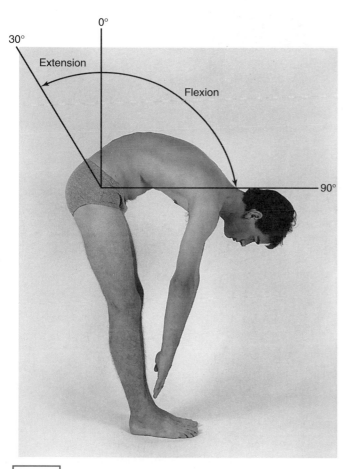

20–42

If you suspect a spinal curvature during inspection, this may be more clearly seen when the person touches the toes. While the person is bending over, mark a dot on each spinous process. When the person resumes standing, the dots should form a straight vertical line.

If the dots form a slight S-shape when the person stands, a spinal curve is present.

Stabilize the pelvis with your hands. Check ROM (Fig. 20–43) by asking the person to do the following:

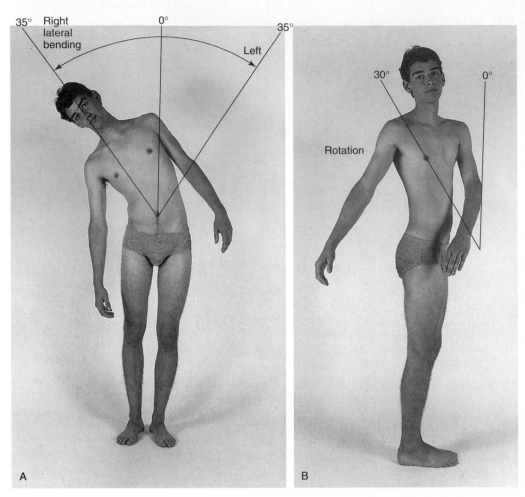

20–43

INSTRUCTIONS TO PERSON	MOTION AND EXPECTED RANGE
● Bend sideways.	Lateral bending of 35 degrees (Fig. 20–43A).
● Bend backward.	Hyperextension of 30 degrees.
● Twist shoulders to one side, then the other.	Rotation of 30 degrees, bilaterally (Fig. 20–43B).

Limited ROM.

Pain with motion.

These maneuvers reveal only gross restriction. Movement is still possible even if some spinal fusion has occurred.

Straight Leg Raising or LaSegue's Test. These maneuvers reproduce back and leg pain and help confirm the presence of a herniated nucleus pulposus. Straight leg raising while keeping the knee extended normally produces no pain. Raise the affected leg just short of the point where it produces pain. Then dorsiflex the foot (Fig. 20–44).

Positive if the test reproduces sciatic pain. If lifting the affected leg reproduces sciatic pain, it confirms the presence of a herniated nucleus pulposus.

► Normal Range of Findings	Abnormal Findings

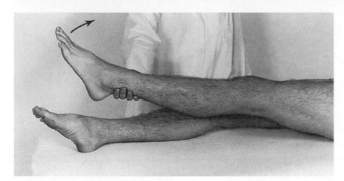

20-44

Raise the unaffected leg while leaving the other leg flat. Inquire about the involved side.

Measure Leg Length Discrepancy. Perform this measurement if you need to determine if one leg is shorter than the other. For *true leg length,* measure between *fixed* points, from the anterior iliac spine to the medial malleolus, crossing the medial side of the knee (Fig. 20–45). Normally, these measurements are equal or within 1 cm, indicating no true bone discrepancy.

Sometimes the true leg length is equal, but the legs still look unequal. For *apparent leg length,* measure from a nonfixed point (the umbilicus) to a fixed point (medial malleolus) on each leg.

If lifting the unaffected leg reproduces sciatic pain, it strongly suggests a herniated nucleus pulposus.

Unequal leg lengths.

True leg lengths are equal, but apparent leg lengths unequal—this condition occurs with pelvic obliquity or adduction or flexion deformity in the hip.

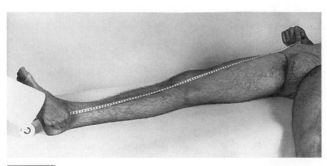

20-45

 DEVELOPMENTAL CONSIDERATIONS

Review the developmental milestones discussed in Chapter 2. Keep handy a concise chart of the usual sequence of motor development so that you can refer to expected findings for the age of each child you are examining. Use the Denver II to screen the fine and gross motor skills for the child's age.

Since some overlap exists between the musculoskeletal and neurologic examinations, assessment of muscle tone, resting posture, and motor activity are discussed in the next chapter.

► Normal Range of Findings	Abnormal Findings

Infants

Examine the infant fully undressed and lying on the back. Take care to place the newborn on a warming table to maintain body temperature.

Feet and Legs. Start with the feet and work your way up the extremities. Note any *positional deformities,* a residual of fetal positioning. Often the newborn's feet are not held straight but in a varus (apart) or valgus (together) position. It is important to distinguish whether this position is flexible (and thus usually self-correctable) or fixed. Scratch the outside of the bottom of the foot. If the deformity is self-correctable, the foot assumes a normal right angle to the lower leg. Or, immobilize the heel with one hand and gently push the forefoot to the neutral position with the other hand. If you can move it to neutral position, it is flexible.

> A true deformity is fixed and assumes a right angle only with forced manipulation or not at all.

Note the relationship of the forefoot to the hindfoot. Commonly, the hindfoot is in alignment with the lower leg and just the forefoot angles inward. This forefoot adduction is *metatarsus adductus.* It is usually present at birth and usually resolves spontaneously by age 3 years.

> Metatarsus varus—adduction and inversion of forefoot.
> Talipes equinovarus (see Table 20–10).

Check for *tibial torsion,* a twisting of the tibia. Place both feet flat on the table, and push to flex up the knees. With the patella and the tibial tubercle in a straight line, place your fingers on the malleoli. In an infant, note that a line connecting the four malleoli is parallel to the table.

Tibial torsion may originate from intrauterine positioning and then may be exacerbated at a later age by continuous sitting in a reverse tailor position, the "TV squat." This is sitting with the buttocks on the floor and the lower legs splayed back and out on either side.

> More than 20 degrees of deviation; or if lateral malleolus is anterior to medial malleolus, it indicates tibial torsion.

Hips. Check the hips for *congenital dislocation.* The most reliable method is the **Ortolani maneuver,** which should be done at every professional visit until the infant is 1 year old (Fig. 20–46). With the infant supine, flex the knees holding your thumbs on the inner mid-thighs, and your fingers outside on the hips touching the greater trochanters. Adduct the legs until your thumbs touch (Fig. 20–46A). Then gently lift and *abduct,* moving the knees apart and down so their lateral aspects touch the table (Fig. 20–46B). This normally feels smooth and has no sound.

> With a dislocated hip, the head of the femur is not cupped in the acetabulum but rests posterior to it.
> Hip instability feels like a clunk as the head of the femur pops back into place. This is a *positive Ortolani sign* and warrants referral.

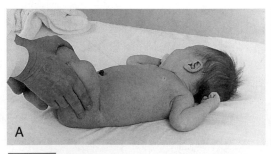 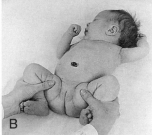

20–46

Ortolani Maneuver

The **Allis test** also is used to check for hip dislocation by comparing leg lengths (Fig. 20–47). Place the baby's feet flat on the table and flex the knees up. Scan the tops of the knees; normally, they are at the same elevation.

> Finding one knee significantly lower than the other is a positive indication of Allis' sign and suggests hip dislocation.

Normal Range of Findings	Abnormal Findings

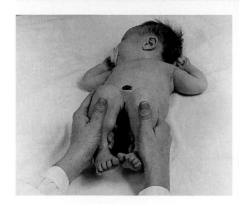

20–47

Allis Test

Note the gluteal folds. Normally, they are equal on both sides. However, some asymmetry may occur in normal children.

Unequal gluteal folds may accompany hip dislocation after 2 to 3 months of age.

Hands and Arms. Inspect the hands, noting shape, number, and position of fingers and palmar creases.

Polydactyly is the presence of extra fingers or toes. Syndactyly is webbing between adjacent fingers or toes (see Table 20–6).

A simian crease is a single palmar crease that occurs with Down syndrome, accompanied by short broad fingers, incurving of little fingers, and low-set thumbs.

Palpate the length of the clavicles because the clavicle is the bone most frequently fractured during birth. The clavicles should feel smooth, regular, and without crepitus. Also note equal ROM of arms during the Moro reflex.

Fractured clavicle—Note irregularity at the fracture site, crepitus, and angulation. The site has rapid callus formation with a palpable lump within a few weeks. Observe limited arm ROM and unilateral response to the Moro reflex.

Back. Lift up the infant and examine the back. Note the normal single C curve of the newborn's spine (Fig. 20–48). By 2 months of age, the infant can lift the head while prone. This builds the concave cervical spinal curve, and indicates normal forearm strength. Inspect the length of the spine for any tuft of hair, dimple in midline, cyst, or mass. Normally, none are present.

A tuft of hair over a dimple in the midline may indicate spina bifida.

A small dimple in the midline, anywhere from the head to the coccyx, suggests dermoid sinus.

Mass, e.g., meningocele.

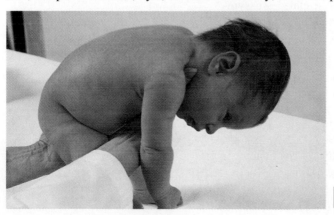

20–48

Normal Range of Findings	Abnormal Findings

Observe ROM through spontaneous movement of extremities.

Test muscle strength by lifting up the infant with your hands under the axillae (Fig. 20–49). A baby with normal muscle strength wedges securely between your hands.

A baby who starts to "slip" between your hands shows weakness of the shoulder muscles.

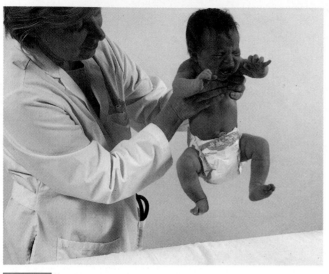

20–49

Preschool- and School-Age Children

Once the infant learns to crawl and then to walk, the waking hours show perpetual motion. This is convenient for your musculoskeletal assessment—You can observe the muscles and joints during spontaneous play before a table-top examination. Most young children enjoy showing off their physical accomplishments. For specific motions, coax the toddler: "Show me how you can walk to Mom," ". . . climb the step stool." Ask the preschooler to hop on one foot or to jump.

Back. While the child is standing, note the posture. From behind, you should note a "plumb line" from the back of the head, along the spine, to the middle of the sacrum. Shoulders are level within 1 cm, and scapulae are symmetric. From the side, lordosis is common throughout childhood, appearing more pronounced in children with a protuberant abdomen.

Lordosis is marked with muscular dystrophy and rickets.

Legs and Feet. Anteriorly, note the leg position. A "bow-legged" stance *(genu varum)* is a lateral bowing of the legs (Fig. 20–50A). It is present when you measure a persistent space of more than 2.5 cm between the knees when the medial malleoli are together. Genu varum is normal for 1 year after the child begins walking. "Knock knees" *(genu valgum)* are present when there is more than 2.5 cm between the medial malleoli when the knees are together (Fig. 20–50B). It occurs normally between 2 and 3½ years of age. (Note: To remember the two conditions, remember to link the r's and g's, i.e., genu varum—knees apart; genu valgum—knees together.)

Genu varum also occurs with rickets.

Genu valgum also occurs with rickets, poliomyelitis, and syphilis.

▶ Normal Range of Findings	Abnormal Findings

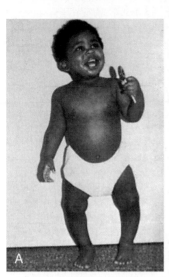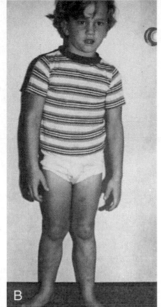

20-50

A, Genu Varum;   *B*, Genu Valgum

Often, parents tell you they are concerned about the child's foot development. The most common questions are about "flatfeet" and "pigeon toes." Flatfoot *(pes planus)* is pronation, or turning in, of the medial side of the foot. The young child may look flatfooted because the normal longitudinal arch is concealed by a fat pad until age 3 years. When standing begins, the child takes a broad-based stance, which causes pronation. Thus, pronation is common between 12 and 30 months. You can see it best from behind the child, where the medial side of the foot drops down and in.

Pronation beyond 30 months.

Pigeon toes, or toeing in, are demonstrated when the child tends to walk on the lateral side of the foot, and the longitudinal arch looks higher than normal. It often starts as a forefoot adduction, which usually corrects spontaneously by age 3 years, as long as the foot is flexible.

Toeing in from forefoot adduction that is fixed, or lasts beyond age 3 years.
Toeing in from tibial torsion.

Check the child's gait while walking away from and returning to you. Let the child wear socks, because a cold tile floor will distort the usual gait. From 1 to 2 years of age, expect a broad-based gait, with arms out for balance. Weight-bearing falls on the inside of the foot. From 3 years of age, the base narrows and the arms are closer to the sides. Inspect the shoes for spots of greatest wear to aid your judgment of the gait. Normally, the shoes wear more on the outside of the heel and the inside of the toe.

Limp; usually caused by trauma, fatigue, or hip disease.

Abnormal gait patterns (see Chapter 21).

Normal Range of Findings	Abnormal Findings

Check the **Trendelenburg sign** to screen progressive subluxation of the hip (Fig. 20–51). Watching from behind, ask the child to stand on one leg, then the other. Watch the iliac crests; they should stay level when weight is shifted.

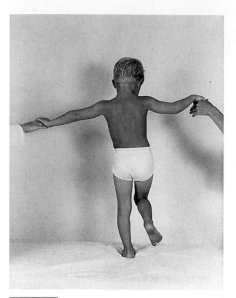

20–51

The child may sit for the remainder of the examination. Start with the feet and hands of the child from 2 to 6 years of age because the child is happy to show these off, and proceed through the examination described earlier.

Particularly, check the arm for full ROM and presence of pain. Look for subluxation of the elbow (head of the radius). This occurs most often between 2 and 4 years of age as a result of forceful removal of clothing or dangling while adults suspend the child by the hands.

Palpate the bones, joints, and muscles of the extremities as described in the adult examination.

The sign occurs with subluxation of one hip. When the child stands on the good leg, the pelvis looks level. When the child stands on the affected leg, the pelvis drops toward the "good" side.

Inability to supinate the hand while the arm is flexed, together with pain in elbow, indicates subluxation of the head of the radius.

Pain or tenderness in extremities usually is caused by trauma or infection.

Fractures are usually due to trauma and are exhibited as an inability to use the area, a deformity, or an excess motion in the involved bone with pain and crepitation.

Enlargement of the tibial tubercles with tenderness suggests Osgood-Schlatter disease (see Table 20–7).

▶ | Normal Range of Findings | Abnormal Findings

Adolescents

Proceed with the musculoskeletal examination you provide for the adult, except pay special note to spinal posture. Kyphosis is common during adolescence because of chronic poor posture. **Screen for scoliosis** with the *forward bend test* starting at age 10 to 12 (Fig. 20–52). Seat yourself behind the standing child, and ask the child to stand with the feet shoulder-width apart and bend forward slowly to touch the toes. Expect a straight vertical spine while standing and also while bending forward. Posterior ribs should be symmetric, with equal elevation of shoulders, scapulae, and iliac crests. You may wish to mark each spinous process with a felt marker. The line-up of ink dots highlights even a subtle curve.

Scoliosis is most apparent during the preadolescent growth spurt. Asymmetry suggests scoliosis—ribs hump up on one side as child bends forward, and with an equal landmark elevation (see Table 20–9).

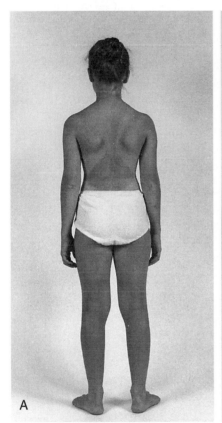
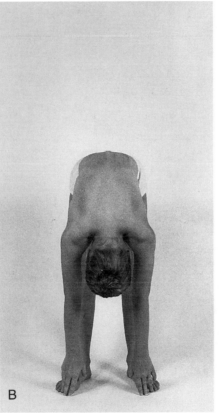

20–52

Be aware of the risk of sports-related injuries with the adolescent, because sports participation and competition often peak with this age group.

▶ Normal Range of Findings   Abnormal Findings

The Pregnant Female

Proceed through the examination described in the adult section. Expected postural changes in pregnancy include progressive lordosis and, toward the third trimester, anterior cervical flexion, kyphosis, and slumped shoulders (Fig. 20–53A). When the pregnancy is at term, the protuberant abdomen and the relaxed mobility in the joints create the characteristic "waddling" gait (Fig. 20–53B).

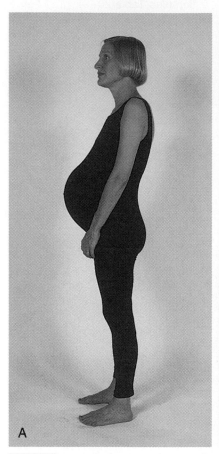
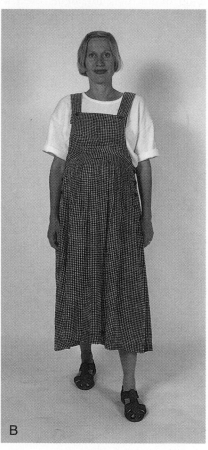

20–53

▶ Normal Range of Findings	Abnormal Findings

The Aging Adult

Postural changes include a decrease in height, more apparent in the eighth and ninth decades (Fig. 20–54). "Lengthening of the arm-trunk axis" describes this shortening of the trunk with comparatively long extremities. Kyphosis is common, with a backward head tilt to compensate. This creates the outline of a figure 3 when you view this older adult from the left side. Slight flexion of hips and knees also is common.

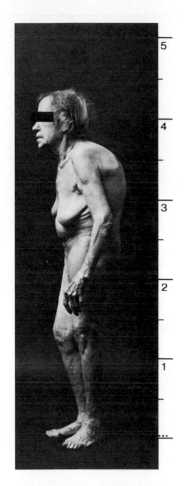

20–54

Contour changes include a decrease of fat in the body periphery and fat deposition over the abdomen and hips. The bony prominences become more marked.

For most older adults, ROM testing proceeds as described earlier. ROM and muscle strength are much the same as with the younger adult, provided no musculoskeletal illnesses or arthritic changes are present.

Functional Assessment

For those with advanced aging changes, arthritic changes, or musculoskeletal disability, perform a **functional assessment for ADL.** This applies the ROM and muscle strength assessments to the accomplishment of specific activities. You need to determine adequate and safe performance of functions essential for independent home life.

▶ Normal Range of Findings   Abnormal Findings

INSTRUCTIONS TO PERSON	COMMON ADAPTATION FOR AGING CHANGES*
1. Walk (with shoes on).	Shuffling pattern; swaying; arms out to help balance; broader base of support; person may watch feet.
2. Climb up stairs.	Person holds hand rail; may haul body up with it; may lead with favored (stronger) leg.
3. Walk down stairs.	Holds hand rail, sometimes with both hands.
	If the person is weak, he or she may descend sideways lowering the weaker leg first. If the person is unsteady, he or she may watch feet.
4. Pick up object from floor.	Person often bends at waist instead of bending knees; holds furniture to support while bending and straightening.
5. Rise up from sitting in chair.	Person uses arms to push off chair arms, upper trunk leans forward before body straightens, feet planted wide in broad base of support.
6. Rise up from lying in bed.	May roll to one side, push with arms to lift up torso, grab bedside table to increase leverage.

*Data from Bowers AC, Thompson JM: Clinical Manual of Health Assessment, 4th ed. St. Louis, C. V. Mosby, 1992.

SUMMARY CHECKLIST: Musculoskeletal Exam

For each joint to be examined:

1: Inspection
Size and contour of joint
Skin color and characteristics

2: Palpation of joint area
Skin
Muscles
Bony articulations
Joint capsule

3: ROM
Active
Passive (if limitation in active ROM is present)
Measure with goniometer (if abnormality in ROM is present)

4: Muscle testing

APPLICATION AND CRITICAL THINKING

SAMPLE CHARTING

 Subjective

States no joint pain, stiffness, swelling, or limitation. No muscle pain or weakness. No history of bone trauma or deformity. Able to manage all usual daily activities with no physical limitations. Occupation involves no musculoskeletal risk factors. Exercise pattern is brisk walk 1 mile 5×/week.

Objective

Joints and muscles symmetric; no swelling, masses, deformity; normal spinal curvature. No tenderness to palpation of joints; no heat, swelling, or masses. Full ROM; movement smooth, no crepitance, no tenderness. Muscle strength—able to maintain flexion against resistance and without tenderness.

CLINICAL CASE STUDY

M.T. is a 45-year-old white female salesperson with a diagnosis of rheumatoid arthritis 3 years PTA, who seeks care now for "swelling and burning pain in my hands" for 1 day.

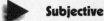 **Subjective**

M.T. was diagnosed as having rheumatoid arthritis at age 41, by staff at this agency. Since that time, her "flare-ups" seem to come every 6 to 8 months. Acute episodes involve hand joints, and are treated with aspirin, which gives relief. Typically experiences morning stiffness, lasting ½ to 1 hour. Joints feel warm, swollen, tender. Has had weight loss of 15 pounds over last 4 years, and feels fatigued much of the time. States should rest more, but "I can't take the time." Daily exercises have been prescribed but doesn't do them regularly. Takes aspirin for acute flare-ups, feels better in a few days, decreases dose by herself.

 Objective

Body joints within normal limits with exception of joints of wrist and hands. Radiocarpal, metacarpophalangeal, and proximal interphalangeal joints are red, swollen, tender to palpation. Spindle-shaped swelling of proximal interphalangeal joints of third digit right hand and second digit left hand; ulnar deviation of metacarpophalangeal joints.

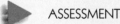 ASSESSMENT

Acute pain R/T inflammation
Impaired physical mobility R/T inflammation
Knowledge deficit about aspirin treatment R/T lack of exposure
Noncompliance with exercise program R/T lack of perceived benefits of treatment
Noncompliance with advised rest periods R/T lack of perceived benefits of treatment

NURSING DIAGNOSES COMMONLY ASSOCIATED WITH THE MUSCULOSKELETAL DISORDERS

Diagnosis	Related Factors (Etiology)	Defining Characteristics (Symptoms and Signs)
Impaired physical mobility	Neuromuscular impairment Sensory-perceptual impairment Fatigue, decreased strength and endurance Intolerance to activity Effects of trauma or surgery Inflammation Pain Obesity Side effects of sedatives, narcotics, or tranquilizers Depression Severe anxiety Fear of movement Architectural barriers Lack of assistive devices	Reluctance to attempt movement Imposed restrictions on movement Limited range of motion Decreased muscle strength, control, or mass Inability to move purposefully within the environment Impaired coordination Falling or stumbling

Continued

Diagnosis	Related Factors (Etiology)	Defining Characteristics (Symptoms and Signs)

Risk for disuse syndrome		Presence of risk factors such as:
		  Paralysis
		  Mechanical immobilization
		  Prescribed immobilization
		  Severe pain
		  Altered level of consciousness

Risk for trauma	Balancing difficulties
	Pain
	Reduced large, small muscle coordination
	Reduced mobility of arms, legs
	Weakness
	Insufficient finances to purchase safety equipment or to make repairs
	Lack of safety precautions, safety education
	Fatigue
	Visual, hearing impairment
	History of
	  Previous trauma
	  Substance abuse	

Pain	Inflammation
	Muscle spasm
	Effects of surgery or trauma
	Immobility
	Pressure points
	Infectious process
	Overactivity
	Obstructive processes
		Clutching of painful area
		Trembling
		Facial mask of pain
		Changes in posture or gait
		Change in muscle tone: listless to rigid
		Reports of pain
		Anxiety
		Immobilization
		Positive response to palpation
		Withdrawal reflex
		Autonomic responses
		  Increased blood pressure, pulse, respirations
		  Diaphoresis
		  Dilated pupils
		Crying or moaning
		Fatigue
		Distraction behavior—pacing, restlessness
		Focused on self
		Depression

Other Related Nursing Diagnoses

ACTUAL

Activity intolerance (see Chapter 16)
Altered growth and development
Body image disturbance
Chronic pain
Diversional activity deficit
Impaired home maintenance management (see Chapter 12)
Impaired skin integrity (see Chapter 10)
Self-care deficit
Sleep pattern disturbance

RISK/WELLNESS

Risk

Risk for altered growth
Risk for disuse syndrome
Risk for impaired skin integrity
Risk for injury

Wellness

Health-seeking behavior R/T knowledge about community resources
Health-seeking behavior R/T knowledge about disease process
Increasing own responsibility for self-care
Maintaining current mobility
Progressing toward previous mobility status

ASSESSMENT VIDEO CRITICAL THINKING QUESTIONS

The Saunders *Physical Examination and Health Assessment* Video Series—MUSCULO-SKELETAL SYSTEM—will direct you to consider the following:

1. What other assessment findings can you expect to see in a patient who reports joint pain?

2. What abnormal findings may commonly be detected during assessment of the wrists and hands?

3. When are genu varum and genu valgum considered normal? What abnormal conditions may also cause them?

4. How does musculoskeletal assessment of an adolescent differ from that of an adult?

Table 20–3   ABNORMALITIES AFFECTING MULTIPLE JOINTS

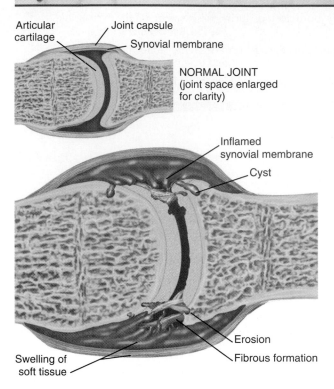

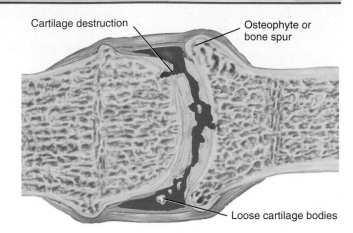

INFLAMMATORY CONDITIONS

Rheumatoid Arthritis (RA)

This is a chronic, systemic inflammatory disease of joints and surrounding connective tissue. Inflammation of synovial membrane leads to thickening; then to fibrosis, which limits motion; and finally to bony ankylosis. The disorder is symmetric and bilateral and is characterized by heat, redness, swelling, and painful motion of the affected joints. RA is associated with fatigue, weakness, anorexia, weight loss, low-grade fever, and lymphadenopathy. Associated signs are described in the following tables, especially Table 20–6.

Ankylosing Spondylitis (not illustrated)

Chronic progressive inflammation of spine, sacroiliac, and larger joints of the extremities, leading to bony ankylosis and deformity. A form of RA, this affects primarily men by a 10 : 1 ratio, in late adolescence or early adulthood. Spasm of paraspinal muscles pulls spine into forward flexion, obliterating cervical and lumbar curves. Thoracic curve exaggerated into single kyphotic rounding. Also includes flexion deformities of hips and knees.

DEGENERATIVE CONDITIONS

Osteoarthritis (Degenerative Joint Disease)

Noninflammatory, localized, progressive disorder involving deterioration of articular cartilages and subchondral bone, and formation of new bone (osteophytes) at joint surfaces. Aging increases incidence; nearly all adults over 60 have some radiographic signs of osteoarthritis. Asymmetric joint involvement commonly affects hands, knees, hips, and lumbar and cervical segments of the spine. Affected joints have stiffness, swelling with hard, bony protuberances, pain with motion, and limitation of motion (see Table 20–6).

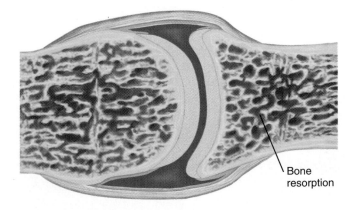

Osteoporosis

Decrease in skeletal bone mass occurring when rate of bone resorption is greater than that of bone formation. The weakened bone state increases risk for stress fractures, especially at wrist, hip, and vertebrae. Occurs primarily in postmenopausal white women. Osteoporosis risk also is associated with smaller height and weight, younger age at menopause, lack of physical activity, and lack of estrogen replacement therapy.

Table 20–4   ABNORMALITIES OF THE SHOULDER

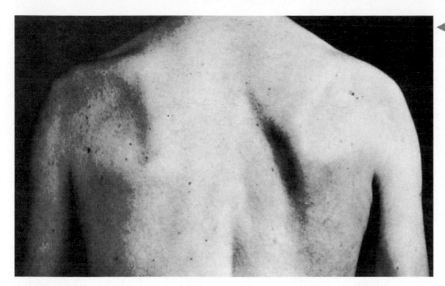

Atrophy

Loss of muscle mass is exhibited as a lack of fullness surrounding the scapulae, here greater on the left side than on the right. In this case, atrophy is due to cervical radiculitis. Atrophy also occurs from disuse, muscle tissue damage, or motor nerve damage.

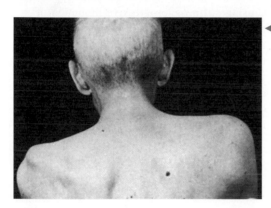

Dislocated Shoulder

Anterior dislocation (95 percent) is exhibited as a hollow where normally it would look rounded. It occurs with trauma involving abduction, extension, and rotation, e.g., falling on an outstretched arm or diving into a pool.

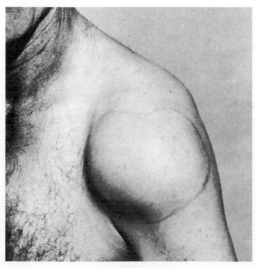

Joint Effusion

Swelling from excess fluid in the joint capsule, here from rheumatoid arthritis. Best observed anteriorly. Fluctuant to palpation. Considerable fluid must be present to cause a visible distention because the capsule normally is so loose.

Table continued on following page

Table 20–4   ABNORMALITIES OF THE SHOULDER *Continued*

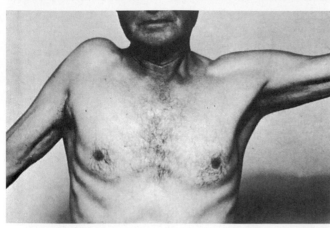

◀ Tear of Rotator Cuff

Characteristic "hunched" position and limited abduction of arm. Occurs from traumatic adduction while arm is held in abduction, or from fall on shoulder, throwing, or heavy lifting. Positive drop arm test: If the arm is passively abducted at the shoulder, the person is unable to sustain the position and the arm falls to the side.

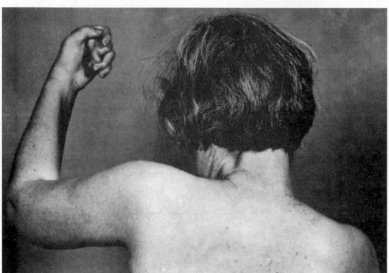

◀ Frozen Shoulder—Adhesive Capsulitis

Fibrous tissues form in the joint capsule, causing stiffness, progressive limitation of motion, and pain. Motion limited in abduction and external rotation; unable to reach overhead. It may lead to atrophy of shoulder girdle muscles. Gradual onset; unknown cause. It is associated with prolonged bedrest or shoulder immobility. May resolve spontaneously.

Subacromial Bursitis (not illustrated)

Inflammation and swelling of subacromial bursa over the shoulder cause limited ROM and pain with motion. Localized swelling under deltoid muscle may increase by partial passive abduction of the arm. Caused by direct trauma, strain during sports, local or systemic inflammatory process, or repetitive motion with injury.

Table 20–5 ABNORMALITIES OF THE ELBOW

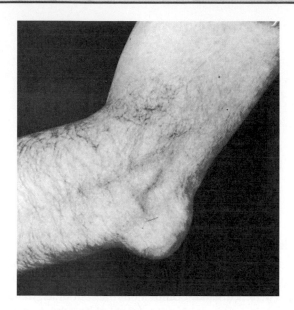

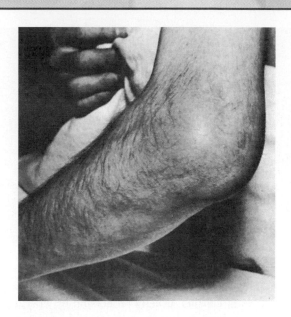

Olecranon Bursitis

Large knob, or "goose egg," and redness due to inflammation of olecranon bursa. Localized and easy to see because bursa lies just under skin.

Gouty Arthritis

Joint effusion or synovial thickening, seen first as bulge or fullness in grooves on either side of olecranon process. Redness and heat can extend beyond area of synovial membrane. Soft, boggy, or fluctuant fullness to palpation. Limited extension of elbow.

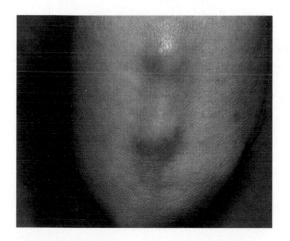

Subcutaneous Nodules

Raised, firm, nontender nodules that occur with rheumatoid arthritis. Common sites are in the olecranon bursa and along extensor surface of arm. The skin slides freely over the nodules.

Epicondylitis—Tennis Elbow (not illustrated)

Chronic disabling pain at lateral epicondyle of humerus, radiates down extensor surface of forearm. Occurs with activities combining excessive pronation and supination of forearm with an extended wrist, e.g., racquet sports or using a screwdriver.

Medial epicondylitis is more rare and is due to activity of forced palmar flexion of wrist against resistance.

Table 20-6   ABNORMALITIES OF THE WRIST AND HAND

ABNORMAL FINDINGS

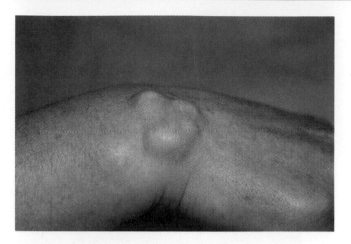

Ganglion Cyst

Round, cystic, nontender nodule overlying a tendon sheath or joint capsule, usually on dorsum of wrist. Flexion makes it more prominent. A common benign tumor; it does not become malignant.

Colles' Fracture (not illustrated)

Nonarticular fracture of distal radius, with or without fracture of ulna at styloid process. Usually from a fall on an outstretched hand; occurs more often in older women. Wrist looks puffy, with "silver fork" deformity, a characteristic hump when viewed from the side.

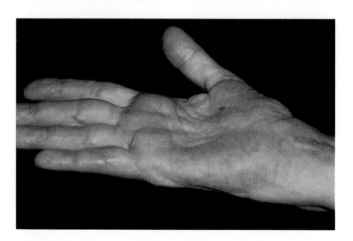

Carpal Tunnel Syndrome With Atrophy of Thenar Eminence

Atrophy occurs from interference with motor function, due to compression of the median nerve inside the carpal tunnel. Caused by chronic repetitive motion; occurs between 30 and 60 years of age and is five times more common in women than in men. Symptoms of carpal tunnel syndrome include pain, burning and numbness, positive findings on Phalen's test, positive indication of Tinel's sign, and often atrophy of thenar muscles.

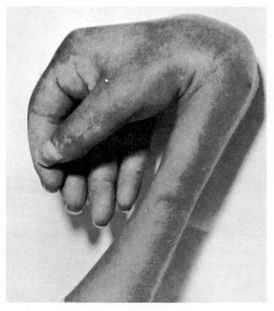

Ankylosis

Wrist in extreme flexion, due to severe rheumatoid arthritis. This is a functionally useless hand, because when the wrist is palmar flexed, a good deal of power is lost from the fingers, and the thumb cannot oppose the fingers.

Table 20–6   ABNORMALITIES OF THE WRIST AND HAND *Continued*

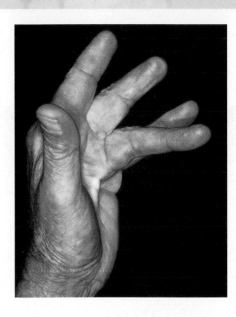

Dupuytren's Contracture

Chronic hyperplasia of the palmar fascia causes flexion contractures of the digits, first in the fourth digit, then the fifth digit, and then the third digit. Note the bands that extend from the mid-palm to the digits, and the puckering of palmar skin. The condition occurs commonly in men past 40 years of age and is usually bilateral. It occurs with diabetes, epilepsy, and alcoholic liver disease, and as an inherited trait. The contracture is painless but impairs hand function.

Reprinted from the Clinical Slide Collection on the Rheumatic Diseases, © 1991, 1995, 1997. Used by permission of the American College of Rheumatology.

CONDITIONS CAUSED BY CHRONIC RHEUMATOID ARTHRITIS

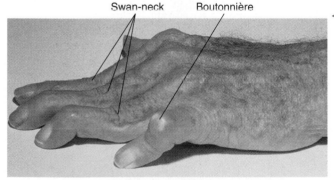

Swan-neck   Boutonnière

Swan-Neck and Boutonnière Deformity

Flexion contracture resembles curve of a **swan's neck.** Note flexion contracture of metacarpophalangeal joint, then hyperextension of the proximal interphalangeal joint, and flexion of the distal interphalangeal joint. It occurs with chronic rheumatoid arthritis and is often accompanied by ulnar drift of the fingers.

In **boutonnière deformity,** the knuckle looks as if it is being pushed through a buttonhole. It is a relatively common deformity and includes flexion of proximal interphalangeal joint with compensatory hyperextension of distal interphalangeal joint.

Reprinted from the Clinical Slide Collection on the Rheumatic Diseases, © 1991, 1995, 1997. Used by permission of the American College of Rheumatology.

Ulnar Deviation or Drift

Fingers drift to the ulnar side because of stretching of the articular capsule and muscle imbalance. Also note subluxation and swelling in the joints, and muscle atrophy on the dorsa of the hands. This is caused by chronic rheumatoid arthritis.

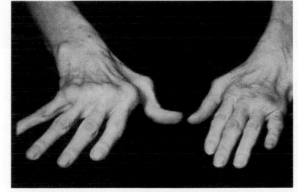

Table continued on following page

679

Table 20-6 ABNORMALITIES OF THE WRIST AND HAND *Continued*

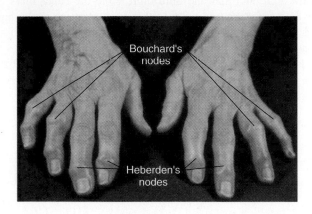

Degenerative Joint Disease or Osteoarthritis

Osteoarthritis is characterized by hard, nontender nodules, 2 to 3 mm or more. These osteophytes (bony overgrowths) of the distal interphalangeal joints are called Heberden's nodes, and those of the proximal interphalangeal joints are called Bouchard's nodes.

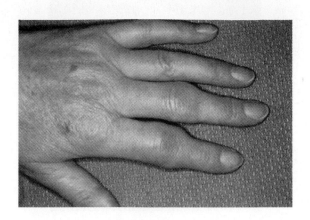

Acute Rheumatoid Arthritis

Painful swelling and stiffness of joints, with fusiform or spindle-shaped swelling of the soft tissue of proximal interphalangeal joints. Fusiform swelling is usually symmetric, the hands are warm, and the veins are engorged. The inflamed joints have a limited range of motion.

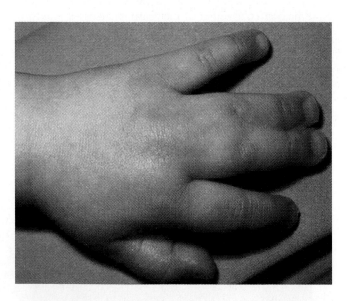

Syndactyly

Webbed fingers are a congenital deformity, usually requiring surgical separation. The metacarpals and phalanges of the webbed fingers are different lengths, and the joints do not line up. To leave the fingers fused would thus limit their flexion and extension.

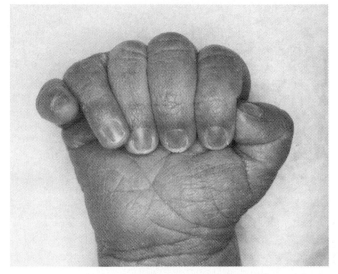

Polydactyly

Extra digits are a congenital deformity, usually occurring at the fifth finger or the thumb. Surgical removal is considered for cosmetic appearance. The sixth finger shown here was not removed, because it had full ROM and sensation and a normal appearance.

Table 20–7 ABNORMALITIES OF THE KNEE

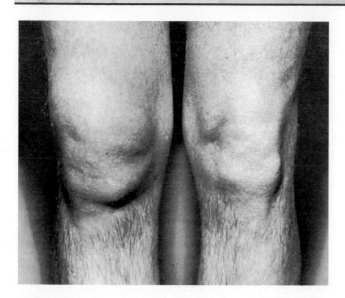

Mild Synovitis

Loss of normal hollows on either side of the patella, which are replaced by mild distention. Occurs with synovial thickening or effusion (excess fluid). Also note mild distention of the suprapatellar pouch.

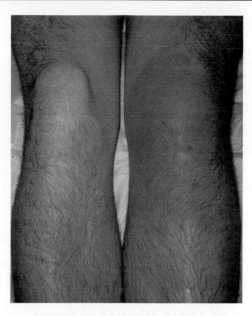

Prepatellar Bursitis

Localized swelling on anterior knee between patella and skin. A tender fluctuant mass indicates swelling; in this case, infection has spread to surrounding soft tissue. The condition is limited to the bursa, and the knee joint itself is not involved. Overlying skin may be red, shiny, atrophic, or coarse and thickened.

Reprinted from the Clinical Slide Collection on the Rheumatic Diseases, © 1991, 1995, 1997. Used by permission of the American College of Rheumatology.

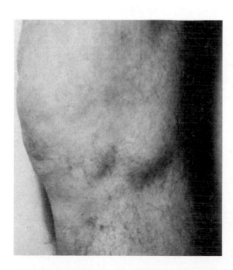

Swelling of Menisci

Localized soft swelling due to cyst in medial meniscus shows at the midpoint of the anteromedial joint line. Flexion of the knee makes swelling more prominent.

Osgood-Schlatter Disease (not illustrated)

Painful swelling of the tibial tubercle just below the knee, probably due to repeated stress on the patellar tendon. Occurs most in puberty during rapid growth and most often in males. Pain increases with kicking, running, bike-riding, stair-climbing, or kneeling. The condition is usually self-limited, and symptoms resolve with rest.

Chondromalacia Patellae (not illustrated)

Degeneration of articular surface of patellae. The condition occurs most often in females, and its cause is unknown. May produce mild effusion. Joint motion is painless, but crepitus may be present. Pain starts with kneeling.

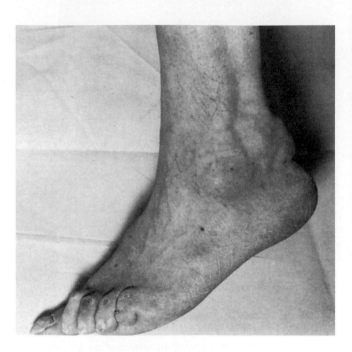

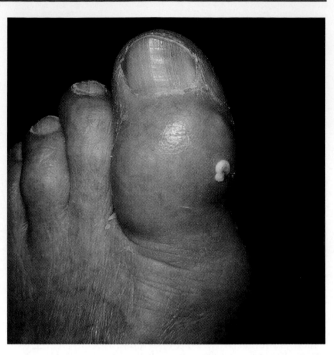

Achilles Tenosynovitis

Inflammation of a tendon sheath near the ankle (here, the Achilles tendon) produces a superficial linear swelling and a localized tenderness along the route of the sheath. Movement of the involved tendon usually causes pain.

Tophi With Chronic Gout

Hard, painless nodule (tophi) over metatarsophalangeal joint of first toe. Tophi are collections of sodium urate crystals due to chronic gout in and around the joint that cause extreme swelling and joint deformity. They sometimes burst with a chalky discharge.

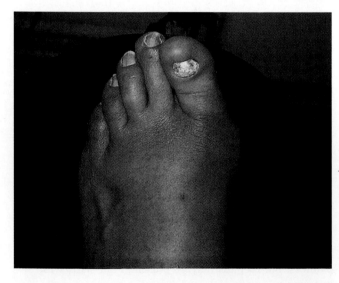

◀ Acute Gout

Acute episode of gout usually involves first the metatarsophalangeal joint. Clinical findings consist of redness, swelling, heat, and extreme tenderness. Gout is a metabolic disorder of disturbed purine metabolism, associated with elevated serum uric acid. It occurs primarily in men over 40 years of age.

Table 20-8 ABNORMALITIES OF THE ANKLE AND FOOT *Continued*

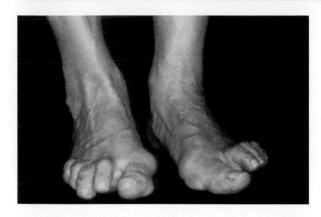

Hallux Valgus With Bunion and Hammer Toes

Hallux valgus is a common deformity from rheumatoid arthritis. It is a lateral or outward deviation of the toe with medial prominence of the head of the first metatarsal. The **bunion** is the inflamed bursa that forms at the pressure point. The great toe loses power to push off while walking; this stresses the second and third metatarsal heads, and they develop calluses and pain. Chronic sequelae include corns, calluses, hammer toes, and joint subluxation.

Note the **hammer toe** deformities in the second, third, fourth, and fifth toes. Often associated with hallux valgus, hammer toe includes hyperextension of the metatarsophalangeal joint and flexion of the proximal interphalangeal joint.

Corns (thickening of soft tissue) develop on the dorsum over the bony prominence owing to prolonged pressure from shoes.

Callus (not illustrated)

Hypertrophy of the epithelium develops because of prolonged pressure, commonly on the plantar surface of the first metatarsal head in the hallux valgus deformity. The condition is not painful.

Plantar Wart (not illustrated)

Vascular papillomatous growth probably is due to a virus and occurs on the sole of the foot, commonly at the ball. The condition is extremely painful.

Ingrown Toenail (not illustrated)

A misnomer; the nail does not grow in, but the soft tissue grows over the nail and obliterates the groove. It occurs almost always on the great toe on the medial or lateral side. It is due to trimming the nail too short or toe-crowding in tight shoes. The area becomes infected when the nail grows and its corner penetrates the soft tissue.

Table 20-9   ABNORMALITIES OF THE SPINE

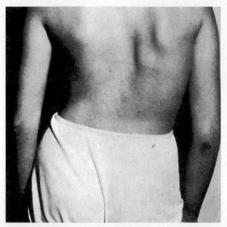

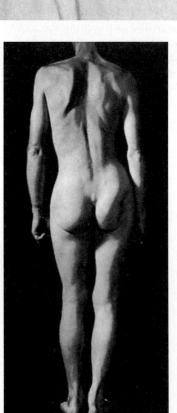

◄ Scoliosis

Lateral curvature of thoracic and lumbar segments of the spine, usually with some rotation of involved vertebral bodies.

Functional scoliosis is flexible; it is apparent with standing and disappears with forward bending. It may be compensatory for other abnormalities such as leg length discrepancy.

Structural scoliosis is fixed; the curvature shows both on standing and on bending forward. Note rib hump with forward flexion. When the person is standing, note unequal shoulder elevation, unequal scapulae, obvious curvature, unequal elbow level, and unequal hip level. At greatest risk are females 10 years of age through adolescence during the peak of the growth spurt.

◄ Herniated Nucleus Pulposus

The nucleus pulposus (at the center of the intervertebral disc) ruptures into the spinal canal and puts pressure on the local spinal nerve root. Usually occurs from stress, e.g., lifting, twisting, continuous flexion with lifting, or fall on buttocks. Occurs mostly in men 20 to 45 years of age. Lumbar herniations occur mainly in interspaces L4 to L5 and L5 to S1. Note: sciatic pain, numbness, and paresthesia of involved dermatome; listing away from affected side; decreased mobility; low back tenderness; and decreased motor and sensory function in leg. Straight leg raising tests reproduce sciatic pain.

Table 20–10   COMMON CONGENITAL OR PEDIATRIC ABNORMALITIES

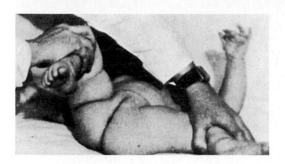

Congenital Dislocated Hip

Head of the femur is displaced out of the cup-shaped acetabulum.

The degree of the condition varies; subluxation may occur as stretched ligaments allow partial displacement of femoral head, and acetabular dysplasia may develop because of excessive laxity of hip joint capsule.

Occurrence is 1 : 500 to 1 : 1000 births more frequently in girls by 7 : 1 ratio. Signs include limited abduction of flexed thigh, positive indications of Ortolani's and Barlow's signs, asymmetric skin creases or gluteal folds, limb length discrepancy, and positive indication of Trendelenburg's sign in older children.

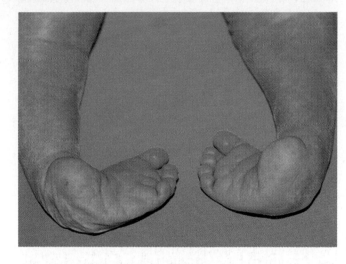

Talipes Equinovarus (Clubfoot)

Congenital, rigid, and fixed malposition of foot including (1) inversion, (2) forefoot adduction, and (3) foot pointing downward (equinus). A common birth defect, with an incidence of 1 : 1000 to 3 : 1000 live births. Males are affected twice as frequently as females.

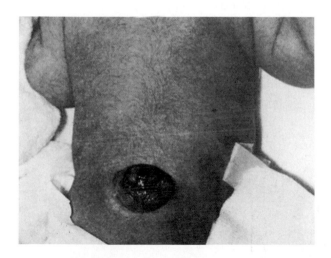

Spina Bifida

Incomplete closure of posterior part of vertebrae results in a neural tube defect. Seriousness varies from skin defect along the spine to protrusion of the sac containing meninges, spinal fluid, or malformed spinal cord. The most serious type is myelomeningocele (shown here), in which the meninges and neural tissue protrude. In these cases, the child is usually paralyzed below the level of the lesion.

Coxa Plana (Legg-Calvé-Perthes Syndrome)

(not illustrated)

Avascular necrosis of the femoral head, occurring primarily in males between 3 and 12 years of age, with peak at age 6 years. In initial inflammatory stage, interruption of blood supply to femoral epiphysis occurs, halting growth. Revascularization and healing occur later, but significant residual deformity and dysfunction may be present.

Bibliography

Alexander M, Kuo KN: Musculoskeletal assessment of the newborn. Orthop Nurs 16(1):21–31, Jan–Feb 1997.

Allison M, Keller C: Physical activity in the elderly: Benefits and intervention strategies. Nurse Pract 22(8):53–69, Aug 1997.

Anonymous: Fibromyalgia: An important diagnosis to consider. Nurse Pract 22(8):27–28, Aug 1997.

Ballas MT, Tytko J, Cookson D: Common overuse running injuries: Diagnosis and management. Am Fam Physician 55(7):2473–2484, 1997.

Behrman RE, Vaughan VC (Eds): Nelson Textbook of Pediatrics, 15th ed. Philadelphia, W.B. Saunders Company, 1996.

Benetti MC, Marchese T: Management of common musculoskeletal disorders. J Nurse Midwifery 41(2):173–187, Mar–Apr 1996.

Bowers AC, Thompson JM: Clinical Manual of Health Assessment, 4th ed. St. Louis, C.V. Mosby, 1992.

Bynum DT: Gout. Am J Nurs 97(7):36–37, July 1997.

Campbell-Giovaniello KJ: Plantar fasciitis. Am J Nurs 97(9):38–39, Sep 1997.

Cline MG, Meredith KE, Boyer JT, Burrows B: Decline of height with age in adults in a general population sample: Estimating maximum height and distinguishing birth cohort effects from actual loss of stature with aging. Hum Biol 61(3):415–425, June 1989.

Cote P, Kreitz BG, Cassidy JD, et al: A study of the diagnostic accuracy and reliability of the scoliometer and Adam's forward bend test. Spine 23(7):796–803, Apr 1, 1998.

Crumrine PK: Gait disorders in children. Emerg Med 26(13):16–32, Nov 1994.

Dodds TA, Martin DP, Stolov WC, Deyo RA: A validation of the Functional Independence Measurement and its performance among rehabilitation inpatients. Arch Phys Rehabil 74:531–536, 1993.

Duffield P: Tibialis posterior tendon rupture. Adv Nurse Pract 5(8):39–40, 78, Aug 1997.

Ebrahim S, Thompson PW, Baskaran V, Evans K: Randomized placebo-controlled trial of brisk walking in the prevention of postmenopausal osteoporosis. Age Aging 26(4):253–260, May 1997.

Ensrud KE, Black DM, Harrit F, et al: Correlates of kyphosis in older women. J Am Geriatr Soc 45(6):682–687, June 1997.

Farrally MR, Moore WJ: Anatomical differences in the femur and tibia between Negroes and Caucasians and their effect on locomotion. Am J Phys Anthropol 43(1):63–69, 1975.

File P, Wood JP, Kreplick LW: Diagnosis of hip fracture by the auscultatory percussion technique. Am J Emerg Med 16(2):173–176, Mar 1998.

Garn SM: Compact bone in Chinese and Japanese. Science 143(3613):1439–1441, 1964.

Granger CV, Ottenbacher KJ, Baker JG, Sehgal A: Reliability of a brief outpatient functional outcome assessment measure. Am J Phys Med Rehabil 74(6):469–475, Nov–Dec 1995.

Gregg EW, Cauley JA, Seeley DG, et al: Physical activity and osteoporotic fracture risk in older women. Ann Intern Med 129(2):81–88, Jul 15, 1998.

Huston CJ: Ruptured Achilles tendon. Am J Nurs 94(12):37, 1994.

Jones AK: Primary care management of acute low back pain. Nurse Pract 22(7):50–68, June 1997.

Kelley WN, Harris ED, Ruddy S, Sledge CB: Textbook of Rheumatology, 5th ed. Philadelphia, W.B. Saunders Company, 1997.

Kessenich CR: Preventing and managing osteoporosis. Am J Nurs 97(1): 16B–16D, Jan 1997.

LeCompte CM: Post polio syndrome: An update for the primary health care provider. Nurse Pract 22(6):133–154, June 1997.

Maldonado A: Comprehensive assessment of common musculoskeletal disorders. J Nurse Midwifery 40(2):202–215, Mar–Apr 1995.

McDowell LD, Seymour SF: Diagnosis and treatment of ankle sprains. Nurs Pract 19(3):36–43, 1994.

McIntosh E: Low back pain in adults: Guidelines for the history and physical exam. Adv Nurse Pract 5(8):16–25, Aug 1997.

Melton LJ: Epidemiology of spinal osteoporosis. Spine 22(24S):2S–11S, Dec 15, 1997.

Muscari ME: Preventing sports injuries. Am J Nurs 98(7):58–60, July 1998.

Neal L: Basic musculoskeletal assessment: Tips for the home health nurse. Home Healthcare Nurse 15(4):227–234, 1997.

Newland JA: Ankle injury. Am J Nurs 96(7):16E, July 1996.

O'Hanlon-Nichols T: A review of the adult musculoskeletal system. Am J Nurs 98(6):48–52, June 1998.

Philip PA, Traisman ES, Philip M: Musculoskeletal injuries in child abuse. Phys Med Rehabil 9(1):251–268, Feb 1995.

Ross C: A comparison of osteoarthritis and rheumatoid arthritis: Diagnosis and treatment. Nurse Pract 22(9):20–41, Sep 1997.

U.S. Preventive Services Task Force: Screening for adolescent idiopathic scoliosis. Nurse Pract 19(9):39–45, 1994.

Van Heest AE: Congenital disorders of the hand and upper extremity. Pediatr Clin North Am 43(5):1113–1133, Oct 1996.

Winzeler S: Orthopedic problems of the upper extremities. AAOHN J 45(4):188–203, Apr 1997.

Woodhead GA, Moss MM: Osteoporosis: Diagnosis and prevention. Nurse Pract 23(11):18–37, Nov 1998.

CHAPTER TWENTY ONE

Neurologic System

The nervous system can be divided into two parts—central and peripheral. The **central nervous system** (CNS) includes the brain and spinal cord. The **peripheral nervous system** includes the 12 pairs of cranial nerves, the 31 pairs of spinal nerves, and all their branches. The peripheral nervous system carries sensory messages *to* the CNS from sensory receptors, motor messages *from* the CNS out to muscles and glands, as well as autonomic messages that govern the internal organs and blood vessels.

THE CENTRAL NERVOUS SYSTEM (CNS)

Cerebral Cortex. The cerebral cortex is the cerebrum's outer layer of nerve cell bodies, which looks like "gray matter" because it lacks myelin. The cerebral cortex is the center for humans' highest functions, governing thought, memory, reasoning, sensation, and voluntary movement (Fig. 21–1). Each half of the cerebrum is a **hemisphere;** the left hemisphere is dominant in most (95 percent) people, including those who are left handed.

Each hemisphere is divided into four **lobes:** frontal, parietal, temporal, and occipital. The lobes have certain areas that mediate specific functions.

- The **frontal** lobe has areas concerned with personality, behavior, emotions, and intellectual function.
- The precentral gyrus of the frontal lobe initiates voluntary movement.
- The **parietal** lobe's postcentral gyrus is the primary center for sensation.
- The **occipital** lobe is the primary visual receptor center.
- The **temporal** lobe behind the ear has the primary auditory reception center.
- **Wernicke's area** in the temporal lobe is associated with language comprehension. When damaged in the person's dominant hemisphere, *receptive aphasia* results. The person hears sound, but it has no meaning, like hearing a foreign language.
- **Broca's area** in the frontal lobe mediates motor speech. When injured in the dominant hemisphere, *expressive aphasia* results; the person cannot talk. The person can understand language and knows what he or she wants to say, but can produce only a garbled sound.

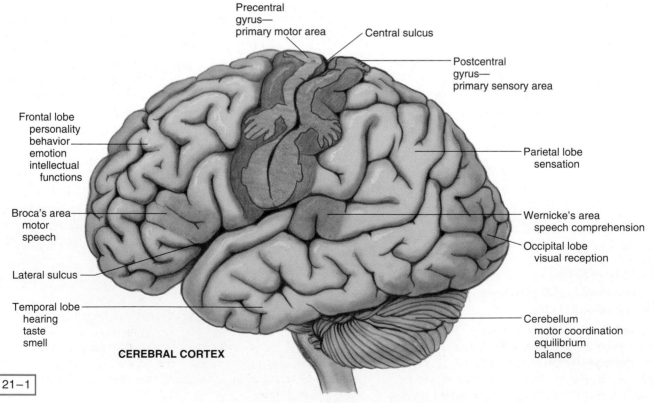

Precentral gyrus— primary motor area

Central sulcus

Postcentral gyrus— primary sensory area

Frontal lobe personality behavior emotion intellectual functions

Parietal lobe sensation

Broca's area motor speech

Wernicke's area speech comprehension

Occipital lobe visual reception

Lateral sulcus

Temporal lobe hearing taste smell

Cerebellum motor coordination equilibrium balance

CEREBRAL CORTEX

21–1

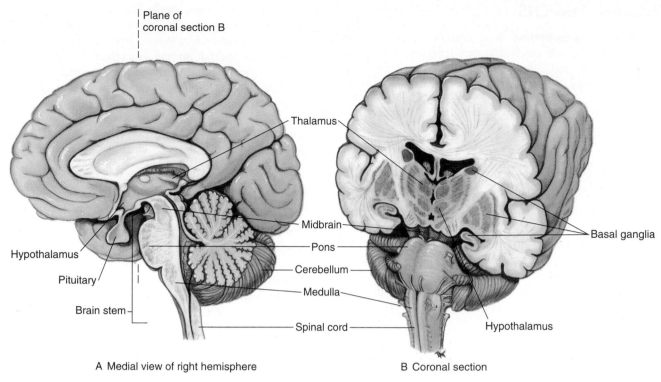

Plane of coronal section B

Thalamus

Midbrain

Pons

Cerebellum

Medulla

Spinal cord

Hypothalamus

Pituitary

Brain stem

Basal ganglia

Hypothalamus

A Medial view of right hemisphere

B Coronal section

COMPONENTS OF THE CENTRAL NERVOUS SYSTEM

21–2

Damage to any of these specific cortical areas produces a corresponding loss of function: motor weakness, paralysis, loss of sensation, or impaired ability to understand and process language. Damage occurs when the highly specialized neurologic cells are deprived of their blood supply, such as when a cerebral artery becomes occluded, or when vascular bleeding or vasospasm occurs.

Basal Ganglia. The basal ganglia are bands of gray matter buried within the two cerebral hemispheres that form the subcortical associated motor system (the extrapyramidal system) (Fig. 21–2). They control automatic associated movements of the body, e.g., the arm swing alternating with the legs during walking.

Thalamus. The thalamus is the main relay station for the nervous system. Sensory pathways of the spinal cord and brain stem form **synapses** (sites of contact between two neurons) on their way to the cerebral cortex.

Hypothalamus. The hypothalamus is a major control center with many vital functions: temperature, heart rate, and blood pressure control, sleep center, anterior and posterior pituitary gland regulator, and coordinator of autonomic nervous system activity and emotional status.

Cerebellum. The cerebellum is a coiled structure located under the occipital lobe that is concerned with motor coordination of voluntary movements, equilibrium, and muscle tone. It does not initiate movement but coordinates and smooths it, e.g., the complex and quick coordination of many different muscles needed in playing the piano, swimming, or juggling. It is like a "black box" in that it adjusts and corrects the voluntary movements, but operates entirely below the conscious level.

Brain Stem. The brain stem is the central core of the brain consisting of mostly nerve fibers. It has three areas:

1. **Midbrain**—the most anterior part of the brain stem that still has the basic tubular structure of the spinal cord. It merges into the thalamus and hypothalamus. It contains many motor neurons and tracts.
2. **Pons**—the enlarged area containing ascending and descending fiber tracts.
3. **Medulla**—the continuation of the spinal cord in the brain that contains all ascending and descending fiber tracts connecting the brain and spinal cord. It has vital autonomic centers (respiration, heart, gastrointestinal function), as well as nuclei for cranial nerves VIII through XII. Pyramidal decussation (crossing of the motor fibers) occurs here (see p. 691).

Spinal Cord. The spinal cord is the long cylindrical structure about as big around as the little finger that occupies the upper two thirds of the vertebral canal. It is the main highway for ascending and descending fiber tracts that connect the brain to the spinal nerves, and it mediates reflexes. Its nerve cell bodies, or gray matter, are arranged in a butterfly shape with anterior and posterior "horns."

Pathways of the CNS

Crossed representation is a notable feature of the nerve tracts; the *left* cerebral cortex receives sensory information from and controls motor function to the *right* side of the body, while the *right* cerebral cortex likewise interacts with the *left* side of the body. Knowledge of where the fibers cross the midline will help you interpret clinical findings.

Sensory Pathways

Millions of sensory receptors are embroidered into the skin, mucous membranes, muscles, tendons, and viscera. They monitor conscious sensation, internal organ functions, body position, and reflexes. Sensation travels in the afferent fibers in the peripheral nerve, then through the posterior (dorsal) root, and then into the spinal cord. There, it may take one of two routes—the spinothalamic tract or the posterior (dorsal) columns (Fig. 21–3).

Spinothalamic Tract. The spinothalamic tract contains sensory fibers that transmit the sensations of pain, temper-ature, and crude or light touch. The fibers enter the dorsal root of the spinal cord and synapse with a second sensory neuron. The second-order neuron fibers cross to the opposite side and ascend up the spinothalamic tract to the thalamus. Fibers carrying pain and temperature sensations ascend the *lateral* spinothalamic tract, whereas those of crude touch form the *anterior* spinothalamic tract. At the thalamus, the fibers synapse with a third sensory neuron, which carries the message to the sensory cortex for full interpretation.

Posterior (Dorsal) Columns. These fibers conduct the sensations of position, vibration, and finely localized touch.

- **Position** (proprioception)—Without looking, you know where your body parts are in space and in relation to each other
- **Vibration**—Feeling vibrating objects
- **Finely localized touch** (stereognosis)—Without look-ing, you can identify familiar objects by touch

These fibers enter the dorsal root and proceed immedi-ately up the same side of the spinal cord to the brain

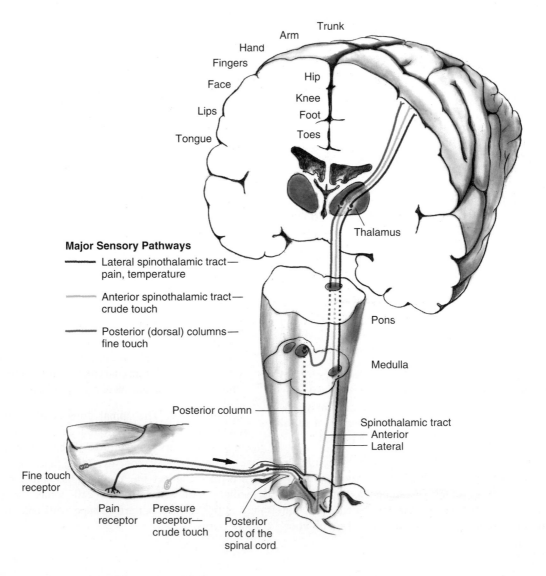

Trunk
Arm
Hand
Fingers
Hip
Face
Knee
Lips
Foot
Tongue
Toes

Thalamus

Major Sensory Pathways

—— Lateral spinothalamic tract—
pain, temperature

—— Anterior spinothalamic tract—
crude touch

—— Posterior (dorsal) columns—
fine touch

Pons

Medulla

Posterior column

Spinothalamic tract
Anterior
Lateral

Fine touch
receptor

Pain
receptor

Pressure
receptor—
crude touch

Posterior
root of the
spinal cord

21–3

stem. At the medulla, they synapse with a second sensory neuron and then cross. They travel to the thalamus, synapse again, and proceed to the sensory cortex, which localizes the sensation and makes full discrimination.

The sensory cortex is arranged in a specific pattern forming a corresponding "map" of the body. Pain in the right hand is perceived at its specific spot on the left cortex map. Some organs are absent from the brain map, such as the heart, liver, or spleen. You know you have one but you have no "felt image" of it. Pain originating in these organs is referred, because no felt image exists in which to have pain. Pain is felt "by proxy" by another body part that does have a felt image. For example, pain in the heart is referred to the chest, shoulder, and left arm, which were its neighbors in fetal development. Pain originating in the spleen is felt on the top of the left shoulder.

Motor Pathways

Corticospinal or Pyramidal Tract (Fig. 21–4). The area has been named "pyramidal" because it crosses through the pyramids of the medulla. Motor nerve fibers originate in the motor cortex and travel to the brain stem, where they cross to the opposite side *(pyramidal decussation)* and then pass down in the lateral column of the spinal cord. At each cord level, they synapse with a lower motor neuron contained in the anterior horn of the spinal cord. Ten percent of corticospinal fibers do *not* cross, and these descend in the anterior column of the spinal cord. Corticospinal fibers mediate voluntary movement, particularly very skilled, discrete, purposeful movements, such as writing.

The corticospinal tract is a newer, "higher," motor system that humans have that permits very skilled and purposeful movements. The tract's origin in the motor cortex is arranged in a specific pattern called *somatotopic organization.* It is another body map, this one of a person, or *homunculus,* hanging "upside down" (see Fig. 21–1). Body parts are not equally represented on the map, and the homunculus looks distorted. It is more like an electoral map than a geographic map. That is, body parts whose movements are relatively more important to humans (e.g., the hand) occupy proportionally more space on the brain map.

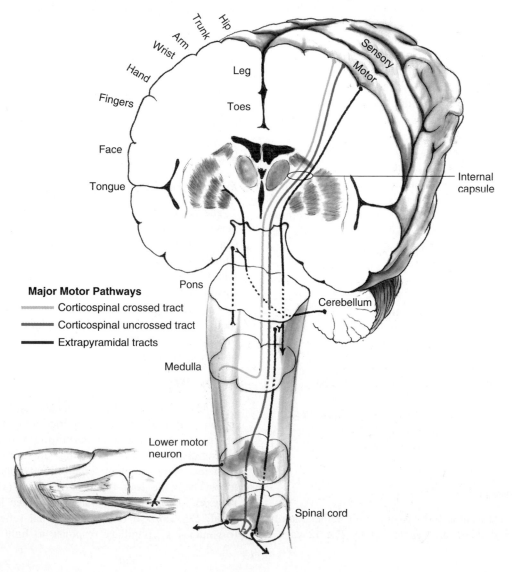

Major Motor Pathways
- Corticospinal crossed tract
- Corticospinal uncrossed tract
- Extrapyramidal tracts

21–4

Extrapyramidal Tracts. The extrapyramidal tracts include all the motor nerve fibers originating in the motor cortex, basal ganglia, brain stem, and spinal cord that are *outside* the pyramidal tract. This is a phylogenetically older, "lower," more primitive motor system. These subcortical motor fibers maintain muscle tone and control body movements, especially gross automatic movements, such as walking.

Cerebellar System. This complex motor system coordinates movement, maintains equilibrium, and helps maintain posture. The cerebellum receives information about the position of muscles and joints, the body's equilibrium, and what kind of motor messages are being sent from the cortex to the muscles. The information is integrated, and the cerebellum uses feedback pathways to exert its control back on the cortex or down to lower motor neurons in the spinal cord. This entire process occurs on a subconscious level.

Upper and Lower Motor Neurons

Upper motor neurons are a complex of all the descending motor fibers that can influence or modify the lower motor neurons. Upper motor neurons are located completely within the CNS. The neurons convey impulses from motor areas of the cerebral cortex to the lower motor neurons in the anterior horn cells of the spinal cord. Examples of upper motor neurons are corticospinal, corticobulbar, and extrapyramidal tracts. Examples of upper motor neuron diseases are cerebrovascular accident, cerebral palsy, and multiple sclerosis.

Lower motor neurons are located mostly in the peripheral nervous system. The cell body of the lower motor neuron is located in the anterior gray column of the spinal cord, but the nerve fiber extends from here to the muscle. The lower motor neuron is the "final common pathway," because it funnels many neural signals here, and it provides the final direct contact with the muscles. Any movement must be translated into action by lower motor neuron fibers. Examples of lower motor neurons are cranial nerves and spinal nerves of the peripheral nervous system. Examples of lower motor neuron diseases are spinal cord lesions, poliomyelitis, and amyotrophic lateral sclerosis.

THE PERIPHERAL NERVOUS SYSTEM

A **nerve** is a bundle of fibers *outside* the CNS. The peripheral nerves carry input to the CNS via their sensory afferent fibers and deliver output from the CNS via the efferent fibers.

Cranial Nerves

Cranial nerves enter and exit the brain rather than the spinal cord (Fig. 21–5 and Table 21–1). The 12 pairs of cranial nerves supply primarily the head and neck, except the vagus nerve (Lat. vagus, or wanderer, as in "vagabond"), which travels to the heart, respiratory muscles, stomach, and gallbladder.

Spinal Nerves

The 31 pairs of **spinal nerves** arise from the length of the spinal cord and supply the rest of the body. They are named for the region of the spine from which they exit: 8 cervical, 12 thoracic, 5 lumbar, 5 sacral, and 1 coccygeal. They are "mixed" nerves because they contain both sensory and motor fibers. The nerves enter and exit the cord through roots—sensory afferent fibers through the posterior or dorsal roots, and motor efferent fibers through the anterior or ventral roots.

The nerves exit the spinal cord in an orderly ladder. Each nerve innervates a particular segment of the body. **Dermal segmentation** is the cutaneous distribution of the various spinal nerves.

A **dermatome** is a circumscribed skin area that is supplied mainly from one spinal cord segment through a particular spinal nerve (Fig. 21–6). The dermatomes overlap, which is a form of biologic insurance. That is, if one nerve is severed, most of the sensations can be transmitted by the one above and the one below. While you may not need to memorize all dermatome territories, the following are useful landmarks:

- The **thumb, middle finger,** and **fifth finger** are each in the dermatomes of **C6, C7, and C8.**
- The **nipple** is at the level of **T4.**
- The **umbilicus** is at the level of **T10.**
- The **groin** is in the region of **L1.**

Autonomic Nervous System

The peripheral nervous system is composed of cranial nerves and spinal nerves. These nerves carry fibers that can be divided functionally into two parts—somatic and autonomic. The somatic fibers innervate the skeletal (voluntary) muscles; the autonomic fibers innervate smooth (involuntary) muscles, cardiac muscle, and glands. The autonomic system mediates unconscious activity. Although a description of the autonomic system is beyond the scope of this book, its overall function is to maintain homeostasis of the body.

Reflex Arc

Reflexes are basic defense mechanisms of the nervous system. They are involuntary, operating below the level of conscious control and permitting a quick reaction to potentially painful or damaging situations. Reflexes also help the body maintain balance and appropriate muscle tone. There are four types of reflexes: (1) **deep tendon reflexes** (myotatic), e.g., patellar or knee jerk; (2) **superficial,** e.g., corneal reflex, abdominal reflex; (3) **visceral** (organic), e.g., pupillary response to light and accommo-

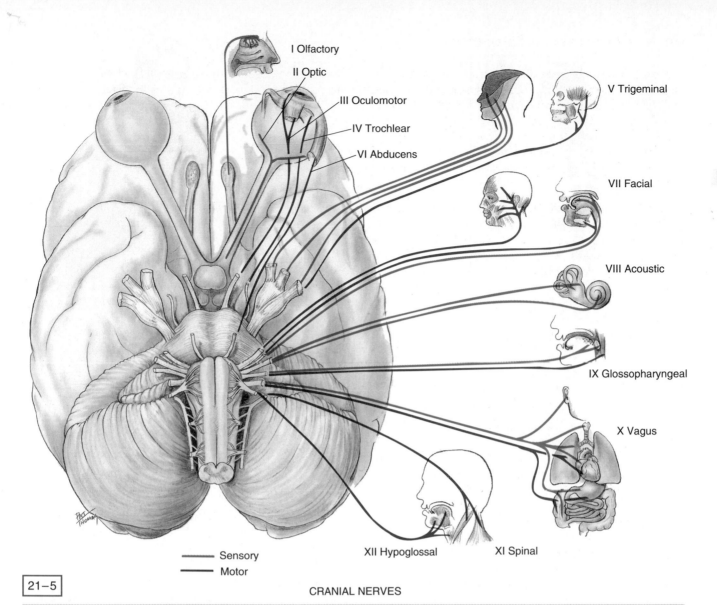

I Olfactory
II Optic
III Oculomotor
IV Trochlear
VI Abducens

V Trigeminal

VII Facial

VIII Acoustic

IX Glossopharyngeal

X Vagus

XII Hypoglossal   XI Spinal

—— Sensory
—— Motor

21–5 CRANIAL NERVES

Table 21–1 • Cranial Nerves

Cranial Nerve	Type	Function
I: Olfactory	Sensory	Smell
II: Optic	Sensory	Vision
III: Oculomotor	Mixed*	Motor—most EOM movement, raise eyelids
		Parasympathetic—pupil constriction, lens shape
IV: Trochlear	Motor	Down and inward movement of eye
V: Trigeminal	Mixed	Motor—muscles of mastication
		Sensory—sensation of face and scalp, cornea, mucous membranes of mouth and nose
VI: Abducens	Motor	Lateral movement of eye
VII: Facial	Mixed	Motor—facial muscles, close eye, labial speech
		Sensory—taste (sweet, salty, sour, bitter) on anterior two-thirds of tongue
		Parasympathetic—saliva and tear secretion
VIII: Acoustic	Sensory	Hearing and equilibrium
IX: Glossopharyngeal	Mixed	Motor—pharynx (phonation and swallowing)
		Sensory—taste on posterior one-third of tongue, pharynx (gag reflex)
		Parasympathetic—parotid gland, carotid reflex
X: Vagus	Mixed	Motor—pharynx and larynx (talking and swallowing)
		Sensory—general sensation from carotid body, carotid sinus, pharynx, viscera
		Parasympathetic—carotid reflex
XI: Spinal	Motor	Movement of trapezius and sternomastoid muscles
XII: Hypoglossal	Motor	Movement of tongue

*Mixed refers to a nerve carrying a combination of fibers: motor + sensory; motor + parasympathetic; or motor + sensory + parasympathetic.

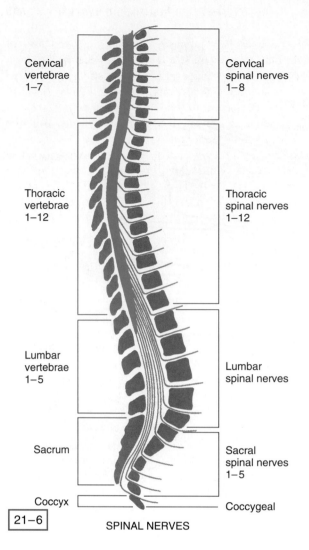

Cervical
vertebrae
1–7

Cervical
spinal nerves
1–8

Thoracic
vertebrae
1–12

Thoracic
spinal nerves
1–12

Lumbar
vertebrae
1–5

Lumbar
spinal nerves

Sacrum

Sacral
spinal nerves
1–5

Coccyx

Coccygeal

21–6

SPINAL NERVES

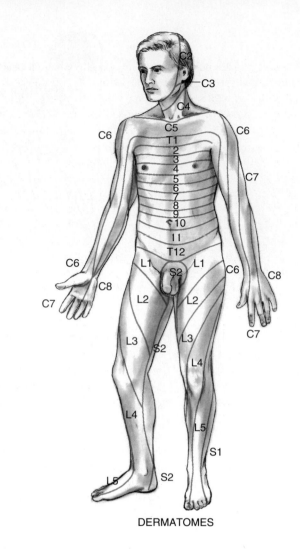

DERMATOMES

dation; and (4) **pathologic** (abnormal), e.g., Babinski's or extensor plantar reflex.

The fibers that mediate the reflex are carried by a specific spinal nerve. In the most simple reflex, tapping the tendon stretches the muscle spindles in the muscle, which activates the sensory afferent nerve. The sensory afferent fibers carry the message from the receptor and travel through the dorsal root into the spinal cord (Fig. 21–7). They synapse in the cord with the motor neuron in the anterior horn. Motor efferent fibers leave via the ventral root and travel to the muscle.

The deep tendon (myotatic or stretch) reflex has five components: (1) an intact sensory nerve (afferent); (2) a functional synapse in the cord; (3) an intact motor nerve fiber (efferent); (4) the neuromuscular junction; and (5) a competent muscle.

DEVELOPMENTAL CONSIDERATIONS

Infants

The neurologic system is not completely developed at birth. Motor activity in the newborn is under the control of the spinal cord and medulla. Very little cortical control

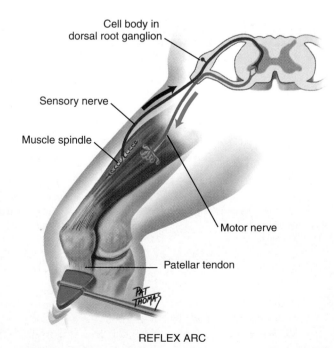

Cell body in
dorsal root ganglion

Sensory nerve

Muscle spindle

Motor nerve

Patellar tendon

REFLEX ARC

21–7

694

exists, and the neurons are not yet myelinated. Movements are directed primarily by primitive reflexes. As the cerebral cortex develops during the 1st year, it inhibits these reflexes, and they disappear at predictable times. Persistence of the primitive reflexes is an indication of CNS dysfunction.

The infant's sensory and motor development proceeds along with the gradual acquisition of myelin, because myelin is needed to conduct most impulses. The process of myelinization follows a cephalocaudal and proximodistal order (head, neck, trunk, and extremities). This is just the order we observe the infant gaining motor control (lifts head, lifts head and shoulders, rolls over, moves whole arm, uses hands, walks). As the milestones are achieved, each is more complex and coordinated. Milestones occur in an orderly sequence, although the exact age of occurrence may vary.

Sensation also is rudimentary at birth. The newborn needs a strong stimulus and then responds by crying and with whole body movements. As myelinization develops, the infant is able to localize the stimulus more precisely and to make a more accurate motor response.

The Aging Adult

The aging process causes a general atrophy with a steady loss of neurons in the brain and spinal cord. The loss of neurons causes a decrease in weight and volume so that by 80 years, the brain has decreased in weight by 15 percent (Waxman, 1996). Neuron loss leads many people over 65 to show signs that, in the younger adult, would be considered abnormal, such as general loss of muscle bulk, loss of muscle tone in the face, in the neck, and around the spine, decreased muscle strength, impaired fine coordination and agility, loss of vibratory sense at the ankle, decreased or absent Achilles reflex, loss of position sense at the big toe, pupillary miosis, irregular pupil shape, and decreased pupillary reflexes.

The velocity of nerve conduction decreases between 5 and 10 percent with aging, making the reaction time slower in some older persons. An increased delay at the synapse also occurs, so the impulse takes longer to travel. As a result, touch and pain sensation, taste, and smell may be diminished.

The motor system may show a general slowing down of movement. Muscle strength and agility decrease. A generalized decrease occurs in muscle bulk, which is most apparent in the dorsal hand muscles. Muscle tremors may occur in the hands, head, and jaw, along with possible repetitive facial grimacing (dyskinesias).

Aging has a progressive decrease in cerebral blood flow and oxygen consumption. In some people this causes dizziness and a loss of balance with position change. These people need to be taught to get up slowly. Otherwise they have an increased risk for falls and resulting injuries. Additionally, older people may forget they fell, which makes it hard to diagnose the cause of the injury.

When they are in good health, aging people walk about as well as they did during their middle and younger years, except more slowly and more deliberately. Some survey the ground for obstacles or uneven terrain. Some show a hesitation and a slightly wayward path.

SUBJECTIVE DATA

1. Headache
2. Head injury
3. Dizziness/vertigo
4. Seizures
5. Tremors
6. Weakness
7. Incoordination

8. Numbness or tingling
9. Difficulty swallowing
10. Difficulty speaking
11. Significant past history
12. Environmental/occupational hazards

Examiner Asks	Rationale

1 **Headache.** Any unusually frequent or severe headaches?
● When did this start? How often does it occur?
● Where in your head do you feel the headaches? Do the headaches seem to be associated with anything? (Headache history fully discussed in Chapter 11.)

Examiner Asks	Rationale

(**Pain in body part.** Although pain is a neurologic phenomenon, it usually does not come up during the history in relation to the neurologic system. Pain is usually mentioned in relation to the body system in which it occurs. Pain arising from neurologic dysfunction is usually mentioned during the review of systems for the head, back, or extremities.)

2 Head injury. Ever had any **head injury?** Please describe.
- What part of your head was hit?
- Did you have a loss of consciousness? For how long?

3 Dizziness/vertigo. Ever feel lightheaded, a swimming sensation, like feeling faint?
- When have you noticed this? How often does it occur? Does it occur with activity, change in position?
- Do you ever feel a sensation called **vertigo,** a rotational spinning sensation? (Note—Distinguish vertigo from dizziness.) Do you feel as if the room spins (objective vertigo)? Or do you feel that you are spinning (subjective vertigo)? Did this come on suddenly or gradually?

Syncope is a sudden loss of strength, a temporary loss of consciousness due to lack of cerebral blood flow, a faint.

True vertigo is rotational spinning caused by neurologic dysfunction or a problem in the vestibular apparatus or the vestibular nuclei in the brain stem.

4 Seizures. Ever had any convulsions? When did they start? How often do they occur?

Seizures occur with epilepsy, a paroxysmal disease characterized by altered or loss of consciousness, involuntary muscle movements, and sensory disturbances.

Aura is a subjective sensation that precedes a seizure; it could be auditory, visual, or motor.

- Course and duration—When a seizure starts, do you have any warning sign? What type of sign?
- Motor activity—Where in your body do the seizures begin? Do the seizures travel through your body? On one side or both? Does your muscle tone seem tense or limp?
- Any associated signs: color change in face or lips, loss of consciousness, for how long, automatisms (eyelid fluttering, eye rolling, lip smacking), incontinence?
- Postictal phase—After the seizure, are you told you spend time sleeping or have any confusion, weakness, headache, or muscle ache?
- Precipitating factors—Does anything seem to bring on the seizures: activity, discontinuing medication, fatigue, stress?
- Are you on any medication?
- Coping strategies—How have the seizures affected daily life, occupation?

5 Tremors. Any shakes or **tremors** in the hands or face? When did these start?
- Do they seem to grow worse with anxiety, intention, or rest?
- Are they relieved with rest, activity, alcohol? Do they affect daily activities?

Tremor is an involuntary shaking, vibrating, or trembling.

6 Weakness. Any **weakness** or problem moving any body part? Is this generalized or local? Does it occur with anything?

Paresis is a slight paralysis.

Paralysis is a loss of motor function due to a lesion in the neurologic or muscular system or loss of sensory innervation.

Examiner Asks	Rationale
7 **Incoordination.** Any problem with **coordination?** Any problem with balance when walking? Do you list to one side? Any falling? Which way? Do your legs seem to give way? Any clumsy movement?	Dysmetria is the inability to control range of motion of muscles.
8 **Numbness or tingling.** Any **numbness or tingling** in any body part? Does it feel like pins and needles? When did this start? Where do you feel it? Does it occur with activity?	Paresthesia is an abnormal sensation, e.g., burning, tingling.
9 **Difficulty swallowing.** Any problem **swallowing?** Occur with solids or liquids? Have you experienced excessive saliva, drooling?	
10 **Difficulty speaking.** Any problem **speaking:** with forming words or with saying what you intended to say? When did you first notice this? How long did it last?	
11 **Significant past history. Past history** of: stroke (cerebrovascular accident), spinal cord injury, meningitis or encephalitis, congenital defect, or alcoholism?	
12 **Environmental/occupational hazards.** Are you exposed to any environmental/occupational hazards: insecticides, organic solvents, lead? ● Are you taking any medications now? ● How much alcohol do you drink? Each week? Each day? ● How about other mood-altering drugs: marijuana, cocaine, barbiturates, tranquilizers?	Review especially anticonvulsants, antitremor, antivertigo, pain medication.

ADDITIONAL HISTORY FOR INFANTS AND CHILDREN

1 Did you (the mother) have any health problems during the pregnancy: any infections or illnesses, medications taken, toxemia, hypertension, alcohol or drug use, diabetes?	Prenatal history may affect infant's neurologic development.
2 Please tell me about this baby's birth. Was the baby at term or premature? Birth weight? ● Any birth trauma? Did the baby breathe immediately? ● Were you told the baby's Apgar scores? ● Any congenital defects?	
3 Reflexes—What have you noticed about the baby's behavior? Do the baby's sucking and swallowing seem coordinated? When you touch the cheek, does the baby turn his or her head toward touch? Does the baby startle with a loud noise or shake of crib? Does the baby grasp your finger?	
4 Does the child seem to have any problem with balance? Have you noted any unexplained falling, clumsy or unsteady gait, progressive muscular weakness, problem with going up or down stairs, problem with getting up from lying position?	If occurs, may not be noticed until starts to walk in late infancy. Screens for muscular dystrophy.
5 Has this child had any seizures? Please describe. Did the seizure occur with a high fever? Did any loss of consciousness occur—how long? How many seizures occurred with this same illness (if occurred with high fever)?	Seizures may occur with high fever in infants and toddlers. Or seizures may be sign of neurologic disease.

Examiner Asks	Rationale
6 Did this child's motor or developmental milestones seem to come at about the right age? Does this child seem to be growing and maturing normally to you? How does this child's development compare to siblings or to age-mates?	
7 Do you know if your child has had any environmental exposure to lead?	Chronically elevated lead levels may cause a developmental delay, a loss of a newly acquired skill, or no clinical signs may be present.
8 Have you been told about any learning problems in school: problems with attention span, cannot concentrate, hyperactive?	
9 Any family history of: seizure disorder, cerebral palsy, muscular dystrophy?	

ADDITIONAL HISTORY FOR THE AGING ADULT

1 Any problem with dizziness? Does this occur when you first sit or stand up, when you move your head, when you get up and walk just after eating?	Diminished cerebral blood flow and diminished vestibular response may produce staggering with position change, which increases risk of falls.
• (For men) Do you ever get up at night and then feel faint while standing to urinate?	Micturition syncope.
• How does dizziness affect your daily activities? Are you able to drive safely and to maneuver within your house safely?	
• What safety modifications have you applied at home?	
2 Have you noticed any decrease in memory, change in mental function? Have you felt any confusion? Did this seem to come on suddenly or gradually?	
3 Have you ever noticed any tremor? Is this in your hands or face? Is this worse with: anxiety, activity, rest? Does the tremor seem to be relieved with: alcohol, activity, rest? Does the tremor interfere with daily or social activities?	Senile tremor is relieved by alcohol, although this is not a recommended treatment. Assess if the person is abusing alcohol in effort to relieve tremor.
4 Have you ever had any sudden vision change, fleeting blindness? Did this occur along with weakness? Did you have any loss of consciousness?	Screen symptoms of stroke.

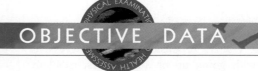

OBJECTIVE DATA

Preparation

Perform a **screening neurologic examination** (items identified in following sections) on seemingly well persons who have no significant subjective findings from the history.

Perform a **complete neurologic examination** on persons who have neurologic concerns (e.g., headache, weakness, loss of coordination) or who have shown signs of neurologic dysfunction.

Perform a **neurologic recheck** examination on persons with demonstrated neurologic deficits who require periodic assessments (e.g., hospitalized persons or those in extended care), using the examination sequence beginning on page 729.

Integrate the steps of the neurologic examination with the examination of each particular part of the body, as much as you are able. For example, test cranial nerves while assessing the head and neck (recall Chapters 11 through 14) and superficial abdominal reflexes while assessing the abdomen. When recording your findings, however, consider all neurologic data as a functional unit, and record them all together.

Use the following sequence for the complete neurologic examination.

1. Mental status (see Chapter 6)
2. Cranial nerves
3. Motor system
4. Sensory system
5. Reflexes

Position the person sitting up with the head at your eye level.

Equipment Needed

Penlight
Tongue blade
Cotton swab
Cotton ball
Tuning fork (128 Hz or 256 Hz)
Percussion hammer
(Possibly) familiar aromatic substances, e.g., peppermint, coffee, vanilla

Normal Range of Findings	Abnormal Findings

CRANIAL NERVES

Test cranial nerves
Cranial Nerve I—Olfactory Nerve

Do not test routinely. Test the sense of smell in those who report loss of smell, those with head trauma, and those with abnormal mental status, and when the presence of an intracranial lesion is suspected. First, assess patency by occluding one nostril at a time and asking the person to sniff. Then, with the person's eyes closed, occlude one nostril and present an aromatic substance. Use familiar, conveniently obtainable, and non-noxious smells, such as coffee, toothpaste, orange, vanilla, soap, or peppermint. Alcohol swabs smell familiar and are easy to find but are irritating.

Normally, a person can identify an odor on each side of the nose. Smell normally is decreased bilaterally with aging. Any asymmetry in the sense of smell is important.

One cannot test smell when air passages are occluded with upper respiratory infection or with sinusitis.

Anosmia—decrease or loss of smell occurs bilaterally with tobacco smoking, allergic rhinitis, and cocaine use.

Unilateral loss of smell in the absence of nasal disease is *neurogenic anosmia* (see Table 21–3).

Cranial Nerve II—Optic Nerve

Test visual acuity and test visual fields by confrontation (see Chapter 12).

Using the ophthalmoscope, examine the ocular fundus to determine the color, size, and shape of the optic disc (see Chapter 12).

Visual field loss (see Table 12–2).

Papilledema with increased intracranial pressure; optic atrophy (see Table 12–11).

|

Cranial Nerves III, IV, and VI—Oculomotor, Trochlear, and Abducens Nerves

Palpebral fissures are usually equal in width or nearly so.

Check pupils for size, regularity, equality, direct and consensual light reaction, and accommodation (see Chapter 12).

Assess extraocular movements by the cardinal positions of gaze (see Chapter 12).

Nystagmus is a back-and-forth oscillation of the eyes. End-point nystagmus, a few beats of horizontal nystagmus at extreme lateral gaze, occurs normally. Assess any other nystagmus carefully, noting:

- Presence of nystagmus in one or both eyes.
- *Pendular* movement (oscillations move equally left to right) or *jerk* (a quick phase in one direction, then a slow phase in the other). Classify the jerk nystagmus in the direction of the quick phase.
- Amplitude. Judge whether the degree of movement is fine, medium, or coarse.
- Frequency. Is it constant, or does it fade after a few beats?
- Plane of movement: horizontal, vertical, rotary, or a combination.

Cranial Nerve V—Trigeminal Nerve

Motor Function. Assess the muscles of mastication by palpating the temporal and masseter muscles as the person clenches the teeth (Figs. 21–8 and 21–9). Muscles should feel equally strong on both sides.

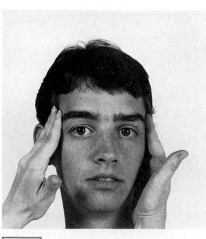

21–8

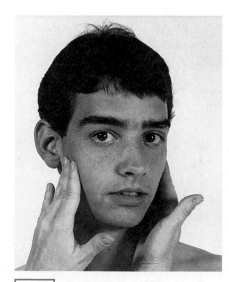

21–9

Try to separate the jaws by pushing down on the chin; normally you cannot.

Abnormal Findings

Ptosis (drooping) occurs with myasthenia gravis, dysfunction of cranial nerve III, or Horner's syndrome (see Table 12–4).
(See Table 12–9.)

Strabismus (deviated gaze) or limited movement (see Table 12–3).

Nystagmus occurs with disease of the vestibular system, cerebellum, or brain stem.

Decreased strength on one or both sides.

Asymmetry in jaw movement.

Pain with clenching of teeth.

► Normal Range of Findings	Abnormal Findings

Sensory Function. With the person's eyes closed, test light touch sensation by touching a cotton wisp to these designated areas on person's face: forehead, cheeks, and chin (Fig. 21–10). Ask the person to say "Now," whenever the touch is felt. This tests all three divisions of the nerve: (1) ophthalmic, (2) maxillary, and (3) mandibular.

Decreased or unequal sensation.

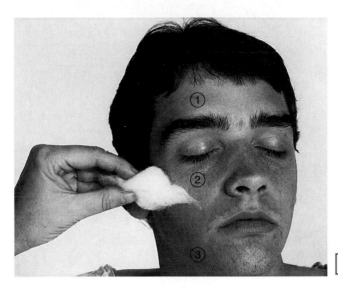

21–10

Corneal Reflex. (Omit this test, unless the person has abnormal facial sensation or abnormalities of facial movement.) Remove any contact lenses. With the person looking forward, bring a wisp of cotton in from the side (to minimize defensive blinking) and lightly touch the cornea, not the conjunctiva (Fig. 21–11). Normally, the person will blink bilaterally. The corneal reflex may be decreased or absent in those who have worn contact lenses. This procedure tests the sensory afferent in cranial nerve V and the motor efferent in cranial nerve VII.

No blink occurs with a lesion of cranial nerve V or cranial nerve VII paralysis.

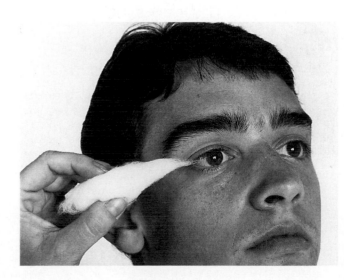

21–11

Cranial Nerve VII—Facial Nerve

Motor Function. Note mobility and facial symmetry as the person responds to these requests: smile, frown, close eyes tightly (against your attempt to open them), lift eyebrows, show teeth (Fig. 21–12), and puff cheeks. Then, press the person's puffed cheeks in, and note that the air should escape equally from both sides.

Muscle weakness is shown by loss of the nasolabial fold, drooping of one side of the face, lower eyelid sagging, and escape of air from only one cheek that is pressed in.

Loss of movement and asymmetry of movement occur with both central nervous system lesions (e.g., brain attack or stroke) and peripheral nervous system lesions (e.g., Bell's palsy).

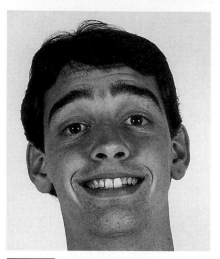

21–12

Sensory Function. Do not test routinely. Test only when you suspect facial nerve injury. When indicated, test sense of taste by applying to the tongue a cotton applicator covered with a solution of sugar, salt, or lemon juice (sour). Ask the person to identify the taste.

Cranial Nerve VIII—Acoustic (Vestibulocochlear) Nerve

Test hearing acuity by the ability to hear normal conversation, by the whispered voice test, and by Weber and Rinne tuning fork tests (see Chapter 13).

Cranial Nerves IX and X—Glossopharyngeal and Vagus Nerves

Motor Function. Depress the tongue with a tongue blade, and note pharyngeal movement as the person says "ahhh" or yawns; the uvula and soft palate should rise in the midline, and the tonsillar pillars should move medially.

Absence or asymmetry of soft palate movement.
Uvula deviates to side.
Asymmetry of tonsillar pillar movement.

Touch the posterior pharyngeal wall with a tongue blade, and note the gag reflex. Also note that the voice sounds smooth and not strained.

Hoarse or brassy voice occurs with vocal cord dysfunction; nasal twang occurs with weakness of soft palate.

Sensory Function. Cranial nerve IX does mediate taste on the posterior one third of the tongue, but technically this sensation is too difficult to test.

Normal Range of Findings	Abnormal Findings

Cranial Nerve XI—Spinal Accessory Nerve

Examine the sternomastoid and trapezius muscles for equal size. Check equal strength by asking the person to rotate the head forcibly against resistance applied to the side of the chin (Fig. 21–13). Then ask the person to shrug the shoulders against resistance (Fig. 21–14). These movements should feel equally strong on both sides.

Atrophy.
Muscle weakness or paralysis.

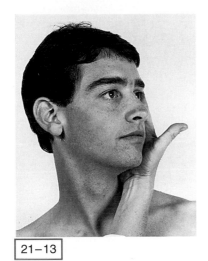

21–13

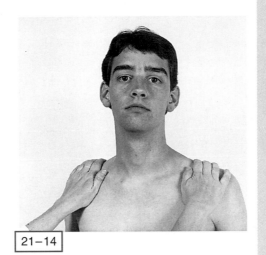

21–14

Cranial Nerve XII—Hypoglossal Nerve

Inspect the tongue. No wasting or tremors should be present. Note the forward thrust in the midline as the person protrudes the tongue. Also ask the person to say "light, tight, dynamite," and note that lingual speech (sounds of letters l, t, d, n) is clear and distinct.

Atrophy. Fasciculations.
Tongue deviates to side with lesions of the hypoglossal nerve (when this occurs, deviation is toward the paralyzed side).

THE MOTOR SYSTEM

Inspect and palpate the motor system
Muscles

Size. As you proceed through the examination, inspect all muscle groups for size. Compare the right side with the left. Muscle groups should be within the normal size limits for age and should be symmetric bilaterally. When muscles in the extremities look asymmetric, measure each in centimeters and record the difference. A difference of 1 cm or less is not significant. Note that it is difficult to assess muscle mass in very obese people.

Atrophy—abnormally small muscle with a wasted appearance; occurs with disuse, injury, lower motor neuron disease such as polio, diabetic neuropathy.
Hypertrophy—increased size and strength; occurs with isometric exercise.

Strength. (See Chapter 20, Musculoskeletal System.) Test the power of homologous muscles simultaneously. Test muscle groups of the extremities, neck, and trunk.

Paresis or weakness is diminished strength; paralysis or plegia is absence of strength.

▶ N o r m a l R a n g e o f F i n d i n g s	A b n o r m a l F i n d i n g s

Tone. Tone is the normal degree of tension (contraction) in voluntarily relaxed muscles. It shows as a mild resistance to passive stretch. To test muscle tone, move the extremities through a passive range of motion. First, persuade the person to relax completely, to "go loose like a rag doll." Move each extremity smoothly through a full range of motion. Support the arm at the elbow and the leg at the knee (Fig. 21–15). Normally, you will note a mild, even resistance to movement.

Limited range of motion.
Pain with motion.
Flaccidity—decreased resistance, hypotonic.
Spasticity and rigidity—types of increased resistance (see Table 21–4).

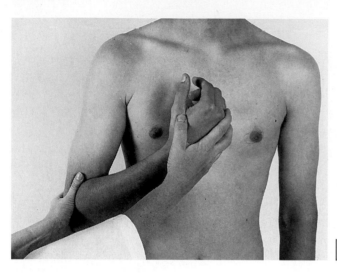

21-15

Involuntary Movements. Normally, no involuntary movements occur. If they are present, note their location, frequency, rate, and amplitude. Note if the movements can be controlled at will.

Tic, tremor, fasciculation, myoclonus, chorea, and athetosis (see Table 21–5).

Cerebellar Function

Balance Tests

Gait. Observe as the person walks 10 to 20 feet, turns, and returns to the starting point. Normally, the person moves with a sense of freedom. The gait is smooth, rhythmic, and effortless; the opposing arm swing is coordinated; the turns are smooth. The step length is about 15 inches from heel to heel.

Stiff, immobile posture. Staggering or reeling. Wide base of support.
Lack of arm swing or rigid arms.
Unequal rhythm of steps. Slapping of foot. Scraping of toe of shoe.
Ataxia—uncoordinated or unsteady gait (see Table 21–6).

Ask the person to walk a straight line in a heel-to-toe fashion (tandem walking) (Fig. 21–16). This decreases the base of support and will accentuate any problem with coordination. Normally, the person can walk straight and stay balanced.

Crooked line of walk.
Widens base to maintain balance.
Staggering, reeling, loss of balance.
An ataxia that did not appear with regular gait may appear now. Inability to tandem walk is sensitive for an upper motor neuron lesion, such as multiple sclerosis.

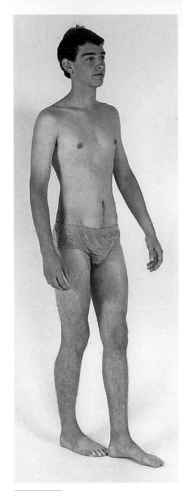

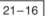

Tandem Walking

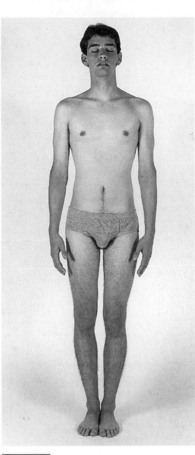

21–17

Romberg Test

The Romberg Test. Ask the person to stand up with feet together and arms at the sides. Once in a stable position, ask the person to close the eyes and to hold the position (Fig. 21–17). Wait about 20 seconds. Normally, a person can maintain posture and balance even with the visual orienting information blocked, although slight swaying may occur. (Stand close to catch the person in case he or she falls.)

Sways, falls, widens base of feet to avoid falling.

Positive Romberg sign is loss of balance that occurs when closing the eyes. You eliminate the advantage of orientation with the eyes, which had compensated for sensory loss. A positive Romberg sign occurs with cerebellar ataxia (multiple sclerosis, alcohol intoxication), loss of proprioception, and loss of vestibular function.

Ask the person to perform a shallow knee bend or to hop in place, first on one leg, then the other (Fig. 21–18). This demonstrates normal position sense, muscle strength, and cerebellar function. Note that some individuals cannot hop owing to aging or obesity.

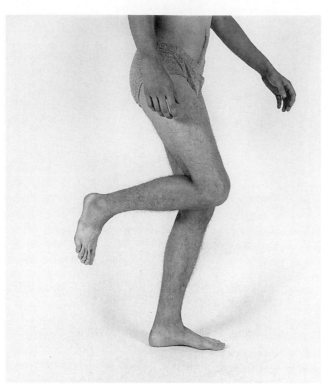

21–18

Coordination and Skilled Movements

Rapid Alternating Movements (RAM). Ask the person to pat the knees with both hands, lift up, turn hands over, and pat the knees with the backs of the hands (Fig. 21–19). Then ask the person to do this faster. Normally, this is done with equal turning and a quick rhythmic pace.

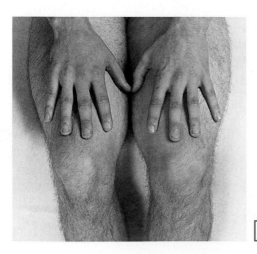

21–19

Lack of coordination.

Slow, clumsy, and sloppy response is termed *dysdiadochokinesia* and occurs with cerebellar disease.

Normal Range of Findings	Abnormal Findings

Alternatively, ask the person to touch the thumb to each finger on the same hand, starting with the index finger, then reverse direction (Fig. 21–20). Normally, this can be done quickly and accurately.

Lack of coordination.

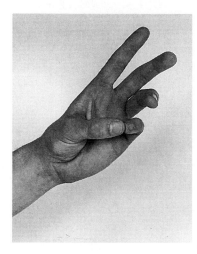

21–20

Finger-to-Finger Test. With the person's eyes open, ask that he or she use the index finger to touch your finger, then his or her own nose (Fig. 21–21). After a few times move your finger to a different spot. The person's movement should be smooth and accurate.

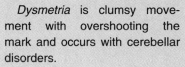

Dysmetria is clumsy movement with overshooting the mark and occurs with cerebellar disorders.

Past-pointing is a constant deviation to one side.

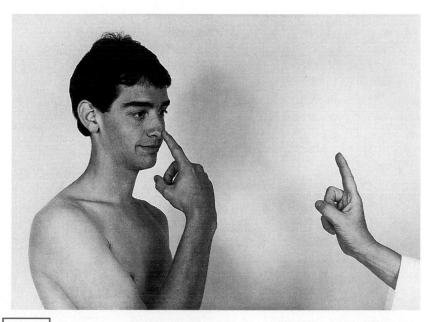

21–21

Normal Range of Findings	Abnormal Findings

Finger-to-Nose Test. Ask the person to close the eyes and to stretch out the arms. Ask the person to touch the tip of his or her nose with each index finger, alternating hands and increasing speed. Normally this is done with accurate and smooth movement.

Misses nose. Worsening of coordination when the eyes are closed occurs with cerebellar disease.

Heel-to-Shin Test. Test lower extremity coordination by asking the person, who is in a supine position, to place the heel on the opposite knee, and run it down the shin from the knee to the ankle (Fig. 21–22). Normally, the person moves the heel in a straight line down the shin.

Lack of coordination. Heel falls off shin.

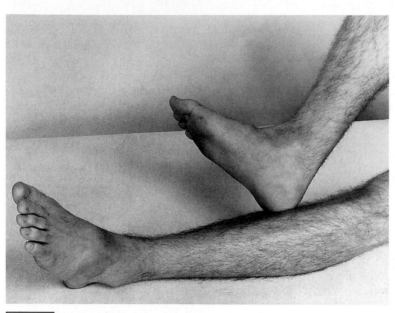

21–22

THE SENSORY SYSTEM

Assess the sensory system

Ask the person to identify various sensory stimuli in order to test the intactness of the peripheral nerve fibers, the sensory tracts, and higher cortical discrimination.

Ensure validity of sensory system testing by making sure the person is alert, cooperative, and comfortable and has an adequate attention span. Otherwise, you may get misleading and invalid results. Testing of the sensory system can be fatiguing. You may need to repeat the examination later or to break it into parts when the person is tired.

You do not need to test the entire skin surface for every sensation. Routine screening procedures include testing superficial pain, light touch, and vibration in a few distal locations, and testing stereognosis. This will suffice for all who have not demonstrated any neurologic symptoms or signs. Complete testing of the sensory system is warranted in those with neurologic symptoms (e.g., localized pain, numbness, and tingling) or when you discover abnormalities (e.g., motor deficit). Then, test all sensory modalities and cover most dermatomes of the body.

Normal Range of Findings	Abnormal Findings

Compare sensations on symmetric parts of the body. When you find a definite decrease in sensation, map it out by systematic testing in that area. Proceed from the point of decreased sensation toward the sensitive area. By asking the person to tell you where the sensation changes, you can map the exact borders of the deficient area. Draw your results on a diagram.

Note if the topographic pattern of sensory loss is distal, i.e., over the hands and feet in a "glove and stocking" distribution, or if it is over a specific dermatome.

Avoid asking leading questions, "Can you feel this pin prick?" This creates an expectation of how the person should feel the sensation, which is called *suggestion*. Instead, use unbiased directions.

The person's eyes should be closed during each of the tests. Take time to explain what will be happening and exactly how you expect the person to respond.

Spinothalamic Tract

Pain. Pain is tested by the person's ability to perceive a pin prick. Break a tongue blade lengthwise, forming a sharp point at the fractured end and a dull spot at the rounded end. Lightly apply the sharp point or the dull end to the person's body in a random, unpredictable order (Fig. 21–23). Ask the person to say "sharp" or "dull," depending on the sensation felt. (Note that the sharp edge is used to test for pain; the dull edge is used as a general test of the person's responses.)*

Hypalgesia—decreased pain sensation.

Analgesia—absent pain sensation.

Hyperalgesia—increased pain sensation.

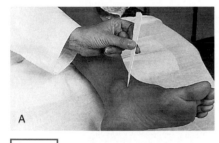
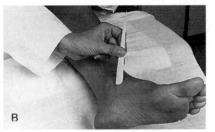

21–23

Let at least 2 seconds elapse between each stimulus to avoid *summation*. With summation, frequent consecutive stimuli are perceived as one strong stimulus.

Temperature. Test temperature sensation only when pain sensation is abnormal; otherwise, you may omit it because the fiber tracts are much the same. Fill two test tubes, one with hot water and one with cold water, and apply the bottom ends to the person's skin in a random order. Ask the person to say which temperature is felt. Alternatively, you could place the flat side of the tuning fork on the skin; its metal always feels cool.

---

*Alternatively, you could use a sterile needle to test the pin prick. To prevent any possible contagion, do not reuse a needle or sharp tool on another person. Dispose of needles or any sharp tool in a special impenetrable container.

Light Touch. Apply a wisp of cotton to the skin. Stretch a cotton ball to make a long end and brush it over the skin in a random order of sites and at irregular intervals (Fig. 21–24). This prevents the person from responding just from repetition. Include the arms, forearms, hands, chest, thighs, and legs. Ask the person to say "now" or "yes" when touch is felt. Compare symmetric points.

Hypoesthesia—decreased touch sensation.

Anesthesia—absent touch sensation.

Hyperesthesia—increased touch sensation.

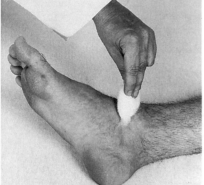

21–24

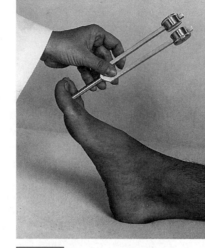

21–25

Posterior Column Tract

Vibration. Test the person's ability to feel vibrations of a tuning fork over bony prominences. Use a low-pitch tuning fork (128 Hz or 256 Hz) because its vibration has a slower decay. Strike the tuning fork on the heel of your hand, and hold the base on a bony surface of the fingers and great toe (Fig. 21–25). Ask the person to indicate when the vibration starts and stops. If the person feels the normal vibration or buzzing sensation on these distal areas, you may assume proximal spots are normal and proceed no further. If no vibrations are felt, move proximally and test ulnar processes, and ankles, patellae, and iliac crests. Compare the right side with the left side. If you find a deficit, note whether it is gradual or abrupt.

Unable to feel vibration. Loss of vibration sense occurs with peripheral neuropathy, e.g., diabetes and alcoholism. Often, this is the first sensation lost.

Peripheral neuropathy is worse at the feet and gradually improves as you move up the leg, as opposed to a specific nerve lesion, which has a clear zone of deficit for its dermatome.

Position (Kinesthesia). Test the person's ability to perceive passive movements of the extremities. Move a finger or the big toe up and down, and ask the person to tell you which way it is moved (Fig. 21–26). The test is done with the eyes closed, but to be sure it is understood, have the person watch a few trials first. Vary the order of movement up or down. Hold the digit by the sides, since upward or downward pressure on the skin may provide a clue as to how it has been moved. Normally, a person can detect movement of a few millimeters.

Loss of position sense.

Normal Range of Findings	Abnormal Findings

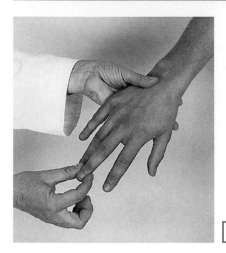

21-26

Tactile Discrimination (Fine Touch). The following tests also measure the discrimination ability of the sensory cortex. As a prerequisite, the person needs a normal or near-normal sense of touch and position sense.

Stereognosis. Test the person's ability to recognize objects by feeling their forms, sizes, and weights. With the eyes closed, place a familiar object (paper clip, key, coin, cotton ball, or pencil) in the person's hand and ask the person to identify it (Fig. 21–27). Normally, a person will explore it with the fingers and correctly name it. Test a different object in each hand; testing the left hand assesses right parietal lobe functioning.

Problems with tactile discrimination occur with lesions of the sensory cortex or posterior column.

Astereognosis—inability to identify object correctly. Occurs in sensory cortex lesions, e.g., brain attack (stroke).

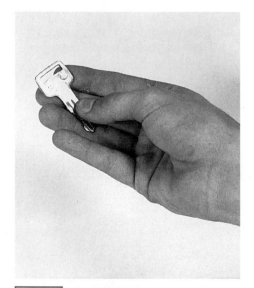

21-27 **Stereognosis**

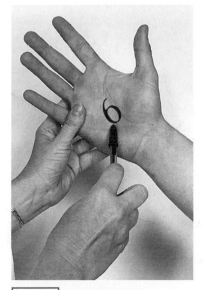

21-28 **Graphesthesia**

Graphesthesia. Graphesthesia is the ability to "read" a number by having it traced on the skin. With the person's eyes closed, use a blunt instrument to trace a single digit number or a letter on the palm (Fig. 21–28). Ask the person to tell you what it is. Graphesthesia is a good measure of sensory loss if the person cannot make the hand movements needed for stereognosis, as occurs in arthritis.

Inability to distinguish number occurs with lesions of the sensory cortex.

Two-Point Discrimination. Test the person's ability to distinguish the separation of two simultaneous pin pricks on the skin. Apply two sterile needles or the two points of an opened paper clip lightly to the skin in ever-closing distances. Note the distance at which the person no longer perceives two separate points. The level of perception varies considerably with the region tested; it is most sensitive in the fingertips (2 to 8 mm) (Fig. 21–29) and least sensitive on the upper arms, thighs, and back (40 to 75 mm).

An increase in the distance it normally takes to identify two separate points occurs with sensory cortex lesions.

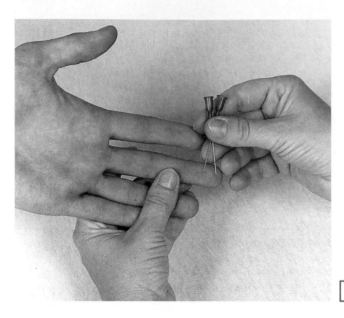

21–29

Extinction. Simultaneously touch both sides of the body at the same point. Ask the person to state how many sensations are felt and where they are. Normally, both sensations are felt.

The ability to recognize only one of the stimuli occurs with sensory cortex lesion; the stimulus is extinguished on the side *opposite* the cortex lesion.

Point Location. Touch the skin, and withdraw the stimulus promptly. Tell the person, "Put your finger where I touched you." You can perform this test simultaneously with light touch sensation.

With a sensory cortex lesion, the person cannot localize the sensation accurately, even though light touch sensation may be retained.

REFLEXES

Test the reflexes
Stretch, or Deep Tendon Reflexes (DTRs)

Measurement of the stretch reflexes reveals the intactness of the reflex arc at specific spinal levels as well as the normal override on the reflex of the higher cortical levels.

For an adequate response, the limb should be relaxed and the muscle partially stretched. Stimulate the reflex by directing a short, snappy blow of the reflex hammer onto the muscle's insertion tendon. Use a relaxed hold on the hammer. As with the percussion technique, the action takes place at the wrist. Strike a brief, well-aimed blow, and bounce up promptly; do not let the hammer rest on the tendon. Use the pointed end of the reflex hammer when aiming at a

▶ **Normal Range of Findings**   **Abnormal Findings**

smaller target such as your thumb on the tendon site; use the flat end when the target is wider or to diffuse the impact and prevent pain.

Use just enough force to get a response. Compare right and left sides—The responses should be equal. The reflex response is graded on a 4-point scale:

4+ Very brisk, hyperactive with clonus, indicative of disease
3+ Brisker than average, may indicate disease
2+ Average, normal
1+ Diminished, low normal
0   No response

This is a subjective scale and requires some clinical practice. Even then the scale is not completely reliable because no standard exists to say *how* brisk a reflex should be to warrant a grade of 3+. Also, a wide range of normal exists in reflex responses. Healthy people may have diminished reflexes or they may have brisk ones. Your best plan is to interpret the DTRs *only* within the context of the rest of the neurologic exam.

Sometimes the reflex response fails to appear. Try further encouragement of relaxation, varying the person's position or increasing the strength of the blow. **Reinforcement** is another technique to relax the muscles and enhance the response (Fig. 21–30). Ask the person to perform an isometric exercise in a muscle group somewhat away from the one being tested. For example, to enhance a patellar reflex, ask the person to lock the fingers together and "pull." To enhance a biceps response, ask the person to clench the teeth or to grasp the thigh with the opposite hand.

Clonus is a set of short jerking contractions of the same muscle.
Hyperreflexia is the exaggerated reflex seen when the monosynaptic reflex arc is released from the influence of higher cortical levels. This occurs with upper motor neuron lesions, e.g., a brain attack.
Hyporeflexia, which is the absence of a reflex, is a lower motor neuron problem. It occurs with interruption of sensory afferents or destruction of motor efferents and anterior horn cells, e.g., spinal cord injury.

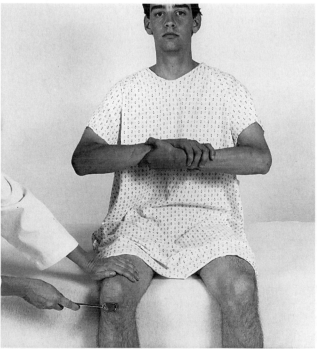

21–30

Reinforcement

Biceps Reflex (C5 to C6). Support the person's forearm on yours; this position relaxes, as well as partially flexes, the person's arm. Place your thumb on the biceps tendon and strike a blow on your thumb. You can feel as well as see the normal response, which is contraction of the biceps muscle and flexion of the forearm (Fig. 21–31).

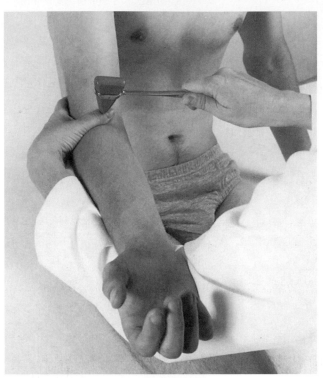

21–31

Triceps Reflex (C7 to C8). Tell the person to let the arm "just go dead" as you suspend it by holding the upper arm. Strike the triceps tendon directly just above the elbow (Fig. 21–32). The normal response is extension of the forearm. Alternately, hold the person's wrist across the chest to flex the arm at the elbow, and tap the tendon.

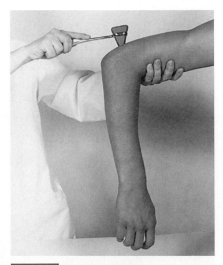

21–32 **Triceps Reflex**

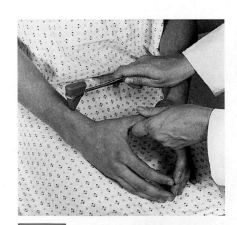

21–33 **Brachioradialis Reflex**

Brachioradialis Reflex (C5 to C6). Hold the person's thumbs to suspend the forearms in relaxation. Strike the forearm directly, about 2 to 3 cm above the radial styloid process (Fig. 21–33). The normal response is flexion and supination of the forearm.

Quadriceps Reflex ("Knee Jerk") (L2 to L4). Let the lower legs dangle freely to flex the knee and stretch the tendons. Strike the tendon directly just below the patella (Fig. 21–34). Extension of the lower leg is the expected response. You also will palpate contraction of the quadriceps.

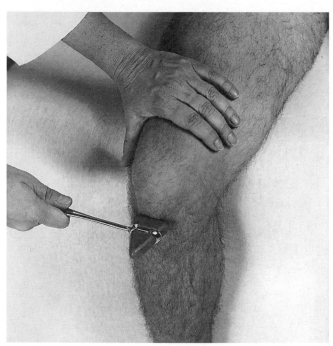

21–34

For the person in the supine position, use your own arm as a lever to support the weight of one leg against the other leg (Fig. 21–35). This maneuver also flexes the knee.

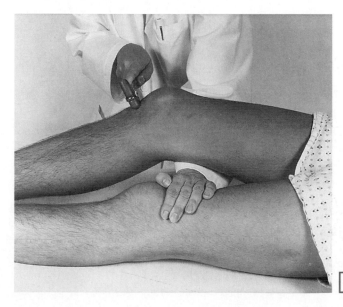

21–35

Achilles Reflex ("Ankle Jerk") (L5 to S2). Position the person with the knee flexed and the hip externally rotated. Hold the foot in dorsiflexion, and strike the Achilles tendon directly (Fig. 21–36). Feel the normal response as the foot plantar flexes against your hand.

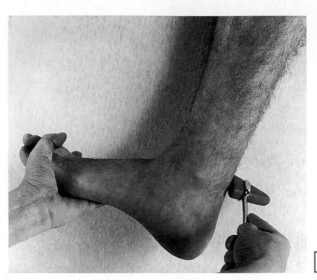

21–36

For the person in the supine position, flex one knee and support that lower leg against the other leg so that it falls "open." Dorsiflex the foot and tap the tendon (Fig. 21–37).

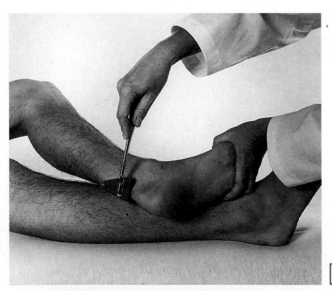

21–37

Clonus. Test for clonus, particularly when the reflexes are hyperactive. Support the lower leg in one hand. With your other hand, move the foot up and down a few times to relax the muscle. Then stretch the muscle by briskly dorsiflexing the foot. Hold the stretch (Fig. 21–38). With a normal response, you feel no further movement. When clonus is present, you will feel and see rapid rhythmic contractions of the calf muscle and movement of the foot.

Clonus is repeated reflex muscular movements. A hyperactive reflex with sustained clonus (lasting as long as the stretch is held) occurs with upper motor neuron disease.

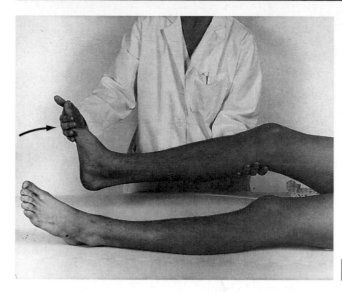

21–38

Superficial Reflexes

Here, the receptors are in the skin rather than the muscles.

Abdominal Reflexes—Upper (T8 to T10), Lower (T10 to T12). Have the person assume a supine position, with the knees slightly bent. Use the handle end of the reflex hammer, a wood applicator tip, or the end of a split tongue blade to stroke the skin. Move from the side of the abdomen toward the midline at both the upper and lower abdominal levels (Fig. 21–39). The normal response is ipsilateral contraction of the abdominal muscle with an observed deviation of the umbilicus toward the stroke. When the abdominal wall is very obese, pull the skin to the opposite side, and feel it contract toward the stimulus.

Cremasteric Reflex (L1 to L2). On the male, lightly stroke the inner aspect of the thigh with the reflex hammer or tongue blade (Fig. 21–39). Note elevation of the ipsilateral testicle.

Superficial reflexes are absent with diseases of the pyramidal tract, e.g., they are absent on the contralateral side with brain attack.

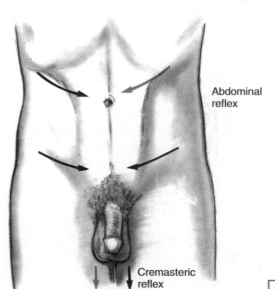

Abdominal reflex

Cremasteric reflex

21–39

Normal Range of Findings	Abnormal Findings

Plantar Reflex (L4 to S2). Position the thigh in slight external rotation. With the reflex hammer, draw a light stroke up the lateral side of the sole of the foot and inward across the ball of the foot, like an upside-down J (Fig. 21–40). The normal response is plantar flexion of all the toes and inversion and flexion of the forefoot.

Except in infancy, the abnormal response is dorsiflexion of the big toe and fanning of all toes, which is a **positive Babinski sign,** also called "upgoing toes." This occurs with upper motor neuron disease of the corticospinal (or pyramidal) tract.

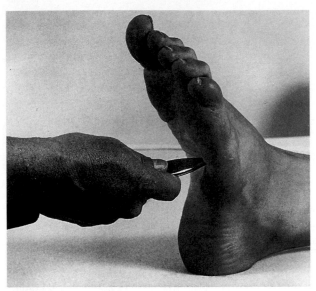

21–40

Plantar Reflex

 DEVELOPMENTAL CONSIDERATIONS

Infants (Birth to 12 Months)

The neurologic system shows dramatic growth and development during the 1st year of life. Assessment includes noting that milestones you normally would expect for each month have indeed been achieved, and that the early, more primitive reflexes are eliminated from the baby's repertory when they are supposed to be.

At birth, the newborn is very alert, with the eyes open, and demonstrates strong, urgent sucking. The normal cry is loud, lusty, and even angry. The next 2 or 3 days may be spent mostly sleeping as the baby recovers from the birth process. After that, the pattern of sleep and waking activity is highly variable; it depends on the baby's individual body rhythm as well as external stimuli.

The behavioral assessment should include your observations of the infant's spontaneous waking activity, responses to environmental stimuli, and social interaction with the parents and others.

By 2 months of age, the baby smiles responsively and recognizes the parent's face. Babbling occurs at 4 months, and one or two words (mama, dada) are used nonspecifically after 9 months.

The cranial nerves cannot be tested directly, but you can infer their proper functioning by the maneuvers shown in Table 21–2.

Failure to attain a skill by expected time.

Persistence of reflex behavior beyond the normal time.

A high-pitched, shrill cry or cat-sounding screech occurs with CNS damage.

A weak, groaning cry or expiratory grunt occurs with respiratory distress.

Lethargy, hyporeactivity, hyperirritability, and parent's report of significant change in behavior all warrant referral.

► **Normal Range of Findings**

Abnormal Findings

Table 21–2 • Testing Cranial Nerve Function of Infants

Cranial Nerve	Response
II, III, IV, VI	Optical blink reflex—shine light in open eyes, note rapid closure
	Size, shape, equality of pupils
	Regards face or close object
	Eyes follow movement
V	Rooting reflex, sucking reflex
VII	Facial movements (e.g., wrinkling forehead and nasolabial folds) symmetric when crying or smiling
VIII	Loud noise yields Moro reflex (until 4 mo)
	Acoustic blink reflex—infant blinks in response to a loud hand clap 30 cm (12 in) from head (avoid making air current)
	Eyes follow direction of sound
IX, X	Swallowing, gag reflex
	Coordinated sucking and swallowing
XII	Pinch nose, infant's mouth will open and tongue rise in midline

The Motor System

Observe spontaneous motor activity for smoothness and symmetry. Smoothness of movement suggests proper cerebellar function, as does the coordination involved in sucking and swallowing. To screen gross and fine motor coordination, use the Denver II with its age-specific developmental milestones. You also can assess movement by testing the reflexes listed in the following section. Note their smoothness of response and symmetry. Also, note whether their presence or absence is appropriate for the infant's age.

Assess muscle tone by first observing resting posture. The newborn favors a flexed position; extremities are symmetrically folded inward, the hips are slightly abducted, and the fists are tightly flexed (Fig. 21–41). Infants born by breech delivery, however, do not have flexion in the lower extremities.

Delay in motor activity occurs with brain damage, mental retardation, peripheral neuromuscular damage, prolonged illness, and parental neglect.

Abnormal postures:

Frog position—hips abducted and almost flat against the table, externally rotated (only normal after breech delivery).
Opisthotonos—head arched back, stiffness of neck, and extension of arms and legs; occurs with meningeal or brain stem irritation and kernicterus (see Table 21–10).
Extension of limbs may occur with intracranial hemorrhage.

Any type of continual asymmetry, e.g., asymmetry of upper limbs occurs with brachial plexus palsy.

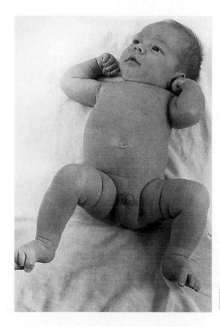

21–41

▶ Normal Range of Findings	Abnormal Findings

After 2 months of age, flexion gives way to gradual extension, beginning with the head and continuing in a cephalocaudal direction. Now is the time to check for spasticity; none should be present. Test for spasticity by flexing the infant's knees onto the abdomen and then quickly releasing them. They will unfold but not too quickly. Also, gently push the head forward—The baby should comply.

The fists normally are held in tight flexion for the first 3 months. Then the fists open for part of the time. A purposeful reach for an object with both hands occurs around 4 months of age, a transfer of an object from hand to hand at 7 months of age, a grasp using fingers and opposing thumb at 9 months of age, and a purposeful release at 10 months of age. Babies are normally ambidextrous for the first 18 months.

Head control is an important milestone in motor development. You can incorporate the following two movements into every infant assessment to check the muscle tone necessary for head control.

First, with the baby supine, pull to a sit holding the wrists and note head control (Fig. 21–42). The newborn will hold the head almost in the same plane as the body, and it will balance briefly when the baby reaches a sitting position, then flop forward. (Even a premature infant shows some head flexion.) At 4 months of age, the head stays in line with the body and does not flop.

Spasticity is an early sign of cerebral palsy. After releasing flexed knees, legs will quickly extend and adduct, even to a "scissoring" motion when spasticity is present. Also, the baby often resists head flexion and extends back against your hand when spasticity is present.

Note persistent one-hand preference in children younger than 18 months of age. The condition may indicate a motor deficit on the opposite side.

Because development progresses in a cephalocaudal direction, head lag is an early sign of brain damage.

After 6 months of age, refer any baby with failure to hold head in midline when sitting.

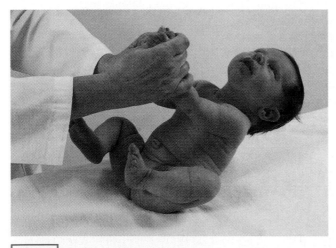

21–42

▶ Normal Range of Findings	Abnormal Findings

Second, lift up the baby in a prone position, with one hand supporting the chest (Fig. 21–43). The term newborn holds the head at an angle of 45 degrees or less from horizontal, the back is straight or slightly arched, and the elbows and knees are partly flexed. At 3 months of age, the baby raises the head and arches the back, as in a swan dive. This is the *Landau reflex*, which persists until 1½ years of age.

Head lag, a limp, floppy trunk, and dangling arms and legs.

Absence of the reflex indicates motor weakness, upper motor neuron disease, or mental retardation.

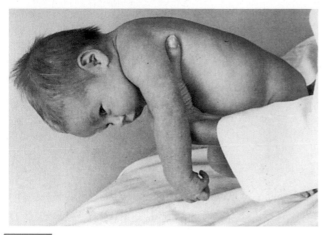

21–43

Assess muscle strength by noting the strength of sucking and of spontaneous motor activity. Normally, no tremors are present, and no continual overshooting of the mark occurs when reaching.

The Sensory System

You will perform very little sensory testing with infants and toddlers. The newborn normally has hypoesthesia and requires a strong stimulus to elicit a response. The baby responds to pain by crying and a general reflex withdrawal of all limbs. By 7 to 9 months of age, the infant can localize the stimulus and shows more specific signs of withdrawal. Other sensory modalities are not tested.

Unusually rapid withdrawal is *hyperesthesia,* which occurs with spinal cord lesions, CNS infections, increased intracranial pressure, peritonitis.

No withdrawal is decreased sensation, which occurs with decreased consciousness, mental deficiency, spinal cord or peripheral nerve lesions.

Reflexes

Infantile automatisms are reflexes that have a predictable timetable of appearance and departure. The reflexes most commonly tested are listed in the following section. For the screening examination, you can just check the rooting, grasp, tonic neck, and Moro reflexes.

▶ Normal Range of Findings | Abnormal Findings

Rooting Reflex. Brush the infant's cheek near the mouth. Note whether the infant turns the head toward that side and opens the mouth (Fig. 21–44). Appears at birth and disappears at 3 to 4 months.

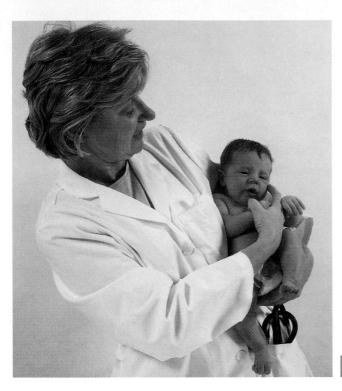

21–44

Sucking Reflex. Touch the lips and offer your gloved little finger to suck. Note strong sucking reflex. The reflex is present at birth and disappears at 10 to 12 months.

Palmar Grasp. Place the baby's head midline to ensure symmetric response. Offer your finger from the baby's ulnar side, away from the thumb. Note tight grasp of all the baby's fingers (Fig. 21–45). Sucking enhances grasp. Often, you can pull baby to a sit from grasp. The reflex is present at birth, is strongest at 1 to 2 months, and disappears at 3 to 4 months.

The palmar grasp reflex is absent with brain damage and with local muscle or nerve injury.

Persistence of palmar grasp reflex after 4 months of age occurs with frontal lobe lesion.

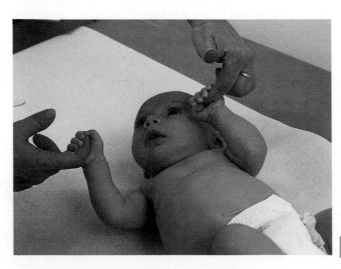

21–45

Normal Range of Findings	Abnormal Findings

Plantar Grasp. Touch your thumb at the ball of the baby's foot. Note that the toes curl down tightly (Fig. 21–46). The reflex is present at birth and disappears at 8 to 10 months.

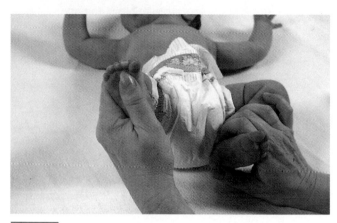

21–46

Babinski's Reflex. Stroke your finger up the lateral edge and across the ball of the infant's foot. Note fanning of toes (positive Babinski's reflex) (Fig. 21–47). The reflex is present at birth and disappears (changes to the adult response) by 24 months of age (variable).

Positive Babinski's reflex after 2 or 2½ years of age occurs with pyramidal tract disease.

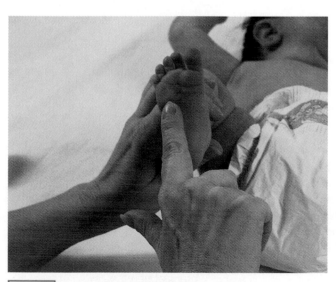

21–47

▶ Normal Range of Findings   Abnormal Findings

Tonic Neck Reflex. With the baby supine, relaxed, or sleeping, turn the head to one side with the chin over shoulder. Note ipsilateral extension of the arm and leg, and flexion of the opposite arm and leg; this is the "fencing" position. If you turn the infant's head to the opposite side, positions will reverse (Fig. 21–48). The reflex appears by 2 to 3 months, decreases at 3 to 4 months, and disappears by 4 to 6 months.

Persistence later in infancy occurs with brain damage.

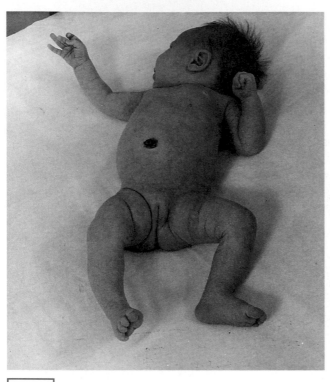

21–48

Moro Reflex. Startle the infant by jarring the crib, making a loud noise, or supporting the head and back in a semi-sitting position and quickly lowering the infant to 30 degrees. The baby looks as if he or she is hugging a tree. That is, symmetric abduction and extension of the arms and legs, fanning fingers, and curling of the index finger and thumb to C position occur. The infant then brings in both arms and legs (Fig. 21–49). The reflex is present at birth, and disappears at 1 to 4 months.

Absence of the Moro reflex in the newborn or persistence after 5 months of age indicates severe CNS injury.

Absence of movement in just one arm occurs with fracture of the humerus or clavicle and with brachial nerve palsy.

Absence in one leg occurs with a lower spinal cord problem or a dislocated hip.

A hyperactive Moro reflex occurs with tetany or CNS infection.

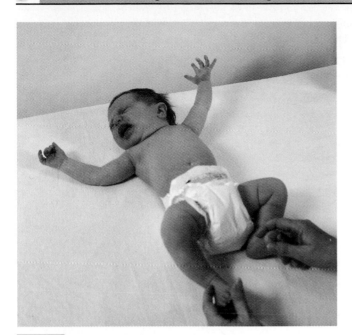

21–49   **Moro reflex**

Placing Reflex. Hold the infant upright under the arms, close to a table. Let the dorsal "top" of foot touch the underside of table (Fig. 21–50). Note flexing of hip and knee, followed by extension at the hip, to place foot on table. Reflex appears at 4 days after birth.

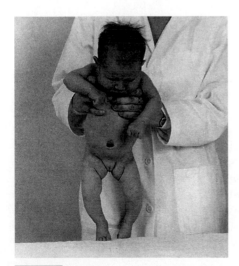

21–50

▶ Normal Range of Findings	Abnormal Findings

Stepping Reflex. Hold the infant upright under the arms, with the feet on a flat surface. Note regular alternating steps (Fig. 21–51). The reflex disappears before voluntary walking.

Extensor thrust, or "scissoring"; crossing of lower extremities.

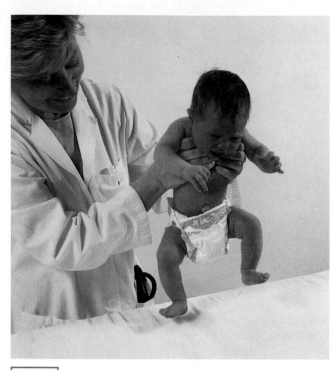

21–51

Preschool- and School-Age Children

Use the same sequence of neurologic assessment as with the adult, with the omissions or modifications mentioned in the following section.

Assess the child's general behavior during play activities, reaction to parent, and cooperation with parent and with you. Complete details are described in Chapter 6, Mental Status Assessment.

Smell and taste are almost never tested, but if you need to test the child's sense of smell (cranial nerve I), use a scent familiar to the child such as peanut butter or orange peel. When testing visual fields (cranial nerve II) and cardinal positions of gaze (cranial nerves III, IV, VI), you often need to gently immobilize the head, or the child will track with the whole head. Make a game out of asking the child to imitate your funny "faces" (cranial nerve VII); thus, the child has fun and you win a friend.

Much of the motor assessment can be derived from watching the child undress and dress and manipulate buttons. This indicates muscle strength, symmetry, joint range of motion, and fine motor skills. Use the Denver II to screen gross and fine motor skills that are appropriate for the child's specific age. Be familiar with developmental milestones described in Chapter 2 for each age.

Muscle hypertrophy or atrophy occurs with muscular dystrophy.
Muscle weakness.
Incoordination.

▶ Normal Range of Findings	Abnormal Findings

Note the child's gait during both walking and running. Allow for the normal wide-based gate of the toddler and the normal knock-kneed walk of the preschooler. Normally, the child can balance on one foot for about 5 seconds by 4 years of age, can balance for 8 to 10 seconds at 5 years of age, and can hop at 4 years. Children enjoy performing these tests (Fig. 21–52).

Causes of motor delay are listed earlier in the infant section.

Staggering, falling.

Weakness climbing up or down stairs occurs with muscular dystrophy.

Broad-based gait beyond toddlerhood, scissor gait (see Table 21–6).

Failure to hop after 5 years of age indicates incoordination of gross motor skill.

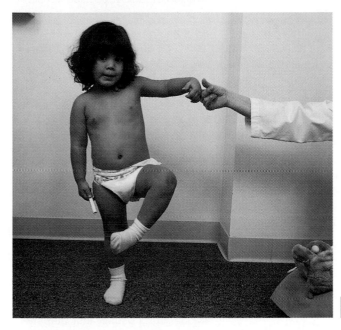

21–52

Observe the child as he or she rises from a supine position on the floor to a sitting position, and then to a stand. Note the muscles of the neck, abdomen, arms, and legs. Normally, the child curls up in the midline to sit up, then pushes off with both hands against the floor to stand (Fig. 21–53A).

Weak pelvic muscles are a sign of muscular dystrophy; from the supine position, the child will roll to one side, bend forward to all four extremities, plant hands on legs, and literally "climb" up him- or herself. This is *Gower's sign* (Fig. 21–53B).

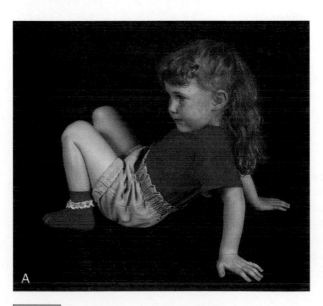

A

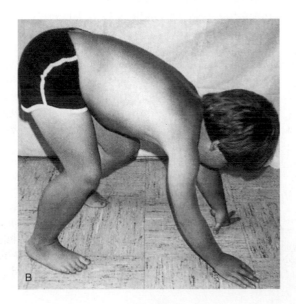

B

21–53

Assess fine coordination by using the finger-to-nose test if you can be sure the young child understands your directions. Demonstrate the procedure first, then ask the child to do the test with the eyes open, then with the eyes closed. Fine coordination is not fully developed until the child has reached 4 or 6 years of age. Consider it normal if a younger child can bring the finger to within 2 to 5 cm (1 to 2 in) of the nose.

Testing sensation is very unreliable in toddlers and preschoolers. You may test light touch by asking the child to close the eyes and then to point to the spot where you touch or tickle. Testing of vibration, position, stereognosis, graphesthesia, or two-point discrimination usually is not done on a child younger than 6 years of age. Also, do not test for perception of superficial pain because the child has a natural fear of needles. In children older than 6 years of age, you may perform sensory testing as with adults. Use a fractured tongue blade instead of a needle if you need to test superficial pain.

The DTRs usually are not tested in children younger than 5 years of age due to lack of cooperation in relaxation. When you need to test DTRs in a young child, use your finger to percuss the tendon. Use a reflex hammer only with an older child. Coax the child to relax, or distract and percuss discreetly when the child is not paying attention. The knee jerk is present at birth, then the ankle jerk and brachial reflex appear, and the triceps reflex is present at 6 months.

Failure of the finger-to-nose test with the eyes open indicates gross incoordination; failure of the test with the eyes closed indicates minor incoordination or lack of position sense.

Sensory loss occurs with decreased consciousness, mental deficiency, or spinal cord or peripheral nerve dysfunction.

Hyperactivity of DTRs occurs with upper motor neuron lesion, hypocalcemia, and hyperthyroidism, and with muscle spasm associated with early poliomyelitis.

Decreased or absent reflexes occur with a lower motor neuron lesion, muscular dystrophy, and flaccidity or flaccid paralysis.

Clonus may occur with fatigue, but it usually indicates hyperreflexia.

The Aging Adult

Use the same examination as used with the younger adult. Be aware that some aging adults show a slower response to your requests, especially to those calling for coordination of movements. The conditions discussed in the following sections are normal variants due to aging.

Although the cranial nerves mediating taste and smell are not usually tested, they may show some decline in function.

Any decrease in muscle bulk is most apparent in the hand, as seen by guttering between the metacarpals. These dorsal hand muscles often look wasted, even with no apparent arthropathy. The grip strength remains relatively good.

Senile tremors occasionally occur. These benign tremors include an intention tremor of the hands, head nodding (as if saying yes or no), and tongue protrusion. *Dyskinesias* are the repetitive stereotyped movements in the jaw, lips, or tongue that may accompany senile tremors. No associated rigidity is present.

The gait may be slower and more deliberate than that in the younger person, and it may deviate slightly from a midline path.

The rapid alternating movements, e.g., pronating and supinating the hands on the thigh, may be more difficult to perform by the aging adult.

After 65 years of age, loss of the sensation of vibration at the ankle malleolus is common and is usually accompanied by loss of the ankle jerk. Position sense in the big toe may be lost, although this is less common than vibration loss. Tactile sensation may be impaired. The aging person may need stronger stimuli for light touch and especially for pain.

Hand muscle atrophy is worsened with disuse and degenerative arthropathy.

Distinguish senile tremors from tremors of parkinsonism. The latter includes rigidity and slowness and weakness of voluntary movement.

Absence of a rhythmic reciprocal gait pattern is seen in parkinsonism and hemiparesis (see Table 21-6).

Note any difference in sensation between right and left sides, which may indicate a neurologic deficit.

Normal Range of Findings	Abnormal Findings

The DTRs are less brisk. Those in the upper extremities are usually present, but the ankle jerks are commonly lost. Knee jerks may be lost, but this occurs less often. Because aging people find it difficult to relax their limbs, always use reinforcement when eliciting the DTRs.

The plantar reflex may be absent or difficult to interpret. Often, you will not see a definite normal flexor response. However, you still should consider a definite extensor response to be abnormal.

The superficial abdominal reflexes may be absent, probably because of stretching of the musculature through pregnancy or obesity.

NEUROLOGIC RECHECK

Some hospitalized persons have head trauma or a neurologic deficit due to a systemic disease process. These people must be monitored closely for any improvement or deterioration in neurologic status and for any indication of increasing intracranial pressure. Signs of increasing intracranial pressure signal impending cerebral disaster and death and require early and prompt intervention.

Use an abbreviation of the neurologic examination in the following sequence:

1. Level of consciousness
2. Motor function
3. Pupillary response
4. Vital signs

Level of Consciousness. A *change* in the level of consciousness is the single most important factor in this examination. It is the earliest and most sensitive index of change in neurologic status. Note the ease of *arousal* and the state of awareness, or *orientation*. Assess orientation by asking questions about:

- Person—own name, occupation, names of workers around person, their occupations
- Place—where person is, nature of building, city, state
- Time—day of week, month, year

Vary the questions during repeat assessments so that the person is not merely memorizing answers. Note the quality and the content of the verbal response; articulation, fluency, manner of thinking, and any deficit in language comprehension or production (see Chapter 6).

When the person is intubated and cannot speak, you will have to ask questions that require a nod or shake of the head, "Is this a hospital?" "Are you at home?" "Are we in Texas?"

A person is fully alert when his or her eyes open at your approach or spontaneously; when he or she is oriented to person, place, and time; and when he or she is able to follow verbal commands appropriately.

If the person is not fully alert, increase the amount of stimulus used in this order:

1. Name called
2. Light touch on person's arm
3. Vigorous shake of shoulder
4. Pain applied (pinch nail bed, pinch trapezius muscle, rub your knuckles on the person's sternum)

Record the stimulus used as well as the person's response to it.

Abnormal Findings column:

A change in consciousness may be subtle. Note any decreasing level of consciousness, disorientation, memory loss, uncooperative behavior, or even complacency in a previously combative person.

Review Table 6–3, Levels of Consciousness, Chapter 6.

Motor Function. Check the voluntary movement of each extremity by giving the person specific commands. (This procedure also tests level of consciousness by noting the person's ability to follow commands.)

Ask the person to lift the eyebrows, frown, bare teeth. Note symmetric facial movements and bilateral nasolabial folds (cranial nerve VII).

You can check upper arm strength by checking hand grasps. Ask the person to squeeze your fingers. Offer your two fingers, one on top of the other, so that a strong hand grasp does not hurt your knuckles (Fig. 21–54). Be judicious about asking the person to squeeze your hands; some persons with diffuse brain damage, especially frontal lobe injury, have a grasp that is a reflex only.

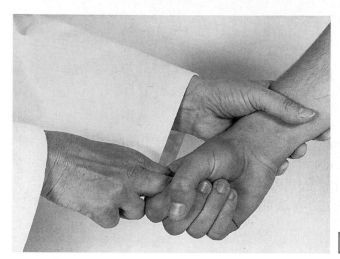

21–54

Alternatively, ask the person to lift each hand or to hold up one finger. You also can check upper extremity strength by palmar drift. Ask the person to extend both arms forward or halfway up, palms up, eyes closed, and hold for 10 to 20 seconds (Fig. 21–55). Normally, the arms stay steady with no downward drift.

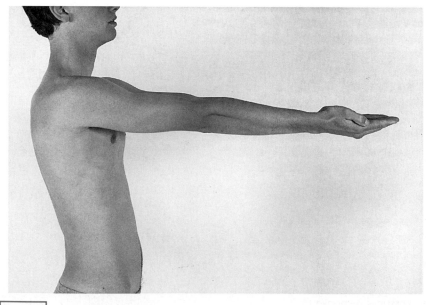

21–55

Normal Range of Findings	Abnormal Findings

Check lower extremities by asking the person to do straight leg raises. Ask the person to lift one leg at a time straight up off the bed (Fig. 21–56). Full strength allows the leg to be lifted 90 degrees. If multiple trauma, pain, or equipment preclude this motion, ask the person to push one foot at a time against your hand's resistance, "like putting your foot on the gas pedal of your car" (Fig. 21–57).

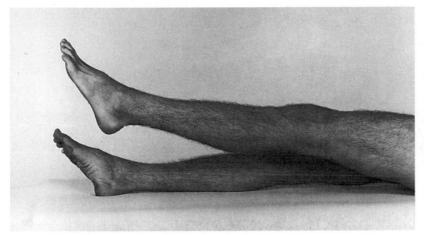

21–56

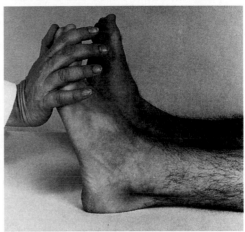

21–57

For the person with decreased level of consciousness, note if movement occurs spontaneously and as a result of noxious stimuli such as pain or suctioning. An attempt to push away your hand after such stimuli is called *localizing* and is characterized as purposeful movement.

Pupillary Response. Note the size, shape, and symmetry of both pupils. Shine a light into each pupil and note the direct and consensual light reflex. Both pupils should constrict briskly. (Allow for the effects of any medication that could affect pupil size and reactivity.) When recording, pupil size is best expressed in millimeters. Tape a millimeter scale onto a tongue blade and hold it next to the person's eyes for the most accurate measurement (Fig. 21–58).

Any abnormal posturing, decorticate rigidity, or decerebrate rigidity indicates diffuse brain injury (see Table 21–10).

In a brain-injured person, a sudden, unilateral, dilated and nonreactive pupil is ominous. Cranial nerve III runs parallel to the brain stem. When increasing intracranial pressure pushes the brain stem down (uncal herniation), it puts pressure on cranial nerve III, causing pupil dilatation.

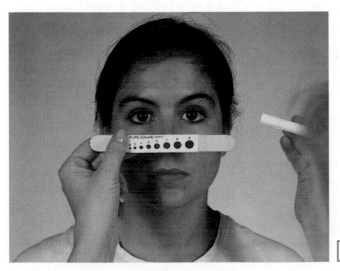

21–58

▶ Normal Range of Findings

Abnormal Findings

Vital Signs. Measure the temperature, pulse, respiration, and blood pressure as often as the person's condition warrants. Although they are vital to the overall assessment of the critically ill person, pulse and blood pressure are notoriously unreliable parameters of CNS deficit. Any changes are late consequences of rising intracranial pressure.

The **Cushing reflex** shows signs of increasing intracranial pressure: blood pressure—sudden elevation with widening pulse pressure; pulse—decreased rate, slow and bounding.

The Glasgow Coma Scale (GCS). Since the terms describing levels of consciousness are ambiguous, the Glasgow Coma Scale was developed as an accurate and reliable *quantitative* tool (Fig. 21–59). The GCS is a standardized, objective assessment that defines the level of consciousness by giving it a numeric value.

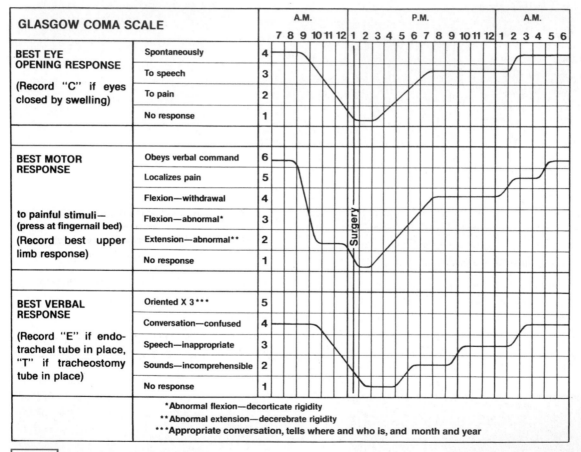

21–59

The scale is divided into three areas: eye opening, verbal response, and motor response. Each area is rated separately, and a number is given for the person's best response. The three numbers are added; the total score reflects the brain's functional level. A fully alert, normal person has a score of 15, whereas a score of 7 or less reflects coma. Serial assessments can be plotted on a graph to illustrate visually whether the person is stable, improving, or deteriorating.

The GCS assesses the functional state of the brain as a whole, not of any particular site in the brain. The scale is easy to learn and master, has good interrater reliability (Juarez and Lyons, 1995), and enhances interprofessional communication by providing a common language.

► **SUMMARY CHECKLIST:** Neurologic Exam

Neurologic Screening Examination

1: Mental status

2: Cranial nerves
II: Optic
III, IV, VI: Extraocular muscles
V: Trigeminal
VII: Facial mobility

3: Motor function
Gait and balance
Knee flexion—hop or shallow knee
    bend

4: Sensory function
Superficial pain and light touch—
    arms and legs
Vibration—arms and legs

5: Reflexes
Biceps
Triceps
Patellar
Achilles

Neurologic Complete Examination

1: Mental status

2: Cranial nerves II through XII

3: Motor system
Muscle size, strength, tone
Gait and balance
Rapid alternating movements

4: Sensory function
Superficial pain and light touch
Vibration
Position sense
Stereognosis, graphesthesia, two-
    point discrimination

5: Reflexes
DTRs: biceps, triceps, brachioradi-
    alis, patellar, Achilles
Superficial: abdominal, plantar

APPLICATION AND CRITICAL THINKING

SAMPLE CHARTING

Subjective

No unusually frequent or severe headaches, no head injury, dizziness or vertigo, seizures or tremors. No weakness, numbness or tingling, difficulty swallowing or speaking. Has no past history of stroke, spinal cord injury, meningitis, or alcoholism.

Objective

Mental status: appearance, behavior, and speech appropriate; alert and oriented to person, place, and time; recent and remote memory intact.

Cranial nerves:
I: Identifies coffee and peppermint.
II: Vision 20/20 OS, 20/20 OD, peripheral fields intact by confrontation, fundi normal.

Continued

III, IV, VI: EOMs intact, no ptosis or nystagmus; pupils equal, round, react to light and accommodation (PERRLA).

V: Sensation intact and equal bilaterally, jaw strength equal bilaterally.

VII: Facial muscles intact and symmetric.

VIII: Hearing—whispered words heard bilaterally, Weber test—tone is heard midline without lateralization.

IX, X: Swallowing intact, gag reflex present, uvula rises in midline on phonation.

XI: Shoulder shrug, head movement intact and equal bilaterally.

XII: Tongue protrudes midline, no tremors.

Motor: no atrophy, weakness, or tremors. Gait smooth and coordinated, able to tandem walk, negative Romberg. Rapid alternating movements (RAM)—finger-to-nose smoothly intact.

Sensory: pin prick, light touch, vibration intact. Stereognosis—able to identify key.

Reflexes: normal abdominal, no Babinski's sign, DTRs 2+ and = bilaterally with down going toes, see drawing below:

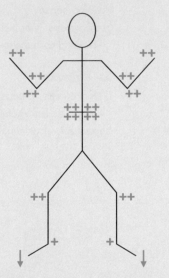

CLINICAL CASE STUDY

J.T. is a 61-year-old white male carpenter with a large building firm who is admitted to the Rehabilitation Institute with a diagnosis of right hemiplegia and aphasia following a brain attack (CVA) 4 weeks PTA.

 Subjective

Because of J.T.'s speech dysfunction, history provided by wife.

4 weeks PTA—complaint of severe headache, then sudden onset of collapse and loss of consciousness while at work. Did not strike head as fell. Transported by ambulance to Memorial Hospital where admitting physician said J.T. "probably had a stroke." Right arm and leg were limp, and he remained unconscious. Admitted to critical care unit. Regained consciousness day 3 after admission, unable to move right side, unable to speak clearly or write. Remained in ICU 4 more days until "doctors were sure heart and breathing were steady."

3 weeks PTA—transferred to medical floor where care included physical therapy twice per day, and passive ROM 4 ×/day.

Now—some improvement in right motor function. Bowel control achieved with use of commode same time each day (after breakfast). Bladder control improved with some occasional incontinence, usually when cannot tell people he needs to urinate.

Objective

Mental status: dressed in jogging suit, sitting in wheel chair, appears alert with appropriate eye contact, listening intently to history. Speech is slow, requires great effort, able to give one-word answers that are appropriate but lack normal tone. Seems to understand all language spoken to him. Follows requests appropriately, within limits of motor weakness.

Cranial nerves:

II: Acuity normal, fields by confrontation—right homonymous hemianopsia, fundi normal.

III, IV, VI: EOMs intact, no ptosis or nystagmus, PERRLA.

V: Sensation intact to pin prick and light touch. Jaw strength weak on right.

VII: Flat nasolabial fold on right, motor weakness on right lower face. Able to wrinkle forehead bilaterally, but unable to smile or bare teeth on right.

VIII: Hearing intact.

IX, X: Swallowing intact, gag reflex present, uvula rises midline on phonation.

XI: Shoulder shrug, head movement weaker on right.

XII: Tongue protrudes midline, no tremors.

Sensory:

Pin prick and light touch present but diminished on right arm and leg. Vibration intact. Position sense impaired on right side. Stereognosis intact.

Motor: Right hand grip weak, right arm drifts, right leg weak, unable to support weight. Spasticity in right arm and leg muscles, limited range of motion on passive motion. Unable to stand up and walk unassisted. Unable to perform finger-to-nose or heel-to-shin on right side, left side smoothly intact.

Reflexes: Hyperactive 4+ with clonus, and upgoing toes in right leg. Abdominal and cremasteric reflexes absent on right.

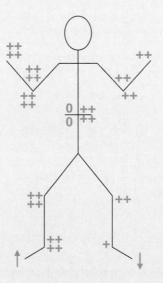

 ASSESSMENT

Impaired verbal communication R/T effects of CVA

Impaired physical mobility R/T neuromuscular impairment

Body image disturbance R/T effects of loss of body function

Self-care deficits: feeding, bathing, toileting, dressing/grooming R/T muscular weakness

Sensory-perceptual alteration (absent right visual fields) R/T neurologic impairment

Risk for injury R/T visual field deficit

Continued

NURSING DIAGNOSES COMMONLY ASSOCIATED WITH NEUROLOGIC DISORDERS

Diagnosis	Related Factors (Etiology)	Defining Characteristics (Symptoms and Signs)
Sensory perceptual alteration: kinesthetic	Effects of inner ear inflammation Neurologic impairment Side effects of tranquilizers, sedatives, muscle relaxants, or antihistamines Sleep deprivation	Falling Vertigo Stumbling Nausea Motion sickness Motor incoordination Alteration in posture Inability to sit or stand

Impaired verbal communication	Altered thought processes
	Auditory impairment
	Decreased circulation to the brain
	Effects of surgery or trauma
	Physical barriers of
	   Intubation
	   Tracheostomy
	Inability to read or write
	Language barrier
	Psychological barriers
	   Anxiety
	   Fear
	Inflammation
	Mental retardation
	Oral deformities
	Respiratory embarrassment
	Speech pattern dysfunction
		Difficulty with phonation
		Disorientation
		Dyspnea
		Flight of ideas
		Impaired articulation
		Inability to
		   Find words
		   Identify objects
		   Modulate speech
		   Name words
		Incessant verbalization
		Lack of desire to speak
		Loose association of ideas
		Stuttering or slurring

Reflex incontinence	Neurologic impairment
	   Cerebral loss
	   Interruption of spinal nerve impulse above the level of S3
		Lack of awareness of
		   Being incontinent
		   Bladder filling
		Lack of urge to void or feelings of fullness
		Somewhat unpredictable voiding pattern
		Uninhibited bladder contractions and spasms at regular intervals
		Voiding in large amounts

Unilateral neglect	Effects of disturbed perceptual abilities, e.g., hemianopsia, one-sided blindness Effects of neurologic illness or trauma	Does not look toward affected side Consistent inattention to stimuli on affected side Leaves food on plate on the affected side Inadequate self-care, positioning, and/or safety precautions in regard to affected side

Other Related Nursing Diagnoses

ACTUAL	RISK/WELLNESS
Activity intolerance (see Chapter 16) Anxiety Body image disturbance Diversional activity deficit Dysreflexia Fear Impaired bed mobility Impaired home maintenance management	**Risk** Risk for aspiration Risk for autonomic dysreflexia Risk for caregiver role strain Risk for constipation Risk for trauma (see Chapter 20) Risk for impaired skin integrity (see Chapter 10)

Other Related Nursing Diagnoses

ACTUAL	RISK/WELLNESS
Impaired walking Hopelessness Impaired physical mobility (see Chapter 20) Reflex urinary incontinence Sensory perceptual alteration: tactile, visual Sexual dysfunction Social isolation Thought processes, altered Total incontinence Altered urinary elimination	**Wellness** Improving activity tolerance Maintaining effective communication

 ASSESSMENT VIDEO CRITICAL THINKING QUESTIONS

The Saunders *Physical Examination and Health Assessment* Video Series—NEUROLOGIC SYSTEM—will direct you to consider the following:

1. Which cranial nerve and sensory system assessments would you include in a neurologic screening examination?

2. Describe abnormal assessment findings that occur with lower motor neuron dysfunction of cranial nerve VII.

3. How would you modify your techniques when assessing an older adult's sensory system?

4. Which nursing diagnoses are appropriate for individuals with cranial nerve or sensory deficits?

5. Which motor system and reflex assessments would you include in a neurologic screening examination?

6. What abnormal findings may commonly be detected when assessing a child's gait?

7. What findings would you expect to see when assessing gait and balance in an older adult?

8. What techniques can you use to elicit deep tendon reflexes?

▼ Table 21-3   ABNORMALITIES IN CRANIAL NERVES

Nerve	Test	Abnormal Findings	Possible Causes
I: Olfactory	Identify familiar odors	Anosmia	Upper respiratory infection (temporary); tobacco or cocaine use; fracture of cribriform plate or ethmoid area; frontal lobe lesion; tumor in olfactory bulb or tract
II: Optic	Visual acuity	Defect or absent central vision	Congenital blindness, refractive error, acquired vision loss from numerous diseases (e.g., cerebrovascular accident, diabetes), trauma to globe or orbit (see discussion of cranial nerve III)
	Visual fields	Defect in peripheral vision, hemianopsia	
	Shine light in eye	Absent light reflex	
	Direct inspection	Papilledema	Increased intracranial pressure
		Optic atrophy	Glaucoma
		Retinal lesions	Diabetes
III: Oculomotor	Inspection	Dilated pupil, ptosis, eye turns out and slightly down	Paralysis in cranial nerve III from internal carotid aneurysm, tumor, inflammatory lesions, uncal herniation with increased intracranial pressure
	Extraocular muscle movement	Failure to move eye up, in, down	Ptosis from myasthenia gravis, oculomotor nerve palsy, Horner's syndrome
	Shine light in eye	Absent light reflex	Blindness, drug influence, increased intracranial pressure, CNS injury, circulatory arrest, CNS syphilis
IV: Trochlear	Extraocular muscle movement	Failure to turn eye down or out	Fracture of orbit, brain stem tumor
V: Trigeminal	Superficial touch—three divisions	Absent touch and pain, paresthesias	Trauma, tumor, pressure from aneurysm, inflammation, sequelae of alcohol injection for trigeminal neuralgia
	Corneal reflex	No blink	
	Clench teeth	Weakness of masseter or temporalis muscles	Unilateral weakness with cranial nerve V lesion; bilateral weakness with upper or lower motor neuron disorder
VI: Abducens	Extraocular muscle movement to right and left sides	Failure to move laterally, diplopia on lateral gaze	Brain stem tumor or trauma, fracture of orbit

Table 21-3   ABNORMALITIES IN CRANIAL NERVES *Continued*

Nerve	Test	Abnormal Findings	Possible Causes
VII: Facial	Wrinkle forehead, close eyes tightly	Absent or asymmetric facial movement	Bell's palsy (lower motor neuron lesion) causes paralysis of entire half of face
	Smile, puff cheeks		
	Identify tastes	Loss of taste	Upper motor neuron lesions (cerebrovascular accident, tumor, inflammatory) cause paralysis of lower half of face, leaving forehead intact
			Other lower motor neuron causes of paralysis: swelling from ear or meningeal infections
VIII: Acoustic	Hearing acuity	Decrease or loss of hearing	Inflammation, occluded ear canal, otosclerosis, presbycusis, drug toxicity, tumor
IX: Glossopharyngeal	Gag reflex	See cranial nerve X	
X: Vagus	Phonates "ahh"	Uvula deviates to side	Brain stem tumor, neck injury, cranial nerve X lesion
	Gag reflex	No gag reflex	Vocal cord weakness
	Note voice quality	Hoarse or brassy	Soft palate weakness
		Nasal twang	Unilateral cranial nerve X lesion
		Husky	
	Note swallowing	Dysphagia, fluids regurgitate through nose	Bilateral cranial nerve X lesion
XI: Spinal accessory	Turn head, shrug shoulders against resistance	Absent movement of sternomastoid or trapezius muscles	Neck injury, torticollis
XII: Hypoglossal	Protrude tongue	Deviates to side	Lower motor neuron lesion
	Wiggle tongue from side to side	Slowed rate of movement	Bilateral upper motor neuron lesion

 Table 21-4   ABNORMALITIES IN MUSCLE TONE

Condition	Description	Associated With
Flaccidity	Decreased muscle tone or hypotonia; muscle feels limp, soft, and flabby; muscle is weak and easily fatigued	Lower motor neuron injury (peripheral neuritis, poliomyelitis, Guillain-Barré syndrome). Early cerebrovascular accident and spinal cord injury are flaccid at first.
Spasticity	Increased tone; increased resistance to passive lengthening; then may suddenly give way (clasp-knife phenomenon)	Injury to corticospinal motor tract, e.g., paralysis with cerebrovascular accident (chronic stage)
Rigidity	Constant state of resistance; resists passive movement in any direction; dystonia	Injury to extrapyramidal motor tracts, e.g., parkinsonism
Cogwheel rigidity	Type of rigidity in which the increased tone is released by degrees during passive range of motion so it feels like small regular jerks	Parkinsonism

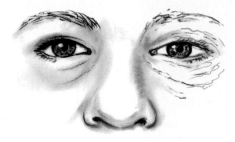

Table 21-5 ABNORMALITIES IN MUSCLE MOVEMENT

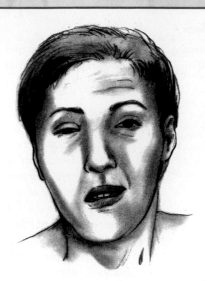

Paralysis

Decreased or loss of motor power due to problem with motor nerve or muscle fibers. Causes: acute—trauma, spinal cord injury, brain attack, poliomyelitis, polyneuritis, Bell's palsy; chronic—muscular dystrophy, diabetic neuropathy, multiple sclerosis; episodic—myasthenia gravis.

Patterns of paralysis: *hemiplegia*—spastic or flaccid paralysis of one side (right or left) of body and extremities; *paraplegia*—symmetric paralysis of both lower extremities; *quadriplegia*—paralysis in all four extremities; *paresis*—weakness of muscles rather than paralysis.

Fasciculation

Rapid, continuous twitching of resting muscle or part of muscle, without movement of limb, that can be seen or palpated. Types: fine—occurs with lower motor neuron disease, associated with atrophy and weakness; coarse—occurs with cold exposure or fatigue and is not significant.

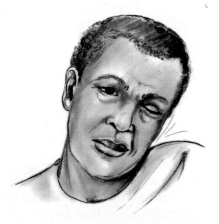

Tic

Repetitive twitching of a muscle group at inappropriate times, e.g., wink, grimace, head movement, shoulder shrug; due to a neurologic cause, e.g., tardive dyskinesias; emotional cause; or may be under voluntary control.

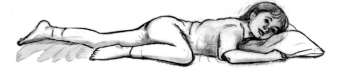

Myoclonus

Rapid, sudden jerk or a short series of jerks at fairly regular intervals. A hiccup is a myoclonus of diaphragm. Single myoclonic arm or leg jerk is normal when the person is falling asleep; myoclonic jerks are severe with grand mal seizures.

Tremor

Involuntary contraction of opposing muscle groups. Results in rhythmic, back-and-forth movement of one or more joints. May occur at rest or with voluntary movement. All tremors disappear while sleeping. Tremors may be slow (3 to 6 per second) or rapid (10 to 20 per second).

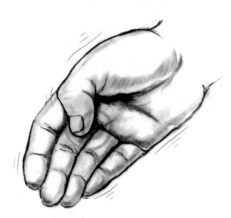

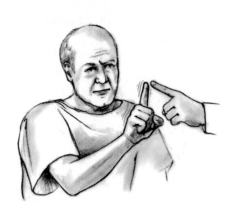

Rest Tremor

Coarse and slow (3 to 6 per second); partly or completely disappears with voluntary movement, e.g., "pill rolling" tremor of parkinsonism, with thumb and opposing fingers.

Intention Tremor

Rate varies; worse with voluntary movement. Occurs with cerebellar disease and multiple sclerosis.

Essential tremor (familial)—a type of intention tremor; most common tremor with older people. Benign (no associated disease) but causes emotional stress in business or social situations. Improves with the administration of sedatives, propranolol, alcohol, but use of alcohol is discouraged because of the risk of addiction.

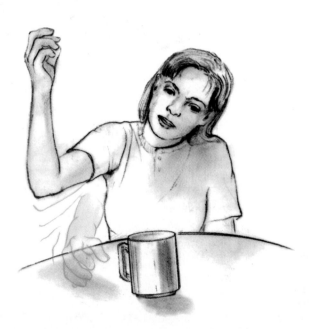

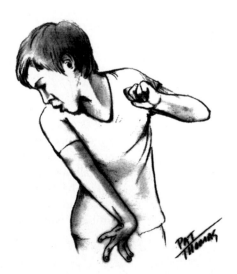

Chorea

Sudden, rapid, jerky, purposeless movement involving limbs, trunk, or face.

Occurs at irregular intervals, not rhythmic or repetitive, more convulsive than a tic. Some are spontaneous, and some are initiated; all are accentuated by voluntary acts. Disappears with sleep. Common with Sydenham's and Huntington's disease.

Athetosis

Slow, twisting, writhing, continuous movement, resembling a snake or worm. Involves distal part of limb more than the proximal part. Occurs with cerebral palsy. Disappears with sleep. "Athetoid" hand—Some fingers are flexed and some are extended.

Table 21–6 ABNORMAL GAITS

Type	Characteristic Appearance	Possible Causes
Spastic hemiparesis 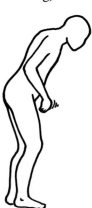	Arm is immobile against the body, with flexion of the shoulder, elbow, wrist, fingers, and adduction of shoulder. The leg is stiff and extended and circumducts with each step (drags toe in a semicircle)	Upper motor neuron lesion of the corticospinal tract, e.g., cerebrovascular accident, trauma
Cerebellar ataxia 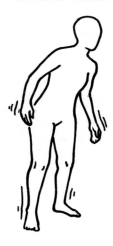	Staggering, wide-based gait; difficulty with turns; uncoordinated movement with positive Romberg sign	Alcohol or barbiturate effect on cerebellum; cerebellar tumor; multiple sclerosis
Parkinsonian (festinating)	Posture is stooped; trunk is pitched forward; elbows, hips, and knees are flexed. Steps are short and shuffling. Hesitation to begin walking, and difficult to stop suddenly. The person holds the body rigid. Walks and turns body as one fixed unit. Difficulty with any change in direction.	Parkinsonism

Table 21-6   ABNORMAL GAITS *Continued*

Type	Characteristic Appearance	Possible causes
Scissors	Knees cross or are in contact, like holding an orange between the thighs. The person uses short steps, and walking requires effort	Paraparesis of legs, multiple sclerosis
Steppage or foot-drop	Slapping quality—looks as if walking up stairs and finds no stair there. Lifts knee and foot high and slaps it down hard and flat to compensate for footdrop	Weakness of peroneal and anterior tibial muscles; due to lower motor neuron lesion at the spinal cord, e.g., poliomyelitis, Charcot-Marie-Tooth disease
Waddling	Weak hip muscles—when the person takes a step, the opposite hip drops, which allows compensatory lateral movement of pelvis. Often, the person also has marked lumbar lordosis and a protruding abdomen	Hip girdle muscle weakness due to muscular dystrophy, dislocation of hips

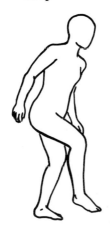
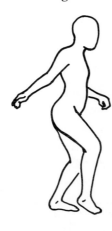

Table continued on following page

▼ Table 21–6   ABNORMAL GAITS *Continued*

Type	Characteristic Appearance	Possible Causes
Short leg	Leg length discrepancy >2.5 cm (1 in). Vertical telescoping of affected side, which dips as the person walks. Appearance of gait varies depending on amount of accompanying muscle dysfunction	Congenital dislocated hip; acquired shortening due to disease, trauma

▼ Table 21–7   CHARACTERISTICS OF UPPER AND LOWER MOTOR NEURON LESIONS

	Upper Motor Neuron Lesion	Lower Motor Neuron Lesion
Weakness/paralysis	In muscles corresponding to distribution of damage in pyramidal tract lesion; usually in hand grip, arm extensors, leg flexors	In specific muscles served by damaged spinal segment, ventral root, or peripheral nerve
Location	Descending motor pathways that originate in the motor areas of cerebral cortex and carry impulses to the anterior horn cells of the spinal cord	Nerve cells that originate in the anterior horn of spinal cord or in brain stem, and carry impulses by the spinal nerves or cranial nerves to the muscles, the "final common pathway"
Example	Brain attack or cerebrovascular accident	Poliomyelitis, herniated intervertebral disc
Muscle tone	Increased tone; spasticity	Loss of tone, flaccidity
Bulk	May have some atrophy from disuse; otherwise normal	Atrophy (wasting), may be marked
Abnormal movements	None	Fasciculations
Reflexes	Hyperreflexia, ankle clonus; diminished or absent superficial abdominal reflexes; positive Babinski's sign	Hyporeflexia or areflexia; no Babinski's sign, no pathologic reflexes
Possible nursing diagnoses	Risk for contractures; impaired physical mobility	Impaired physical mobility

Table 21–8   COMMON PATTERNS OF MOTOR SYSTEM DYSFUNCTION

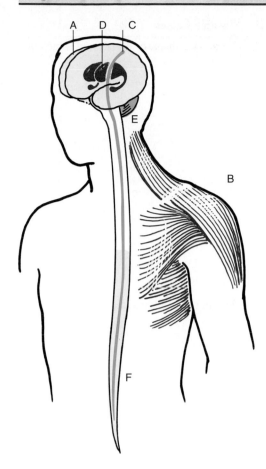

A—Cerebral palsy. Mixed group of paralytic neuromotor disorders of infancy and childhood; due to damage to cerebral cortex caused by a developmental defect, intrauterine meningitis or encephalitis, birth trauma, anoxia, or kernicterus.

B—Muscular dystrophy. Chronic, progressive wasting of skeletal musculature, which produces weakness, contractures, and in severe cases, respiratory dysfunction and death. Onset of symptoms occurs in childhood. Many types exist; the most severe is Duchenne's dystrophy, characterized by the waddling gait described in Table 21–6.

C—Hemiplegia. Damage to corticospinal tract. Initially flaccid when the lesion is acute; later, the muscles become spastic, and abnormal reflexes appear. Characteristic posture: arm—shoulder adducted, elbow flexed, wrist pronated; leg extended; face—weakness only in lower muscles. Hyperreflexia and possible clonus occur on the involved side; loss of corneal, abdominal, and cremasteric reflexes; positive Babinski's and Hoffman's reflexes.

D—Parkinsonism. Defect of extrapyramidal tracts, in the region of the basal ganglia, with loss of the neurotransmitter dopamine. Classic triad of symptoms: tremor, rigidity, akinesia. Also slower monotonous speech and diminutive writing. Body tends to stay immobile; facial expression is flat, staring, expressionless; excessive salivation occurs; reduced eye blinking. Posture is stooped; equilibrium is impaired; loses balance easily; gait is described in Table 21–6. Parkinsonian tremor; cogwheel rigidity on passive range of motion.

E—Cerebellar. A lesion in one hemisphere produces motor abnormalities on the ipsilateral side. Characterized by ataxia, lurching forward of affected side while walking, rapid alternating movements are slow and arrhythmic, finger-to-nose test reveals ataxia and tremor with overshoot or undershoot, and eyes display coarse nystagmus.

F—Paraplegia. Caused by spinal cord injury. A severe injury or complete transection initially produces "spinal shock," which is defined as no movement or reflex activity below the level of the lesion. Gradually, deep tendon reflexes reappear and become increased, flexor spasms of legs occur; and finally, extensor spasms of legs occur; these spasms lead to prevailing extensor tone.

Table 21–9   COMMON PATTERNS OF SENSORY LOSS

Type	Characteristics	Possible Causes
Peripheral neuropathy 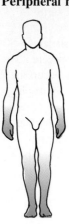	Loss of sensation involves all modalities. Loss is most severe distally (feet and hands); response improves as stimulus is moved proximally (glove-and-stocking anesthesia). Anesthesia zone gradually merges into a hypoesthesia zone, then gradually becomes normal.	Metabolic disease, nutritional deficiency
Individual nerves or roots 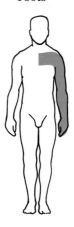	Decrease or loss of all sensory modalities. Area of sensory loss corresponds to distribution of the involved nerve.	Trauma, vascular occlusion
Spinal cord hemisection (Brown-Séquard syndrome) 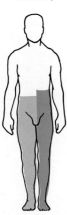	Loss of pain and temperature, contralateral side, starting one to two segments below the level of the lesion. Loss of vibration and position discrimination on the ipsilateral side, below the level of the lesion.	Meningioma, neurofibroma, cervical spondylosis, multiple sclerosis

Table 21–9 COMMON PATTERNS OF SENSORY LOSS *Continued*

Type	Characteristics	Possible Causes
Complete transection of the spinal cord 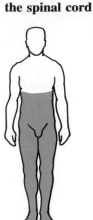	Complete loss of *all* sensory modalities below the level of the lesion. Condition is associated with motor paralysis and loss of sphincter control.	Trauma, demyelinating disorders, tumor
Thalamus 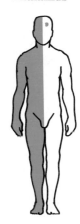	Loss of *all* sensory modalities on the face, arm, and leg on the side contralateral to the lesion.	Vascular occlusion
Cortex 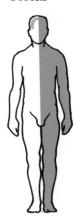	Since pain, vibration, and crude touch are mediated by thalamus, little loss of these sensory functions occurs with a cortex lesion. Loss of discrimination occurs on the contralateral side. Loss of graphesthesia, stereognosis, recognition of shapes and weights, finger finding.	Cerebral cortex, parietal lobe lesion

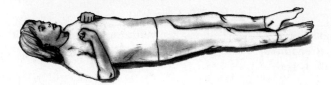

Table 21–10   ABNORMAL POSTURES

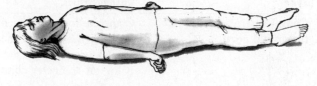

Decorticate Rigidity

Upper extremities—flexion of arm, wrist, and fingers; adduction of arm. Lower extremities—extension, internal rotation, plantar flexion. This indicates hemispheric lesion of cerebral cortex.

Decerebrate Rigidity

Upper extremities stiffly extended, adducted, internal rotation, palms pronated. Lower extremities stiffly extended, plantar flexion; teeth clenched; hyperextended back. More ominous than decorticate rigidity; indicates lesion in brain stem at midbrain or upper pons.

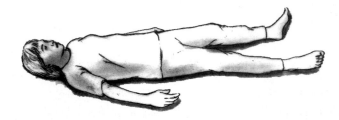

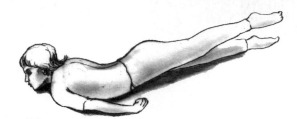

Flaccid Quadriplegia

Complete loss of muscle tone and paralysis of all four extremities, indicating completely nonfunctional brain stem.

Opisthotonos

Prolonged arching of the back, with head and heels bent backward. This indicates meningeal irritation.

Table 21–11   PATHOLOGIC REFLEXES

Reflex	Method of Testing	Abnormal Response (Reflex Is Present)	Indications
Babinski	Stroke lateral aspect and across ball of foot	Extension of great toe, fanning of toes	Corticospinal (pyramidal) tract disease
Oppenheim	Stroke anterior medial tibial muscle	Same as above	Same
Gordon	Firmly squeeze calf muscles	Same as above	Same
Hoffman	Flick distal phalanx of middle or index finger	Clawing of fingers and thumb	Same
Kernig	Raise leg straight or flex thigh on abdomen, then extend knee	Resistance to straightening, pain down posterior thigh	Meningeal irritation
Brudzinski	Flex chin on chest, watch hips and knees	Resistance and pain in neck, with flexion of hips and knees	Meningeal irritation

Table 21-12   FRONTAL RELEASE SIGNS

Reflex

Snout

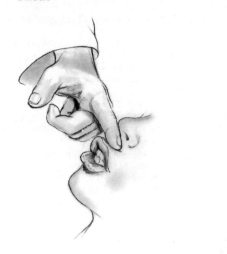

Method of Testing
Gently percuss oral region
Abnormal Response (Reflex Is Present)
Puckers lips
Indications
Frontal lobe disease, cerebral degenerative disease (Alzheimer's)

Sucking

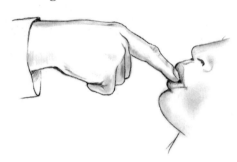

Method of Testing
Touch oral region
Abnormal Response (Reflex Is Present)
Sucking movement of lips, tongue, jaw
Indications
Same as for snout reflex

Grasp

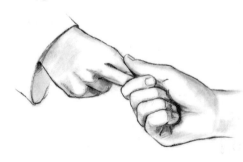

Method of Testing
Touch palm with your finger
Abnormal Response (Reflex Is Present)
Uncontrolled, forced grasping (grasp is usually last of these signs to appear, so its presence indicates severe disease)
Indications
Same as for snout reflex

Bibliography

Barker S, Grant A, Hodnicki DR: Parkinson's disease—A holistic approach. Am J Nurs 98(11):48A–48H, Nov 1998.

Beatty WW, Scott JG, Moreland VJ, Rankin EJ: Head injury effects on a new measure of remote memory: The famous tunes test. J Head Trauma Rehabil 10(3):59–66, June 1995.

Benson C, Lusardi P: Neurologic antecedents to patient falls. J Neurosci Nurs 27(6):331–337, Dec 1995.

Bernstein S, Heimler R, Sasidharan P: Approaching the management of the neonatal intensive care unit graduate through history and physical assessment. Pediatr Clin North Am 45(1):79–105, Feb 1998.

Beveridge DL: Back to basics. Axone 17(1):6–8, Sep 1995.

Callahan SW: Arteriovenous malformations. Am J Nurs 96(12):30–31, Dec 1996.

Cammermeyer M, Prendergast V: Profiles of cognitive functioning in subjects with neurological disorders. J Neurosci Nurs 29(3):163–169, June 1997.

Carey BE: Physical assessment of the newborn: Neurologic assessment. Mother-Baby J 1(3):33–38, May 1996.

Carter AB: The neurologic aspects of aging. In Rossman I (Ed): Clinical Geriatrics. Philadelphia, J.B. Lippincott Company, 1986.

Chiocca EM: Meningococcal meningitis. Am J Nurs 95(12):25, Dec 1995.

Criger N, Forbes W: Assessing neurologic function in older patients. Am J Nurs 97(3):37–40, March 1997.

DeLorenzo RA: Demystifying the neurological examination. JEMS: J Emerg Med Serv 22(9):68–78, Sep 1997.

Duffy JD: The neurology of alcoholic denial: Implications for assessment and treatment. Can J Psychiatry 40(5):257–263, June 1995.

Fenichel GM: Clinical Pediatric Neurology, 3rd ed. Philadelphia, W.B. Saunders Company, 1996.

Frozena C: Multiple sclerosis. Am J Nurs 97(11):48–49, Nov 1997.

Gallegos SJ, Michalec DL: Neurologic assessment of the orthopaedic patient. Orthop Nurs 15(5):23–29, Sep–Oct 1996.

Gawande A: The pain perplex. The New Yorker 74:86–94, Sep 21, 1998.

Goldsmith C: Parkinson's disease. Am J Nurs 99(2):46–47, Feb 1999.

Gross SB: Transient ischemic attacks (TIA): Current issues in diagnosis and management. J Am Acad Nurs Pract 7(7):329–338, July 1995.

Hajek VE, Gagnon S, Ruderman JE: Cognitive and functional assessments of stroke patients: An analysis of their relation. Arch Phys Med Rehabil 78(12):1331–1337, Dec 1997.

Halper J, Holland N: Meeting the challenge of multiple sclerosis. Part I. Am J Nurs 98(10):26–31, Oct 1998.

Halper J, Holland N: Meeting the challenge of multiple sclerosis. Part II. Am J Nurs 98(11):39–45, Nov 1998.

Harrahill M: Glasgow Coma Scale: A quick review. J Emerg Nurs 22(1):81–83, Feb 1996.

Harrahill M: Upper extremity nerve assessment: A quick review. J Emerg Nurs 21(4):360–362, Aug 1995.

Herf C, Nichols J, Fruh S: Meningococcal disease: Recognition, treatment, and prevention. Nurs Pract 23(8):30–46, Aug 1998.

Hickey JV: The clinical practice of neurological and neurosurgical nursing, 4th ed. Philadelphia, J.B. Lippincott Company, 1997.

Hudak CM, Gallo BM: Quick review of neurodiagnostic testing. Am J Nurs 97(7):16cc–16ff, July 1997.

Jaweed MM, Monga TN: Neuromuscular function assessment. Phys Med Rehabil 11(1):205–237, Feb 1997.

Juarez VJ, Lyons M: Interrater reliability of the Glasgow Coma Scale. J Neurosci Nurs 27(5):283–286, Oct 1995.

Kelly M: Transient ischemic attack. Am J Nurs 95(9):42–43, Sep 1995.

Kongable GL: Code stroke: Using t-PA to prevent ischemic brain injury. Am J Nurs 97(11):16BB–16HH, Nov 1997.

Kuhlman KA, Hennessey WJ: Sensitivity and specificity of carpal tunnel syndrome signs. Am J Phys Med Rehabil 76(6):451–457, Nov–Dec 1997.

Lemke DM: Defining assessment parameters in dual injuries: Spinal cord injury and traumatic brain injury. SCI Nurs 12(2):40–47, June 1995.

Nance PW, Hoy CSG: Assessment of the autonomic nervous system. Phys Med Rehabil State Art Rev 10(1):15–35, Feb 1996.

Neuman J: Certified neuroscience registered nurses' use of neuroassessment tools in their practice: Perceived strengths and weaknesses of these tools. Prairie-Rose 64(4):4–6, Dec 1995–Feb 1996.

Newton HB: Common neurologic complications of HIV-1 infection and AIDS. Am Fam Physician 51(2):387–398, Feb 1, 1995.

Nolan MF, Brownlee HJ: Neurologic examination: A strategy to enhance the diagnostic yield. Consultant 36(2):323–330, Feb 1996.

O'Hanlon-Nichols T: Intracranial tumors. Am J Nurs 96(4):38–39, Apr 1996.

Pieper DR, Valadka AB, Marsh C: Surgical management of patients with severe head injuries. AORN J 63(5):854–864, May 1996.

Prerssler JL, Helworth JT: Newborn neurologic screening using NBAS reflexes. Neonat Network 16(6):33–46, Sep 1997.

Pressman EK, Zeidman SM, Summers L: Comprehensive assessment of the neurologic system. J Nurse Midwifery 40(2):163–171, Mar–Apr 1995.

Price RW: Neurological complications of HIV infection. Lancet 348: 445–452, Aug 17, 1996.

Schaff D: Common questions about transient ischemic attacks. Am J Nurs 97(10):16BB–16DD, Oct 1997.

Schwartz B, Klima RR: Vibration sensation: Measurement techniques and applications. Crit Rev Phys Rehabil Med 7(2):113–130, 1995.

Shpritz DW: Understanding neurological assessment. J Post Anesth Nurs 10(4):216–219, Aug 1995.

Tapper VJ: Pathophysiology, assessment, and treatment of Parkinson's disease. Nurs Pract 22(7):76–95, July 1997.

Waxman SG: Correlative Neuroanatomy, 23rd ed. Stamford, CT, Appleton & Lange, 1996.

Wooten C: The top 10 ways to detect deteriorating central neurological status. J Trauma Nurs 3(1):25–27, Jan–Mar 1996.

CHAPTER TWENTY TWO

Male Genitalia

THE MALE GENITALIA

The male genital structures include the penis and scrotum externally and the testis, epididymis, and vas deferens internally. Glandular structures accessory to the genital organs (the prostate, seminal vesicles, and bulbo-urethral glands) are discussed in Chapter 23.

Penis

The **penis** is composed of three cylindrical columns of erectile tissue: the two corpora cavernosa on the dorsal side and the corpus spongiosum ventrally (Fig. 22–1). At the distal end of the shaft, the corpus spongiosum expands into a cone of erectile tissue, the **glans.** The shoulder where the glans joins the shaft is the **corona.** The **urethra** transverses the corpus spongiosum, and its meatus forms a slit at the glans tip. Over the glans, the skin folds in and back on itself forming a hood or flap. This is the **foreskin** or **prepuce.** Often, it is surgically removed shortly after birth by circumcision. The **frenulum** is a fold of the foreskin extending from the urethral meatus ventrally.

Scrotum

The **scrotum** is a loose protective sac, which is a continuation of the abdominal wall (Fig. 22–2). After adolescence, the scrotal skin is deeply pigmented and has large sebaceous follicles. The scrotal wall consists of thin skin lying in folds, or **rugae,** and the underlying cremaster muscle. The **cremaster muscle** controls the size of the scrotum by responding to ambient temperature. This is to keep the testes at 3° C below abdominal temperature, the best temperature for producing sperm. When it is cold, the muscle contracts, raising the sac and bringing the testes closer to the body to absorb heat necessary for sperm viability. As a result, the scrotal skin looks corrugated. When it is warmer, the muscle relaxes, the scrotum lowers, and the skin looks smoother.

Inside, a septum separates the sac into two halves. In each scrotal half is a **testis,** which produces sperm. The testis has a solid oval shape, which is compressed laterally and measures 4 to 5 cm long by 3 cm wide in the adult. The testis is suspended vertically by the spermatic cord. The left testis is lower than the right because the left spermatic cord is longer. Each testis is covered by a

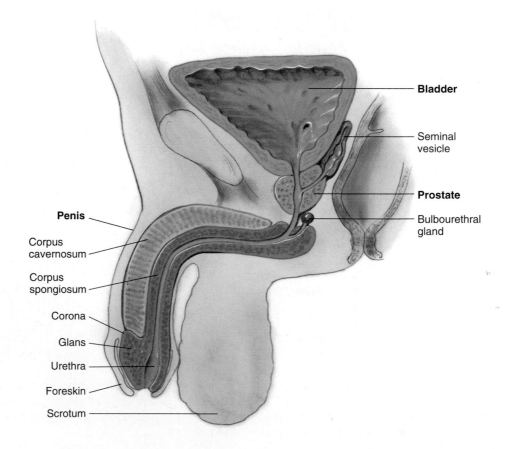

Penis

Corpus cavernosum

Corpus spongiosum

Corona

Glans

Urethra

Foreskin

Scrotum

Bladder

Seminal vesicle

Prostate

Bulbourethral gland

22–1

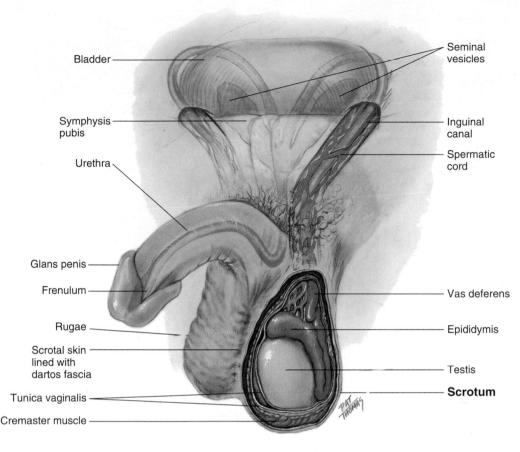

Bladder

Seminal vesicles

Symphysis pubis

Inguinal canal

Spermatic cord

Urethra

Glans penis

Frenulum

Vas deferens

Rugae

Epididymis

Scrotal skin lined with dartos fascia

Testis

Tunica vaginalis

Scrotum

Cremaster muscle

22–2

MALE GENITAL STRUCTURES

double-layered membrane, the tunica vaginalis, which separates it from the scrotal wall. The two layers are lubricated by fluid so that the testis can slide a little within the scrotum; this helps prevent injury.

Sperm are transported along a series of ducts. First, the testis is capped by the **epididymis,** which is a markedly coiled duct system and the main storage site of sperm. It is a comma-shaped structure, curved over the top and the posterior surface of the testis. Occasionally (in 6 to 7 percent of males), the epididymis is anterior to the testis.

The lower part of the epididymis is continuous with a muscular duct, the **vas deferens.** This duct approximates with other vessels (arteries and veins, lymphatics, nerves) to form the **spermatic cord.** The spermatic cord ascends along the posterior border of the testis and runs through the tunnel of the inguinal canal into the abdomen. Here, the vas deferens continues back and down behind the bladder, where it joins the duct of the seminal vesicle to form the **ejaculatory duct.** This duct empties into the urethra.

The **lymphatics** of the penis and scrotal surface drain into the inguinal lymph nodes, whereas those of the testes drain into the abdomen. Abdominal lymph nodes are inaccessible to clinical examination.

Inguinal Area

The **inguinal area,** or groin, is the juncture of the lower abdominal wall and the thigh (Fig. 22–3). Its diagonal borders are the anterior superior iliac spine and the symphysis pubis. Between these landmarks lies the **inguinal ligament** (Poupart's ligament). Superior to the ligament lies the **inguinal canal,** a narrow tunnel passing obliquely between layers of abdominal muscle. It is 4 to 6 cm long in the adult. Its openings are an internal ring, located 1 to 2 cm above the midpoint of the inguinal ligament, and an external ring, located just above and lateral to the pubis.

Inferior to the inguinal ligament is the **femoral canal.** It is a potential space located 3 cm medial to and parallel with the femoral artery. You can use the artery as a landmark to find this space.

Knowledge of these anatomic areas in the groin is useful because they are potential sites for a hernia, which is a loop of bowel protruding through a weak spot in the musculature.

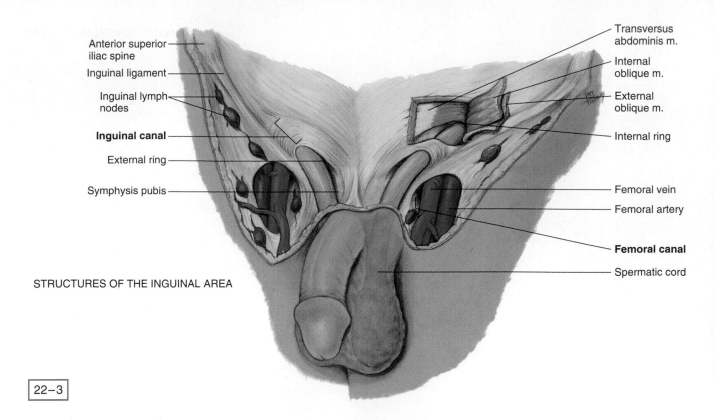

Anterior superior
iliac spine

Inguinal ligament

Inguinal lymph
nodes

Inguinal canal

External ring

Symphysis pubis

Transversus
abdominis m.

Internal
oblique m.

External
oblique m.

Internal ring

Femoral vein

Femoral artery

Femoral canal

Spermatic cord

STRUCTURES OF THE INGUINAL AREA

22-3

 DEVELOPMENTAL CONSIDERATIONS

Infants

Prenatally, the testes develop in the abdominal cavity near the kidneys. During the later months of gestation the testes migrate, pushing the abdominal wall in front of them and dragging the vas deferens, the blood vessels, and nerves behind. The testes descend along the inguinal canal into the scrotum before birth. At birth, each testis measures 1.5 to 2 cm long and 1 cm wide. Only a slight increase in size occurs during the prepubertal years.

Adolescents

Puberty begins sometime between the ages of 9½ and 13½. The first sign is enlargement of the testes. Next, pubic hair appears, then penis size increases. The stages of development are documented in Tanner's sexual maturity ratings (SMR) (Table 22-1).

The complete change in development from a preadolescent to an adult takes around 3 years, although the normal range is 2 to 5 years (Fig. 22-4). The chart shown in Figure 22-4 is useful in teaching a boy the expected sequence of events and in reassuring him about the wide range of normal ages when these events are experienced.

Although Tanner's studies were based on data from post World War II British youth, Tanner's results are corroborated by the U.S. Health Examination Survey, which studied close to 7000 youths from 1966 to 1970 (Harlan et al., 1979). This study found concordance between Tanner's stages for pubic hair and genitalia. It also found that sexual characteristics developed similarly for

black and white boys, and that development was not influenced by socioeconomic status.

Adults and Aging Adults

The level of sexual development at the end of puberty remains constant through young and middle adulthood, with no further genital growth and no change in circulating sex hormone.

The male does not experience a definite end to fertility as the female does. Around age 40 years, the production of sperm begins to decrease, although it continues into the 80s and 90s. After age 55 to 60 years, testosterone production declines. This decline proceeds very gradually

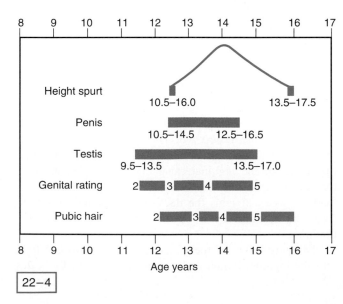

22-4

Table 22–1 • Sex Maturity Ratings (SMR) in Boys

Developmental Stage	Pubic Hair	Penis	Scrotum
1	No pubic hair. Fine body hair on abdomen (vellus hair) continues over pubic area	Preadolescent, size, and proportion the same as during childhood	Preadolescent, size, and proportion the same as during childhood
2	Few straight slightly darker hairs at base of penis. Hair is long and downy	Little or no enlargement	Testes and scrotum begin to enlarge. Scrotal skin reddens and changes in texture
3	Sparse growth over entire pubis. Hair darker, coarser, and curly	Penis begins to enlarge, especially in length	Further enlarged
4	Thick growth over pubic area but not on thighs. Hair coarse and curly as in adult	Penis grows in length and diameter, with development of glans	Testes almost fully grown, scrotum darker
5	Growth spread over medial thighs, although not yet up toward umbilicus*	Adult size and shape	Adult size and shape

*After puberty, pubic hair growth continues until the mid-20s, extending up the abdomen toward the umbilicus.
Adapted from Tanner JM: Growth at Adolescence. Oxford, England, Blackwell Scientific Publications, 1962.

so that resulting physical changes are not evident until later in life. Aging changes also are due to decreased muscle tone, decreased subcutaneous fat, and decreased cellular metabolism.

In the aging male, the amount of pubic hair decreases, and the remaining hair turns gray. Penis size decreases. Due to decreased tone of the dartos muscle, the scrotal contents hang lower, the rugae decrease, and the scrotum looks pendulous. The testes decrease in size and are less firm to palpation. Increased connective tissue is present in the tubules, so these become thickened and produce less sperm.

In general, declining testosterone production leaves the older male with a slower and less intense sexual response. Although a wide range of individual differences can occur, the older male may find that an erection takes longer to develop and that it is less full or firm. Once obtained, the erection may be maintained for longer periods without ejaculation. Ejaculation is shorter and less forceful, and the volume of seminal fluid is less than when the man was younger. After ejaculation, rapid detumescence (return to the flaccid state) occurs, especially after 60 years of age. This occurs in a few seconds as compared with minutes or hours in the younger male. The refractory state (when the male is physiologically unable to ejaculate) lasts longer, from 12 to 24 hours as compared with 2 minutes in the younger male.

Sexual Expression in Later Life. Chronologic age by itself should not mean a halt in sexual activity. The above-mentioned physical changes need not interfere with the libido and pleasure from sexual intercourse. The older male is capable of sexual function as long as he is in reasonably good health and has an interested, willing partner. Even chronic illness does not mean a complete end to sexual desire or activity.

The danger is in the male misinterpreting normal age changes as a sexual failure. Once this idea occurs, it may demoralize the man and place undue emphasis on performance rather than on pleasure. In the absence of disease, a withdrawal from sexual activity may be due to

- Loss of spouse
- Depression

- Preoccupation with work
- Marital or family conflict
- Side effects of medications such as antihypertensives, psychotropics, antidepressants, antispasmodics, sedatives, tranquilizers or narcotics, and estrogens
- Heavy use of alcohol
- Lack of privacy (living with adult children or in a nursing home)
- Economic or emotional stress
- Poor nutrition
- Fatigue

TRANSCULTURAL CONSIDERATIONS

Circumcision. Occasionally, during pregnancy or the immediate neonatal period, parents will ask you about whether or not to circumcise the male infant. Indications for circumcision include cultural reasons, the prevention of phimosis and inflammation of the glans penis and foreskin, decreasing the incidence of cancer of the penis, and slightly decreasing the incidence of urinary tract infections in infancy. However, there is no difference in risk of contracting sexually transmitted diseases (STDs) between circumcised and uncircumcised men (Laumann, Masi, and Zuckerman, 1997). Circumcision carries a very small but possible risk of complications, such as sepsis, amputation of the distal edge of the glans, removal of an excessive amount of foreskin, urethrocutaneous fistula (Behrman, 1996), and significant pain, about which the parents should know.

The decision to circumcise is culturally based. In the United States, 70 to 80 percent of newborn males are circumcised, while in Canada, Great Britain, Australia, and Sweden, circumcision is considered unnecessary, and less than 20 percent of newborn boys are circumcised (Cornell, 1997). Some groups, such as Jews and Muslims, practice circumcision as part of their religious value system. Other groups, such as Native Americans and Hispanics, have no tradition to practice circumcision. However, many parents in the United States who are not part of these groups also believe in circumcision because it conforms to dominant cultural values.

SUBJECTIVE DATA

1. Frequency, urgency, and nocturia
2. Dysuria
3. Hesitancy and straining
4. Urine color
5. Past genitourinary history

6. Penis—pain, lesion, discharge
7. Scrotum, self-care behaviors, lump
8. Sexual activity and contraceptive use
9. STD contact

Examiner Asks	Rationale
1 **Frequency, urgency, and nocturia.** Urinating more often than usual?	**Frequency.** Average adult voids five to six times per day, varying with fluid intake, individual habits. Polyuria—excessive quantity. Oliguria—diminished quantity, <400 ml/24 hours. **Urgency.** **Nocturia** occurs together with frequency and urgency in urinary tract disorders. Other origins: cardiovascular, habitual, diuretic medication.
• Feel as if you cannot wait to urinate? • Awaken during the night because you need to urinate? How often? Is this a recent change?	
2 **Dysuria.** Any pain or burning with urinating?	**Dysuria.** Burning is common with acute cystitis, prostatitis, urethritis.
3 **Hesitancy and straining.** Any trouble starting the urine stream? • Need to strain to start or maintain stream? • Any change in force of stream: narrowing, becoming weaker? • Dribbling, such that you must stand closer to the toilet? • Afterward, do you still feel you need to urinate? • Ever had any urinary tract infections?	**Hesitancy.** Straining. Loss of force and decreased caliber. Terminal dribbling. Sense of residual urine. Recurrent episodes of acute cystitis. Above-mentioned symptoms (i.e., hesitancy, and so on) suggest progressive prostatic obstruction.
4 **Urine color.** Is the usual **urine** clear or discolored, cloudy, foul-smelling, bloody?	As in urinary tract infection. Hematuria—a danger sign that warrants further workup.
5 **Past genitourinary history.** Any difficulty controlling your urine?	True incontinence—loss of urine without warning. Urgency incontinence—sudden loss, as with acute cystitis. Stress incontinence—loss of urine with physical strain due to weakness of sphincters.
• Accidentally urinate when you sneeze, laugh, cough, or bear down?	
• Any **history** of kidney disease, kidney stones, flank pain, urinary tract infections, prostate trouble?	
6 **Penis.** Any problem with penis—**pain, lesions?** • Any **discharge?** How much? Has that increased or decreased since start? • The color? Any odor? Discharge associated with pain or with urination?	Urethral discharge occurs with infection.
7 **Scrotum, self-care behaviors.** Any problem with the scrotum or testicles? • Do you perform testicular self-examination? • Noticed any **lump or swelling** on testes? • Noted any change in size of the scrotum? • Noted any bulge or swelling in the scrotum? For how long? Ever been told you have a hernia? Any dragging, heavy feeling in scrotum?	**Self-care behaviors.** Possible hernia.
8 **Sexual activity and contraceptive use.** Are you in a relationship involving sexual intercourse now? • Are aspects of sex satisfactory to you and your partner?	Questions about **sexual activity** should be routine in review of body systems for these reasons:

Examiner Asks	Rationale

- Are you satisfied with the way you and your partner communicate about sex?
- Occasionally a man notices a change in ability to have an erection when aroused. Have you noticed any changes?*
- Do you and your partner use a contraceptive? Which method? Is this satisfactory? Any questions about this method?
- How many sexual partners have you had in the last 6 months?

- What is your sexual preference—relationship with a woman, a man, both?

9 **STD contact.** Any sexual contact with a partner having a sexually transmitted disease, such as gonorrhea, herpes, AIDS, chlamydia, venereal warts, syphilis?
- When was this contact? Did you get the disease?
- How was it treated? Any complications?
- Do you use condoms to help prevent STDs?
- Any questions or concerns about any of these diseases?

Rationale:
- Communicates that you accept individual's sexual activity and believe it is important
- Your comfort with discussion prompts person's interest and possibly relief that topic has been introduced
- Establishes a data base for comparison with any future sexual activities
- Provides opportunity to screen sexual problems
  Your questions should be objective and matter-of-fact.
  Gay and bisexual men need to feel acceptance to discuss their health concerns.

ADDITIONAL HISTORY FOR INFANTS AND CHILDREN

1 Does your child have any problem urinating? Urine stream look straight?
- Any pain with urinating, crying, or holding the genitals?
- Any urinary tract infection?

2 (If child older than 2 to 2½ years of age.) Has toilet training started? How is it progressing?
- Wet the bed at night? Is this a problem for child or for you (parents)? What have you done? How does the child feel about it?

3 Any problem with child's penis or scrotum: sores, swelling, discoloration?
- Told if his testes are descended?
- Ever had a hernia or hydrocele?
- Swelling in his scrotum during crying or coughing?

4 (Ask directly to preschooler or young school-age child.) Has anyone ever touched your penis or in between your legs and you did not want them to?
  Sometimes that happens to children and it's not okay. They should remember that they have not been bad. They should try to tell a big person about it. Can you tell me three different big people you trust who you could talk to?

Screen for sexual abuse. For prevention, teach the child that it's not okay for someone to look at or touch their private parts while telling them it's a secret. Naming three trusted adults will include someone outside the family—important, since most molestation is by a parent (Brown, 1997).

*At times, phrase your questions so that it is all right for the person to acknowledge a problem.

Examiner Asks	Rationale

ADDITIONAL HISTORY FOR PREADOLESCENTS AND ADOLESCENTS

Use the following questions regarding sexual growth and development and sexual behavior. First

- Ask questions that seem appropriate for boy's age but be aware that norms vary widely. When you are in doubt, it is better to ask too many questions than to omit something. Children obtain information, often misinformation, from the media and from peers at surprisingly early ages. You may be sure your information will be more thoughtful and accurate.
- Ask direct, matter-of-fact questions. Avoid sounding judgmental.
- Start with a *permission statement,* "Often boys your age experience . . ." This conveys that it is normal and all right to think or feel a certain way.
- Try the *ubiquity approach,* "When did you . . ." rather than "Do you . . ." This method is less threatening because it implies that the topic is normal and unexceptional.
- Do not be concerned if a boy will not discuss sexuality with you or respond to your offers for more information. He may not wish to let on that he needs or wants more information. You do well to "open the door." The adolescent may come back at a future time.

1 Around age 12 to 13 years, but sometimes earlier, boys start to change and grow around the penis and scrotum. What changes have you noticed?

Have you ever seen charts and pictures of normal growth patterns for boys? Let us go over these now.

Who can you talk to about your body changes and about sex information? How do these talks go? Do you think you get enough information? What about sex education classes at school? How about your parents? Is there a favorite teacher, nurse, doctor, minister, or counselor to whom you can talk?

2 Boys around age 12 to 13 years (SMR3) have a normal experience of fluid coming out of the penis at night, called nocturnal emissions, or "wet dreams." Have you had this?

An occasional boy confuses this with a sign of STD or feels guilty.

3 Teenage boys have other normal experiences and wonder if they are the only ones who ever had them, like having an erection at embarrassing times, having sexual fantasies, or masturbating. Also, a boy might have a thought about touching another boy's genitals and wonder if this thought means he might be homosexual. Would you like to talk about any of these things?

A boy may feel guilty about experiencing these things if not informed that they are normal.

4 Often boys your age have questions about sexual activity. What questions do you have? How about things like birth control, or STDs such as gonorrhea or herpes? Any questions about these?

- Are you dating? Someone steady? Have you had intercourse? Are you using birth control? What kind?

Assess level of knowledge. Many boys will not admit they need more knowledge.

Avoid the term "having sex." It is ambiguous, and teens can take it to mean anything from foreplay to intercourse.

- What kind of birth control did you use the *last* time you had intercourse?

This particular question often reveals that the teen is not using any method of birth control.

Examiner Asks	Rationale

5 Has a nurse or doctor ever taught you how to examine your own testicles to make sure they are healthy?

Assess knowledge of testicular self-examination.

6 Has anyone ever touched your genitals and you did not want them to? Another boy, or an adult, even a relative? Sometimes that happens to teenagers. They should remember it is not their fault. They should tell another adult about it.

ADDITIONAL HISTORY FOR THE AGING ADULT

1 Any difficulty urinating? Any hesitancy and straining? A weakened force of stream? Any dribbling? Or any incomplete emptying?

Early symptoms of enlarging prostate may be tolerated or ignored. Later symptoms are more dramatic: hematuria, urinary tract infection.

2 Do you need to get up at night to urinate? What medications are you taking? What fluids do you drink in the evening?

Nocturia may be due to diuretic medication, habit, or fluid ingestion 3 hours before bedtime, especially coffee and alcohol, which have a specific diuretic effect.

Also, fluid retention from mild heart failure or varicose veins produces nocturia; recumbency at night mobilizes fluid.

3 A man in his 70s, 80s, or 90s may notice changes in his sexual relationship or in his sexual response and wonder if it is normal. For example, it is normal for an erection to develop slowly at this age. This is not a sign of impotence, but a man might wonder if it is.

Excluding physical illness, an older man is fully capable of sexual function. But some men assume normal changes mean that they are "old men" and voluntarily withdraw from sexual activity. The older person is not reluctant to discuss sexual activity, and most welcome the opportunity.

Depressants to sexual desire and function include antihypertensives, sedatives, tranquilizers, estrogens, and alcohol. Alcohol decreases the sexual response even more dramatically in the older person.

OBJECTIVE DATA

Preparation

Position the male standing with undershorts down and appropriate draping. The examiner should be sitting. Alternatively, the male may be supine for the first part of the examination and stand to check for a hernia.

It is normal for a male to feel apprehensive about having his genitalia examined, especially by a female examiner. Younger adolescents usually have more anxiety than older adolescents. But any male may have difficulty

▶ ## Equipment Needed

Gloves—Wear gloves during every male genitalia examination

Occasionally: glass slide for urethral specimen

Materials for cytology

Flashlight

dissociating a necessary, matter-of-fact step in the physical examination from the feeling this is an invasion of his privacy. His concerns are similar to those experienced by the female during the examination of the genitalia: modesty, fear of pain, cold hands, negative judgment, or memory of previously uncomfortable examinations. Additionally, he may fear comparison to others, or fear having an erection during the examination and that this would be misinterpreted by the examiner.

This normal apprehension becomes manifested in different behaviors. Many act resigned and embarrassed and avoid eye contact. An occasional man will laugh and make jokes to cover embarrassment. Also, a man may refuse examination by a female and insist on a male examiner.

Take time to consider these feelings, as well as to explore your own. It is normal for you to feel embarrassed and apprehensive too. You may worry about your age, lack of clinical experience, causing pain, or even that your movements might "cause" an erection. Some examiners feel guilty when this occurs. You need to accept these feelings and work through them so that you can examine the male in a professional way. Discussing these concerns in a group with other beginning examiners works best. Your demeanor is important. Your unresolved discomfort magnifies any discomfort the man may have.

Your demeanor should be *confident* and relaxed, unhurried yet businesslike. Do not discuss genitourinary history or sexual practices while you are performing the examination. This may be perceived as judgmental. Use a firm deliberate touch, not a soft, stroking one. If an erection does occur, do *not* stop the examination or leave the room. This only focuses more attention on the erection and increases embarrassment. Reassure the male that this is only a normal physiologic response to touch, just as when the pupil constricts in response to bright light. Proceed with the rest of the examination.

▶ **Normal Range of Findings**   **Abnormal Findings**

PENIS

Inspect and palpate the penis
The skin normally looks wrinkled, hairless, and without lesions. The dorsal vein may be apparent (Fig. 22–5).

Inflammation.

Lesions: nodules, solitary ulcer (chancre), grouped vesicles or superficial ulcers, wartlike papules (see Table 22–2).

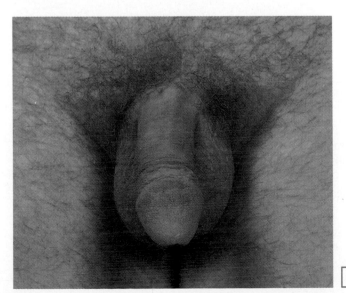

22–5

▶ Normal Range of Findings

Abnormal Findings

The glans looks smooth and without lesions. Ask the uncircumcised male to retract the foreskin, or you retract it. It should move easily. Some cheesy smegma may have collected under the foreskin. After inspection, slide the fore-skin back to the original position.

The urethral meatus is positioned just about centrally.

At the base of the penis, pubic hair distribution is consistent with age. Hair is without pest inhabitants.

Compress the glans anteroposteriorly between your thumb and forefinger (Fig. 22–6). The meatus edge should appear pink, smooth, and without dis-charge.

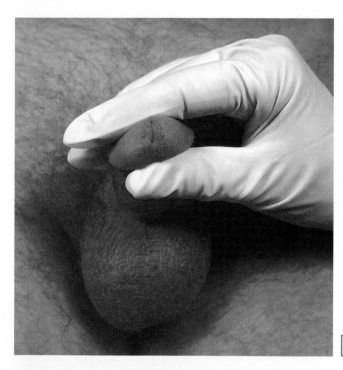

22–6

If you note urethral discharge, collect a smear for microscopic examination and a culture. If no discharge shows but the person gives a history of it, ask him to milk the shaft of the penis. This should produce a drop of discharge.

Palpate the shaft of the penis between your thumb and first two fingers. Normally, the penis feels smooth, semifirm, and nontender.

Inflammation. Lesions on glans or corona.

Phimosis—unable to retract the foreskin.

Paraphimosis—unable to re-turn foreskin to original position.

Hypospadias—ventral loca-tion of meatus.

Epispadias—dorsal location of meatus (see Table 22–3).

Pubic lice or nits. Excoriated skin usually accompanies.

Stricture—narrowed opening.

Edges that are red, everted, edematous, along with purulent discharge, suggest urethritis (see Table 22–2).

Nodule or induration.

Tenderness.

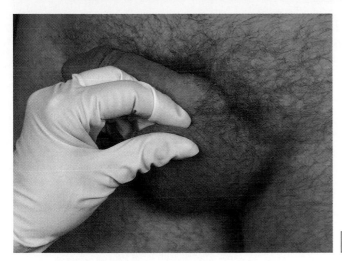

22–7

SCROTUM

Inspect and palpate the scrotum

Inspect the scrotum as male holds the penis out of the way. Alternatively, you hold the penis out of the way with the back of your hand (Fig. 22–7). Scrotal size varies with ambient room temperature. Asymmetry is normal, with the left scrotal half usually lower than the right.

Spread rugae out between your fingers. Lift the sac to inspect the posterior surface. Normally, no scrotal lesions are present, except for the commonly found sebaceous cysts. These are yellowish, 1-cm nodules and are firm, nontender, and often multiple.

Palpate gently each scrotal half between your thumb and first two fingers (Fig. 22–8). The scrotal contents should slide easily. Testes normally feel oval, firm and rubbery, smooth, and equal bilaterally, and are freely movable and slightly tender to moderate pressure. Each epididymis normally feels discrete, softer than the testis, smooth, and nontender.

Scrotal swelling (edema) may be taut and pitting. This occurs with congestive heart failure, renal failure, or local inflammation.

Lesions.

Inflammation.

Absent testis—may be a temporary migration or true cryptorchidism (see Table 22–4).

Atrophied testes—small and soft.

Fixed testes.

Nodules on testes or epididymides.

Marked tenderness.

An indurated, swollen, and tender epididymis indicates epididymitis.

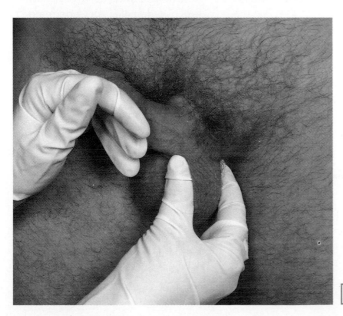

22–8

Normal Range of Findings	Abnormal Findings

Palpate each spermatic cord between your thumb and forefinger, along its length from the epididymis up to the external inguinal ring (Fig. 22–9). You should feel a smooth, nontender cord.

Thickened cord.

Soft, swollen, and tortuous— see the discussion of varicocele, Table 22–4.

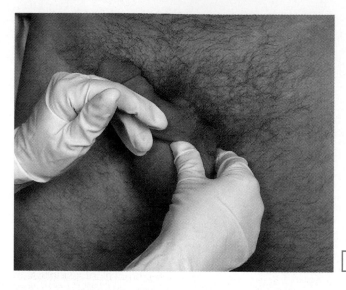

22–9

Normally, no other scrotal contents are present. If you do find a mass, note:

- Any tenderness?
- Is the mass distal or proximal to testis?
- Can you place your fingers over it?
- Does it reduce when person lies down?
- Can you auscultate bowel sounds over it?

Abnormalities in the scrotum: hernia, tumor, orchitis, epididymitis, hydrocele, spermatocele, varicocele (see Table 22–4).

Transillumination. Perform this maneuver if you note a swelling or mass. Darken the room. Shine a strong flashlight from behind the scrotal contents. Normal scrotal contents do not transilluminate.

Serous fluid does transilluminate and shows as a red glow, e.g., hydrocele, or spermatocele. Solid tissue and blood do not transilluminate, e.g., hernia, epididymitis, or tumor (see Table 22–4).

HERNIA

Inspect and palpate for hernia

Inspect the inguinal region for a bulge as the person stands and as he strains down. Normally, none is present.

Bulge at external inguinal ring or at femoral canal. (A hernia may be present but easily reduced and may appear only intermittently with an increase in intraabdominal pressure.)

Normal Range of Findings	Abnormal Findings

Palpate the inguinal canal (Fig. 22–10). For the right side, ask the male to shift his weight onto the left (unexamined) leg. Place your right index finger low on the right scrotal half. Palpate up the length of the spermatic cord, invaginating the scrotal skin as you go, to the external inguinal ring. It feels like a triangular slitlike opening, and it may or may not admit your finger. If it will admit your finger, gently insert it into the canal and ask the person to "bear down."* Normally, you feel no change. Repeat the procedure on the left side.

Palpate the femoral area for a bulge. Normally you feel none.

Palpable herniating mass bumps your fingertip or pushes against the side of your finger (see Table 22–5).

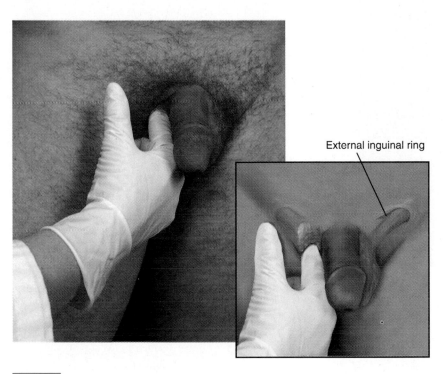

External inguinal ring

22–10

---

*Avoid the old direction, "turn your head and cough." For one thing, a brief cough does not give the steady, increased intraabdominal pressure you need. For another, the person is likely to cough right in your face.

INGUINAL LYMPH NODES

Palpate the horizontal chain along the groin inferior to the inguinal ligament and the vertical chain along the upper inner thigh.

It is normal to palpate an isolated node on occasion; it then feels small (<1 cm), soft, discrete, and movable (Fig. 22–11).

Enlarged, hard, matted, fixed nodes.

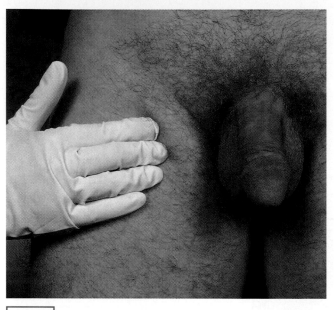

22–11

SELF-CARE—TESTICULAR SELF-EXAMINATION (TSE)

Encourage self-care by teaching every male (from 13 to 14 years old through adulthood) how to examine his own testicles every month. The overall incidence of testicular cancer is still rare, but testicular cancer is the most common cancer in young men age 15 to 35 (Murphy et al., 1997). Males with undescended testicles are at greatest risk, and white males are four times more likely to contract testicular cancer than nonwhites. This tumor has no early symptoms. If detected early by palpation and treated, the cure rate is almost 100 percent.

Early detection is enhanced if the male is familiar with his normal consistency. Points to include during health teaching are

- **T** = timing, once a month
- **S** = shower, warm water relaxes scrotal sac
- **E** = examine, check for changes, report changes immediately

Normal Range of Findings	Abnormal Findings

Phrase your teaching something like this:

A good time to examine the testicles is during the shower or bath, when your hands are warm and soapy and the scrotum is warm. Cold hands stimulate a muscle (cremasteric) reflex, retracting the scrotal contents. The procedure is simple. Hold the scrotum in the palm of your hand and gently feel each testicle using your thumb and first two fingers. If it hurts, you are using too much pressure. The testicle is egg-shaped and movable. It feels rubbery with a smooth surface, like a hard-boiled egg. The epididymis is on top and behind the testicle; it feels a bit softer. If you ever notice a firm, painless lump, a hard area, or an overall enlarged testicle, call your physician for a further check.

 DEVELOPMENTAL CONSIDERATIONS

Infants and Children

For an infant or toddler, perform this procedure right after the abdominal examination. In a preschool-age to young school-age child (3 to 8 years of age), leave underpants on until just before the examination. In an older school-age child or adolescent, offer an extra drape, as with the adult. Reassure child and parents of normal findings.

Inspect the penis and scrotum. Penis size is usually small in infants (2 to 3 cm) (Fig. 22–12) and in young boys until puberty. In the obese boy, the penis looks even smaller because of folds of skin covering the base.

Rarely, a very small penis may be an enlarged clitoris in a genetically female infant.

Enlarged penis—precocious puberty.

Redness, swelling, lesions.

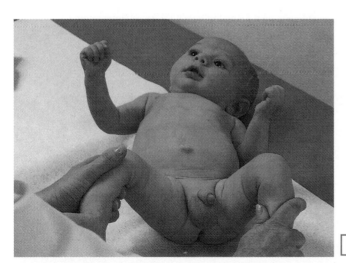

22–12

In the circumcised infant, the glans looks smooth with the meatus centered at the tip. While the child wears diapers, the meatus may become ulcerated from ammonia irritation. This is more common in circumcised infants.

Hypospadias, epispadias (see Table 22–3).

Stricture—narrowed opening.

Discharge.

▶ Normal Range of Findings

Abnormal Findings

If possible, observe the newborn's first voiding to assess strength and direction of stream.

If uncircumcised, the foreskin is normally tight during the first 3 months and should not be retracted because of the risk of tearing the membrane attaching the foreskin to the shaft. This leads to scarring and, possibly, to adhesions later in life. In infants older than 3 months of age, retract the foreskin gently to check the glans and meatus. It should return to its original position easily.

The scrotum looks pink in white infants and dark brown in dark-skinned infants. Rugae are well formed in the full-term infant. Size varies with ambient temperature, but overall, the infant's scrotum looks large in relation to the penis. No bulges, either constant or intermittent, are present.

Palpate the scrotum and testes. The cremasteric reflex is strong in the infant, pulling the testes up into the inguinal canal and abdomen from exposure to cold, touch, exercise, or emotion. Take care not to elicit the reflex: (1) Keep your hands warm and palpate from the external inguinal ring down; (2) block the inguinal canals with the thumb and forefinger of your other hand to prevent the testes from retracting (Fig. 22–13).

Occasionally, ulceration may produce a stricture, shown by a pinpoint meatus and a narrow stream. This increases the risk of urine obstruction.

Poor stream is significant, because it may indicate a stricture or neurogenic bladder.

Phimosis—unable to retract the foreskin.

Paraphimosis—the foreskin cannot be slipped forward once it is retracted.

Dirt and smegma collecting under foreskin.

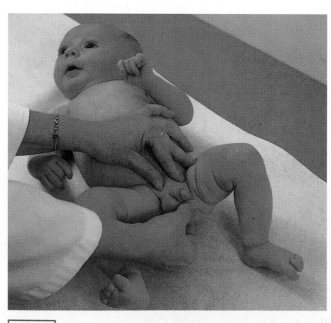

22–13

Normal Range of Findings	Abnormal Findings

Normally, the testes are descended and are equal in size bilaterally (1.5 to 2 cm until puberty). It is important to document that you have palpated the testes. Once palpated, they are considered descended, even if they have retracted momentarily at the next visit.

If the scrotal half feels empty, search for the testes along the inguinal canal and try to milk them down. Ask the toddler or child to squat with the knees flexed up; this pressure may force the testes down. Or, have the young child sit cross-legged to relax the reflex (Fig. 22–14).

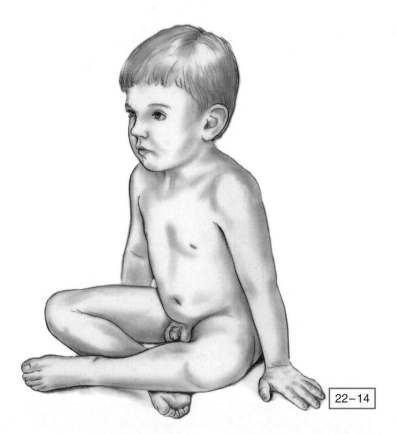

22–14

Migratory testes (physiologic cryptorchidism) are common because of the strength of the cremasteric reflex and the small mass of the prepubertal testes. Note that the affected side has a normally developed scrotum (with true cryptorchidism, the scrotum is atrophic) and that the testis can be milked down. These testes descend at puberty and are normal.

Palpate the epididymis and spermatic cord as described in the adult section. A common scrotal finding in the boy under 2 years of age is a *hydrocele*, or fluid in the scrotum. It appears as a large scrotum and transilluminates as a faint pink glow. It usually disappears spontaneously.

Cryptorchidism: undescended testes (those that have never descended). Undescended testes are common in premature infants. They occur in 3 to 4 percent of term infants, although most have descended by 3 months of age. Age at which child should be referred differs among physicians (see Table 22–4).

A hydrocele is a cystic collection of serous fluid in the tunica vaginalis, surrounding the testis. (See Table 22–4.)

▶ Normal Range of Findings	Abnormal Findings

Inspect the inguinal area for a bulge. If you do not see a bulge but the parent gives a positive history of one, try to elicit it by increasing intraabdominal pressure. Ask the boy to hold his breath and strain down or have him blow up a balloon.

If a hernia is suspected, palpate the inguinal area. Use your little finger to reach the external inguinal ring.

The Adolescent

The adolescent shows a wide variation in normal development of the genitals. Using the SMR charts, note: (1) enlargement of the testes and scrotum; (2) pubic hair growth; (3) darkening of scrotal color; (4) roughening of scrotal skin; (5) increase in penis length and width; and (6) axillary hair growth.

Be familiar with the normal sequence of growth.

The Aging Adult

In the older male, you may note thinner, graying pubic hair and the decreased size of the penis. The size of the testes may be decreased and may feel less firm. The scrotal sac is pendulous with less rugae. The scrotal skin may become excoriated if the man continually sits on it.

▶ SUMMARY CHECKLIST: Male Genitalia Exam

1: Inspect and palpate the penis

2: Inspect and palpate the scrotum

3: If a mass exists, transilluminate it

4: Palpate for an inguinal hernia

5: Palpate the inguinal lymph nodes

APPLICATION AND CRITICAL THINKING

SAMPLE CHARTING

▶ **Subjective**

Urinates four to five times/day, clear, straw-colored. No nocturia, dysuria, or hesitancy. No pain, lesions, or discharge from penis. Does not do testicular self-examination. No history of genitourinary disease. Sexually active in a monogamous relationship. Sexual life satisfactory to self and partner. Uses birth control via barrier method (partner uses diaphragm). No known STD contact.

Objective

No lesions, inflammation, or discharge from penis. Scrotum—testes descended, symmetric, no masses. No inguinal hernia.

CLINICAL CASE STUDY

Subjective

R.C. is a 19-year-old student who 2 days PTA noted acute onset of painful urination, frequency, and urgency. Noted some thick penile discharge. States has no side pain, no abdominal pain, no fever, or genital skin rash. R.C. is concerned he has an STD because of episode of unprotected intercourse with a new partner 6 days PTA. Has no known allergies.

Objective

Vital signs 37° C-72-16. No lesions or inflammation around penis or scrotum. Urethral meatus has mild edema with purulent urethral discharge. No pain on palpation of genitalia. Testes symmetric with no masses. No lymphadenopathy.

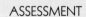

ASSESSMENT

Urethral discharge
Knowledge deficit about STD prevention R/T lack of information recall

NURSING DIAGNOSES COMMONLY ASSOCIATED WITH THE MALE GENITALIA AND RELATED DISORDERS

Diagnosis	Related Factors (Etiology)	Defining Characteristics (Symptoms and Signs)
Altered sexuality patterns	Effects of illness or medical treatment Drugs Radiation Anomalies Extreme fatigue Obesity Pain Performance anxiety Knowledge/skill deficit about alternative responses to health-related transitions Pregnancy Surgery Recent childbirth Trauma Menopause Impaired relationship with a significant other Fear of pregnancy or of acquiring a sexually transmitted disease Conflicts with sexual orientation or variant preferences Ineffective or absent role models Loss of job or ability to work Separation from or loss of significant other	Identification of sexual difficulties, limitations, or changes

Continued

| Urinary retention | Diminished or absent sensory and/or motor impulses
Effects of medications
　Anesthetics
　Opiates
　Psychotropics
Strong sphincter
Urethral blockage associated with
　Fecal impaction
　Prostate hypertrophy
　Surgical swelling
　Postpartum edema
Anxiety (fear of postoperative pain) | Bladder distention
Diminished force of urinary stream
Dribbling
Dysuria
Hesitancy
High residual urine
Nocturia
Sensation of bladder fullness
Small, frequent voiding or absence of urine output |
| Impaired skin integrity | Infection
Allergy
Chemical substances on skin
Autoimmune dysfunction
Decreased circulation
Edema
Effects of aging or medications
Excretions/secretions
Immobility
Insect bites
Parasites
Pressure
Radiation
Shearing force
Stress
Surgery | Blisters
Chafing
Disruption of skin surface or layers
Lesions
Pruritus
Bruising
Cyanosis
Denuded skin
Erythema
Induration |

Other Related Nursing Diagnoses

ACTUAL	RISK/WELLNESS
Altered growth and development Altered sexuality patterns Altered urinary elimination Anxiety Impaired skin integrity Incontinence Pain Sexual dysfunction (see Chapter 24) Rape trauma syndrome (see Chapter 24) Rape trauma syndrome: compound reaction Rape trauma syndrome: silent reaction Urinary retention	**Risk** Risk for infection Risk for trauma **Wellness** Health-seeking behavior for instruction on testicular self-examination

 ASSESSMENT VIDEO CRITICAL THINKING QUESTIONS

The Saunders *Physical Examination and Health Assessment* Video Series—MALE GENITALIA—will direct you to consider the following:

1. Which presenting symptoms are associated with abnormalities of the male genitalia?
2. What abnormal findings may be detected during inspection of the penis?
3. How do genitalia assessment findings in a male infant compare to those in a male adolescent?

Table 22-2 MALE GENITAL LESIONS

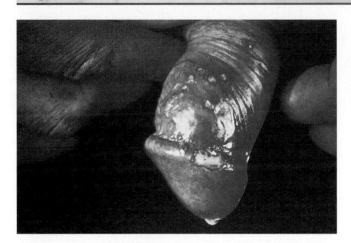

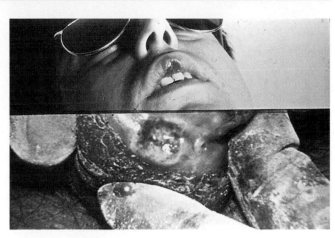

Herpes Progenitalis

Clusters of small vesicles with surrounding erythema, which are often painful, erupt on the glans or foreskin. These rupture to form superficial ulcers. A sexually transmitted disease (STD), the initial infection lasts 7 to 10 days. The virus remains dormant indefinitely; recurrent infections last 3 to 10 days with milder symptoms.

Syphilitic Chancre

Begins as a small, solitary, silvery papule that erodes to a red, round or oval, superficial ulcer with a yellowish serous discharge. Palpation reveals a nontender indurated base that can be lifted like a button between the thumb and the finger. Lymph nodes enlarge early but are nontender. This is an STD.

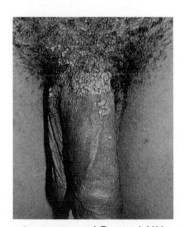

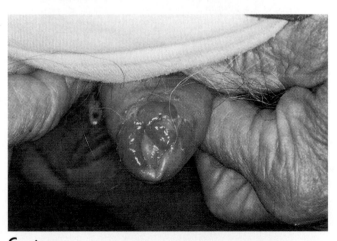

Condylomata Acuminata (Genital Warts)

Soft, pointed, moist, fleshy, painless papules may be single or multiple in a cauliflowerlike patch. Color may be gray, pale yellow, or pink in white males, and black or translucent gray-black in black males. They occur on shaft of penis, behind corona, or around the anus where they may grow into large grapelike clusters.

These are caused by the human papillomavirus (HPV) and are one of the most common STDs. The HPV infection is correlated with early onset of sexual activity, infrequent use of contraception, and multiple sexual partners.

Carcinoma

Begins as red, raised warty growth or as an ulcer, with watery discharge. As it grows, may necrose and slough. Usually painless. Almost always on glans or inner lip of foreskin and following chronic inflammation. Enlarged lymph nodes are common.

Table continued on following page

▼ Table 22–2 MALE GENITAL LESIONS *Continued*

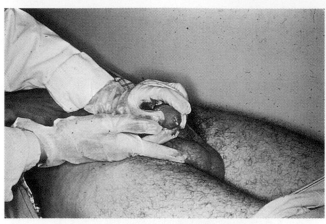

◀ Urethritis (Urethral Discharge and Dysuria)

Infection of urethra causes painful burning urination. Meatus edges are reddened, everted, and swollen. Purulent urethral discharge is present. Urine is cloudy with discharge and mucous shreds. Cause determined by culture: (1) gonococcal urethritis has thick, profuse, yellow or gray-brown discharge; (2) nonspecific urethritis (NSU) may have similar discharge but often has scanty, mucoid discharge. Of these, about 50 percent are caused by chlamydia infection. This is important to differentiate because antibiotic treatment is different.

▼ Table 22–3 ABNORMALITIES ON THE PENIS

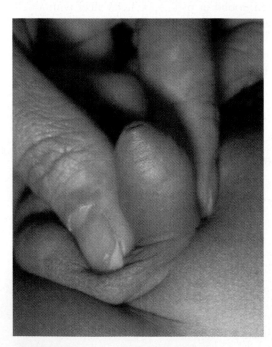

Phimosis

Foreskin is advanced and fixed so tight it is impossible to retract over glans. May be congenital or acquired from adhesions secondary to infection. Poor hygiene leads to retained dirt and smegma, which increases risk of inflammation or calculus formation.

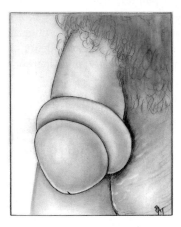

Paraphimosis

Foreskin is retracted and fixed. Once retracted behind glans, a tight or inflamed foreskin cannot return to its original position. Constriction impedes circulation, so glans swells. If untreated, it may compromise arterial circulation.

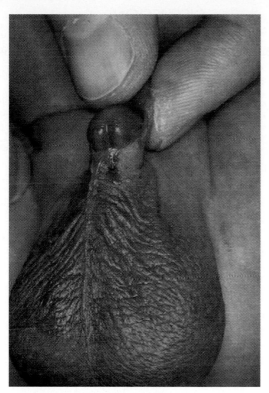

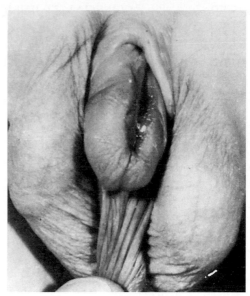

Hypospadias

Urethral meatus opens on the ventral (under-) side of glans, shaft, or at the penoscrotal junction. A groove extends from the meatus to the normal location at the tip. This is a congenital defect that is important to recognize at birth. The newborn should not be circumcised because surgical correction may use foreskin tissue to extend urethral length.

Epispadias

Meatus opens on the dorsal (upper) side of glans or shaft. Rare; less common than hypospadias but more disabling because of associated urinary incontinence and separation of pubic bones.

Urethral Stricture (not illustrated)

Pinpoint, constricted opening at meatus or inside along urethra. Occurs congenitally or secondary to urethral injury. Gradual decrease in force and caliber of urine stream is most common symptom. Shaft feels indurated along ventral aspect at the site of the stricture.

Peyronie's Disease ▶

Hard, nontender, subcutaneous plaques palpated on dorsal or lateral surface of penis. May be single or multiple and asymmetric. They are associated with painful bending of the penis during erection. Plaques are fibrosis of covering of corpora cavernosa. Usually occurs after 45 years. Its cause is unknown. Ten to 20 percent of those afflicted also have Dupuytren's contracture of the palm.

Priapism (not illustrated)

Prolonged painful erection of penis without sexual desire. Rare condition occurs with sickle-cell trait or disease; leukemia where increased numbers of white blood cells produce engorgement; malignancy; or local trauma or spinal cord injuries with autonomic nervous system dysfunction.

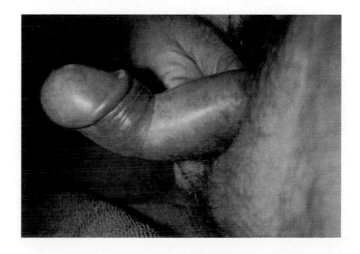

▼ Table 22-4 ABNORMALITIES IN THE SCROTUM

DISORDER	CLINICAL FINDINGS	DISCUSSION
Absent Testis Cryptorchidism 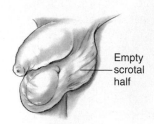 Empty scrotal half	S: Empty scrotal half O: Inspection—in true maldescent, atrophic scrotum on affected side Palpation—no testis A: Absent testis	True cryptorchidism—testes that have never descended. Incidence at birth is 3 to 4 percent, one-half of these descend in first month. Incidence with premature infants is 30 percent; in the adult 0.7 to 0.8 percent. True undescended testes have a histologic change by 6 years, causing decreased spermatogenesis and infertility
Small Testis 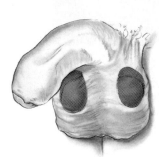	S: (None) O: Palpation—small and soft (rarely may be firm) A: Small testis	Small and soft (< 3.5 cm) indicates atrophy as with cirrhosis, hypopituitarism, following estrogen therapy, or as a sequelae of orchitis. Small and firm (< 2 cm) occurs with Klinefelter's syndrome (hypogonadism)
Testicular Torsion 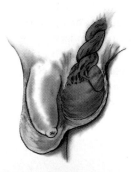	S: Excruciating pain in testicle of sudden onset, often during sleep or following trauma. May also have lower abdominal pain, nausea and vomiting, no fever O: Inspection—red, swollen scrotum, one testis (usually left) higher owing to rotation and shortening Palpation—cord feels thick, swollen, tender, epididymis may be anterior, cremasteric reflex is absent on side of torsion	Sudden twisting of spermatic cord. Occurs in late childhood, early adolescence, rare after age of 20 years. Torsion occurs usually on the left side. Faulty anchoring of testis on wall of scrotum allows testis to rotate. The anterior part of the testis rotates medially toward the other testis. Blood supply is cut off, resulting in ischemia and engorgement. This is an emergency requiring surgery; testis can become gangrenous in a few hours
Epididymitis 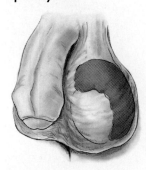	S: Severe pain of sudden onset in scrotum, somewhat relieved by elevation (a positive Phren's sign); also rapid swelling, fever O: Inspection—enlarged scrotum; reddened Palpation—exquisitely tender; epididymis enlarged, indurated; may be hard to distinguish from testis. Overlying scrotal skin may be thick and edematous Laboratory—white blood cells and bacteria in urine A: Tender swelling of epididymis	Acute infection of epididymis commonly caused by prostatitis, after prostatectomy because of trauma of urethral instrumentation, or due to chlamydia, gonorrhea, or other bacterial infection. Often difficult to distinguish between epididymitis and testicular torsion.

S = subjective data; O = objective data; A = assessment.

DISORDER	CLINICAL FINDINGS	DISCUSSION
Spermatic Cord Varicocele 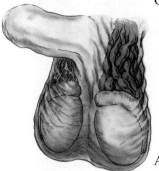	S: Dull pain; constant pulling or dragging feeling; or may be asymptomatic O: Inspection—usually no sign. May show bluish color through light scrotal skin Palpation—when standing, feel soft, irregular mass posterior to and above testis; collapses when supine, refills when upright. Feels distinctive, like a "bag of worms" The testis on the side of the varicocele may be smaller owing to impaired circulation A: Soft mass on spermatic cord	A varicocele is dilated, tortuous varicose veins in the spermatic cord due to incompetent valves within the vein, which permit reflux of blood. Most often on left side, perhaps because left spermatic vein is longer and inserts at a right angle into left renal vein. Common in young males. Screen at early adolescence; early treatment important to prevent potential infertility when an adult. Treatment is relatively easy; surgical ligation of spermatic vein
Spermatocele 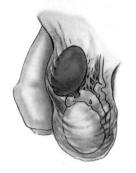	S: Painless, usually found on examination O: Inspection—does transilluminate higher in the scrotum than a hydrocele, and the sperm may fluoresce Palpation—round, freely movable mass lying above and behind testis. If large, feels like a third testis A: Free cystic mass on epididymis	Retention cyst in epididymis. Cause unclear but may be obstruction of tubules. Filled with thin, milky fluid that contains sperm. Most spermatoceles are small (< 1 cm); occasionally, they may be larger and then mistaken for hydrocele
Early Testicular Tumor 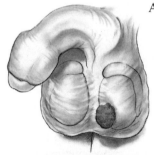	S: Painless, found on examination O: Palpation—firm nodule or harder than normal section of testicle A: Solitary nodule	Most testicular tumors occur between the ages of 18 and 35. Practically all are malignant. Occur in whites; relatively rare in blacks, Mexican Americans, and Asians. Must biopsy to confirm. Most important risk factor is undescended testis, even those surgically corrected. Early detection important in prognosis, but practice of testicular self-examination is currently low
Diffuse Tumor 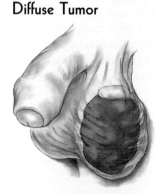	S: Enlarging testis (most common symptom). When enlarges, has feel of increased weight O: Inspection—enlarged, does not transilluminate Palpation—enlarged, smooth, ovoid, firm. Important—firm palpation does *not* cause usual sickening discomfort as with normal testis A: Nontender swelling of testis	Diffuse tumor maintains shape of testis

S = subjective data; O = objective data; A = assessment.

Table continued on following page

Table 22-4   ABNORMALITIES IN THE SCROTUM *Continued*

ABNORMAL FINDINGS

DISORDER
Hydrocele

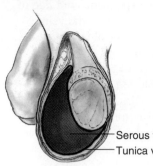

—Serous fluid
—Tunica vaginalis

Scrotal Hernia

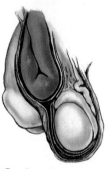

Orchitis

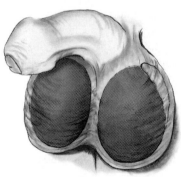

Scrotal Edema

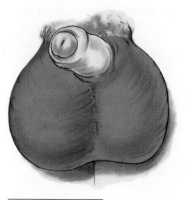

CLINICAL FINDINGS

S: Painless swelling, although person may complain of weight and bulk in scrotum
O: Inspection—enlarged, mass does transilluminate with a pink or red glow (in contrast to a hernia)
Palpation—nontender mass, able to get fingers above mass (in contrast to scrotal hernia)
A: Nontender swelling of testis

S: Swelling, may have pain with straining
O: Inspection—enlarged, may reduce when supine, does not transilluminate
Palpation—soft mushy mass, palpating fingers cannot get above mass. Mass is distinct from testicle that is normal
A: Nontender swelling of scrotum

S: Acute or moderate pain of sudden onset, swollen testis, feeling of weight, fever
O: Inspection—enlarged, edematous, reddened; does not transilluminate
Palpation—swollen, congested, tense, and tender; hard to distinguish testis from epididymis
A: Tender swelling of testis

S: Tenderness
O: Inspection—enlarged, may be reddened (with local irritation)
Palpation—taut with pitting
Probably unable to feel scrotal contents
A: Scrotal edema

DISCUSSION

Cystic. Circumscribed collection of serous fluid in tunica vaginalis, surrounding testis. May occur following epididymitis, trauma, hernia, tumor of testis, or spontaneously in the newborn

Scrotal hernia usually due to indirect inguinal hernia (see Table 22-5)

Acute inflammation of testis. Most common cause is mumps; can occur with any infectious disease
May have associated hydrocele that does transilluminate

Accompanies marked edema in lower half of body, e.g., congestive heart failure, renal failure, and portal vein obstruction. Occurs with local inflammation: epididymitis, torsion of spermatic cord. Also obstruction of inguinal lymphatics produces lymphedema of scrotum

S = subjective data; O = objective data; A = assessment.

▼ **Table 22–5   INGUINAL AND FEMORAL HERNIAS**

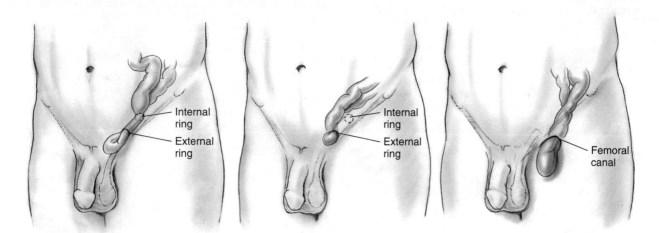

	INDIRECT INGUINAL	DIRECT INGUINAL	FEMORAL
Course	Sac herniates through internal inguinal ring; can remain in canal or pass into scrotum	Directly behind and through external inguinal ring, above inguinal ligament; rarely enters scrotum	Through femoral ring and canal, below inguinal ligament, more often on right side
Clinical Symptoms and Signs	Pain with straining; soft swelling that increases with increased intraabdominal pressure; may decrease when lying down	Usually painless; round swelling close to the pubis in area of internal inguinal ring; easily reduced when supine.*	Pain may be severe, may become strangulated
Frequency	Most common; 60 percent of all hernias. More common in infants < 1 year and in males 16 to 20 years of age	Less common, occurs most often in men > 40, rare in women	Least common, 4 percent of all hernias; more common in women
Cause	Congenital or acquired	Acquired weakness; brought on by heavy lifting, muscle atrophy, obesity, chronic cough, or ascites	Acquired; due to increased abdominal pressure, muscle weakness, or frequent stooping

*Reducible—contents will return to abdominal cavity by lying down or gentle pressure. **Incarcerated**—herniated bowel cannot be returned to abdominal cavity. **Strangulated**—blood supply to hernia is shut off. Accompanied by nausea, vomiting, and tenderness.

Bibliography

Behrman RE: Nelson Textbook of Pediatrics, 15th ed. Philadelphia, WB Saunders Company, 1996.

Best DL, Davis SW, Vaz RM, Kaiser M: Testicular cancer education: A comparison of teaching methods. Am J Health Behav 20(4):229–241, Jul–Aug 1996.

Brown MS: Pediatric genital exam. Nurs Pract 22(7):160, July 1997.

Cornell S: Controversies in circumcision: Examining a cultural norm. Adv Nurs Pract 5(10):49–52, Oct 1997.

Douglas T, Claman F: Teens and sex: Sensitive issues demand sensitive skills. Adv Nurs Pract 3(8):28–32, Aug 1995.

Duffield P: Managing urinary tract infections. Am J Nurs 96(10):16I–16L, Oct 1996.

Editorial. Male reproductive health and environmental estrogens. Lancet 345(8955):933–935, Apr 15, 1995.

Harlan W, Grillo GP, Corroni-Huntley J, et al: Secondary sex characteristics of boys 12 to 17 years of age. The U.S. Health Examination Survey. J Pediatr 95:293, 1979.

Irwin R: Sexual health promotion and nursing. J Adv Nurs 25(1):170–177, Jan 1997.

Kurgan A, Nunnelee JD, Zilberman M: The importance of the early detection of varicocele in adolescent males. Nurs Pract 19(10):36–37, 1994.

Laumann EO, Masi CM, Zuckerman MA: Circumcision in the United States: Prevalence, prophylactic effects, and sexual practice. JAMA 277(13):1052–1057, Apr 2, 1997.

LeMone P, Weber J: Validating gender-specific defining characteristics of altered sexuality. Nurs Diagn 6(2):64–69, Apr–June 1995.

Marshall W, Tanner J: Variations in the pattern of pubertal changes in boys. Arch Dis Child 45:13, 1970.

Meadus RJ: Testicular self-examination (TSE). Can Nurse 91(8):41–44, Sep 1995.

Misener TR, Fuller SG: Testicular versus breast and colorectal cancer screening. Cancer Pract 3(5):310–316, Sep–Oct 1995.

Moser R: Genitourinary problems in adolescent boys. Adv Nurs Pract 3(8):37–39, Aug 1995.

Murphy GP, Morris LB, Lange D: Informed Decisions. New York, American Cancer Society, Penguin Group, 1997.

Peate I: Testicular cancer: The importance of effective health education. Br J Nurs 6(6):311–316, Mar 27, 1997.

Rossiter K, Diehl S: Gender reassignment in children: Ethical conflicts in surrogate decision making. Pediatr Nurs 24(1):59–62, Jan–Feb 1998.

Schaffner RJ: Knowledge of testicular self-exam. Nurs Pract 20(8):10–11, Aug 1995.

Smith M: Pediatric sexuality: Promoting normal sexual development in children. Nurs Pract 18(8):37–44, 1993.

Sugar EC, Firlit CF, Reisman M: Pediatric hypospadias surgery. Pediatr Nurs 19(6):585–615, 1993.

Tanner J: Growth at Adolescence, 2nd ed. Oxford, Blackwell Scientific Publications, 1962.

Thayer D: How to assess and control urinary incontinence. Am J Nurs 94(10):42–48, 1994.

Van Howe RS: Circumcision and infectious diseases revisited. Pediatr Infec Dis J 17(1):1–6, Jan 1998.

Walsh PC, Retik AB, Wein AJ, et al: Campbell's Urology, 7th ed. Philadelphia, WB Saunders Company, 1998.

CHAPTER TWENTY THREE

Anus, Rectum, and Prostate

ANUS AND RECTUM

The **anal canal** is the outlet of the gastrointestinal tract, and it is about 3.8 cm long in the adult. It is lined with modified skin (having no hair or sebaceous glands) that merges with rectal mucosa at the anorectal junction. The canal slants forward toward the umbilicus, forming a distinct right angle with the rectum, which rests back in the hollow of the sacrum. Although the rectum contains only autonomic nerves, numerous somatic sensory nerves are present in the anal canal and external skin, so a person feels sharp pain from any trauma to the anal area.

The anal canal is surrounded by two concentric layers of muscle, the **sphincters** (Fig. 23–1). The internal sphincter is under involuntary control by the autonomic nervous system. The external sphincter surrounds the in-

ternal sphincter but also has a small section overriding the tip of the internal sphincter at the opening. It is under voluntary control. Except for the passing of feces and gas, the sphincters keep the anal canal tightly closed. The **intersphincteric groove** separates the internal and external sphincters and is palpable.

The **anal columns** (or columns of Morgagni) are folds of mucosa. These extend vertically down from the rectum and end in the **anorectal junction** (also called the muco-cutaneous junction, pectinate, or dentate line). This junction is not palpable, but it is visible on proctoscopy. Each anal column contains an artery and a vein. Under conditions of chronic increased venous pressure, the vein may enlarge, forming a hemorrhoid. At the lower end of each column is a small crescent fold of mucous membrane, the **anal valve.** The space above the anal valve (between the columns) is a small recess, the **anal crypt.**

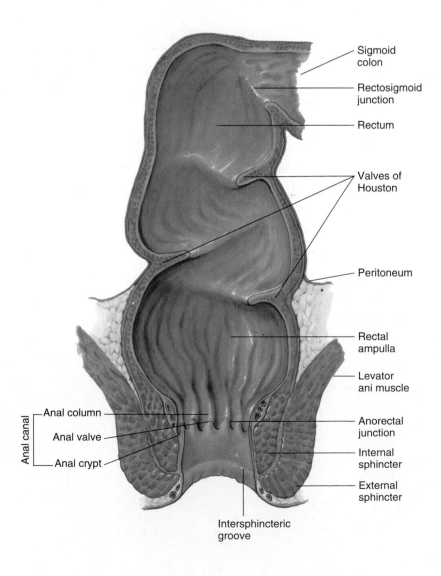

Sigmoid colon

Rectosigmoid junction

Rectum

Valves of Houston

Peritoneum

Rectal ampulla

Levator ani muscle

Anorectal junction

Internal sphincter

External sphincter

Intersphincteric groove

Anal canal

Anal column

Anal valve

Anal crypt

23–1

The **rectum,** which is 12 cm long, is the distal portion of the large intestine. It extends from the sigmoid colon, at the level of the third sacral vertebra, and ends at the anal canal. Just above the anal canal, the rectum dilates and turns posteriorly, forming the rectal ampulla. The rectal interior has three semilunar transverse folds called the **valves of Houston.** These cross one-half the circumference of the rectal lumen. Their function is unclear, but they may serve to hold feces as the flatus passes. The lowest is within reach of palpation, usually on the person's left side, and must not be mistaken for an intrarectal mass.

Peritoneal Reflection. The peritoneum covers only the upper two-thirds of the rectum. In the male, the anterior part of the peritoneum reflects down to within 7.5 cm of the anal opening, forming the **rectovesical pouch** (Fig. 23–2) and then covers the bladder. In the female, this is termed the **rectouterine pouch,** and extends down to within 5.5 cm of the anal opening.

PROSTATE

In the male, the **prostate gland** lies in front of the anterior wall of the rectum and 2 cm behind the symphysis pubis. It surrounds the bladder neck and the urethra

and has 15 to 30 ducts that open into the urethra. The prostate secretes a thin, milky alkaline fluid that helps sperm viability. It is a bilobed structure with a round or heart shape. It measures 2.5 cm long and 4 cm in diameter. The two lateral lobes are separated by a shallow groove called the **median sulcus.**

The two **seminal vesicles** project like rabbit ears above the prostate. The seminal vesicles secrete a fluid that is rich in fructose, which nourishes the sperm, and contains prostaglandins. The two **bulbourethral** (Cowper's) glands are each the size of a pea and are located inferior to the prostate on either side of the urethra (see Fig. 23–5). They secrete a clear, viscid mucus.

Regional Structures

In the female, the uterine cervix lies in front of the anterior rectal wall and may be palpated through it.

The combined length of the anal canal and the rectum is about 16 cm in the adult. The average length of the examining finger is from 6 cm to 10 cm, bringing many rectal structures within reach.

The sigmoid colon is named from its S-shaped course in the pelvic cavity. It extends from the iliac flexure of the descending colon and ends at the rectum. It is 40 cm long and is accessible to examination only through the colonoscope. The flexible fiberoptic scope in current use provides a view of the entire mucosal surface of the sigmoid, as well as the colon.

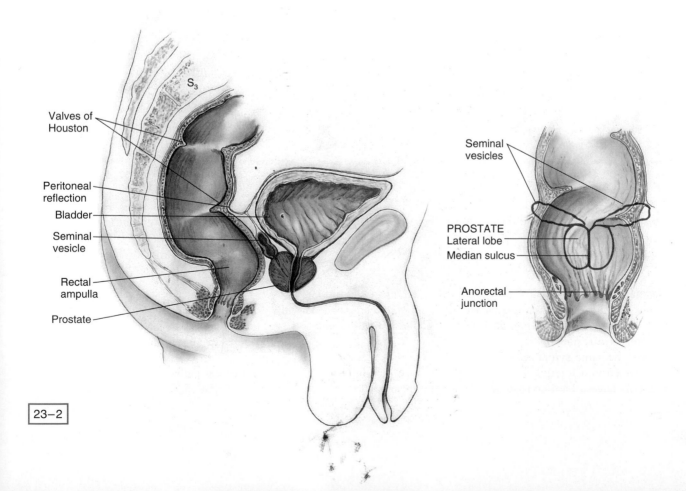

23–2

DEVELOPMENTAL CONSIDERATIONS

The first stool passed by the newborn is dark green meconium and occurs within 24 to 48 hours of birth, indicating anal patency. From that time on, the infant usually has a stool after each feeding. This response to eating is a wave of peristalsis called the gastrocolic reflex. It continues throughout life, although children and adults usually produce no more than one or two stools per day.

The infant passes stools by reflex. Voluntary control of the external anal sphincter cannot occur until the nerves supplying the area have become fully myelinated, usually around 1½ to 2 years of age. Toilet training usually starts after age 2 years.

At male puberty, the prostate gland undergoes a very rapid increase to more than twice its prepubertal size. During young adulthood its size remains fairly constant.

The prostate gland commonly starts to enlarge during the middle adult years. This *benign prostatic hypertrophy*

(BPH) is present in 1 of 10 males at the age of 40 years and increases with age. It is thought that the hypertrophy is caused by hormonal imbalance that leads to the proliferation of benign adenomas. These gradually impede urine output because they obstruct the urethra.

TRANSCULTURAL **CONSIDERATIONS**

Prostate cancer is more common in North America and northwestern Europe and is rare in Central and South America, Africa, and Asia. The incidence rates of prostate cancer are two times higher for black-American men than white men, with black Americans having the highest incidence rates in the world (American Cancer Society, 1998). Reasons for this are not yet known. However, an inherited predisposition may account for 5 to 10 percent of prostate cancers, and dietary fat may also be a factor (American Cancer Society, 1998).

SUBJECTIVE DATA

1. Usual bowel routine
2. Change in bowel habits
3. Rectal bleeding, blood in the stool
4. Medications (laxatives, stool softeners, iron)
5. Rectal conditions (pruritus, hemorrhoids, fissure, fistula)
6. Family history
7. Self-care behaviors (diet of high-fiber foods, most recent examinations)

Examiner Asks	Rationale
① **Usual bowel routine.** Bowels move regularly? How often? Usual color? Hard or soft? Pain while passing a bowel movement?	Assess **usual bowel routine.** Dyschezia. Pain may be due to a local condition (hemorrhoid, fissure) or constipation.
② **Change in bowel habits.** Any **change** in usual **bowel habits?** Loose stools, or diarrhea? When did this start? Is the diarrhea associated with nausea and vomiting, abdominal pain, something you ate recently? • Eaten at a restaurant recently? Anyone else in your group or family have the same symptoms? • Traveled to a foreign country during the last 6 months? • Stools have a hard consistency? When did this start?	Diarrhea occurs with gastroenteritis, colitis, irritable colon syndrome. Consider food poisoning. Consider parasitic infection. Constipation.

Examiner Asks	Rationale
3 **Rectal bleeding, blood in the stool.** Ever had black or bloody stools? When did you first notice blood in the stools? What is the color, bright red or dark red-black? How much blood: spotting on the toilet paper or outright passing of blood with the stool? Do the bloody stools have a particular smell?	Melena. Black stools may be tarry due to occult blood (melena) from gastrointestinal bleeding, or nontarry from ingestion of iron medications. Red blood in stools occurs with gastrointestinal bleeding or localized bleeding around the anus. Rectal bleeding and blood in the stool occur with colon and rectal cancer. Clay color indicates absent bile pigment. Steatorrhea is excessive fat in the stool as in malabsorption of fat. Flatulence.
• Ever had clay-colored stools? • Ever had mucus or pus in stool? • Frothy stool? • Need to pass gas frequently?	
4 **Medications.** What medications do you take—prescription and over-the-counter? Laxatives or stool softeners? Which ones? How often? Iron pills? Do you ever use enemas to move your bowels? How often?	
5 **Rectal conditions.** Any problems in rectal area: itching, pain or burning, hemorrhoids? How do you treat these? Any hemorrhoid preparations? Ever had a fissure, or fistula? How was this treated? • Ever had a problem controlling your bowels?	Pruritus. Fecal incontinence. Mucoid discharge and soiled underwear occur with prolapsed hemorrhoids.
6 **Family history.** Any **family history:** polyps or cancer in colon or rectum, inflammatory bowel disease, prostate cancer?	Risk factors for colon cancer, rectal cancer, prostate cancer.
7 **Self-care behaviors.** What is the usual amount of **high-fiber foods** in your daily diet: cereals, apples or other fruits, vegetables, whole-grain breads? How many glasses of water do you drink each day?	High-fiber foods of the soluble type (beans, prunes, barley, carrots, broccoli, cabbage) have been shown to lower cholesterol, while insoluble fiber foods (cereals, wheat germ) reduce the risk of colon cancer. Also, fiber foods help fight obesity, stabilize blood sugar, and may help certain gastrointestinal disorders.
• Date last: digital rectal examination, stool blood test, colonoscopy, (for men) prostate-specific antigen blood test.	Early detection for cancer: digital rectal examination performed annually after age 50; fecal occult blood test annually after age 50; sigmoidoscopy every 5 years or colonoscopy every 10 years after age 50; prostate-specific antigen blood test annually for men over 50, except black men beginning at age 45 (American Cancer Society, 1998).

Examiner Asks	Rationale

ADDITIONAL HISTORY FOR INFANTS AND CHILDREN

 1 Have you ever noticed any irritation in your child's anal area: redness, raised skin, frequent itching?

In children, pinworms are a common cause of intense itching and irritated anal skin.

OBJECTIVE DATA

Preparation

Perform a rectal examination on all adults and particularly for those in middle and late years. Help the person assume one of the following positions (Fig. 23–3): Examine the male in the left lateral decubitus or standing position. Instruct the standing male to point his toes together; this relaxes the regional muscles, making it easier to spread the buttocks.

Place the female in the lithotomy position if examining genitalia as well; use the left lateral decubitus position for the rectal area alone.

Equipment Needed
Penlight
Lubricating jelly
Glove
Guaiac test container

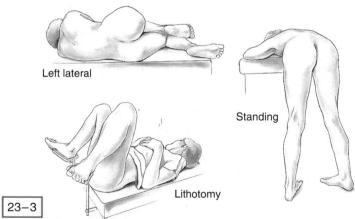

Left lateral

Standing

Lithotomy

23–3

Normal Range of Findings	Abnormal Findings

INSPECTION OF THE PERIANAL AREA

Spread the buttocks wide apart and observe the perianal region. The anus normally looks moist and hairless, with coarse folded skin that is more pigmented than the perianal skin. The anal opening is tightly closed. No lesions are present.

Inflammation. Lesions or scars.

Linear split—fissure.

▶ | Normal Range of Findings | Abnormal Findings

Flabby skin sac—hemorrhoid. Shiny blue skin sac—thrombosed hemorrhoid.

Small round opening in anal area—fistula (see Table 23–1).

Inflammation or tenderness, swelling, tuft of hair, or dimple at tip of coccyx may indicate pilonidal cyst (see Table 23–1).

Appearance of fissure.

Appearance of hemorrhoids.

Circular red doughnut of tissue—rectal prolapse.

Inspect the sacrococcygeal area. Normally, it appears smooth and even.

Instruct the person to hold the breath and bear down by performing a Valsalva maneuver. No break in skin integrity or protrusion through the anal opening should be present. Describe any abnormality in clock-face terms, with 12:00 as the anterior point toward the symphysis pubis and 6:00 toward the coccyx.

PALPATION OF THE ANUS AND RECTUM

Don a glove and drop lubricating jelly onto your index finger. Instruct the person that palpation is not painful but may feel like needing to move the bowels. Place the pad of your index finger gently against the anal verge (Fig. 23–4). You will feel the sphincter tighten, then relax. As it relaxes, flex the tip of your finger and slowly insert it into the anal canal in a direction toward the umbilicus. *Never* approach the anus at right angles with your index finger extended. Such a jabbing motion does not promote sphincter relaxation and is painful.

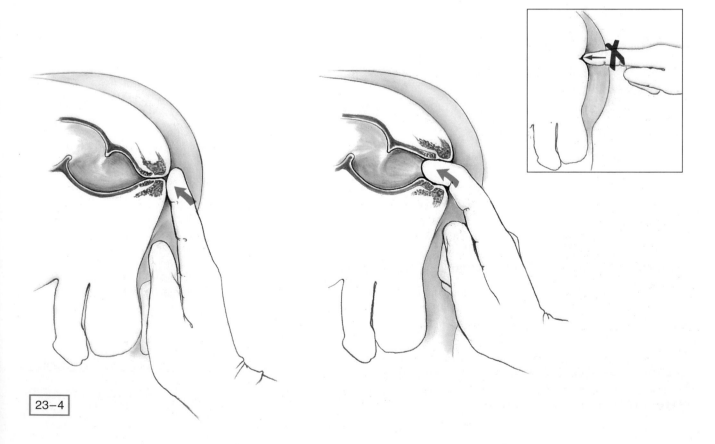

23–4

Rotate your examining finger to palpate the entire muscular ring. The canal should feel smooth and even. Note the intersphincteric groove circling the canal wall. To assess tone, ask the person to tighten the muscle. The sphincter should tighten evenly around your finger with no pain to the person.

Use a bidigital palpation with your thumb against the perianal tissue (Fig. 23–5). Press your examining finger toward it. This maneuver highlights any swelling or tenderness and helps assess the bulbourethral glands.

Decreased tone.

Increased tone occurs with inflammation and anxiety.

Tenderness.

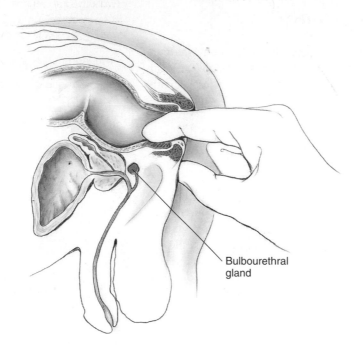

Bulbourethral gland

23–5

Above the anal canal, the rectum turns posteriorly, following the curve of the coccyx and sacrum. Insert your finger farther and explore all around the rectal wall. It normally feels smooth with no nodularity. Promptly report any mass you discover for further examination.

Internal hemorrhoid above anorectal junction is not palpable unless thrombosed.

A soft, slightly movable mass may be a polyp.

A firm or hard mass with irregular shape or rolled edges may signify carcinoma (see Table 23–2).

Prostate Gland. On the anterior wall in the male, note the elastic, bulging prostate gland (Fig. 23–6). Palpate the entire prostate in a systematic manner. Press *into* the gland at each location, because when a nodule occurs, it will not project into the rectal lumen. The surface should feel smooth and muscular; search for any distinct nodule or diffuse firmness. Note these characteristics:

- **Size**—2.5 cm long by 4 cm wide; should not protrude more than 1 cm into the rectum
- **Shape**—heart shape, with palpable central groove
- **Surface**—smooth
- **Consistency**—elastic, rubbery
- **Mobility**—slightly movable
- **Sensitivity**—nontender to palpation

Enlarged, or atrophied gland.

Flat with no groove.

Nodular.

Hard; or boggy, soft, fluctuant.

Fixed.

Tender.

Normal Range of Findings	Abnormal Findings

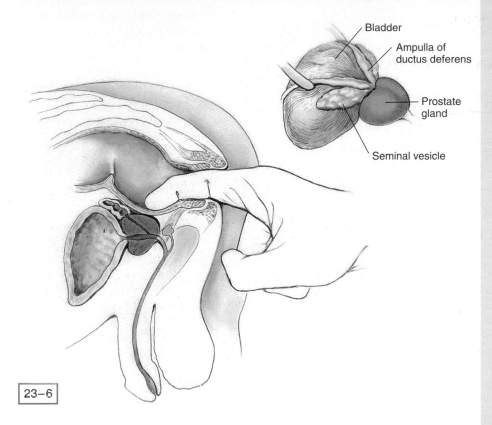

Bladder

Ampulla of
ductus deferens

Prostate
gland

Seminal vesicle

23–6

In the female, palpate the cervix through the anterior rectal wall. It normally feels like a small round mass. You also may palpate a retroverted uterus or a tampon in the vagina. Do not mistake the cervix or a tampon for a tumor.

Withdraw your examining finger; normally, no bright red blood or mucus is on the glove. To complete the examination, offer the person tissues to remove the lubricant and help the person to a more comfortable position.

Examination of Stool. Inspect any feces remaining on the glove. Normally, the color is brown and the consistency is soft.

Test any stool on the glove for **occult blood** using the specimen container that your agency directs. A negative response is normal. If the stool is *hematest* positive, it indicates occult blood. Note that a false-positive finding may occur if the person has ingested significant amounts of red meat within 3 days of the test.

Abnormal Findings

Enlarged, firm smooth gland with central groove obliterated suggests benign prostatic hypertrophy.

Swollen, exquisitely tender gland accompanies prostatitis.

Any stone-hard, irregular, fixed nodule indicates carcinoma (see Table 23–3).

Jelly-like mucus shreds mixed in stool indicate inflammation.

Bright red blood on stool surface indicates rectal bleeding. Bright red blood mixed with feces indicates possible colonic bleeding.

Black tarry stool with distinct malodor indicates upper gastrointestinal bleeding with blood partially digested. (Must lose more than 50 cc from upper gastrointestinal tract to be considered melena.)

Normal Range of Findings	Abnormal Findings

Prostate Cancer Risk factors
Age >50
blacks; family History, Diet high in Animal fat.
Common finding in aging males

Colon Cancer Risk factors (Peak 65- 70 yo.)
Age >40; Personal history of colon polyps; Cohn disease
Deit high in beef + animal fat, ↓ fiber
Exposure to Asbestos, acrylics, carcinogens.

DEVELOPMENTAL CONSIDERATIONS

Infants and Children

For the newborn, hold the feet with one hand and flex the knees up onto the abdomen. Note the presence of the anus. Confirm a patent rectum and anus by noting the first meconium stool passed within 24 to 48 hours of birth. To assess sphincter tone, check the *anal reflex.* Gently stroke the anal area and note a quick contraction of the sphincter.

For each infant and child, note that the buttocks are firm and rounded with no masses or lesions. Recall that the *mongolian spot* is a common variation of hyperpigmentation in black, Native American, Mediterranean, and Asian newborns (see Chapter 10).

The perianal skin is free of lesions. However, diaper rash is common in children younger than 1 year of age and is exhibited as a generalized reddened area with papules or vesicles.

Omit palpation unless the history or symptoms warrant. When internal palpation is needed, position the infant or child on the back with the legs flexed, and gently insert a gloved, well-lubricated finger into the rectum. Your fifth finger usually is long enough, and its smaller size is more comfortable for the infant or child. However, you may need to use the index finger because of its better control and increased tactile sensitivity. On withdrawing the finger, scant bleeding or protruding rectal mucosa may occur.

Inspect the perianal region of the school-aged child and adolescent during examination of the genitalia. Internal palpation is not performed routinely.

The Aging Adult

As an aging person performs the Valsalva maneuver, you may note relaxation of the perianal musculature and decreased sphincter control. Otherwise, the full examination proceeds as that described earlier for the younger adult.

Black stool—also occurs with ingesting iron or bismuth preparations.

Gray, tan stool—absent bile pigment, e.g., obstructive jaundice.

Pale yellow, greasy stool—increased fat content (steatorrhea), as occurs with malabsorption syndrome.

Occult bleeding usually indicates cancer of colon.

Imperforate anus.

Flattened buttocks in cystic fibrosis or celiac syndrome.

Coccygeal mass.

Meningocele (sac containing meninges that protrude through a defect in the bony spine).

Tuft of hair or pilonidal dimple.

Pustules indicate secondary infection of diaper rash.

Signs of physical or sexual abuse.

Fissure—common cause of constipation or rectal bleeding in child. (Painful, so the child does not defecate.)

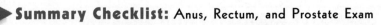

Summary Checklist: Anus, Rectum, and Prostate Exam

1: Inspect anus and perianal area

2: Inspect during Valsalva maneuver

3: Palpate anal canal and rectum on all adults

4: Test stool for occult blood

APPLICATION AND CRITICAL THINKING

SAMPLE CHARTING

▶ **Subjective**

Has one BM daily, soft, brown, no pain, no change in bowel routine. On no medications. Has no history of pruritus, hemorrhoids, fissure, or fistula. Diet includes one to two servings daily each of fresh fruits and vegetables but no whole-grain cereals or breads.

▶ **Objective**

No fissure, hemorrhoids, fistula, or skin lesions in perianal area. Sphincter tone good, no prolapse. Rectal walls smooth, no masses or tenderness. Prostate not enlarged, no masses or tenderness. Stool brown, hematest negative.

CLINICAL CASE STUDY

▶ **Subjective**

C.M. is a 62-year-old white male with chronic obstructive pulmonary disease for 15 years, who today has "diarrhea for 3 days."

7 days PTA: C.M. seen at this agency for acute respiratory infection that was diagnosed as acute bronchitis and treated with oral ampicillin. Took medication as directed.

3 days PTA: symptoms of respiratory infection improved. Ingesting usual diet. Onset of four to five loose, unformed, brown stools a day. No abdominal pain or cramping. No nausea.

Now: diarrhea continues. No blood or mucus noticed in stool. No new foods or restaurant food in past 3 days. Wife not ill.

▶ **Objective**

Vital signs: 37° C-88-18. B/P 142/82.

Respiratory. Respirations unlabored. Barrel chest. Hyperresonant to percussion. Lung sounds clear but diminished. No crackles or rhonchi today.

Abdomen. Flat. Bowel sounds present. No organomegaly or tenderness to palpation.

Rectal. No lesions in perianal area. Sphincter tone good. Rectal walls smooth, no mass or tenderness. Prostate smooth and firm, no median sulcus palpable, no masses or tenderness. Stool brown, hematest negative.

▶ ASSESSMENT

Diarrhea R/T effects of antibiotic medication

Continued

NURSING DIAGNOSES COMMONLY ASSOCIATED WITH ANAL AND RECTAL DISORDERS

Diagnosis	Related Factors (Etiology)	Defining Characteristics (Symptoms and Signs)

Constipation	Less than adequate dietary intake and bulk
	Neuromuscular or musculoskeletal impairment
	Pain and discomfort on defecation
	Effects of
	   Diagnostic procedures
	   Pregnancy
	   Aging
	   Medication
	   Stress or anxiety
	Weak abdominal musculature
	Immobility or less than adequate physical activity
	Chronic use of laxatives and enemas
	Ignoring the urge to defecate
	Fear of rectal or cardiac pain
	Gastrointestinal lesions
		Frequency less than usual pattern
		Hard, formed stools
		Palpable mass
		Straining at stool
		Less than usual amount of stool
		Decreased bowel sounds
		Gas pain and flatulence
		Abdominal or back pain
		Reported feeling of abdominal or rectal fullness or pressure
		Impaired appetite
		Headache
		Nausea
		Irritability
		Palpable hard stool on rectal examination

Bowel incontinence	Diarrhea
	Impaction
	Impairment
	   Cognitive
	   Neuromuscular
	   Perceptual
	Large stool volume
	Depression
	Severe anxiety
	Physical or psychological barriers that prevent access to an acceptable toileting area
	Effects of medications
	Excessive use of laxatives
		Involuntary passage of stool
		Lack of awareness of need to defecate
		Lack of awareness of passage of stool
		Rectal oozing of stool
		Urgency

Other Related Nursing Diagnoses

ACTUAL	RISK/WELLNESS
Colonic constipation Diarrhea (see Chapter 19) Impaired skin integrity Perceived constipation	**Risk** Risk for constipation Risk for fluid imbalance **Wellness** Health-seeking behavior for information on high-fiber diet

ASSESSMENT VIDEO CRITICAL THINKING QUESTION

The Saunders *Physical Examination and Health Assessment* Video Series—ANUS, RECTUM, and PROSTATE—will direct you to consider the following:
1. Describe abnormal findings that may be noted on inspection of the perianal canal of an infant or child.

▼ **Table 23–1   ABNORMALITIES OF THE ANUS AND PERIANAL REGION**

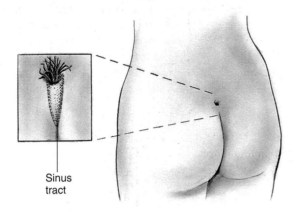

Sinus
tract

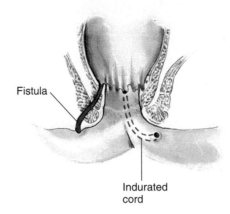

Fistula

Indurated
cord

Pilonidal Cyst or Sinus

A hair-containing cyst or sinus located in the midline
over the coccyx or lower sacrum. Often opens as a dimple with visible tuft of hair and, possibly, an erythematous halo. Or, may appear as a palpable cyst. When
advanced, has a palpable sinus tract. Although it is a
congenital disorder, the lesion is first diagnosed between
the ages of 15 and 30 years.

Anorectal Fistula

A chronically inflamed gastrointestinal tract creates an
abnormal passage from inner anus or rectum out to skin
surrounding anus. Usually originates from a local abscess.
The red, raised tract opening may drain serosanguineous
or purulent matter when pressure is applied. Bidigital
palpation may reveal an indurated cord.

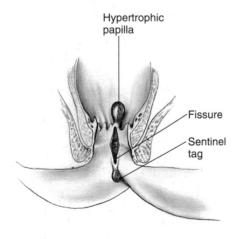

Hypertrophic
papilla

Fissure

Sentinel
tag

◀ ## Fissure

A painful longitudinal tear in the superficial mucosa at
the anal margin. Most fissures (>90 percent) occur in the
posterior midline area. They are frequently accompanied
by a papule of hyperplastic skin, called a *sentinel tag,* on
the anal margin below. Fissures often result from trauma,
e.g., passing a large, hard stool or from irritant diarrheal
stools. The person has itching, bleeding, and exquisite
pain. A resulting spasm in the sphincters makes the area
painful to examine; local anesthesia may be indicated.

Table continued on following page

Table 23-1   ABNORMALITIES OF THE ANUS AND PERIANAL REGION
Continued

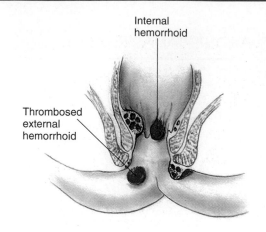

Internal hemorrhoid

Thrombosed external hemorrhoid

◄ **Hemorrhoids**

These painless, flabby papules are due to a varicose vein of the hemorrhoidal plexus. An *external hemorrhoid* originates below the anorectal junction and is covered by anal skin. When *thrombosed,* it contains clotted blood and becomes a painful, swollen, shiny blue mass that itches and bleeds with defecation. When it resolves, it leaves a painless, flabby skin sac around the anal orifice. An *internal hemorrhoid* originates above the anorectal junction, and is covered by mucous membrane. When the person performs a Valsalva maneuver, it may appear as a red mucosal mass. It is not palpable. All hemorrhoids result from increased portal venous pressure, as occurs with straining at stool, chronic constipation, pregnancy, obesity, chronic liver disease, or the low-fiber diet common in Western society.

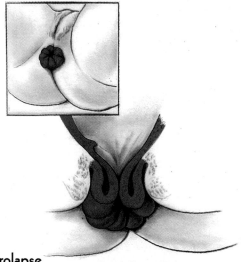

Rectal Prolapse

The rectal mucous membrane protrudes through the anus, appearing as a moist red doughnut with radiating lines. When prolapse is incomplete, only the mucosa bulges. When complete, it includes the anal sphincters. Occurs following a Valsalva maneuver, such as straining at stool, or with exercise.

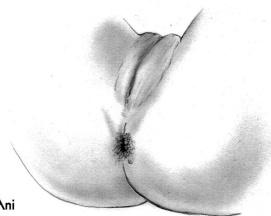

Pruritus Ani

Intense perianal itching is manifested by red, raised, thickened, excoriated skin around the anus. Common causes are pinworms in children and fungal infections in adults. The area is swollen and moist, and with a fungal infection, it appears dull grayish-pink. The skin is dry and brittle with psychosomatic itching.

Table 23-2   ABNORMALITIES OF THE RECTUM

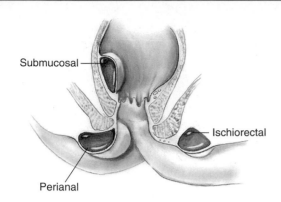

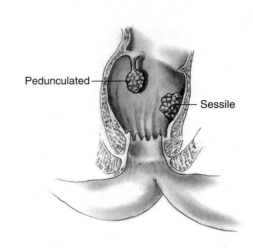

Abscess

A localized cavity of pus from infection in a pararectal space. Infection usually extends from an anal crypt. Characterized by persistent throbbing rectal pain. Termed by the space it occupies, e.g., a perianal abscess is superficial around the anal skin, and appears red, hot, swollen, indurated, and tender. An ischiorectal abscess is deep and tender to bidigital palpation. It occurs laterally between the anus and ischial tuberosity and is uncommon.

Rectal Polyp

A protruding growth from the rectal mucous membrane that is fairly common. The polyp may be *pedunculated* (on a stalk) or *sessile* (a mound on the surface, close to the mucosal wall). The soft nodule is difficult to palpate. Proctoscopy is needed as well as biopsy to screen for a malignant growth.

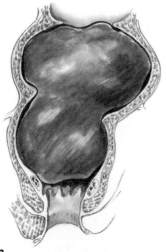

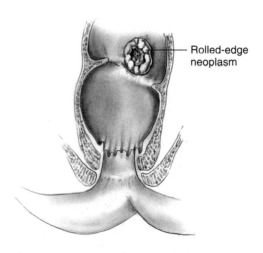

Fecal Impaction

A collection of hard, desiccated feces in the rectum. The obstruction often results from decreased bowel motility, in which more water is reabsorbed from the stool. Also occurs with retained barium from gastrointestinal x-ray examination. The person may complain of constipation or of diarrhea as a fecal stream passes around the impaction.

Carcinoma

A malignant neoplasm in the rectum is asymptomatic, thus the importance of routine rectal palpation. An early lesion may be a single firm nodule. You may palpate an ulcerated center with rolled edges. As the lesion grows, it has an irregular cauliflower shape and is fixed and stone-hard. Refer a person with any rectal lesion for further study because about half are malignant.

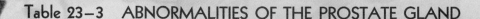

Table 23-3 ABNORMALITIES OF THE PROSTATE GLAND

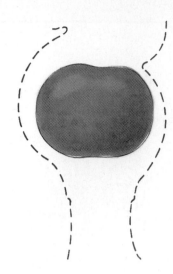

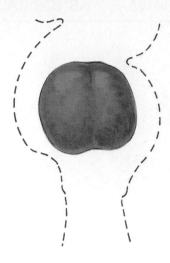

Benign Prostatic Hypertrophy (BPH)

S: Urinary frequency, urgency, hesitancy, straining to urinate, weak stream, intermittent stream, sensation of
incomplete emptying, nocturia.

O: A symmetric nontender enlargement, commonly occurs in males beginning in the middle years. The
prostate surface feels smooth, rubbery, or firm (like
the consistency of the nose), with the median sulcus
obliterated.

Prostatitis

S: Fever, chills, malaise, urinary frequency and urgency,
dysuria, urethral discharge, dull, aching pain in perineal and rectal area.

O: An exquisitely tender enlargement is *acute* inflammation of the prostate gland yielding a swollen, slightly
asymmetric gland that is quite tender to palpation.

With a chronic inflammation the signs can vary from
tender enlargement with a boggy feel to isolated firm
areas due to fibrosis. Or the gland may feel normal.

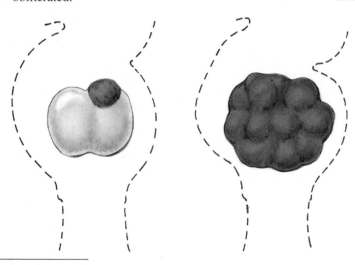

Carcinoma

S: Frequency, nocturia, hematuria, weak stream,
hesitancy, pain or burning on urination, continuous pain in lower back, pelvis, thighs.

O: A malignant neoplasm often starts as a single
hard nodule on the posterior surface, producing asymmetry and a change in consistency.
As it invades normal tissue, multiple hard nodules appear, or the entire gland feels stone-
hard and fixed. The median sulcus is obliterated.

S = subjective data; O = objective data.

Bibliography

American Cancer Society: Cancer facts & figures—1998. Atlanta, GA,
American Cancer Society, Inc., 1998.

Feldman M, Scharschmidt BF, Sleisenger MH: Sleisenger and Fordtran's Gastrointestinal and Liver Disease, 6th ed. Philadelphia, WB
Saunders Company, 1997.

Frydenberg M, Stricker PD, Kaye KW: Prostate cancer diagnosis and
management. Lancet 349(9066):1681–1687, June 7, 1997.

Gambert SR: The crucial prostate exam. Emerg Med 29(1):45–52, Jan
1997.

Gelfand DE, Parzuchowski J, Cort M, Powel I: Digital rectal examinations and prostate cancer screening: Attitudes of African American
men. Oncol Nurs Forum 22(8):1253–1255, Sep 1995.

Goolsby M: Screening, diagnosis, and management of prostate cancer:

Improving primary care outcomes. Nurs Pract 23(3):11–36, Mar
1998.

Holmes A, Webb V: Prostate disease: Expanding the nurse's role. Com-
mun Nurse 4(4):23–24, May 1998.

Macchia RJ: Benign prostatic hyperplasia: Clinical pearls for diagnosis
and therapy. Consultant 37(2):336–345, Feb 1997.

Moul JW, Sesterhenn IA, Connelly RR, et al: Prostate-specific antigen
values at the time of prostate cancer diagnosis in African-American
men. JAMA 274(16):1277–1281, Oct 1995.

Stern S, Altkorn D, Levinson W: Detection of prostate and colon cancer. JAMA 280(2):117–118, July 8, 1998.

Von Eschenback A, Ho R, Murphy GP, et al: American Cancer Society
guideline for the early detection of prostate cancer: Update 1997.
CA Cancer J Clin 47(5):261–264, Sep–Oct 1997.

Weinrich SP, Weinrich MC, Boyd MD, Atkinson C: The impact of
prostate cancer knowledge on cancer screening. Oncol Nurs Forum
25(3):527–534, Apr 1998.

CHAPTER TWENTY FOUR

Female Genitalia

EXTERNAL GENITALIA

The external genitalia are called the **vulva,** or pudendum (Fig. 24–1). The **mons pubis** is a round, firm pad of adipose tissue covering the symphysis pubis. After puberty, it is covered with hair in the pattern of an inverted triangle. The **labia majora** are two rounded folds of adipose tissue extending from the mons pubis down and around to the perineum. After puberty, hair covers the outer surfaces of the labia, while the inner folds are smooth and moist, and contain sebaceous follicles.

Inside the labia majora are two smaller, darker folds of skin, the **labia minora.** These are joined anteriorly at the clitoris where they form a hood, or prepuce. The labia minora are joined posteriorly by a transverse fold, the **frenulum** or fourchette. The **clitoris** is a small, pea-shaped erectile body, homologous with the male penis and highly sensitive to tactile stimulation.

The labial structures encircle a boat-shaped space, or cleft, termed the **vestibule.** Within it are numerous openings. The **urethral meatus** appears as a dimple 2.5 cm posterior to the clitoris. Surrounding the urethral meatus are the tiny, multiple **paraurethral (Skene's) glands.** Their ducts are not visible but open posterior to the urethra at the 5 and 7 o'clock positions.

The **vaginal orifice** is posterior to the urethral meatus. It appears either as a thin median slit or as a large opening with irregular edges, depending on the presentation of the membranous **hymen.** The hymen is a thin, circular or crescent-shaped fold that may cover part of the vaginal orifice or may be absent completely. On either side and posterior to the vaginal orifice are two **vestibular (Bartholin's) glands,** which secrete a clear lubricating mucus during intercourse. Their ducts are not visible but open in the groove between the labia minora and the hymen.

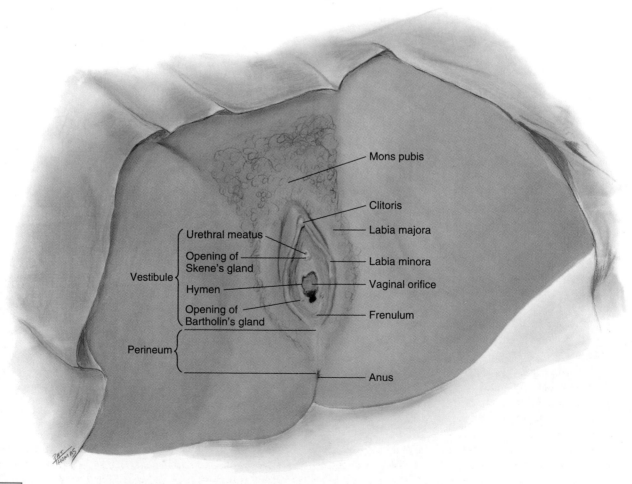

Mons pubis

Clitoris

Labia majora

Urethral meatus

Opening of Skene's gland

Labia minora

Vestibule

Vaginal orifice

Hymen

Opening of Bartholin's gland

Frenulum

Perineum

Anus

24–1

ANTERIOR VIEW OF ADNEXA

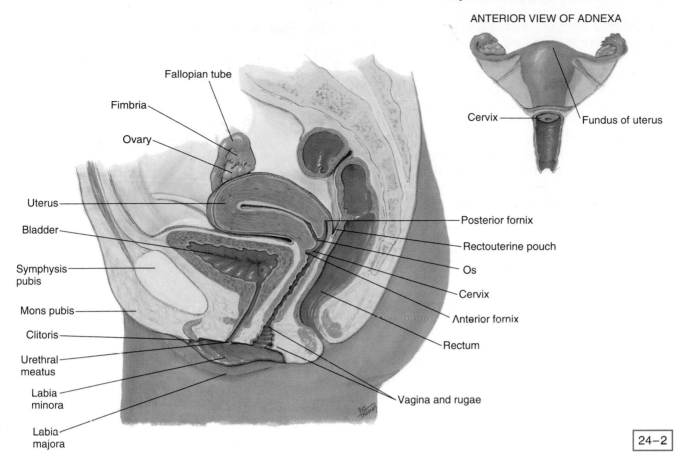

24–2

INTERNAL GENITALIA

The internal genitalia include the **vagina,** a flattened, tubular canal extending from the orifice up and backward into the pelvis (Fig. 24–2). It is 9 cm long and sits between the rectum posteriorly and the bladder and urethra anteriorly. Its walls are in thick transverse folds, or **rugae,** enabling the vagina to dilate widely during childbirth.

At the end of the canal, the uterine **cervix** projects into the vagina. In the nulliparous female, the cervix appears as a smooth doughnut-shaped area with a small circular hole, or **os.** After childbirth, the os is slightly enlarged and irregular. The cervical epithelium is of two distinct types. The vagina and cervix are covered with smooth, pink, stratified squamous epithelium. Inside the os, the endocervical canal is lined with columnar epithelium that looks red and rough. The point where these two tissues meet is the **squamocolumnar junction** and is not visible.

A continuous recess is present around the cervix, termed the **anterior fornix** in front and the **posterior fornix** in back. Behind the posterior fornix, another deep recess is formed by the peritoneum. It dips down between the rectum and cervix to form the **rectouterine pouch,** or **cul-de-sac of Douglas.**

The **uterus** is a pear-shaped, thick-walled, muscular organ. It is flattened anteroposteriorly, measuring 5.5 to 8 cm long by 3.5 to 4 cm wide and 2 to 2.5 cm thick. It is freely movable, not fixed, and usually tilts forward and superior to the bladder (a position labeled as anteverted and anteflexed, see p. 819).

The **fallopian tubes** are two pliable, trumpet-shaped tubes, 10 cm in length, extending from the uterine fundus laterally to the brim of the pelvis. There, they curve posteriorly, their fimbriated ends located near the **ovaries.** The two ovaries are located one on each side of the uterus at the level of the anterior superior iliac spine. Each is oval shaped, 3 cm long by 2 cm wide by 1 cm thick, and serves to develop ova (eggs) as well as the female hormones.

 DEVELOPMENTAL CONSIDERATIONS

Infants and Adolescents

At birth, the external genitalia are engorged because of the presence of maternal estrogen. The structures recede in a few weeks, remaining small until puberty. The ovaries are located in the abdomen during childhood. The uterus is small with a straight axis and no anteflexion.

At puberty, estrogens stimulate the growth of cells in the reproductive tract and the development of secondary sex characteristics. The first signs of puberty are breast and pubic hair development, beginning between the ages of 8½ and 13 years. These signs are usually concurrent, but it is not abnormal if they do not develop together. They take about 3 years to complete.

Menarche occurs during the latter half of this sequence, just after the peak of growth velocity. Irregularity of the menstrual cycle is common during adolescence because of the girl's occasional failure to ovulate. With menarche, the uterine body flexes on the cervix. The ovaries now are in the pelvic cavity.

Tanner's table on the five stages of pubic hair development (sex maturity rating [SMR]) is helpful in teaching girls the expected sequence of sexual development (Table 24–1).

These data are derived from Tanner's study of white British females and may not necessarily generalize to all other racial groups. For example, mature Asian women normally have fine sparse pubic hair. However, the U.S. Health Examination Survey (Harlan et al., 1980) studied girls representative of the contemporary United States population. Its findings correlate closely with Tanner's SMR results. One significant difference is that black girls tend to develop breasts and pubic hair earlier than white girls of the same age.

The Pregnant Female

Shortly after the first missed menstrual period in the pregnant female, the genitalia show signs of the growing fetus. The cervix softens (*Goodell's sign*) at 4 to 6 weeks, and the vaginal mucosa and cervix look cyanotic (*Chadwick's sign*) at 8 to 12 weeks. These changes occur because of increased vascularity and edema of the cervix and hypertrophy and hyperplasia of the cervical glands. The isthmus of the uterus softens (*Hegar's sign*) at 6 to 8 weeks.

The greatest change is in the uterus itself. It increases in capacity by 500 to 1000 times its nonpregnant state, at first owing to hormone stimulation, and then owing to the increasing size of its contents (Cunningham et al., 1997). The nonpregnant uterus has a flattened pear shape. Its early growth encroaches on the space occupied by the bladder, which produces the symptom of urinary frequency. By 10 to 12 weeks gestation, the uterus becomes globular in shape and is too large to stay in the pelvis. At 20 to 24 weeks, the uterus has an oval shape. It rises almost to the liver, displacing the intestines superiorly and laterally.

A clot of thick, tenacious mucus forms in the spaces of the cervical canal (the mucus plug), which protects the fetus from infection. The mucus plug dislodges when

Table 24–1 • Sex Maturity Ratings (SMR) in Girls

Stage 1 Preadolescent. No pubic hair. Mons and labia covered with fine vellus hair as on abdomen.

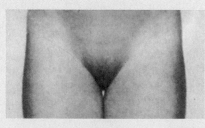

Stage 2 Growth sparse and mostly on labia. Long, downy hair, slightly pigmented, straight or only slightly curly.

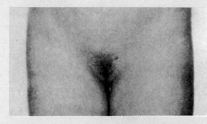

Stage 3 Growth sparse and spreading over mons pubis. Hair is darker, coarser, curlier.

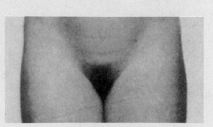

Stage 4 Hair is adult in type but over smaller area; none on medial thigh.

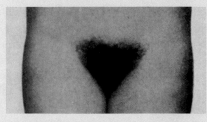

Stage 5 Adult in type and pattern; inverse triangle. Also on medial thigh surface.

labor begins at the end of term, producing a sign of labor called "bloody show." Cervical and vaginal secretions increase during pregnancy and are thick, white, and more acidic. The increased acidity occurs because of the action of *Lactobacillus acidophilus,* which changes glycogen into lactic acid. The acidic pH keeps pathogenic bacteria from multiplying in the vagina, but the increase in glycogen increases the risk of candidiasis (commonly called a yeast infection) during pregnancy.

The Aging Female

In contrast to the slowly declining hormones in the aging male, the female's hormonal milieu decreases rapidly. *Menopause* is cessation of the menses. Usually this occurs around the ages of 48 to 51 years, although a wide normal variation of ages from 35 to 60 years exists. The stage of menopause includes the preceding 1 to 2 years of decline in ovarian function, shown by irregular menses that gradually become farther apart and produce a lighter flow than usual. The ovaries stop producing progesterone and estrogen. Since cells in the reproductive tract are estrogen dependent, decreased estrogen levels during menopause bring dramatic physical changes.

The uterus shrinks in size because of its decreased myometrium. The ovaries atrophy to 1 to 2 cm and are not palpable after menopause. Ovulation still may occur sporadically after menopause. The sacral ligaments relax, and the pelvic musculature weakens, so the uterus droops. Sometimes it may protrude, or prolapse, into the vagina. The cervix shrinks and looks paler with a thick, glistening epithelium.

The vagina becomes shorter, narrower, and less elastic because of increased connective tissue. Without sexual activity, the vagina atrophies to one half its former length and width. The vaginal epithelium atrophies, becoming thinner, drier, and itchy. This results in a fragile mucosal surface that is at risk for bleeding and vaginitis. Decreased vaginal secretions leave the vagina dry and at risk for irritation and pain with intercourse (dyspareunia). The vaginal pH becomes more alkaline, and a decreased glycogen content occurs from the decreased estrogen. These factors also increase the risk of vaginitis because they create a suitable medium for pathogens.

Externally, the mons pubis looks smaller because the fat pad atrophies. The labia and clitoris gradually decrease in size. Pubic hair becomes thin and sparse.

Declining estrogen levels produce some physiologic changes in the female sexual response cycle (Table 24–2). However, these changes do not affect sexual pleasure and function. Sexual desire and the need for full sexual expression continue. As with the male, the older female is capable of sexual function given reasonably good health and an interested partner. The problem for many older women is finding a socially acceptable sexual partner. Aging women greatly outnumber their male counterparts. And, aging women are more likely to be single while males their same age are more likely to be married.

Table 24–2 • Aging Changes in Sexual Response Cycle

Phase	Physiologic Change
Excitement	Reduced amount of vaginal secretion and lubrication
Plateau	Less expansion of vagina
	Labia majora do not elevate against perineum
	No color change in labia minora (was from pink to cardinal-red or dark red)
	Size of clitoris decreases after age 60
Orgasm	Shorter duration
Resolution	Occurs more rapidly

Data from Masters WH, Johnson VE: Human Sexual Response. Boston, Little, Brown, and Company, 1966.

SUBJECTIVE DATA

1. Menstrual history
2. Obstetric history
3. Menopause
4. Self-care behaviors
5. Urinary symptoms
6. Vaginal discharge
7. Past history
8. Sexual activity
9. Contraceptive use
10. Sexually transmitted disease (STD) contact
11. STD risk reduction

Examiner Asks	Rationale

1 **Menstrual history.** Tell me about your menstrual periods:
 	
• Date of your last menstrual period?
• Age at first period?
 	
• How often are your periods?
 	
• How many days does your period last?
• Usual amount of flow: light, medium, heavy? How many pads or tampons do you use each day or hour?
• Any clotting?
 	
• Any pain or cramps before or during period? How do you treat it? Interfere with daily activities? Any other associated symptoms: bloating, cramping, breast tenderness, moodiness? Any spotting between periods?
	Menstrual history is usually nonthreatening, thus it is a good place to start history.
	    LMP—last menstrual period.
	    Menarche—onset between 12 and 14 years indicates normal growth; onset between 16 and 17 years suggests an endocrine problem.
	    Cycle—normally varies every 18 to 45 days.
	    Amenorrhea—absent menses.
	    Duration—average 3 to 7 days.
	    Menorrhagia—heavy menses.
	
	Clotting indicates heavy flow or vaginal pooling.
	    Dysmenorrhea.

2 **Obstetric history.** Have you ever been pregnant?
• How many times?
• How many babies have you had?
• Any miscarriage or abortion?
 	
• For each pregnancy, describe: duration, any complication, labor and delivery, baby's sex, birth weight, condition.
• Do you think you may be pregnant now? What symptoms have you noticed?
	Obstetric history.
	    Gravida—number of pregnancies.
	    Para—number of births.
	    Abortions—interrupted pregnancies, including elective abortions and spontaneous miscarriages.

3 **Menopause.** Have your periods slowed down or stopped?
• Any associated symptoms of menopause, e.g., hot flash, numbness and tingling, headache, palpitations, drenching sweats, mood swings, vaginal dryness, itching? Any treatment?
• If hormone replacement, how much? How is it working? Any side effects?
 	
• How do you feel about going through menopause?
	Menopause—cessation of menstruation.
	    Perimenopausal period, from 40 to 55 years of age, has hormone shifts, resulting in vasomotor instability.
	    Side effects of estrogen replacement therapy include fluid retention, breast pain or enlargement, vaginal bleeding.
	    Although this is a normal life stage, reaction varies from acceptance to feelings of loss.

4 **Self-care behaviors.** How often do you have a gynecologic checkup? • Last Papanicolaou smear? Results? • Has your mother ever mentioned taking hormones while pregnant with you?	Assess **self-care behaviors.** Maternal ingestion of DES (diethylstilbestrol) causes cervical and vaginal abnormalities in female offspring requiring frequent follow-up.

Examiner Asks	Rationale
5 **Urinary symptoms.** Any problems with urinating? Frequently and small amounts? Cannot wait to urinate?	**Urinary symptoms.** Frequency. Urgency.
• Any burning or pain on urinating?	Dysuria.
• Awaken during night to urinate?	Nocturia.
• Blood in the urine?	Hematuria.
• Urine dark, cloudy, foul smelling?	Bile in urine or urinary tract infection.
• Any difficulty controlling urine or wetting yourself?	True incontinence—loss of urine without warning. Urgency incontinence—sudden loss, as with acute cystitis.
• Urinate with a sneeze, laugh, cough, bearing down?	Stress incontinence—loss of urine with physical strain due to muscle weakness.
6 **Vaginal discharge.** Any unusual **vaginal discharge?** Increased amount?	Normal discharge is small, clear or cloudy, and always nonirritating.
• Character or color: white, yellow-green, gray, curdlike, foul smelling?	Suggests vaginal infection; character of discharge often suggests causative organism (see Table 24–6).
• When did this begin?	Acute versus chronic problem.
• Is the discharge associated with vaginal itching, rash, pain with intercourse?	Occurs secondary to irritation from discharge. Dyspareunia occurs with vaginitis of any cause.
• Taking any medications?	Factors that increase the risk of vaginitis:
	• Oral contraceptives increase glycogen content of vaginal epithelium, providing fertile medium for some organisms.
	• Broad-spectrum antibiotics alter balance of normal flora.
• Family history of diabetes?	• Diabetes increases glycogen content.
• What part of your menstrual cycle are you in now?	• Menses, postpartum, menopause have a more alkaline vaginal pH.
• Use a vaginal douche? How often?	• Frequent douching alters pH.
• Use feminine hygiene spray?	• Spray has risk of contact dermatitis.
• Wear nonventilating underpants, pantyhose?	• Local irritation.
• Treated the discharge with anything? Result?	
7 **Past history.** Any other problems in the genital area? Sores or lesions—now or in the past? How were these treated?	
• Any abdominal pain?	
• Any past surgery on uterus, ovaries, vagina?	Assess feelings about surgery. Some fear loss of sexual response following hysterectomy. This belief may cause problems in intimate relationships.

Examiner Asks	Rationale

8 Sexual activity. Often women have a question about their **sexual relationship** and how it affects their health. Do you?
- Are you in a relationship involving sex now?
- Are aspects of sex satisfactory to you and your partner?
- Satisfied with the way you and partner communicate about sex?
- Satisfied with your ability to respond sexually?
- Do you have more than one sexual partner?

Begin with open-ended question to assess individual needs. Include appropriate questions as a routine part of history:
- Communicates that you accept individual's sexual activity and believe it is important.
- Your comfort with discussion prompts person's interest and possibly relief that the topic has been introduced.
- Establishes a data base for comparison with any future sexual activities.
- Provides opportunity to screen sexual problems.

Lesbians and bisexual women need to feel acceptance to discuss their health concerns.

- What is your sexual preference: relationship with a man, with a woman, both?

9 Contraceptive use. Currently planning a pregnancy, or avoiding pregnancy?
- Do you and your partner use a **contraceptive?** Which method? Is this satisfactory? Do you have any questions about method?

If oral contraceptives are used, assess smoking history. Cigarettes increase cardiovascular side effects of oral contraceptives.

- Which methods have you used in the past? Have you and partner discussed having children?
- Have you ever had any problems becoming pregnant?

Infertility is considered after 1 year of engaging in unprotected sexual intercourse without conceiving.

10 Sexually transmitted disease (STD) contact. Any sexual contact with partner having a sexually transmitted disease, such as gonorrhea, herpes, AIDS, chlamydial infection, venereal warts, syphilis? When? How was this treated? Were there any complications?

11 STD risk reduction. Any precautions to reduce risk of STDs? Use condoms at each episode of sexual intercourse?

ADDITIONAL HISTORY FOR INFANTS AND CHILDREN

1 Does your child have any problem urinating? Pain with urinating, crying, holding genitals? Urinary tract infection?
- (If the child is older than 2 to 2½ years of age) Has toilet training started? How is it progressing?
- Does the child wet bed at night? Is this a problem for child or you (parents)? What have you (parents) done?

2 Problem with genital area: itching, rash, vaginal discharge?

Occurs with poor perineal hygiene or insertion of foreign body in vagina.

Examiner Asks	Rationale

3 (To child) Has anyone ever touched you in between your legs and you did not want them to? Sometimes that happens to children. They should remember they have not been bad. They should try to tell a big person about it. Can you tell me three different big people you trust who you could talk to?

Screen for sexual abuse. For prevention, teach the child that it's not okay for someone to look at or touch their private parts while telling them it's a secret. Naming three trusted adults will include someone outside the family — important since most molestation is by a parent (Brown, 1997).

ADDITIONAL HISTORY FOR PREADOLESCENTS AND ADOLESCENTS

Use the following questions, as appropriate, to assess sexual growth and development and sexual behavior. First
- Ask questions that seem appropriate for girl's age but be aware that norms vary widely. When in doubt, it is better to ask too many questions than to omit something. Children obtain information, often misinformation, from the media and from peers at surprisingly early ages. You can be sure your information will be more thoughtful and accurate.
- Ask direct, matter-of-fact questions. Avoid sounding judgmental.
- Start with a *permission statement,* "Often girls your age experience . . ." This conveys that it is normal to think or feel a certain way.
- Try the open-ended, "When did you . . ." rather than "Do you . . ." This is less threatening because it implies that the topic is normal and unexceptional.

1 Around age 11, but sometimes earlier, girls start to develop breasts and pubic hair. Have you ever seen charts and pictures of normal growth patterns for girls? Let us go over these now.

2 Have your periods started? How did you feel? Were you prepared or surprised?

Assess attitude of girl and parents. Note inadequate preparation or attitude of distaste.

3 Who in your family do you talk to about your body changes and about sex information? How do these talks go? Do you think you get enough information? What about sex education classes at school? Is there a teacher, a nurse or doctor, a minister, a counselor to whom you can talk?

Often girls your age have questions about sexual activity. Do you have questions? Are you dating? Someone steady?

Do you and your boyfriend have intercourse? Are you using condoms? What method of protection did you use the last time you had sex?

Avoid the term "sexually active," which is ambiguous.

4 Has anyone ever talked to you about sexually transmitted diseases, such as herpes, gonorrhea, or AIDS?

Teach STD risk reduction.

5 Sometimes it happens that a person touches a girl in a way that she does not want them to. Has that ever happened to you? If that happens, the girl should remember it is not her fault. She should tell another adult about it.

Screen for sexual abuse.

Examiner Asks	Rationale

ADDITIONAL HISTORY FOR THE AGING ADULT

1 After menopause, noted any vaginal bleeding?

Postmenopausal bleeding warrants further workup and referral.

2 Any vaginal itching, discharge, pain with intercourse?

Associated with atrophic vaginitis.

3 Any pressure in genital area, loss of urine with cough or sneeze, back pain, or constipation?

Occurs with weakened pelvic musculature and uterine prolapse.

4 Are you in a relationship involving sex now? Are aspects of sex satisfactory to you and your partner? Is there adequate privacy for a sexual relationship?

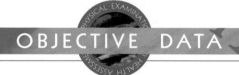

OBJECTIVE DATA

Assemble these items before helping the woman into position. Arrange within easy reach.

Equipment Needed

Gloves

Protective clothing for examiner

Goose-necked lamp with a strong light

Vaginal speculum of appropriate size (Fig. 24–3)

    Graves' speculum—useful for most adult women, available in varying lengths and widths

    Pederson speculum—narrow blades, useful for virginal or postmenopausal women with narrowed introitus

Large cotton-tipped applicators (rectal swabs)

Materials for cytologic study:

    Glass slide with frosted end

    Sterile Cytobrush or cotton-tipped applicator

    Ayre's spatula

    Spray fixative

    Specimen container for gonorrhea culture (GC)/*Chlamydia*

    Small bottle of normal saline, potassium hydroxide (KOH), and acetic acid (white vinegar)

Lubricant

Preparation

Familiarize yourself with the vaginal speculum before the examination. Practice opening and closing the blades, locking them into position, and releasing them. Try both metal and plastic types. Note that the plastic speculum locks and unlocks with a resounding click that can be alarming to the uninformed woman.

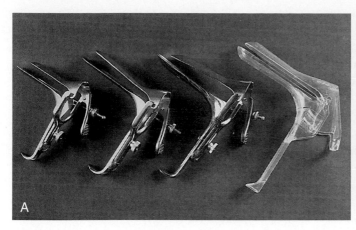
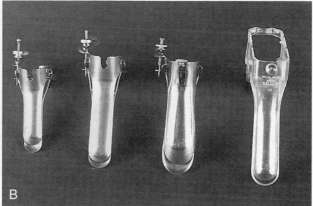

24-3

POSITION

Initially, the woman should be sitting up. An equal status position is important to establish trust and rapport before the vaginal examination.

For the examination, the woman should be placed in the lithotomy position, with the examiner sitting on a stool. Help the woman into lithotomy position, with the body supine, feet in stirrups and knees apart, and buttocks at edge of examining table (Fig. 24–4). Ask the woman to lift her hips as you guide them to the edge of the table. Some women prefer to leave their shoes or socks on. Or, you can place an exam glove over each of the stirrups to warm the stirrups and keep her feet from slipping.

The arms should be at the woman's sides or across the chest, not over the head, because this position only tightens the abdominal muscles. The traditional mode is to drape the woman fully, covering the stomach and legs, exposing only the vulva to your view. Be sure to push down the drape between the woman's legs so that you can see her face.

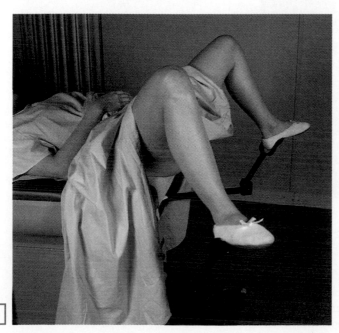

24-4

The lithotomy position leaves many women feeling helpless and vulnerable. Indeed, many women tolerate the pelvic examination because they consider it basic for health care, yet they find it embarrassing and uncomfortable. Previous examinations may have been painful, or the previous examiner's attitude hurried and patronizing.

The examination need not be this way. You can help the woman relax, decrease her anxiety, and retain a sense of control by employing these measures:

- Have her empty the bladder before the examination.
- Position the exam table so that her perineum is not exposed to an inadvertent open door.
- Ask if she would like a friend, family member, or chaperone present. Position this person by the woman's head to maintain privacy.
- Elevate her head and shoulders to a semi-sitting position to maintain eye contact.
- Place the stirrups so the legs are not abducted too far.
- Explain each step in the examination before you do it.
- Assure the woman she can stop the examination at any point should she feel any discomfort.
- Use a gentle, firm touch, and gradual movements.
- Communicate throughout the examination. Maintain a dialogue to share information.
- Use the techniques of the *educational* or *mirror pelvic examination* (Fig. 24–5). This is a routine examination with some modifications in attitude, position, and communication. First, the woman is considered an active participant, one who is interested in learning and in sharing decisions about her own health care. The woman props herself up on one elbow, or the head of the table is raised. Her other hand holds a mirror between her legs, above the examiner's hands. The woman can see all that the examiner is doing and has a full view of her genitalia.

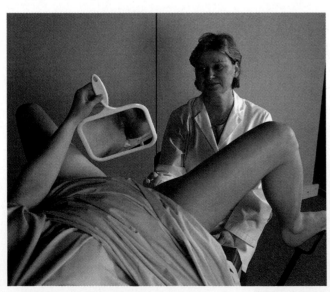

24–5

The mirror works well for teaching normal anatomy and its relation to sexual behavior. Even women who are in a sexual relationship or who have had children may be surprisingly uninformed about their own anatomy. You will find the woman's enthusiasm on seeing her own cervix is rewarding too.

The mirror pelvic examination also works well when abnormalities arise because the woman can see the rationale for treatment and can monitor progress at the next appointment. She is more willing to comply with treatment when she shares in the decision.

▶ | Normal Range of Findings | Abnormal Findings

EXTERNAL GENITALIA

Inspection

Note:

- Skin color (Fig. 24–6).

- Hair distribution is in the usual female pattern of inverted triangle, although it normally may trail up the abdomen toward the umbilicus.

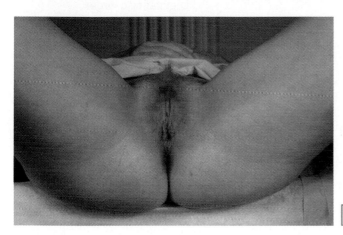

24–6

- Labia majora normally are symmetric, plump, and well formed. In the nulliparous woman, labia meet in the midline; following a vaginal delivery, the labia are gaping and slightly shriveled.
- No lesions should be present, except for occasional sebaceous cysts. These are yellowish, 1-cm nodules that are firm, nontender, and often multiple.

    With your gloved hand, separate the labia majora to inspect:

- Clitoris (Fig. 24–7).
- Labia minora are dark pink and moist, usually symmetric.
- Urethral opening appears stellate or slitlike and is midline.
- Vaginal opening, or introitus, may appear as a narrow vertical slit or as a larger opening.

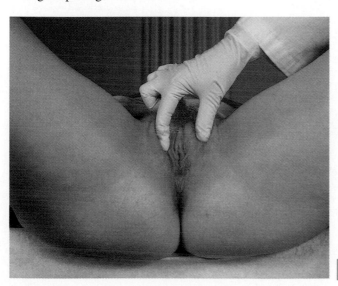

24–7

Abnormal Findings column:

Refer any suspicious pigmented lesion for biopsy.

Consider delayed puberty if no pubic hair or breast development has occurred by age 13.

Nits or lice at the base of pubic hair.

Swelling.

Excoriation, nodules, rash, or lesions (see Table 24–3).

Inflammation or lesions.
Polyp.
Foul-smelling, irritating discharge.

- Perineum is smooth. A well-healed episiotomy scar, midline or mediolateral, may be present following a vaginal birth.
- Anus has coarse skin of increased pigmentation (see Chapter 23 for assessment).

Palpation

Assess the urethra and Skene's glands (Fig. 24–8). Dip your gloved finger in a bowl of warm water to lubricate. Then insert your index finger into the vagina, and gently milk the urethra by applying pressure up and out. This procedure should produce no pain. If any discharge appears, culture it.

Tenderness.

Induration along urethra.

Urethral discharge.

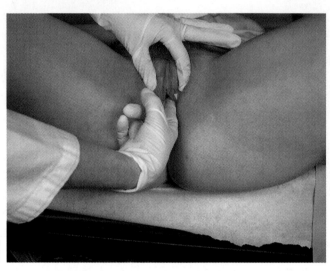

24–8

Assess Bartholin's glands. Palpate the posterior parts of the labia majora with your index finger in the vagina and your thumb outside (Fig. 24–9). Normally, the labia feel soft and homogeneous.

Swelling (see Table 24–3).

Induration.

Pain with palpation.

Erythema around or discharge from duct opening.

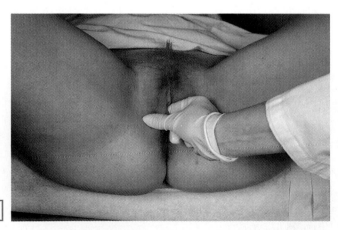

24–9

▶ Normal Range of Findings	Abnormal Findings

Assess the support of pelvic musculature by using these maneuvers:

1. Palpate the perineum. Normally, it feels thick, smooth, and muscular in the nulliparous woman, and thin and rigid in the multiparous woman.
2. Ask the woman to squeeze the vaginal opening around your fingers; it should feel tight in the nulliparous woman and have less tone in the multiparous woman.
3. Using your index and middle fingers, separate the vaginal orifice and ask the woman to strain down. Normally, no bulging of vaginal walls or urinary incontinence occurs.

Tenderness.
Paper-thin perineum.
Absent or decreased tone may diminish sexual satisfaction.
Bulging of the vaginal wall indicates cystocele, rectocele, or uterine prolapse (see Table 24–4).
Urinary incontinence.

INTERNAL GENITALIA

Speculum Examination

Select the proper-sized speculum. Warm and lubricate the speculum under warm running water. Avoid gel lubricant at this point because it is bacteriostatic and would distort cells in the cytology specimen you will collect.

A good technique is to dedicate one hand to the patient and the other hand to picking up equipment in the room. For example, hold the speculum in your left hand (the equipment hand), with the index and the middle fingers surrounding the blades and your thumb under the thumbscrew. This prevents the blades from opening painfully during insertion. With your right index and middle fingers (the patient hand), push the introitus down and open to relax the pubococcygeal muscle (Fig. 24–10). Tilt the width of the blades obliquely and insert the speculum past your right fingers, applying any pressure downward. This avoids pressure on the sensitive urethra above it.

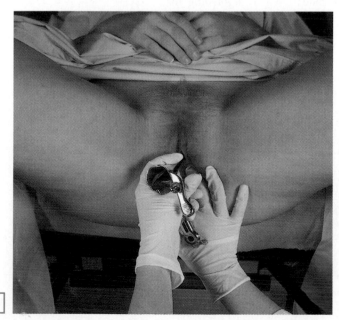

24–10

Ease insertion by asking the woman to bear down. This method relaxes the perineal muscles and opens the introitus. (With experience, you can combine speculum insertion with assessing the support of the vaginal muscles.) As the blades pass your right fingers, withdraw your fingers. Now change the hand holding the speculum to your right hand and turn the width of the blades horizontally. Continue to insert in a 45-degree angle downward toward the small of the woman's back (Fig. 24–11). This matches the natural slope of the vagina.

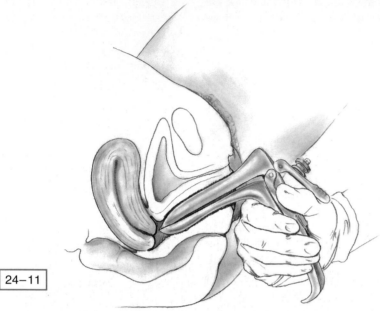

24–11

After the blades are fully inserted, open them by squeezing the handles together (Fig. 24–12). The cervix should be in full view. Sometimes this does not occur (especially with beginning examiners), because the blades are angled above the location of the cervix. Try closing the blades, withdrawing about halfway, and reinserting in a more *downward* plane. Then slowly sweep upward. Once you have the cervix in full view, lock the blades open by tightening the thumbscrew.

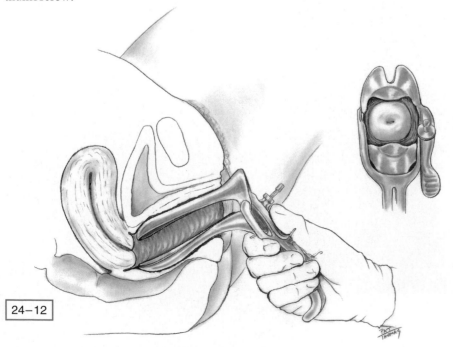

24–12

► **Normal Range of Findings**   **Abnormal Findings**

Inspect the cervix and its os

Note:

- **Color.** Normally the cervical mucosa is pink and even. During the 2nd month of pregnancy it looks blue (Chadwick's sign), and after menopause it is pale.

- **Position.** Midline, either anterior or posterior. Projects 1 to 3 cm into the vagina.

- **Size.** Diameter is 2.5 cm (1 inch).

- **Os.** This is small and round in the nulliparous woman. In the parous woman, it is a horizontal irregular slit and also may show healed lacerations on the sides (Fig. 24–13).

- **Surface.** This is normally smooth, but **cervical eversion,** or ectropion, may occur normally after vaginal deliveries. The endocervical canal is everted or "rolled out." It looks like a red, beefy halo inside the pink cervix surrounding the os. It is difficult to distinguish this normal variation from an abnormal condition (e.g., erosion, or carcinoma), and biopsy may be needed.

Redness, inflammation.
Pallor with anemia.
Cyanotic other than with pregnancy (see Table 24–5).
Lateral position may be due to adhesion or tumor. Projection of more than 3 cm may be a prolapse.
Hypertrophy of more than 4 cm occurs with inflammation or tumor.

Surface reddened, granular, and asymmetric, particularly around os.
Friable, bleeds easily.
Any lesions: white patch on cervix; strawberry spot.
Refer any suspicious red, white, or pigmented lesion for biopsy (see erosion, ulceration, and carcinoma, Table 24–5).

NORMAL VARIATIONS OF THE CERVIX

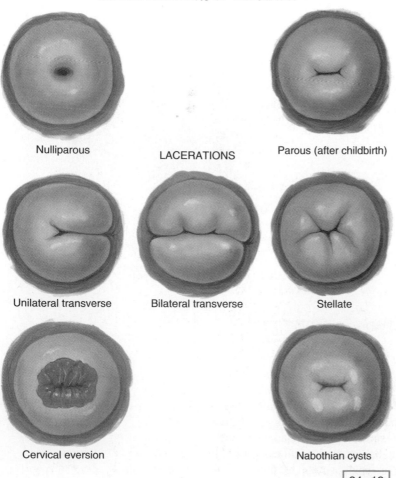

Nulliparous   LACERATIONS   Parous (after childbirth)

Unilateral transverse   Bilateral transverse   Stellate

Cervical eversion   Nabothian cysts

24–13

|

Nabothian cysts are benign growths that commonly appear on the cervix after childbirth. They are small, smooth, yellow nodules that may be single or multiple. Less than 1 cm, they are retention cysts due to obstruction of cervical glands.

- **Note the cervical secretions.** Depending on the day of the menstrual cycle, secretions may be clear and thin, or thick, opaque, and stringy. Always they are odorless and nonirritating.

  If secretions are copious, swab the area with a thick-tipped rectal swab. This method sponges away secretions, and you have a better view of the structures.

Obtain cervical smears and cultures

The Papanicolaou, or Pap, smear screens for cervical cancer. Do not obtain during the woman's menses or if a heavy infectious discharge is present. Instruct the woman not to douche, have intercourse, or put anything into the vagina within 24 hours before collecting the specimens. Obtain the Pap smear before other specimens so you will not disrupt or remove cells. Laboratories may vary in method, but usually the test consists of three specimens:

Vaginal Pool. Gently rub the blunt end of an Ayre spatula over the vaginal wall under and lateral to the cervix (Fig. 24–14). Wipe the specimen on a slide and spray with fixative immediately. If the mucosa is very dry (as in a postmenopausal woman), moisten a sterile swab with normal saline to collect this specimen.

Cervical polyp—bright red growth protruding from the os (see Table 24–5).

Foul-smelling, irritating, with yellow, green, white, or gray discharge (see Table 24–6).

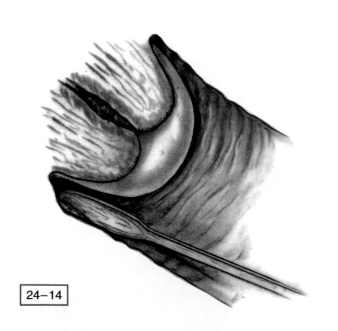

24–14

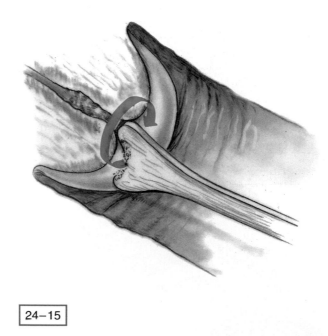

24–15

Ectocervical Scrape (Fig. 24–15). Reverse the Ayre spatula and insert the bifid end into the vagina with the more pointed bump into the cervical os. Rotate it 360 to 720 degrees, using firm pressure. The rounded cervix fits snugly into the spatula's groove. The spatula scrapes the surface of the squamocolumnar junction and cervix as you turn the instrument. Spread the specimen from both sides of the spatula onto a glass slide. Use a single stroke to thin out the specimen, not a back-and-forth motion.

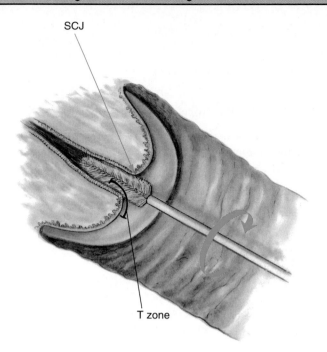

SCJ

T zone

24–16

Endocervical Specimen (Fig. 24–16). Insert a Cytobrush (instead of a cotton applicator) into the os. A Cytobrush gives a higher yield of endocervical cells at the squamocolumnar junction, or SCJ, and safety for use during pregnancy has been shown (Foster and Smith, 1996; Stillson, Knight, and Elswick, 1997). The woman may feel a slight pinch with the brush and scant bleeding may occur. For this reason, collect the endocervical specimen last so that bleeding will not obscure cytologic evaluation.

Rotate the brush 720 degrees in ONE direction in the endocervical canal, either clockwise or counterclockwise. Then rotate the brush gently on a slide to deposit all the cells. Rotate in the opposite direction from the one in which you obtained the specimen. Avoid leaving a thick specimen that would be hard to read under the microscope. Immediately (within 2 seconds) spray the slide with fixative to avoid drying.

For the woman following hysterectomy whose cervix has been removed, collect a scrape from the end of the vagina and a vaginal pool.

Immediately spray the slides with fixative. The frosted ends of the slides should be labeled with the woman's name. Send these to the laboratory with the following necessary data:

- Date of specimen
- Woman's date of birth
- Date of last menstrual period
- Hormone administration if any
- If pregnant, with estimated date of delivery
- Known infections
- Prior surgery or radiation
- Prior abnormal cytology
- Abnormal findings on physical examination

These data are important for accurate interpretation; e.g., a specimen may be interpreted as positive unless the laboratory technicians know the woman has had prior radiation treatment.

To screen for STDs, or if you note any abnormal vaginal discharge, obtain the following samples:

Saline Mount, or "Wet Prep." Spread a sample of the discharge onto a glass slide and add one drop of normal saline and a coverslip.

KOH Prep. To a sample of the discharge on a glass slide, add one drop potassium hydroxide and a coverslip.

Gonorrhea (GC)/*Chlamydia* Culture. Insert a sterile cotton applicator into the os, rotate it 360 degrees, and leave it in place 10 to 20 seconds for complete saturation. Insert into specimen container and label immediately. Note that newer specimen containers from many laboratories combine the GC/*Chlamydia* culture and do not require incubation.

Anal Culture. Insert a sterile cotton swab into the anal canal about 1 cm. Rotate it, and move it side to side. Leave in place 10 to 20 seconds. If the swab collects feces, discard it and begin again. Insert into specimen container.

Five Percent Acetic Acid Wash. Acetic acid (white vinegar) screens for asymptomatic human papilloma virus (HPV), which causes genital warts. After all other specimens are gathered, soak a thick-tipped cotton rectal swab with acetic acid and "paint" the cervix. Acetic acid dissolves mucus and temporarily causes intracellular dehydration and coagulation of protein. A normal response (indicating no HPV infection) is no change in the cervical epithelium.

Rapid acetowhitening or blanching, especially with irregular borders, suggests HPV infection (see Table 24–3).

Inspect the vaginal wall

Loosen the thumbscrew but continue to hold the speculum blades open. Slowly withdraw the speculum, rotating it as you go, to fully inspect the vaginal wall. Normally, the wall looks pink, deeply rugated, moist and smooth, and is free of inflammation or lesions. Normal discharge is thin and clear, or opaque and stringy, but always odorless.

Inflammation or lesions.

Leukoplakia, appears as spot of dried white paint.

Vaginal discharge: thick, white, and curdlike with candidiasis; profuse, watery, gray-green, and frothy with trichomoniasis; or any gray, green-yellow, white, or foul-smelling discharge (see Table 24–6).

When the blade ends near the vaginal opening, let them close, but be careful not to pinch the mucosa or catch any hairs. Turn the blades obliquely to avoid stretching the opening. Place the metal speculum in a basin to be cleaned later and soaked in a sterilizing and disinfecting solution; discard the plastic variety. Discard your gloves and wash hands.

Bimanual Examination

Rise to a stand, and have the woman remain in lithotomy position. Drop lubricant onto the first two fingers of your gloved intravaginal hand (Fig. 24–17). Assume the "obstetric" position with the first two fingers extended, the last two flexed onto the palm, and the thumb abducted. Insert your fingers into the vagina, with any pressure directed posteriorly. Wait until the vaginal walls relax, then insert your fingers fully.

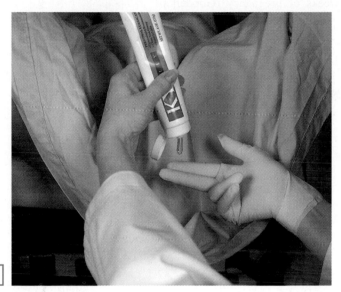

24–17

You will use both hands to palpate the internal genitalia to assess their location, size, and mobility, and to screen for any tenderness or mass. One hand is on the abdomen while the other (often the dominant, more sensitive hand) inserts two fingers into the vagina (Fig. 24–18). It does not matter which you choose as the intravaginal hand; try each way, and settle on the most comfortable method for you.

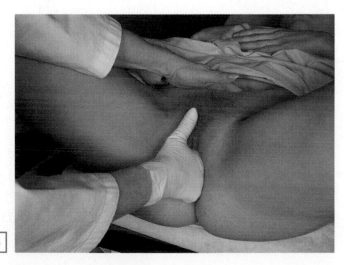

24–18

Normal Range of Findings	Abnormal Findings

Palpate the vaginal wall. Normally, it feels smooth and has no area of induration or tenderness.

Nodule.
Tenderness.

Cervix. Locate the cervix in the midline, often near the anterior vaginal wall. The cervix points in the opposite direction of the fundus of the uterus. Palpate using the palmar surface of the fingers. Note these characteristics of a normal cervix:

- **Consistency**—feels smooth and firm, as the consistency of the tip of the nose. It softens and feels velvety at 5 to 6 weeks of pregnancy (Goodell's sign).
- **Contour**—evenly rounded.
- **Mobility**—With a finger on either side, move the cervix gently from side to side. Normally, this produces no pain (Fig. 24–19).

Palpate all around the fornices; the wall should feel smooth.

Hard with malignancy.
Nodular.

Irregular.
Immobile with malignancy.

Painful with inflammation or ectopic pregnancy.

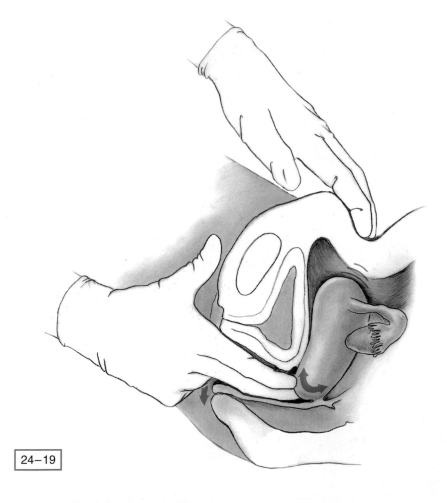

24–19

Next, use your abdominal hand to push the pelvic organs closer for your intravaginal fingers to palpate. Place your hand midway between the umbilicus and the symphysis; push down in a slow, firm manner, fingers together and slightly flexed. Brace the elbow of your pelvic arm against your hip, and keep it horizontal. The woman must be relaxed.

▶

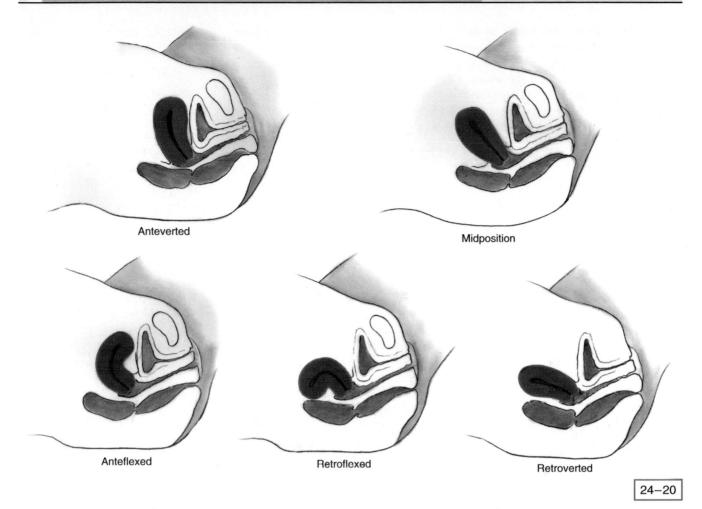

Anteverted

Midposition

Anteflexed

Retroflexed

Retroverted

24–20

Uterus. With your intravaginal fingers in the anterior fornix, assess the uterus. Determine the position, or *version,* of the uterus (Fig. 24–20). This compares the long axis of the uterus with the long axis of the body. In many women, the uterus is anteverted; you palpate it at the level of the pubis with the cervix pointing posteriorly. Two other positions occur normally (midposition and retroverted), as well as two aspects of flexion, where the long axis of the uterus is not straight but is flexed.

Palpate the uterine wall with your fingers in the fornices. Normally, it feels firm and smooth, with the contour of the fundus rounded. It softens during pregnancy. Bounce the uterus gently between your abdominal and intravaginal hand. It should be freely movable and nontender.

Enlarged uterus (see Table 24–7).
Lateral displacement.
Nodular mass. Irregular, asymmetric uterus. Fixed and immobile.
Tenderness.

Adnexa. Move both hands to the right to explore the adnexa. Place your abdominal hand on the lower quadrant just inside the anterior iliac spine and your intravaginal fingers in the lateral fornix (Fig. 24–21). Push the abdominal hand in and try to capture the ovary. Often, you cannot feel the ovary. When you can, it normally feels smooth, firm, and almond shaped, and is highly movable, sliding through the fingers. It is slightly sensitive but not painful. The fallopian tube is not palpable normally. No other mass or pulsation should be felt.

Enlarged adnexa. Nodules or mass in adnexa.

Immobile.

Markedly tender (see Table 24–8).

Pulsation or palpable fallopian tube suggests ectopic pregnancy; this warrants immediate referral.

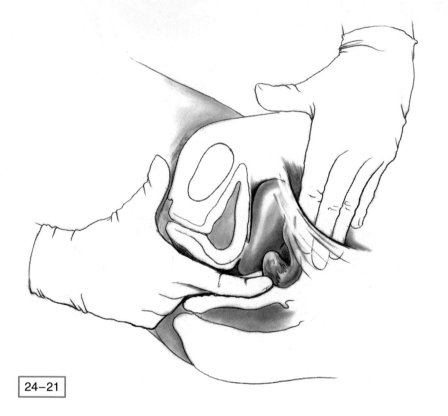

24–21

A note of caution—Normal adnexal structures often are not palpable. Be careful not to mistake an abnormality for a normal structure. To be safe, consider abnormal any mass that you cannot *positively* identify, and refer the woman for further study.

Move to the left to palpate the other side. Then, withdraw your hand and check secretions on the fingers before discarding the glove. Normal secretions are clear or cloudy and odorless.

Rectovaginal Examination

Use this technique to assess the rectovaginal septum, posterior uterine wall, cul-de-sac, and rectum. Change gloves to avoid spreading any possible infection. Lubricate the first two fingers. Instruct the woman that this may feel uncomfortable and will mimic the feeling of moving her bowels. Ask her to bear down as you insert your index finger into the vagina and your middle finger gently into the rectum (Fig. 24–22).

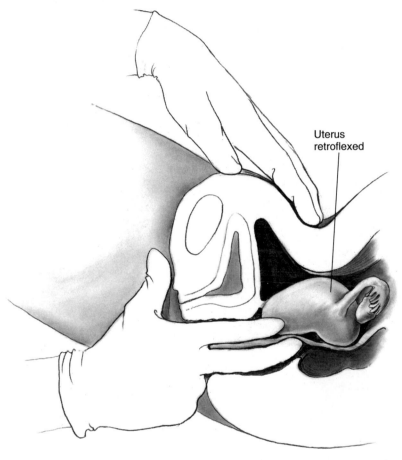

Uterus retroflexed

RECTOVAGINAL PALPATION

24–22

While pushing with the abdominal hand, repeat the steps of the bimanual examination. Try to keep the intravaginal finger on the cervix so the intrarectal finger does not mistake the cervix for a mass. Note:

- Rectovaginal septum should feel smooth, thin, firm, and pliable.
- Rectovaginal pouch, or cul-de-sac, is a potential space and usually not palpated.
- Uterine wall and fundus feel firm and smooth.

Nodular or thickened.

Rotate the intrarectal finger to check the rectal wall and anal sphincter tone. (See Chapter 23 for assessment of anus and rectum.) Check your gloved finger as you withdraw; test any adherent stool for occult blood.

Give the woman tissues to wipe the area and help her up. Remind her to slide her hips back from the edge before sitting up so she will not fall.

Normal Range of Findings	Abnormal Findings

DEVELOPMENTAL CONSIDERATIONS

Infants and Children

Preparation

- **Infant**—place on examination table.
- **Toddler/preschooler**—place on parent's lap.
    Frog-leg position—hips flexed, soles of feet together and up to bottom.
    Preschool child may want to separate her own labia.
    No drapes—the young girl wants to see what you are doing.
- **School-age child**—place on examination table, frog-leg position, no drapes.

During childhood, a routine screening is limited to inspection of the external genitalia to determine that (1) the structures are intact, (2) the vagina is present, and (3) the hymen is patent.

The newborn's genitalia are somewhat engorged. The labia majora are swollen, the labia minora are prominent and protrude beyond the labia majora, the clitoris looks relatively large, and the hymen appears thick. Because of transient engorgement, the vaginal opening is more difficult to see now than it will be later. Place your thumbs on the labia majora. Push laterally while pushing the perineum down, and try to note the vaginal opening above the hymenal ring. Do not palpate the clitoris because it is very sensitive.

A sanguineous vaginal discharge and/or leukorrhea (mucoid discharge) are normal during the first few weeks because of the maternal estrogen effect. (This also may cause transient breast engorgement and secretion.) During the early weeks, the genital engorgement resolves, and the labia minora atrophy and remain small until puberty (Fig. 24–23).

Ambiguous genitalia are rare but are suggested by a markedly enlarged clitoris, fusion of the labia (resembling scrotum), and palpable mass in fused labia (resembling testes) (see Table 24–9).

Imperforate hymen warrants referral.

Lesions, rash.

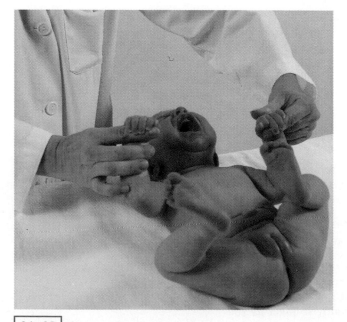

24–23

▶ Normal Range of Findings	Abnormal Findings

Between the ages of 2 months and 7 years, the labia majora are flat, the labia minora are thin, the clitoris is relatively small, and the hymen is tissue-paper thin. Normally, no irritation or foul-smelling discharge is present.

Poor perineal hygiene. Pest inhabitants. Excoriations. During and after toddler age, foul-smelling discharge occurs with lodging of foreign body, pinworms, or infection.

In the young school-age girl (7 to 10 years), the mons pubis thickens, the labia majora thicken, and the labia minora become slightly rounded. Pubic hair appears beginning around age 11, although sparse pubic hair may occur as early as age 8 years. Normally, the hymen is perforate.

Absence of pubic hair by 13 years indicates delayed puberty.

Amenorrhea in adolescent, together with bluish and bulging hymen, indicates imperforate hymen and warrants referral.

Almost always in these age groups, an external examination will suffice. If needed, an internal pelvic examination is best performed by a pediatric gynecologist using specialized instruments.

The Adolescent

The adolescent girl has special needs during the genitalia examination. Examine her alone, without the mother present. Assure her of privacy and confidentiality. Allow plenty of time for health education and discussion of pubertal progress. Assess her growth velocity and menstrual history, and use the SMR charts to teach breast and pubic hair development. Assure her that increased vaginal fluid (physiologic *leukorrhea*) is normal because of the estrogen effect.

A pelvic examination is indicated when contraception is desired, when the girl's sexual activity includes intercourse, or at age 18 years in virgins. Periodic Pap smears also are started when intercourse begins. Although the techniques of the examination are listed in the adult section, you will need to provide additional time and psychological support for the adolescent having her first pelvic examination.

The experience of the first pelvic examination determines how the adolescent will approach future care. Your accepting attitude and gentle, unhurried approach are important. You have a unique teaching opportunity here. Take the time to teach, using the girl's own body as illustration. Your frank discussion of anatomy and sexual behavior communicates that these topics are acceptable to discuss and not taboo with health care providers. This affirms the girl's self-concept.

During the bimanual examination, note that the adnexa are not palpable in the adolescent.

Pelvic or adnexal mass.

The Pregnant Female

Depending on the week of gestation of the pregnancy, inspection shows the enlarging abdomen (see Fig. 25–1 in the following chapter). The height of the fundus ascends gradually as the fetus grows. At 16 weeks, the fundus is palpable halfway between the symphysis and umbilicus; at 20 weeks, at the lower edge of the umbilicus; at 28 weeks, halfway between the umbilicus and the xiphoid; and at 34 to 36 weeks, almost to the xiphoid. Then close to term, the fundus drops as the fetal head engages in the pelvis.

The external genitalia show hyperemia of the perineum and vulva because of increased vascularity. Varicose veins may be visible in the labia or legs. Hemorrhoids may show around the anus. Both are caused by interruption in venous return from the pressure of the fetus.

Normal Range of Findings | Abnormal Findings

Internally, the walls of the vagina appear violet or blue (Chadwick's sign) owing to hyperemia. The vaginal walls are deeply rugated and the vaginal mucosa thickens. The cervix looks blue, feels velvety, and feels softer than in the nonpregnant state, making it a bit more difficult to differentiate from the vaginal walls.

During bimanual examination, the isthmus of the uterus feels softer and is more easily compressed between your two hands (Hegar's sign). The fundus balloons between your two hands; it feels connected to, but distinct from, the cervix because the isthmus is so soft.

Search the adnexal area carefully during early pregnancy. Normally, the adnexal structures are not palpable.

An ectopic pregnancy has serious consequences (see Table 24–8).

The Aging Adult

Natural lubrication is decreased; to avoid a painful examination, take care to lubricate instruments and the examining hand adequately. Use the Pedersen speculum (rather than the Graves) because its narrower, flatter blades are more comfortable in women with vaginal stenosis or dryness.

Menopause and the resulting decrease in estrogen production cause numerous physical changes. Pubic hair gradually decreases, becoming thin and sparse in later years. The skin is thinner and fat deposits decrease, leaving the mons pubis smaller and the labia flatter. Clitoris size also decreases after age 60.

Internally, the rugae of the vaginal walls decrease, and the walls look pale pink because of the thinned epithelium. The cervix shrinks and looks pale and glistening. It may retract, appearing to be flush with the vaginal wall. In some, it is hard to distinguish the cervix from the surrounding vaginal mucosa. Alternately, the cervix may protrude into the vagina if the uterus has prolapsed.

With the bimanual examination, you may need to insert only one gloved finger if vaginal stenosis exists. The uterus feels smaller and firmer, and the ovaries are not palpable normally.

Prior surgery for hysterectomy does not preclude the need for routine gynecologic care, including the Pap smear. The Pap smear can help detect gynecologic malignancies even when the cervix has been removed. Be aware that older women may have special needs and will appreciate the following plans of care: for those with arthritis, taking a mild analgesic or anti-inflammatory before the appointment may ease joint pain in positioning; schedule appointment times when joint pain or stiffness is at its least; allow extra time for positioning and "unpositioning" after the examination; and be careful to maintain dignity and privacy (Blesch and Prohaska, 1991).

Refer any suspicious red, white, or pigmented lesion for biopsy.
Vaginal atrophy increases the risk of infection and trauma.

Refer any mass for prompt evaluation.

 SUMMARY CHECKLIST: Female Genitalia Exam

1: Inspect external genitalia

2: Palpate labia, Skene's and Bartholin's glands

3: Using vaginal speculum, inspect cervix and vagina

4: Obtain specimens for cytologic study

5: Perform bimanual examination: cervix, uterus, adnexa

6: Perform rectovaginal examination

7: Test stool for occult blood

SAMPLE CHARTING

▶ **Subjective**

Menarche age 12, cycle usually q 28 days, duration 5 days, flow moderate, no dysmenor-rhea, LMP April 3. Grav 0/Para 0/Ab 0. Gyne checkups yearly. Last Pap test 1 year PTA, negative.

No urinary problems, no irritating or foul-smelling vaginal discharge, no sores or lesions, no history pelvic surgery. Satisfied with sexual relationship with husband, uses vaginal diaphragm for birth control, no plans for pregnancy at this time. Aware of no STD contact to self or husband.

▶ **Objective**

External genitalia—no swelling, lesions, or discharge. No urethral swelling or discharge. Internal—vaginal walls have no bulging or lesions, cervix pink with no lesions, scant clear mucoid discharge.

Bimanual—no pain on moving cervix, uterus anteflexed and anteverted, no enlargement or irregularity. Adnexa—ovaries not enlarged. Rectal—no hemorrhoids, fissures or lesions, no masses or tenderness, stool brown with guaiac test negative.

CLINICAL CASE STUDY 1

J.K., 27-year-old, white, married newspaper reporter, Grav 0/Para 0/Ab 0. Presents at clinic with "urinary burning, vaginal itching, and discharge $\times$ 4 days."

▶ **Subjective**

3 weeks PTA: treated at clinic for bronchitis with erythromycin. Improved within 5 days.

4 to 5 days PTA: noted burning on urination, intense vaginal itching, thick, white, "smelly" discharge. Warm water douche—no relief.

No previous history vaginal infection, urinary tract infection, or pelvic surgery. Monog-amous sexual relationship, has used low-estrogen birth control pills for 3 years with no side effects.

▶ **Objective**

Vulva and vagina erythematous and edematous. Thick, white, curdlike discharge clinging to vaginal walls. Cervix pink, no lesions. Bimanual examination—no pain on palpating cervix, uterus not enlarged, ovaries not enlarged.

Specimens: Pap smear, GC/*Chlamydia* to lab. KOH prep shows mycelia and spores of *Candida albicans*.

▶ ASSESSMENT

Candida vaginitis
Pain R/T infectious process

Continued

CLINICAL CASE STUDY 2

Brenda, 17-year-old, white high school student, comes to clinic for pelvic examination.

 Subjective

Menarche 12 years, cycle q 30 days, duration 6 days, mild cramps relieved by acetaminophen. LMP March 10. No dysuria, vaginal discharge, vaginal itching. Relationship involving intercourse with one boyfriend for 8 months PTA. For birth control boyfriend uses condoms "sometimes." Wants to start birth control pills. Never had pelvic examination. No knowledge of breast self-examination. No knowledge of STDs except AIDS. Smokes cigarettes, ½ PPD, started age 11.

 Objective

Breasts—symmetric, no lesions or discharge, palpation reveals no mass or tenderness.

External genitalia—no redness, lesions, or discharge. Internal genitalia—vaginal walls and cervix pink with no lesions or discharge. Specimens obtained. Acetic acid wash shows no acetowhitening.

Bimanual—no tenderness to palpation, uterus anteverted with no enlargement, ovaries not enlarged. Rectum—no masses, fissure, or tenderness. Stool brown and guaiac test negative.

Specimens—GC, *Chlamydia,* Pap smear to lab.

 ASSESSMENT

Breast and pelvic structures appear healthy.

Knowledge deficit regarding: breast self-examination; birth control measures; STD prevention; cigarette smoking R/T lack of exposure

NURSING DIAGNOSES COMMONLY ASSOCIATED WITH THE FEMALE GENITALIA AND RELATED DISORDERS

Diagnosis	Related Factors (Etiology)	Defining Characteristics (Symptoms and Signs)
Sexual dysfunction	Depression Disturbance in self-esteem or body image Lack of significant other Lack of privacy Effects of actual or perceived limitation imposed by disease and/or therapy Substance abuse Physical or psychosocial abuse Dysfunctional interpersonal relationships Ineffective or absent role models Failure to identify satisfactorily with same-sex parent Cultural norms regarding male/female roles Values conflict Knowledge deficit	Decreased or absent sexual desire Impotence Delayed development of secondary sex characteristics Sexual promiscuity Exhibitionism Guilt Alterations in achieving perceived sex role or sexual satisfaction Verbalization about the problem Conflicts involving values Changes in interest in self and others Seeking confirmation of desirability Voyeurism Transsexualism Transvestism Masochism/sadism
Functional incontinence	Deficits 　Cognitive 　Motor 　Sensory Altered environment	Unpredictable voiding pattern Unrecognized signals of bladder fullness Urge to void or bladder contractions sufficiently strong to result in loss of urine before reaching an appropriate site or receptacle

Rape-trauma syndrome	Rape event	**Acute Phase**
		Emotional reactions
		Anger
		Crying
		Overcontrol
		Panic
		Denial
		Self-blame
		Emotional shock
		Embarrassment
		Fear of being alone
		Humiliation
		Fear of physical violence and death
		Mistrust of the opposite sex
		Desire for revenge
		Change in sexual behavior
		Multiple physical symptoms
		Muscle tension
		Pain
		Sleep pattern disturbance
		Gastrointestinal irritability
		Genitourinary discomfort
		Long-Term Phase
		Mentally reliving rape
		Depression
		Loss of self-confidence
		Changes in lifestyle
		Changes in residence
		Dealing with repetitive nightmares and phobias
		Anxiety
		Ambivalence about own sexuality

Other Related Nursing Diagnoses

ACTUAL	RISK/WELLNESS
Altered sexuality patterns (see Chapter 22)	**Risk**
Impaired skin integrity (see Chapters 10 and 22)	Risk for urinary urge incontinence
Pain	Risk for infection
Stress incontinence	Risk for post-trauma syndrome
Reflex incontinence	
Total incontinence	**Wellness**
Urge incontinence	Health seeking behavior for information on STD risk reduction

 ## ASSESSMENT VIDEO CRITICAL THINKING QUESTIONS

The Saunders *Physical Examination and Health Assessment* Video Series—FEMALE GEN-ITALIA—will direct you to consider the following:

1. What presenting complaint would lead you to assess the female genitalia?

2. How may you adapt the female genitalia assessment to allow for health education?

3. How do normal genitalia assessment findings differ between nulliparous women and parous women who gave birth vaginally?

4. What normal and abnormal assessment findings may commonly be detected by a recto-vaginal examination?

▼ Table 24–3   ABNORMALITIES OF THE EXTERNAL GENITALIA

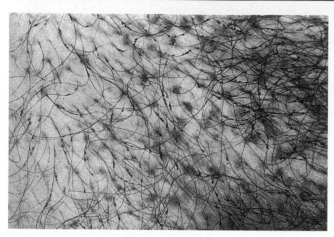

Pediculosis Pubis (Crab Lice)

S: Severe perineal itching.

O: Excoriations and erythematous areas. May see little dark spots (lice are small), nits (eggs) adherent to pubic hair near roots. Usually localized in pubic hair, occasionally in eyebrows or eyelashes.

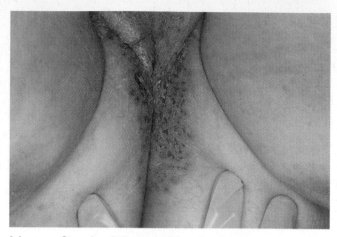

Herpes Simplex Virus—Type 2 (Herpes Genitalis)*

S: Episodes of local pain, dysuria, fever.

O: Clusters of small, shallow vesicles with surrounding erythema; erupt on genital areas and inner thigh. Also, inguinal adenopathy, edema. Vesicles on labia rupture in 1 to 3 days, leaving painful ulcers. Initial infection lasts 7 to 10 days. Virus remains dormant indefinitely; recurrent infections last 3 to 10 days with milder symptoms.

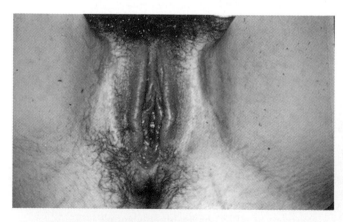

Red Rash—Contact Dermatitis

S: History of skin contact with allergenic substance in environment, intense pruritus.

O: Primary lesion—red, swollen, vesicles. Then may have weeping of lesions, crusts, scales, thickening of skin, excoriations from scratching. May result from reaction to feminine hygiene spray or synthetic underclothing.

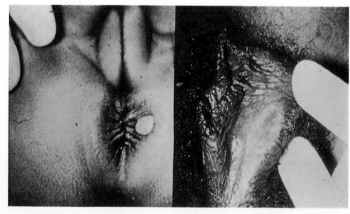

Syphilitic Chancre*

O: Begins as a small, solitary silvery papule that erodes to a red, round or oval, superficial ulcer with a yellowish serous discharge. Palpation—nontender indurated base; can be lifted like a button between thumb and finger. Nontender inguinal lymphadenopathy.

Table 24–3 ABNORMALITIES OF THE EXTERNAL GENITALIA *Continued*

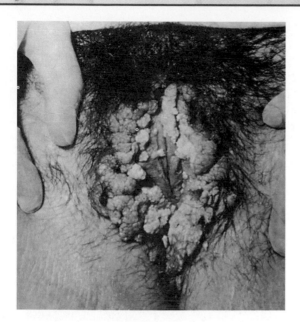

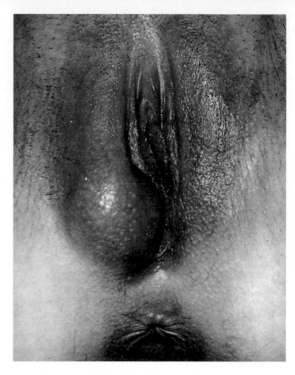

Genital Human Papillomavirus (HPV, Condylomata Acuminata, Genital Warts)*

S: Painless warty growths, may be unnoticed by woman.

O: Pink or flesh-colored, soft, pointed, moist, warty papules. Single or multiple in a cauliflowerlike patch. Occur around vulva, introitus, anus, vagina, cervix.

HPV infection is common among sexually active women, especially adolescents, regardless of ethnicity or socioeconomic status. Risk factors include early age at menarche and multiple sexual partners. The long incubation period (6 weeks to 8 months) makes it difficult to establish history of exposure. A strong association of HPV infection and abnormal cervical cytology exists.

Abscess of Bartholin's Gland

S: Local pain, can be severe.

O: Overlying skin red and hot. Posterior part of labia swollen; palpable fluctuant mass and tenderness. Mucosa shows red spot at site of duct opening; can express purulent discharge. Often secondary to gonococcal infection.*

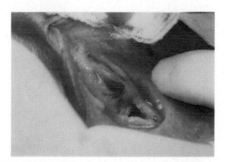

Urethritis (not illustrated)

S: Dysuria.

O: Palpation of anterior vaginal wall shows erythema, tenderness, induration along urethra, purulent discharge from meatus. Caused by *Neisseria gonorrhoeae, Chlamydia,* or *Staphylococcus* infection.

Urethral Caruncle

S: Tender, painful with urination, urinary frequency, hematuria, dyspareunia, or asymptomatic.

O: Small, deep red mass protruding from meatus; usually secondary to urethritis or skenitis; lesion may bleed on contact.

---

*This condition is a sexually transmitted disease (STD). The classic term, *venereal disease,* a disease transmitted only by sexual intercourse, now is obsolete. A broader category, STDs, includes all conditions that are *usually* or *can be* transmitted during sexual intercourse or intimate sexual contact with an infected partner. Although not inclusive of all STDs, the conditions described in this table encompass more common conditions.

S = subjective data; O = objective data.

Table 24–4   ABNORMALITIES OF THE PELVIC MUSCULATURE

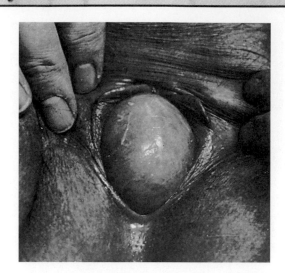

Cystocele

S: Feeling of pressure in vagina, stress incontinence.
O: With straining or standing, note introitus widening and the presence of a soft, round anterior bulge. The bladder, covered by vaginal mucosa, prolapses into vagina.

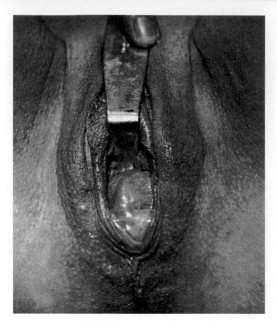

Rectocele

S: Feeling of pressure in vagina, possibly constipation.
O: With straining or standing, note introitus widening and the presence of a soft, round bulge from posterior. Here, part of the rectum, covered by vaginal mucosa, prolapses into vagina.

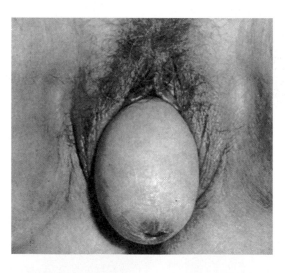

Uterine Prolapse

O: With straining or standing, uterus protrudes into vagina. Prolapse is graded: first degree, cervix appears at introitus with straining; second degree, cervix bulges outside introitus with straining; third degree, whole uterus protrudes even without straining—essentially, uterus is inside out.

Enterocele (not illustrated)

O: With straining, a bulge appears from posterior fornix, as cul-de-sac (pouch of Douglas) protrudes into the vagina.

S = subjective data; O = objective data.

Table 24–5   ABNORMALITIES OF THE CERVIX

ABNORMAL FINDINGS

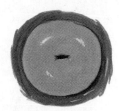

Bluish Cervix—Cyanosis

O: Bluish discoloration of the mucosa occurs normally in pregnancy (Chadwick's sign at 6 to 8 weeks gestation) and with any other condition causing hypoxia or venous congestion, e.g., congestive heart failure, pelvic tumor.

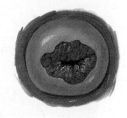

Erosion

O: Cervical lips inflamed and eroded. Reddened granular surface is superficial inflammation, with no ulceration (loss of tissue). Usually secondary to purulent or mucopurulent cervical discharge. Biopsy needed to distinguish erosion from carcinoma; cannot rely on inspection.

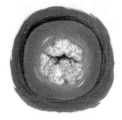

Human Papillomavirus (HPV, Condylomata)

O: Virus can appear in various forms when affecting cervical epithelium. Here warty growth appears as abnormal thickened white epithelium. Visibility of lesion is enhanced by acetic acid (vinegar) wash, which dissolves mucus and temporarily causes intracellular dehydration and coagulation of protein.

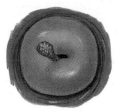

Polyp

S: May have mucoid discharge or bleeding.

O: Bright red, soft, pedunculated growth emerges from os. It is a benign lesion, but this must be determined by biopsy.

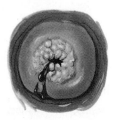

Carcinoma

S: Bleeding between menstrual periods or after menopause, unusual vaginal discharge.

O: Chronic ulcer and induration are early signs of carcinoma, although the lesion may or may not show on the exocervix. Diagnosed by Papanicolaou smear and biopsy. Risk factors for cervical cancer are early age at first intercourse, multiple sex partners, cigarette smoking, certain sexually transmitted diseases.

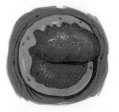

Diethylstilbestrol (DES) Syndrome

S: Prenatal exposure to DES causes cervical and vaginal abnormalities.

O: Red, granular patches of columnar epithelium extend beyond normal squamocolumnar junction onto cervix and into fornices (vaginal adenosis). Also cervical abnormalities: circular groove, transverse ridge, protuberant anterior lip, "cocks-comb" formation. Warrants monitoring by physician.

Table 24-6 VULVOVAGINAL INFLAMMATIONS

ABNORMAL FINDINGS

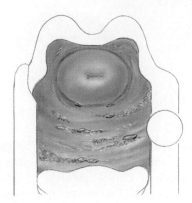

Atrophic Vaginitis

S: Postmenopausal vaginal itching, dryness, burning sensation, dyspareunia, mucoid discharge (may be flecked with blood).

O: Pale mucosa with abraded areas that bleed easily; may have bloody discharge.

An opportunistic infection related to chronic estrogen deficiency.

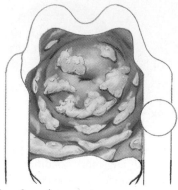

Candidiasis (Moniliasis)

S: Intense pruritus, thick whitish discharge.

O: Vulva and vagina are erythematous and edematous. Discharge is usually thick, white, curdy, "like cottage cheese." Diagnose by microscopic examination of discharge on potassium hydroxide wet mount.

Predisposing causes—use of oral contraceptives or antibiotics, more alkaline vaginal pH (as with menstrual periods, postpartum, menopause), also pregnancy from increased glycogen and diabetes.

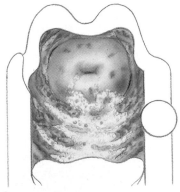

Trichomoniasis*

S: Pruritus, watery and often malodorous vaginal discharge, urinary frequency, terminal dysuria. Symptoms are worse during menstruation when the pH becomes optimal for the organism's growth.

O: Vulva may be erythematous. Vagina diffusely red, granular, occasionally with red raised papules and petechiae ("strawberry" appearance). Frothy, yellow-green, foul-smelling discharge. Microscopic examination of saline wet mount specimen shows characteristic flagellated cells.

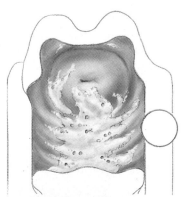

Bacterial Vaginosis (*Gardnerella vaginalis, Haemophilus vaginalis,* or Nonspecific Vaginitis)*

S: Profuse discharge, "constant wetness" with "foul, fishy, rotten" odor.

O: Thin, creamy, gray-white, malodorous discharge. No inflammation on vaginal wall or cervix because this is a surface parasite. Microscopic view of saline wet mount specimen shows typical "clue cells."

---

*This condition is considered an STD.

S = subjective data; O = objective data.

Table 24—6 VULVOVAGINAL INFLAMMATIONS *Continued*

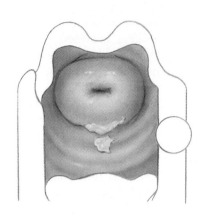

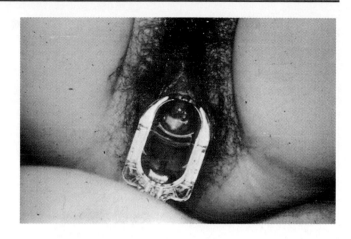

Chlamydia*

S: (Mimics gonorrhea.) Three of four infected women have no symptoms. May have urinary frequency, dysuria, or vaginal discharge, postcoital bleeding.

O: May have yellow or green mucopurulent discharge, friable cervix, cervical motion tenderness. Signs are subtle, easily mistaken for gonorrhea. The two are important to distinguish because antibiotic treatment is different; if the wrong drug is given or if the condition is untreated, chlamydia can ascend the reproductive tract to cause pelvic inflammatory disease (PID), and result in infertility. This is the most common STD in the United States; the highest prevalence is among sexually active adolescent girls, with an incidence of almost 30 percent in some settings (Burstein et al., 1998). Clinicians are urged to screen all sexually active girls every 6 months, regardless of symptoms or risk.

Gonorrhea*

S: Variable: vaginal discharge, dysuria, abnormal uterine bleeding, abscess in Bartholin's or Skene's glands; the majority of cases are asymptomatic.

O: Often no signs are apparent. May have purulent vaginal discharge. Diagnose by positive culture of organism. If the condition is untreated, it may progress to acute salpingitis, pelvic inflammatory disease (PID).

 ## Table 24—7 CONDITIONS OF UTERINE ENLARGEMENT

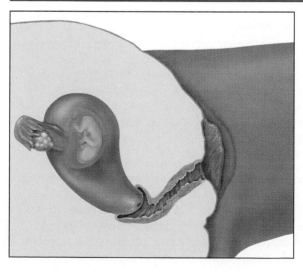

◀ ### Pregnancy

Obviously a normal condition, pregnancy is included here for comparison.

S: Amenorrhea, fatigue, breast engorgement, nausea, change in food tolerance, weight gain.

O: Early signs: cyanosis of vaginal mucosa and cervix (Chadwick's sign). Palpation—soft consistency of cervix, enlarging uterus with compressible fundus and isthmus (Hegar's sign at 10 to 12 weeks).

Table continued on following page

Table 24–7   CONDITIONS OF UTERINE ENLARGEMENT *Continued*

ABNORMAL FINDINGS

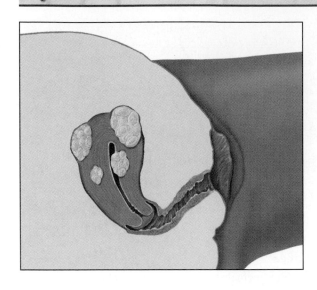

◀ Myomas (Leiomyomas, Uterine Fibroids)

S: Varies, depending on size and location. Often no symptoms. When symptoms do occur, include vague discomfort, bloating, heaviness, pelvic pressure, dyspareunia, urinary frequency, backache, or hypermenorrhea if myoma disturbs endometrium. Heavy bleeding produces anemia.

O: Uterus irregularly enlarged, firm, mobile, and nodular with hard, painless nodules in the uterine wall.

They are usually benign. Highest incidence between the ages of 30 and 45 years and in blacks. Myomas are estrogen dependent; after menopause, the lesions usually regress but do not disappear. Surgery may be indicated.

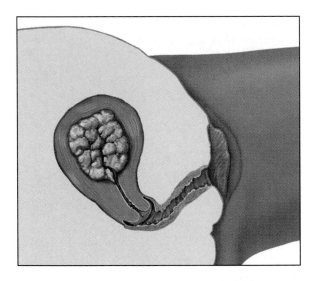

◀ Carcinoma of the Endometrium

S: Abnormal and intermenstrual bleeding before menopause; postmenopausal bleeding or mucosanguineous discharge. Pain and weight loss occur late in the disease.

O: Uterus may be enlarged.

The Pap smear is rarely effective in detecting endometrial cancer. Women at high risk should have an endometrial tissue sample evaluated at menopause and periodically thereafter (American Cancer Society, 1998). Risk factors for endometrial cancer are early menarche, late menopause, history of infertility, failure to ovulate, tamoxifen, unopposed estrogen therapy (which continually stimulates the endometrium, causing hyperplasia), and obesity (which increases endogenous estrogen).

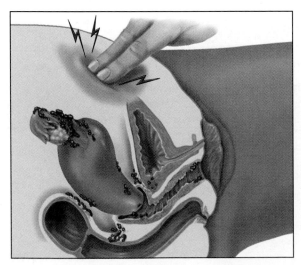

◀ Endometriosis

S: Cyclic or chronic pelvic pain, occurring as dysmenorrhea, or dyspareunia, low backache. Also may have irregular uterine bleeding or hypermenorrhea or may be asymptomatic.

O: Uterus fixed, tender to movement. Small, firm nodular masses tender to palpation on posterior aspect of fundus, uterosacral ligaments, ovaries, sigmoid colon. Ovaries often enlarged.

Masses are aberrant growths of endometrial tissue scattered throughout pelvis due to transplantation of tissue by retrograde menstruation. Ectopic tissue responds to hormone stimulation; builds up between periods, sloughs during menstruation. May cause infertility due to pelvic adhesions, tubal obstruction, decreased ovarian function.

S = subjective data; O = objective data.

Table 24-8 ADNEXAL ENLARGEMENT

Fallopian Tube Mass—Acute Salpingitis (Pelvic Inflammatory Disease [PID]) ▶

S: Sudden fever >38° C or 100.4° F, suprapubic pain and tenderness.

O: Acute—rigid boardlike lower abdominal musculature. May have purulent discharge from cervix. Movement of uterus and cervix causes intense pain. Pain in lateral fornices and adnexa. Bilateral adnexal masses difficult to palpate owing to pain and muscle spasm. Chronic—bilateral, tender, fixed adnexal masses.

Complications include ectopic pregnancy, infertility, and reinfection. PID usually caused by *Neisseria gonorrhoeae* and *Chlamydia trachomatis.*

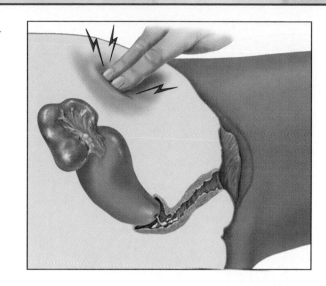

Fallopian Tube Mass—Ectopic Pregnancy ▶

S: Amenorrhea or irregular vaginal bleeding, pelvic pain.

O: Softening of cervix and fundus; movement of cervix and uterus causes pain; palpable tender pelvic mass, which is solid, mobile, unilateral.

This has potential for serious sequelae; seek gynecologic consultation immediately before the mass ruptures or shows signs of acute peritonitis.

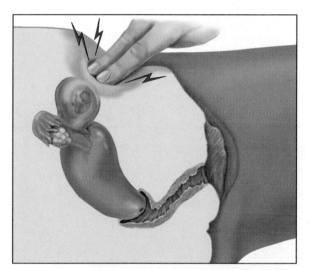

Fluctuant Ovarian Mass—Ovarian Cyst ▶

S: Usually asymptomatic.

O: Smooth, round, fluctuant, mobile, nontender mass on ovary. Some cysts resolve spontaneously within 60 days but must be followed closely.

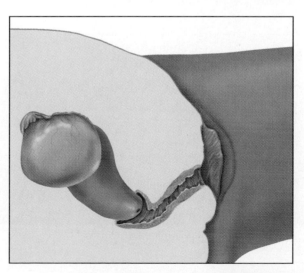

Table continued on following page

Table 24–8   ADNEXAL ENLARGEMENT *Continued*

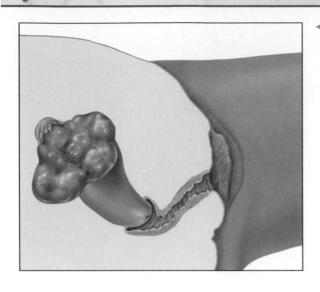

◀ **Solid Ovarian Mass—Ovarian Cancer**

S: Usually asymptomatic. May have abdominal enlargement from fluid accumulation.

O: Solid tumor palpated on ovary. Heavy, solid, fixed, poorly defined mass suggests malignancy; benign mass may feel mobile and solid.

Biopsy necessary to distinguish the two types of masses. The Pap smear does not detect ovarian cancer. Women over age 40 should have a thorough pelvic examination every year.

S = subjective data; O = objective data.

 Table 24–9   ABNORMALITIES IN PEDIATRIC GENITALIA

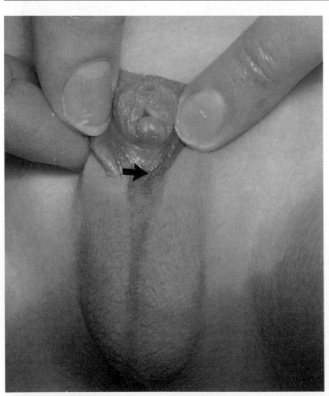

◀ **Ambiguous Genitalia**

Female pseudohermaphroditism is a congenital anomaly resulting from hyperplasia of the adrenal glands, which exposes the female fetus to excess amounts of androgens. This causes masculinized external genitalia, here shown as enlargement of the clitoris and fusion of the labia. Ambiguous means the enlarged clitoris here may look like a small penis with hypospadias, and the fused labia look like an incompletely formed scrotum with absent testes. Other forms of intersexual conditions occur, and the family must be referred for diagnostic evaluation.

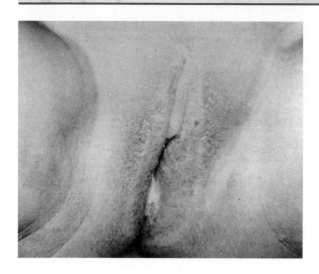

◀ **Vulvovaginitis in Child**

This infection is caused by *Candida albicans* in a diabetic child. Symptoms include pruritus and burning when urine touches excoriated area. Examination shows red, shiny, edematous vulva, vaginal discharge, excoriated area from scratching.

Other, more common causes of vulvovaginitis in the prepubertal child include infection from a respiratory or bowel pathogen, sexually transmitted disease, or presence of a foreign body.

Bibliography

Abercrombie PD: Multifocal lower genital tract neoplasia in women with HIV disease. Nurse Pract 20(5):68–76, May 1995.

Abercrombie PD: Women living with HIV infection. Nurs Clin North Am 31(1):97–106, Mar 1996.

Alexander LL, Treiman K, Clarke P: A national survey of nurse practitioner *Chlamydia* knowledge and treatment practices of female patients. Nurs Pract 21(5):48–54, May 1996.

American Cancer Society: Cancer Facts & Figures—1998. Atlanta, GA, American Cancer Society, 1998.

Andrist LC: Genital herpes: Overcoming barriers to diagnosis and treatment. Am J Nurs 97(10):16AAA–16DDD, Oct 1997.

Bader T, Bowes WA, Hochbaum SR, et al.: When minutes count: Responding to Ob/Gyn emergencies. Patient Care 31(13):138–148, Aug 15, 1997.

Baldwin D, Landa HM: Evaluating pediatric gynecologic problems. Patient Care 30(12):89–106, July 15, 1996.

Blesch KS, Prohaska TR: Cervical cancer screening in older women. Cancer Nurs 14(3):141–147, 1991.

Bromberger JT, Matthews KA: Prospective study of the determinants of age at menopause. Am J Epidemiol 145(2):124–133, Jan 1997.

Brown MS: Pediatric genital exam. Nurs Pract 22(7):160, July 1997.

Burstein GR, Gaydos CA, Diener-West M, et al.: Incident *Chlamydia trachomatis* infections among inner-city adolescent females. JAMA 280(6):521–526, Aug 12, 1998.

Corwin EJ: Endometriosis: Pathophysiology, diagnosis, and treatment. Nurs Pract 22(10):35–51, Oct 1997.

Cunningham FG, MacDonald PC, Gant NF: Williams' Obstetrics, 20th ed. Stamford, CT, Appleton & Lange, 1997.

Dumesic DA: Pelvic examination: What to focus on in menopausal women. Consultant 36(8):39–46, Jan 1996.

Ferreira N: Sexually transmitted *Chlamydia trachomatis*. Nurs Pract Forum 8(2):70–76, June 1997.

Foster JC, Smith HL: Use of the Cytobrush for Papanicolaou smear screens in pregnant women. J Nurse Midwifery 41(3):211–217, May–June 1996.

Harlan WR, Harlan EA, Grillo GP: Secondary sex characteristics of girls 12 to 17 years of age—The U.S. Health Examination Survey. J Pediatr 96:1074–1078, 1980.

Hook EW, Sondheimer S, Zenilman J: Today's treatment for STDs. Patient Care 29(4):40–56, Feb 28, 1995.

Kelsey B, Freeman S: Identifying and treating pelvic inflammatory disease. Am J Nurs 97(11 Suppl.):17–22, Nov 1997.

Khosla RK: Detecting sexually transmitted disease: A new role for urinalysis in the preparticipation exam? Phys Sports Med 23(1):77–104, Jan 1995.

Marshall WA, Tanner JM: Variations in pattern of pubertal changes in girls. Arch Dis Child 44:291–303, 1969.

Masters WH, Johnson VE: Human Sexual Response. Boston, Little Brown, 1966.

Mayeaux EJ, Spigener SD: Treatment of human genital papillomavirus infections. Hosp Pract 32(12):87–90, Dec 15, 1997.

McCarthy V: The first pelvic examination. J Pediatr Health Care 11(5):247–249, Sep–Oct 1997.

Mehring P: Dysfunctional uterine bleeding. Adv Nurs Pract 5(11):27–32, Nov 1997.

Moran G: Diagnosing STDs: Part 1. Ulcerating diseases. Emerg Med 29(1):58–70, Jan 1997.

Moran G: Diagnosing STDs: Part 2. Lesionless disorders. Emerg Med 29(2):20–31, Feb 1997.

Morgan KW, Deneris A: Emergency contraception: Preventing unintended pregnancy. Nurs Pract 22(11):34–48, Nov 1997.

Newland JA: Cystitis in women. Am J Nurs 98(1):16AAA, Jan 1998.

Newland JA: Gonorrhea in women. Am J Nurs 97(8):16AA, Aug 1997.

Office of Disease Prevention and Health Promotion: Cancer detection by physical examination: Breast and pelvic organ examination. *In* Clinician's Handbook of Preventive Services 1994. Washington, D.C., U.S. Government Printing Office, 1994.

Orr DP: Screening adolescents for sexually transmitted infections. JAMA 280(6):564–565, Aug 12, 1998.

Orr DP: Urine-based diagnosis of sexually transmitted infections using amplified DNA techniques: A shift in paradigms? J Adol Health 20(1):3–5, Jan 1997.

Patel K: Sexually transmitted diseases in adolescents: Focus on gonorrhea, chlamydia, and trichomoniasis. J Pediatr Health Care 12(4):211–217, Jul–Aug 1998.

Penn C, Lekan-Rutledge D, Joers AM, et al: Assessment of urinary incontinence. J Gerontol Nurs 2(1):8–19, Jan 1996.

Reifsnider E: Common adult infectious skin conditions. Nurs Pract 22(11):17–33, Nov 1997.

Rose PG: Endometrial carcinoma. N Engl J Med 335(9):640–649, Aug 29, 1996.

Shafer M: Lower abdominal pain and the adolescent girl. Emerg Med 29(2):91–99, Feb 1997.

Stevens-Simon C: Clinical applications of adolescent female sexual development. Nurse Pract 18(12):18–29, Dec 1993.

Stillson T, Knight AL, Elswick RK: The effectiveness and safety of two cervical cytologic techniques during pregnancy. J Fam Pract 45(2):159–163, Aug 1997.

Swanson JM, Dibble SL, Chenitz C: Clinical features and psychosocial factors in young adults with genital herpes. Image 27(1):16–22, Spring 1995.

Tagg PI: Chlamydia: What you should know. Nurs Pract 21(2):133–134, Feb 1996.

Thylan S: Endometriosis link disputed. Nurs Pract 21(10):8, Oct 1996.

Wasaha S, Angelopoulos FM: What every woman should know about menopause. Am J Nurs 96(1):24–33, Jan 1996.

CHAPTER TWENTY FIVE

The Pregnant Female

PREGNANCY AND THE ENDOCRINE PLACENTA

The first day of the menses is day 1 of the menstrual cycle. For the first 14 days of the cycle, one or more follicles in the ovary develop and mature. One follicle grows faster than the others, and on day 14 of the menstrual cycle, this dominant follicle ruptures and ovulation occurs. If the ovum meets viable sperm, fertilization occurs somewhere in the oviduct (fallopian tube). The remaining cells in the follicle form the **corpus luteum,** or "yellow body," which makes important hormones. Chief among these is progesterone, which prevents the sloughing of the endometrial wall, ensuring a rich vascular network into which the fertilized ovum will implant.

The fertilized ovum, now called the **blastocyst,** continues to divide, differentiate, and grow rapidly. Specialized cells in the blastocyst produce human chorionic gonadotropin (hCG), which stimulates the corpus luteum to continue making progesterone. Between days 20 and 24, the blastocyst implants into the wall of the uterus, which may cause a small amount of vaginal bleeding. A specialized layer of cells around the blastocyst becomes the **placenta.** The placenta starts to produce progesterone to support the pregnancy at 7 weeks, and takes over this function completely from the corpus luteum at about 10 weeks.

The placenta functions as an endocrine organ and produces several hormones. These hormones help in the growth and maintenance of the fetus, and they direct changes in the woman's body to prepare for birth and lactation. The hCG stimulates the rise in progesterone during pregnancy. Progesterone maintains the endometrium around the fetus, increases the alveoli in the breast, and keeps the uterus in a quiescent state. Estrogen stimulates the duct formation in the breast, increases the weight of the uterus, and increases certain receptors in the uterus that are important at birth.

The average length of pregnancy is 280 days from the first day of the last menstrual period (LMP), which is equal to 40 weeks, 10 lunar months, or 9 calendar months. Note that this includes the 2 weeks when the follicle was maturing but before conception actually occurred. Pregnancy is divided into three trimesters: (1) the first 12 weeks; (2) from 13 to 27 weeks; and (3) from 28 weeks to delivery. A woman who is pregnant for the first time is called a **primigravida.** After she delivers, she is called a **primipara.** The **multigravida** is a pregnant woman who has previously carried a fetus to the point of viability. She is a **multipara** after delivery. Any pregnant woman might be called a gravida.

CHANGES DURING NORMAL PREGNANCY

Pregnancy is diagnosed by three types of signs and symptoms. **Presumptive signs** are those the woman experiences, such as amenorrhea and nausea. **Probable signs** are those detected by the examiner, such as an enlarged uterus. **Positive signs** of pregnancy are those that are direct evidence of the fetus, such as the auscultation of fetal heart tones (FHTs).

First Trimester

Conception occurs on approximately the 14th day of the menstrual cycle. The blastocyst (developing fertilized ovum) implants in the uterus 6 to 10 days after conception, sometimes accompanied by a small amount of painless bleeding, which may be interpreted as a menstrual period (Cunningham et al., 1997). The serum hCG becomes positive after implantation. The following menstrual period is missed. At the time of the missed menses, hCG can be detected in the urine (Cunningham et al., 1997). Breast tingling and tenderness begin as the rising estrogen levels promote mammary growth and development of the ductal system; progesterone stimulates the alveolar system as well as the mammary growth. Chorionic somatomammotropin (also called human placental lactogen or hPL), also produced by the placenta, stimulates breast growth and exerts lactogenic properties (Varney, 1997). More than half of all pregnant women experience nausea and vomiting. The cause is unclear but may involve the hormonal changes of pregnancy, low blood sugar, gastric overloading, slowed peristalsis, an enlarging uterus, and emotional factors. Fatigue is common and may be related to the initial fall in metabolic rate that occurs in early pregnancy (Varney, 1997).

Estrogen, and possibly progesterone, cause hypertrophy of the uterine muscle cells, and uterine blood vessels and lymphatics enlarge. The uterus becomes globular in shape, softens, and flexes easily over cervix (**Hegar's sign**). This causes compression of the bladder, which results in urinary frequency. Increased vascularity, congestion, and edema cause the cervix to soften (**Goodell's sign**) and become bluish purple (**Chadwick's sign**) (Varney, 1997).

Early first-trimester blood pressures reflect prepregnancy values. In the 7th gestational week, blood pressure begins to drop as a result of falling peripheral vascular resistance. Systemic vascular resistance decreases due to the vasodilatory effect of progesterone and prostaglandins, and possibly because of the low resistance of the placental bed (Creasy and Resnick, 1994).

At the end of 9 weeks, the embryonic period of fetal development ends, at which time major structures are present (Varney, 1997). FHTs can be heard by Doppler ultrasound between 9 and 12 weeks. The uterus may be palpated just above the symphysis pubis at approximately 12 weeks. See Figure 25–1 for growth of the uterine fundus during the first trimester.

Second Trimester

By weeks 12 to 16, the nausea, vomiting, fatigue, and urinary frequency of the first trimester improve. The woman recognizes fetal movement ("quickening") at approximately 18 to 20 weeks (the multigravida earlier). As breast enlargement continues, the veins of the breast enlarge and are more visible through the skin of lightly pigmented women. **Colostrum,** the precursor of milk, may be expressed from the nipples. Colostrum is yellow in color, and contains more minerals and protein but less sugar and fat than mature milk. Colostrum also contains antibodies, which are protective for the newborn during its first days of life until mature milk production begins (Cunningham et al., 1997). The areola and nipples darken, it is thought, because estrogen and progesterone have a melanocyte-stimulating effect, and melanocyte-stimulating hormone levels escalate from the 2nd month of pregnancy until delivery. For the same reason, the midline of the abdominal skin becomes pigmented and is called the **linea nigra.** **Striae gravidarum** ("stretch marks") may be noted on the breast, abdomen, and areas of weight gain.

During the second trimester, systolic blood pressure may be 2 to 8 mm Hg lower and diastolic blood pressure 5 to 15 mm Hg lower than prepregnancy levels (Cunningham et al., 1997). This drop is most pronounced at 20 weeks, and may cause symptoms of dizziness and faintness, particularly after rising quickly. Stomach displacement due to the enlarging uterus, and altered esophageal sphincter and gastric tone as a result of progesterone, predispose the woman to heartburn (Cunningham et al., 1997). Intestines are also displaced by the growing uterus, and tone and motility are decreased due to the action of progesterone, often causing constipation. The gallbladder, possibly due to the action of progesterone on its smooth muscle, empties sluggishly and may become distended. The stasis of bile, together with the increased cholesterol saturation of pregnancy, predisposes some women to gallstone formation.

Progesterone and, to a lesser degree, estrogen cause increased respiratory effort during pregnancy by increasing tidal volume. Hemoglobin, and therefore oxygen carrying capacity, also increases. Increased tidal volume causes a slight drop in partial pressure of arterial carbon dioxide ($PaCO_2$), causing the woman to occasionally experience dyspnea (Cunningham et al., 1997).

The high level of estrogen during pregnancy causes an increase in the major thyroxine transport protein, thyroxine-binding globulin. Several thyroidal stimulating factors of placental origin are produced. The thyroid gland enlarges due to hyperplasia and increased vascularity (Cunningham et al., 1997).

Cutaneous blood flow is augmented during pregnancy due to decreased vascular resistance, presumably helping to dissipate heat generated by increased metabolism. Gums may hypertrophy and bleed easily. This condition is called **gingivitis** or **epulis of pregnancy,** and occurs due to growth of the capillaries of the gums (Cunningham et al., 1997). For the same reason, nosebleeds may occur more frequently than usual.

FHTs are audible by fetoscope (as opposed to Doppler) at approximately 17 to 19 weeks. The fetal outline is palpable through the abdominal wall at approximately 20 weeks. A multicenter study lists the following expected survival rates: 15.5 percent of neonates born at 25 weeks gestation survive; 54.7 percent at 26 weeks; 67 percent at 27 weeks; 77.4 percent at 28 weeks; and 85.2 percent at 29 weeks, increasing slowly to 33 weeks, when 97.9 percent of the neonates survive (Creasy and Resnick, 1994). Figure 25–1 illustrates the growth of the uterine fundus during the second trimester.

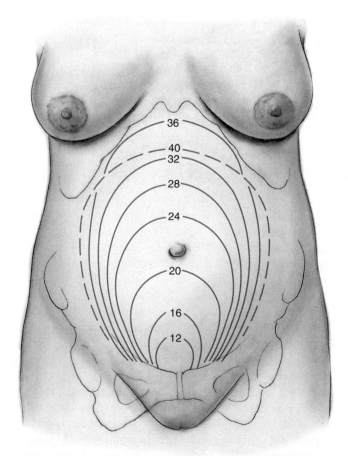

HEIGHT OF FUNDUS AT WEEKS OF GESTATION

25–1

Third Trimester

Blood volume, which increased rapidly during the second trimester, peaks in the middle of the third trimester at approximately 45 percent greater than the prepregnancy level and plateaus thereafter (Creasy and Resnick, 1994). Erythrocyte mass increases by 20 to 30 percent (caused by an increase in erythropoiesis, mediated by progesterone, estrogen, and placental chorionic somatomammotropin), while plasma volume increases slightly more, causing a slight hemodilution and a small drop in hematocrit. Blood pressure slowly rises again to approximately the prepregnant level (Cunningham et al., 1997).

Uterine enlargement causes the diaphragm to rise and the shape of the rib cage to widen at the base. Decreased space for lung expansion may cause a sense of shortness of breath. The rising diaphragm displaces the heart up and to the left. Cardiac output, stroke volume, and force of contraction are increased. The pulse rate rises 15 to 20 beats per minute (Creasy and Resnick, 1994). Due to the increase in blood volume, a functional systolic murmur, grade ii/iv or less, can be heard in more than 95 percent of pregnant women (Creasy and Resnick, 1994).

Edema of the lower extremities may occur due to the enlarging fetus impeding venous return. The edema worsens with dependency, such as prolonged standing. Varicosities, for which many women have a familial tendency, may form or enlarge due to progesterone-induced vascular relaxation as well as engorgement caused by the weight of the full uterus compressing the inferior vena cava and the vessels of the pelvic area, resulting in venous congestion in the legs, vulva, and rectum. Hemorrhoids are varicosities of the rectum that are worsened by constipation, which occurs due to relaxation of the large bowel by progesterone.

Progressive lordosis occurs to compensate for the shifting center of balance caused by the anteriorly bulging uterus, predisposing the woman to backaches. Slumping of the shoulders and anterior flexion of the neck secondary to the increasing weight of the breasts may cause aching and numbness of the arms and hands due to compression of the median and ulnar nerves in the arm (Varney, 1997).

Approximately 2 weeks before going into labor, the primigravida experiences engagement (also called "lightening" or "dropping"), when the fetal head moves down into the pelvis. Symptoms include a lower appearing and smaller measuring fundus, urinary frequency, increased vaginal secretions due to increased pelvic congestion, and increased lung capacity. In the multigravida, the fetus may move down at any time in late pregnancy or often not until labor. The cervix, in preparation for labor, begins to thin (efface) and open (dilate). A thick **mucous plug,** formed in the cervix as a mechanical barrier during pregnancy, is expelled at variable times before or during labor. Between 37 and 42 weeks, the pregnancy is con-

sidered full term (see Fig. 25–1). After 42 weeks, the pregnancy is considered postdates.

Determining Weeks of Gestation

The **expected date of confinement** (EDC) (also less commonly known as the expected date of delivery, or EDD), being 280 days from the first day of the LMP, may be calculated by using **Nägele's rule.** That is, determine the first day of the last normal menstrual period (normal in timing, length, premenstrual symptoms, and amount of flow and cramping). Using the first day of the LMP, add 7 days and subtract 3 months. This date is the EDC. This date can then be used with a pregnancy wheel, on which the EDC arrow is set, then the present date will be pointing to the present weeks gestation (Fig. 25–2). The number of weeks gestation also can be estimated by physical exam, by measurement of the maternal serum hCG, by ultrasound, and by signs such as the first perceived fetal movement.

Weight Gain in Pregnancy

The amount of weight gained by term represents a baby, amniotic fluid, placenta, increased uterine size, increased blood volume, increased extravascular fluid, maternal fat stores, and increased breast size. In 1990, the National Academy of Science made the following recommendation for weight gain during pregnancy, which was later accepted by the American College of Obstetricians and Gynecologists: 28 to 40 lb for underweight women, 25–35 lb for normal weight women, and 15–25 lb for overweight women. A healthy outcome may be expected within a great range of weight gain (Cunningham et al., 1997).

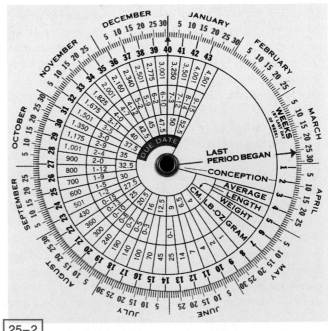

25–2

DEVELOPMENTAL CONSIDERATIONS

The risks for the adolescent who is pregnant are largely psychosocial. This young woman is at risk for the downward cycle of poverty beginning with an incomplete education, failure to limit family size, and continuing with failure to establish a vocation and become independent. She may be unprepared emotionally to be a mother. Her social situation may be stressful. She may not have the support of her family, her partner, or his family. Medical risks for the pregnant adolescent are generally related to poverty, inadequate nutrition, substance abuse, genital infection, and poor health before pregnancy. The adolescent is also at risk for preeclampsia and for bearing a low-birth-weight infant, and it is unclear whether this is due to biologic or social factors (Cunningham et al., 1997). The adolescent, for social reasons, often seeks health care later, and early prenatal care has been shown to provide optimal management.

Since many baby boomers have delayed childbearing, and since the advent of assisted conception, more women older than age 35 are now becoming pregnant. In 1993, there were 357,053 births to American women 35 to 39 years of age; 59,071 to women 40 to 44 years old, and 2329 to women between 45 and 49 years old (Cunningham et al., 1997).

Primigravidae pregnant after the age of 35 years have been referred to as **"elderly primigravidae,"** though many clinicians now consider this to be an unfortunate term. Women over 35 are often more prepared emotionally and financially to parent; however, they are more at risk for infertility. Female fertility declines with maternal age due to ovulation and atresia of follicles, causing anovulation to occur with increasing frequency after the age of 40 (Kennedy, Griffin, and Frishman, 1998; Rousseau, 1998). Once conception is achieved, the older woman is at increased risk for congenital anomalies, particularly Down syndrome, which occurs 1 in every 900 live births at age 30; 1 in every 350 live births at age 35; 1 in every 300 live births at age 40; and 1 in every 25 live births at age 45 (Cunningham et al., 1997).

Women 35 years and older are offered genetic counseling and prenatal testing such as **chorionic villi sampling (CVS)** and **amniocentesis.** For these tests, fetal material is removed from the uterus and analyzed for genetic make-up. At age 35, the risk of testing is approximately the same as the risk that the fetus will be affected with a congenital problem.

Because the incidence of chronic diseases increases with age, women over age 35 who are pregnant more often suffer medical complications such as diabetes and hypertension (Cunningham et al., 1997). The increased incidence of hypertension causes an increase in placental abruption and pregnancy-induced hypertension. Hypertension, in turn, increases the number of babies born small

for gestational age. More older women experience placenta previa, but this occurs with increasing numbers of pregnancies as well, and may occur statistically only because older women have more often had more pregnancies (Cunningham et al., 1997). They experience more spontaneous abortions, in part because of the increase in genetically abnormal embryos. A Centers for Disease Control and Prevention study found that maternal mortality for women older than 35 was four times that of women aged 20 to 24 (Buehler et al., 1986). They more often deliver by primary cesarean section; some studies showed the risk of cesarean section doubled for women older than 35 years (Adashek et al., 1993; Edge and Laros, 1993). Although hypertensive disorders, diabetes, preterm labor, and placental accidents would seem to be causative, one of these studies carefully controlled for other factors and found age to be an independent risk factor. This suggests that increased physician concern for the older woman itself may be an independent factor in this increased risk of cesarean deliver for the older gravida (Cunningham et al., 1997; Peipert and Bracken, 1993).

TRANSCULTURAL CONSIDERATIONS

Some complications of pregnancy occur more frequently among some racial groups than others. One California study showed gestational diabetes occurred in 4.5 percent of Hispanic women compared with 1.5 percent of white women (Hollingsworth, Vaucher, and Yamamoto, 1991). Another study in the Midwest showed an increased risk for gestational diabetes among black, Hispanic, and Asian women (Dooley et al., 1991). Pregnancy-induced hypertension has been noted to occur more frequently among black women (22 percent), followed by Hispanic women (20 percent), and least often among white women (18 percent) (Cunningham and Leveno, 1988). The underlying chronic hypertension seen more commonly among black women—8.5 percent among the multiparas in this study compared with 6.6 percent of Hispanics and 6.2 percent of whites—explains their increased risk for blood pressure complications in pregnancy (Cunningham et al., 1997). The incidence of twinning has been shown to be greater among some populations. White women will carry twins in 1 of 100 pregnancies, whereas women in one Nigerian community carry them in 1 of 20 pregnancies (Cunningham et al., 1997)!

Pregnancy, however, is not only a medical event, but one with profound psychological and social meaning for the woman and also for her family and community. Customs and beliefs regarding childbearing have been developed through the ages in every culture. Pregnancy is intensely personal, and involves such charged issues as spiritual practices and beliefs, sexuality, relationship, contraception, nutritional practices, maternal weight gain, and abortion. You must be sensitive to these issues. You may begin by inquiring whether the woman and/or her significant others have any special requests. This communicates your intention to respect cultural differences and preferences. A continuing rapport will help enable the woman to bring up issues as they develop.

A woman's resistance to an action or a suggestion by the clinician may represent a cultural issue. Such issues may also be held differently by the woman and one or more of her significant others, and such situations must be handled with care. Examples of culturally charged issues are dietary practices, sexuality during and after pregnancy, preference for gender of care provider, preference for gender of infant, and contraceptive usage. Use your skill to understand such preferences within a cultural context and accept rather than judge the person. Whenever safe and possible, respect such wishes. This enhances the success of the birth in its psychological and social dimensions.

SUBJECTIVE DATA

1. Menstrual history
2. Gynecologic history
3. Obstetric history
4. Present pregnancy
5. Past medical history

6. Family history
7. Review of systems
8. Nutritional history
9. Environment/hazards

Examiner Asks	Rationale

❶ Menstrual history
● When was the first day of your last menstrual period that was normal in timing, premenstrual symptoms, length, amount of flow, cramping?

Using Nägele's rule, calculate the EDC using this date. With a pregnancy wheel, determine the present number of weeks gestation.

❷ Gynecologic history
● Ever had surgery of the cervix? Uterus?

Cervical surgery may affect the integrity of the cervix during pregnancy and, during labor, may impede cervical dilation. Uterine surgery may place the woman at risk for uterine rupture during pregnancy and labor.

● Any history of genital herpes?

Onset during pregnancy is potentially *teratogenic,* i.e., causing physical defects in the developing fetus, and a lesion at delivery precludes vaginal birth.

● When your mother was pregnant with you, did she ever take a drug called diethylstilbesterol (DES)?

Prenatal exposure to DES may cause vaginal, cervical, and/or uterine abnormalities in the daughter, which may increase the risk of spontaneous abortion or affect the integrity of the cervix during pregnancy.

❸ Obstetric History
● In earlier pregnancies, any history of hypertension, diabetes, β-hemolytic streptococcus infection, intrauterine growth retardation, congenital anomalies, premature labor, postpartum hemorrhage, or postpartum depression?

The woman who has experienced these complications in the past is at increased risk for them in subsequent pregnancies.

Examiner Asks	Rationale
• How did you experience previous pregnancies and deliveries?	The subjective quality of previous experiences tells a great deal about the woman's emotions regarding the present pregnancy.
• Ever had a cesarean section? If so, what was the indication? At how many centimeters dilation, if any, was the surgery performed? What type of uterine incision was made? (Confirming records of this surgery must be obtained.)	The woman who has had surgery on her uterus is at risk for uterine rupture during pregnancy and labor. The vertical, or "classical," incision carries a higher risk of rupture, and mandates that all subsequent deliveries be by cesarean section. The "low transverse," or horizontal incision carries a low risk, and subsequent deliveries may be vaginal. Note that the direction of the skin scar does not necessarily tell how the uterus was incised. Document the previous surgery to verify the safest route for the present pregnancy's delivery.
• Tell me the weights of your babies at birth.	A small infant may indicate prematurity or intrauterine growth retardation—complications that the woman is at risk to repeat. A large infant may indicate gestational diabetes (also repeatable). Conversely, birth weights of other children may indicate a "constitutional size"—e.g., the tendency of a couple to conceive smaller but normal children. Also, the woman's pelvis has been "proven" to the weight of the largest baby born vaginally, and the birth attendant will bear this number in mind as labor begins, estimating and comparing the weight of the baby about to be born.
• Did you breastfeed the previously born infants? How was that experience for you?	The woman's experience and knowledge base will shape the practitioner's teaching and support.
④ **Present pregnancy** [Having calculated the present number of weeks gestation, you can reassess the probable accuracy of that date when eliciting the following history]	
• What method of contraceptive did you use most recently, and when did you discontinue it?	Recent use of birth control pills or other hormonal contraceptives may have caused delayed ovulation and irregular menses, which must be considered when establishing the EDC. An intrauterine device (IUD) that is still in place requires removal and threatens the pregnancy. Also, this opens topic of whether pregnancy was planned.
• Was the pregnancy planned? How do you feel about it?	Even a planned pregnancy represents loss for the woman—perhaps a loss of freedom, compromise of goals, loss of time with other children or partner. The first trimester is known as the "trimester

Examiner Asks	Rationale
	of ambivalence," and encouraging acceptance and expression of these feelings facilitates resolution.
• How does the baby's father feel about the pregnancy? Other family members?	The woman may need assistance in gathering together her support group. Inviting significant others to future visits affirms their importance and supports their involvement.
• Experienced any vaginal bleeding? When? How much? What color? Accompanied by any pain?	Vaginal bleeding may indicate threatened abortion, cervicitis, or other complications, and must be investigated.
• Experienced abdominal pain? When? Where in your abdomen? Accompanied by vaginal bleeding?	The most common causes of abdominal pain in early pregnancy are spontaneous abortion, ectopic pregnancy, urinary tract infection, and round ligament discomfort. Later in pregnancy, premature labor must be ruled out. Also consider other medical and surgical causes for abdominal pain.
• Experienced any illnesses since being pregnant? Had any x-rays? Taken any medications? Used any recreational drugs or alcohol? Do you smoke cigarettes?	The potential effect of any teratogenic exposure must be discussed with the woman. Refer for expert counseling if necessary.
• Experiencing any visual changes such as the new onset of blurred vision or spots before your eyes?	In the third trimester, this may be a sign of preeclampsia. Evaluate for other signs and symptoms of preeclampsia (see Table 25–2).
• Experiencing any edema? Where and under what circumstances?	In the third trimester, differentiate the normal weight-dependent edema of pregnancy from the edema of preeclampsia.
• Any burning, frequency, or burning with urination? Any blood in your urine? Do you void in small amounts?	Differentiate the normal urinary frequency of the first and third trimesters from urinary tract infection, for which pregnant women are at increased risk. Findings are confirmed by urinalysis.
• Any vaginal burning or itching? Any foul-smelling or colored discharge? Large amount of discharge?	Rule out vaginal infection. If symptoms exist, add cultures or a wet mount to the pelvic examination. Discuss partner treatment if necessary. Educate the woman to the normal increase in vaginal secretions during pregnancy.
• What date did you first feel the baby move?	This sign is compared with the EDC in evaluation of the accuracy of that date. Tell the woman who has not experienced movement to note and report that event at the following prenatal visit.
• How does the baby move on a daily basis?	Fetal movement is an excellent indicator of fetal health. Many clinicians assign women to count fetal movements during the last weeks of their pregnancy.
• Do you have cats in the home?	Educate the woman about toxoplasmosis, a teratogenic disease transmitted

Examiner Asks	Rationale
	through cat feces. To avoid exposure, another person should empty cat litter at frequent intervals.
● Do you plan to breastfeed this baby?	Reading, classes, and other support may be arranged for the woman who is breastfeeding for the first time, or for the woman with an unsuccessful experience.
5 Past medical history	
● Ever had German measles (rubella)?	This mild childhood disease is highly teratogenic, especially during the first trimester. Instruct the woman who has not had rubella to avoid small children who are ill. Check immunity status in the serum prenatal panel as well. The nonimmune woman will be offered immunization after delivery.
● Ever had chickenpox?	Rarely, varicella causes congenital anomalies. The nonimmune woman should avoid exposure.
● Any injury to the back or another weight-bearing part?	The localized and overall weight gain of pregnancy as well as the joint-softening property of progesterone causes lordosis and will aggravate such injuries with increasing gestation.
● Have you been tested for HIV? When? What was the result? Ever had a blood transfusion? Used intravenous drugs? Had a sexual partner who had any HIV risk factors? Are you and your partner mutually monogamous?	HIV status must be addressed to promote the health of the gravida as well as to consider therapies that can decrease the risk of transmission of the virus across the placenta to the fetus. Breastfeeding is contraindicated for the HIV-positive mother because the virus is present in the breast milk. Educate the gravida who practices high-risk activities.
● Do you smoke cigarettes? How many? For how many years? Ever tried to quit? Drink any alcohol? How much of what type? Use any street drugs?	Educate the woman regarding the danger of these substances in pregnancy. Smoking increases the risk of ectopic pregnancy, spontaneous abortion, low birth weight, prematurity, preterm premature rupture of membranes, pregnancy-induced hypertension, placental abruption, and sudden infant death syndrome. Alcohol increases the risk to the fetus of fetal alcohol syndrome (see Table 11–3). Cocaine use during pregnancy is associated with a number of congenital anomalies, a fourfold increased risk for abruptio placenta and the risk of fetal addiction. Narcotic-addicted infants may experience developmental delays or behavioral disturbances

Examiner Asks	Rationale
	(Cunningham et al., 1997). Consider referral to a counseling/support program and periodic toxicology screening.
● Do you take any prescribed medications?	Screen all medications to establish safety during pregnancy.
⑥ **Family history** Anyone in your family have hypertension?	Increases the risk of chronic hypertension and of preeclampsia.
● Diabetes? If so, of juvenile or adult onset? Insulin dependent?	Increases risk of gestational diabetes. A heavy family history might prompt early screening and dietary interventions.
● Mental illness?	Increases risk for postpartum depression (Cunningham et al., 1997).
● Kidney disease?	Increases risk for renal disease, hypertension, and preeclampsia.
● Fraternal twins?	The tendency to ovulate twice in one month is familial, and thus the incidence of twinning is increased.
● Anyone in your family, or in the family of the baby's father had: congenital anomalies?	Some anomalies, such as heart conditions, are familial. Offer genetic counseling if needed.

● Is your racial descent Mediterranean?
  Black?
  Ashkenazi Jewish?
  Irish?
	Increased risk for β-thalassemia.
	Increased risk for sickle-cell disease.
	Increased risk for Tay-Sachs disease.
	Increased risk for spinal malformations (see Table 3–2).

⑦ **Review of Systems** ● Your weight before pregnancy? ● Wear glasses?	Baseline needed to evaluate changes. A transient change in visual correction may occur during pregnancy.
● When did you last see the dentist? Need any dental work?	Gums may be puffy and bleed easily during pregnancy, predisposing the woman to caries. Encourage careful dental hygiene. Suggest any dental care be done, if possible, during the second trimester, and to notify the dentist that she is pregnant.
● Been exposed to tuberculosis (TB)?	Consider TB screening using the tine test.
● Any cardiovascular disease, such as vascular disease, or disease of a heart valve?	The woman with cardiac disease who becomes pregnant must be monitored carefully for signs of cardiac compromise. Blood volume increases by 40 percent, and the demand on the heart is significantly increased.
● Any anemia? What kind? When? Was it treated? How? Did it improve?	Pregnancy worsens any pre-existing anemia, as iron is utilized extensively by the fetus. Identify the need for early supplementation. Sickle-cell anemia may worsen during pregnancy, while sickle-cell carriers experience more urinary tract infections. Screen the latter periodically for bacteriuria.

Examiner Asks	Rationale
• Had a thrombophlebitis?	Pregnancy itself is a hypercoagulable state due to increases in coagulation factors I, VII, VIII, IX, and X. This increases the risk of phlebitis (Cunningham et al., 1997).
• Have you had hypertension or kidney disease?	The woman with renal disease or with chronic hypertension is at increased risk for preeclampsia. Know the baseline BP and renal function to evaluate any changes.
• Ever had hepatitis?	Confirm this with serum testing. Treatment for mother and/or baby when born may be appropriate. Breastfeeding may be contraindicated in some cases.
• Have you had urinary tract infections?	The hormonal milieu of pregnancy predisposes the woman to urinary tract infections (UTIs), so a history of infection before pregnancy may indicate periodic screening. Pregnancy may also mask the symptoms of UTIs. Further, a serious UTI may cause irritability of the uterus, threatening the pregnancy. Educate the woman in measures to prevent such infections.
• Have you experienced depression or any other mental illness?	This woman will be at risk for postpartum depression. Assist her to prepare a support network. Counseling may help her successfully navigate the developmental challenges of becoming a mother.
• Do you have diabetes? Did you have diabetes during a previous pregnancy?	Diabetes is carefully managed during pregnancy to avoid serious complications, such as a macrosomic infant and operative delivery. Consider early screening and nutritional interventions.

8 Nutritional history

Examiner Asks	Rationale
• Do you follow a special diet?	A special diet may put the woman at nutritional risk. Help her achieve adequate nutrition within the confines of her diet.
• Any food intolerance?	A food intolerance might affect the woman's and fetus's nutrition, such as lactose intolerance limiting calcium intake.
• Do you crave nonfoods such as ice, paint chips, dirt, or clay?	Craving for ice and/or dirt is called pica and is associated with anemia.
• Record everything you eat and drink for 3 days, and bring the list to your next prenatal visit so that we can review it.	Assign a 3-day diet history so the woman's baseline diet can be analyzed and nutritional guidance tailored to her needs and practices.

Examiner Asks	Rationale

9 Environment/hazards

- What is your occupation? What are the physical demands of the work? Are you exposed to any strong odors, chemicals, radiation, or other harmful substances?

Hazards? Possible teratogenic exposures? The woman who is rubella nonimmune may be advised not to continue working in a day care center. Suitability for pregnancy? The woman whose job requires long hours of standing may be disabled early if signs of preterm labor occur.

- Do you consider your food and housing adequate?

If appropriate, refer for state and federal programs to assist with food, housing, or other needs.

- Other questions or concerns?

Encourage the woman to write down questions between visits so she does not forget them.

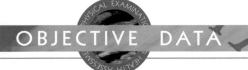

OBJECTIVE DATA

Preparation

The initial exam for pregnancy is often a woman's first pelvic exam, and many women are extremely anxious. Alternatively, the woman may not know for certain if she is pregnant, and she may be anxious about the findings. Verbally prepare the woman for what will happen during the exam before touching her. Save the pelvic exam for last—By that time the woman will be more comfortable with your gentle, informing manner. Communicate all findings as you go along to demonstrate your respectful affirmation of her control and responsibility in her own health and health care and that of her child's.

Ask the woman to empty her bladder before the exam, reserving a specimen for dipping for protein and glucose, and for urinalysis, if required. Ask her to weigh herself before the exam on the office scale.

Give the woman a gown and drape. Begin the examination with the woman sitting on the exam table, wearing the gown, her lap covered by a drape. During the breast exam, help her to lie down. She remains recumbent for the abdominal and extremity exam. Use the lithotomy position for the pelvic exam (see Chapter 24). Help her to a seated position to check her BP at the end of the exam, when, it is hoped, she will be most relaxed.

 Equipment Needed

Stethoscope BP cuff
Centimeter measuring tape
Fetoscope and Doppler
Reflex hammer
Urine collection containers
Chemostix for checking urine for glucose and protein
Equipment needed for pelvic exam as noted in Chapter 24.

Normal Range of Findings	Abnormal Findings

GENERAL SURVEY

Observe the woman's state of nourishment, and her grooming, posture, mood, and affect, which reflect her mental state. Throughout the exam, observe

Undernourished; or obesity.

▶ | Normal Range of Findings | Abnormal Findings

her maturity and ability to attend and learn in order to plan your teaching of the information she needs to successfully complete a healthy pregnancy.

Poor grooming, a slumped posture, and a flat affect may be signs of depression and risk for postpartum depression. Poor grooming may reflect a lack of resources and a need for a social service referral.

A lack of attention may indicate some preoccupation with a concern. The woman who has had learning difficulties may benefit from written and verbal information, special classes, as well as a support person to accompany her. A flat, unclear affect may indicate depression or the influence of drugs.

SKIN

Note any scars (particularly those of previous cesarean section). Many women experience skin changes during pregnancy that may spontaneously resolve after the pregnancy, such as acne or skin tags. Vascular spiders may be present on the upper body. Some women develop **chloasma,** known as the "mask of pregnancy," which is a butterfly-shaped pigmentation of the face. Note the presence of the **linea nigra,** a hyperpigmented line that begins at the sternal notch and extends down the abdomen through the umbilicus to the pubis (Fig. 25–3). Also note **striae,** or stretch marks, in areas of weight gain, particularly on the abdomen and breasts of multiparous women. These marks are bright red when they first form, but they will shrink and lighten to a silvery color (in the lightly pigmented woman) after the pregnancy (Fig. 25–3).

Multiple bruises may suggest physical abuse.

Tracks (scars along easily accessed veins) indicate intravenous drug use.

Palmar erythema in the first trimester may indicate hepatitis, but thereafter is not clinically significant (Varney, 1997).

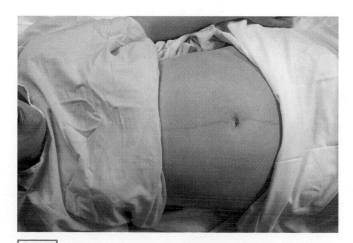

25–3

▶ Normal Range of Findings	Abnormal Findings

MOUTH

Mucous membranes should be red and moist. Gum hypertrophy (surface looks smooth and stippling disappears) may occur normally during pregnancy (pregnancy gingivitis).

Pale mucous membranes are indicative of anemia.

NECK

The thyroid may be palpable and feel full but smooth during the normal pregnancy of a euthyroid woman.

Solitary nodules indicate neoplasm; multiple nodules usually indicate inflammation or a multinodular goiter. Significant diffuse enlargement occurs with hyperthyroidism, thyroiditis, and hypothyroidism.

BREASTS

The breasts are enlarged (Fig. 25–4), perhaps with resulting striae and may be very tender. The areolae and nipples enlarge and darken in pigmentation, the nipples become more erect, and "secondary areolae" (mottling around the areolae) may develop. The blood vessels of the breast enlarge, and may shine blue through a seemingly more translucent than usual chest wall. When auscultating, blood flow through these blood vessels can be heard and may be mistaken for a cardiac murmur. This sound is called the mammary souffle. Montgomery's tubercles, located around the areola and responsible for skin integrity of the areola, enlarge. Colostrum, a thick yellow fluid, may be expressed from the nipples.

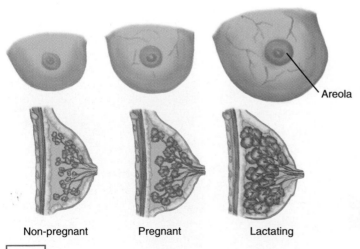

Areola

Non-pregnant   Pregnant   Lactating

25–4

The breast tissue feels nodular as the mammary alveoli hypertrophy. Take this opportunity to teach or reinforce breast self-exam (BSE). The woman should expect changes in the breast tissue during the pregnancy. Due to the lack of menses, instruct her to perform BSE according to the calendar on a monthly basis, on a date familiar to her such as her birth date.

Recall that some women have an embryologic remnant called a supernumerary nipple, which may or may not have breast tissue beneath it. Possibly mistaken previously for a mole, these occur under the arm or in a line directly underneath each nipple on the abdominal wall (see Chapter 15). This nipple and breast tissue may show the same changes of pregnancy. Instruct the woman to check these areas as well during breast self-examination.

HEART

The pregnant woman often develops a functional, soft, blowing, systolic murmur, which occurs due to increased volume. The murmur requires no treatment and will resolve after pregnancy.

Note any other murmur and refer. Valvular disease may necessitate the use of prophylactic antibiotics at delivery. Pregnancy places a large hemodynamic burden on the heart, and the woman with cardiac disease is managed closely.

PERIPHERAL VASCULATURE

The legs may show diffuse, bilateral pitting edema, particularly if the exam is occurring later in the day when the woman has been on her feet and in the third trimester. Varicose veins in the legs are common in the third trimester. The Homans' sign is negative.

Edema, together with increased BP and proteinuria, is a sign of preeclampsia. The pregnant woman is at risk for thrombophlebitis—Carefully evaluate any redness, or red, hot, tender swelling to rule out phlebitis. Varicosities increase the risk of thrombophlebitis, and she should not wear restrictive clothing or sit without moving legs for a long period. Varicosities will worsen with the weight and volume of pregnancy, and support hose help to minimize them.

NEUROLOGIC

Using the reflex hammer, check the biceps, patellar, and ankle deep tendon reflexes (DTRs). Normally these are 1+ to 2+ and equal bilaterally.

Brisk or greater than 2+ DTRs and clonus may be associated with elevated BP and cerebral edema in the preeclamptic woman.

ABDOMEN

Inspect and palpate the abdomen

Observe the shape and contours of the abdomen to discern signs of fetal position. As the woman lifts her head, you may see the **diastasis recti,** the separation of the abdominal muscles, which occurs during pregnancy, with the muscles returning together after pregnancy with abdominal exercise. When palpating, note the abdominal muscle tone, which grows more relaxed with each subsequent pregnancy. Throughout the palpation of the uterus, note any tenderness. The uterus is normally nontender.

The fundus should be palpable abdominally from 12 weeks gestation on. Use the side of your hand and begin palpating centrally on the abdomen higher than you expect the uterus to be. Palpate down until you feel the fundus. Alternatively, stand at the woman's right side facing her head (Fig. 25–5). Place the palm of your right hand on the curve of the uterus in the left lower quadrant; and your left palm on the curve of the uterus in the right lower quadrant. Moving from hand to hand, allowing the curve of the uterus to guide you, "walk" your hands to where they meet centrally at the fundus. Note the fundal location by landmarks and fingerbreadths, as described in Figure 25–1. Note that individual women's variations in location of landmarks as well as examiner's variations in finger width makes this measurement inexact. It is more accurate to use the centimeter measuring tape and measure the height of the fundus in centimeters from the superior border of the symphysis to the fundus (Fig. 25–6). After 20 weeks, the number of centimeters should approximate the number of weeks gestation.

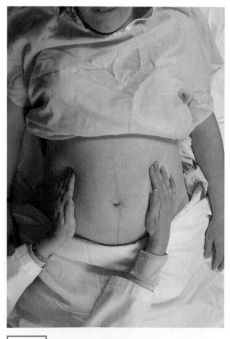

25–5

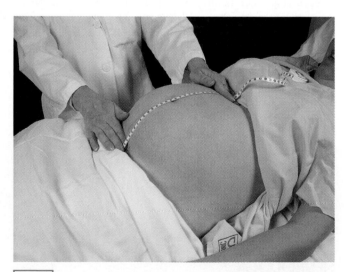

25–6

Beginning at 20 weeks, you may feel fetal movement, and the fetus' head can be ballotted. A gentle, quick palpation with the fingertips can locate a head that is not only hard when you push it away, but is hard as it bobs or bounces back against your fingers.

▶ **N o r m a l   R a n g e   o f   F i n d i n g s**   **A b n o r m a l   F i n d i n g s**

If you suspect the woman to be in labor, palpate for uterine contractions. Palpate the uterus over its entire surface to familiarize yourself with its "indentability." Then rest your hand lightly on the uterus with fingers opened. When the uterus contracts, it rises and pulls together, drawing your fingers closer together. During the contraction, notice that the uterus is less "indentable." When the uterus relaxes, your fingers relax open again. In this way, contractions can be monitored for frequency (from the beginning of one contraction to the beginning of the next), length, and quality. Note that a mild contraction feels like the firmness of the tip of your nose; a moderate contraction feels like your chin; and a hard contraction feels like a forehead. (Make allowance for the amount of soft tissue between your fingers and the uterus.)

Leopold's Maneuvers

In the third trimester, perform Leopold's maneuvers to determine fetal lie, presentation, attitude, position, variety, and engagement. **Fetal lie** is the orientation of the fetal spine to the maternal spine and may be longitudinal, transverse, or oblique. **Presentation** describes the part of the fetus that is entering the pelvis first. **Attitude** is the position of fetal parts in relation to each other, and may be flexed, military (straight), or extended. **Position** designates the location of a fetal part to the right or left of the maternal pelvis. **Variety** is the location of the fetal back to the anterior, lateral, or posterior part of the maternal pelvis. **Engagement** occurs when the widest diameter of the presenting part has descended into the pelvic inlet—specifically, to the imagined plane at the level of the ischial spines.

Leopold's first maneuver is performed by facing the gravida's head, and placing your fingertips around the top of the fundus (Fig. 25–7). Note its size, consistency, and shape. Imagine what fetal part is in the fundus. The breech feels large and firm. Moving it between the thumb and fingers of the hand, because it is attached to the fetus at the waist, results in moving it slowly and with difficulty. In contrast, the fetal head feels large, round, and hard. When it is ballotted, it feels hard as you push it away and hard again as it bobs back against your fingers in an "answer." Note that the "bobbing" or "ballotting" sensation of the movement occurs because the head is attached at the neck and moves easily. If there is no part in the fundus, the fetus is in the transverse lie.

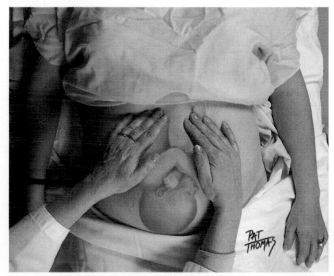

25–7

Leopold's first maneuver

For **Leopold's second maneuver,** move your hands to the sides of the uterus (Fig. 25–8). Note whether small parts or a long, firm surface are palpable on the woman's left or right side. The long, firm surface is the back. Note whether the back is anterior, lateral, or out of reach (posterior). The small parts, or limbs, indicate a posterior position when they are palpable all over the abdomen.

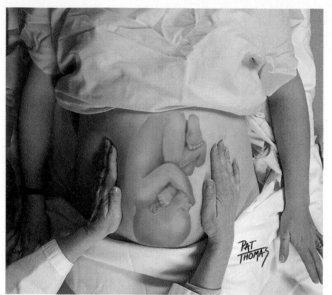

25–8

Leopold's second maneuver

Leopold's third maneuver, also called Pawlik's maneuver, requires the woman to bend her knees up slightly (Fig. 25–9). Grasp the lower abdomen just above the symphysis pubis between the thumb and fingers of one hand and, as you did at the fundus during the first maneuver, determine what part of the fetus is there. If the presenting part is beginning to engage, it will feel "fixed." With this maneuver alone, it may be difficult to differentiate the shoulder from the vertex.

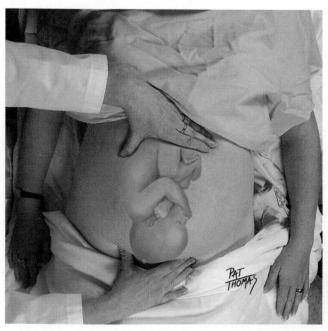

25–9

Leopold's third maneuver

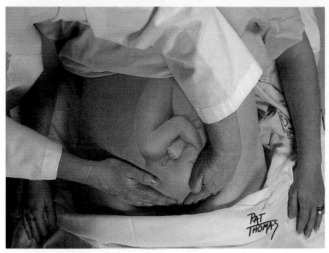

25–10

Leopold's fourth maneuver

The **fourth maneuver** assists you to determine engagement and, in the vertex presentation, to differentiate shoulder from vertex (Fig. 25–10). The woman's knees are still bent. Facing her feet, place your palms, with fingers pointing toward the feet, on either side of the lower abdomen. Pressing your fingers firmly, move slowly down toward the pelvic inlet. If your fingers meet, the presenting part is not engaged. If your fingers diverge at the pelvic rim meeting a hard prominence on one side, this prominence is the occiput. This indicates the vertex is presenting with a deflexed head (the face presenting). If your fingers meet hard prominences on both sides, the vertex is engaged in either a military or a flexed position. If your fingers come to the pelvic brim diverged but with no prominences palpable, the vertex is "dipping" into the pelvis, or is engaged. In this case, the firm object felt above the symphysis pubis in the third maneuver is the shoulder. See Figure 25–11 for various fetal positions and where to auscultate the fetal heart tones for each. At the end of pregnancy, 96 percent of fetal presentations are vertex, 3.5 percent are breech, 0.3 percent are face, and 0.4 percent are shoulder (Cunningham et al., 1997).

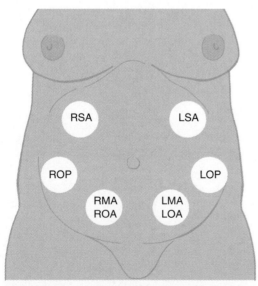

25–11

RSA and LSA = right and left sacral anterior (breech)
RMA and LMA = right and left mentum anterior (face)
ROA and LOA = right and left occiput anterior (vertex)
ROP and LOP= right and left occiput posterior (vertex)

Location of FHTs for various fetal positions

Normal Range of Findings	Abnormal Findings

Auscultate the fetal heart tones

FHTs are a positive sign of pregnancy. They can be heard with the Doppler ultrasound at 8 to 10 weeks gestation and with a fetoscope at 20 weeks. This use of the fetoscope assists in dating the pregnancy. FHTs are auscultated best over the shoulder of the fetus. After identifying the position of the fetus (see Fig. 25–11), use the heart tones to confirm your findings. Count the FHTs for 5 seconds and multiply by 12 to obtain the rate (Fig. 25–12). The normal rate is between 120 and 160 beats per minute. Differentiate the FHTs from the slower rate of the maternal pulse, and the uterine souffle (the soft, swishing sound of the placenta receiving the pulse of maternal arterial blood) by palpating the mother's pulse while you listen. Also, distinguish FHTs from the funic souffle (blood rushing through the umbilical arteries at the same rate as the FHTs). The FHTs are a double sound, like the tick-tock of a watch under a pillow, whereas the funic souffle is a sharp, whistling sound that is heard only 15 percent of the time (Cunningham et al., 1997).

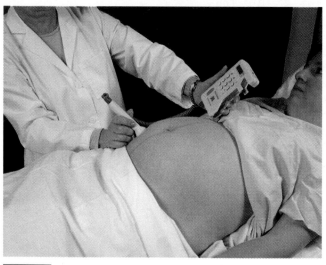

25–12

All of the abdominal findings are of interest to the woman—Share them with her. Often she will want to listen to FHTs with her significant others.

PELVIC EXAMINATION

Genitalia

Use the procedure for the pelvic examination described in Chapter 24. Note the following characteristics. You may note a bluish-purple discoloration of the external genitalia, **Chadwick's sign** of pregnancy. The enlargement of the labia minora is common in multiparous women. The perineum may be scarred from a previous episiotomy or from lacerations. Note the presence of any hemorrhoids of the rectum.

Speculum Examination

When examining the vagina, again you may see **Chadwick's sign,** the bluish-purplish discoloration of the vaginal wall and cervix. Note the vaginal discharge. Vaginal discharge in pregnancy may be heavier in amount, but should be similar in description to the woman's nonpregnant discharge, and should not be associated with itching, burning, or an unusual odor (except that, occasionally, chapping of the vaginal area may be seen due to excessive moisture). Perform a wet mount or culture of the discharge when you are uncertain of its normalcy.

Note whether the cervix appears open. Note whether it is the smooth, round cervix with a dotlike external os of the nulliparous woman, or the irregular multiparous cervix with an external os that appears more like a crooked line, the result of cervical dilation and possibly lacerations in a previous pregnancy.

Bimanual Examination

As described in Chapter 24, palpate the uterus between your internal and external hands. Note its position. The pregnant uterus may be rotated toward the right side as it rises out of the pelvis due to the presence of the descending colon on the left. This is called **dextrorotation.** Irregular enlargement of the uterus may be noted at 8 to 10 weeks and occurs when implantation occurs close to a cornual area of the uterus. This is called **Piskacek's sign.** Also you may note **Hegar's sign,** when the enlarged uterus bends forward on its softened isthmus.

Note the size and consistency of the uterus. The 6-week gestation uterus may seem only slightly enlarged and softened. The 8-week gestation uterus is approximately the size of an avocado, approximately 7 to 8 cm across the fundus. The 10-week gestation uterus is about the size of a grapefruit and may reach to the pelvic brim, but is narrow and does not fill the pelvis from side to side; the 12-week gestation uterus will fill the pelvis. After 12 weeks, the uterus is sized from the abdomen. The multigravid uterus may be larger initially, and early sizing of this uterus may be less reliable for dating.

Softening of the cervix is called **Goodell's sign.** When examining the cervix, note its position (anterior, midposition, or posterior); degree of effacement (or thinning, expressed in percentages assuming a 2-cm long cervix initially); dilation (opening, expressed in centimeters); consistency (soft or firm); and the station of the presenting part (centimeters above or below the ischial plane) (Fig. 25–13).

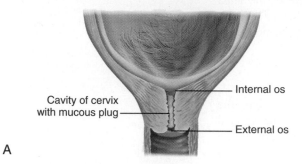

Cavity of cervix with mucous plug — Internal os — External os

A

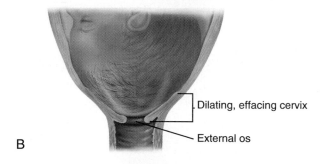

Dilating, effacing cervix — External os

B

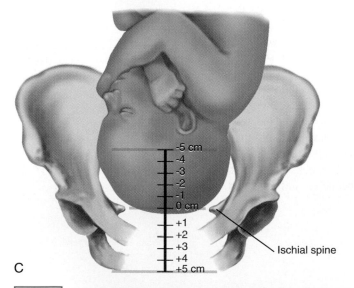

-5 cm
-4
-3
-2
-1
0 cm
+1
+2
+3
+4
+5 cm
Ischial spine

C

25–13 | **A, Cervix before labor   B, Cervix begins to efface and dilate
C, Station height of presenting part in relation to ischial spines.**

The ovaries rise with the growing uterus. Always examine the adnexae to rule out the presence of a mass, such as an ectopic pregnancy.

Ask the woman to squeeze your fingers as they rest in the vagina to determine tone. Take this opportunity to teach Kegel exercise, the squeezing of the vagina, which the woman can do to prepare for and to recover from birth. (The woman can also identify the exercise of these muscles by stopping the flow of urine midstream, although she should only do this once, and should usually let urine flow freely.) Direct the woman to squeeze slowly to a peak at the count of eight and then release slowly to the count of eight. You can prescribe this exercise to be performed 50 to 100 times a day.

The woman will often appreciate palpating her own uterus from the abdomen. If the uterus is small, you can lift it up internally.

Pelvimetry

Assess the bones of the pelvis for shape and size. The dimensions may indicate the favorableness of the bony structure for vaginal delivery. However, the relaxation of the pelvic joints, the widening of the pelvis in the squatting position, as well as the capacity of the fetal head to mold to the shape of the pelvis, may enable a vaginal birth despite seemingly unfavorable measurements.

To aid in visualizing the pelvis, imagine three planes: the pelvic inlet (from the sacral promontory to the upper edge of the pubis), the midpelvis, and the pelvic outlet (from the coccyx to the lower edge of the pubis) (Fig. 25–14). Assessment of each of these pelvic planes, as described in the following techniques, allows you to estimate the adequacy of the pelvis for vaginal delivery.

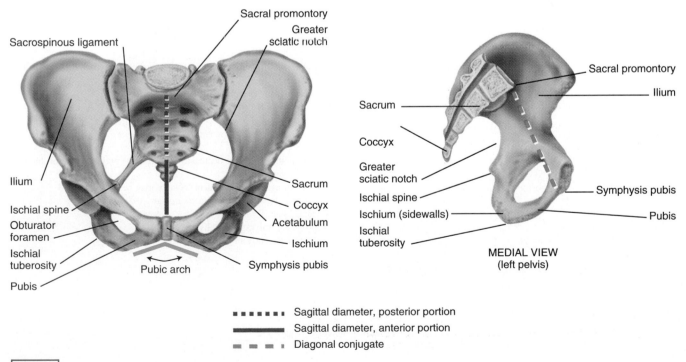

Sacrospinous ligament
Sacral promontory
Greater sciatic notch
Ilium
Ischial spine
Obturator foramen
Ischial tuberosity
Pubis
Pubic arch
Sacrum
Coccyx
Acetabulum
Ischium
Symphysis pubis

Sacrum
Coccyx
Greater sciatic notch
Ischial spine
Ischium (sidewalls)
Ischial tuberosity
Sacral promontory
Ilium
Symphysis pubis
Pubis

MEDIAL VIEW
(left pelvis)

▪▪▪▪▪▪ Sagittal diameter, posterior portion
▬▬▬ Sagittal diameter, anterior portion
▬ ▬ ▬ Diagonal conjugate

25–14

▶ Normal Range of Findings	Abnormal Findings

There are four general types of pelves: gynecoid, anthropoid, android, and platypelloid (Table 25–1). Most commonly, a woman's pelvis will be an "intermediate" or "mixed" type. You may postpone examination of the bony pelvis until the third trimester when the vagina is more distensible. With your two fingers still in the vagina, note the shape and width of the pubic arch (a 90-degree arch, or 2 fingerbreadths, is desirable.) If you are right-handed, move your hand to the woman's right pelvis. If you are left-handed, move it to the left side of the woman's pelvis. Assess the inclination and curve of the side walls,

Table 25–1 · The Four Pelvic Types

The Gynecoid Pelvis	The Android Pelvis
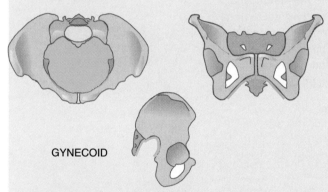	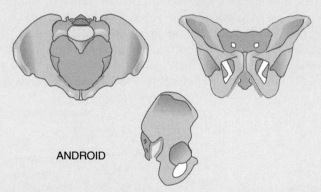
GYNECOID	ANDROID
Inlet round or oval.	Inlet heart-shaped.
Posterior sagittal diameter of inlet only slightly less than anterior sagittal diameter.	Posterior sagittal diameter of inlet less than the anterior sagittal diameter.
Pubic arch wide (90 degrees or more).	Pubic arch narrow (less than 90 degrees).
Spines are not prominent, allowing a transverse diameter at spines 10 cm or more.	Spines are prominent, decreasing transverse diameter at spines.
Sacrosciatic notch round and wide.	Sacrosciatic notch is narrow and highly arched.
Straight side walls.	Side walls converge.
Posterior pelvis is round and wide.	Posterior sagittal diameter decreases from inlet to outlet as sacrum inclines forward.
Sacrum is parallel with the symphysis pubis; hollow and concave.	Sacrum is straight and prominent; coccyx may be prominent.
	Anterior of pelvis is narrow and triangular.
	The "male" pelvis.
Favors vaginal delivery.	Poor prognosis for vaginal delivery.
Seen in 50 percent of all women.	Seen more frequently in Caucasian women.

Data from Varney H: Varney's Midwifery, 3rd ed. Sudbury, MA, Jones and Bartlett, 1997.

▶ | Normal Range of Findings   Abnormal Findings

and the prominence of the ischial spine (refer back to Fig. 25–14 for location of these landmarks). Move your fingers back and forth between the spines to get an impression of the transverse diameter—10 cm is desirable. Sweep your fingers down the sacrum, noting its shape and inclination (hollow, J-shaped, or straight). Assess the coccyx for prominence and mobility. From the sacrum, locate the sacrospinous ligament. Assess the length of the ligament—2½ to 3 finger-breadths is adequate. Assess the shape and width of the sacrospinous notch. Shift to the other side of the pelvis and assess it for similarity to the first.

Table 25–1 • The Four Pelvic Types *Continued*

The Anthropoid Pelvis   **The Platypelloid Pelvis**

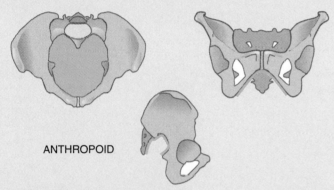

ANTHROPOID

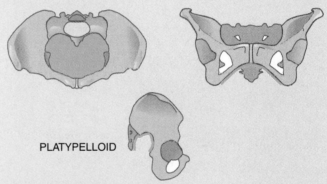

PLATYPELLOID

Inlet oval in shape.
Pubic arch may be somewhat narrow.
Spines usually prominent but not encroaching because of the spaciousness of the posterior segment.
Sacrosciatic notch average height but wide (about 4 fingerbreadths).
Side walls somewhat convergent.
Sacrum posteriorly inclined, with posterior sagittal diameters long throughout the pelvis.
Occurs in 40.5 percent nonwhite women; 23.5 percent white women.
If pelvis somewhat large, adequate for vaginal delivery since posterior pelvis is generous.

Inlet shaped like a flattened gynecoid pelvis.
Pubic arch wide.
Spines usually prominent but not encroaching because of the already wide interspinous diameter.
Sacrosciatic notch wide and flat.
Side walls slightly convergent.
Sacrum inclined posteriorly and hollow, making a short and shallow pelvis.
Occurs in less than 3 percent of all women.

Not conducive to vaginal delivery.

The pelvic inlet cannot be reached by clinical examination, but you can estimate it by the measure of the **diagonal conjugate,** which indicates the anteroposterior diameter of the pelvic inlet. Having measured the length of the second and third fingers of your examining hand, with your fingers still in the vagina, point these fingers toward the sacral promontory (Fig. 25–15). If you cannot reach the promontory, note the measurement as being greater than the centimeters of length of your examining fingers. A measurement of 11.5 to 12.0 cm is desirable.

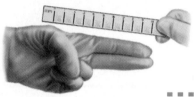

■ ■ ■ Diagonal conjugate

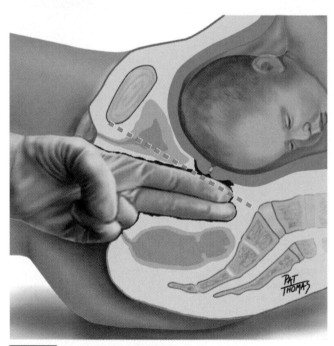

| 25–15 | **Diagonal conjugate**

Remove your fingers from the vagina. Having previously measured the width of your own hand across the knuckles, form your hand into a closed fist and place it across the perineum between the ischial tuberosities. Estimate this diameter, which is the **biischial diameter** (also known as the intertubous diameter and the transverse diameter of the pelvic outlet. A measurement greater than 8 cm is generally adequate (Fig. 25–16).

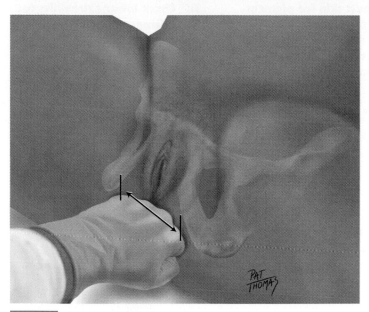

25–16 | **Biischial diameter**

When describing pelvimetry, note all of the above measurements and state the pelvic type. The pelvis may be described as being "proven" to the number of pounds of the largest vaginally born infant. Alternatively, to describe a small pelvis, you may make the assessment, for example, "adequate for a 7-lb baby."

Blood Pressure

After the exam, take the blood pressure when the woman is the most relaxed, in the semi-Fowler's or upright position. An elevated pressure should be rechecked on the right arm with the woman resting on her left side.

ROUTINE LABORATORY AND RADIOLOGIC IMAGING STUDIES

At the onset of pregnancy, order a routine prenatal panel, which usually includes a complete blood count, serology, rubella antibodies, hepatitis B screening, blood type and Rhesus factor, and an antibody screen. Offer the woman an HIV test. Collect a urinalysis. At each prenatal visit, check urine for protein and glucose. A clean-catch specimen is ideal for this dip because a random specimen may include vaginal secretions, which contain protein, skewing the result.

Each agency has a policy regarding the frequency of ultrasound examinations. Although many groups utilize ultrasound only when there is a medical indication, other groups routinely order ultrasounds to confirm dates and fetal normalcy (insofar as ultrasound is able to determine normalcy), as well as for any specific medical indication, such as the fundus's measuring small for dates. The ultrasound also shows placental location and fetal gender.

Summary Checklist: The Pregnant Female

1: Collect historical information.

2: Determine EDC and present number of weeks gestation.

3: Instruct the woman to undress and empty her bladder, saving her urine to dip it for protein and glucose.

4: Measure weight.

5: Perform a physical examination, starting with general survey.

6: Inspect skin for pigment changes, scars.

7: Check oral mucous membranes.

8: Palpate thyroid gland.

9: Inspect breast changes and palpate.

10: Auscultate heart sounds, heart rate, and any murmurs.

11: Check lower extremities for edema, varicosities.

12: The abdomen: Measure fundus height, perform Leopold's maneuvers, auscultate FHTs.

13: The pelvic exam: Note signs of pregnancy, the condition of the cervix, and the size and position of the uterus.

14: Perform pelvimetry.

15: Measure the blood pressure.

APPLICATION AND CRITICAL THINKING

SAMPLE CHARTING

 Subjective

Rosa Gutierrez is a 27-year-old Hispanic Gravida 2/Para 1 who presents with her husband and daughter for her first prenatal visit. She is a full-time homemaker who completed 2 years of college. Last normal menstrual period (LNMP) was April 4 of this year (certain of date), with an expected date of confinement (EDC) of January 11 of next year, making her 10 weeks' gestation today. Her obstetric history includes a normal spontaneous vaginal delivery (NSVD) 3 years ago of a viable 7 lb, 12 oz female infant after an 8-hour labor without anesthesia, midline episiotomy. No complications of pregnancy, delivery, or the postpartum. She breast fed this daughter, Ana, for 1 year. Present pregnancy was planned, and Rosa and her husband are pleased. Rosa is having breast tenderness, and nausea on occasion, which resolves with crackers. No past medical or surgical conditions are present. She denies allergies. Family history is significant only for diet-controlled adult-onset diabetes in two maternal aunts.

 Objective

General: appears well nourished and is carefully groomed. English is second language, and Rosa is fluent. Skin: light tan in color, surface smooth with no lesions, small tattoo noted on left forearm. Mouth: good dentition and oral hygiene. Oral mucosa pink, no gum hypertrophy. Thyroid gland small and smooth.

Chest expansion equal, respirations effortless. Lung sounds clear bilaterally with no adventitious sounds. No CVA tenderness.

Heart: rate 76 bpm, regular rhythm, S_1 and S_2 are normal, not accentuated or diminished, with soft, blowing systolic murmur Gr ii/vi at 2nd left interspace.

Breasts: tender, without masses, with supple, everted nipples. Breast self-exam reviewed.

Abdomen: no masses, bowel sounds present. No hepatosplenomegaly. Uterus nonpalpable. No inguinal lymphadenopathy noted.

Extremities: no varicosities, redness, or edema. Homans' sign negative. DTRs 2+ and equal bilaterally.

BP 110/68 in semi-Fowler's.

Pelvic: Bartholin's, urethra, and Skene's glands (BUS) negative for discharge. Vagina: pink, with white, creamy, nonodorous discharge. Cervix: pink, closed, multiparous, 2 cm long, firm.

Uterus: 10-week size, consistent with dates, nontender, dextrorotated. FHTs heard with Doppler, rate 140s.

Pelvis: pubic arch wide; side walls straight, spines blunt, interspinous diameter > 10 cm. Sacrum hollow; coccyx mobile. Sacrospinous ligament 3 fingerbreadths (FBs) wide. Diagonal conjugate > 12 cm, bituberous diameter > 8 cm. Spacious gynecoid pelvis proven to 7 lb, 12 oz.

ASSESSMENT

Intrauterine pregnancy 10 weeks by good dates, size = dates.

Rosa and husband happy with pregnancy; she feels well.

PLAN

Begin prenatal vitamins.

Prenatal blood screen and urinalysis.

HIV offered and accepted.

Reviewed comfort measures for nausea.

Return visit in 4 weeks.

Three-day diet recall assigned for next visit.

NURSING DIAGNOSES COMMONLY ASSOCIATED WITH PREGNANCY

Diagnosis	Related factors (Etiology)	Defining characteristics (Symptoms and Signs)
Altered parenting	Ineffective role model Effects of physical and psychosocial abuse Unmet social/emotional maturational needs of parenting figure Interruption in bonding process Unrealistic expectations for self, infant, partner Multiple pregnancies Physical or mental handicaps Acute/chronic mental or physical illnesses Limited cognitive functioning Lack of support from significant others Lack of knowledge Lack of role identity Perceived threat to own survival, physical and emotional Presence of stress (financial, legal, cultural move)	Verbalizes disappointment in gender or physical characteristics of infant Verbalizes resentment toward infant Verbalizes role inadequacy Verbalizes frustration Lack of parental attachment behaviors Inattention to infant's/child's needs Noncompliance with health appointments History of child abuse by primary caretaker Compulsively seeks role approval from others

Continued

Other Related Nursing Diagnoses

ACTUAL	RISK/WELLNESS
Altered comfort	**Risk**
Altered health maintenance	Risk for altered nutrition: less than body requirements
Body image disturbance (see Chapter 11)	Risk for altered nutrition: more than body requirements
Constipation	Risk for altered sexual patterns
Fatigue	
Ineffective family coping	**Wellness**
Noncompliance	Potential for effective health management
Sleep pattern disturbance	Potential for effective nutritional-metabolic pattern
	Potential for positive role-relationship pattern

 ASSESSMENT VIDEO CRITICAL THINKING QUESTIONS

The Saunders *Physical Examination and Health Assessment* Video Series—THE PREGNANT WOMAN—will direct you to consider the following:

1. What information does an obstetric history provide and how is it used?
2. Why should you document the patient's position when taking her blood pressure?
3. When is edema in the legs a danger sign in a pregnant patient?
4. Why are the external genitalia examined?
5. Why are pelvic measurements important to a prenatal assessment?
6. What is the significance of a fundal height that is higher or lower than expected for the patient's weeks of gestation?

Table 25–2 PREECLAMPSIA

Preeclampsia is a condition specific to pregnancy. The etiology remains unknown, but it involves vasospasm, hemolysis, and several organ systems. Predisposing conditions include a family history of preeclampsia, nulliparity, age greater than 35 years, chronic vascular disease, renal disease, diabetes, fetal hydrops, multiple fetuses, or hydatidiform mole.

The classic syndrome involves a "triad" of symptoms: elevated blood pressure, proteinuria, and edema. Edema is common in pregnancy and is the least reliable symptom. However, edema of the face that is of sudden onset, associated with sudden weight gain, signals a consideration of preeclampsia. Proteinuria is a late development in preeclampsia and is, therefore, an indicator of the severity of the disease. The BP should be compared with the woman's prenatal or early pregnancy readings. An increase of 15 mm Hg diastolic over the baseline or a BP greater than 140 systolic or 90 diastolic is considered hypertension. Hypertension is necessary for the diagnosis of preeclampsia, but preeclampsia may be seen without the edema or proteinuria.

Preeclampsia is rarely seen before 20 weeks gestation and only then in conjunction with hydatidiform mole. The condition worsens with continuation of pregnancy. Onset and worsening may be sudden. Subjective signs may include headaches, visual changes (spots or blurring), and/or epigastric pain. The liver may become necrotic and hemorrhagic. Liver enzymes become elevated, and edema stretches the liver capsule, which causes pain referred to the epigastric area. Cerebral edema causes the neurologic signs. Hemolysis occurs, in part at least, as a result of vasospasm. A serious variant of preeclampsia, the HELLP syndrome involves hemolysis, elevated liver enzymes, and low platelets, and represents an ominous clinical picture. Untreated preeclampsia may progress to eclampsia, which is manifested by grand mal seizures. Eclampsia may develop as late as 10 days postpartum.

Before the syndrome becomes clinically manifested, it is affecting the placenta through vasospasm and a series of small infarctions. The placenta's capacity to deliver oxygen and nutrients may be seriously diminished, and fetal growth may be stunted.

Table 25–3 FETAL SIZE INCONSISTENT WITH DATES

SIZE SMALL FOR DATES	Fundal height measures smaller than expected for dates
Inaccuracy of Dates	Conception may have occurred later than originally thought. Reconsider the woman's menstrual history, sexual history, contraceptive use, early pregnancy testing, early sizing of the uterus, ultrasound results, timing of pregnancy symptoms, including the date of quickening, and the fundal height measurements. If, after this review, the expected date of delivery is correct, then further investigation is required.
Premature Labor	When premature labor moves the presenting part of the fetus from the abdomen into the pelvis for delivery, the fundus may shorten. Premature or preterm birth occurs before 37 weeks gestation, which happens in 11 percent of births in the United States (Cunningham et al., 1997). The cause of preterm birth usually is multifactorial. Risk factors include history of previous preterm delivery, short stature, occupational factors, hypertensive disorders, infection, multiple gestation, low maternal age, lifestyle behaviors such as cigarette smoking, poor nutrition and weight gain, substance abuse (especially cocaine and alcohol), and prenatal stress of the mother (Cunningham et al., 1997).

Table continued on following page

Intrauterine Growth Retardation (IUGR) or Fetal Growth Restriction	IUGR may occur due to environmental factors such as early exposure to a chemical, an early viral infection, living at high altitudes, maternal anemia, or malnutrition. Fetal factors include congenital malformations or chromosomal abnormalities that affect cellular growth. Placental factors include placental or cord abnormalities, such as chronic placental insufficiency, which may occur with hypertensive disorders. That is, excessive pressure causes the blood vessels of the placenta to wear out prematurely. Areas of the placenta will atrophy, causing a reduced supply of nutrients and oxygen, thus reducing fetal growth. IUGR becomes more threatening as pregnancy advances, as the normal aging of the placenta is accelerated.
Fetal Position	Fetal position varies until about 34 weeks when the vertex should settle into the pelvis and remain there. The fetus occupying a transverse lie, or shoulder presentation, results in the maternal abdomen's widening from side to side and the fundal height's diminishing. Fetal malposition may occur with lax maternal abdominal musculature (simply not holding the baby in close), an abnormality in the fetus (e.g., the enlarged head of the hydrocephalic infant), placenta previa (the placenta being implanted over the cervix, blocking fetal descent), or a restricted maternal pelvis.
SIZE LARGE FOR DATES	Fundal height measures larger than expected for dates
Inaccuracy of Dates	Review the same findings as listed above.
Multiple Fetuses	The frequency of multiple fetuses increases with the use of infertility drugs and may show as a fullness of the uterus. The occurrence of twins is proven when two clinicians count FHTs simultaneously and count different heart rates for the babies during the same minute. Ultrasound examination confirms the diagnosis.
Polyhydramnios	The cause of a larger than normal amount of amniotic fluid usually is idiopathic, but it may be associated with maternal diabetes, multiple fetuses, or fetal abnormalities (Cunningham et al., 1997).
Fetal Macrosomia	This is the condition in which the full-term infant weighs greater than 4000 to 4500 g at birth (Cunningham et al., 1997). Maternal diabetes is the most important risk factor, during which the fetus is exposed to high blood sugar and converts the glucose into soft tissue. Other predisposing factors include maternal obesity, multiparity, prolonged gestation, male fetus, previous delivery of infant weighing more than 4000 g, race, and ethnicity (Cunningham et al., 1997). Risks of macrosomia to the infant include birth injuries due to a more difficult delivery, and greater difficulty with transition to life, such as maintaining blood sugar and temperature.
Leiomyoma (Myoma or "Fibroids")	These are pre-existing benign tumors of the uterine wall, which then are stimulated to enlarge by the estrogen levels of pregnancy. Myomata may be located anywhere in the uterine wall (see Table 24–7). When they grow in the outer uterine wall, the myometrium, they may affect the clinician's judgment of where the fundus of the uterus should be measured. A myoma may grow just underneath the endometrial surface into the uterine cavity, displacing the fetus or preventing its descent into the pelvis.

Table 25-4   MALPRESENTATIONS

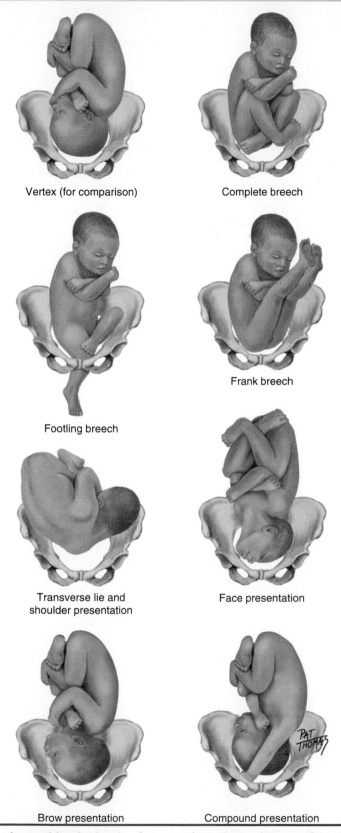

Vertex (for comparison)

Complete breech

Footling breech

Frank breech

Transverse lie and shoulder presentation

Face presentation

Brow presentation

Compound presentation

Malpresentations may be detected by the hands of an experienced examiner, confirmed by the FHT location, and further confirmed by ultrasound. Before 34 weeks gestation, any position is normal. The vertex presentation is desirable thereafter, because spontaneous turning becomes less likely as the fetus grows in proportion to the amount of space and fluid in the uterus and pelvis.

Bibliography

Adashek JA, Peaceman AM, Lopez-Zeno J, et al: Factors contributing to the increased cesarean birth rate in older parturient women. Am J Obstet Gynecol 169:936, 1993.

Ament LA, Whalen E: Sexually transmitted diseases in pregnancy: Diagnosis, impact, and intervention. J Obstet Gynecol Neonatal Nurs 25(8):657–666, Oct 1996.

Bastian LA, Piscitelli, JT: Is this patient pregnant? Can you reliably rule in or out early pregnancy by clinical examination? JAMA 18:586–91, Aug 20, 1997.

Buehler JW, Kaunitz AM, Hogue CJR, et al: Maternal mortality in women aged 35 years or older: United States. JAMA 255:53, 1986.

Creasy RK, Resnick R: Maternal-Fetal Medicine, 3rd ed. Philadelphia, WB Saunders Company, 1994.

Cunningham FG, Leveno KJ: Management of pregnancy induced hypertension. In Rubin PC (Ed): Handbook of Hypertension, Vol X. Hypertension in Pregnancy. Amsterdam, Elsevier, 1988.

Cunningham FG, MacDonald PC, Gant NF, et al: Williams Obstetrics, 20th ed. Stamford, CT, Appleton & Lange, 1997.

Dooley SL, Metzger BE, Cho N, et al: The influence of demographic and phenotypic heterogeneity on the prevalence of gestational diabetes mellitus. Int J Gynecol Obstet 35:13, 1991.

Edge V, Laros RK: Pregnancy outcome on nulliparous women age 35 or older. Am J Obstet Gynecol 168:1881, 1993.

Evans MF: Diagnosing pregnancy. What is the best way? Can Fam Physician 44:287–289, Feb 1998.

Freda MC, Anderson F, Damus K, Merkatz IR: Are there differences in information given to private and public prenatal patients? Am J Obstet Gynecol 169(1):155–160, 1995.

Hollingsworth DR, Vaucher Y, Yamamoto TR: Diabetes in pregnancy in Mexican Americans. Diabetes Care 14:695, 1991.

Kennedy HP, Griffin M, Frishman G: Enabling conception and pregnancy. Midwifery care of women experiencing infertility. J Nurse Midwifery 43(3):190–207, 1998.

Knox G, Morley D: Twinning in Yoruba women. J Obstet Gynaecol Br Emp 67:981, 1960.

Lowe SW, Pruitt RH, Smart PT, Dooley RL: Routine use of ultrasound during pregnancy. Nurse Pract 23(10):60–71, Oct 1998.

Nagey DA. The content of prenatal care. Obstet Gynecol 74(3, Pt 2): 516–528, Sep 1989.

O'Day MP: Cardio-respiratory physiological adaptation of pregnancy. Semin Perinatol 21(4):268–275, Aug 1997.

Peipert JF, Bracken MB: Maternal age: An independent risk factor for cesarean delivery. Obstet Gynecol 81:200, 1993.

Peoples-Sheps MD, Hogan VK, Ng'andu N: Content of prenatal care during the initial workup. Am J Obstet Gynecol 174(1, Pt 1):220–226, Jan 1996.

Perry LE: Preconception care: A health promotion opportunity. Nurse Pract 21:(11)24–41, Nov 1996.

Rousseau ME: Women's midlife health. J Nurse Midwifery 43(3):208–223, 1998.

Varney H: Varney's Midwifery, 3rd ed. Sudbury, MA, Jones and Bartlett, 1997.

UNIT 3

Integration of the Health Assessment

CHAPTER TWENTY SIX

The Complete Health Assessment: Putting It All Together

The choreography of the complete history and physical examination is the art of arranging all the separate steps you have learned so far. Your first examination may seem awkward and contrived; you may have to pause and think of what comes next rather than just gather data. Repeated rehearsals will make the choreography smoother. You will come to the point at which the procedure flows naturally, and even if you forget a step, you will be able to insert it gracefully into the next logical place.

The following examination sequence is one suggested route. It is intended to minimize the number of position changes for the patient and for you. With experience, you may wish to adapt this and arrange a sequence that feels natural for you. Perform all the steps listed here for a complete examination. With experience, you will learn to strike a balance between which steps you must retain to be thorough and which corners you may safely cut when time is pressing.

Have all equipment prepared and accessible before the examination. Review Chapter 8, Assessment Techniques and Approach to the Clinical Setting, for the list of necessary equipment, the setting, the patient's emotional state, your demeanor, and the preparation of the patient considering his or her age.

▶ Sequence   Selected Photos

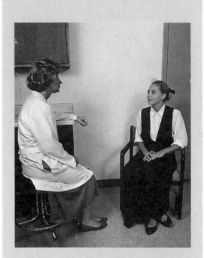

The patient walks into the room, sits; the examiner sits facing the patient; the patient is in street clothes.

THE HEALTH HISTORY

Collect the history, complete or limited as visit warrants. While obtaining the history and throughout the examination, note data on the person's general appearance.

GENERAL APPEARANCE

1. Appears stated age
2. Level of consciousness
3. Skin color
4. Nutritional status
5. Posture and position comfortably erect
6. Obvious physical deformities
7. Mobility
    Gait
    Use of assistive devices
    Range of motion (ROM) of joints
    No involuntary movement
8. Facial expression
9. Mood and affect
10. Speech: articulation, pattern, content
    appropriate, native language
11. Hearing
12. Personal hygiene

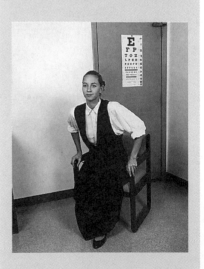

MEASUREMENT

1. Weight
2. Height
3. Skinfold thickness, if indicated
4. Vision using Snellen's eye chart

Sequence	Selected Photos

Ask the person to empty the bladder (save specimen, if needed), disrobe except for underpants, and put on a gown. The person sits with legs dangling off side of the bed or table; you stand in front of the person.

SKIN

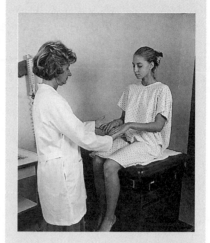

1. Examine both hands and inspect the nails.
2. For the rest of the examination, examine skin with corresponding regional examination.

VITAL SIGNS

1. Radial pulse
2. Respirations
3. Blood pressure
4. Temperature (if indicated)

HEAD AND FACE

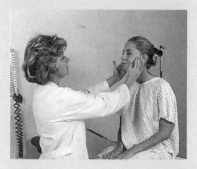

1. Inspect and palpate scalp, hair, and cranium.
2. Inspect face: expression, symmetry (cranial nerve VII).
3. Palpate the temporal artery, then the temporomandibular joint as the person opens and closes the mouth.
4. Palpate the maxillary sinuses and the frontal sinuses; if tender, transilluminate the sinuses.

EYE

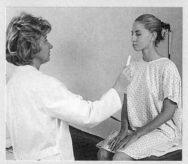

1. Test visual fields by confrontation (cranial nerve II).
2. Test extraocular muscles: corneal light reflex, six cardinal positions of gaze (cranial nerves III, IV, VI).
3. Inspect external eye structures.
4. Inspect conjunctivae, sclerae, corneas, irides.
5. Test pupil: size, response to light and accommodation.

   Darken room

6. Using an ophthalmoscope, inspect ocular fundus: red reflex, disc, vessels, and retinal background.

EAR

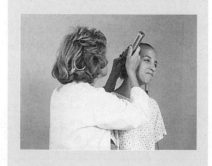

1. Inspect the external ear: position and alignment, skin condition, and auditory meatus.
2. Move auricle and push tragus for tenderness.
3. Using an otoscope, inspect the canal, then the tympanic membrane for color, position, landmarks, and integrity.
4. Test hearing: voice test; tuning fork tests—Weber and Rinne.

Sequence

NOSE

1. Inspect the external nose: symmetry, lesions.
2. Test the patency of each nostril.
3. Using a speculum, inspect the nares: nasal mucosa, septum, and turbinates.

MOUTH AND THROAT

1. Using a penlight, inspect the mouth: buccal mucosa, teeth and gums, tongue, floor of mouth, palate, and uvula.
2. Grade tonsils, if present.
3. Note mobility of uvula as the person phonates "ahh," and test gag reflex (cranial nerves IX, X).
4. Ask the person to stick out the tongue (cranial nerve XII).
5. Don a glove and bimanually palpate the mouth, if indicated.

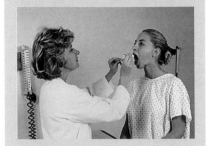

NECK

1. Inspect the neck: symmetry, lumps, and pulsations.
2. Palpate the cervical lymph nodes.
3. Inspect and palpate the carotid pulse, one side at a time. If indicated, listen for carotid bruits.
4. Palpate the trachea in midline.
5. Test ROM and muscle strength against your resistance: head forward and back, head turned to each side, and shoulder shrug (cranial nerve XI).

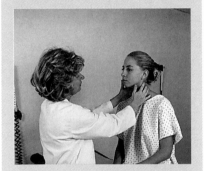

Step behind the person, taking your stethoscope, ruler, and marking pen with you.
6. Palpate thyroid gland.

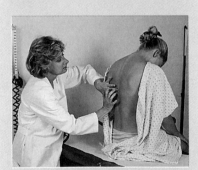

Open the person's gown to expose all of the back for examination of the thorax, but leave gown on shoulders and anterior chest.

CHEST, POSTERIOR AND LATERAL

1. Inspect the posterior chest: configuration of the thoracic cage, skin characteristics, and symmetry of shoulders and muscles.
2. Palpate: symmetric expansion; tactile fremitus; lumps or tenderness.
3. Palpate length of spinous processes.
4. Percuss over all lung fields, percuss diaphragmatic excursion.
5. Percuss costovertebral angle, noting tenderness.
6. Auscultate breath sounds; note adventitious sounds.

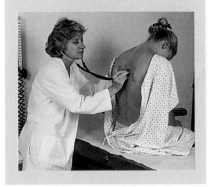

▶ Sequence	Selected Photos

Move around to face the patient; the patient remains sitting. For a female breast examination, ask permission to lift gown to drape on the shoulders, exposing the anterior chest; for a male, lower the gown to the lap.

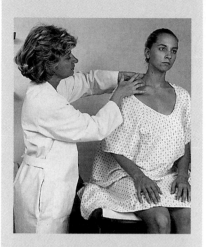

CHEST, ANTERIOR

1. Inspect: respirations and skin characteristics.
2. Palpate: tactile fremitus, lumps, or tenderness.
3. Percuss lung fields.
4. Auscultate breath sounds.

HEART

1. Ask the person to lean forward and exhale briefly; auscultate cardiac base for any murmurs.

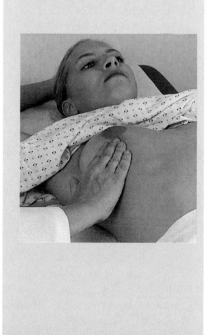

UPPER EXTREMITIES

1. Test ROM and muscle strength of hands, arms, and shoulders.
2. Palpate the epitrochlear nodes.

FEMALE BREASTS

1. Inspect for symmetry, mobility, and dimpling as the woman lifts arms over the head, pushes the hands on the hips, and leans forward.
2. Inspect supraclavicular and infraclavicular areas.

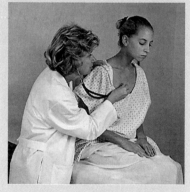

Help the woman to lie supine with head at a 30- to 45-degree angle. Stand at the person's *right* side. Drape the gown up across shoulders and place an extra sheet across lower abdomen.

3. Palpate each breast, lifting the same side arm up over head. Include the tail of Spence and areola.
4. Palpate each nipple for discharge.
5. Support the person's arm and palpate axilla and regional lymph nodes.
6. Teach breast self-examination.

MALE BREASTS

1. Inspect and palpate while palpating the anterior chest wall.
2. Supporting each arm, palpate the axilla and regional nodes.

Sequence   **Selected Photos**

NECK VESSELS

1. Inspect each side of neck for a jugular venous pulse, turning the person's head slightly to the other side.
2. Estimate jugular venous pressure, if indicated.

HEART

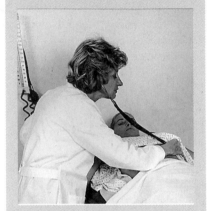

1. Inspect the precordium for any pulsations and/or heave (lift).
2. Palpate the apical impulse and note the location.
3. Palpate precordium for any abnormal thrill.
4. Auscultate apical rate and rhythm.
5. Auscultate with the diaphragm of the stethoscope to study heart sounds, inching from the apex up to the base, or vice versa.
6. Auscultate the heart sounds with the bell of the stethoscope, again inching through all locations.
7. Turn the person over to left side while again auscultating apex with the bell.

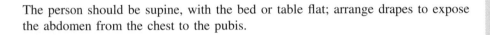

The person should be supine, with the bed or table flat; arrange drapes to expose the abdomen from the chest to the pubis.

ABDOMEN

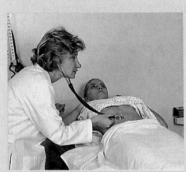

1. Inspect: contour, symmetry, skin characteristics, umbilicus, and pulsations.
2. Auscultate bowel sounds.
3. Auscultate for vascular sounds over the aorta and renal arteries.
4. Percuss all quadrants.
5. Percuss height of the liver span in right midclavicular line.
6. Percuss the location of the spleen.
7. Palpate: light palpation in all quadrants, then deep palpation in all quadrants.
8. Palpate for liver, spleen, kidneys, and aorta.
9. Test the abdominal reflexes, if indicated.

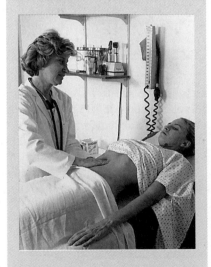

INGUINAL AREA

1. Palpate each groin for the femoral pulse and the inguinal nodes.
   Lift the drape to expose the legs.

Sequence   Selected Photos

LOWER EXTREMITIES

1. Inspect: symmetry, skin characteristics, and hair distribution.
2. Palpate pulses: popliteal, posterior tibial, dorsalis pedis.
3. Palpate for temperature and pretibial edema.
4. Separate toes and inspect.
5. Test ROM and muscle strength of hips, knees, ankles, and feet.

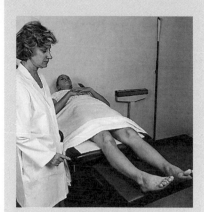

Ask the person to sit up and to dangle the legs off the bed or table. Keep the gown on and the drape over the lap.

MUSCULOSKELETAL

1. Note muscle strength as person sits up.

NEUROLOGIC

1. Test sensation in selected areas on face, arms, hands, legs, and feet: superficial pain, light touch, and vibration.
2. Test position sense of finger, one hand.
3. Test stereognosis.
4. Test cerebellar function of the upper extremities using finger-to-nose test or rapid-alternating-movements test.
5. Test the cerebellar function of the lower extremities by asking the person to run each heel down the opposite shin.
6. Elicit deep tendon reflexes: biceps, triceps, brachioradialis, patellar, and Achilles.
7. Test the Babinski's reflex.

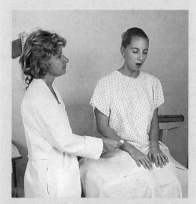

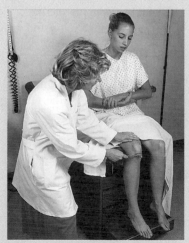

▶ Sequence	Selected Photos

Ask the person to stand with the gown on. Stand close to the person.

LOWER EXTREMITIES

1. Inspect legs for varicose veins.

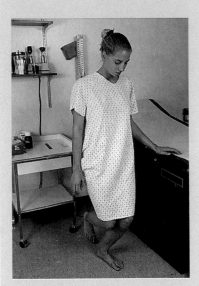

MUSCULOSKELETAL

1. Ask the person to walk across the room in his or her regular walk, turn, then walk back toward you, in heel-to-toe fashion.
2. Ask the person to walk on the toes for a few steps, then to walk on the heels for a few steps.
3. Stand close and check the Romberg's sign.
4. Ask the person to hold the edge of the bed and to perform a shallow knee bend, one for each leg.
5. Stand behind and check the spine as the person touches the toes.
6. Stabilize the pelvis and test the ROM of the spine as the person hyperextends, rotates, and laterally bends.

Sit on a stool in front of a male. The person stands.

MALE GENITALIA

1. Inspect the penis and scrotum.
2. Palpate the scrotal contents. If a mass exists, transilluminate.
3. Check for inguinal hernia.
4. Teach testicular self-examination.

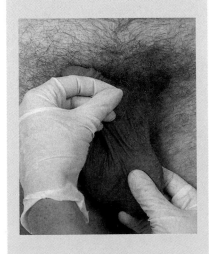

For an adult male, ask him to bend over the examination table, supporting the torso with forearms on the table. Assist the bedfast male to a left lateral position, with the right leg drawn up.

MALE RECTUM

1. Inspect the perianal area.
2. With a gloved lubricated finger, palpate the rectal walls and prostate gland.
3. Save a stool specimen for an occult blood test.

Sequence	Selected Photos

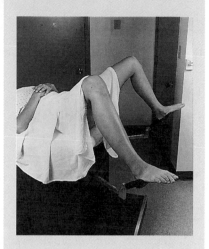

Assist the female back to the examination table, and help her assume the lithotomy position. Drape her appropriately. You sit on a stool at the foot of the table, then stand.

FEMALE GENITALIA

1. Inspect the perineal and perianal areas.
2. Using a vaginal speculum, inspect the cervix and vaginal walls.
3. Procure specimens.
4. Perform a bimanual examination; cervix, uterus, and adnexa.
5. Continue the bimanual examination, checking the rectum and rectovaginal walls.
6. Save a stool specimen for an occult blood test.
7. Provide tissues for the female to wipe the perineal area, and help her up to a sitting position.

Tell the patient you are finished with the examination and that you will leave the room as he or she gets dressed. Return to discuss the examination and further plans and to answer any questions. Thank the person for his or her time.

For the hospitalized person, return the bed and any room equipment to the way you found it. Make sure the call light and telephone are in easy reach.

THE NEONATE AND INFANT

Review Chapter 8, Assessment Techniques and Approach to the Clinical Setting, for the steps on preparation and positioning and on developmental principles of the infant. The 1-minute and 5-minute Apgar results will give important data on the neonate's immediate response to extrauterine life. The following sequence will expand these data. You may reorder this sequence as the infant's sleep and wakefulness state or physical condition warrants.

The infant is supine on a warming table or examination table with an overhead heating element. The infant may be nude except for a diaper over a boy.

Vital Signs

Note pulse, respirations, and temperature.

Measurement

Weight, length, and head circumference are measured and plotted on growth curves for the infant's age.

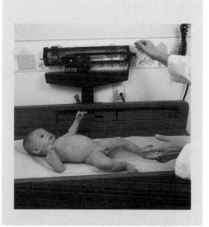

Sequence   **Selected Photos**

General Appearance

1. Body symmetry, spontaneous position, flexion of head and extremities, and spontaneous movement.
2. Skin color and characteristics, any obvious deformities.
3. Symmetry and positioning of the facial features.
4. Alert, responsive affect.
5. Strong, lusty cry.

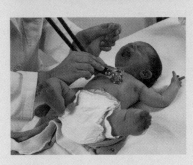

Chest and Heart

1. Inspect the skin condition over the chest and abdomen, chest configuration, and nipples and breast tissue.
2. Note movement of the abdomen with respirations, and any chest retraction.
3. Palpate: apical impulse and note its location; chest wall for thrills; tactile fremitus if the infant is crying.
4. Auscultate: breath sounds, heart sounds in all locations, and bowel sounds in the abdomen and in the chest.

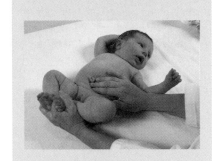

Abdomen

1. Inspect the shape of the abdomen and skin condition.
2. Inspect the umbilicus; count vessels; note condition of cord or stump; any hernia.
3. Palpate skin turgor.
4. Palpate lightly for muscle tone, liver, spleen tip, and bladder.
5. Palpate deeply for kidneys, any mass.
6. Palpate femoral pulses, inguinal lymph nodes.
7. Percuss all quadrants.

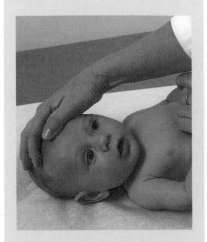

Head and Face

1. Note molding following delivery; any swelling on cranium, bulging of fontanel with crying or at rest.
2. Palpate fontanels, suture lines, and any swellings.
3. Inspect positioning and symmetry of facial features at rest and while the infant is crying.

Sequence	Selected Photos

To open the neonate's eyes, support the head and shoulders and gently lower the baby backward, or ask the parent to hold the baby over his or her shoulder while you stand behind the parent.

Eyes

1. Inspect the lids (edematous in the neonate), palpebral slant, conjunctivae, any nystagmus, and any discharge.
2. Using a penlight: elicit the pupillary reflex, blink reflex, and corneal light reflex; assess tracking of moving light.
3. Using an ophthalmoscope, elicit the red reflex.

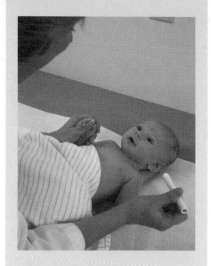

Ears

1. Inspect size, shape, alignment of auricle, patency of auditory canals, any extra skin tags or pits.
2. Note the startle reflex in response to a loud noise.
3. Palpate flexible auricles.

   (Defer otoscopic examination until the end of the complete examination.)

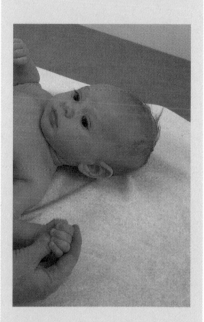

Nose

1. Determine the patency of the nares.
2. Note the nasal discharge, sneezing, and any flaring with respirations.

Mouth and Throat

1. Inspect the lips and gums, high-arched intact palate, buccal mucosa, tongue size, and frenulum of tongue; note absent or minimal salivation in neonate.
2. Note the rooting reflex.
3. Insert a gloved little finger, note the sucking reflex, and palpate palate.

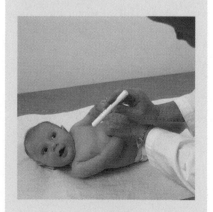

► Sequence	Selected Photos

Neck

1. Lift the shoulders and let the head lag to inspect the neck: Note midline trachea, any skinfolds, and any lumps.
2. Palpate the lymph nodes, the thyroid, and any masses.
3. While the infant is supine, elicit the tonic neck reflex; note a supple neck with movement.

Upper Extremities

1. Inspect and manipulate, noting ROM, muscle tone, and absence of scarf sign (elbow should not reach midline).
2. Count fingers, count palmar creases, and note color of hands and nail beds.
3. Place your thumbs in the infant's palms to note the grasp reflex, then wrap your hands around infant's hands to pull up and note the head lag.

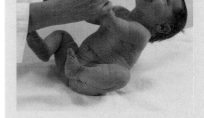

Lower Extremities

1. Inspect and manipulate the legs and feet, noting ROM, muscle tone, and skin condition.
2. Note alignment of feet and toes, look for flat soles, and count toes; note any syndactyly.
3. Test Ortolani's sign for hip stability.

Genitalia

1. Females. Inspect labia and clitoris (edematous in the newborn), vernix caseosa between labia, and patent vagina.
2. Males. Inspect position of urethral meatus (do not retract foreskin), strength of urine stream if possible, and rugae on scrotum.
3. Palpate the testes in the scrotum.

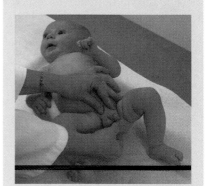

Lift the infant under the axillae, and hold the infant facing you at eye level.

Neuromuscular

1. Note shoulder muscle tone and the infant's ability to stay in your hands without slipping.
2. Rotate the neonate slowly side to side; note the doll's eye reflex.
3. Turn the infant around so his or her back is to you; elicit the stepping reflex and the placing reflex against the edge of the examination table.

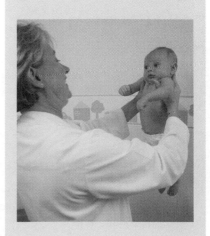

▶ Sequence	Selected Photos

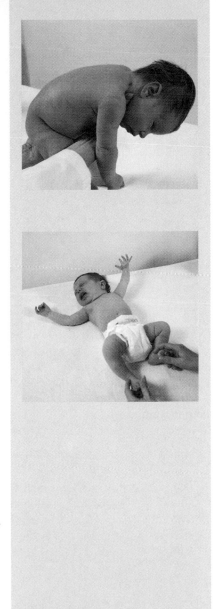

Turn the infant over and hold him or her prone in your hands, or place the infant prone on the examination table.

Spine and Rectum

1. Inspect the length of the spine, trunk incurvation reflex, and symmetry of gluteal folds.
2. Inspect intact skin; note any sinus openings, protrusions, or tufts of hair.
3. Note patent anal opening. Check for passage of meconium stool during the first 24 to 48 hours.

Final Procedures

1. Using an otoscope, inspect the auditory canal and the tympanic membrane.
2. Elicit the Moro reflex by letting the infant's head and trunk drop back a short way, by jarring crib sides, or by making a loud noise.

THE YOUNG CHILD

Review the developmental considerations in preparing for an examination of the toddler and the young child in Chapter 8, Assessment Techniques and Approach to the Clinical Setting. A young child during this time is beset with independence and dependence needs on the parent, is aware of and fearful of a new environment, has a fear of invasive procedures, dislikes being restrained, and may be attached to a security object.

Focus on the parent as the child plays with a toy.

The Health History

1. Collect the history, including developmental data.
   During the history, note data on general appearance.

General Appearance

1. Note child's ability to amuse himself or herself while the parent speaks.
2. Note parent and child interaction.
3. Note gross motor and fine motor skills as the child plays with toys.

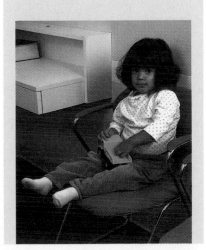

▶ Sequence	Selected Photos

Gradually focus on and involve yourself with the child, at first in a "play" period.

4. Evaluate developmental milestones by using a Denver II test: gait, jumping, hopping, building a tower, and throwing a ball.
5. Evaluate posture while the child is sitting and standing. Evaluate alignment of the legs and feet while the child is walking.
6. Evaluate speech acquisition.
7. Evaluate vision, hearing ability.
8. Evaluate social interaction.

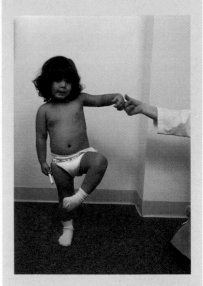

Ask the parent to undress the child to the diaper or the underpants. Position the older infant and young child, 6 months to 2 or 3 years, in the parent's lap. Move your chair to sit knee-to-knee with the parent. A 4- or 5-year old child usually feels comfortable on the examination table.

Measurement

Height, weight, head circumference (may need to defer head circumference until later in the examination).

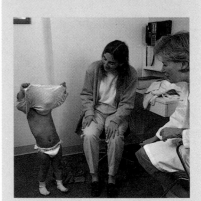

Chest and Heart

1. Auscultate breath sounds and heart sounds in all locations, count respiratory rate, count heart rate, and auscultate bowel sounds.
2. Inspect size, shape, and configuration of chest cage. Assess respiratory movement.
3. Inspect pulsations on the precordium. Note nipple and breast development.
4. Palpate: apical impulse and note location, chest wall for thrills, any tactile fremitus.

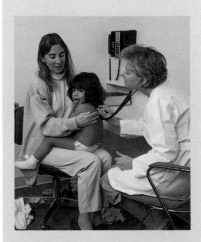

Sequence	Selected Photos

The child should be sitting up in the parent's lap or on examination table, diaper or underpants in place.

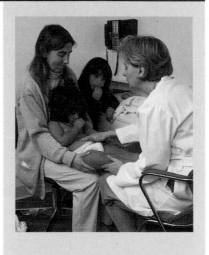

Abdomen

1. Inspect shape of abdomen, skin condition, and periumbilical area.
2. Palpate skin turgor, muscle tone, liver edge, spleen, kidneys, and any masses.
3. Palpate the femoral pulses. Compare strength with radial pulses.
4. Palpate inguinal lymph nodes.

Genitalia

1. Inspect the external genitalia.
2. On males, palpate the scrotum for testes. If masses are present, transilluminate.

Lower Extremities

1. Test Ortolani's sign for hip stability.
2. Note alignment of legs and skin condition.
3. Note alignment of feet. Inspect toes and longitudinal arch.
4. Palpate the dorsalis pedis pulse.
5. Gain cooperation with reflex hammer. Elicit plantar, Achilles, and patellar reflexes.

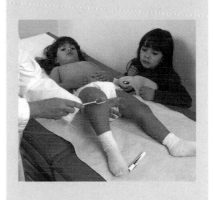

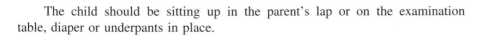

The child should be sitting up in the parent's lap or on the examination table, diaper or underpants in place.

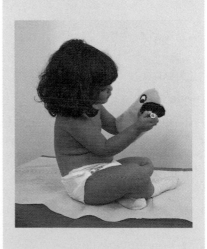

Upper Extremities

1. Inspect arms and hands for alignment, skin condition; inspect fingers and note palmar creases.
2. Palpate and count the radial pulse.
3. Test biceps and triceps reflexes with a reflex hammer.
4. Measure blood pressure.

Sequence   **Selected Photos**

Head and Neck

1. Inspect the size and shape of the head and symmetry of facies.
2. Palpate the fontanels and cranium. Palpate the cervical lymph nodes, trachea, and thyroid gland.
3. Measure the head circumference.

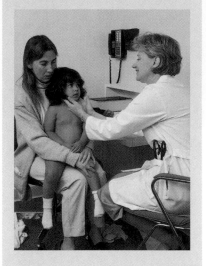

Eyes

1. Inspect the external structures. Note any palpebral slant.
2. Using a penlight, test the corneal light and pupillary light reflexes.
3. Direct a moving penlight for cardinal positions of gaze.
4. If indicated, perform the cover test, covering the eye with your thumb in a young child, or use an index card.
5. Inspect conjunctivae and sclerae.
6. Using an ophthalmoscope, check the red reflex. Inspect the fundus as much as possible.

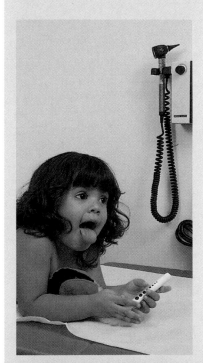

Nose

1. Inspect the external nose and skin condition.
2. Using a penlight, inspect the narcs for foreign body, mucosa, septum, and turbinates.

Mouth and Throat

1. Using a penlight, inspect the mouth, buccal mucosa, teeth and gums, tongue, palate, and uvula in midline. Use a tongue blade as the last resort.

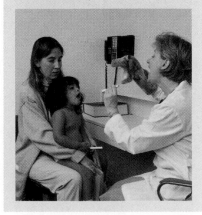

Ears

1. Inspect and palpate the auricle. Note any discharge from the auditory meatus. Check for any foreign body.
2. Using an otoscope, inspect the ear canal and tympanic membrane. Gain cooperation through the use of a puppet, encouraging the child to handle the equipment or to look in the parent's ear as you hold the otoscope. You may need to have the parent help restrain the child.

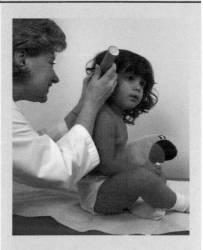

THE SCHOOL-AGE CHILD, THE ADOLESCENT, AND THE AGING ADULT

The sequence of the examination for people in these age groups is the head-to-toe format described in the adult section. However, you should be aware of differences in approach and timing and special developmental considerations. Review Chapter 8, Assessment Techniques and Approach to the Clinical Setting, for a full discussion of these factors.

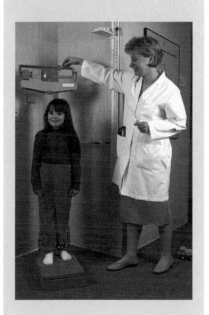

APPLICATION AND CRITICAL THINKING

RECORDING THE DATA

Record the data from the history and physical examination as soon after the event as possible. Memory fades as the day develops, especially when you are responsible for the care of more than one person.

Continued

It is difficult to strike a balance between recording too much data and recording too little. It is important to remember that, from a legal perspective, if it is not documented, it was not done. Data important for the diagnosis and treatment of the person's health should be recorded, as well as data that contribute to your decision-making process. This includes charting relevant normal or negative findings.

On the other hand, a listing of every assessment parameter described in this text yields an unwieldy, unworkable record. One way to keep your record complete yet succinct is to study your writing style. Use short, clear phrases. Avoid redundant introductory phrases such as, "The patient states that . . ." Avoid redundant descriptions such as "no inguinal, femoral, or umbilical hernias." Just write, "no hernias."

Use simple line drawings to describe your findings. You do not need artistic talent; draw a simple sketch of a tympanic membrane, breast, abdomen, or cervix and mark your findings on it. A clear picture is worth many sentences of words.

Study the following complete history and physical examination for a sample write-up. Note that the subject is the same young woman introduced in Chapter 1 of this text.

HEALTH HISTORY

Biographical Data

Name: Ellen K.   *Birth date:* 1/18/
Address: 123 Center St.   *Birthplace:* Springfield
Marital Status: single   *Race:* white

Ellen K. is a 23-year-old, single, white, female cashier at a tavern, currently unemployed for 6 months.

Source. Ellen, seems reliable.

Reason for Seeking Care. "I'm coming in for alcohol treatment."

History of Present Illness. First alcoholic drink, age 16. First intoxication, age 17, drinking one to two times per week, a 6-pack per occasion. Attending high school classes every day, but grades slipping from A − /B + average to C − average. At age 20, drinking two times per week, six to nine beers per occasion. At age 22, drinking two times per week, a 12-pack per occasion, and occasionally a 6-pack the next day to "help with the hangover." During this year, experienced blackouts, failed attempts to cut down on drinking, being physically sick the morning after drinking, and being unable to stop drinking once started. Also, incurred three driving-under-the-influence (DUI) legal offenses. Last DUI 1 month PTA, last alcohol use just before DUI, 18 beers that occasion. Abstinent since that time.

Past Health

Childhood Illnesses. Chicken pox at age 6. No measles, mumps, croup, pertussis. No rheumatic fever, scarlet fever, or polio.

Accidents. 1. Auto accident, age 12, father driving, Ellen thrown from car, right leg crushed. Hospitalized at Memorial, surgery for leg pinning to repair multiple compound fracture. 2. Auto accident, age 21, head hit dashboard, no loss of consciousness, treated and released at Memorial Hospital ED. 3. Auto accident, age 23, "car hit median strip," no injuries, not seen at hospital.

Chronic Illnesses. None.

Hospitalizations. Age 12, Memorial Hospital, surgery to repair right leg as described, Dr. M.J. Carlson, surgeon.

Obstetric History. Gravida 0/Para 0/Abortion 0.

Immunizations. Childhood immunizations up to date. Last tetanus "probably high school." No TB skin test.

Last Examinations. Yearly pelvic examinations at Health Department since age 15, told "normal." High school sports physical as sophomore. Last dental examination as high school junior; last vision test for driver's license age 16, never had ECG, chest x-ray study.

Allergies. No known allergies.

Current Medications. Birth control pills, low-estrogen type, 1/day, for 5 years. No other prescription or over-the-counter medications.

Family History

Ellen is second youngest child, parents divorced 8 years, father has chronic alcoholism. See Family genogram below.

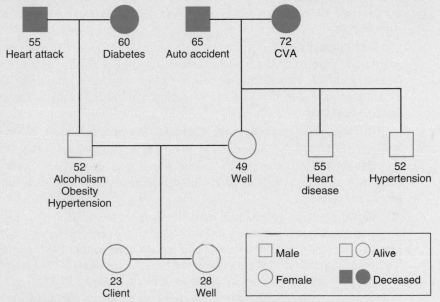

Review of Systems

General Health. Reports usual health "OK." No recent weight change, no fatigue, weakness, fever, sweats.

Skin. No change in skin color, pigmentation, or nevi. No pruritus, rash, lesions. Has bruise now over right eye, struck by boyfriend 1 week PTA. No history skin disease. Hair, no loss, change in texture. Nails, no change. Self-care. Stays in sun "as much as I can." No use of sunscreen. Goes to tanning beds at hair salon twice/week during winter.

Head. No unusually frequent or severe headaches, no head injury, dizziness, syncope, or vertigo.

Eyes. No difficulty with vision or double vision. No eye pain, inflammation, discharge, lesions. No history glaucoma or cataracts. Wears no corrective lenses.

Ears. No hearing loss or difficulty. No earaches, infections now or as child, no discharge, tinnitus, or vertigo. Self-care. No exposure to environmental noise, cleans ears with washcloth.

Nose. No discharge, has two to three colds per year, no sinus pain, nasal obstruction, epistaxis, or allergy.

Mouth and Throat. No mouth pain, bleeding gums, toothache, sores or lesions in mouth, dysphagia, hoarseness, or sore throat. Has tonsils. Self-care. Brushes teeth twice/day, no flossing.

Neck. No pain, limitation of motion, lumps, or swollen glands.

Breast. No pain, lump, nipple discharge, rash, swelling, or trauma. No history breast disease in self, mother, or sister. No surgery. Self-care. Does not do breast self-examination.

Continued

Respiratory. No past history lung disease, no chest pain with breathing, wheezing, shortness of breath. Colds sometimes "go to my chest," treats with over-the-counter cough medicine and aspirin. Occasional early morning cough, nonproductive. Smokes cigarettes 2 PPD × 2 years, prior use 1 PPD × 4 years. Never tried to quit. Works in poorly ventilated tavern, "everybody smokes."

Cardiovascular. No chest pain, palpitation, cyanosis, fatigue, dyspnea with exertion, orthopnea, paroxysmal nocturnal dyspnea, nocturia, edema. No history of heart murmur, hypertension, coronary artery disease, or anemia.

Peripheral Vascular. No pain, numbness or tingling, swelling in legs. No coldness, discoloration, varicose veins, infections, or ulcers. Legs are unequal in length as sequelae of accident age 12. Self-care. Usual work as cashier involves standing for 8-hour shifts, no support hose.

Gastrointestinal. Appetite good with no recent change. No food intolerance, heartburn, indigestion, pain in abdomen, nausea, or vomiting. No history of ulcers, liver or gallbladder disease, jaundice, appendicitis, or colitis. Bowel movement 1/day, soft, brown, no rectal bleeding or pain. Self-care. No use of vitamins, antacids, laxatives. Diet recall—see Functional Assessment.

Urinary. No dysuria, frequency, urgency, nocturia, hesitancy, or straining. No pain in flank, groin, suprapubic region. Urine color yellow, no history kidney disease.

Genitalia. Menarche age 11. Last menstrual period April 18. Cycle usually q 28 days, duration 4 to 5 days, flow moderate, no dysmenorrhea. No vaginal itching or discharge, sores or lesions.

Sexual health. In relationship now that includes intercourse. This boyfriend has been her only sexual partner for 2 years, had one other partner before that. Uses birth control pills to prevent pregnancy, partner uses no condoms. Concerned that boyfriend may be having sex with other women but has not confronted him. Aware of no STD contact. Never been tested for AIDS. Past history of sexual abuse by father from ages 12 to 16 years, abuse did not include intercourse. Ellen is unwilling to discuss further at this time.

Musculoskeletal. No past history arthritis, gout. No joint pain, stiffness, swelling, deformity, limitation of motion. No muscle pain, or weakness. Bone trauma at age 12, has sequela of unequal leg lengths, right leg shorter, walks with limp. Self-care. No walking or running for sport or exercise "because of leg." Able to stand as cashier. Uses lift pad in right shoe to equalize leg length.

Neurologic. No history of seizure disorder, stroke, fainting. Has had blackouts with alcohol use. No weakness, tremor, paralysis, problems with coordination, difficulty speaking or swallowing. No numbness or tingling. Not aware of memory problem, nervousness or mood change, depression. Had counseling for sexual abuse in the past. Denies any suicidal ideation or intent during adolescent years or now.

Hematologic. No bleeding problems in skin, excessive bruising. Not aware of exposure to toxins, never had blood transfusion, never used needles to shoot drugs.

Endocrine. Paternal grandmother with diabetes. No increase in hunger, thirst, or urination; no problems with hot or cold environments; no change in skin, appetite, or nervousness.

Functional Assessment

Self-Concept. Graduated from high school. Trained "on-the-job" as bartender, also worked as cashier in tavern. Unemployed now, on public aid, does not perceive she has enough money for daily living. Lives with older sister. Raised as Presbyterian, believes in God, does not attend church. Believes self to be "honest, dependable." Believes limitations are "smoking, weight, drinking."

Activity-Exercise. Typical day: arises 9:00 AM, light chores or TV, spends day looking for work, running errands, with friends, bedtime at 11:00 PM. No sustained physical exercise. Believes self able to perform all ADLs; limp poses no problem in bathing, dressing, cooking, household tasks, mobility, driving a car, or work as cashier. No mobility aids.

Hobbies are fishing, boating, snowmobiling, although currently has no finances to engage in most of these.

Sleep-Rest. Bedtime 11:00 PM. Sleeps 8 to 9 hours. No sleep aids.

Nutrition. 24-hour recall: breakfast, none; lunch, bologna sandwich, chips, diet soda; dinner, hamburger, french fries, coffee; snacks, peanuts, pretzels, potato chips, "bar food." This menu is typical of most days. Eats lunch at home alone. Most dinners at fast-food restaurants or in tavern. Shares household grocery expenses and cooking chores with sister. No food intolerances.

Alcohol. See present illness. Denies use of street drugs. Cigarettes, smokes 2 PPD $\times$ 2 years, prior use 1 PPD $\times$ 4 years. Never tried to quit. Boyfriend smokes cigarettes.

Interpersonal Relationships. Describes family life growing up as chaotic. Father physically abusive toward mother and sexually abusive toward Ellen. Parents divorced because of father's continual drinking. Few support systems currently. Estranged from mother, "didn't believe me about my father." Father estranged from entire family. Gets along "OK" with sister. Relationship with boyfriend chaotic, has hit her twice in the past. Ellen has never pressed legal charges. No close women friends. Most friends are "drinking buddies" at tavern.

Coping and Stress Management. Believes housing adequate, adequate heat and utilities, and neighborhood safe. Believes home has no safety hazards. Does not use seat belts. No travel outside 60 miles of hometown.

Identifies current stresses to be drinking, legal problems with DUIs, unemployment, financial worries. Considers her drinking to be problematic.

Perception of Health

Identifies alcohol as a health problem for herself, feels motivated for treatment. Never been interested in physical health and own body before, "Now I think it's time I learned." Expects health care providers to "Help me with my drinking. I don't know beyond that." Expects to stay at this agency for 6 weeks, "Then, I don't know what."

PHYSICAL EXAMINATION

Height: 163 cm (5'4")   *Weight:* 68.6 kg (151 lb)
B/P: 142/100 right arm, sitting
140/96 right arm, lying
138/98 left arm, lying
Temp: 37° C Pulse 76, regular   *Respirations:* 16, unlabored

General Survey. Ellen K. is a 23-year-old white female, not currently under the influence of alcohol or other drugs, who articulates clearly, ambulates without difficulty, and is in no distress.

Skin. Uniformly tan-pink in color, warm, dry, intact, turgor good. No lesions, birthmarks, edema. Resolving 2-cm yellow-green hematoma present over right eye, no swelling, ocular structures not involved. Hair, normal distribution and texture, no pest inhabitants. Nails, no clubbing, biting, or discolorations. Nail beds pink and firm with prompt capillary refill.

Head. Normocephalic, no lesions, lumps, scaling, parasites, or tenderness. Face, symmetric, no weakness, no involuntary movements.

Eyes. Acuity by Snellen chart O.D. 20/20, O.S. 20/20 $-$ 1. Visual fields full by confrontation. EOMs intact, no nystagmus. No ptosis, lid lag, discharge, or crusting. Corneal light reflex symmetric, no strabismus. Conjunctivae clear. Sclera white, no lesion or redness. PERRLA. Fundi: discs flat with sharp margins. Vessels present in all quadrants without crossing defects. Background has even color, no hemorrhage or exudates.

Ears. Pinna no mass, lesions, scaling, discharge, or tenderness to palpation. Canals clear. Tympanic membrane pearly gray, landmarks intact, no perforation. Whispered words

Continued

heard bilaterally. Weber test—tone heard midline with lateralization. Rinne test—AC > BC and = bilaterally.

Nose. No deformities or tenderness to palpation. Nares patent. Mucosa pink, no lesions. Septum midline, no perforation. No sinus tenderness.

Mouth. Mucosa and gingivae pink, no lesions or bleeding. Right lower 1st molar missing, multiple dark spots on most teeth, gums receding on lower incisors. Tongue symmetric, protrudes midline, no tremor. Pharynx pink, no exudate. Uvula rises midline on phonation. Tonsils 1 +. Gag reflex present.

Neck. Neck supple with full ROM. Symmetric, no masses, tenderness, lymphadenopathy. Trachea midline. Thyroid nonpalpable, not tender. Jugular veins flat @ 45 degrees. Carotid arteries 2+ and = bilaterally, no bruits.

Spine and Back. Normal spinal profile, no scoliosis. No tenderness over spines, no CVA tenderness.

Thorax and Lungs. AP < transverse diameter. Chest expansion symmetric. Tactile fremitus equal bilaterally. Lung fields resonant. Diaphragmatic excursion 4 cm and = bilaterally. Breath sounds diminished. Expiratory wheeze in posterior chest at both bases, scattered rhonchi in posterior chest at both bases, do not clear with coughing.

Breasts. Symmetric; no retraction, discharge, or lesions. Contour and consistency firm and homogeneous. No masses or tenderness, no lymphadenopathy.

Heart. Precordium, no abnormal pulsations, no heaves. Apical impulse at 5th ics in left MCL, no thrills. S_1–S_2 are not diminished or accentuated, no S_3 or S_4. Systolic murmur, grade ii/vi, loudest at left lower sternal border, no radiation, present supine and sitting.

Abdomen. Flat, symmetric. Skin smooth with no lesions, scars, or striae. Bowel sounds present, no bruits. Tympany predominates in all quadrants. Liver span 7 cm in right MCL. Abdomen soft, no organomegaly, no masses or tenderness, no inguinal lymphadenopathy.

Extremities. Color tan-pink, no redness, cyanosis, lesions other than surgical scar. Scar right lower leg, anterior, 28 cm × 2 cm wide, well healed. No edema, varicosities. No calf tenderness. All peripheral pulses present, 2+ and = bilaterally. Asymmetric leg length, right leg 3 cm shorter than left.

Musculoskeletal. Temporomandibular joint no slipping or crepitation. Neck full ROM, no pain. Vertebral column no tenderness, no deformity or curvature. Full extension, lateral bending, rotation. Arms symmetric, legs measure as above, extremities have full ROM, no pain or crepitation. Muscle strength, able to maintain flexion against resistance and without tenderness.

Neurologic. Mental status. Appearance, behavior, speech appropriate. Alert and oriented to person, place, time. Thought coherent. Remote and recent memories intact. Cranial nerves II through XII intact. Sensory: pin prick, light touch, vibration intact. Stereognosis, able to identify key. Motor: no atrophy, weakness, or tremors. Gait has limp, able to tandem walk with shoes on. Negative Romberg's sign. Cerebellar, finger-to-nose smoothly intact. DTRs (see stick gram).

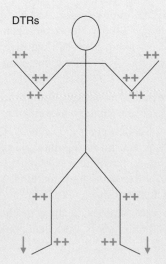

Genitalia. External genitalia has no lesion, discharge. Internal genitalia: vaginal walls pink, no lesion. Cervix pink, nulliparous os, no lesions, small amount nonodorous clear discharge. Specimens for Pap test, GC/chlamydia, trichomoniasis, moniliasis obtained. Swabbing mucosa with acetic acid shows no acetowhitening.

Bimanual, no pain on moving cervix, uterus midline, no enlargement, masses, or tenderness. Adnexa, ovaries not enlarged, no tenderness. Anus, no hemorrhoids, fissures, or lesions. Rectal wall intact, no masses or tenderness. Stool soft, brown; Hematest negative.

ASSESSMENT

Alcohol dependence, severe, with physiologic dependence
Nicotine dependence with physiologic dependence
Elevated blood pressure
Systolic heart murmur
Ineffective airway clearance R/T tracheobronchial secretions and obstruction
Right orbital contusion (resolving)
Risk for trauma
Self-care deficit: oral hygiene R/T lack of motivation
Knowledge deficit about alcoholism disease process, treatment options, support systems R/T lack of exposure
Knowledge deficit about balanced diet R/T lack of exposure and substance abuse
Altered family processes R/T effects of alcoholism and unemployment
Low self-esteem R/T effects of alcoholism, sexual abuse, physical abuse

 ## ASSESSMENT VIDEO CRITICAL THINKING QUESTIONS

The Saunders *Physical Examination and Health Assessment* Video Series—INTEGRATION OF THE HEALTH ASSESSMENT—will direct you to consider the following:

ADULT

1. What information can be gained about the patient's mental status during the health history interview?
2. How would you adapt breast inspection for a woman with pendulous breasts?
3. If you detect a heart murmur during auscultation, what should you do?
4. If the patient were to have abdominal distention, how would you assess his liver span?
5. What alternative techniques might you use to palpate the liver and spleen?
6. If the popliteal pulse is difficult to find, what technique might you use to palpate it?
7. What techniques can you use to elicit a deep tendon reflex, if it does not appear at first?

NEONATE

8. What vital information about a neonate can you obtain from the maternal history?
9. What information can you gain from the gestational age assessment? Why is it important to know the neonate's age at the time of the examination?
10. Why is nasal patency so important to the neonate's health? What other techniques can you use to assess it?
11. What effects can maternal hormone levels have on a neonate's assessment findings?
12. What is an innocent murmur and why is it common in neonates?
13. Which developmental reflexes are commonly present in neonates? Why are they tested?

Continued

CHILD

14. When assessing a child's general appearance, what findings would cause concern?
15. What mistakes may commonly occur when assessing a child's height and weight?
16. What condition should an examiner of a child expect if pain results from pulling on the auricle?
17. What abnormal findings may be found when assessing respirations in a child?
18. Name one common illness in which a child's spleen typically is enlarged?
19. What is the difference between pigeon toes (pes varus) and metatarsus adductus?

AGING ADULT

20. During the health history, how would you assess an older adult patient's risk factors and functional status?
21. What strategies can you use to assess an older adult's understanding of prescribed medications, medication use, and compliance with the prescribed regimen?
22. During an older adult's physical examination, how would you screen for risk factors?
23. How could you adapt the physical examination for an older adult with arthritis?
24. Which assessment findings may indicate a prostate disorder?
25. What physiologic changes occur in the female genitalia as a result of menopause?

CHAPTER TWENTY SEVEN

Critical Thinking in Health Assessment

ASSESSMENT—POINT OF ENTRY IN AN ONGOING PROCESS

Assessment is the collection of data about the individual's health state (Fig. 27–1). Throughout this text, you have been studying the techniques of collecting and analyzing **subjective** data, what the person *says* about himself or herself during history-taking; and **objective** data, what you as the health professional *observe* by inspecting, percussing, palpating, and auscultating during the physical examination. Together with the patient's record and laboratory studies, these elements form the **data base.**

From the data base, you make a clinical judgment or diagnosis about the individual's health state or response to actual or high-risk health problems and life processes. Thus, the purpose of assessment is to make a judgment or diagnosis.

Diagnostic Reasoning—The Key to Clinical Judgment

The step from data collection to diagnosis can be a difficult one. Most beginning examiners perform well in gathering the data, given adequate practice, but then treat

PLANNING
Establish priorities
Develop outcomes
Set time frames for outcomes
Identify interventions
Document plan of care

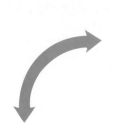

DIAGNOSIS
Interpret data:
    Identify clusters of cues
    Make inferences

Validate inferences

Compare clusters of cues
with definition and
defining characteristics

Identify related factors

Document the diagnosis

ASSESSMENT
Collect data:
    Review of the clinical record
    Interview
    Health history
    Physical examination
    Functional assessment
    Consultation
    Review of the literature

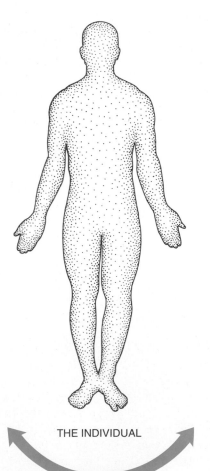

THE INDIVIDUAL

IMPLEMENTATION
Review the planned interventions

Schedule and coordinate the person's
total health care

Collaborate with other team members

Supervise implementation of the
care plan by delegating
appropriate responsibilities

Counsel the person and significant
others

Involve the person in the health care

Refer individuals who require
continuing care

Document the care provided

EVALUATION
Refer to established outcomes

Evaluate the individual's condition and
compare actual outcomes with
expected outcomes

Summarize the results of the
evaluation

Identify reasons for the person's
failure, if indicated, to achieve expected
outcomes stated in the plan of care

Take corrective action to modify the
plan of care as necessary

Document the evaluation of the
person's achievement of outcomes
and the modifications, if any, in the
plan of care

27–1

all the data as being equally important. This makes decision-making slow and labored.

A way of collecting and analyzing information is the model of **diagnostic reasoning** (Elstein, Shulman, and Sparfka, 1978). It has four major components: (1) attending to initially available cues, (2) formulating diagnostic hypotheses, (3) gathering data relative to the tentative hypotheses, and (4) evaluating each hypothesis with the new data collected, thus arriving at a final diagnosis. A cue is a piece of information, a sign or symptom, or a piece of laboratory data. A hypothesis is a tentative explanation for a cue or a set of cues that can be used as a basis for further investigation.

For example, consider Ellen K. who was introduced in Chapter 1 and whose complete health history and physical examination are recorded in Chapter 26. Ellen presents with a number of initial cues, one of which is the resolving hematoma under her eye. (1) You can recognize this cue even before history-taking starts. Is it significant? (2) Ellen says she ran into a door, although she mumbles as she speaks and avoids eye contact. At this point, you formulate a hypothesis of trauma. (3) During the history and physical examination, you gather data to support or reject the tentative hypothesis. (4) You synthesize the new data collected, which support the hypothesis of trauma but eliminate the accidental cause. The final diagnoses are resolving right orbital contusion and risk for trauma.

Diagnostic hypotheses are activated very early in the reasoning process (Hanneman, 1996; Tanner, 1988). This helps diagnosticians adapt to large amounts of information because it clusters cues into meaningful groups and directs subsequent data collection.

Once you complete data collection, develop a preliminary list of significant signs and symptoms and all patient health needs. This is less formal in structure than your final list of diagnoses will be and is in no particular order. Such a list for Ellen is found on page 4 of Chapter 1. In some institutions, it is easier to generate such a list if you use a conceptual model. Examples of conceptual models are described later in this chapter.

Group together the assessment data that appear to be causal or associated. For example, with a person in acute pain, associated data are rapid heart rate and anxiety. Organizing the data into meaningful clusters is slow at first; experienced examiners cluster data more rapidly because they recall proven results of earlier patient situations.

Validate any data you need to. Again, this depends on experience. If you are sure of the blood pressure, validate by repeating it yourself. If you have less experience analyzing breath sounds or heart murmurs, ask an expert to listen. Even with years of clinical experience, some signs always require validation; e.g., a breast lump.

Now study the list of diagnoses (both medical and nursing) derived from Ellen K.'s health history and physical examination in Chapter 26:

- Alcohol dependence, severe, with physiologic dependence
- Nicotine dependence, with physiologic dependence
- Ineffective airway clearance R/T tracheobronchial secretions and obstruction
- Elevated blood pressure
- Systolic heart murmur
- Right orbital contusion (resolving)
- Risk for trauma
- Self-care deficit: oral hygiene R/T lack of motivation
- Knowledge deficit about alcoholism, treatment options, support systems, R/T lack of exposure
- Knowledge deficit about balanced diet R/T lack of exposure and substance abuse
- Altered family processes R/T effects of alcoholism and unemployment
- Low self-esteem R/T effects of alcoholism, sexual abuse, physical abuse
- Inadequate social support
- Inadequate finances

This is a multidisciplinary problem list, with physicians, nurses, and, in Ellen K.'s case, addictions counselors, all working from and contributing to the same problem list. Consider now how diagnoses are ordered and formulated.

In an ambulatory, nonacute care setting, the first problems identified usually are those concerned with the reasons the person has sought care. In Ellen's case, the admission to the agency is for substance abuse, and the initial problems reflect that.

In the hospitalized, acute care setting, the initial problems also are usually related to the reason for admission. However, the acuity of illness often determines the order of priorities of the person's problems (Table 27–1).

For example, **first-level priority problems** are those that are emergent, life threatening, and immediate, e.g., establishing an airway, supporting breathing and ventilation, maintaining circulation, and monitoring severely abnormal vital signs.

Second-level priority problems are those that are next in urgency—those requiring your prompt intervention to forestall further deterioration, e.g., mental status change, acute pain, acute urinary elimination problems, untreated medical problems, abnormal laboratory values, risks of infection, or risk to safety or security. Ellen has abnormal physical signs that fit in the category of untreated medical problems. For example, Ellen's adventitious breath sounds are a cue to further assess respiratory status to determine the final diagnosis. Ellen's mildly elevated blood pressure needs monitoring also.

Third-level priority problems are those that are important to the patient's health but can be addressed in a

Table 27–1 • A Common Approach to Identifying Immediate Priorities

Treatment for first- and second-level priorities is usually initiated in rapid succession or simultaneously. At times, the order of priority might change, depending on the seriousness of the problem and relationship between the problems. For example, if abnormal laboratory values are life-threatening, they become a higher priority; if the patient is having trouble breathing because of acute pain, treating the pain might become the highest priority. It is important to consider the relationship between the problems; for example, if *Problem Y* causes *Problem Z*, *Problem Y* takes priority over *Problem Z*.

1. **First-level priority problems** (immediate priorities; remember the ABCs):
   - Airway problems
   - Breathing problems
   - Cardiac/circulation problems
   - Signs (vital **signs** concerns)
2. **Second-level priority problems** (immediate, after treatment for first-level problems is initiated).
   Note: To help you remember, the mnemonic MAA-U-AR provides the first letter of each of the second-level priority problems):
   - Mental status change
   - Acute pain
   - Acute urinary elimination problems
   - Untreated medical problems requiring immediate attention (e.g., a diabetic who hasn't had insulin)
   - Abnormal laboratory values
   - Risks of infection, safety, or security (for the patient or for others)
3. **Third-level priority problems** (later priorities):
   - Health problems that do not fit into the above categories (e.g., problems with lack of knowledge, activity, rest, family coping)

From Alfaro-LeFevre R: Critical Thinking in Nursing—A Practical Approach, 2nd ed. Philadelphia, W.B. Saunders Company, 1999.

more deliberate manner. In Ellen's case, the diagnoses of knowledge deficit, altered family processes, and low self-esteem fit in this category. Interventions to treat these problems are more long term, and the response to treatment is expected to take more time.

Collaborative problems are those in which the approach to their treatment involves multiple disciplines. With collaborative problems, nurses have the primary responsibility to diagnose the onset and monitor the changes in status (Carpenito, 1997). For example, the diagnosis of *Alcohol dependence, severe, with physiologic dependence* represents a collaborative problem. With this problem, the nurse must be aware of the profound implications that the sudden withdrawal of alcohol has on the central nervous and cardiovascular systems. The nurse must manage Ellen's response to the rebound effects of these systems during detoxification.

Another example of a collaborative problem from Ellen's list is the ineffective airway clearance involving the respiratory system. If the adventitious breath sounds and further laboratory tests lead to a diagnosis of acute bronchitis, antibiotic treatment is indicated. The nurse continues to assess the respiratory and other body systems to determine Ellen's response to treatment. In this case, the nursing diagnoses are judgments about human responses to acute bronchitis. Other potential complications of acute bronchitis for which the nurse must be aware are adverse reactions to medication treatment.

Finally, many nursing diagnoses represent situations in which only nursing will prescribe the definitive treatment to achieve the desired outcome (Carpenito, 1997), for example, *Knowledge deficit,* or *Self-care deficit.* Both nursing diagnoses and collaborative problems involve the steps of the nursing process. Dynamic and flexible, the steps of the nursing process overlap.

From Beginner to Expert in Clinical Judgment

The nursing process alone does not explain the dynamic and interactive processes that actually occur in arriving at a diagnosis and planning treatment (Tanner, 1988). Although the nursing process is a logical problem-solving approach to clinical judgments, it seems that expert nurses vault over the steps and arrive at a judgment in one leap (Benner, Tanner, and Chesla, 1997; Hanneman, 1996). This is true particularly with expert nurses in critical care situations in which patient status changes rapidly and accurate decisions are paramount. The stakes are high, and nursing autonomy is strong. In these cases, the expert focuses on patient responses and prevents complications with vigilant monitoring (Hanneman, 1996). The expert has well-developed physical assessment skills and trusts these physical assessment skills, even if this conflicts with technologically driven data. For example, consider this expert's actions in assessing a woman with a drug overdose who had an endotracheal tube and was receiving mechanical ventilation:

The expert nurse examined the woman's posterior chest during medical rounds. She said to the medical team, "Mrs. Potter has bronchial breath sounds and dullness to percussion here and here (pointing to an area the size of a nickel and to another area the size of a quarter over the right lower lobe). Do you think she aspirated?" The physicians said, "No, her chest x-ray is normal." Three physicians took turns auscultating and percussing Mrs. Potter's chest. None of them could hear the changes, even when the expert drew circles around the areas. The medical conclusion was that Mrs. Potter had not aspirated. Undaunted, the expert nurse initiated a regimen of pulmonary interventions. On rounds the next day, the medical team ordered antibiotics and frequent pulmonary treatments based on the early morning chest x-ray findings of right lower lobe consolidation (Hanneman, 1996, p. 332).

Table 27–2 • Novice Thinking Compared With Expert Thinking

The depth and breadth of expert knowledge, largely gained from opportunities to apply theory *in real situations,* greatly enhance critical thinking ability.

Novice Nurses	Expert Nurses
Knowledge is organized as separate facts; must rely heavily on resources (texts, notes, preceptors); lack knowledge gained from actually *doing* (e.g., listening to breath sounds)	Knowledge is highly organized and structured, making recall of information easier; have a large storehouse of experiential knowledge (e.g., what abnormal breath sounds sound like, what subtle changes look like)
Focus so much on *actions,* they tend to forget to *assess* before acting	*Assess* and think things through before *acting*
Need clear cut rules	Know when to bend the rules
Are often hampered by unawareness of resources	Are aware of resources and how to use them
Are often hindered by anxiety and lack of self-confidence	Are usually more self-confident, less anxious, and therefore more focused
Must be able to rely on step-by-step procedures; tend to focus more on *procedures* than the patient *response* to the procedure	Know when it is safe to skip steps or to do two steps together; are able to focus on both the parts (the procedures) and the whole (the patient response)
Become uncomfortable if patient needs preclude performing procedures exactly as they were learned	Comfortable with rethinking procedure if patient needs require modification of the procedure
Have limited knowledge of suspected problems; therefore, they question and collect data more superficially	Have a better idea of suspected problems, allowing them to question more deeply and to collect more relevant and in-depth data
Tend to follow standards and policies by rote	Analyze standards and policies, looking for ways to improve them
Learn more readily when matched with supportive, knowledgeable preceptor or mentor	Are challenged by novices' questions, clarifying their own thinking when teaching novices

From Alfaro-LeFevre F: Critical Thinking in Nursing—A Practical Approach, 2nd ed. Philadelphia, W.B. Saunders Company, 1999.

Functioning at the level of expert in clinical judgment includes using intuition, i.e., knowledge received as a whole. Intuition is characterized by immediate instantaneous recognition of patterns—Expert practitioners learn to attend to a pattern of assessment data and act without consciously labeling it (Tanner, 1988). Whereas the beginner operates more from a set of defined, structured rules, the expert practitioner uses intuitive links, has the ability to see salient issues in a patient situation, and knows instant therapeutic responses (Benner et al., 1997).

For example, compare the actions of the nonexpert and the expert nurse in this situation of a young man with *Pneumocystis carinii* pneumonia:

> He was banging the side rails, making gurgling sounds, and pointing to his endotracheal tube. He was diaphoretic, gasping, and frantic. The nurse put her hand on his arm and tried to ascertain whether he had a sore throat from the tube. While she was away from the bedside retrieving an analgesic, the expert nurse strolled by, hesitated, listened, went to the man's bedside, reinflated the endotracheal cuff, and accepted the patient's look of gratitude because he was able to breathe again. The nonexpert nurse was distressed that she had misread the situation. The expert reviewed the signs of a leaky cuff with the nonexpert and pointed out that banging the side rails and panic help differentiate acute respiratory distress from pain (Hanneman, 1996, p. 333).

Critical Thinking

Another way of comparing the novice with the expert is by comparing the different levels at which each uses **critical thinking.** The novice thinker needs the familiarity of clear-cut rules to guide actions. The experienced thinker has learned to assess and modify, if indicated, before acting (Alfaro-LeFevre, 1999). Compare the characteristics of these levels of thinking in Table 27–2.

Critical thinking is a process synonymous with the diagnostic reasoning process described earlier. Critical thinking in nursing has these characteristics:

- Entails purposeful, goal-directed thinking
- Aims to make judgments based on evidence (fact) rather than conjecture (guesswork)
- Is based on principles of science and scientific method
- Requires strategies that maximize *human potential* and compensate for problems caused by *human nature* (Alfaro-LeFevre, 1999)

Applying the characteristics of critical thinking to the logical step-by-step format of the nursing process results in a dynamic nursing process (Fig. 27–2).

USING A CONCEPTUAL FRAMEWORK TO GUIDE NURSING PRACTICE

The assessment data listed on p. 5 of Chapter 1 are the standard set by the American Nurses' Association. But the *organization* of assessment data—the data base—varies depending on the conceptual model that is used. A model provides the framework in determining what to observe, how to organize the observations or data, and how to interpret and use the information. Many different conceptual models exist, but they all deal with

Linear nursing process followed
rotely without critical thinking

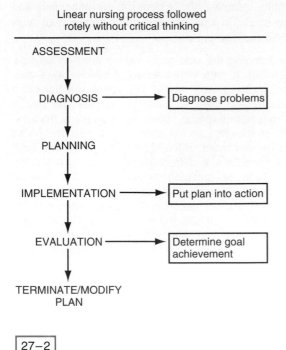

Dynamic nursing process as
used by a critical thinker

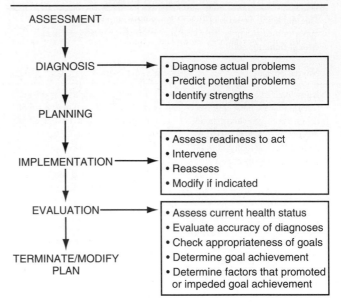

27-2

the same concepts: human beings, environment and society, health and illness, and nursing.

Although all nursing models describe the same four concepts, each one has a different focus or emphasis. For example, the focus of Orem's model (1995) is self-care. The focus of Roy's model (1984) is adaptation. The focus of Leininger's model (1993) is cultural diversity. The focus of Gordon's structural framework (1994) involves functional health patterns.

If you were using Orem's model to collect data, you would focus on the abilities and limitations of the individual for self-care. In using Roy's model, you would focus on data about stimuli in the environment and the individual's adaptation to those stimuli. In using Leininger's model, you would focus on factors that influence care and health patterns for individuals, families, and cultural groups. Although each route is different, all three nursing models should lead to similar nursing diagnoses.

This does not mean nurses must ignore the medical model. A nursing model is used with, not in place of, a medical model. Nurses use the medical model when they work interdependently with the physician in the diagnosis and treatment of disease. A concurrent nursing model is needed to focus assessment on core nursing concerns, such as nutrition, activity, hygiene, skin problems, coping problems, or self-care limitations (Feild and Winslow, 1985).

No *one particular* model is the hallmark of the entire profession. Multiple models exist, some of which are more appropriate in various settings or with certain types of patients. Nursing models currently are being tested in clinical practice and refined. Although subject to refinement, a model is still useful as a framework for assessment and is useful because it leads to the formulation of nursing diagnoses.

As long as no consensus exists on one nursing model, how can we reconcile the various assessment tools called for in each case? Nurses from many institutions must be able to communicate with each other. They must speak a common language so that the health care consumer is assured of consistently efficient care. While the various models are being studied and utilized, nurses can practice with consistency around two points:

1. The list of assessment data (see p. 5 in Chapter 1) deemed standard by the American Nurses' Association. This list provides a consistent data base that is adaptable to any nursing model and allows for nursing diagnoses. Whatever format nurses do use should be holistic, systematic and orderly, and practical.
2. The use of nursing diagnoses (see Table 1–1, p. 6). These diagnoses give nurses a common language with which to communicate nursing findings.

Bibliography

Alfaro-LeFevre R: Critical Thinking in Nursing—A Practical Approach, 2nd ed. Philadelphia, W.B. Saunders Company, 1999.

Bandman EL, Bandman B: Critical Thinking in Nursing. East Norwalk, CT, Appleton & Lange, 1995.

Benner P, Tanner CA, Chesla CA: Becoming an expert nurse. Am J Nurs 97(6):16BBB–16DDD, June 1997.

Benner P, Tanner C, Chesla C: From beginner to expert: Gaining a differentiated clinical world in critical care nursing. Adv Nurs Sci 14(3):13–28, Mar 1992.

Carpenito LJ: Nursing Diagnosis: Application to Clinical Practice, 7th ed. Philadelphia, J.B. Lippincott Company, 1997.

Cohen MZ, Hausner J, Johnson M: Knowledge and presence: Accountability as described by nurses and surgical patients. J Prof Nurs 10: 177–185, 1994.

Elstein A, Shulman L, Sparfka S: Medical Problem-Solving: An Analysis of Clinical Reasoning. Cambridge, MA, Harvard University Press, 1978.

Feild L, Winslow E: Moving to a nursing model. Am J Nurs 85:1100–1101, 1985.

Gordon M: Nursing Diagnosis—Process and Application. St. Louis, Mosby-Year Book, 1994.

Hanneman SK: Advancing nursing practice with a unit-based clinical expert. Image 28(4):331–337, winter 1996.

Leininger M: Transcultural Nursing: Concepts, Theories, and Practice, 2nd ed. Philadelphia, FA Davis, 1993.

Orem DE: Nursing: Concepts of Practice, 5th ed. St. Louis, C.V. Mosby, 1995.

Roy C: Introduction to Nursing: An Adaptation Model, 2nd ed. Englewood Cliffs, NJ, Prentice Hall, 1984.

Tanner CA, Benner P, Chesla C, Gordon DR: The phenomenology of knowing the patient. Image 25(4):273–280, 1993.

Tanner C: Curriculum revolution: The practice mandate. Nurs Health Care 9:427–430, 1988.

Wallace CL, Appleton C: Nursing as the promotion of well-being: The client's experience. J Adv Nurs 22:285–289, 1995.

Age ▶ Vaccine ▼	Birth	1 mo	2 mos	4 mos	6 mos	12 mos	15 mos	18 mos	4–6 yrs	11–12 yrs	14–16 yrs
Hepatitis B[†]	Hep B	Hep B			Hep B					Hep B	
Diphtheria, tetanus, pertussis[‡]			DTaP	DTaP	DTaP		DTaP[‡]		DTaP	Td	
Haemophilus influenzae type b[§]			Hib	Hib	Hib	Hib					
Polio[∥]			IPV	IPV		Polio[∥]			Polio		
Rotavirus[¶]			Rv[¶]	Rv[¶]	Rv[¶]						
Measles, mumps, rubella[#]						MMR			MMR[#]	MMR[#]	
Varicella[**]						Var				Var[¶]	

Approved by the Advisory Committee on Immunization Practices (ACIP), the American Academy of Pediatrics (AAP), and the American Academy of Family Physicians (AAFP).

Vaccines are listed under routinely recommended ages. Bars indicate range of recommended ages for immunization. Any dose not given at the recommended age should be given as a "catch-up" immunization at any subsequent visit when indicated and feasible. Ovals indicate vaccines to be given if previously recommended doses were missed or given earlier than the recommended minimum age.

*This schedule indicates the recommended ages for routine administration of currently licensed childhood vaccines. Combination vaccines may be used whenever any components of the combination are indicated and its other components are not contraindicated. Providers should consult the manufacturers' package inserts for detailed recommendations.

[†]*Infants born to hepatitis B surface antigen–negative mothers* should receive the second dose of hepatitis B (Hep B) vaccine at least 1 month after the first dose. The third dose should be administered at least 4 months after the first dose and at least 2 months after the second dose, but not before 6 months of age for infants.

Infants born to hepatitis B surface antigen–positive mothers should receive hepatitis B vaccine and 0.5 mL hepatitis B immunoglobulin (HBIG) within 12 hours of birth at separate sites. The second dose is recommended at 1–2 months of age and the third dose at 6 months of age.

Infants born to mothers whose hepatitis B surface antigen status is unknown should receive hepatitis B vaccine within 12 hours of birth. Maternal blood should be drawn at the time of delivery to determine the mother's HBsAg status; if the HBsAg test is positive, the infant should receive HBIG as soon as possible (no later than 1 week of age).

All children and adolescents (through 18 years of age) who have not been immunized against hepatitis B may begin the series during any visit. Special efforts should be made to immunize children who were born in or whose parents were born in areas of the world with moderate or high endemicity of hepatitis B virus infection.

[‡]DTaP (diphtheria and tetanus toxoids and acellular pertussis vaccine) is the preferred vaccine for all doses in the immunization series, including completion of the series in children who have received one or more doses of whole-cell DTP vaccine. Whole-cell DTP is an acceptable alternative to DTaP. The fourth dose (DTP or DTaP) may be administered as early as 12 months of age, provided 6 months have elapsed since the third dose and if the child is unlikely to return at age 15–18 months. Td (tetanus and diphtheria toxoids) is recommended at 11–12 years of age if at least 5 years have elapsed since the last dose of DTP, DTaP, or DT. Subsequent routine Td boosters are recommended every 10 years.

[§]Three *Haemophilus influenzae* type b (Hib) conjugate vaccines are licensed for infant use. If PRP-OMP (PedvaxHIB® or ComVax®[Merck]) is administered at 2 and 4 months of age, a dose at 6 months is not required. Because clinical studies in infants have demonstrated that using some combination products may induce a lower immune response to the Hib vaccine component, DTaP/Hib combination products should not be used for primary immunization in infants at 2, 4, or 6 months of age, unless FDA approved for these ages.

[∥]Two poliovirus vaccines currently are licensed in the United States: inactivated poliovirus (IPV) vaccine and oral poliovirus (OPV) vaccine. The ACIP, AAP, and AAFP now recommend that the first two doses of poliovirus vaccine should be IPV. The ACIP continues to recommend a sequential schedule of two doses of IPV administered at ages 2 and 4 months, followed by two doses of OPV at 12–18 months and 4–6 years. Use of IPV for all doses also is acceptable and is recommended for immunocompromised persons and their household contacts. OPV is no longer recommended for the first two doses of the schedule and is acceptable only for special circumstances, such as children of parents who do not accept the recommended number of injections, late initiation of immunization, which would require an unacceptable number of injections, and imminent travel to polio-endemic areas. OPV remains the vaccine of choice for mass immunization campaigns to control outbreaks due to wild poliovirus.

[¶]Rotavirus (Rv) vaccine is shaded and italicized to indicate (1) health care providers may require time and resources to incorporate this new vaccine into practice, and (2) the AAFP feels that the decision to use rotavirus vaccine should be made by the parent or guardian in consultation with their physician or other health care provider. The first dose of Rv vaccine should not be administered before 6 weeks of age, and the minimum interval between doses is 3 weeks. The Rv vaccine series should not be initiated at 7 months of age or older, and all doses should be completed by the first birthday.

[#]The second dose of measles, mumps, and rubella (MMR) vaccine is recommended routinely at 4–6 years of age but may be administered during any visit, provided at least 4 weeks have elapsed since receipt of the first dose and that both doses are administered beginning at or after 12 months of age. Those who have not previously received the second dose should complete the schedule by the 11–12 year old visit.

[**]Varicella (Var) vaccine is recommended at any visit on or after the first birthday for susceptible children, i.e., those who lack a reliable history of chickenpox (as judged by a health care provider) and who have not been immunized. Susceptible persons 13 years of age or older should receive two doses given at least 4 weeks apart.

APPENDIX A-2: Recommended Immunization Schedules for Children Not Immunized in the First Year of Life*

Recommended Time/Age	Immunization(s)[†] [‡]	Comments
	Younger Than 7 Years	
First visit	DTaP (or DTP), Hib, HBV, MMR, OPV[§]	If indicated, tuberculin testing may be done at same visit. If child is 5 yr of age or older, Hib is not indicated in most circumstances.
Interval after first visit		
1 mo (4 wk)	DTaP (or DTP), HBV, Var [‖]	The second dose of OPV may be given if accelerated poliomyelitis vaccination is necessary, such as for travelers to areas where polio is endemic.
2 mo	DTaP (or DTP), Hib, OPV[§]	Second dose of Hib is indicated only if the first dose was received when younger than 15 mo.
≥8 mo	DTaP (or DTP), HBV, OPV[§]	OPV and HBV are not given if the third doses were given earlier.
Age 4–6 yr (at or before school entry)	DTaP (or DTP), OPV,[§] MMR*[¶]	DTaP (or DTP) is not necessary if the fourth dose was given after the fourth birthday; OPV is not necessary if the third dose was given after the fourth birthday.
Age 11–12 yr		
	7–12 Years	
First visit	HBV, MMR, Td, OPV[§]	
Interval after first visit		
2 mo (8 wk)	HBV, MMR,[¶] Var, [‖] Td, OPV[§]	OPV also may be given 1 mo after the first visit if accelerated poliomyelitis vaccination is necessary.
8–14 mo	HBV,[#] Td, OPV[§]	OPV is not given if the third dose was given earlier.
Age 11–12 yr		

*Table is not completely consistent with all package inserts. For products used, also consult manufacturer's package insert for instructions on storage, handling, dosage, and administration. Biologics prepared by different manufacturers may vary, and package inserts of the same manufacturer may change from time to time. Therefore, the physician should be aware of the contents of the current package insert.

Vaccine abbreviations: HBV indicates hepatitis B virus vaccine; Var, varicella vaccine; DTP diphtheria and tetanus toxoids and pertussis vaccine; DTP, diphtheria and tetanus toxoids and acellular pertussis vaccine; Hib, *Haemophilus influenzae* type b conjugate vaccine; OPV, oral poliovirus vaccine; IPV, inactivated poliovirus vaccine; MMR, live measles-mumps-rubella vaccine; Td, adult tetanus toxoid (full dose) and diphtheria toxoid (reduced dose), for children ≥7 years and adults.

[†]If all needed vaccines cannot be administered simultaneously, priority should be given to protecting the child against those diseases that pose the greatest immediate risk. In the United States, these diseases for children younger than 2 years usually are measles and *Haemophilus influenzae* type b infection; for children older than 7 years, they are measles, mumps, and rubella. Before 13 years of age, immunity against hepatitis B and varicella should be ensured.

[‡]DTaP, HBV, Hib, MMR, and Var can be given simultaneously at separate sites if failure of the patient to return for future immunizations is a concern.

[§]IPV is also acceptable. However, for infants and children starting vaccination late (ie, after 6 months of age), OPV is preferred in order to complete an accelerated schedule with a minimum number of injections.

[‖] Varicella vaccine can be administered to susceptible children any time after 12 months of age. Unvaccinated children who lack a reliable history of chicken pox should be vaccinated before their 13th birthday.

[¶]Minimal interval between doses of MMR is 1 month (4 weeks).

[#]HBV may be given earlier in a 0-, 2-, and 4-month schedule.

Modified with permission of the American Academy of Pediatrics. *In* Peter G (Ed): 1997 Red Book: Report of the Committee on Infectious Diseases, 24th ed. Elk Grove Village, IL; American Academy of Pediatrics, 1997, p 20.

APPENDIX B: Recommended Dietary Allowances

Table B-1 • Median Heights and Weights and Recommended Vitamins and Minerals*

		Weight[†]		Height[†]		Protein	Fat-Soluble Vitamins			
Category	Age (yr) or Condition	(kg)	(lb)	(cm)	(in)	(g)	Vitamin A (µg RE)[‡]	Vitamin D (µg)[§]	Vitamin E (mg α-TE) [‖]	Vitamin K (µg)
Infants	0.0–0.5	6	13	60	24	13	375	7.5	3	5
	0.5–1.0	9	20	71	28	14	375	10	4	10
Children	1–3	13	29	90	35	16	400	10	6	15
	4–6	20	44	112	44	24	500	10	7	20
	7–10	28	62	132	52	28	700	10	7	30
Men	11–14	45	99	157	62	45	1000	10	10	45
	15–18	66	145	176	69	59	1000	10	10	65
	19–24	72	160	177	70	58	1000	10	10	70
	25–50	79	174	176	70	63	1000	5	10	80
	51 +	77	170	173	68	63	1000	5	10	80
Women	11–14	46	101	157	62	46	800	10	8	45
	15–18	55	120	163	64	44	800	10	8	55
	19–24	58	128	164	65	46	800	10	8	60
	25–50	63	138	163	64	50	800	5	8	65
	51 +	65	143	160	63	50	800	5	8	65

Table B-1 • Median Heights and Weights and Recommended Vitamins and Minerals* Continued

Pregnant			60	800	10	10	65
Lactating	First 6 mo		65	1300	10	12	65
	Second 6 mo		62	1200	10	11	65

Water-Soluble Vitamins							Minerals						
Vitamin C (mg)	Thiamin (mg)	Riboflavin (mg)	Niacin (mg NE¶)	Vitamin B₆ (mg)	Folate (µg)	Vitamin B₁₂ (µg)	Calcium (mg)	Phosphorus (mg)	Magnesium (mg)	Iron (mg)	Zinc (mg)	Iodine (µg)	Selenium (µg)
30	0.3	0.4	5	0.3	25	0.3	400	300	40	6	5	40	10
35	0.4	0.5	6	0.6	35	0.5	600	500	60	10	5	50	15
40	0.7	0.8	9	1.0	50	0.7	800	800	80	10	10	70	20
45	0.9	1.1	12	1.1	75	1.0	800	800	120	10	10	90	20
45	1.0	1.2	13	1.4	100	1.4	800	800	170	10	10	120	30
50	1.3	1.5	17	1.7	150	2.0	1200	1200	270	12	15	150	40
60	1.5	1.8	20	2.0	200	2.0	1200	1200	400	12	15	150	50
60	1.5	1.7	19	2.0	200	2.0	1200	1200	350	10	15	150	70
60	1.5	1.7	19	2.0	200	2.0	800	800	350	10	15	150	70
60	1.2	1.4	15	2.0	200	2.0	800	800	350	10	15	150	70
50	1.1	1.3	15	1.4	150	2.0	1200	1200	280	15	12	150	45
60	1.1	1.3	15	1.5	180	2.0	1200	1200	300	15	12	150	50
60	1.1	1.3	15	1.6	180	2.0	1200	1200	280	15	12	150	55
60	1.1	1.3	15	1.6	180	2.0	800	800	280	15	12	150	55
60	1.0	1.2	13	1.6	180	2.0	800	800	280	10	12	150	55
70	1.5	1.6	17	2.2	400	2.2	1200	1200	320	30	15	175	65
95	1.6	1.8	20	2.1	280	2.6	1200	1200	355	15	19	200	75
90	1.6	1.7	20	2.1	260	2.6	1200	1200	340	15	16	200	75

*The allowances, expressed as average daily intakes over time, are intended to provide for individual variations among most normal persons as they live in the United States under usual environmental stresses. Diets should be based on a variety of common foods to provide other nutrients for which human requirements have been less well defined. See text for detailed discussion of allowances and of nutrients not tabulated.

†Weights and heights of reference adults are actual medians for the U.S. population of the designated age, as reported by NHANES II. The median weights and heights of those under 19 years of age were taken from Hamill PV, Drizd TA, Johnson CL, et al: Physical Growth: Nutritional Center for Health Statistics Percentiles. Am J Clin Nutr 32:607–629, 1979. The use of these figures does not imply that the height-to-weight ratios are ideal.

‡Retinol equivalents: 1 retinol equivalent = 1 µg retinol or 6 µg β-carotene. See text for calculation of vitamin A activity of diets as retinol equivalents.

§As cholecalciferol. 10 µg cholecalciferol = 400 IU of vitamin D.

‖ α-Tocopherol equivalents. 1 mg d-α tocopherol = 1 α-TE. See text for variation in allowances and calculation of vitamin E activity of the diet as α-tocopherol equivalents.

¶1 NE (niacin equivalent) is equal to 1 mg of niacin or 60 mg of dietary tryptophan.

From Recommended Dietary Allowances, Revised. Washington, D.C., Food and Nutrition Board. National Academy of Sciences, National Research Council, 1989.

Table B-2 • Median Heights and Weights and Recommended Energy Intake

Category	Age (yr) or Condition	Weight (kg)	Weight (lb)	Height (cm)	Height (in)	REE* (kcal/day)	Average Energy Allowance (kcal)† Multiples of REE	Per kg	Per day‡
Infants	0.0–0.5	6	13	60	24	320		180	650
	0.5–1.0	9	20	71	28	500		98	850
Children	1–3	13	29	90	35	740		102	1300
	4–6	20	44	112	44	950		90	1800
	7–10	28	62	132	52	1130		70	2000
Men	11–14	45	99	157	62	1440	1.70	55	2500
	15–18	66	145	176	69	1760	1.67	45	3000
	19–24	72	160	177	70	1780	1.67	40	2900
	25–50	79	174	176	70	1800	1.60	37	2900
	51 +	77	170	173	68	1530	1.50	30	2300
Women	11–14	46	101	157	62	1310	1.67	47	2200
	15–18	55	120	163	64	1370	1.60	40	2200
	19–24	58	128	164	65	1350	1.60	38	2200
	25–50	63	138	163	64	1380	1.55	36	2200
	51 +	65	143	160	63	1280	1.50	30	1900
Pregnant	First trimester								+ 0
	Second trimester								+ 300
	Third trimester								+ 300
Lactating	First 6 mo								+ 500
	Second 6 mo								+ 500

*Calculation based on FAO equations, then rounded.

†In the range of light to moderate activity, the coefficient of variation is ±20%.

‡Figure is rounded.

Reprinted, with permission, from Recommended Dietary Allowances, 10th ed. Copyright 1989 by the National Academy of Sciences. Courtesy of the National Academy Press, Washington, DC.

Table C-1 • Recommended Weight Gain for Pregnant Women Based on Body Mass Index

Weight Category Based on BMI*	Total Weight Gain†		1st Trimester Gain		2nd and 3rd Trimester Weekly Gain	
	(lb)	*(kg)*	*(lb)*	*(kg)*	*(lb)*	*(kg)*
Underweight (BMI < 19.8)	28–40	12.5–18	5	2.3	1.07	0.49
Normal weight (BMI = 19.8–26)	25–35	11.5–16	3.5	1.6	0.97	0.44
Overweight (BMI > 26–29)	15–25	7–11.5	2	0.9	0.67	0.3
Obese (BMI > 29)	≥15	6				

*Body mass index (BMI).

†Young adolescents and black women should strive for gains at the upper end of the recommended range. Short women (<62 in or <157 cm) should strive for gains at the lower end of the range.

Data from Subcommittee on Nutritional Status and Weight Gain During Pregnancy and Subcommittee on Dietary Intake and Nutrient Supplements During Pregnancy, Food and Nutrition Board, National Academy of Sciences: Nutrition During Pregnancy, Parts I and II. Washington, DC, National Academy Press, 1990.

From Mahan LK, Escott-Stump S: Krause's Food, Nutrition & Diet Therapy, 9th ed. Philadelphia, W.B. Saunders Company, 1996, p. 183.

The Weighting Game Weight Graph

Your Beginning Weight _____ lbs.

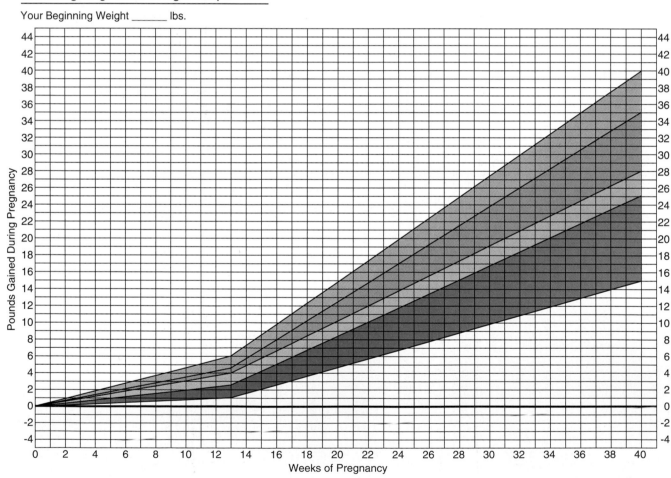

Key: The colored areas represent weight gain ranges that can be expected during a normal pregnancy. Ask your health care provider in which category you belong. This is not the time to lose weight. Try to gain weight at a steady pace. Report any sudden and/or unexplained weight changes to your health care provider.

If your weight was normal before you became pregnant, try to keep your weight in the yellow/orange range.

If you were underweight before you became pregnant, your weight gain should be in the orange/pink area.

If your weight was much higher than ideal, your weight gain should be in the blue-green range.

APPENDIX D: Selected Percentiles of Triceps Skinfold Thickness and Bone-Free Upper Arm Area by Height in U.S. Men, Age 25 to 54 yr, with Small, Medium, and Large Frames

Height		Triceps (mm)							Bone-Free MAMA (cm²)						
		5	10	15	50	85	90	95	5	10	15	50	85	90	95
Small frame															
in	cm														
62	157				11							52			
63	160			6	10	17					32	48	54		
64	163		5	5	10	16	18			37	38	49	58	63	
65	165	4	5	6	11	17	19	21	31	35	37	47	60	63	71
66	168	5	6	6	11	18	18	20	31	36	38	49	60	62	71
67	170	5	6	6	11	18	20	22	35	39	41	49	58	60	62
68	173	5	6	6	10	15	16	20	33	37	40	49	59	62	69
69	175		6	6	11	17	20			36	40	58	61	63	
70	178			7	10	17					35	48	57		
71	180			7	10	16					39	47	52		
72	183				10							45			
73	185														
74	188														
Medium frame															
in	cm														
62	157				15							58			
63	160				11							55			
64	163		6	6	12	18	20			43	47	56	67	71	
65	165	5	7	8	12	20	22	25	40	43	45	56	67	69	70
66	168	5	6	7	11	16	18	22	38	42	44	55	69	72	78
67	170	5	7	7	13	21	23	28	39	42	44	53	66	69	73
68	173	4	5	7	11	18	20	24	41	44	45	55	67	71	76
69	175	5	6	7	12	18	20	24	38	41	44	54	66	69	73
70	178	5	6	7	12	18	20	23	39	42	43	55	65	68	72
71	180	4	5	7	12	19	21	25	37	41	44	54	67	68	73
72	183	5	7	7	12	20	22	26	40	42	44	56	65	67	74
73	185	6	7	8	12	20	24	27	39	42	43	55	67	69	73
74	188		6	9	13	21	23			43	43	55	62	63	
Large frame															
in	cm														
62	157														
63	160														
64	163														
65	165				14							62			
66	168		9		14	30					48	58	76		
67	170		7	7	11	23	27			50	52	61	73	78	
68	173		9	10	14	22	23			51	53	65	78	86	
69	175	6	7	8	15	25	29	31	46	48	49	61	73	78	83
70	178	7	7	7	14	23	25	30	43	47	50	61	75	77	86
71	180	6	8	10	15	25	27	31	47	48	50	62	75	81	83
72	183	5	6	7	12	20	22	25	45	48	50	61	77	80	86
73	185	5	6	7	13	19	22	31	47	49	51	66	79	83	86
74	188			8	12	19					53	66	78		

MAMA = mid-arm muscle area. Adapted from Frisancho AR: New standards of weight and body composition by frame size and height for assessment of nutritional status of adults and the elderly. Am J Clin Nutr Assoc 40:808–819, 1984 © American Society for Clinical Nutrition.

APPENDIX E: Selected Percentiles of Triceps Skinfold Thickness and Bone-Free Upper Arm Area by Height in U.S. Women, Age 25 to 54 yr, with Small, Medium, and Large Frames

Height		Triceps (mm)							Bone-Free MAMA (cm²)						
in	cm	5	10	15	50	85	90	95	5	10	15	50	85	90	95
Small frame															
58	147		12	13	24	30	33			22	24	29	36	44	
59	150	8	11	14	21	29	36	37	17	20	22	28	38	39	43
60	152	8	11	12	21	28	29	33	19	21	22	28	36	40	44
61	155	11	12	14	21	28	31	34	20	21	23	28	28	39	42
62	157	10	12	14	20	28	31	34	20	21	21	27	33	35	37
63	160	10	11	13	20	27	30	36	20	21	22	27	33	35	38
64	163	10	13	13	20	28	30	34	22	23	23	28	34	38	42
65	165	12	13	14	22	29	31	34	21	22	23	28	37	39	47
66	168			12	19	30					23	27	35		
67	170				18							26			
68	173				20							25			
69	175														
70	178														
Medium frame															
58	147			20	25	40				24		35	42		
59	150	15	19	21	30	37	40	40	23	24	26	33	43	45	49
60	152	14	15	17	26	35	37	41	22	25	25	32	42	45	49
61	155	11	14	15	25	34	36	42	21	24	25	31	42	45	51
62	157	12	14	16	24	34	36	40	21	23	25	31	40	43	48
63	160	12	13	15	24	33	35	38	22	23	25	32	41	43	50
64	163	11	14	15	23	33	36	40	21	23	24	31	40	43	48
65	165	12	14	15	22	31	34	38	21	23	24	31	40	43	49
66	168	11	13	14	22	31	33	37	21	23	24	30	39	41	44
67	170	12	13	15	21	29	30	35	22	24	25	30	40	43	48
68	173	10	14	15	22	31	32	36	22	24	25	30	37	38	39
69	175		11	12	19	29	31			23	24	30	36	39	
70	178				19							32			
Large frame															
58	147														
59	150				36							45			
60	152				38							44			
61	155		25	26	36	48	50			29	33	41	62	74	
62	157	16	19	22	34	48	48	50	26	28	31	44	56	63	72
63	160	18	20	22	34	48	48	50	27	30	32	43	60	65	77
64	163	16	20	21	32	43	45	49	26	28	29	39	50	55	63
65	165	17	20	21	31	43	46	48	27	28	29	39	56	59	67
66	168	13	17	18	27	40	43	45	23	24	27	35	49	53	69
67	170	13	16	17	30	41	43	49	25	28	30	37	50	53	55
68	173		16	20	29	37	40			28	30	38	51	54	
69	175			21	30	42					27	35	49		
70	178				20							37			

MAMA = mid-arm muscle area. Adapted from Frisancho AR: New standards of weight and body composition by frame size and height for assessment of nutritional status of adults and the elderly. Am J Clin Nutr Assoc 40:808–819, 1984 © American Society for Clinical Nutrition.

APPENDIX F: Percentiles of Upper Arm Circumference (mm) and Estimated Upper Arm Muscle Circumference (mm)

Age (yr)	Arm Circumference (mm)							Arm Muscle Circumference (mm)						
	5	10	25	50	75	90	95	5	10	25	50	75	90	95
Males														
1–1.9	142	146	150	159	170	176	183	110	113	119	127	135	144	147
2–2.9	141	145	153	162	170	178	185	111	114	122	130	140	146	150
3–3.9	150	153	160	167	175	184	190	117	123	131	137	143	148	153
4–4.9	149	154	162	171	180	186	192	123	126	133	141	148	156	159
5–5.9	153	160	167	175	185	195	204	128	133	140	147	154	162	169
6–6.9	155	159	167	179	188	209	228	131	135	142	151	161	170	177
7–7.9	162	167	177	187	201	223	230	137	139	151	160	168	177	190
8–8.9	162	170	177	190	202	220	245	140	145	154	162	170	182	187
9–9.9	175	178	187	200	217	249	257	151	154	161	170	183	196	202
10–10.9	181	184	196	210	231	262	274	156	160	166	180	191	209	221
11–11.9	186	190	202	223	244	261	280	159	165	173	183	195	205	230
12–12.9	193	200	216	232	254	282	303	167	171	182	195	210	223	241
13–13.9	194	211	228	247	263	286	301	172	179	196	211	226	238	245
14–14.9	220	226	237	253	283	303	322	189	199	212	223	240	260	264
15–15.9	222	229	244	264	284	311	320	199	204	218	237	254	266	272
16–16.9	244	248	262	278	303	324	343	213	225	234	249	269	287	296
17–17.9	246	253	267	285	308	336	347	224	231	245	258	273	294	312
18–18.9	245	260	276	297	321	353	379	226	237	252	264	283	298	324
19–24.9	262	272	288	308	331	355	372	238	245	258	273	289	309	321
25–34.9	271	282	300	319	342	362	375	243	250	264	279	298	314	326
35–44.9	278	287	305	326	345	363	374	247	255	269	286	302	318	327
45–54.9	267	281	301	322	342	362	376	239	249	265	281	300	315	326
55–64.9	258	273	296	317	336	355	269	236	245	260	278	295	310	320
65–74.9	248	263	285	307	325	344	355	223	235	251	268	284	298	306
Females														
1–1.9	138	142	148	156	164	172	177	105	111	117	124	132	139	143
2–2.9	142	145	152	160	167	176	184	111	114	119	126	133	142	147
3–3.9	143	150	158	167	175	183	189	113	119	124	132	140	146	152
4–4.9	149	154	160	169	177	184	191	115	121	128	136	144	152	157
5–5.9	153	157	165	175	185	203	211	125	128	134	142	151	159	165
6–6.9	156	162	170	176	187	204	211	130	133	138	145	154	166	171
7–7.9	164	167	174	183	199	216	231	129	135	142	151	160	171	176
8–8.9	168	172	183	195	214	247	261	138	140	151	160	171	183	194
9–9.9	178	182	194	211	224	251	260	147	150	158	167	180	194	198
10–10.9	174	182	193	210	228	251	265	148	150	159	170	180	190	197
11–11.9	185	194	208	224	248	276	303	150	158	171	181	196	217	223
12–12.9	194	203	216	237	256	282	294	162	166	180	191	201	214	220
13–13.9	202	211	223	243	271	301	338	169	175	183	198	211	226	240
14–14.9	214	223	237	252	272	304	322	174	179	190	201	216	232	247
15–15.9	208	221	239	254	279	300	322	175	178	189	202	215	228	244
16–16.9	218	224	241	258	283	318	334	170	180	190	202	216	234	249
17–17.9	220	227	241	264	295	324	350	175	183	194	205	221	239	257
18–18.9	222	227	241	258	281	312	325	174	179	191	202	215	237	245
19–24.9	221	230	247	265	290	319	345	179	185	195	207	221	236	249
25–34.9	233	240	256	277	304	342	368	183	188	199	212	228	246	264
35–44.9	241	251	267	290	317	356	378	186	192	205	218	236	257	272
45–54.9	242	256	274	299	328	362	384	187	193	206	220	238	260	274
55–64.9	243	257	280	303	335	367	385	187	196	209	225	244	266	280
65–74.9	240	252	274	299	326	356	373	185	195	208	225	244	264	279

From Frisancho AR: New norms of upper limb fat and muscle areas for assessment of nutritional status. Am J Clin Nutr 30:2540–2548, 1981 © American Society for Clinical Nutrition.

APPENDIX G: Frame Size by Elbow Breadth of Male and Female Adults in the United States

Age (yr)	Frame Size (cm)		
	Small	*Medium*	*Large*
Males			
18–24	≤6.6	>6.6 and <7.7	≥7.7
25–34	≤6.7	>6.7 and <7.9	≥7.9
35–44	≤6.7	>6.7 and <8.0	≥8.0
45–54	≤6.7	>6.7 and <8.1	≥8.1
55–64	≤6.7	>6.7 and <8.1	≥8.1
65–74	≤6.7	>6.7 and <8.1	≥8.1
Females			
18–24	≤5.6	>5.6 and <6.5	≥6.5
25–34	≤5.7	>5.7 and <6.8	≥6.8
35–44	≤5.7	>5.7 and <7.1	≥7.1
45–54	≤5.7	>5.7 and <7.2	≥7.2
55–64	≤5.8	>5.8 and <7.2	≥7.2
65–74	≤5.8	>5.8 and <7.2	≥7.2

From Frisancho AR: New standards of weight and body composition by frame size and height for assessment of nutritional status of adults and the elderly. Am J Clin Nutr 40:808–819, 1984, 1981 © American Society for Clinical Nutrition.

APPENDIX H-1: Standard Precautions

Synopsis of Types of Precautions and Patients Requiring the Precautions

Standard Precautions

Use Standard Precautions for the care of all patients

Airborne Precautions

In addition to Standard Precautions, use Airborne Precautions for patients known or suspected to have serious illnesses transmitted by airborne droplet nuclei. Examples of such illnesses include:

1. Measles
2. Varicella (including disseminated zoster)*
3. Tuberculosis†

Droplet Precautions

In addition to Standard Precautions, use Droplet Precautions for patients known or suspected to have serious illnesses transmitted by large-particle droplets. Examples of such illnesses include:

1. Invasive *Haemophilus influenzae* type b disease, including meningitis, pneumonia, epiglottitis, and sepsis
2. Invasive *Neisseria meningitidis* disease, including meningitis, pneumonia, and sepsis
3. Other serious bacterial respiratory infections spread by droplet transmission, including:
   a) Diphtheria (pharyngeal)
   b) Mycoplasma pneumonia
   c) Pertussis
   d) Pneumonic plague
   e) Streptococcal pharyngitis, pneumonia, or scarlet fever in infants and young children
4. Serious viral infections spread by droplet transmission, including:
   a) Adenovirus*
   b) Influenza
   c) Mumps
   d) Parvovirus B19
   e) Rubella

Contact Precautions

In addition to Standard Precautions, use Contact Precautions for patients known or suspected to have serious illnesses easily transmitted by direct patient contact or by contact with items in the patient's environment. Examples of such illnesses include:

1. Gastrointestinal, respiratory, skin, or wound infections or colonization with multi-drug-resistant bacteria judged by the infection control program, based on current state, regional, or national recommendations, to be of special clinical and epidemiologic significance

Synopsis of Types of Precautions and Patients Requiring the Precautions

2. Enteric infections with a low infectious dose or prolonged environmental survival, including:
   a) *Clostridium difficile*
   b) For diapered or incontinent patients: enterohemorrhagic *Escherichia coli* O157:H7, *Shigella,* hepatitis A, or rotavirus
3. Respiratory syncytial virus, parainfluenza virus, or enteroviral infections in infants and young children
4. Skin infections that are highly contagious or that may occur on dry skin, including:
   a) Diphtheria (cutaneous)
   b) Herpes simplex virus (neonatal or mucocutaneous)
   c) Impetigo
   d) Major (noncontained) abscesses, cellulitis, or decubiti
   e) Pediculosis
   f) Scabies
   g) Staphylococcal furunculosis in infants and young children
   h) Zoster (disseminated or in the immunocompromised host)*
5. Viral/hemorrhagic conjunctivitis
6. Viral hemorrhagic infections (Ebola, Lassa, or Marburg)

Adapted from Garner JS: Guideline for Isolation Precautions in Hospitals. Atlanta, GA, Public Health Service, U.S. Department of Health and Human Services; Centers for Disease Control and Prevention, 1996.
*Certain infections require more than one type of precaution.
†See CDC "Guidelines for Preventing the Transmission of Tuberculosis in Health-Care Facilities."

APPENDIX H-2: Transmission-based Precautions

AIRBORNE PRECAUTIONS

In addition to Standard Precautions, use Airborne Precautions, or the equivalent, for patients known or suspected to be infected with microorganisms transmitted by airborne droplet nuclei (small-particle residue [5 μm or smaller in size] of evaporated droplets containing microorganisms that remain suspended in air and that can be dispersed widely by air currents within a room or over a long distance).

A. Patient Placement

Place the patient in a private room that has (1) monitored negative air pressure in relation to the surrounding areas, (2) 6 to 12 air changes per hour, and (3) appropriate discharge of air outdoors or monitored high-efficiency filtration of room air before the air is circulated to other areas in the hospital. Keep the room door closed and the patient in the room. When a private room is not available, place the patient in a room with a patient who has active infection with the same microorganism, unless otherwise recommended, but with no other infection.

B. Respiratory Protection

Wear respiratory protection when entering the room of a patient with known or suspected infectious pulmonary tuberculosis. Susceptible persons should not enter the room of patients known or suspected to have measles (rubeola) or varicella (chickenpox) if other immune caregivers are available. If susceptible persons must enter the room of a patient known or suspected to have measles (rubeola) or varicella, they should wear respiratory protection. Persons immune to measles (rubeola) or varicella need not wear respiratory protection.

C. Patient Transport

Limit the movement and transport of the patient from the room to essential purposes only. If transport or movement is necessary, minimize patient dispersal of droplet nuclei by placing a surgical mask on the patient, if possible.

D. Additional Precautions for Preventing Transmission of Tuberculosis

Consult CDC "Guidelines for Preventing the Transmission of Tuberculosis in Health-Care Facilities" for additional prevention strategies.

DROPLET PRECAUTIONS

In addition to Standard Precautions, use Droplet Precautions, or the equivalent, for a patient known or suspected to be infected with microorganisms transmitted by droplets (large-particle droplets [larger than 5 μm in size] that can be generated by the patient during coughing, sneezing, talking, or the performance of procedures).

A. Patient Placement

Place the patient in a private room. When a private room is not available, place the patient in a room with a patient(s) who has active infection with the same microorganism but with no other infection (cohorting). When a private room is not available and cohorting is not achievable, maintain spatial separation of at least 3 ft between the infected patient and other patients and visitors. Special air handling and ventilation are not necessary, and the door may remain open.

B. Mask

In addition to Standard Precautions, wear a mask when working within 3 ft of the patient. (Logistically, some hospitals may want to implement the wearing of a mask to enter the room.)

C. Patient Transport

Limit the movement and transport of the patient from the room to essential purposes only. If transport or movement is necessary, minimize patient dispersal of droplets by masking the patient, if possible.

CONTACT PRECAUTIONS

In addition to Standard Precautions, use Contact Precautions, or the equivalent, for specified patients known or suspected to be infected or colonized with epidemiologically important microorganisms that can be transmitted by direct contact with the patient (hand or skin-to-skin contact that occurs when performing patient-care activities that require touching the patient's dry skin) or indirect contact (touching) with environmental surfaces or patient-care items in the patient's environment.

A. Patient Placement

Place the patient in a private room. When a private room is not available, place the patient in a room with a patient(s) who has active infection with the same microorganism but with no other infection (cohorting). When a private room is not available and cohorting is not achievable, consider the epidemiology of the microorganism and the patient population when determining patient placement.

B. Gloves and Handwashing

In addition to wearing gloves as outlined under Standard Precautions, wear gloves (clean, nonsterile gloves are adequate) when entering the room. During the course of providing care for a patient, change gloves after having contact with infective material that may contain high concentrations of microorganisms (fecal material and wound drainage). Remove gloves before leaving the patient's environment and wash hands immediately with an antimicrobial agent or a waterless antiseptic agent. After glove removal and handwashing, ensure that hands do not touch potentially contaminated environmental surfaces or items in the patient's room to avoid transfer of microorganisms to other patients or environments.

C. Gown

In addition to wearing a gown as outlined under Standard Precautions, wear a gown (a clean, nonsterile gown is adequate) when entering the room if you anticipate that your clothing will have substantial contact with the patient, environmental surfaces, or items in the patient's room, or if the patient is incontinent or has diarrhea, an ileostomy, a colostomy, or wound drainage not contained by a dressing. Remove the gown before leaving the patient's environment. After gown removal, ensure that clothing does not contact potentially contaminated environmental surfaces to avoid transfer of microorganisms to other patients or environments.

D. Patient Transport

Limit the movement and transport of the patient from the room to essential purposes only. If the patient is transported out of the room, ensure that precautions are maintained to minimize the risk of transmission of microorganisms to other patients and contamination of environmental surfaces or equipment.

E. Patient-Care Equipment

When possible, dedicate the use of noncritical patient-care equipment to a single patient (or cohort of patients infected or colonized with the pathogen requiring precautions) to avoid sharing between patients. If use of common equipment or items is unavoidable, then adequately clean and disinfect them before use for another patient.

F. Additional Precautions for Preventing the Spread of Vancomycin Resistance

Consult the HICPAC report on preventing the spread of vancomycin resistance for additional prevention strategies.

Adapted from Garner JS; Hospital Infection Control Practices Advisory Committee: *Guideline for Isolation Precautions in Hospitals.* Atlanta, GA, Public Health Service, US Dept. of Health and Human Services, Centers for Disease Control and Prevention, 1996.

APPENDIX I: Sample Growth Charts for Girls and Boys (Height and Weight)

GIRLS: BIRTH TO 36 MONTHS; PHYSICAL GROWTH NCHS PERCENTILES*

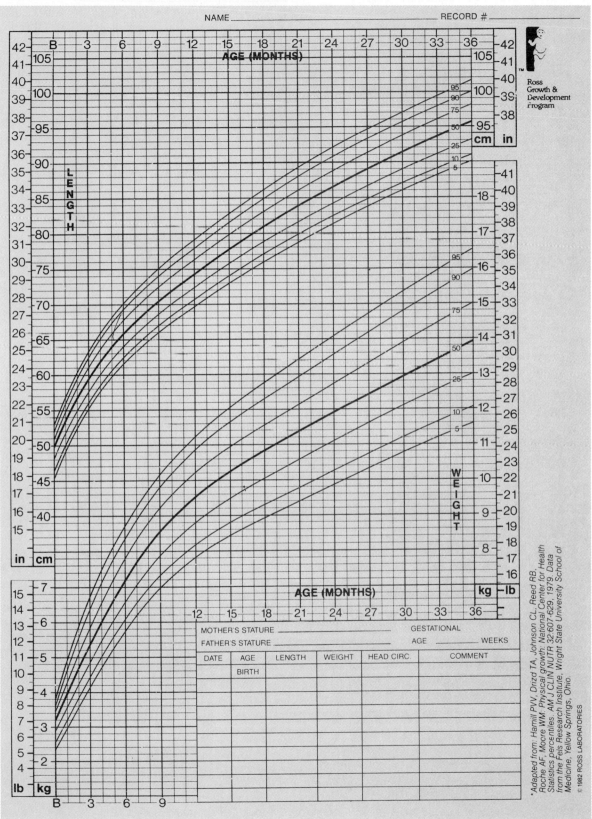

GIRLS: BIRTH TO 36 MONTHS; PHYSICAL GROWTH NCHS PERCENTILES*

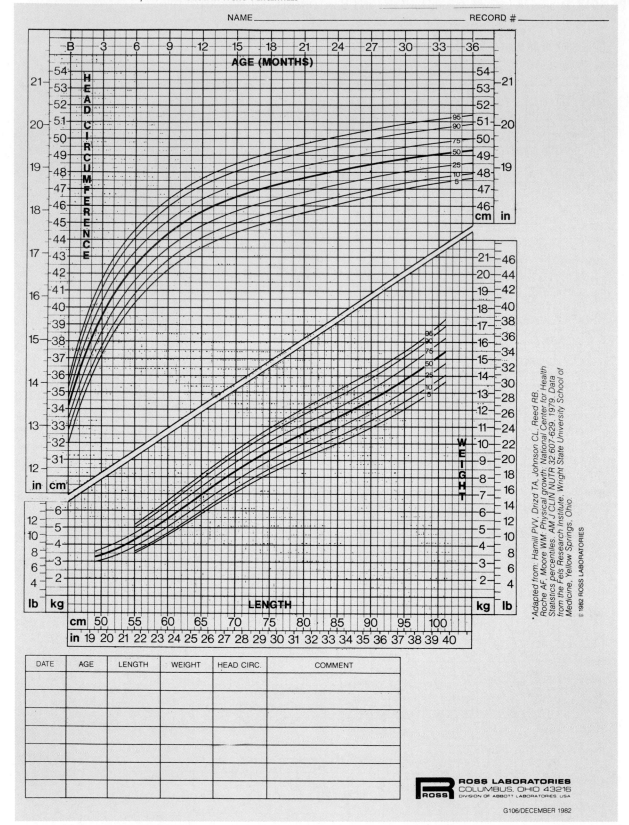

*Adapted from: Hamill PVV, Drizd TA, Johnson CL, Reed RB, Roche AF, Moore WM. Physical growth: National Center for Health Statistics percentiles. AM J CLIN NUTR 32:607-629, 1979. Data from the Fels Research Institute, Wright State University School of Medicine, Yellow Springs, Ohio.

© 1982 ROSS LABORATORIES

DATE	AGE	LENGTH	WEIGHT	HEAD CIRC.	COMMENT

ROSS LABORATORIES
COLUMBUS, OHIO 43216
DIVISION OF ABBOTT LABORATORIES USA

G106/DECEMBER 1982

GIRLS: 2 TO 18 YEARS; PHYSICAL GROWTH NCHS PERCENTILES*

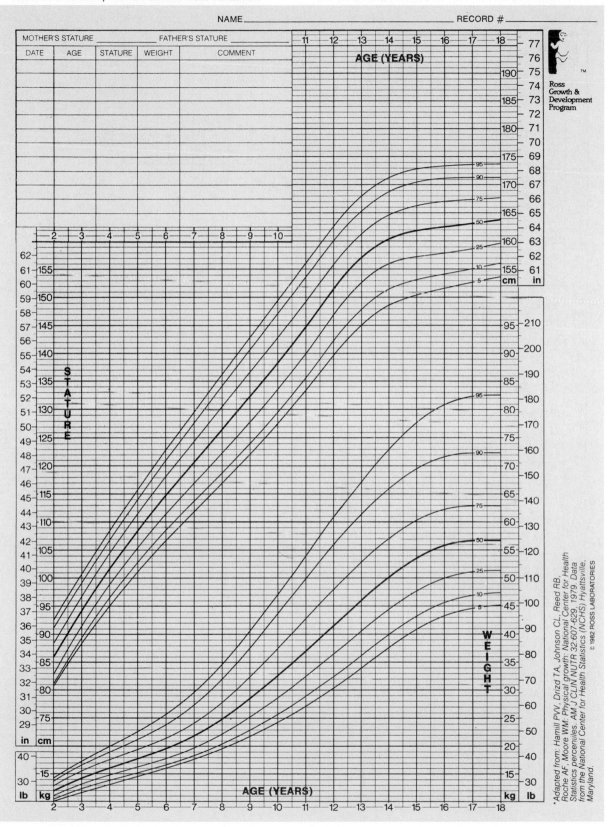

*Adapted from: Hamill PVV, Drizd TA, Johnson CL, Reed RB, Roche AF, Moore WM: Physical growth: National Center for Health Statistics percentiles. AM J CLIN NUTR 32:607-629, 1979. Data from the National Center for Health Statistics (NCHS) Hyattsville, Maryland.

© 1982 ROSS LABORATORIES

Boys: Birth to 36 Months; Physical Growth NCHS Percentiles*

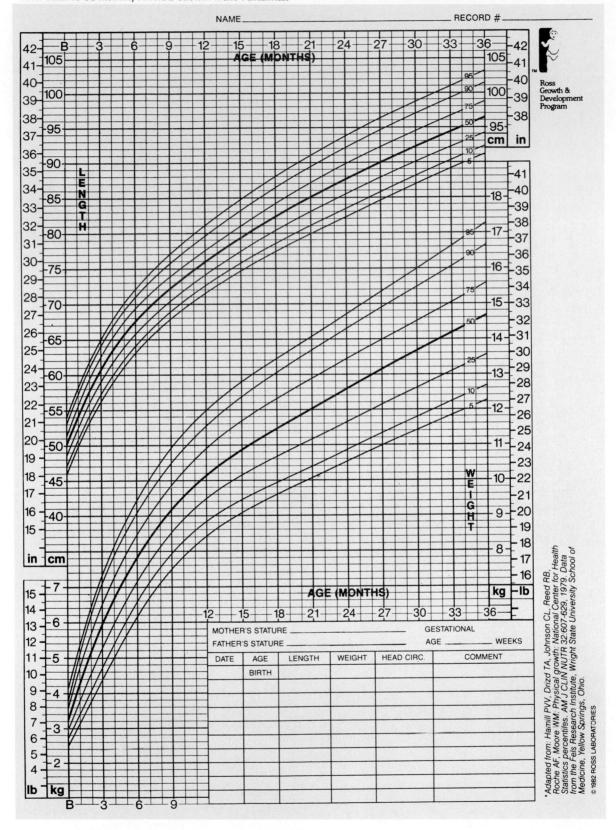

*Adapted from: Hamill PVV, Drizd TA, Johnson CL, Reed RB, Roche AF, Moore WM: Physical growth: National Center for Health Statistics percentiles. AM J CLIN NUTR 32:607-629, 1979. Data from the Fels Research Institute, Wright State University School of Medicine, Yellow Springs, Ohio.

© 1982 ROSS LABORATORIES

BOYS: BIRTH TO 36 MONTHS; PHYSICAL GROWTH NCHS PERCENTILES*

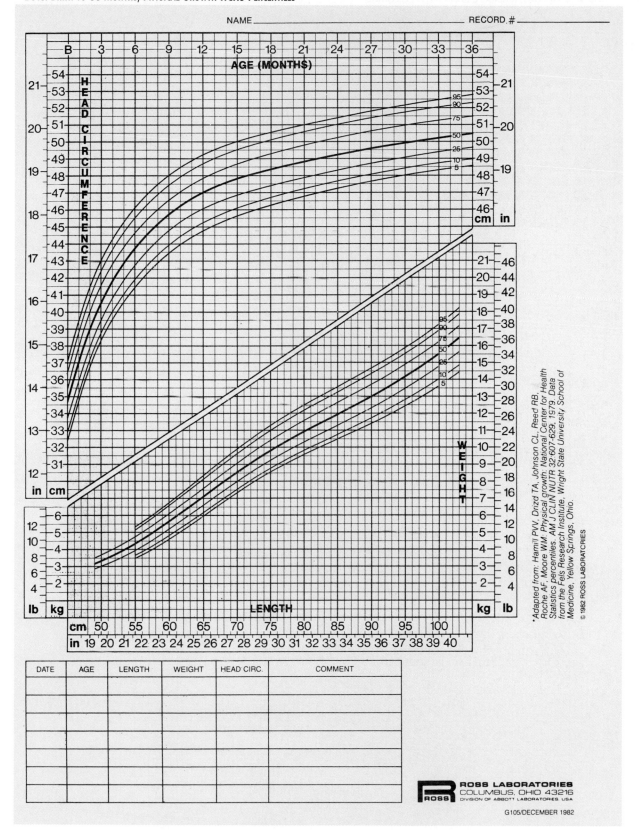

*Adapted from: Hamill PVV, Drizd TA, Johnson CL, Reed RB, Roche AF, Moore WM: Physical growth: National Center for Health Statistics percentiles. AM J CLIN NUTR 32:607-629, 1979. Data from the Fels Research Institute, Wright State University School of Medicine, Yellow Springs, Ohio.
© 1982 ROSS LABORATORIES

DATE	AGE	LENGTH	WEIGHT	HEAD CIRC.	COMMENT

ROSS LABORATORIES
COLUMBUS, OHIO 43216
DIVISION OF ABBOTT LABORATORIES, USA
G105/DECEMBER 1982

BOYS: 2 TO 18 YEARS; PHYSICAL GROWTH NCHS PERCENTILES*

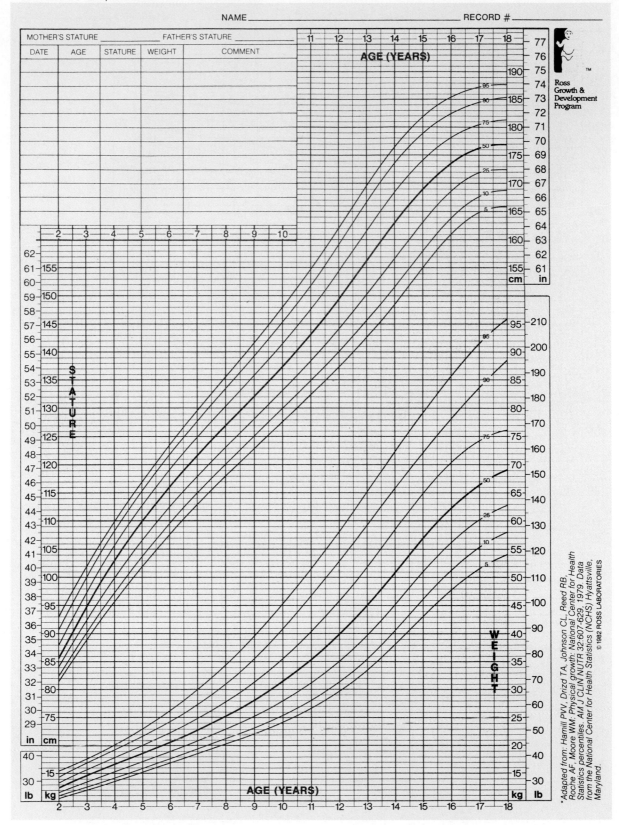

*Adapted from: Hamill PVV, Drizd TA, Johnson CL, Reed RB,
Roche AF, Moore WM: Physical growth: National Center for Health
Statistics percentiles. AM J CLIN NUTR 32:607-629, 1979. Data
from the National Center for Health Statistics (NCHS) Hyattsville,
Maryland.

© 1982 ROSS LABORATORIES

Ross
Growth &
Development
Program

APPENDIX J-1: Maturational Assessment of Gestational Age (New Ballard Score)
MATURATIONAL ASSESSMENT OF GESTATIONAL AGE (New Ballard Score)

NAME _____   SEX _____

HOSPITAL NO. _____   BIRTH WEIGHT _____

RACE _____   LENGTH _____

DATE/TIME OF BIRTH _____   HEAD CIRC. _____

DATE/TIME OF EXAM _____   EXAMINER _____

AGE WHEN EXAMINED _____

APGAR SCORE: 1 MINUTE _____ 5 MINUTES _____ 10 MINUTES _____

NEUROMUSCULAR MATURITY

NEUROMUSCULAR MATURITY SIGN	SCORE							RECORD SCORE HERE
	-1	0	1	2	3	4	5	
POSTURE								
SQUARE WINDOW (Wrist)	>90°	90°	60°	45°	30°	0°		
ARM RECOIL		180°	140°-180°	110°-140°	90°-110°	<90°		
POPLITEAL ANGLE	180°	160°	140°	120°	100°	90°	<90°	
SCARF SIGN								
HEEL TO EAR								

TOTAL NEUROMUSCULAR MATURITY SCORE

PHYSICAL MATURITY

PHYSICAL MATURITY SIGN	SCORE							RECORD SCORE HERE
	-1	0	1	2	3	4	5	
SKIN	sticky friable transparent	gelatinous red translucent	smooth pink visible veins	superficial peeling &/or rash, few veins	cracking pale areas rare veins	parchment deep cracking no vessels	leathery cracked wrinkled	
LANUGO	none	sparse	abundant	thinning	bald areas	mostly bald		
PLANTAR SURFACE	heel-toe 40-50 mm:-1 <40 mm:-2	>50 mm no crease	faint red marks	anterior transverse crease only	creases ant. 2/3	creases over entire sole		
BREAST	imperceptible	barely perceptible	flat areola no bud	stippled areola 1-2 mm bud	raised areola 3-4 mm bud	full areola 5-10 mm bud		
EYE/EAR	lids fused loosely: -1 tightly: -2	lids open pinna flat stays folded	sl. curved pinna; soft; slow recoil	well-curved pinna; soft but ready recoil	formed & firm instant recoil	thick cartilage ear stiff		
GENITALS (Male)	scrotum flat, smooth	scrotum empty faint rugae	testes in upper canal rare rugae	testes descending few rugae	testes down good rugae	testes pendulous deep rugae		
GENITALS (Female)	clitoris prominent & labia flat	prominent clitoris & small labia minora	prominent clitoris & enlarging minora	majora & minora equally prominent	majora large minora small	majora cover clitoris & minora		

TOTAL PHYSICAL MATURITY SCORE

SCORE

Neuromuscular _____

Physical _____

Total _____

MATURITY RATING

score	weeks
-10	20
-5	22
0	24
5	26
10	28
15	30
20	32
25	34
30	36
35	38
40	40
45	42
50	44

GESTATIONAL AGE (weeks)

By dates _____

By ultrasound _____

By exam _____

Reference
Ballard JL, Khoury JC, Wedig K, et al: New Ballard Score, expanded to include extremely premature infants. J Pediatr 1991; 119:417-423. Reprinted by permission of Dr. Ballard and Mosby - Year Book, Inc.

CLASSIFICATION OF NEWBORNS (BOTH SEXES)
BY INTRAUTERINE GROWTH AND GESTATIONAL AGE [1,2]

NAME _____   DATE OF EXAM _____   LENGTH _____

HOSPITAL NO. _____   SEX _____   HEAD CIRC. _____

RACE _____   BIRTH WEIGHT _____   GESTATIONAL AGE _____

DATE OF BIRTH _____

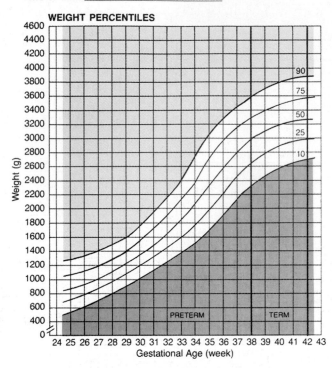

WEIGHT PERCENTILES

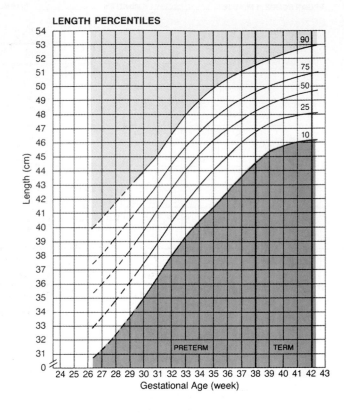

LENGTH PERCENTILES

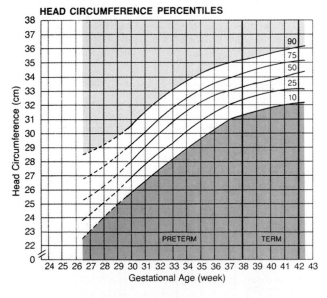

HEAD CIRCUMFERENCE PERCENTILES

CLASSIFICATION OF INFANT*	Weight	Length	Head Circ.
Large for Gestational Age (LGA) (>90th percentile)			
Appropriate for Gestational Age (AGA) (10th to 90th percentile)			
Small for Gestational Age (SGA) (<10th percentile)			

*Place an "X" in the appropriate box (LGA, AGA or SGA) for weight, for length and for head circumference.

References
1. Battaglia FC, Lubchenco LO: A practical classification of newborn infants by weight and gestational age. *J Pediatr* 1967; 71:159-163.
2. Lubchenco LO, Hansman C, Boyd E: Intrauterine growth in length and head circumference as estimated from live births at gestational ages from 26 to 42 weeks. *Pediatrics* 1966; 37:403-408.

Reprinted by permission from Dr. Battaglia, Dr. Lubchenco, *Journal of Pediatrics and Pediatrics.*

A service of **SIMILAC® WITH IRON** Infant Formula

The Ross Hospital Formula System

ROSS PRODUCTS DIVISION
ABBOTT LABORATORIES
COLUMBUS, OHIO 43215-1724

LITHO IN USA

APPENDIX K-1: Blood Pressure Levels for the 90th and 95th Percentiles of Blood Pressure for Girls Aged 1 to 17 Years by Percentiles of Height

Age (yr)	Blood Pressure Percentile*	Systolic Blood Pressure by Percentile of Height, (mm Hg)†							Diastolic Blood Pressure by Percentile of Height, (mm Hg)†						
		5%	10%	25%	50%	75%	90%	95%	5%	10%	25%	50%	75%	90%	95%
1	90th	97	98	99	100	102	103	104	53	53	53	54	55	56	56
	95th	101	102	103	104	105	107	107	57	57	57	58	59	60	60
2	90th	99	99	100	102	103	104	105	57	57	58	58	59	60	61
	95th	102	103	104	105	107	108	109	61	61	62	62	63	64	65
3	90th	100	100	102	103	104	105	106	61	61	61	62	63	63	64
	95th	104	104	105	107	108	109	110	65	65	65	66	67	67	68
4	90th	101	102	103	104	106	107	108	63	63	64	65	65	66	67
	95th	105	106	107	108	109	111	111	67	67	68	69	69	70	71
5	90th	103	103	104	106	107	108	109	65	66	66	67	68	68	69
	95th	107	107	108	110	111	112	113	69	70	70	71	72	72	73
6	90th	104	105	106	107	109	110	111	67	67	68	69	69	70	71
	95th	108	109	110	111	112	114	114	71	71	72	73	73	74	75
7	90th	106	107	108	109	110	112	112	69	69	69	70	71	72	72
	95th	110	110	112	113	114	115	116	73	73	73	74	75	76	76
8	90th	108	109	110	111	112	113	114	70	70	71	71	72	73	74
	95th	112	112	113	115	116	117	118	74	74	75	75	76	77	78
9	90th	110	110	112	113	114	115	116	71	72	72	73	74	74	75
	95th	114	114	115	117	118	119	120	75	76	76	77	78	78	79
10	90th	112	112	114	115	116	117	118	73	73	73	74	75	76	76
	95th	116	116	117	119	120	121	122	77	77	77	78	79	80	80
11	90th	114	114	116	117	118	119	120	74	74	75	75	76	77	77
	95th	118	118	119	121	122	123	124	78	78	79	79	80	81	81
12	90th	116	116	118	119	120	121	122	75	75	76	76	77	78	78
	95th	120	120	121	123	124	125	126	79	79	80	80	81	82	82
13	90th	118	118	119	121	122	123	124	76	76	77	78	78	79	80
	95th	121	122	123	125	126	127	128	80	80	81	82	82	83	84
14	90th	119	120	121	122	124	125	126	77	77	78	79	79	80	81
	95th	123	124	125	126	128	129	130	81	81	82	83	83	84	85
15	90th	121	121	122	124	125	126	127	78	78	79	79	80	81	82
	95th	124	125	126	128	129	130	131	82	82	83	83	84	85	86
16	90th	122	122	123	125	126	127	128	79	79	79	80	81	82	82
	95th	125	126	127	128	130	131	132	83	83	83	84	85	86	86
17	90th	122	123	124	125	126	128	128	79	79	79	80	81	82	82
	95th	126	126	127	129	130	131	132	83	83	83	84	85	86	86

*Blood pressure percentile was determined by a single reading.
†Height percentile was determined by standard growth curves.

APPENDIX K-2: Blood Pressure Levels for the 90th and 95th Percentiles of Blood Pressure for Boys Aged 1 to 17 Years by Percentiles of Height

Age (yr)	Blood Pressure Percentile*	Systolic Blood Pressure by Percentile of Height, (mm Hg)†							Diastolic Blood Pressure by Percentile of Height, (mm Hg)†						
		5%	10%	25%	50%	75%	90%	95%	5%	10%	25%	50%	75%	90%	95%
1	90th	94	95	97	98	100	102	102	50	51	52	53	54	54	55
	95th	98	99	101	102	104	106	106	55	55	56	57	58	59	59
2	90th	98	99	100	102	104	105	106	55	55	56	57	58	59	59
	95th	101	102	104	106	108	109	110	59	59	60	61	62	63	63
3	90th	100	101	103	105	107	108	109	59	59	60	61	62	63	63
	95th	104	105	107	109	111	112	113	63	63	64	65	66	67	67
4	90th	102	103	105	107	109	110	111	62	62	63	64	65	66	66
	95th	106	107	109	111	113	114	115	66	67	67	68	69	70	71
5	90th	104	105	106	108	110	112	112	65	65	66	67	68	69	69
	95th	108	109	110	112	114	115	116	69	70	70	71	72	73	74
6	90th	105	106	108	110	111	113	114	67	68	69	70	70	71	72
	95th	109	110	112	114	115	117	117	72	72	73	74	75	76	76
7	90th	106	107	109	111	113	114	115	69	70	71	72	72	73	74
	95th	110	111	113	115	116	118	119	74	74	75	76	77	78	78
8	90th	107	108	110	112	114	115	116	71	71	72	73	74	75	75
	95th	111	112	114	116	118	119	120	75	76	76	77	78	79	80
9	90th	109	110	112	113	115	117	117	72	73	73	74	75	76	77
	95th	113	114	116	117	119	121	121	76	77	78	79	80	80	81
10	90th	110	112	113	115	117	118	119	73	74	74	75	76	77	78
	95th	114	115	117	119	121	122	123	77	78	79	80	80	81	82
11	90th	112	113	115	117	119	120	121	74	74	75	76	77	78	78
	95th	116	117	119	121	123	124	125	78	79	79	80	81	82	83
12	90th	115	116	117	119	121	123	123	75	75	76	77	78	78	79
	95th	119	120	121	123	125	126	127	79	79	80	81	82	83	83
13	90th	117	118	120	122	124	125	126	75	76	76	77	78	79	80
	95th	121	122	124	126	128	129	130	79	80	81	82	83	83	84
14	90th	120	121	123	125	126	128	128	76	76	77	78	79	80	80
	95th	124	125	127	128	130	132	132	80	81	81	82	83	84	85
15	90th	123	124	125	127	129	131	131	77	77	78	79	80	81	81
	95th	127	128	129	131	133	134	135	81	82	83	83	84	85	86
16	90th	125	126	128	130	132	133	134	79	79	80	81	82	82	83
	95th	129	130	132	134	136	137	138	83	83	84	85	86	87	87
17	90th	128	129	131	133	134	136	136	81	81	82	83	84	85	85
	95th	132	133	135	136	138	140	140	85	85	86	87	88	89	89

*Blood pressure percentile was determined by a single measurement.
†Height percentile was determined by standard growth curves.
From the National High Blood Pressure Education Program: Update on the 1987 Task Force report on high blood pressure in children and adolescents. Pediatrics 98(4): 649–667, 1997.

Illustration Credits

Inside front cover Spanish/English assessment tool is modified from Black JM, Matassarin-Jacobs E: Luckmann and Sorensen's Medical-Surgical Nursing: A Psychophysiologic Approach, 4th ed. Philadelphia, W.B. Saunders Company, 1993. Adapted from Taber's Cyclopedic Dictionary, 16th ed. Philadelphia, F.A. Davis, 1989.

Chapter 1

Figure 1–1: Redrawn from the *Democrat and Chronicle,* Gannett Rochester Newspapers, Rochester, NY, 1992.

Chapter 2

Figure 2–1: From Gorrie TM, McKinney ES, Murray SS: Foundations of Maternal-Newborn Nursing, 2nd ed. Philadelphia, W.B. Saunders Company, 1998, p 463.

Figure 2–9: Reprinted with permission from Denver Developmental Materials, Inc., Denver, CO, 1990.

Chapter 7

Figure 7–1: From Nutrition Screening Initiative: Implementing Nutrition Screening and Intervention Strategies. Washington, DC, Nutrition Screening Initiative, 1993. (Reprinted with permission by the Nutrition Screening Initiative, a project of the American Academy of Family Physicians, the American Dietetic Association and the National Council on Aging, Inc., and funded in part by a grant from Ross Products Divisions, Abbott Laboratories.)

Art for Table 7–7: (marasmus) With permission from George Comerci, MD.

Art for Table 7–8: (pellagra) From Latham MC, McGandy RB, McCann MB, Stare FJ: Scope Manual on Nutrition. Kalamazoo, MI: The Upjohn Company, 1980, copyright by Thomas Spies, MD; (scorbutic gums) from Taylor KB, Anthony LE: Clinical Nutrition. New York, McGraw-Hill, 1983, copyright by The Upjohn Company; (follicular hyperkeratosis) from Taylor KB, Anthony LE: Clinical Nutrition. New York, McGraw-Hill, 1983, copyright by Harold H. Sandstead, MD; (Bitot's spots) from Taylor KB, Anthony LE: Clinical Nutrition. New York, McGraw-Hill, 1983, copyright by Helen Keller International, Inc.; (kwashiorkor) from Latham MC, et al.: Scope Manual on Nutrition. Kalamazoo, MI, The Upjohn Company, 1980, copyright by Michael C. Latham, MD; (HIV infection) from Friedman-Kien AE, Cockerell CJ: Color Atlas of AIDS, 2nd ed. Philadelphia, W.B. Saunders Company, 1996; (magenta tongue) from McLaren DS: Color Atlas of Nutritional Disorders. London, Wolfe Medical, Ltd, 1981 copyright by C. E. Butterworth, Jr; (rickets) from Latham MC, et al.: Scope Manual on Nutrition. Kalamazoo, MI. The Upjohn Company, 1980, copyright by Rosa Lee Nemir, MD.

Chapter 9

Figure 9–16: From Rossman I: Clinical Geriatrics, 3rd ed. Philadelphia, J.B. Lippincott Company, 1986, p 6.

Art for Table 9–8: (hypopituitary dwarfism) From Wilson JD, Foster DW: Williams' Textbook of Endocrinology, 7th ed. Philadelphia, W.B. Saunders Company, 1985, p 599; (gigantism) from Jacob SW, Francone CA, Lossow WJ: Structure and Function, 5th ed. Philadelphia, W.B. Saunders Company, 1982, p 550; (achondroplastic dwarfism) from Moore KL: The Developing Human, 4th ed. Philadelphia, W.B. Saunders Company, 1988, p 142; (anorexia nervosa) Courtesy of George D. Comerci, MD; (Marfan's syndrome) from Manusov EG, Martucci E: The Marfan syndrome. Arch Fam Med 3:824, Sept 1994. (Cushing's syndrome) from Wenig BM, Heffess CS, Adair CF: Atlas of Endocrine Pathology. Philadelphia, W.B. Saunders Company, 1997, p 282.

Chapter 10

Figure 10–3B: From Lookingbill DP, Marks JG: Principles of Dermatology, 2nd ed. Philadelphia, W.B. Saunders Company, 1993, p 208.

Figure 10–4A: From Hurwitz S: Clinical Pediatric Dermatology: A Textbook of Skin Disorders of Childhood and Adolescence, 2nd ed. Philadelphia, W.B. Saunders Company, 1993, p 212.

Figure 10–4B: From Hurwitz S: Clinical Pediatric Dermatology: A Textbook of Skin Disorders of Childhood and Adolescence, 2nd ed. Philadelphia, W.B. Saunders Company, 1993, p 200.

Figure 10–4C: From Lookingbill DP, Marks JG: Principles of Dermatology, 2nd ed. Philadelphia, W.B. Saunders Company, 1993, p 91.

Figure 10–6: From Lookingbill DP, Marks JG: Principles of Dermatology, 2nd ed. Philadelphia, W.B. Saunders Company, 1993, p 103.

Figure 10–9: From Callen JP, Greer KE, Hood AF, et al: Color Atlas of Dermatology. Philadelphia, W.B. Saunders Company, 1993, p 349.

Figure 10–10: From Hurwitz S: Clinical Pediatric Dermatology: A Textbook of Skin Disorders of Childhood and Adolescence, 2nd ed. Philadelphia, W.B. Saunders Company, 1993, p 509.

Figure 10–12: Courtesy of Jane Deacon, RNC, MS, NNP, The Children's Hospital, Denver, Colorado.

Figure 10–13: From Bowden VR, Dickey SB, Greenberg CS: Children and Their Families. Philadelphia, W.B. Saunders Company, 1998, p 1716.

Figure 10–14: From Hurwitz A: Clinical Pediatric Dermatology: A Textbook of Skin Disorders of Childhood and Adolescence, 2nd ed. Philadelphia, W.B. Saunders Company, 1993, p 13.

Figure 10–15: From Hurwitz A: Clinical Pediatric Dermatology: A Textbook of Skin Disorders of Childhood and Adolescence, 2nd ed. Philadelphia, W.B. Saunders Company, 1993. p 9.

Figure 10–16: From Gorrie TM, McKinney ES, Murray SS: Foundations of Maternal-Newborn Nursing, 2nd ed. Philadelphia, W.B. Saunders Company, 1998, p 536.

Figure 10–17: From Hurwitz A: Clinical Pediatric Dermatology: A Textbook of Skin Disorders of Childhood and Adolescence, 2nd ed. Philadelphia, W.B. Saunders Company, 1993, p 249.

Figure 10–18: From Gorrie TM, McKinney ES, Murray SS: Foundations of Maternal-Newborn Nursing, 2nd ed. Philadelphia, W.B. Saunders Company, 1998, p 536.

Figure 10–19: From Hurwitz A: Clinical Pediatric Dermatology: A Textbook of Skin Disorders of Childhood and Adolescence, 2nd ed. Philadelphia, W.B. Saunders Company, 1993, p 137.

Figure 10–20: From Lookingbill DP, Marks JG: Principles of Dermatology, 2nd ed. Philadelphia, W.B. Saunders Company, 1993, p 89.

Figure 10–21: From Lookingbill DP, Marks JG: Principles of Dermatology, 2nd ed. Philadelphia, W.B. Saunders Company, 1993, p 74.

Figure 10–22: From Lookingbill DP, Marks JG: Principles of Dermatology, 2nd ed. Philadelphia, W.B. Saunders Company, 1993, p 77.

Figure 10–23: From Lookingbill DP, Marks JG: Principles of Dermatology, 2nd ed. Philadelphia, W.B. Saunders Company, 1993, p 75.

Figure 10–24: From Callen JP, Greer KE, Hood AF, et al: Color Atlas of Dermatology. Philadelphia, W.B. Saunders Company, 1993, p 103.

Art for Table 10–6: (port-wine stain): From Hurwitz S: Clinical Pediatric Dermatology: A Textbook of Skin Disorders of Childhood and Adolescence, 2nd ed. Philadelphia, W.B. Saunders Company, 1993, p 250; (strawberry mark): from Lookingbill DP, Marks JG: Principles of Dermatology, 2nd ed. Philadelphia, W.B. Saunders Company, 1993, p 102; (cavernous hemangioma): from Hurwitz S: Clinical Pediatric Dermatology: A Textbook of Skin Disorders of Childhood and Adolescence, 2nd ed. Philadelphia, W.B. Saunders Company, 1993, p 244; (telangiectases): from Hurwitz S: Clinical Pediatric Dermatology: A Textbook of Skin Disorders of Childhood and Adolescence, 2nd ed. Philadelphia, W.B. Saunders Company, 1993, p 266; (venous lake) from Dockery GL: Cutaneous Disorders of the Lower Extremity. Philadelphia, W.B. Saunders Company, 1997, p 114. (petechiae): from Dockery GL: Cutaneous Disorders of the Lower Extremity. Philadelphia, W.B. Saunders Company 1997, p 119. (purpura): from Hurwitz S: Clinical Pediatric Dermatology: A Textbook of Skin Disorders of Childhood and Adolescence, 2nd ed. Philadelphia, W.B. Saunders Company, 1993, p 269.

Art for Table 10–7: (diaper dermatitis): From Hurwitz S: Clinical Pediatric Dermatology: A Textbook of Skin Disorders of Childhood and Adolescence, 2nd ed. Philadelphia, W.B. Saunders Company, 1993, p 37; (impetigo): from Hurwitz S: Clinical Pediatric Dermatology: A Textbook of Skin Disorders of Childhood and Adolescence, 2nd ed. Philadelphia, W.B. Saunders Company, 1993, p 280; (intertrigo): from Hurwitz S: Clinical Pediatric Dermatology: A Textbook of Skin Disorders of Childhood and Adolescence, 2nd ed. Philadelphia, W.B. Saunders Company, 1993, p 36; (atopic dermatitis): from Hurwitz S: Clinical Pediatric Dermatology: A Textbook of Skin Disorders of Childhood and Adolescence, 2nd ed. Philadelphia, W.B. Saunders Company, 1993, p 49; (measles in dark skin): from Feigin RD, Cherry JD: Textbook of Pediatric Infectious Diseases, 4th ed. Philadelphia, W.B. Saunders Company, 1998, p 725; (measles in light skin): from Hurwitz S: Clinical Pediatric Dermatology: A Textbook of Skin Disorders of Childhood and Adolescence, 2nd ed. Philadelphia, W.B. Saunders Company, 1993, p 350; (German measles): from Hurwitz S: Clinical Pediatric Dermatology: A Textbook of Skin Disorders of Childhood and Adolescence, 2nd ed. Philadelphia, W.B. Saunders Company, 1993, p 356; (chickenpox): from Callen JP, Greer, KE, Hood AF et al: Color Atlas of Dermatology. Philadelphia, W.B. Saunders Company, 1993, p 170.

Art for Table 10–8: (primary contact dermatitis): From Lookingbill DP, Marks JG: Principles of Dermatology, 2nd ed. Philadelphia, W.B. Saunders Company, 1993, p 124; (tinea corporis): from Hurwitz S: Clinical Pediatric Dermatology: A Textbook of Skin Disorders of Childhood and Adolescence, 2nd ed. Philadelphia, W.B. Saunders Company, 1993, p 380; (allergic drug reaction): from Lookingbill DP, Marks JG: Principles of Dermatology, 2nd ed. Philadelphia, W.B. Saunders Company, 1993, p 218; (tinea pedis): from Feigin RD, Cherry JD: Textbook of Pediatric Infectious Diseases, 3rd ed. Philadelphia, W.B. Saunders Company, 1992, p 776; (psoriasis): from Lookingbill DP, Marks JG: Principles of Dermatology, 2nd ed. Philadelphia, W.B. Saunders Company, 1993, p 138; (herpes simplex): from Hurwitz S: Clinical Pediatric Dermatology: A Textbook of Skin Disorders of Childhood and Adolescence, 2nd ed. Philadelphia, W.B. Saunders Company, 1993, p 321; (tinea versicolor): from Lookingbill DP, Marks JG: Principles of Dermatology, 2nd ed. Philadelphia, W.B. Saunders Company, 1993, p 206; (herpes zoster): from Hurwitz S: Clinical Pediatric Dermatology: A Textbook of Skin Disorders of Childhood and Adolescence, 2nd ed. Philadelphia, W.B. Saunders Company, 1993, p 325.

Art for Table 10–9: (basal cell carcinoma): From Lookingbill DP, Marks JG: Principles of Dermatology, 2nd ed. Philadelphia, W.B. Saunders Company, 1993, p 81; (malignant melanoma): from Lookingbill DP, Marks JG: Principles of Dermatology, 2nd ed. Philadelphia, W.B. Saunders Company, 1993, p 94; (squamous cell carcinoma): from Lookingbill DP, Marks JG: Principles of Dermatology, 2nd ed. Philadelphia, W.B. Saunders Company, 1993, p 79.

Art for Table 10–10: (epidemic Kaposi's sarcoma, patch stage; epidemic Kaposi's sarcoma, plaque stage; and epidemic Kaposi's sarcoma, advanced stage): From Friedman-Kien AE: Color Atlas of AIDS. Philadelphia, W.B. Saunders Company, 1989, pp 25, 32, and 37, respectively.

Art for Table 10–11: (seborrheic dermatitis): From Hurwitz S: Clinical Pediatric Dermatology, 2nd ed. Philadelphia, W.B. Saunders Company, 1993, p 17; (toxic alopecia): from Hurwitz S: Clinical Pediatric Dermatology, 2nd ed. Philadelphia, W.B. Saunders Company, 1993, p 485; (tinea capitis): from Lookingbill DP, Marks JG: Principles of Dermatology, 2nd ed. Philadelphia, W.B. Saunders Company, 1993, p 282; (alopecia areata): from Hurwitz S: Clinical Pediatric Dermatology, 2nd ed. Philadelphia, W.B. Saunders Company, 1993, p 486; (traumatic alopecia): from Hurwitz S: Clinical Pediatric Dermatology. 2nd ed. Philadelphia, W.B. Saunders Company, 1993, p 490; (pediculosis capitas): from Callen JP, Greer KE, Hood AF, et al: Color Atlas of Dermatology. Philadelphia, W.B. Saunders Company, 1993, p 373; (furuncle and abscess): from Lookingbill DP, Marks JG: Principles of Dermatology, 2nd ed. Philadelphia, W.B. Saunders Company, 1993, p 234; (trichotillomania): from Callen JP, Greer KE, Hood AF, et al: Color Atlas of Dermatology. Philadelphia, W.B. Saunders Company, 1993, p 363; (hirsutism): from Wenig BM, Heffess CS, Adair CF: Atlas of Endocrine Pathology. Philadelphia, W.B. Saunders Company, 1997, p 282.

Art for Table 10–12: (koilonychia): From Callen JP, Greer KE, Hood AF, et al: Color Atlas of Dermatology. Philadelphia, W.B. Saunders Company, 1993, p 354. (Beau's line): from Callen JP, Greer KE, Hood AF, et al: Color Atlas of Dermatology. Philadelphia, W.B. Saunders Company, 1993, p 343; (paronychia): from Lookingbill DP, Marks JG: Principles of Dermatology, 2nd ed. Philadelphia, W.B. Saunders Company, 1993, p. 288; (splinter hemorrhages): from Callen JP, Greer KE, Hood AF, et al: Color Atlas of Dermatology. Philadelphia, W.B. Saunders Company, 1993, p 350; (habit-tic dystrophy): from Hurwitz S: Clinical Pediatric Dermatology: A Textbook of Skin Disorders of Childhood and Adolescence, 2nd ed. Philadelphia, W.B. Saunders Company, 1993, p 506; (onycholysis): from Arndt KA, Wintroub BU, Robinson JK, et al: Primary Care Dermatology. Philadelphia, W.B. Saunders Company, 1997, plate 15; (pitting): from Lookingbill DP, Marks JG: Principles of Dermatology, 2nd ed. Philadelphia, W.B. Saunders Company, 1993, p 287.

Chapter 11

Figure 11–16: From Gorrie TM, McKinney ES, Murray SS: Foundations of Maternal-Newborn Nursing, 2nd ed. Philadelphia, W.B. Saunders Company, 1998, p 514.

Figure 11–17a: From Gorrie TM, McKinney ES, Murray SS: Foundations of Maternal-Newborn Nursing, 2nd ed. Philadelphia, W.B. Saunders Company, 1998, p 515.

Figure 11–19: From Behrman RE, Vaughn VC: Nelson Textbook of Pediatrics, 13th ed. Philadelphia, W.B. Saunders Company, 1987, p 1303.

Art for Table 11–1: (hydrocephalus): From Bowden VR, Dickey SB, Greenberg CS: Children and Their Families. Philadelphia, W.B. Saunders Company, 1998, p 1321; (craniosynostosis): from Laurence KM, Weeks R: In Norman AP (Ed): Congenital Abnormalities of Infancy, 2nd ed. Oxford, England, Blackwell Scientific Publications Ltd, 1971; (acromegaly): from Damjanov I: Pathology for the Health-Related Professions. Philadelphia, W.B. Saunders Company, 1996, p 417.

Art for Table 11–2: (pilar cyst): from Callen JP, Greer KE, Hood AF, et al: Color Atlas of Dermatology. Philadelphia, W.B. Saunders Company, 1993, p 127; (parotid gland enlargement): from Swartz MH: Textbook of Physical Diagnosis, 3rd ed. Philadelphia, W.B. Saunders Company, 1998, p 237; (thyroid, multiple nodules): from Swartz MH: Textbook of Physical Diagnosis, 3rd ed. Philadelphia, W.B. Saunders Company, 1998, p 140; (torticollis): from Liebert PS: Color Atlas of Pediatric Surgery, 2nd ed. Philadelphia, W.B. Saunders Company, 1996, p 59.

Art for Table 11–3: (Down syndrome): From Bartalos M, Baramki TA: Medical Cytogenics, Baltimore, Williams & Wilkins, 1967; (fetal alcohol syndrome): from Streissguth AP, Landesman-Dwyer S, Martin JC, et al: Teratogenic effects of alcohol in humans and laboratory animals. Science 209:353–361 (photograph) and Streissguth AP, Little RE: "Unit 5: Alcohol, Pregnancy, and the Fetal Alcohol Syndrome: Second Edition," Project Cork Institute Medical School Curriculum (slide lecture series) on Biomedical Education: Alcohol Use and Its Medical Consequences, produced by Dartmouth Medical School (illustration); (cretinism): from Behrman RE, et al.: Nelson Textbook of Pediatrics, 15th ed. Philadelphia, W.B. Saunders Company 1996, p 1592.

Art for Table 11–4: (atopic facies): From Bierman CW, Pearlman DS: Allergic Diseases from Infancy to Adulthood, 2nd ed. Philadelphia, W.B. Saunders Company, 1988, p 399, (allergic salute): from Bierman CW, Pearlman DS: Allergic Diseases from Infancy to Adulthood, 2nd ed. Philadelphia, W.B. Saunders Company, 1988, p 399.

Art for Table 11–5: (hyperthyroidism): From Swartz MH: Textbook of Physical Diagnosis, 3rd ed. Philadelphia, W.B. Saunders Company, 1998, p 140; (Cushing's syndrome): from Braverman IM: Skin Signs of Systemic Disease, 3rd ed. Philadelphia, W.B. Saunders Company, plate 49: (myxedema): from Jacob SW, Francone CA, Lossow, WJ: Structure and Function in Man, 5th ed. Philadelphia, W.B. Saunders Company, 1982, p 555. (Bell's palsy): from Swartz

MH: Textbook of Physical Diagnosis, 3rd ed. Philadelphia, W.B. Saunders Company, 1998, p 519.

Chapter 12

Figure 12–23: Courtesy of Heather Boyd-Monk and Wills Eye Hospital, Philadelphia.

Figure 12–24: Courtesy of Heather Boyd-Monk and Wills Eye Hospital, Philadelphia.

Figure 12–29: From Friedman N, Pineda R: The Massachusetts Eye and Ear Infirmary Illustrated Manual of Ophthalmology. Philadelphia, W.B. Saunders, Company 1998, p 15.

Figure 12–30: From Albert DM, Jakobiec FA: Atlas of Clinical Ophthalmology. Philadelphia, W.B. Saunders Company, 1996, p 374.

Figure 12–31: From Friedman N, Pineda R: The Massachusetts Eye and Ear Infirmary Illustrated Manual of Ophthalmology. Philadelphia, W.B. Saunders Company, 1998, p 272.

Figure 12–32: From Swartz MH: Textbook of Physical Diagnosis, 3rd ed. Philadelphia, W.B. Saunders Company, 1998, p 169.

Figure 12–33: From Albert DM, Jakobiec FA: Principles and Practice of Ophthalmology. Vol. 3. Philadelphia, W.B. Saunders Company, 1994, p 1720.

Figure 12–34: From Friedman N, Pineda R: The Massachusetts Eye and Ear Infirmary Illustrated Manual of Ophthalmology. Philadelphia, W.B. Saunders Company, 1998, p 535.

Art for Table 12–2: (pseudostrabismus, esotropia, exotropia): Friedman N, Pineda R: The Massachusetts Eye and Ear Infirmary Illustrated Manual of Ophthalmology. Philadelphia: W.B. Saunders, 1998, pp. 15, 20, 21, respectively.

Art for Table 12–3: (periorbital edema): From Ibsen OAC, Phelan JA: Oral Pathology for the Dental Hygienist, 2nd ed. Philadelphia, W.B. Saunders Company, 1996, slide 13; (exophthalmos): from Scheie HG, Albert DM: Textbook of Ophthalmology, 9th ed. Philadelphia, W.B. Saunders Company, 1977, p 427; (ptosis): courtesy of Heather Boyd-Monk and Wills Eye Hospital, Philadelphia; (ectropion): from Albert DM, Jakobiec FA: Principles and Practice of Ophthalmology. Vol. 3. Philadelphia, W.B. Saunders Company, 1994, p 1849; (entropion): from Albert DM, Jakobiec FA: Principles and Practice of Ophthalmology. Vol. 3. Philadelphia, W.B. Saunders Company, 1994, p 1849.

Art for Table 12–4: (blepharitis): From Friedman N, Pineda R: The Massachusetts Eye and Ear Infirmary Illustrated Manual of Ophthalmology. Philadelphia, W.B. Saunders Company, 1998, p 59; (chalazion): courtesy of Heather Boyd-Monk and Wills Eye Hospital, Philadelphia; (hordeolum): from Albert DM, Jakobiec FA: Principles and Practice of Ophthalmology. Vol. 1. Philadelphia, W.B. Saunders Company, 1994, p 102; (basal cell carcinoma): from Scheie HG, Albert DM: Textbook of Ophthalmology, 9th ed. Philadelphia, W.B. Saunders Company, 1977, p 449; (dacrocystitis): from Friedman N, Pineda R: The Massachusetts Eye and Ear Infirmary Illustrated Manual of Ophthalmology. Philadelphia, W.B. Saunders Company, 1998, p 82.

Art for Table 12–5: (conjunctivitis): From Albert DM, Jakobiec FA: Principles and Practice of Ophthalmology. Vol. 1. Philadelphia, W.B. Saunders Company, 1994, p 151; (iritis): from Scheie HG, Albert DM: Textbook of Ophthalmology, 9th ed. Philadelphia, W.B. Saunders Company, 1977, p 13; (subconjunctival hemorrhage): courtesy of Heather Boyd-Monk and Wills Eye Hospital, Philadelphia; (acute glaucoma): from Scheie HG, Albert DM: Textbook of Ophthalmology, 9th ed. Philadelphia, W.B. Saunders Company, 1977, p 536.

Art for Table 12–6: (pterygium): From Albert DM, Jakobiec FA: Principles and Practice of Ophthalmology. Vol. 1. Philadelphia, W.B. Saunders Company, 1994, p 280; (corneal abrasion): courtesy of Heather Boyd-Monk and Wills Eye Hospital, Philadelphia; (hyphema): from Scheie HG, Albert DM: Textbook of Ophthalmology, 9th ed. Philadelphia, W.B. Saunders Company, 1977, p 561; (hypopyon): from Scheie HG, Albert DM: Textbook of Ophthalmology, 9th ed. Philadelphia, W.B. Saunders Company, 1977, p 391.

Art for Table 12–8: (cataract a, b): From Friedman N, Pineda R: The Massachusetts Eye and Ear Infirmary Illustrated Manual of Ophthalmology. Philadelphia, W.B. Saunders Company, 1998, pp 220, 221.

Art for Table 12–9: (optic atrophy): From Friedman N, Pineda R: The Massachusetts Eye and Ear Infirmary Illustrated Manual of Ophthalmology. Philadelphia, W.B. Saunders Company, 1998, p 351; (papilledema): courtesy of Heather Boyd-Monk and Wills Eye Hospital, Philadelphia; (excessive cup-disc ratio): Friedman N, Pineda R: The Massachusetts Eye and Ear Infirmary Illustrated Manual of Ophthalmology. Philadelphia, W.B. Saunders Company, 1998, p 363.

Art for Table 12–10: (arteriovenous crossing, vessel nicking): From Friedman N, Pineda R: The Massachusetts Eye and Ear Infirmary Illustrated Manual of Ophthalmology. Philadelphia, W.B. Saunders Company, 1998, p 268; (narrowed arteries): from Wu G: Ophthalmology for Primary Care. Philadelphia, W.B. Saunders, 1997, plate fig. 4–3.

Art for Table 12–11: (microaneurysms, dot-shaped hemorrhages, soft exudates, hard exudates): From Friedman N, Pineda R: The Massachusetts Eye and Ear Infirmary Illustrated Manual of Ophthalmology. Philadelphia, W.B. Saunders Company, 1998, p 264.

Chapter 13

Figure 13–8: From Adams GL, Boies LR Jr, Hilger PA: Boies Fundamentals of Otolaryngology: A Textbook of Ear, Nose and Throat Diseases, 6th ed. Philadelphia, W.B. Saunders Company, 1989, p 6.

Art for Table 13–1: (branchial remnant and near deformity): From Liebert PS: Color Atlas of Pediatric Surgery, 2nd ed. Philadelphia, W.B. Saunders Company, 1996, p 31; (otitis externa): from DeWeese DD, et al.: Otolaryngology—Head and Neck Surgery, 7th ed. St. Louis, C.V. Mosby, 1988, p 397.

Art for Table 13–2: (sebaceous cyst): from Liebert PS: Color Atlas of Pediatric Surgery, 2nd ed. Philadelphia, W.B. Saunders Company, 1996, p 29; (chondrodermatitis): from Callen JP, Greer KE, Hood AF, et al: Color Atlas of Dermatology. Philadelphia, W.B. Saunders, 1993, p 124; (keloid): from Liebert PS: Color Atlas of Pediatric Surgery, 2nd ed. Philadelphia, W.B. Saunders Company, 1996, p 18; (carcinoma): from Callen JP, Greer KE, Hood AF, et al: Color Atlas of Dermatology. Philadelphia, W.B. Saunders Company, 1993, p 111.

Art for Table 13–5: (retracted drum): From Adams JL, Boies LR Jr, Hilger PA: Boies Fundamentals of Otolaryngology: A Textbook of Ear, Nose, and Throat Diseases, 6th ed. Philadelphia. W.B. Saunders Company, 1989, p 6; (serous otitis media): Swartz MH: Textbook of Physical Diagnosis, 3rd ed. Philadelphia, W.B. Saunders Company, p 216; (acute purulent otitis media, early and late stages): from Adams JL, Boies LR Jr, Hilger PA: Boies Fundamentals of Otolaryngology: A Textbook of Ear, Nose, and Throat Diseases, 6th ed. Philadelphia, W.B. Saunders Company, p 6; (perforation): from Swartz MH: Textbook of Physical Diagnosis, 3rd ed. Philadelphia, W.B. Saunders Company, p 214; (cholesteatoma): from Swartz MH: Textbook of Physical Diagnosis, 3rd ed. Philadelphia, W.B. Saunders Company, p 214.

Chapter 14

Figure 14–10: From McCarthy JG: Plastic Surgery, Vol. 3. Philadelphia, W.B. Saunders Company, 1990, p 1868.

Figure 14–17: From Ibsen OAC, Phelan JA: Oral Pathology for the Dental Hygienist, 2nd ed. Philadelphia, W.B. Saunders Company, 1996, slide 106.

Figure 14–18: (torus palatinus): From Ibsen OAC, Phelan JA: Oral Pathology for the Dental Hygienist, 2nd ed. Philadelphia, W.B. Saunders, 1996, slide 284.

Figure 14–24: From Moore ML: Realities in Childbearing, 2nd ed. Philadelphia, W.B. Saunders Company, 1983, p. 642.

Art for Table 14–2: (cleft lip): From Ibsen OAC, Phelan JA: Oral Pathology for the Dental Hygienist, 2nd ed. Philadelphia, W.B. Saunders Company, 1996, slide 294. (herpes simplex 1): from Callen JP, Greer KE, Hood AF, et al: Color Atlas of Dermatology. Philadelphia, W.B. Saunders Company, 1993, p 168; (perleche): from Callen JP, Greer KE, Hood AF, et al: Color Atlas of Dermatology. Philadelphia, W.B. Saunders Company, 1993, p 326; (retention cyst or "mucocele"): from Ibsen OAC, Phelan JA: Oral Pathology for the Dental Hygienist, 2nd ed. Philadelphia, W.B. Saunders

Company, 1996, slide 199; (carcinoma): from Wenig BM: Atlas of Head and Neck Pathology. Philadelphia, W.B. Saunders Company, 1993, p. 165.

Art for Table 14–3: (baby bottle tooth decay): Courtesy of F. Ferguson, Department of Children's Dentistry, School of Dental Medicine, SUNY at Stony Brook, Stony Brook, NY 11733; (dental caries): Courtesy of A. McWhorter, Pediatric Dentistry, Baylor College of Dentistry, The Texas A & M University System, Dallas, TX; (epulis): from Ibsen OAC, Phelan JA: Oral Pathology for the Dental Hygienist, 2nd ed. Philadelphia, W.B. Saunders, 1996, slide 92; (gingival hyperplasia): from Ibsen OAC, Phelan JA: Oral Pathology for the Dental Hygienist, 2nd ed. Philadelphia, W.B. Saunders Company, 1996, slide 119; (gingivitis): from Callen JP, Greer KE, Hood AF, et al.: Color Atlas of Dermatology. Philadelphia, W.B. Saunders Company, 1993, p 385.

Art for Table 14–4: (aphthous ulcers): From Sleisinger MH, Fordtran JS: Gastrointestinal Diseases: Pathophysiology, Diagnosis, and Management, 5th ed. Vol. 1. Philadelphia, W.B. Saunders Company, 1993, color plate XVII-B; (Koplik's spots): from Feigin RD, Cherry JD: Textbook of Pediatric Infectious Diseases, 2nd ed. Vol. II. Philadelphia, W.B. Saunders Company, 1992, p 773; (leukoplakia): from Sleisinger MH, Fordtran JS: Gastrointestinal Diseases: Pathophysiology, Diagnosis, and Management, 5th ed. Vol. 1. Philadelphia, W.B. Saunders Company, 1993, color plate XVII-A; (candidiasis): from Callen JR Greer KE, Hood AF, et al.: Color Atlas of Dermatology. Philadelphia, W.B. Saunders Company, p 386.

Art for Table 14–5: (ankyloglossia): From Ibsen OAC, Phelan JA: Oral Pathology for the Dental Hygienist, 2nd ed. Philadelphia, W.B. Saunders Company, 1996, slide 28; (fissured or scrotal tongue): from Callen JP, Greer KE, Hood AF, et al.: Color Atlas of Dermatology. Philadelphia, W.B. Saunders Company, p 387; (geographic tongue): from Callen JP, Greer KE, Hood AF, et al.: Color Atlas of Dermatology. Philadelphia, W.B. Saunders Company, 1993, p 386; (black hairy tongue): from Callen JP, Greer KE, Hood AF, et al.: Color Atlas of Dermatology. Philadelphia, W.B. Saunders Company, 1993, p 387; (smooth glossy tongue): from Adams JL, Boies LR Jr, Hilger PA: Boies Fundamentals of Otolaryngology: A Textbook of Ear, Nose, and Throat Diseases, 6th ed. Philadelphia, W.B. Saunders Company, 1989, p 302; (enlarged tongue): from Behrman RE, Kliegman RM, Nelson WE, et al.: Nelson Textbook of Pediatrics, 14th ed. Philadelphia, W.B. Saunders Company, 1992, p 283; (carcinoma): from Wenig BM: Atlas of Head and Neck Pathology. Philadelphia, W.B. Saunders Company, 1993, p 165.

Art for Table 14–6: (cleft palate): From Adams JL, Boies LR JR, Hilger PA: Boies Fundamentals of Otolaryngology: A Textbook of Ear, Nose, and Throat Diseases, 6th ed. Philadelphia, W.B. Saunders Company, 1989, p 287; (bifid uvula): from DeWeese DD, et al.: Otolaryngology—Head and Neck Surgery, 7th ed. St. Louis, C.V. Mosby, 1988, p 397; (oral Kaposi's sarcoma): from Friedman-Kien AE: Color Atlas of AIDS. Philadelphia, W.B. Saunders Company, 1989, p 38.

Chapter 15

Figure 15–6: Redrawn from Tanner JM: Growth at Adolescence. Oxford, England, Blackwell Scientific, 1962, p 36.

Figure 15–8: From Callen JP, Greer KE, Hood AF, et al: Color Atlas of Dermatology. Philadelphia, W.B. Saunders Company, 1993, p 133.

Figure 15–21: From Moore KL, Persaud TVN: Before We Are Born, 5th ed. Philadelphia, W.B. Saunders Company, 1998, p 159.

Art for Table 15–1: From Tanner JM: Growth at Adolescence, Oxford, England, Blackwell Scientific, 1962.

Art for Table 15–3: (dimpling, nipple retraction): From Evans AJ, Wilson ARM, Blarney RW, et al: Atlas of Breast Disease Management. Philadelphia, W.B. Saunders Company, Ltd, 1998, p 23; (fixation): from Haagensen CD: Diseases of the Breast, 3rd ed. Philadelphia, W.B. Saunders Company, 1986, p 542; (edema): from Haagensen CD: Diseases of the Breast, 3rd ed. Philadelphia, W.B. Saunders Company, 1986, p 521; (deviation in nipple pointing): from Haagensen CD: Diseases of the Breast, 3rd ed. Philadelphia, W.B. Saunders Company, 1986, p 529.

Art for Table 15–6: (intraductal papilloma): From Bland KI, Copeland EM III: The Breast: Comprehensive Management of Benign and Malignant Diseases. Philadelphia, W.B. Saunders Company, 1991; (carcinoma): from Evans AJ, Wilson ARM, Blarney RW, et al: Atlas of Breast Disease Management. Philadelphia, W.B. Saunders Company, Ltd, 1998, p 29; (Paget's disease): from Evans AJ, Wilson ARM, Blarney RW, et al: Atlas of Breast Disease Management. Philadelphia, W.B. Saunders Company, Ltd, 1998, p 53.

Art for Table 15–8: (gynecomastia): From Evans AJ, Wilson ARM, Blarney RW, et al: Atlas of Breast Disease Management. Philadelphia, W.B. Saunders Company, Ltd, 1998, p 85, (carcinoma): from Haagensen CD: Diseases of the Breast, 3rd ed. Philadelphia, W.B. Saunders Company, 1986, p 980.

Chapter 16

Figure 16–12. From Nichols FH, Zwelling E. Maternal-Newborn Nursing. Philadelphia, W.B. Saunders Company, 1998, p. 702.

Chapter 17

Figure 17–15: From Lakatta EG: Cardiovascular function in later life. Cardiovasc Med 10:37–40, 1985.

Figure 17–16: From Office of Minority Health, Washington, DC, 1990.

Chapter 18

Figure 18–7: From Behrman RE, Vaughn VC: Nelson Textbook of Pediatrics, 14th ed. Philadelphia, W.B. Saunders Company, 1992, p 37 (after Scammon: The measurement of the body in childhood. *In* Harris et al [Eds]: The Measurement of Man. Minneapolis, University of Minnesota Press, 1930.)

Figure 18–20B: From Delp MH, Manning RT: Major's Physical Diagnosis: An Introduction to the Clinical Process, 9th ed. Philadelphia, W.B. Saunders, 1981, p 327.

Art for Table 18–2: (Raynaud's syndrome): From Walker JM, Helewa A: Physical Therapy in Arthritis. Philadelphia, W.B. Saunders Company, 1996, plate 4; (lymphedema): Mason PB, Allen EV: Congenital familial lymphagiectasis (lymphedema). Am J Dis Child 50:945–953, 1935. Copyright 1935, American Medical Association.

Art for Table 18–4: (ischemic ulcer): From Dockery GL: Cutaneous Disorders of the Lower Extremity. Philadelphia, W.B. Saunders Company, 1997, p 104; (stasis ulcer): from Lookingbill DP, Marks JG: Principles of Dermatology, 2nd ed. Philadelphia, W.B. Saunders Company, 1993, p 267; (superficial varicose veins): from Dockery GL: Cutaneous Disorders of the Lower Extremity. Philadelphia, W.B. Saunders Company, 1997, p 113; (deep vein thrombophlebitis): from Dockery GL: Cutaneous Disorders of the Lower Extremity. Philadelphia, W.B. Saunders Company, 1997, p 108.

Chapter 19

Figure 19–9: From Swartz MH: Textbook of Physical Diagnosis, 3rd ed. Philadelphia, W.B. Saunders Company, p 367.

Art for Table 19–4: From Liebert PS: Color Atlas of Pediatric Surgery, 2nd ed. Philadelphia, W.B. Saunders Company, 1996, p 112.

Chapter 20

Figure 20–50: From McDade W: Bow legs and knock knees. Pediatr Clin North Am, 24:830, 1977.

Figure 20–54: Copyright held by DeWayne Dalrymple.

Art for Table 20–4: (atrophy): From Polley HF, Hunder GG: Physical Examination of the Joints, 2nd ed. Philadelphia, W.B. Saunders Company, 1978, p 66; (dislocated shoulder): from Rossman I: Clinical Geriatrics, 3rd ed. Philadelphia, J.B. Lippincott Company, 1986, p 588; (joint effusion): from Polley HF, Hunder GG: Physical Examination of the Joints, 2nd ed. Philadelphia, W.B. Saunders Company, 1978, p 66; (tear of rotator cuff): from Polley HF,

Hunder GG: Physical Examination of the Joints, 2nd ed. Philadelphia, W.B. Saunders Company, 1978, p 76; (frozen shoulder): from Polley HF, Hunder GG: Physical Examination of the Joints, 2nd ed. Philadelphia, W.B. Saunders Company, 1978, p 71.

Art for Table 20–5: (olecranon bursitis): From Polley HF, Hunder GG: Physical Examination of the Joints, 2nd ed. Philadelphia, W.B. Saunders Company, 1978, p 83; (subcutaneous nodules): from Callen JP, Greer KE, Hood AF, et al: Color Atlas of Dermatology. Philadelphia, W.B. Saunders Company, 1993, p 130 (gouty arthritis): from Polley HF, Hunder GG: Physical Examination of the Joints, 2nd ed. Philadelphia, W.B. Saunders Company, 1978, p 85.

Art for Table 20–6: (ganglion): From Callen JP, Greer KE, Hood AF, et al: Color Atlas of Dermatology. Philadelphia, W.B. Saunders Company, 1993, p 127; (ankylosis): from Polley HF, Hunder GG: Physical Examination of the Joints, 2nd ed. Philadelphia, W.B. Saunders Company, 1978, p 97; (ulnar deviation or drift): from Walker JM, Helewa A: Physical Therapy in Arthritis. Philadelphia, W.B. Saunders Company, 1996, plate 1; (degenerative joint disease): from Walker JM, Helewa A: Physical Therapy in Arthritis. Philadelphia, W.B. Saunders Company, 1996, plate 3; (syndactyly): from Liebert PS: Color Atlas of Pediatric Surgery, 2nd ed. Philadelphia, W.B. Saunders Company, 1996, p 35.

Art for Table 20–7: (mild synovitis): From Polley HF, Hunder GG: Physical Examination of the Joints, 2nd ed. Philadelphia, W.B. Saunders Company, 1978, p 215; (swelling of menisci): from Polley HF, Hunder GG: Physical Examination of the Joints, 2nd ed. Philadelphia, W.B. Saunders Company, 1978, p 217.

Art for Table 20–8: (Achilles tenosynovitis): From Polley HF, Hunder GG: Physical Examination of the Joints, 2nd ed. Philadelphia, W.B. Saunders Company, 1978, p 264; (acute gout): from Dockery GL: Cutaneous Disorders of the Lower Extremity. Philadelphia, W.B. Saunders Company, 1997, p 184; (tophi with chronic gout): from Dockery GL: Cutaneous Disorders of the Lower Extremity. Philadelphia, W.B. Saunders Company, 1997, p 184; (hallux valgus): from Walker JM, Helewa A: Physical Therapy in Arthritis. Philadelphia, W.B. Saunders Company, 1996, p 53.

Art for Table 20–9: (scoliosis): From Delp MH, Manning RT: Major's Physical Diagnosis: An Introduction to the Clinical Process, 9th ed. Philadelphia, W.B. Saunders Company, 1981, p 450; (herniated nucleus pulposus): from Polley HF, Hunder GG: Physical Examination of the Joints, 2nd ed. Philadelphia, W.B. Saunders Company, 1978, p 159.

Art for Table 20–10: (congenital dislocated hip): From Behrman RE, Vaughn VC: Nelson Textbook of Pediatrics, 14th ed. Philadelphia, W.B. Saunders Company, p 1706; (spina bifida): from Walsh PC, Retik AB, Stamey TA, et al.: Campbell's Urology, 5th ed. Philadelphia, W.B. Saunders Company, 1986, p 2194; (talipes equinovarus): courtesy of Dr. A.E. Chudley, Section of Genetics and Metabolism, Department of Pediatrics and Child Health, Children's Hospital and University of Manitoba, Winnipeg, Manitoba, Canada.

Chapter 21

Figure 21–53B: From Fenichel GM: Clinical Pediatric Neurology. Philadelphia, W.B. Saunders Company, 1988, p 171.

Figure 21–59: From Hickey JV: Neurological and Neurosurgical Nursing, 2nd ed. Philadelphia, J.B. Lippincott Company, 1986, p 121.

Chapter 22

Figure 22–4: Redrawn from Marshall WA and Tanner JM: Variations in the pattern of pubertal changes in boys. Arch Dis Child 45:22, 1970.

Art for Table 22–2: (herpes progenitalis): Courtesy of Pfizer Laboratories Division, Pfizer Inc, New York. From "A Close Look at VD: A Slide Presentation Produced as a Public Service"; (syphilitic chancre): courtesy of Pfizer Laboratories Division, Pfizer Inc, New York. From "A Close Look at VD: A Slide Presentation Produced as a Public Service"; (condylomata acuminata): from Coldiron BM, Jacobson C: Common Penile Lesions. Urol Clin North Am 15:673, 1988; (carcinoma): from Callen JP, Greer KE, Hood AF, et al: Color Atlas of Dermatology. Philadelphia, W.B. Saunders Company, 1993, p 235; (urethritis): courtesy of Pfizer Laboratories Division, Pfizer Inc, New York. From "A Close Look at VD: A Slide Presentation Produced as a Public Service."

Art for Table 22–3: (phimosis): From Liebert PS: Color Atlas of Pediatric Surgery, 2nd ed. Philadelphia, W.B. Saunders Company, 1996, p 289; (hypospadias): from Liebert PS: Color Atlas of Pediatric Surgery, 2nd ed. Philadelphia, W.B. Saunders Company, 1996, p 264; (Peyronic's disease): courtesy of Dr. Hans Stricker, Department of Urology, Henry Ford Hospital, Detroit, MI; (epispadias): from Walsh PC, Gittes RF, Perlmutter AD, et al.: Campbell's Urology, 5th ed. Philadelphia, W.B. Saunders Company, 1986, p 1875.

Chapter 24

Art for Table 24–1: From Tanner JM: Growth at Adolescence, 2nd ed. Oxford, England, Blackwell Scientific, 1962.

Art for Table 24–3: (pediculosis pubis): From Callen JP, Greer KE, Hood AF, et al: Color Atlas of Dermatology. Philadelphia, W.B. Saunders Company, 1993, p 332; (red rash): courtesy of Pfizer Laboratories Division, Pfizer Inc, New York. From "A Close Look at VD: A Slide Presentation Produced as a Public Service"; (herpes simplex virus, type 2): from Callen JP, Greer KE, Hood AF, et al: Color Atlas of Dermatology. Philadelphia, W.B. Saunders Company, 1993, p 169; (syphilitic chancre): courtesy of Pfizer Laboratories Division, Pfizer Inc, New York. From "A Close Look at VD: A Slide Presentation Produced as a Public Service"; (genital human papilloma virus): from Feigin RD, Cherry JD: Textbook of Pediatric Infectious Diseases, 4th ed. Vol. 1. Philadelphia, W.B. Saunders Company, 1998, p 531; (abscess of Bartholin's gland): from Feigin RD, Cherry JD: Textbook of Pediatric Infectious Diseases, 4th ed. Vol.1. Philadelphia, W.B. Saunders Company, 1998, p 524; (urethral caruncle): from Rimsza ME: An illustrated guide to adolescent gynecology. Pediatr Clin North Am 36(3):641, 1989.

Art for Table 24–4: (cystocele): From Huffman JW: Gynecology and Obstetrics. Philadelphia, W.B. Saunders Company, 1962; (rectocele): from Huffman JW: Gynecology and Obstetrics. Philadelphia, W.B. Saunders Company, 1962; (uterine prolapse): from Parsons L, Sommers SC: Gynecology, 2nd ed. Philadelphia, W.B. Saunders Company, 1978, p 1443.

Art for Table 24–6: (gonorrhea): Courtesy of Pfizer Laboratories Division, Pfizer Inc, New York. From "A Close Look at VD: A Slide Presentation Produced as a Public Service."

Art for Table 24–9: (ambiguous genitalia):From Moore KL, Persaud TVN: Before We Are Born, 5th ed. Philadelphia, W.B. Saunders Company, 1998, p 318 (vulvovaginitis): from Feigin RD, Cherry JD: Textbook of Pediatric Infectious Diseases, 4th ed. Vol. 1 Philadelphia, W.B. Saunders Company, 1998, p 518.

Chapter 27

Figure 27–1: From Alfaro-LeFevre R: Critical Thinking in Nursing: A Practical Approach. Philadelphia, W.B. Saunders Company, 1995, p 45.

Index

Note: Page numbers in *italics* refer to illustrations; page numbers followed by t refer to tables.

ASSESSMENT TERMS: ENGLISH AND SPANISH

English	Spanish	English	Spanish
History Taking			
How do you feel?	¿Cómo se siente?	Since when has your eyesight failed you?	¿Desde cuándo ha disminuido su visión?
Good	Bien		
Bad	Mal	Do you sometimes see things double?	¿Ve las cosas doble algunas veces?
Let me see . . .	Déjeme ver . . .		
Let me feel your pulse.	Déjeme tomarle el pulso.	Tell me what number it is.	Dígame qué número es éste.
How does your head feel?	¿Cómo siente la cabeza?	Tell me what letter it is.	Dígame qué letra es ésta.
Your memory	Su memoria	Do you see things through a mist?	¿Ve las cosas nubladas?
Is it good?	¿Es buena?	Can you see clearly?	¿Puede ver claramente?
Have you any pain in the head?	¿Le duele la cabeza?		
Did you fall and how did you fall?	¿Se cayó, y cómo se cayó?	Better at a distance?	¿Mejor a cierta distancia?
Did you faint?	¿Se desmayó?	Nausea	Náusea
Have you ever had fainting spells?	¿Ha tenido desmayos alguna vez?	Does eating make you vomit?	¿El comer le hace vomitar?
Have you slept well?	¿Ha dormido bien?	How are your stools?	¿Cómo son sus defecaciones?
Have you any difficulty in breathing?	¿Tiene dificultad al respirar?	Are they regular?	¿Son regulares?
Since when do you cough?	¿Desde cuándo tose Ud?	Have you noticed their color?	¿Se ha fijado en el color?
You cough a little?	¿Tose poco?	Are you constipated?	¿Está estreñido?
Do you expectorate much?	Escupe mucho?	Do you have diarrhea?	¿Tiene diarrea?
What is the color of your expectorations?	De qué color es el esputo?	Have you any difficulty passing water?	¿Tiene dificultad en orinar?
The hearing	El oído	Do you pass water involuntarily?	¿Orina sin querer?
Is it affected?	¿Está afectado?	Are any of your limbs swollen?	¿Están hinchados algunos de sus miembros?
Do you have ringing in the ears?	¿Le Zumban los oídos?	How long have they been swollen like this?	¿Desde cuándo están hinchados así?